DIAGNOSTIC IMAGING
PEDIATRICS

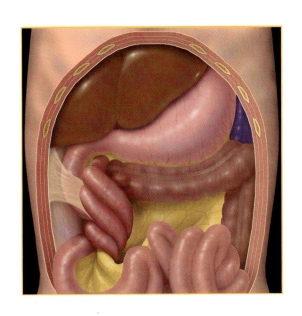

DIAGNOSTIC IMAGING
PEDIATRICS

Lane F. Donnelly, MD
Radiologist-in-Chief
Cincinnati Children's Hospital Medical Center

Professor, Radiology and Pediatrics
University of Cincinnati College of Medicine
Cincinnati, Ohio

Blaise V. Jones, MD
Division Chief, Neuroradiology
Cincinnati Children's Hospital Medical Center

Associate Professor, Radiology and Pediatrics
University of Cincinnati College of Medicine
Cincinnati, Ohio

Sara M. O'Hara, MD
Division Chief, Ultrasound
Cincinnati Children's Hospital Medical Center

Associate Professor, Radiology and Pediatrics
University of Cincinnati College of Medicine
Cincinnati, Ohio

Christopher G. Anton, MD
Staff Radiologist
Cincinnati Children's Hospital Medical Center

Assistant Professor, Radiology
University of Cincinnati College of Medicine
Cincinnati, Ohio

Corning Benton, MD, FACR
Emeritus Staff Radiologist
Cincinnati Children's Hospital Medical Center

Emeritus Professor, Radiology and Pediatrics
University of Cincinnati College of Medicine
Cincinnati, Ohio

Sjirk J. Westra, MD
Pediatric Radiologist
Pediatric Radiology Fellowship Director
Massachusetts General Hospital

Associate Professor, Radiology
Harvard Medical School
Boston, Massachusetts

Steven J. Kraus, MD, MS
Division Chief, Fluoroscopy and Radiography
Cincinnati Children's Hospital Medical Center

Associate Professor, Radiology and Pediatrics
University of Cincinnati College of Medicine
Cincinnati, Ohio

Janet L. Strife, MD, FACR
Staff Radiologist
Cincinnati Children's Hospital Medical Center

Professor, Radiology and Pediatrics
University of Cincinnati College of Medicine
Cincinnati, Ohio

Bernadette L. Koch, MD
Associate Director, Radiology
Cincinnati Children's Hospital Medical Center

Associate Professor, Radiology and Pediatrics
University of Cincinnati College of Medicine
Cincinnati, Ohio

Karin L. Hoeg, MD
Staff Radiologist
Cincinnati Children's Hospital Medical Center

Assistant Professor, Radiology
University of Cincinnati College of Medicine
Cincinnati, Ohio

Eric J. Crotty, MD
Staff Radiologist
Pediatric Radiology Fellowship Director
Cincinnati Children's Hospital Medical Center

Assistant Professor, Radiology
University of Cincinnati College of Medicine
Cincinnati, Ohio

Robert B. Fortuna, MD
Radiology Resident
University of Cincinnati College of Medicine
Cincinnati, Ohio

AMIRSYS®
Names you know, content you trust®

AMIRSYS®
Names you know, content you trust®

First Edition

Text - Copyright Lane F. Donnelly, MD 2005

Drawings - Copyright Amirsys Inc 2005

Compilation - Copyright Amirsys Inc 2005

All rights reserved. No part of this publication may be reproduced, stored in a retrieval system, or transmitted, in any form or media or by any means, electronic, mechanical, photocopying, recording, or otherwise, without prior written permission from Amirsys Inc.

Composition by Amirsys Inc, Salt Lake City, Utah

Printed by Friesens, Altona, Manitoba, Canada

ISBN: 1-4160-2333-X
ISBN: 0-8089-2324-2 (International English Edition)

Notice and Disclaimer

The information in this product ("Product") is provided as a reference for use by licensed medical professionals and no others. It does not and should not be construed as any form of medical diagnosis or professional medical advice on any matter. Receipt or use of this Product, in whole or in part, does not constitute or create a doctor-patient, therapist-patient, or other healthcare professional relationship between Amirsys Inc. ("Amirsys") and any recipient. This Product may not reflect the most current medical developments, and Amirsys makes no claims, promises, or guarantees about accuracy, completeness, or adequacy of the information contained in or linked to the Product. The Product is not a substitute for or replacement of professional medical judgment. Amirsys and its affiliates, authors, contributors, partners, and sponsors disclaim all liability or responsibility for any injury and/or damage to persons or property in respect to actions taken or not taken based on any and all Product information.

In the cases where drugs or other chemicals are prescribed, readers are advised to check the Product information currently provided by the manufacturer of each drug to be administered to verify the recommended dose, the method and duration of administration, and contraindications. It is the responsibility of the treating physician relying on experience and knowledge of the patient to determine dosages and the best treatment for the patient.

To the maximum extent permitted by applicable law, Amirsys provides the Product AS IS AND WITH ALL FAULTS, AND HEREBY DISCLAIMS ALL WARRANTIES AND CONDITIONS, WHETHER EXPRESS, IMPLIED OR STATUTORY, INCLUDING BUT NOT LIMITED TO, ANY (IF ANY) IMPLIED WARRANTIES OR CONDITIONS OF MERCHANTABILITY, OF FITNESS FOR A PARTICULAR PURPOSE, OF LACK OF VIRUSES, OR ACCURACY OR COMPLETENESS OF RESPONSES, OR RESULTS, OF AND LACK OF NEGLIGENCE OR LACK OF WORKMANLIKE EFFORT. ALSO, THERE IS NO WARRANTY OR CONDITION OF TITLE, QUIET ENJOYMENT, QUIET POSSESSION, CORRESPONDENCE TO DESCRIPTION OR NON-INFRINGEMENT, WITH REGARD TO THE PRODUCT. THE ENTIRE RISK AS TO THE QUALITY OF OR ARISING OUT OF USE OR PERFORMANCE OF THE PRODUCT REMAINS WITH THE READER.

Amirsys disclaims all warranties of any kind if the Product was customized, repackaged or altered in any way by any third party.

Library of Congress Cataloging-in-Publication Data

Diagnostic imaging. Pediatrics / Lane F. Donnelly ... [et al.]. — 1st ed.
  p. ; cm.
  Includes index.
  ISBN 1-4160-2333-X
  1. Pediatric diagnostic imaging—Handbooks, manuals, etc.
 I. Donnelly, Lane F. II. Title: Pediatrics.
  [DNLM: 1. Diagnostic Imaging—methods—Child—Handbooks.
 2. Diagnostic Imaging—methods—Infant—Handbooks.   WN 39 D536
2005]
RJ51.D5D54 2005
618.92'00754—dc22
                                2005019410

I would like to dedicate this book to all the families of the *Diagnostic Imaging: Pediatrics* authors, and those family members who had to put up with us working on this text instead of spending more time with them. In addition, I would like to acknowledge all of the mentors that inspired us to go into academic pediatric radiology and participate in projects such as this textbook.
Thanks to all.

Lane F. Donnelly, MD

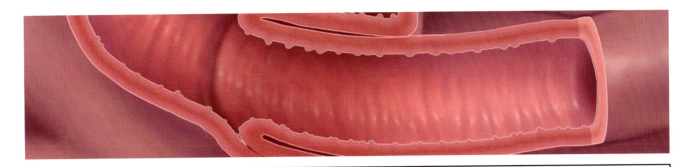

DIAGNOSTIC IMAGING: PEDIATRICS

We at Amirsys and Elsevier are proud to present **Diagnostic Imaging: Pediatrics**, the seventh volume in our acclaimed *Diagnostic Imaging (DI)* series. This precedent-setting, image- and graphic-packed series began with David Stoller's DI: Orthopaedics. The first five volumes, DI: Brain, DI: Head & Neck, DI: Spine, and DI: Abdomen are now joined by Lane Donnelly's superb textbook DI: Pediatrics. The current practice of imaging in pediatrics covers all areas of the human body from the pediatric perspective. Dealing with this range of topics is a challenge facing most radiologists on a daily basis. Dr. Lane Donnelly, one of the world's preeminent authorities in pediatric imaging and his team of experts have covered this area in a logical, in depth fashion that gives the practicing radiologist just the help he/she needs in their practice.

Again, the unique bulleted format of the *Diagnostic Imaging* series allows our authors to present approximately twice the information and four times the images per diagnosis compared to the old-fashioned traditional prose textbook. All the *Diagnostic Imaging* books follow the same format, which means the same information is in the same place: Every time! In every organ system. The innovative visual differential diagnosis "thumbnail" that provides an at-a-glance look at entities that can mimic the diagnosis in question has been highly popular. "Key Facts" boxes provide a succinct summary for quick, easy review.

In summary, **Diagnostic Imaging: Pediatrics** is a product designed with you, the reader, in mind. Today's typical practice settings demand efficiency in both image interpretation and learning. We think you'll find this new *DI: Pediatrics* volume a highly efficient and wonderfully rich resource that will significantly enhance your practice.   Enjoy!

Anne G. Osborn, MD
Executive Vice President & Editor-in-Chief, Amirsys Inc.

H. Ric Harnsberger, MD
CEO & Chairman, Amirsys Inc.

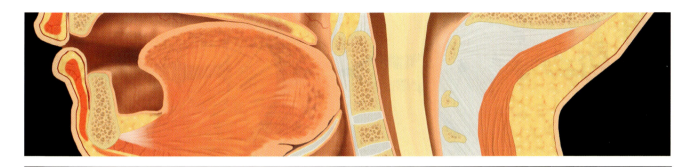

FOREWORD

There are two recognized challenges in the imaging evaluation of children. The first is to have an understanding of the variety of illnesses and injury that are often unique to this population. The second challenge is to be familiar with those findings which are normal variations or developmental appearances which may masquerade as potentially significant pathology. Together with the increasing demands of the daily practice of radiology, it is no wonder that there is a range from uneasiness or discomfort to frank anxiety when it comes to pediatric imaging. Fortunately, this text, Diagnostic Imaging: Pediatrics is carefully and thoughtfully sculpted to address these issues.

Dr. Lane Donnelly, Radiologist-in-Chief at Children's Hospital in Cincinnati is clearly the right individual to orchestrate this effort. Throughout this work and together with an outstanding and internationally recognized team of expert authors, Dr. Donnelly conveys a mastery of the subspecialty of pediatric imaging. This results from a combination of the strengths of the Diagnostic Imaging series and the style of one the most influential leaders in the care of children. Dr. Donnelly is above all else a clinician and teacher. His talents in education, particularly for the practice of pediatric radiology, are outstanding. These serve as the foundation for this volume, providing a comprehensive, clinically relevant work in a form that is organized, efficient and straightforward... another signature accomplishment.

This Diagnostic Imaging volume is the right partnership. As has been recognized with the previous works in this series, the material is a comfortable balance of informative text, superb image figures, and excellent supportive illustrations. The material is presented in a consistent manner which offers the option of either a thorough review of the clinical, imaging, and management continuum, or a directed search for specific information. Chapters are divided into a practical organ-based format, with an overview of the clinical issues, pertinent terminology and anatomy, and a familiar pattern-oriented approach for the differential considerations. This overview serves as a backdrop to subsequent distilled discussion of this material. Ample "break out" boxes of key facts and issues, including salient normal variations and developmental considerations, underscore the distinctive value of this volume for the radiologist confronted with the demands of pediatric imaging.

Who is this work suited for? The answer is simple: anyone who is involved in imaging evaluation of children. The work has layers of information included in the text and figures that serve the spectrum of imagers. For the resident, the information is a complete review of pediatric imaging that can serve as a study guide or day-to-day reference. For more advanced trainees, it is easy to identify material that supplements an existing knowledge base, including references which are both current and pertinent, offering opportunities for additional study. For the practitioner, this work provides a straightforward reference, and can serve as teaching aide or in the preparation of educational material.

Diagnostic Imaging: Pediatrics is written with the special needs of the radiology audience and with the unique considerations of pediatric imaging in mind. There is a rare, harmonious balance of informative text and superb figures that, in a carefully scripted fashion, minimizes or eliminates many of the challenges of imaging and image interpretation of children.

Donald P. Frush, MD
Professor of Radiology
Chief, Division of Pediatric Radiology
Duke University Medical Center

PEDIATRIC IMAGING

Key Facts

Patient And Family Centered Care
- Unique relationship of imager to children/families
- Importance of professionalism and communication
- Child friendly surroundings

Techniques For Enhancing Child's Ability To Cooperate
- Distraction
- Child friendly surroundings
- Minimizing pain
- Immobilization
- Adjusting parameters to decrease length of imaging study
- Sedation

Unique Aspects Of Imaging Children
- Variable size and physiologic parameters
  - Techniques must be adjusted for such changes
- Increased radiosensitivity
  - Infants 10x more radiosensitive than adults
  - Use minimum dose necessary
- Differences in "normal" appearance at different ages
  - Lack of knowledge of normal imaging appearance leads to errors in interpretation
- Differences in differential diagnosis of imaging finding based on age
  - Differential for same imaging finding may be very different in 2 day old vs. 2 year old vs. 20 year old

---

- Cites examples of both behaviors to model and behaviors to avoid
- Family satisfaction surveys
  - Conducted continuously and stress issues of communication and professionalism
- Department scorecard
  - Department scorecard updated quarterly and available to radiology employees on intra-net
  - Measures followed in six areas of which one is professionalism and communication
  - Each measure has current value and goal
- Annual faculty evaluations
  - Section of annual faculty evaluation form dedicated to professionalism and communication
  - Fellow evaluation of faculty form has areas for: Role model for professionalism, effective communication, interaction with referring physicians, interaction with families, and teamwork
- CARES standards: Guidelines for employee behavior posted throughout our medical center, with awards given to individuals who represent CARES standards
  - Courteous, Attentive, Respectful, Enthusiastic, Safe

Child Friendly Surroundings
- Reduces child stress levels
  - Physical spaces
    - Child friendly hallways and waiting areas
    - Kid friendly murals and decorations, particularly in imaging examination areas and on equipment
    - Computer games and other toys in areas
  - Personnel
    - Child friendly behavior
    - Attempt to include child in discussions

Inability Of Child To Cooperate

- Infants and young children are often unable to cooperate and fulfill requirements that are typically easily met by adults
  - Unable to keep still, concentrate for more than a brief moment, hold breath
- Different aged children have unique limitations
  - Infants and toddlers unable to keep still
  - 3 year old often unable/refuses to cooperate
- Limitations affect almost all imaging studies
- Number of potential solutions/tactics can be helpful

Distraction
- Child life specialists
  - Employees trained to coach and distract children so that they are less intimidated and more likely able to cooperate with instructions such as lying still, holding breath, drinking contrast, etc.
  - Also markedly increases family satisfaction
- Distraction toys: Rattles, noise-makers, gameboys and computer games
  - Video/movies in ultrasound, fluoroscopy, nuclear medicine and CT areas
    - Amazing how children will cooperate when watching TV
  - MR compatible video goggles in MR areas
- We have found that by using such distraction techniques that our sedation rates have been able to be reduced for children less than 7 years of age and undergoing CT/MRI by approximately 25%

Child Friendly Surroundings
- As above, child friendly surroundings help ease anxiety and improve cooperation

Dealing With Painful Procedures
- Elimination of painful portions of procedures
  - Topical analgesic for IV line placement
- Isolation of painful portion of procedure
  - Placement of IV in room other than where imaging test will occur may improve cooperation in examination room
- Sequencing of imaging exams with most painful last
  - Urinary tract imaging work-ups may be best with ultrasound exam prior to voiding cystourethrogram: Better cooperation for ultrasound exam

PEDIATRIC IMAGING

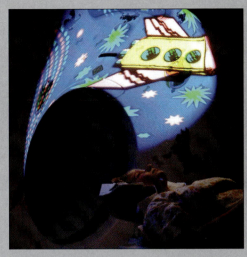

Photograph shows use of a light show projected on the CT gantry. Particularly in infants, this can distract the child long enough to obtain a CT examination.

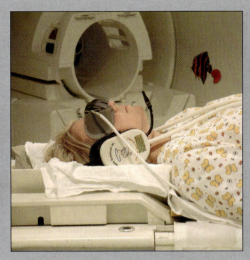

Photograph shows utilization of MR video goggles so child can watch movie during MR. In our experience, many children under 7 years of age with goggles can be imaged without sedation.

Immobilization
- Infants who are bundled or "papoosed" in a blanket are more apt to stay still
- Commercially available immobilization devices for fluoroscopy and radiographic procedures

Imaging Technology Adjustments
- Faster imaging acquisition times
- Less motion sensitive techniques
- Motion reduction software/filters/techniques

Sedation
- When all else fails, the child may need to be sedated in order to complete examination
- Need for sedation most common for MRI examinations (long acquisition time, confining tube, need to be completely still)
- Must have a defined and organized sedation program that meets regulatory requirements in order to provide sedation services

Variable Size And Physiology
- Children vary remarkably in size from several kilogram preterm infants to adult size teenagers
- Adaptations in relation to size must be considered
  - Radiographs need to be coned down to appropriate size and area of interest
  - Contrast and medications should be given on a per kilogram basis
  - On cross sectional imaging slice thickness should be adjusted to patient size and size of anatomic area
    - 5mm images may be sufficient to image a 12 year old's chest but not look for a double aortic arch in a newborn
- Example: IV contrast administration for CT
  - In small children, largest IV to be placed may be a 22 or 24 gauge
  - IV may be in hand or foot
  - Length of region of interest may be variable depending upon patient size
  - Length of patient's veins variable
  - Cardiac output and heart rate very variable

Radiosensitivity
- Infants > 10 times more radiosensitive than adults
- Need appropriate shielding
- Weight based adjusted tube current (mAs)

Age Related Normal Anatomy
- Additional challenge in imaging children is that imaging appearance of "normal" continuously changes with age for multiple organ systems
  - Ultrasound appearance of kidneys is different in a neonate than a 1 year old
  - Developing brain demonstrates differences in signal at different ages, related to myelination stages
  - Normal thymus may very large in young children but not in teenagers
  - Skeletal system has changing imaging appearance related to cartilaginous structures ossifying with age
- Knowledge of normal age-related appearance of these organ systems is vital to appropriate interpretation of imaging studies
  - Conversely, lack of this knowledge is a common cause of errors in imaging children

Age Related Differential Diagnosis
- Types of diseases affecting children are vastly different from those that affect adults
  - Differential diagnoses for similar imaging findings are vastly different
- Differential diagnoses are also very different for similar findings depending on age of child

Related References
1. Donnelly LF: Fundamentals of Pediatric Radiology. W.B. Saunders Company, Philadelphia, 2001

PEDIATRIC IMAGING

IMAGE GALLERY

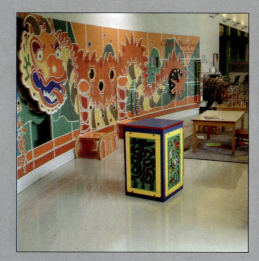
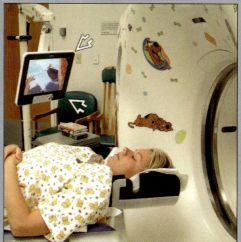

(Left) Photograph shows child oriented welcome corridor. Note wall murals and child oriented furniture. *(Right)* Photograph shows flat screen (arrows) on multi-jointed arm so that children in CT scanner can watch videos, regardless of type of positioning in CT gantry.

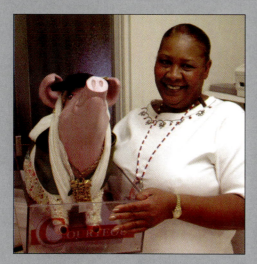
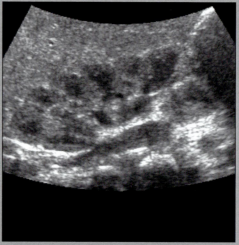

(Left) Photograph shows radiology employee receiving "CARES Pig Award" for "courteous". Awards are given on rotating basis to stress importance of family centered care. *(Right)* Sagittal oblique ultrasound of neonatal kidney shows age specific normal appearance with prominent fetal lobulation and prominent hypoechoic renal pyramids.

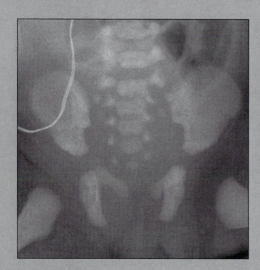
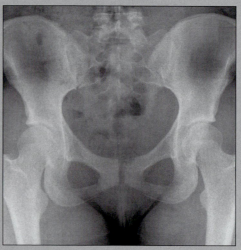

(Left) Anteroposterior radiograph of pelvis in newborn shows age-dependent "normal" appearance. Note large areas of non-ossified cartilaginous bony structures. Compare with right. *(Right)* of pelvis in 16 year old shows age-dependent "normal" appearance. Note ossified structures and striking difference in appearance compared to left image.

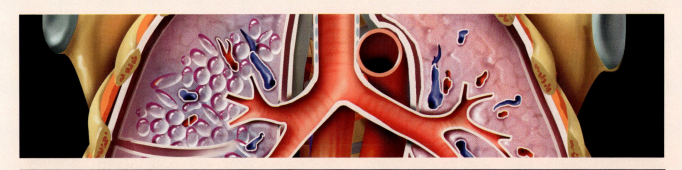

SECTION 1: Airway

Introduction and Overview
Airway 1-2

Acute Upper Airway
Epiglottitis 1-6
Croup 1-10
Exudative Tracheitis 1-14
Retropharyngeal Abscess 1-18

Obstructive Sleep Apnea
Enlarged Pharyngeal Tonsils, OSA 1-22
Glossoptosis 1-26

Lower Central Airway Obstruction
Double Aortic Arch 1-30
Pulmonary Sling 1-34
Subglottic Hemangioma 1-38
Innominate Artery Compression Syndrome 1-42
Right Arch with Aberrant Left SCA 1-46
Midline Descending Aorta 1-50
Airway Compression, Thoracic Deformity 1-54
Tracheomalacia 1-56

"Small" Airway Abnormalities
Bronchial Foreign Body 1-60
Asthma 1-64

AIRWAY

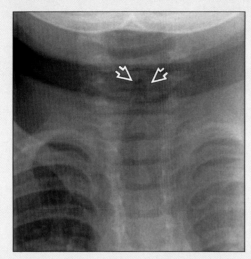

Anteroposterior radiograph of normal airway shows normal "shoulders" or lateral convexities (arrows) in the subglottic region.

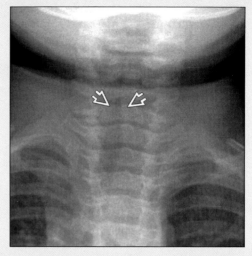

Anteroposterior radiograph in contrast to image on left shows symmetric subglottic narrowing (arrows), as is seen in croup. Note loss of normal shoulders. Appearance has been likened to a "steeple".

Acute Upper Airway Compromise

Clinical Issues
- Most causes inflammatory in origin
- Present with inspiratory stridor
  - Children with distal airway compromise (beyond carina) present with expiratory wheezing
    - Separating a child with noisy breathing into one of these two groups may be difficult

Differential Diagnosis: Acute Stridor
- Croup, epiglottitis, exudative tracheitis, retropharyngeal abscess, laryngeal/tracheal foreign body, chronic esophageal foreign body, subglottic hemangioma, subglottic granuloma, pseudothickening of retropharyngeal soft tissues (inadequate extension)

Age Related Differential Considerations
- Croup
  - Disease of young infants
  - Mean age of presentation: 1 year
  - Age range: 6 months to 3 years
- Epiglottitis
  - "Classic" mean age of presentation: 3.5 years
  - Now with vaccine, mean age: 14.6 years
- Exudative tracheitis
  - Mean age of presentation: 6-10 years
- Retropharyngeal abscess
  - Mean age of presentation 6-12 months
- If subject age > 3 years, much more concerning
  - Consider: Exudative tracheitis, epiglottitis

Anatomic Considerations
- Subglottic trachea
  - On frontal view, subglottic trachea should have lateral convexities (shoulders)
    - With edema or mass, the convexity becomes concave, the shoulder is lost, and the airway becomes narrowed
    - With symmetrical subglottic narrowing, the narrowed airway appears "pointed" and has been likened to a "steeple"
    - Look for subglottic narrowing at same superior to inferior level as inferior aspect of piriform sinuses
  - On the lateral view, the subglottic trachea should not be narrower than the airway above or below
- Epiglottis
  - The epiglottis normally has very thin borders
  - Marked thickened epiglottis = "thumb" appearance
  - Omega epiglottis: Normal variant
    - If epiglottis is obliquely imaged, because of its half cylinder shape, the left and right sides of the epiglottis may be depicted next to each other and cause "omega" appearance
- Aryepiglottic folds
  - Mucosal folds that extend from epiglottis superiorly to arytenoid cartilage posteroinferiorly
  - On lateral view, normally have thin and convex inferior appearance
  - With inflammation seen in epiglottitis, can become markedly thickened and convex superiorly
  - Swollen aryepiglottic folds are what typically obstruct airway in epiglottitis
- Retropharyngeal soft tissues
  - Soft tissues between posterior aspect of aerated pharynx and anterior aspect of vertebral column should not exceed diameter of the cervical vertebral bodies
  - Measured transversely somewhere between level of adenoids superiorly and base of epiglottis inferiorly
    - Below level of epiglottis, esophagus is present and soft tissues are normally thicker
  - "Pseudo-thickening": In young children, if neck is not adequately extended, retropharyngeal soft tissues can appear artificially thickened
    - If tissues thick and neck not extended, repeat with adequate extension

Technical Imaging Considerations
- Imaging evaluation of children with stridor is often limited to radiography
  - High kV technique
  - Quality frontal and lateral radiographs
  - If child has difficulty breathing in supine position, obtain radiographs upright

AIRWAY

Differentials And Key Facts

Acute Upper Airway Compression
- Croup, epiglottitis, exudative tracheitis, retropharyngeal abscess, tracheal foreign body, chronic esophageal foreign body, subglottic hemangioma, subglottic granuloma, pseudothickening

Obstructive Sleep Apnea
- Enlarged palatine and adenoid tonsils, enlarged lingual tonsils, glossoptosis, hypopharyngeal collapse, recurrent adenoid tonsils, enlarged soft palate

Extrinsic Lower Airway Compression
- Double aortic arch, right arch with aberrant left subclavian artery, pulmonary sling, midline descending aorta, complete tracheal rings, tracheomalacia, mediastinal mass, thoracic deformity

Key Anatomic Concepts
- Retropharyngeal "pseudothickening"
- Omega epiglottis
- Subglottic narrowing = "steeple" sign
- Normal airway moves very little during sleep
- Normal trachea round on axial images, posterior wall may flat

Imaging Tests Of Choice
- Acute upper airway compromise: Frontal and lateral radiographs
- Obstructive sleep apnea: Cine MRI
- Extrinsic lower airway compression: CT

- Placing a patient with epiglottitis supine when they are not comfortable may lead to respiratory arrest
  ○ Make sure that the neck is fully extended so that the retropharyngeal soft tissues do not appear artificially thickened on lateral view
- If serious inflammatory condition suspected, next step is usually endoscopic evaluation
- Exception: In cases of suspected retropharyngeal abscess, contrast enhanced CT: Phlegmon versus drainable abscess

Obstructive Sleep Apnea (OSA)

Clinical Issues
- Obstructive sleep apnea (OSA) is a relatively common clinical presentation in children, affecting up to 3% of children
- Most children with OSA are otherwise normal children with enlargement of the adenoid and palatine tonsils
- There are other groups of children with other more complex anatomical and dynamic (increased airway wall collapsibility) conditions that are more difficult to treat
  ○ Down syndrome, micrognathia (Pierre-Robin syndrome), neurologically impaired

Differential Diagnosis: OSA
- Enlarged palatine and/or adenoid tonsils
- Glossoptosis
- Hypopharyngeal collapse

Differential Diagnosis: Persistent OSA After Palatine/Adenoid Tonsillectomy
- Recurrent adenoid tonsils, enlarged lingual tonsils, glossoptosis, hypopharyngeal collapse, enlarged soft palate

Age Related Differential Considerations
- Children who present with OSA tend to be older than those who present with causes of stridor
- Uncommon in infants

Anatomic Considerations
- Adenoid tonsils
  ○ On lateral radiograph, appear as soft tissue pad in posterior nasopharynx
  ○ On MRI, all tonsillar tissue high on T2W
  ○ Rarely visible radiographically < 6 months of age
  ○ Rapid proliferation during infancy
  ○ Peak size between 2-10 years
  ○ Upper limits of normal = 12 mm
  ○ Supportive finding of enlargement: Encroachment on soft palate with obstruction of nasopharynx
  ○ May grow back after resection = recurrent OSA
- Palatine tonsils
  ○ Seen on lateral radiograph as round, prominent soft tissue overlying soft palate
  ○ No defined size criteria for enlargement
  ○ Do not grow back post resection
- Lingual tonsils
  ○ Normally seen as slit-like areas of high T2W signal at base of tongue bilaterally
  ○ Enlargement uncommon cause of OSA
  ○ Typically only seen after tonsillectomy and adenoidectomy
  ○ Most commonly seen in Down syndrome
  ○ Large high T2W masses seen at base of tongue
  ○ On lateral radiograph, prominent, irregular soft tissue encroaching into valleculae
- Normal pharyngeal motion
  ○ On cine imaging, the normal airway is relatively stationary
    ▪ Pharyngeal walls should not move more than several mm
    ▪ Never normally completely collapses
  ○ Collapse of hypopharynx at level of tongue indicative of glossoptosis or pharyngeal collapse

Technical Imaging Issues
- Lateral airway radiograph to evaluate for adenoid enlargement
- Cine MRI techniques in complex cases that fail surgical management

AIRWAY

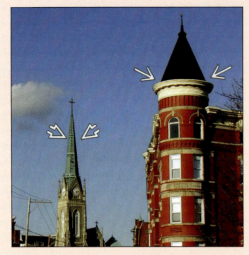

Photograph shows steeple resembling "steeple" sign of narrow airway (open arrows). However, don't be confused. Some steeples look like the normal subglottic airway (arrows)!

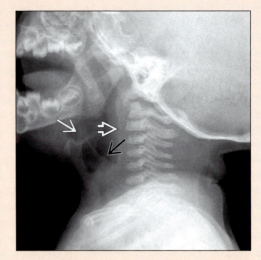

Lateral radiograph of normal airway shows "thin" epiglottis (white arrow). Note normal retropharyngeal soft tissue width (open arrow) and thin aryepiglottic folds (black arrow).

Extrinsic Compression Of Lower Airway

Clinical Issues
- Present with stridor, often worse with feeding
- Apneic attacks, noisy breathing, "seal bark" cough, recurrent infections

Differential Diagnosis: Chronic Lower Airway Compression
- Double aortic arch, right arch, aberrant left subclavian artery, aberrant left pulmonary artery (pulmonary sling), complete tracheal rings, midline descending aorta, thoracic deformity, middle mediastinal mass, large anterior mediastinal mass, tracheomalacia

Age Related Differential Considerations
- Entities associated with severe airway compression present soon after birth
  - Double aortic arch, pulmonary sling
- Airway compression from thoracic deformity typically later related to increasing deformity with age

Anatomic Considerations
- Normal intrathoracic trachea on cross sectional imaging
  - Should be round or oval in configuration (greater in anterior to posterior diameter)
  - Posterior aspect of trachea (non-cartilaginous portion) may have a linear or "flat" appearance
  - If trachea very small and very round, indicative of complete tracheal rings
  - If trachea pancake shaped with normal left to right diameter and small anterior to posterior diameter, indicative of extrinsic compression or tracheomalacia
    - If structure adjacent and "pushing" on = extrinsic compression
    - If no structure adjacent to narrowed area = more likely tracheomalacia
- Normal trachea on radiography
  - Lateral: Tracheal column should be consistent in diameter for entire length
    - Narrowing abnormal
    - Patterns of narrowing on lateral indicative of type of vascular ring
  - Frontal: Trachea should be well visualized
  - Normal left arch pushes trachea towards right and indents on left
    - Straight or leftward trachea raises possibility of arch anomaly

Technical Imaging Issues
- CT currently test of choice
  - Often can be performed without sedation because of rapid acquisition
    - MRI can give same information but infants typically need to be sedated
  - Thin collimation (1.25 or 2.5 mm) to identify small vessels in infants
  - As with CT for all pediatric indications, use low dose technique
    - Because of thin collimation, greater mA may be needed than shown on most weight based tables
  - Contrast bolus timing key to quality exam
    - Empiric timing vs. bolus tracking

Related References

1. Donnelly LF et al: Upper airway motion depicted at cine MR imaging performed during sleep: comparison between young Patients with and those without obstructive sleep apnea. Radiology. 227(1):239-45, 2003
2. Donnelly LF et al: Defining normal upper airway motion in asymptomatic children during sleep by means of cine MR techniques. Radiology. 223(1):176-80, 2002
3. Donnelly LF: Fundamentals of Pediatric Radiology. Philadelphia; W.B. Saunders, 2001
4. Donnelly LF et al: The spectrum of extrinsic lower airway compression in children: MR imaging. AJR Am J Roentgenol. 168(1):59-62, 1997

AIRWAY

IMAGE GALLERY

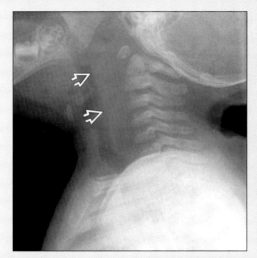
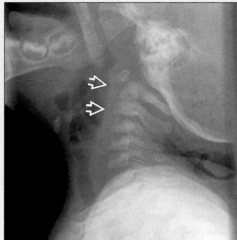

(Left) Lateral radiograph shows apparent thickening of retropharyngeal soft tissues (arrows) which are wider than vertebral body width. Note neck position is not well extended. Film was repeated. (Right) Lateral radiograph was repeated in same patient as on left shows good extension. Now retropharyngeal soft tissues (arrows) appear normal. Thickening was artifactual.

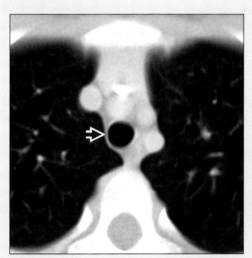
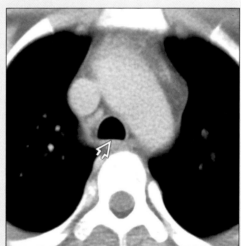

(Left) Axial CECT of normal trachea shows normal round to oval appearance of the trachea (arrow). (Right) Axial CECT of normal trachea shows round appearance. Note non-cartilaginous posterior portion of trachea (arrow) is flat, which is a normal appearance.

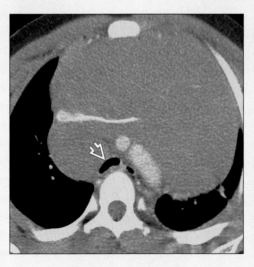
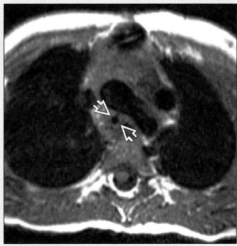

(Left) Axial CECT in child with lymphoma shows large mediastinal mass with flattened, "pancake" appearance of trachea (arrow), consistent with extrinsic compression of trachea. (Right) Axial T1WI MR shows trachea (arrows) to be very round and very small, consistent with complete tracheal rings.

EPIGLOTTITIS

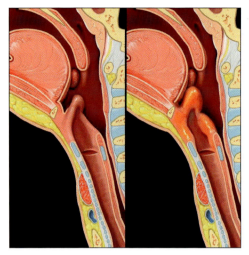

Lateral graphic shows epiglottitis (right) as compared to normal epiglottis (left). Epiglottis and aryepiglottic folds are swollen and diffusely enlarged.

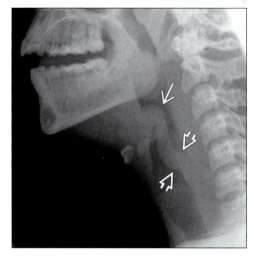

Lateral radiograph shows "thumb sign" secondary to edematous epiglottis (arrow) with markedly thickened aryepiglottic folds (open arrows).

TERMINOLOGY

Definitions
- Airway obstruction secondary to infectious inflammation of the epiglottis and surrounding tissues

IMAGING FINDINGS

General Features
- Best diagnostic clue
  - Classic imaging appearance: Lateral radiograph shows enlargement of epiglottis and thickening of the aryepiglottic folds
  - Not to be confused with "omega" epiglottis: Normal variant when epiglottis imaged obliquely
- Location: Serious, life threatening infection resulting in inflammation and swelling of the epiglottis and surrounding tissues (i.e. the aryepiglottic folds)
- Size: Diffuse enlargement and swelling of the epiglottis
- Morphology: Infectious inflammation of the epiglottitis results in "thumb sign" appreciated on the lateral radiograph

Radiographic Findings
- Radiography
  - Lateral radiograph
    - Should be obtained with patient upright in comfortable position
    - Marked thickening of the epiglottis
    - Aryepiglottic folds: Become markedly thickened
    - Extend from the epiglottis anterosuperiorly to the arytenoid cartilage posteroinferiorly
    - Normally are thin and convex inferiorly
    - When thickened become convex superiorly
    - It is the swelling of these folds that actually leads to airway obstruction
    - Ballooning of the hypopharynx
  - Frontal radiograph
    - Only a lateral radiograph should be obtained when epiglottitis is highly suspected
    - Symmetric subglottic narrowing, similar to as seen in croup, may be seen on frontal radiograph when obtained
    - Swelling of epiglottis and aryepiglottic folds not seen on frontal view

CT Findings
- NECT
  - Rarely indicated, but will show edematous, enlarged epiglottis with involvement of the aryepiglottic folds

DDx: Stridor

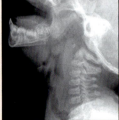
Omega Epiglottis

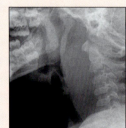
RPA

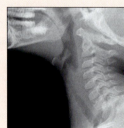
Tracheitis

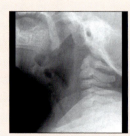
Croup

EPIGLOTTITIS

Key Facts

Terminology
- Airway obstruction secondary to infectious inflammation of the epiglottis and surrounding tissues

Imaging Findings
- Classic imaging appearance: Lateral radiograph shows enlargement of epiglottis and thickening of the aryepiglottic folds
- Not to be confused with "omega" epiglottis: Normal variant when epiglottis imaged obliquely

Pathology
- Typically older than patients with croup
- Since vaccine for Haemophilus influenzae (Hib) is available, incidence of epiglottitis has markedly decreased
- More cases of epiglottitis resulting from other bacterial organisms, viral or combined viral-bacterial infections are now seen since the introduction of Hib vaccination
- With the introduction of the Hib vaccine, the epidemiology has shifted toward significantly older patients
- Epiglottitis may be seen in older patients and even those previously immunized against Hib

Clinical Issues
- Increased respiratory distress when recumbent (reason why radiographs obtained upright or whatever way patient comfortable)
- Life threatening disease often requiring emergent intubation

---

   - May also note that due to the extensive inflammation and edema that the epiglottis is slightly lower in attenuation when compared to other soft tissue
- CECT
   - In rare cases may see a phlegmonous collection within the adjacent soft tissues associated with the epiglottis
   - May be helpful in evaluating for complications such as deep neck space infection

Imaging Recommendations
- Best imaging tool
   - Due to the serious, life-threatening infection and an airway emergency, most cases may go directly for direct laryngoscopy and bronchoscopy with intubation as indicated
   - If the patient is not unstable, only a lateral radiograph should be obtained in cases suspecting epiglottis
- Protocol advice
   - The child should be upright and comfortable
   - The patient may be drooling due to difficulty handling oral secretions and should not be agitated or placed supine
   - A patient with suspected epiglottis should be accompanied by a physician with readily available supportive equipment to secure the airway if necessary
   - Obtaining a lateral radiograph should never interfere with securing the airway given the potential rapid and fatal outcome

DIFFERENTIAL DIAGNOSIS

Omega epiglottis (normal variant)
- If epiglottis obliquely imaged, can appear artificially wide because left and right sides of epiglottis are being imaged adjacent to each other causing an "omega" shaped appearance
- Thickening of aryepiglottic folds is absent

Aspirated bronchial foreign body
- Radiopaque foreign body seen in minority of cases
- Asymmetric lung aeration on chest radiographs

Croup
- Benign, self-limited condition
- Most common acute airway condition encountered
- Symmetric subglottic narrowing

Exudative tracheitis
- Children typically older than those with croup
- Intraluminal filling defect (membrane), tracheal wall plaque-like irregularity, asymmetric subglottic narrowing

Retropharyngeal abscess (RPA)
- Pyogenic infection of the retropharyngeal space

PATHOLOGY

General Features
- General path comments
   - Typically older than patients with croup
   - Since vaccine for Haemophilus influenzae (Hib) is available, incidence of epiglottitis has markedly decreased
   - Can also rarely occur from noninfectious etiologies such as angioneurotic edema, trauma, Stevens-Johnson syndrome, caustic ingestion, bee stings
- Etiology
   - Most common etiologic agent remains Haemophilus influenzae
   - More cases of epiglottitis resulting from other bacterial organisms, viral or combined viral-bacterial infections are now seen since the introduction of Hib vaccination

CROUP

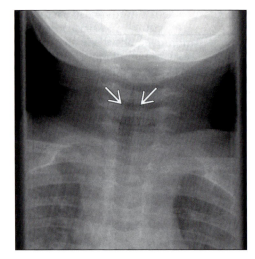

Anteroposterior radiograph shows a steeple appearance of the subglottic trachea due to symmetric subglottic narrowing with loss of the normal shoulders of the upper airway (arrows).

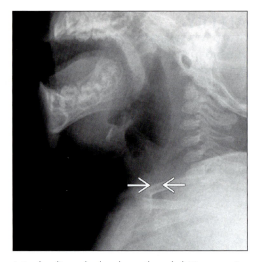

Lateral radiograph also shows the subglottic narrowing of the cervical trachea (arrows). Ballooning of the hypopharynx is also present.

TERMINOLOGY

Abbreviations and Synonyms
- Acute laryngotracheobronchitis

Definitions
- Self-limited viral inflammation of the airways resulting in symmetric subglottic edema and croupy cough

IMAGING FINDINGS

General Features
- Best diagnostic clue: Symmetric subglottic narrowing on the anteroposterior (AP) projection with loss of normal shoulders of the subglottic trachea
- Location: Subglottic airway
- Size: Subglottic narrowing which extends beyond the inferior extent of the pyriform sinuses
- Morphology: "Steeple sign", "pencil tip", or inverted "V" on frontal radiograph

Radiographic Findings
- Radiography
  - Frontal radiograph
    - Purpose of radiographs is to exclude more serious causes of stridor
    - Loss of normal shoulders (lateral convexities) of the subglottic trachea secondary to subglottic edema: "Steeple sign" or inverted "V"
    - Symmetric, subglottic narrowing with narrow portion of airway extending more inferiorly than level of the pyriform sinuses
    - Findings on frontal often more revealing than on lateral radiograph
  - Lateral radiograph
    - Narrowing of the subglottic trachea
    - Loss of definition of the subglottic trachea
    - Hypopharyngeal overdistention
    - Normal epiglottis and aryepiglottic folds
    - Hypopharynx may be collapsed with distention of the lower cervical trachea if expiratory image

Imaging Recommendations
- Best imaging tool
  - Conventional frontal and lateral radiographs
  - Diagnosis can typically be made by frontal radiograph alone
  - Lateral radiograph may show overdistention of the hypopharynx and helps exclude other diagnoses
- Protocol advice: Ensure that the neck is extended and avoid imaging while the child is swallowing

DDx: Other Causes Of Acute Stridor

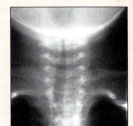

Hemangioma

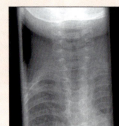

Subglottic Stenosis

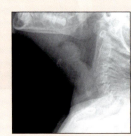

Epiglottitis

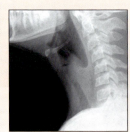

Tracheitis

CROUP

Key Facts

Terminology
- Acute laryngotracheobronchitis
- Self-limited viral inflammation of the airways resulting in symmetric subglottic edema and croupy cough

Imaging Findings
- Loss of normal shoulders (lateral convexities) of the subglottic trachea secondary to subglottic edema: "Steeple sign" or inverted "V"
- Symmetric, subglottic narrowing with narrow portion of airway extending more inferiorly than level of the pyriform sinuses

Top Differential Diagnoses
- Aspirated bronchial foreign body
- Epiglottitis
- Exudative tracheitis

Pathology
- Benign, self-limited condition secondary to viral illness
- Most common cause of upper airway obstruction in young children

Clinical Issues
- Most common signs/symptoms: Acute clinical syndrome characterized by barky ("croupy") cough, inspiratory stridor, and hoarseness
- Peak age: 1 year
- Managed supportively as outpatients
- Oral or inhaled corticosteroids have become more routinely used as therapy for all children with croup

DIFFERENTIAL DIAGNOSIS

Aspirated bronchial foreign body
- Radiopaque foreign body seen in minority of cases
- Most common foreign body in main bronchi
- Tracheal foreign bodies rare
- Asymmetric lung aeration on chest radiographs

Epiglottitis
- Typically older than croup: Mean age of epiglottitis = 3 years
- Severe, life-threatening condition
- Marked enlargement of epiglottis and aryepiglottic folds
- May cause symmetric subglottic narrowing on frontal view: Similar in appearance to croup

Exudative tracheitis
- Children typically older than those with croup
- Intraluminal filling defect (membrane)
- Tracheal wall plaque-like irregularity
- Asymmetric subglottic narrowing

PATHOLOGY

General Features
- General path comments
  - Inflammation and edema of subglottic airway
  - Secondary to viral infection
  - Redundant mucosa in this region predisposes to edema and narrowing
  - Swelling of the vocal cords results in hoarseness
  - Barky cough results from the inflammation of the larynx and trachea
  - Inspiratory stridor results because small children have proportionately small subglottic trachea which is predisposed to obstruction with edema
    - Same viral infections and edema does not compromise adult sized airway
- Etiology
  - Benign, self-limited condition secondary to viral illness
  - Parainfluenza virus types 1 and 2 account for the majority of cases
  - Influenza virus
  - Respiratory syncytial virus
  - Metapneumovirus
  - Adenovirus
  - Rhinovirus
  - Enterovirus and rarely herpes simplex virus types 1 and 2 and measles virus have been described
- Epidemiology
  - Most common cause of upper airway obstruction in young children
  - Seasonal occurrence with viral disease
  - Most prevalent in the fall and winter months

Gross Pathologic & Surgical Features
- Characterized by inflammatory edema of the subglottic airway walls

CLINICAL ISSUES

Presentation
- Most common signs/symptoms: Acute clinical syndrome characterized by barky ("croupy") cough, inspiratory stridor, and hoarseness
- Other signs/symptoms: May be preceded by a prodrome consisting of low-grade fever, mild cough, and rhinorrhea
- Symptoms are characteristically worse at night and are aggravated by agitation and crying
- Barky ("croupy") or seal-like cough
- Occurs with other symptoms of lower respiratory tract infection
- May be febrile
- Typically child able to manage oral secretions

Demographics
- Age
  - Disease of young infants
  - Age range: 6 months to 3 years
  - Peak age: 1 year

CROUP

- Age > 3 years, other cause of stridor should be highly suspected
- Gender: M:F = 3:2

Natural History & Prognosis
- Benign, self-limited disease
- Resolution within several days
- If persistence of symptoms → suspect other cause
- Radiographs obtained to exclude other disease such as
  - Aspirated foreign body
  - Epiglottitis
  - Exudative tracheitis
  - Subglottic hemangioma

Treatment
- Managed supportively as outpatients
- Parents "managed" with reassurance
- Oral or inhaled corticosteroids have become more routinely used as therapy for all children with croup
- Use of corticosteroids has significantly reduced the severity of symptoms, hospital admissions, and rates of return visit to the health care practitioner
- Only in severe cases is nebulized epinephrine or intubation required

DIAGNOSTIC CHECKLIST

Consider
- Best imaging modality is a frontal radiograph
- Bronchoscopy may be helpful in further evaluating children who present with atypical, prolonged or recurrent symptoms or who do not respond to medical therapy
- Younger age of presentation than seen with epiglottitis and exudative tracheitis

Image Interpretation Pearls
- Croup results in symmetric subglottic narrowing

SELECTED REFERENCES

1. Bjornson CL et al: A randomized trial of a single dose of oral dexamethasone for mild croup. N Engl J Med. 351(13):1306-13, 2004
2. Fisher JD: Out-of-hospital cardiopulmonary arrest in children with croup. Pediatr Emerg Care. 20(1):35-6, 2004
3. Hammer J: Acquired upper airway obstruction. Paediatr Respir Rev. 5(1):25-33, 2004
4. Henrickson KJ et al: National disease burden of respiratory viruses detected in children by polymerase chain reaction. Pediatr Infect Dis J. 23(1 Suppl):S11-8, 2004
5. Leung AK et al: Viral croup: a current perspective. J Pediatr Health Care. 18(6):297-301, 2004
6. Knutson D et al: Viral croup. Am Fam Physician. 69(3):535-40, 2004
7. Parker R et al: How long does stridor at rest persist in croup after the administration of oral prednisolone? Emerg Med Australas. 16(2):135-8, 2004
8. Principi N et al: Burden of influenza in healthy children and their households. Arch Dis Child. 89(11):1002-7, 2004
9. Rittichier KK: The role of corticosteroids in the treatment of croup. Treat Respir Med. 3(3):139-45, 2004
10. Russell K et al: Glucocorticoids for croup. Cochrane Database Syst Rev. (1):CD001955, 2004
11. Fitzgerald DA et al: Croup: assessment and evidence-based management. Med J Aust. 179(7):372-7, 2003
12. Yang TY et al: Clinical manifestations of parainfluenza infection in children. J Microbiol Immunol Infect. 36(4):270-4, 2003
13. Zoorob RJ et al: Acute dyspnea in the office. Am Fam Physician. 68(9):1803-10, 2003
14. Brown JC: The management of croup. Br Med Bull. 61:189-202, 2002
15. Chin R et al: Effectiveness of a croup clinical pathway in the management of children with croup presenting to an emergency department. J Paediatr Child Health. 38(4):382-7, 2002
16. Infosino A: Pediatric upper airway and congenital anomalies. Anesthesiol Clin North America. 20(4):747-66, 2002
17. Lichenstein R et al: Respiratory viral infections in hospitalized children: implications for infection control. South Med J. 95(9):1022-5, 2002
18. Neto GM et al: A randomized controlled trial of mist in the acute treatment of moderate croup. Acad Emerg Med. 9(9):873-9, 2002
19. Peltola V et al: Clinical courses of croup caused by influenza and parainfluenza viruses. Pediatr Infect Dis J. 21(1):76-8, 2002
20. Stannard W et al: Management of croup. Paediatr Drugs. 4(4):231-40, 2002
21. Wright RB et al: New approaches to respiratory infections in children. Bronchiolitis and croup. Emerg Med Clin North Am. 20(1):93-114, 2002
22. John SD et al: Stridor and upper airway obstruction in infants and children. RadioGraphics. 12:625-43, 1992
23. Dunbar JS: Upper respiratory tract obstruction in infants and children. AJR 109:227-46, 1970
24. Capitanio MA et al: Obstruction of the upper airway in infants and children. Radiol Clin N Amer. 6:265-77, 1968

CROUP

IMAGE GALLERY

Typical

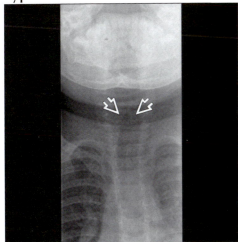
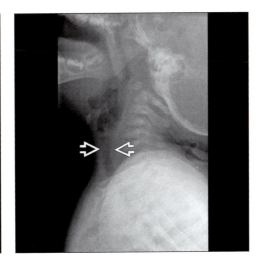

(Left) Anteroposterior radiograph shows the expected normal shouldering (lateral convexities) of the subglottic airway *(arrows)*. *(Right)* Lateral radiograph shows normal appearance of the cervical trachea with non-narrowed subglottic airway *(arrows)*.

Typical

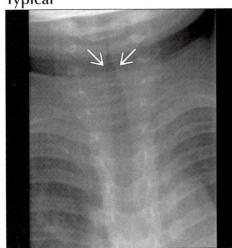
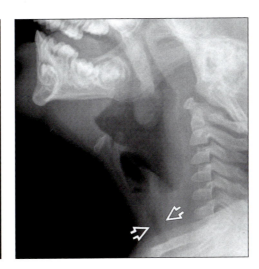

(Left) Anteroposterior radiograph shows symmetric subglottic narrowing resulting in steeple appearance to the subglottic airway *(arrows)*. *(Right)* Lateral radiograph shows overdistention of the hypopharynx and subglottic narrowing *(arrows)*.

Typical

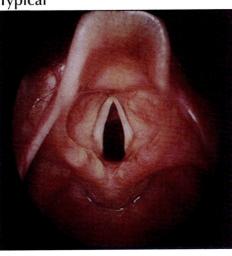
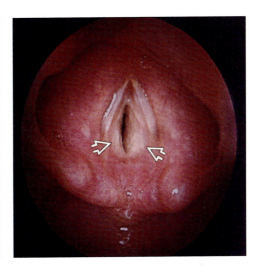

(Left) Endoscopic photograph shows a normal subglottic airway. *(Right)* Endoscopic photograph shows edematous subglottic mucosa *(arrows)* and narrowing of the subglottic airway.

EXUDATIVE TRACHEITIS

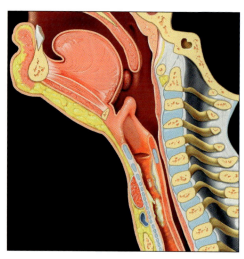

Graphic shows inflammation of trachea with formation of inflammatory plaques (membranes) along tracheal walls. These membranes may detach from the tracheal wall and form an intraluminal filling defect.

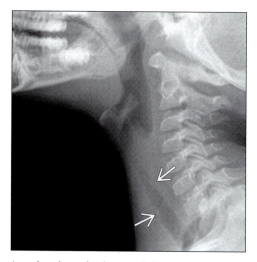

Lateral radiograph shows subglottic narrowing and multiple plaques along the anterior and posterior walls of the cervical trachea (arrows).

TERMINOLOGY

Abbreviations and Synonyms
- Bacterial tracheitis, membranous croup, membranous laryngotracheobronchitis

Definitions
- Purulent infection of trachea that results in exudative plaques that form along tracheal walls and can slough and occlude airway

IMAGING FINDINGS

General Features
- Best diagnostic clue: Radiography demonstrates plaque-like irregularity of tracheal wall or linear filling defect (membrane) within the trachea
- Location: Purulent infection of the trachea which may extend to involve the larynx and bronchi
- Size: Variable
- Morphology: Soft tissue irregularities of the tracheal walls (plaques) and linear filling defects (membranes)

Radiographic Findings
- Radiography
  - Best diagnostic sign or clue: Presence of linear, soft tissue, filling defect within the airway (visualized membrane)
  - Plaque-like irregularity or loss of smooth contours of the tracheal walls seen on frontal or lateral is suggestive
  - Symmetric or asymmetric subglottic narrowing in a child older than typically seen with croup raises possibility of exudative tracheitis
  - Non-adherent mucus can mimic membranes but clears if patient coughs and film repeated

Imaging Recommendations
- Best imaging tool: Plaques and membranes can be detected on the lateral or frontal radiograph: Obtain both lateral and frontal when evaluating for suspected exudative tracheitis
- Protocol advice: If adherent mucus is suspected, radiograph should be repeated after the child has coughed to allow for clearing of the airway

DIFFERENTIAL DIAGNOSIS

Aspirated bronchial foreign body
- Radiopaque foreign body seen in minority of cases
- Asymmetric lung aeration on chest radiographs

DDx: Acute Stridor

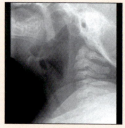
Croup

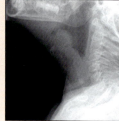
Epiglottitis

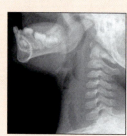
Subglottic Stenosis

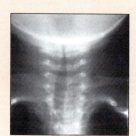
Hemangioma

EXUDATIVE TRACHEITIS

Key Facts

Terminology
- Bacterial tracheitis, membranous croup, membranous laryngotracheobronchitis
- Purulent infection of trachea that results in exudative plaques that form along tracheal walls and can slough and occlude airway

Imaging Findings
- Best diagnostic clue: Radiography demonstrates plaque-like irregularity of tracheal wall or linear filling defect (membrane) within the trachea
- Morphology: Soft tissue irregularities of the tracheal walls (plaques) and linear filling defects (membranes)

Pathology
- Uncommon but potentially life-threatening cause of acute upper airway obstruction

- Inflamed mucosa forms exudative plaques that can slough and lead to obstruction of the airway (much like airway obstruction seen in diphtheria)
- Has replaced epiglottitis as the most common life-threatening acute inflammatory airway disease since Haemophilus influenzae vaccine
- Affected children typically older and more ill than those with croup

Clinical Issues
- Because illness can lead to airway obstruction, respiratory failure and death, children are treated aggressively

Epiglottitis
- Severe, life-threatening condition
- Marked enlargement of epiglottis and aryepiglottic folds
- May cause symmetric subglottic narrowing on frontal view - similar in appearance to croup
- Similar age group to exudative tracheitis

Croup
- Benign, self-limited condition
- Most common such airway condition encountered
- Symmetric subglottic narrowing
- Younger age than exudative tracheitis
- Mean age of patients with croup = 1 year

PATHOLOGY

General Features
- General path comments
  - Purulent infection of the larynx, trachea, and bronchi
  - Uncommon but potentially life-threatening cause of acute upper airway obstruction
  - Inflamed mucosa forms exudative plaques that can slough and lead to obstruction of the airway (much like airway obstruction seen in diphtheria)
- Etiology
  - Debate over whether infection is primary bacterial infection or super infection following compromise of the respiratory mucosa secondary to viral illness
  - Initial descriptions of disease suggested Staphylococcus aureus as most common etiology
  - More recent reports suggest that polymicrobial infection is often present, supporting the etiology of secondary infection
  - Hemophilus influenzae, Streptococcus pneumoniae, and Moraxella catarrhalis have been reported in cases of bacterial tracheitis
- Epidemiology
  - Has replaced epiglottitis as the most common life-threatening acute inflammatory airway disease since Haemophilus influenzae vaccine
  - Affected children typically older and more ill than those with croup

Gross Pathologic & Surgical Features
- Infectious inflammation of the trachea with purulent exudates producing plaques and membranes within the airway

Microscopic Features
- Infectious inflammation

CLINICAL ISSUES

Presentation
- Most common signs/symptoms: High grade fever, severe stridor and respiratory distress
- Other signs/symptoms: Usually preceded by several day history of viral upper respiratory tract infection, low grade fever, and cough
- Patients present with stridor often accompanied by fever
- Initial descriptions described patients as severely toxic in appearance
- More recently encountered patients are not always severely ill
- If symptoms of croup are seen in child older than typical, exudative tracheitis should be suspected
- Child typically able to handle oral secretions and tolerates a supine position, unlike appearance in epiglottitis

Demographics
- Age: Typical age is 6-10 years, much older than patients who present with classic croup
- Gender: No predilection

Natural History & Prognosis
- Endoscopy showing subglottic edema, ulcerations, copious secretions and pseudomembrane formation is diagnostic

EXUDATIVE TRACHEITIS

- Children suspected to have exudative tracheitis usually undergo further evaluation with endoscopy and possible intervention
- Severe systemic complications of bacterial tracheitis such as toxic shock syndrome, septic shock, pulmonary edema, and acute respiratory distress syndrome (ARDS) have been described

Treatment

- Because illness can lead to airway obstruction, respiratory failure and death, children are treated aggressively
- If exudative tracheitis is suspected clinically or radiographically, the child is evaluated with a flexible nasopharyngeal scope
- If membranes are visualized within the trachea, the patients undergo rigid bronchoscopy and "stripping" of the membranes
- The child is then observed under prophylactic tracheal intubation for several days while on antibiotics

DIAGNOSTIC CHECKLIST

Consider
- Repeat radiograph after the child has coughed, if adherent mucus is suspected

Image Interpretation Pearls
- Linear filling defects (membranes) and soft tissue irregularity of the tracheal walls (plaques) are very suggestive of the diagnosis

SELECTED REFERENCES

1. Hammer J: Acquired upper airway obstruction. Paediatr Respir Rev. 5(1):25-33, 2004
2. Rotta AT et al: Respiratory emergencies in children. Respir Care. 48(3):248-58; discussion 258-60, 2003
3. Steinman MA et al: Predictors of broad-spectrum antibiotic prescribing for acute respiratory tract infections in adult primary care. JAMA. 289(6):719-25, 2003
4. Ward MA: Emergency department management of acute respiratory infections. Semin Respir Infect. 17(1):65-71, 2002
5. Stroud RH et al: An update on inflammatory disorders of the pediatric airway: epiglottitis, croup, and tracheitis. Am J Otolaryngol. 22(4):268-75, 2001
6. Damm M et al: Management of acute inflammatory childhood stridor. Otolaryngol Head Neck Surg. 121(5):633-8, 1999
7. Bernstein T et al: Is bacterial tracheitis changing? A 14-month experience in a pediatric intensive care unit. Clin Infect Dis. 27(3):458-62, 1998
8. Brody AS et al: Membranous tracheitis: how accurate is the plain film diagnosis? Pediatr Radiol (Abstr). 27:705, 1997
9. Brook I: Aerobic and anaerobic microbiology of bacterial tracheitis in children. Pediatr Emerg Care. 13(1):16-8, 1997
10. Fayon MJ et al: Nosocomial pneumonia and tracheitis in a pediatric intensive care unit: a prospective study. Am J Respir Crit Care Med. 155(1):162-9, 1997
11. Britto J et al: Systemic complications associated with bacterial tracheitis. Arch Dis Child. 74(3):249-50, 1996
12. Gold SM et al: Radiological case of the month. Membranous laryngotracheobronchitis. Arch Pediatr Adolesc Med. 150(1):97-8, 1996
13. Horowitz IN: Staphylococcal tracheitis, pneumonia, and adult respiratory distress syndrome. Pediatr Emerg Care. 12(4):288-90, 1996
14. Bank DE et al: New approaches to upper airway disease. Emerg Med Clin North Am. 13(2):473-87, 1995
15. Eid NS et al: Bacterial tracheitis as a complication of tonsillectomy and adenoidectomy. J Pediatr. 125(3):401-2, 1994
16. Cox PN: Current management of laryngotracheobronchitis, bacterial tracheitis and epiglottitis. Intensive Care World. 10(1):8-12, 1993
17. Eckel HE et al: Airway endoscopy in the diagnosis and treatment of bacterial tracheitis in children. Int J Pediatr Otorhinolaryngol. 27(2):147-57, 1993
18. Seigler RS: Bacterial tracheitis: recognition and treatment. J S C Med Assoc. 89(2):83-7, 1993
19. John SD et al: Stridor and upper airway obstruction in infants and children. RadioGraphics. 12:625-43, 1992
20. Tan AK et al: Hospitalized croup (bacterial and viral): the role of rigid endoscopy. J Otolaryngol. 21(1):48-53, 1992
21. Walker P et al: Croup, epiglottitis, retropharyngeal abscess, and bacterial tracheitis: evolving patterns of occurrence and care. Int Anesthesiol Clin. 30(4):57-70, 1992
22. Han BK et al: Membranous Laryngotracheobronchitis (membranous croup). AJR. 133:53-8, 1979

EXUDATIVE TRACHEITIS

IMAGE GALLERY

Typical

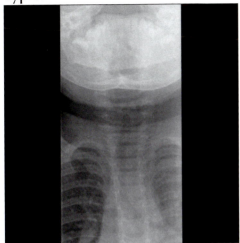
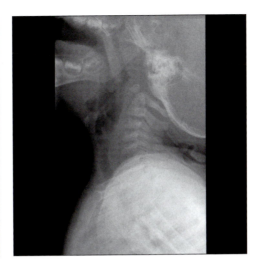

(Left) Anteroposterior radiograph shows normal tracheal air column. *(Right)* Lateral radiograph shows an example of the normal smooth tracheal wall contours.

Typical

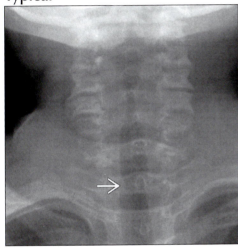
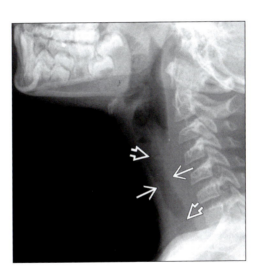

(Left) Anteroposterior radiograph shows an exudative plaque along the right tracheal wall (arrow). *(Right)* Lateral radiograph shows a second example of plaques (arrows) and membranes (open arrows) within the cervical tracheal air column resulting in irregular and obscured tracheal wall contours. These plaques and membranes can detach and lead to airway obstruction and potentially death.

Typical

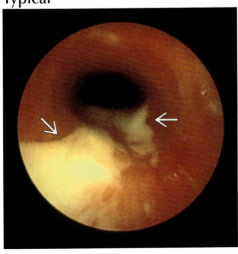
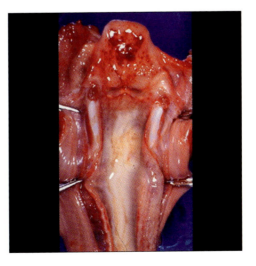

(Left) Endoscopic photograph shows purulent exudative material along the tracheal walls (arrows). This purulent material represents the intraluminal filling defects appreciated on radiographs. *(Right)* Gross pathology shows exudative material along the entire subglottic trachea. Airway compromise and obstruction may result as this exudative material sloughs.

RETROPHARYNGEAL ABSCESS

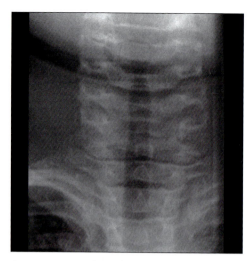

Anteroposterior radiograph shows normal tracheal air column.

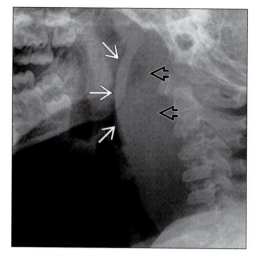

Lateral radiograph shows marked thickening of the retropharyngeal soft tissues (arrows) with several areas containing soft tissue gas (open arrows).

TERMINOLOGY

Abbreviations and Synonyms
- Retropharyngeal abscess (RPA)

Definitions
- Pyogenic infection of the retropharyngeal space

IMAGING FINDINGS

General Features
- Best diagnostic clue
  - Classic imaging appearance: Widening of the retropharyngeal soft tissues
  - Gas within soft tissues diagnostic of abscess
- Location
  - Retropharyngeal soft tissues typically extend from the skull base into the mediastinum to the fourth thoracic vertebral body or tracheal bifurcation and laterally to the parapharyngeal spaces
  - The anterior border is the buccopharyngeal fascia and posterior is the alar or prevertebral fascia
  - The retropharyngeal soft tissues typically contain lymph nodes and fat
- Size: Variable
- Morphology: Well-defined, phlegmonous collection with peripheral enhancing rim

Radiographic Findings
- Radiography
  - Lateral radiograph shows thickening of retropharyngeal soft tissues
  - Soft tissues between posterior aspect of aerated pharynx and anterior aspect of vertebral column should not exceed the diameter of the cervical vertebral bodies
  - "Pseudothickening" can be seen in infants (who have short necks) when radiograph is taken without the neck extended: If question, repeat radiograph with full extension
  - True widening may also demonstrate apex anterior convexity of the retropharyngeal soft tissues
  - Displacement of the airway by enlarged soft tissues
  - Loss of the normal cervical lordosis
  - Identification of gas within soft tissues is diagnostic of abscess in addition to cellulites
  - If there is no gas, radiography cannot distinguish between cellulitis and drainable abscess

CT Findings
- CECT
  - Performed to define extent of disease and help predict cases in which a drainable fluid collection is present
  - Thickening of retropharyngeal soft tissue identified

DDx: Stridor

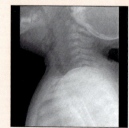
Pseudothickening

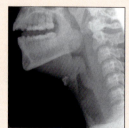
Epiglottitis

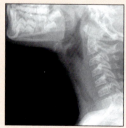
Tracheitis

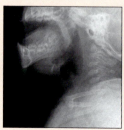
Croup

RETROPHARYNGEAL ABSCESS

Key Facts

Terminology
- Pyogenic infection of the retropharyngeal space

Imaging Findings
- Classic imaging appearance: Widening of the retropharyngeal soft tissues
- Gas within soft tissues diagnostic of abscess
- Well-defined, low-attenuation area with enhancing rim is suspicious for a drainable fluid collection
- Color Doppler: May be used in the evaluation for complications of deep neck infections such as jugular vein thrombosis
- CT performed to define extent of disease and help predict cases in which a drainable fluid collection is present
- If cross sectional imaging is performed, contrast-enhanced CT should be obtained

Pathology
- Retropharyngeal cellulitis much more common than abscess
- Typically follows pharyngitis or upper respiratory tract infection with contiguous spread to the retropharyngeal lymph nodes
- Much less common now with the widespread use of antibiotics

Clinical Issues
- Age: Typical age 6-12 months
- Airway compromise from mass effect on the pharynx/posterior trachea can develop
- A high mortality rate is associated with descending mediastinitis

---

- Mass effect and obliteration of the fat planes can be appreciated
- Often associated with inflamed palatine tonsil
- CT performed with IV contrast-enhancement
- Well-defined, low-attenuation area with enhancing rim is suspicious for a drainable fluid collection

MR Findings
- T1WI
  - MR is rarely obtained
  - CT is the cross sectional imaging of choice
  - Low signal intensity well-defined purulent fluid collection
- T2WI: High signal intensity well-defined collection
- T1 C+: Peripheral rim of enhancement

Ultrasonographic Findings
- Grayscale Ultrasound: May be useful in the evaluation of superficial neck infections or fluid collections
- Color Doppler: May be used in the evaluation for complications of deep neck infections such as jugular vein thrombosis

Imaging Recommendations
- Best imaging tool
  - Gas within soft tissues diagnostic of abscess
  - CT performed to define extent of disease and help predict cases in which a drainable fluid collection is present
  - CT is also helpful with defining the relationship of the abscess and the great vessels of the neck
- Protocol advice
  - Obtain lateral radiograph during inspiration with the neck held in extension
  - If cross sectional imaging is performed, contrast-enhanced CT should be obtained

DIFFERENTIAL DIAGNOSIS

"Pseudothickening" of retropharyngeal soft tissues (normal variant)
- In infants when radiograph is taken without the neck extended: If questionable, repeat radiograph with full extension

Vascular malformation (lymphatic)
- Lymphatic malformation can extend into retropharyngeal soft tissues
- Typically also components of cystic mass present in other soft tissue spaces of cervical or mediastinal regions

Aspirated bronchial foreign body
- Radiopaque foreign body seen in minority of cases
- Asymmetric lung aeration on chest radiographs

Croup
- Benign, self-limited condition
- Most common such airway condition encountered
- Symmetric subglottic narrowing

Exudative tracheitis
- Children typically older than those with croup
- Intraluminal filling defect (membrane), tracheal wall plaque-like irregularity, asymmetric subglottic narrowing

Epiglottitis
- Severe, life-threatening condition
- Marked enlargement of epiglottis and aryepiglottic folds
- May cause symmetric subglottic narrowing on frontal view: Similar in appearance to croup

PATHOLOGY

General Features
- General path comments

RETROPHARYNGEAL ABSCESS

- ○ Lymph nodes in retropharyngeal space drain the posterior nasal passage, nasopharynx, middle ear, and palatine tonsils
- ○ Pyogenic infection can spread from any of these areas to the retropharyngeal tissues
- ○ RPA can also develop following penetrating trauma
- ○ Retropharyngeal cellulitis much more common than abscess
- ○ Bacterial cause variable
- Etiology
  - ○ Typically follows pharyngitis or upper respiratory tract infection with contiguous spread to the retropharyngeal lymph nodes
  - ○ Cellulitis more common than discrete abscess
- Epidemiology
  - ○ Much less common now with the widespread use of antibiotics
  - ○ The most common causative organisms are Staphylococcus aureus and group A beta-hemolytic Streptococcus
  - ○ Other common organisms such as Haemophilus parainfluenzae, Peptostreptococcus, Fusobacterium, and Bacteroides species have been reported

Gross Pathologic & Surgical Features
- Well-defined purulent or phlegmonous fluid collection with surrounding mature wall

Microscopic Features
- Purulent fluid collection

CLINICAL ISSUES

Presentation
- Most common signs/symptoms: Sudden onset of fever, stiff neck, dysphagia, stridor
- Other signs/symptoms: It is a disease of young children with typical age 6-12 months
- Typically follows pharyngitis, middle ear infection, or upper respiratory tract infection
- A neck mass may be a presenting symptom
- Cervical lymphadenopathy is common

Demographics
- Age: Typical age 6-12 months
- Gender: Slightly higher preponderance in boys

Natural History & Prognosis
- May resolve with intravenous and oral antibiotics or may need surgical debridement
- Airway compromise from mass effect on the pharynx/posterior trachea can develop
- Potential complications include mediastinal extension and jugular vein thrombosis
- Sepsis, epidural abscess, osteomyelitis and cervical subluxation have been described
- A high mortality rate is associated with descending mediastinitis

Treatment
- Intravenous and oral antibiotics
- Surgical drainage when abscess present
- May also be treated with aspiration

DIAGNOSTIC CHECKLIST

Consider
- Contrast-enhanced CT if the patient is not improving with initial therapy to determine extent and possible complications from RPA
- CT may be helpful in distinguishing between abscess and cellulitis

Image Interpretation Pearls
- Do not confuse with "pseudothickening" seen in infants when radiograph obtained without neck extended
- Repeat radiograph with full extension

SELECTED REFERENCES
1. Coticchia JM et al: Age-, site-, and time-specific differences in pediatric deep neck abscesses. Arch Otolaryngol Head Neck Surg. 130(2):201-7, 2004
2. Swischuk LE: Stiff and sore neck. Pediatr Emerg Care. 19(4):282-4, 2003
3. Tuerlinckx D et al: Retropharyngeal and mediastinal abscess following adenoidectomy. Pediatr Pulmonol. 36(3):257-8, 2003
4. Hari MS et al: Retropharyngeal abscess presenting with upper airway obstruction. Anaesthesia. 58(7):714-5, 2003
5. Craig FW et al: Retropharyngeal abscess in children: clinical presentation, utility of imaging, and current management. Pediatrics. 111(6 Pt 1):1394-8, 2003
6. Vural C et al: Accuracy of computerized tomography in deep neck infections in the pediatric population. Am J Otolaryngol. 24(3):143-8, 2003
7. Rotta AT et al: Respiratory emergencies in children. Respir Care. 48(3):248-58; discussion 258-60, 2003
8. Wang LF et al: Characterizations of life-threatening deep cervical space infections: a review of one hundred ninety-six cases. Am J Otolaryngol. 24(2):111-7, 2003
9. Cmejrek RC et al: Presentation, diagnosis, and management of deep-neck abscesses in infants. Arch Otolaryngol Head Neck Surg. 128(12):1361-4, 2002
10. Wang LF et al: Space infection of the head and neck. Kaohsiung J Med Sci. 18(8):386-92, 2002
11. Dawes LC et al: Retropharyngeal abscess in children. ANZ J Surg. 72(6):417-20, 2002
12. Kirse DJ et al: Surgical management of retropharyngeal space infections in children. Laryngoscope. 111:1413-22, 2001
13. Parhiscar A et al: Deep neck abscess: a retrospective review of 210 cases. Ann Otol Rhinol Laryngol. 110(11):1051-4, 2001
14. Plaza Mayor G et al: Is conservative treatment of deep neck space infections appropriate? Head Neck. 23(2):126-33, 2001
15. Tan PT et al: Deep neck infections in children. J Microbiol Immunol Infect. 34(4):287-92, 2001
16. Weber AL et al: CT and MR imaging evaluation of neck infections with clinical correlations. Radiol Clin North Am. 38(5):941-68, ix, 2000
17. Chong VF et al: Radiology of the retropharyngeal space. Clin Radiol. 55(10):740-8, 2000
18. Boucher C et al: Retropharyngeal abscesses: a clinical and radiologic correlation. J Otolaryngol. 28:134-7, 1999
19. Stone ME et al: Correlation between computed tomography and surgical findings in retropharyngeal inflammatory processes in children. Int J Pediatr Otorhinolarygol. 49:121-5, 1999

RETROPHARYNGEAL ABSCESS

IMAGE GALLERY

Typical

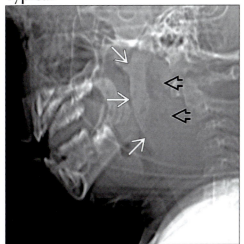
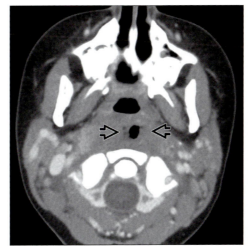

(Left) Lateral radiograph (scout image) shows the gas collections (open arrows) within the markedly increased retropharyngeal soft tissues (arrows) extending from the skull base to the mid cervical spine. Also note the focal kyphosis at the C3-4 level. *(Right)* Axial CECT shows the retropharyngeal soft tissue gas (arrows) tracking up into the nasopharynx.

Typical

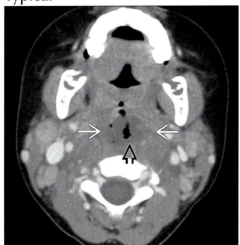
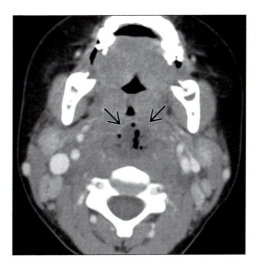

(Left) Axial CECT shows a well defined phlegmonous abscess collection (arrows) with foci of gas (open arrow) within the retropharyngeal soft tissues and peripheral enhancement. *(Right)* Axial CECT again shows the abscess collection with peripheral rim of enhancement (arrows).

Typical

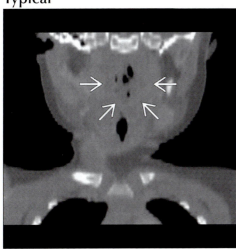
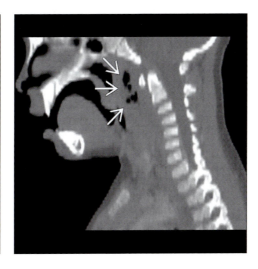

(Left) Coronal CECT reformatted image shows the large abscess collection with peripheral rim of enhancement (arrows). *(Right)* Sagittal CECT reformatted image shows abscess (arrows) and focal kyphosis of the neck centered at the C3-4 level.

ENLARGED PHARYNGEAL TONSILS, OSA

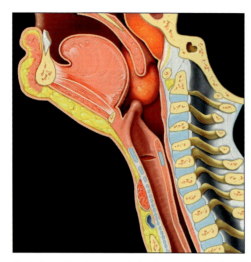

Sagittal graphic shows marked enlargement of adenoid tonsils that completely obstruct nasopharynx. Palatine tonsils are enlarged & appear as a soft tissue mass extending inferiorly, superimposed over soft palate.

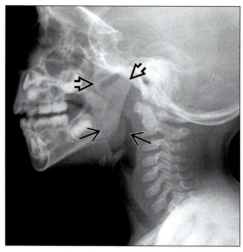

Lateral radiograph shows enlargement of the adenoid (open arrows) and palatine (arrows) tonsils.

TERMINOLOGY

Abbreviations and Synonyms
- Enlarged tonsillectomy and adenoidectomy (T & A)

Definitions
- Enlargement of the palatine and/or adenoid tonsils (and rarely lingual tonsils) that can cause a number of medical problems
- Obstructive sleep apnea (OSA) increasingly recognized as public health problem and major contributor to childhood learning disabilities such as attention deficit disorder

IMAGING FINDINGS

General Features
- Best diagnostic clue: Enlargement of the adenoid or palatine tonsils seen on lateral radiograph of airway

Radiographic Findings
- Radiography
  - Lateral radiograph of the pharynx often obtained as part of OSA work-up
    - Main goal is to evaluate whether adenoid tonsils enlarged and encroaching upon nasopharynx
    - Palatine tonsils can be evaluated on physical exam by looking in mouth
  - Adenoids appear as soft tissue in posterior nasopharynx
    - Considered enlarged when size exceeds diameter criteria for age or adenoids encroach upon or obstruct nasopharynx
    - Debate concerning size criteria for abnormal adenoid: Size variable in healthy children
    - Ratio between size of adenoid tonsils and nasopharynx has also been described.
  - Age dependent size
    - Adenoids rarely visible radiographically < 6 months
    - Rapid proliferation during infancy
    - Peak size between 2-10 years of age
    - Size begins to decrease during second decade
    - Upper limits of normal: 12 mm
  - Size: Adenoid greater than 12 mm should be considered abnormal
  - Palatine tonsils
    - Enlarged palatine tonsils appear as prominent soft tissue mass overlying posterior inferior aspect of soft palate
    - No defined size criteria for enlargement
  - Lingual tonsils
    - Enlargement of lingual tonsils an uncommon cause of OSA

DDx: Cause Of OSA In Children

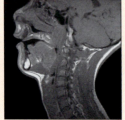
Glossoptosis

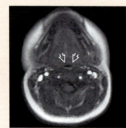
Glossoptosis

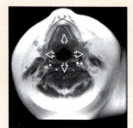
P Collapse (Open)

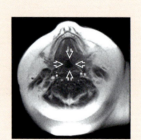
P Collapse (Closed)

ENLARGED PHARYNGEAL TONSILS, OSA

Key Facts

Terminology
- Enlargement of the palatine and/or adenoid tonsils (and rarely lingual tonsils) that can cause a number of medical problems
- Obstructive sleep apnea (OSA) increasingly recognized as public health problem and major contributor to childhood learning disabilities such as attention deficit disorder

Imaging Findings
- Palatine tonsils can be evaluated on physical exam by looking in mouth
- Size: Adenoid greater than 12 mm should be considered abnormal
- Enlarged palatine tonsils appear as prominent soft tissue mass overlying posterior inferior aspect of soft palate
- Tonsillar tissue appears as bright tissue on dark background on STIR or T2 weighted images
- Recurrent and enlarged adenoid tonsils one of the most common causes of recurrent OSA following T & A
- Unlike the adenoids which frequently recur after T & A, palatine tonsils tend to not grow back after resection

Pathology
- Approximately 3% of children affected by OSA

Clinical Issues
- OSA can be associated with excessive daytime sleepiness, hyperactivity, attention deficit disorder, poor hearing, physical debilitation, and failure to thrive

---

- Seen almost exclusively after palatine T & A
- Most often seen in Down syndrome
- Enlarged lingual tonsils seen as prominent soft tissue at inferior posterior tongue
- Irregular and lobulated posterior border

CT Findings
- CT not often utilized as diagnostic tool in evaluation for enlarged tonsils
- However, enlarged palatine and lingual tonsils often seen on CT exams obtained for other reasons such as evaluation of sinus disease or possible retropharyngeal abscess

MR Findings
- Dynamic imaging with MRI
  - Indications for dynamic MR sleep imaging: Persistent OSA despite previous T & A or other airway surgery, OSA and predisposition to obstruction at multiple sites (craniofacial anomalies, Down syndrome), evaluation of any patient with OSA prior to any complex airway surgery, OSA and severe obesity
  - Dynamic imaging studies that evaluate airway motion during real time are used to demonstrate abnormal airway motion in addition to anatomic causes of obstruction
  - Protocol includes
    - Sagittal and axial T1 weighted images
    - Sagittal midline MR cine (fast gradient echo imaging)
    - Axial MR cine (at level of mid tongue, from superior to inferior)
    - Axial and sagittal STIR
  - MR cine images: Fast gradient echo series: Flip angle 80, TR 8.2, E 3.6, slice thickness 8-12 mm, 128 consecutive images, imaging time 2 minutes, displayed in cine mode
  - Tonsillar tissue appears as bright tissue on dark background on STIR or T2 weighted images
  - Adenoids
    - Often, MR cine studies obtained after initial T & A has failed to correct OSA
    - Recurrent and enlarged adenoid tonsils one of the most common causes of recurrent OSA following T & A
    - Recurrent adenoid tonsils often have a wedge shaped defect in the anterior center portion of adenoids from previous resection and tend to proliferate from lateral aspects initially
    - Appear as prominent bright soft tissue mass in posterior nasopharynx
    - Size criteria same as on radiographs
    - When adenoids significantly enlarged, cine images will demonstrate intermittent obstruction of the posterior inferior nasopharynx against enlarged adenoids
    - Cine images may also demonstrate secondary hypopharyngeal collapse more inferiorly secondary to the negative pressure created during inspiration from the more superior obstruction
  - Palatine tonsils
    - Palatine tonsils often absent on MR cine studies because of previous T & A
    - Unlike the adenoids which frequently recur after T & A, palatine tonsils tend to not grow back after resection
    - Appear as bilateral enlarged, round high signal masses on STIR or T2 weighted images
    - No size criteria established for when palatine tonsils considered enlarged
    - When enlarged, cine images will show palatine tonsils to intermittently move centrally and inferiorly with inspiration and lead to intermittent pharyngeal obstruction
  - Lingual tonsils
    - Seen as prominent, high signal masses at level of base of tongue on STIR or T2 weighted images
    - Often, enlarged lingual tonsils will grow centrally and appear as one single oblong shaped mass, rather than two discrete tonsils
    - In normal asymptomatic children, lingual tonsils often inseparable at MRI

ENLARGED PHARYNGEAL TONSILS, OSA

- When enlarged, cine images show obstruction at level of base of tongue secondary to the enlarged lingual tonsils

DIFFERENTIAL DIAGNOSIS

Glossoptosis
- Posterior motion of the posterior aspect of the tongue leading to obstruction of the hypopharynx
- Anterior to posterior motion of the tongue
- Associated with disorders causing macroglossia (Down syndrome), micrognathia (small mandible), or decreased muscular tone (cerebral palsy, Down syndrome)

Hypopharyngeal collapse
- Cylindrical collapse of the hypopharynx
- Anterior, posterior, and lateral walls of hypopharynx all move centrally
- Associated with disorders with decreased muscular tone

Prominent soft palate
- Increases soft palate length and thickness reported to cause OSA

PATHOLOGY

General Features
- General path comments
  - Association of enlarged adenoid/palatine tonsils and OSA controversial in adults
  - In children, association between OSA and enlarged tonsils much more readily accepted
  - Symptoms of OSA shown to resolve in most children with OSA treated with T & A
- Epidemiology
  - Approximately 3% of children affected by OSA
  - Most of these children affected by OSA have enlarged palatine and adenoid tonsils
- Associated abnormalities: Down syndrome associated with increased incidence of enlarged tonsils, recurrence of adenoids, and enlarged lingual tonsils

Gross Pathologic & Surgical Features
- Processes contributing to lymphatic proliferation cause tonsils to increase in size
- Enlargement of tonsils may cause
  - Intermittent obstruction of airway leading to OSA
  - Intermittent obstruction of Eustachian tube leading to otitis media
  - Serve as a source of infection/inflammation leading to recurrent upper respiratory tract and pharyngeal infections

Microscopic Features
- Lymph cell proliferation in tonsils

CLINICAL ISSUES

Presentation
- Most common signs/symptoms
  - Obstructive sleep apnea
  - Recurrent otitis media
  - Recurrent upper respiratory tract infections
  - Recurrent pharyngitis
- Other signs/symptoms
  - OSA being increasingly recognized as a significant cause of morbidity in the pediatric population
  - OSA can be associated with excessive daytime sleepiness, hyperactivity, attention deficit disorder, poor hearing, physical debilitation, and failure to thrive

Demographics
- Age
  - Not common in infants
  - May affect children of all ages

Treatment
- Adenoidectomy and tonsillectomy is one of the more common surgeries performed in children
- The population which does not respond to adenoidectomy and tonsillectomy is one of the populations in which dynamic MR cine studies may be helpful in demonstrating other factors contributing to OSA

SELECTED REFERENCES

1. Donnelly LF et al: Causes of persistent obstructive sleep apnea despite previous tonsillectomy and adenoidectomy in children with down syndrome as depicted on static and dynamic cine MRI. AJR Am J Roentgenol. 183(1):175-81, 2004
2. Erler T et al: Obstructive sleep apnea syndrome in children: a state-of-the-art review. Treat Respir Med. 3(2):107-22, 2004
3. Guilleminault C et al: Sleep disordered breathing: surgical outcomes in prepubertal children. Laryngoscope. 114(1):132-7, 2004
4. Rosen CL: Obstructive sleep apnea syndrome in children: controversies in diagnosis and treatment. Pediatr Clin North Am. 51(1):153-67, vii, 2004
5. Arens R et al: Upper airway size analysis by magnetic resonance imaging of children with obstructive sleep apnea syndrome. Am J Respir Crit Care Med. 167(1):65-70, 2003
6. Donnelly LF et al: Upper airway motion depicted at cine MR imaging performed during sleep: comparison between young Patients with and those without obstructive sleep apnea. Radiology. 227(1):239-45, 2003
7. Friedman BC et al: Adenotonsillectomy improves neurocognitive function in children with obstructive sleep apnea syndrome. Sleep. 26(8):999-1005, 2003
8. Uong EC et al: Magnetic resonance imaging of the upper airway in children with Down syndrome. Am J Respir Crit Care Med. 163(3 Pt 1):731-6, 2001

ENLARGED PHARYNGEAL TONSILS, OSA

IMAGE GALLERY

Typical

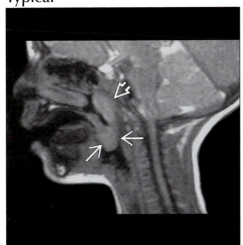
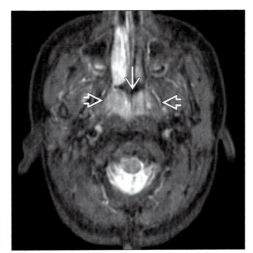

(Left) Sagittal MR cine shows enlarged adenoid (open arrow) and palatine (arrows) tonsils. (Right) Axial T2WI MR in a child with persistent OSA despite T & A shows recurrent and enlarged adenoid tonsils (open arrows). Note wedge shaped defect (arrow) typical of recurrent adenoids.

Typical

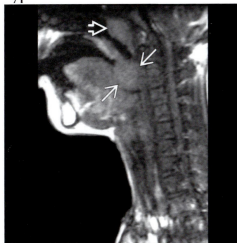
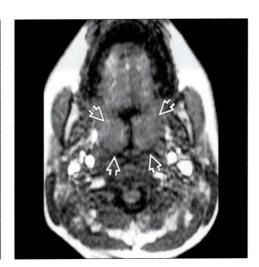

(Left) Sagittal MR cine shows enlargement of the palatine tonsils (arrows) obstructing the hypopharynx. Adenoids (open arrow) are also slightly enlarged. (Right) Axial MR cine in same patient as on left shows enlarged palatine tonsils (arrows) which at cine were shown to move centrally and inferiorly with inspiration leading to obstruction.

Typical

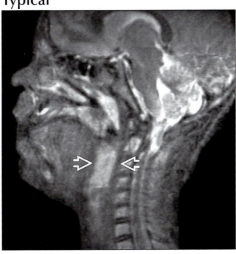
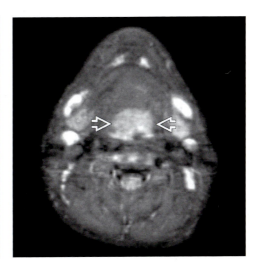

(Left) Sagittal STIR MR in a patient with Down syndrome S/P T & A shows enlarged lingual tonsils (arrows) obstructing hypopharynx. (Right) Axial STIR MR in same patient as on left shows enlarged lingual tonsils (arrows) obstructing hypopharynx. Lingual tonsils are seen as one conglomerate mass, rather than 2 distinct tonsils.

GLOSSOPTOSIS

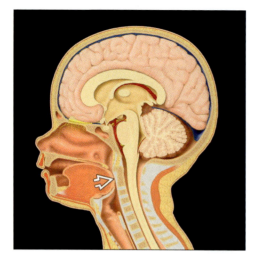
Graphic shows glossoptosis with posterior position of posterior tongue (arrow) abutting both soft palate and posterior pharyngeal wall causing obstruction of airway.

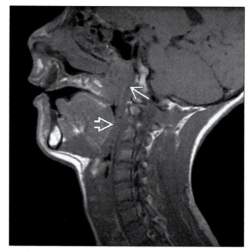
Sagittal T1WI MR shows tongue positioned posterior such that the posterior border (open arrow) abuts the posterior pharyngeal wall. Adenoids (arrow) are also enlarged.

TERMINOLOGY

Definitions
- Abnormal posterior motion of the tongue during sleep leading to obstructive sleep apnea (OSA)
- Glossoptosis almost unheard of in otherwise healthy children
- Typically associated with underlying hypotonia, macroglossia, or micrognathia

IMAGING FINDINGS

General Features
- Best diagnostic clue: Tongue "falls" posteriorly such that the posterior border of tongue abuts the velum (soft palate) and posterior wall of the hypopharynx leading to obstruction of the airway

Radiographic Findings
- Radiography
  - Lateral view of the airway/soft tissues obtained to evaluate for adenoids may show
    - Macroglossia
    - Micrognathia

Fluoroscopic Findings
- Dynamic sleep fluoroscopy
  - Patients sedated and evaluated with lateral fluoroscopy during times of oxygen desaturation or noisy breathing
  - Posterior motion of the tongue with associated obstruction of the hypopharynx
  - More typically, MR cine techniques now utilized

MR Findings
- Dynamic imaging with MRI
  - Indications for dynamic sleep imaging: Persistent obstructive sleep apnea despite previous tonsillectomy/adenoidectomy or other airway surgery, obstructive sleep apnea and predisposition to obstruction at multiple sites (craniofacial anomalies, Down syndrome), evaluation of any patient with OSA prior to any complex airway surgery, and obstructive sleep apnea and severe obesity
  - Dynamic imaging studies that evaluate airway motion during real time are used to demonstrate abnormal airway motion as well as demonstrating anatomic abnormalities
  - Patients sedated and placed in head and neck vascular coil
  - Sagittal midline MR cine (fast gradient echo series: Flip angle 80, TR 8.2, TE 3.6, slice thickness 8 mm, 128 consecutive images, imaging time 2 minutes, displayed in cine mode)

DDx: OSA Causes At Level Of Tongue

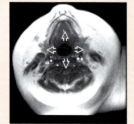
P Collapse (Open)

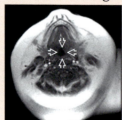
P Collapse (Closed)

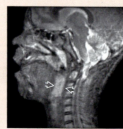
Lingual Tonsil

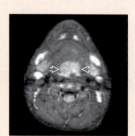
Lingual Tonsils

GLOSSOPTOSIS

Key Facts

Terminology
- Abnormal posterior motion of the tongue during sleep leading to obstructive sleep apnea (OSA)
- Glossoptosis almost unheard of in otherwise healthy children
- Typically associated with underlying hypotonia, macroglossia, or micrognathia

Imaging Findings
- Best diagnostic clue: Tongue "falls" posteriorly such that the posterior border of tongue abuts the velum (soft palate) and posterior wall of the hypopharynx leading to obstruction of the airway
- Dynamic imaging studies that evaluate airway motion during real time are used to demonstrate abnormal airway motion as well as demonstrating anatomic abnormalities
- MR cine studies
- The tongue "falls" posteriorly such that the posterior border of the tongue abuts the velum (soft palate) and posterior wall of the hypopharynx leading to obstruction of the airway
- Posterior and lateral walls of hypopharynx stay stationary differentiating glossoptosis from hypopharyngeal collapse
- Hypopharynx obstructs during inspiration and opens during expiration
- Macroglossia and fatty infiltration of the tongue may also be present

Top Differential Diagnoses
- Hypopharyngeal collapse and glossoptosis best differentiated on axial cine image

---

- MR cine studies
  - The tongue "falls" posteriorly such that the posterior border of the tongue abuts the velum (soft palate) and posterior wall of the hypopharynx leading to obstruction of the airway
  - Posterior and lateral walls of hypopharynx stay stationary differentiating glossoptosis from hypopharyngeal collapse
  - Hypopharynx obstructs during inspiration and opens during expiration
  - Macroglossia and fatty infiltration of the tongue may also be present

Imaging Recommendations
- Best imaging tool
  - MR imaging with MR cine technique
  - Dynamic imaging shows dynamic motion of tongue not shown on static imaging
- Protocol advice
  - MR sleep protocol includes
    - Sagittal and axial T1 weighted images
    - Sagittal midline MR cine (fast gradient echo imaging)
    - Axial MR cine (at level of mid tongue, from superior to inferior)
    - Axial and sagittal STIR (tonsillar tissue seen as high signal on low signal background)

DIFFERENTIAL DIAGNOSIS

Hypopharyngeal collapse
- Often related to decreased muscular tone
- In contrast to glossoptosis in which collapse of the hypopharynx is related primarily to the tongue moving posteriorly, with hypopharyngeal collapse, there is cylindrical collapse of the hypopharynx
- Anterior, posterior, left, and right pharyngeal (P) walls all collapse to center of airway
- Can be primary problem or secondary to negative pressure generated by more superior obstruction (such as enlarged tonsils)
- Hypopharyngeal collapse and glossoptosis best differentiated on axial cine image

Enlarged adenoid and palatine tonsils
- Adenoids > 12-15 mm with cine evidence of associated nasopharyngeal airway collapse
- Tonsillar tissue high in signal on T2W and STIR images

Enlarged lingual tonsils
- Occurs almost exclusively after tonsillectomy and adenoidectomy
- Most commonly seen in patients with Down syndrome
- Enlarged tissue at posterior base of tongue
- Tissue high in signal on T2W and STIR images

PATHOLOGY

General Features
- General path comments
  - Posterior motion of the tongue typically related to one or more of the following features
    - Hypotonia of the pharyngeal and glossal musculature leading to a "droopy" tongue in patients with decreased muscular tone: Down syndrome, cerebral palsy, muscular dystrophy
    - Micrognathia such as seen in Pierre-Robin syndrome
    - Macroglossia such as with Down syndrome, mucopolysaccharidoses
  - The tongue "falls" posteriorly such that the posterior border of the tongue abuts the velum (soft palate) and posterior wall of the hypopharynx leading to obstruction of the airway
- Epidemiology: Uncommon in otherwise healthy children
- Associated abnormalities
  - Down syndrome

GLOSSOPTOSIS

- Down syndrome patients with OSA are problematic to manage as multiple anatomic abnormalities can be present and patients also have decreased muscular tone
- In patients with Down syndrome who have persistent OSA despite previous tonsillectomy and adenoidectomy, most common causes of OSA include
  - Glossoptosis (63%)
  - Recurrent and enlarged adenoid tonsils (63%)
  - Enlarged lingual tonsils (30%)
  - Macroglossia (74%)

Gross Pathologic & Surgical Features
- Enlarged and often floppy tongue

CLINICAL ISSUES

Presentation
- Most common signs/symptoms: Obstructive sleep apnea
- Up to 3% of all children, approximately 2 million in the U.S. alone, are affected by OSA
- Most common cause of OSA is enlarged adenoid and palatine tonsils in otherwise healthy children
- Glossoptosis typically seen in small sub-groups of patients with OSA
- Most children with glossoptosis have complex medical problems including underlying syndromes or neurologic abnormalities
- Glossoptosis is, however, common cause (25%) of OSA in cases referred for dynamic MR imaging

Treatment
- Positive pressure ventilation (C-PAP) first treatment of choice but often poorly tolerated in children
- Radiofrequency ablation of posterior tongue to scar and decrease the size of the tongue
- Geniogiossis suspension
- Surgical interventions to reduce the volume of the tongue
- Surgical advancement of the mandible to pull tongue forward

SELECTED REFERENCES

1. Abbott MB et al: Obstructive sleep apnea: MR imaging volume segmentation analysis. Radiology. 232(3):889-95, 2004
2. Donnelly LF et al: Causes of persistent obstructive sleep apnea despite previous tonsillectomy and adenoidectomy in children with down syndrome as depicted on static and dynamic cine MRI. AJR Am J Roentgenol. 183(1):175-81, 2004
3. Erler T et al: Obstructive sleep apnea syndrome in children: a state-of-the-art review. Treat Respir Med. 3(2):107-22, 2004
4. Guilleminault C et al: Sleep disordered breathing: surgical outcomes in prepubertal children. Laryngoscope. 114(1):132-7, 2004
5. Kaditis AG et al: Sleep-disordered breathing in 3,680 Greek children. Pediatr Pulmonol. 37(6):499-509, 2004
6. Nour SG et al: Percutaneous MR imaging-guided radiofrequency interstitial thermal ablation of tongue base in porcine models: implications for obstructive sleep apnea syndrome. Radiology. 230(2):359-68, 2004
7. Rosen CL: Obstructive sleep apnea syndrome in children: controversies in diagnosis and treatment. Pediatr Clin North Am. 51(1):153-67, vii, 2004
8. Shott SR et al: Cine magnetic resonance imaging: evaluation of persistent airway obstruction after tonsil and adenoidectomy in children with Down syndrome. Laryngoscope. 114(10):1724-9, 2004
9. Abbott MB et al: Using volume segmentation of cine MR data to evaluate dynamic motion of the airway in pediatric patients. AJR Am J Roentgenol. 181(3):857-9, 2003
10. Arens R et al: Upper airway size analysis by magnetic resonance imaging of children with obstructive sleep apnea syndrome. Am J Respir Crit Care Med. 167(1):65-70, 2003
11. Blunden S et al: Symptoms of sleep breathing disorders in children are underreported by parents at general practice visits. Sleep Breath. 7(4):167-76, 2003
12. de Miguel-Diez J et al: Prevalence of sleep-disordered breathing in children with Down syndrome: polygraphic findings in 108 children. Sleep. 26(8):1006-9, 2003
13. Donnelly LF et al: Upper airway motion depicted at cine MR imaging performed during sleep: comparison between young Patients with and those without obstructive sleep apnea. Radiology. 227(1):239-45, 2003
14. Faber CE et al: Available techniques for objective assessment of upper airway narrowing in snoring and sleep apnea. Sleep Breath. 7(2):77-86, 2003
15. Fregosi RF et al: Sleep-disordered breathing, pharyngeal size and soft tissue anatomy in children. J Appl Physiol. 95(5):2030-8, 2003
16. Friedman BC et al: Adenotonsillectomy improves neurocognitive function in children with obstructive sleep apnea syndrome. Sleep. 26(8):999-1005, 2003
17. Macey PM et al: Functional magnetic resonance imaging responses to expiratory loading in obstructive sleep apnea. Respir Physiol Neurobiol. 138(2-3):275-90, 2003
18. Maheshwari PR et al: MRI in sleep apnoea. J Postgrad Med. 49(2):177-8, 2003
19. de Miguel-Diez J et al: Magnetic resonance imaging of the upper airway in children with Down syndrome. Am J Respir Crit Care Med. 165(8):1187; author reply 1187, 2002
20. Arens R et al: Magnetic resonance imaging of the upper airway structure of children with obstructive sleep apnea syndrome. Am J Respir Crit Care Med. 164(4):698-703, 2001
21. Donnelly LF et al: Is sedation safe during dynamic sleep fluoroscopy of children with obstructive sleep apnea? AJR Am J Roentgenol. 177(5):1031-4, 2001
22. Uong EC et al: Magnetic resonance imaging of the upper airway in children with Down syndrome. Am J Respir Crit Care Med. 163(3 Pt 1):731-6, 2001
23. Don GW et al: Site and mechanics of spontaneous, sleep-associated obstructive apnea in infants. J Appl Physiol. 89(6):2453-62, 2000
24. Donnelly LF et al: Glossoptosis (posterior displacement of the tongue) during sleep: a frequent cause of sleep apnea in pediatric patients referred for dynamic sleep fluoroscopy. AJR. 175:1557-59, 2000
25. Donnelly LF et al: Imaging of pediatric tongue abnormalities. AJR. 175;489-93, 2000
26. Gibson SE et al: Sleep fluoroscopy for localization of upper airway obstruction in children. Ann Otol Rhinol Laryngol. 105:678-83, 1996
27. Gonsalez S et al: Treatment of obstructive sleep apnoea using nasal CPAP in children with craniofacial dysostoses. Childs Nerv Syst. 12(11):713-9, 1996

GLOSSOPTOSIS

IMAGE GALLERY

Typical

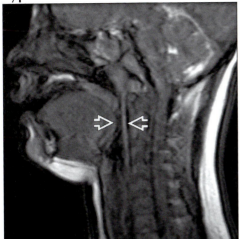
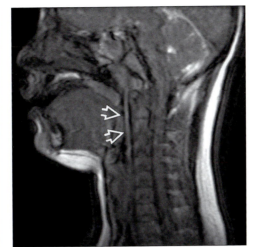

(Left) Sagittal MR cine of child with Down syndrome (same child next four images) during expiration shows tongue positioned such that pharynx (arrows) is patent. *(Right)* Sagittal MR cine in same patient as on left during inspiration shows tongue to have moved posterior (arrows) and abut the posterior pharyngeal wall.

Typical

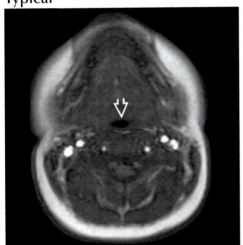
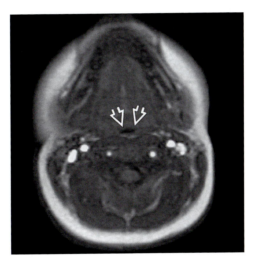

(Left) Axial MR cine in same patient as above shows hypopharynx (arrow) patent during inspiration. *(Right)* Axial MR cine in same patient as on left during expiration shows tongue to have moved posteriorly and narrowed the hypopharynx (arrows).

Typical

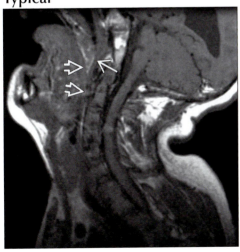
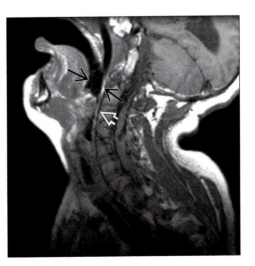

(Left) Sagittal MR cine in a patient with micrognathia shows severe glossoptosis with posterior tongue (open arrows) abutting posterior pharyngeal wall and displacing soft palate (arrow) posteriorly. *(Right)* Sagittal T1WI MR on same patient as on left shows oral airway (arrows) placed pulling tongue anterior but inferior tongue (open arrow) below tube still obstructs hypopharynx.

DOUBLE AORTIC ARCH

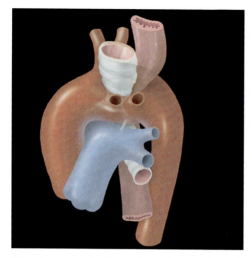

Graphic shows double aortic arch anomaly, with complete vascular ring encircling and compressing trachea and esophagus.

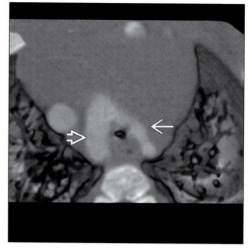

Axial CECT shows dominant right arch (open arrow) and smaller left arch (arrow), with associated focal tracheal stenosis.

TERMINOLOGY

Definitions
- Congenital aortic arch anomaly related to persistence of both the left and right fourth aortic arches

IMAGING FINDINGS

General Features
- Best diagnostic clue: Severe compression of trachea with evidence of right and left aortic arches
- On cross-sectional imaging, both left and right arches are identified arising from ascending aorta and joining to form descending aorta
- Each arch gives rise to a ventral carotid and a dorsal subclavian artery (symmetric "four artery sign")
- Right arch commonly larger and more superior and posterior extending than left
- Right arch typically runs behind esophagus to join left arch, to form left-sided descending aorta
- Part of left arch may be atretic but patent portions remain connected by fibrous band, completing the compressive ring around trachea and esophagus

Radiographic Findings
- Radiography
  - Prominent soft tissue on either side of the trachea
  - Bilateral tracheal indentations, mid-tracheal stenosis
  - Trachea is deviated from dominant arch, or may be in abnormal midline position (normally trachea is slightly deviated to right by left arch)
  - Right arch indentation commonly somewhat higher and more prominent than left
  - On lateral view, anterior and posterior compression of trachea at level of arch
  - Symmetric aeration, no unilateral air trapping
    - Pulmonary sling only vascular ring to be associated with asymmetric aeration

Fluoroscopic Findings
- Anteroposterior (AP) view: Bilateral indentations on contrast-filled upper esophagus, often at different levels
- Lateral view: Prominent oblique or nearly horizontal posterior indentation

CT Findings
- CTA
  - Four artery sign: Symmetric take-off of four aortic branches on axial image at thoracic inlet: 2 ventral carotids and 2 dorsal subclavians
  - Two arches are seen, completely encircling trachea and esophagus, leading to severe mid-tracheal compression
  - Smaller of two arches may be partially atretic
  - Severe tracheal compression at level of double arch

DDx: Tracheal Narrowing

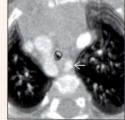
R Arch Aberrant LSA

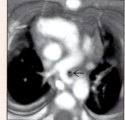
Left PA Sling

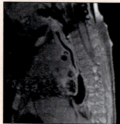
Tracheomalacia

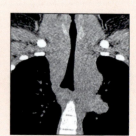
Lymphoma

DOUBLE AORTIC ARCH

Key Facts

Terminology
- Congenital aortic arch anomaly related to persistence of both the left and right fourth aortic arches

Imaging Findings
- Each arch gives rise to a ventral carotid and a dorsal subclavian artery (symmetric "four artery sign")
- Right arch commonly larger and more superior and posterior extending than left
- Trachea is deviated from dominant arch, or may be in abnormal midline position (normally trachea is slightly deviated to right by left arch)

Pathology
- Epidemiology: Most common symptomatic vascular ring anomaly (55%)

- True complete vascular ring with trachea and esophagus encircled
- Dominant right arch, left descending aorta: 75%
- Dominant left arch, right descending aorta: 20%

Clinical Issues
- Most common signs/symptoms: Inspiratory stridor, worsening with feeding
- Determination of which arch is smaller on cross-sectional imaging will determine on which side thoracotomy is performed

Diagnostic Checklist
- Look for signs of atretic segments of the double arch anomaly (will not be opacified on CTA or MRA, and show no flow voids on spin echo MRI)

- Coronal 3D images are very helpful to demonstrate arch anatomy in relation to trachea

MR Findings
- Axial and coronal images most helpful
- Findings comparable with CTA

Echocardiographic Findings
- Echocardiogram
  - Suprasternal notch view most helpful, showing two separate aortic arches, each giving rise to separate carotid and subclavian arteries (no common brachiocephalic trunk)
  - Often insufficient for pre-operative diagnosis (does not show airway compression)

Angiographic Findings
- Conventional: Rarely required with use of cross-sectional imaging

Imaging Recommendations
- Best imaging tool
  - Radiography remains primary diagnostic test
    - If radiography demonstrates lack of tracheal compression, vascular ring excluded
  - Barium swallow rarely obviates need for cross-sectional imaging and therefore many feel is not useful in workup of suspected arch anomaly
    - However many asymptomatic arch anomalies are first diagnosed by barium swallow
  - Cross-sectional imaging (CT or MR) performed to confirm diagnosis and define anatomic variations for pre-surgical planning
- Protocol advice
  - Axial and coronal images/renditions
  - Multidetector-row CTA faster to perform that MR, with generally no need for sedation and endotracheal intubation
  - CT shows airway compromise somewhat better than MR

DIFFERENTIAL DIAGNOSIS

Right arch with aberrant left subclavian artery (LSA) and other arch abnormalities
- Generally not possible to differentiate without cross-sectional imaging

Left pulmonary artery (PA) sling
- Compression on anterior aspect of esophagus and posterior aspect of trachea on radiography
- Often associated with tracheomalacia

Innominate artery compression syndrome
- Compression on anterior aspect of trachea, no esophageal compression

Nonvascular masses
- Small middle mediastinal masses or larger anterior or posterior masses that compress trachea

PATHOLOGY

General Features
- General path comments
  - Related to embryological persistence of the right and left fourth aortic arches
  - Pathophysiology: Severe airway and esophageal compression by vascular ring
  - Underlying tracheomalacia is frequently associated
  - Hemodynamics: No hemodynamic sequelae, unless associated with congenital heart disease
- Genetics: No specific genetic defect identified
- Epidemiology: Most common symptomatic vascular ring anomaly (55%)
- Associated abnormalities
  - Typically an isolated lesion without associated abnormalities
    - 20% Associated with congenital heart disease (tetralogy of Fallot, ventricular septal defect, coarctation, patent ductus arteriosus, transposition of great arteries, truncus arteriosus)

DOUBLE AORTIC ARCH

Gross Pathologic & Surgical Features
- True complete vascular ring with trachea and esophagus encircled
  - Dominant right arch, left descending aorta: 75%
  - Dominant left arch, right descending aorta: 20%
  - Arches equal in size: 5%
- Smaller of two arches may be partially atretic

CLINICAL ISSUES

Presentation
- Most common signs/symptoms: Inspiratory stridor, worsening with feeding
- Other signs/symptoms: Apneic attacks, noisy breathing, "seal bark" cough

Demographics
- Age: Typically presents early in life, soon after birth

Treatment
- Thoracotomy with division of smaller of two arches, atretic segments and ligamentum arteriosum
  - Rare complication of surgery: Aortoesophageal fistula
- Determination of which arch is smaller on cross-sectional imaging will determine on which side thoracotomy is performed
- < 30% of post-operative patients: Persistent airway symptoms, due to tracheobronchomalacia and/or persistent extrinsic airway compression
  - Caused by midline/circumflex descending aorta or previously ligated arch
- 11% of patients require a second operation to relieve airway symptoms: Aortopexy or other vascular suspension procedures, cartilaginous tracheal ring resection followed by airway reconstruction

DIAGNOSTIC CHECKLIST

Consider
- Look for signs of atretic segments of the double arch anomaly (will not be opacified on CTA or MRA, and show no flow voids on spin echo MRI)

Image Interpretation Pearls
- "Four artery sign" on axial slice at thoracic inlet

SELECTED REFERENCES
1. Greil GF et al: Diagnosis of vascular rings and slings using an interleaved 3D double-slab FISP MR angiography technique. Pediatr Radiol. 2005
2. Backer CL: Vascular rings and pulmonary artery sling. In: Mavroudis C, Backer CL ed. Pediatric cardiac surgery. 3rd ed. Philadelphia, Mosby. 234-250, 2003
3. Subramanyan R et al: Vascular rings: an important cause of persistent respiratory symptoms in infants and children. Indian Pediatr. 40(10):951-7, 2003
4. Yilmaz M et al: Vascular anomalies causing tracheoesophageal compression: a 20-year experience in diagnosis and management. Heart Surg Forum. 6(3):149-52, 2003
5. Fleck RJ et al: Imaging findings in pediatric patients with persistent airway symptoms after surgery for double aortic arch. AJR Am J Roentgenol. 178(5):1275-9, 2002
6. Park SC et al: Vascular ring and pulmonary sling. In: Anderson RH et al, ed. Pediatric cardiology. vol 2. 2nd ed. London, Churchill Livingstone. 1559-75, 2002
7. Skinner LJ et al: Complete vascular ring detected by barium esophagography. Ear Nose Throat J. 81(8):554-5, 2002
8. Brockes C et al: Double aortic arch: diagnosis missed for 29 years. Vasa. 29(1):77-9, 2000
9. Gustafson LM et al: Spiral CT versus MRI in neonatal airway evaluation. Int J Pediatr Otorhinolaryngol. 52(2):197-201, 2000
10. McMahon CJ et al: Double aortic arch in D-transposition of the great arteries: confirmation of dominant arch by magnetic resonance imaging. Tex Heart Inst J. 27(4):398-400, 2000
11. Krinsky GA et al: Thoracic aorta: comparison of single-dose breath-hold and double-dose non-breath-hold gadolinium-enhanced three-dimensional MR angiography. AJR Am J Roentgenol. 173(1):145-50, 1999
12. Beghetti M et al: Double aortic arch. J Pediatr. 133(6):799, 1998
13. Donnelly LF et al: The spectrum of extrinsic lower airway compression in children: MR imaging. AJR. 168:59-62, 1997
14. Fattori R et al: Intramural posttraumatic hematoma of the ascending aorta in a patient with a double aortic arch. Eur Radiol. 7(1):51-3, 1997
15. Hopkins KL et al: Pediatric great vessel anomalies: initial clinical experience with spiral CT angiography. Radiology. 200(3):811-5, 1996
16. Murdison KA: Ultrasonic Imaging of Vascular Rings and Other Anomalies Causing Tracheobronchial Compression. Echocardiography. 13(3):337-356, 1996
17. Othersen HB Jr et al: Aortoesophageal fistula and double aortic arch: two important points in management. J Pediatr Surg. 31(4):594-5, 1996
18. Ito K et al: A case of the incomplete double aortic arch diagnosed in adulthood by MR imaging. Radiat Med. 13(5):263-7, 1995
19. Katz M et al: Spiral CT and 3D image reconstruction of vascular rings and associated tracheobronchial anomalies. J Comput Assist Tomogr. 19(4):564-8, 1995
20. Simoneaux SF et al: MR imaging of the pediatric airway. Radiographics. 15(2):287-98; discussion 298-9, 1995
21. Tuma S et al: Double aortic arch in d-transposition of the great arteries complicated by tracheobronchomalacia. Cardiovasc Intervent Radiol. 18(2):115-7, 1995
22. van Son JA et al: Demonstration of vascular ring anatomy with ultrafast computed tomography. Thorac Cardiovasc Surg. 43(2):120-1, 1995
23. van Son JA et al: Imaging strategies for vascular rings. Ann Thorac Surg. 57(3):604-10, 1994
24. Kramer LA et al: Rare case of double aortic arch with hypoplastic right dorsal segment and associated tetralogy of Fallot: MR findings. Magn Reson Imaging. 11(8):1217-21, 1993
25. Chun K et al: Diagnosis and management of congenital vascular rings: a 22-year experience. Ann Thorac Surg. 53(4):597-602; discussion 602-3, 1992
26. Formanek AG et al: Anomaly of the descending aorta: a case of persistent double dorsal aorta. AJR Am J Roentgenol. 156(5):1033-5, 1991
27. Jaffe RB: Radiographic manifestations of congenital anomalies of the aortic arch. Radiol Clin North Am. 29(2):319-34, 1991
28. Lowe GM et al: Vascular rings: 10-year review of imaging. Radiographics. 11(4):637-46, 1991

DOUBLE AORTIC ARCH

IMAGE GALLERY

Typical

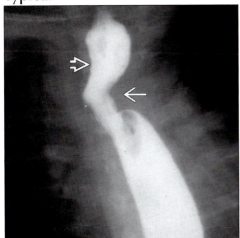
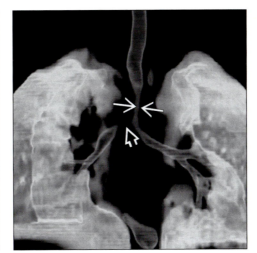

(Left) Anteroposterior upper GI shows characteristic esophageal indentations by dominant higher right arch (open arrow) and lower left arch (arrow) (Right) Coronal CECT airway rendition shows trachea in abnormal midline position, compressed on both sides by the two arches (arrows). Note obliteration of lumen of right mainstem bronchus (open arrow), indicative of bronchomalacia.

Variant

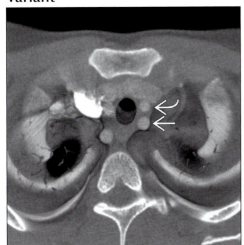
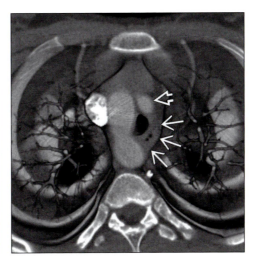

(Left) Axial CTA at thoracic inlet just above both arches shows separate take-off of both carotid (curved arrow, left carotid) and subclavian (arrow, left subclavian) arteries (four-artery sign). (Right) Axial CTA shows dominant right arch and patent portion of smaller left arch (open arrow). Arrows indicate location of atretic cord of distal left arch (between take-off of left subclavian and aorta), completing the constricting vascular ring.

Variant

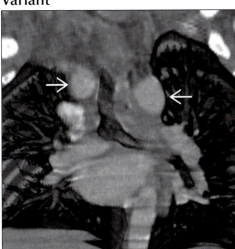
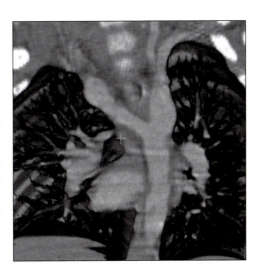

(Left) Coronal CTA 3D rendition shows loose vascular ring from both aortic arches (arrows), with dominant left arch. Note absence of tracheal narrowing. (Right) Oblique CTA 3D volume rendition shows junction of both arches posteriorly. This 7 year old boy was asymptomatic of this incidentally-noted double aortic arch.

PULMONARY SLING

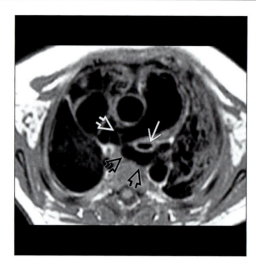

Axial T1WI MR shows type IA left pulmonary artery sling (open arrows) encircling and compressing distal trachea (arrow).

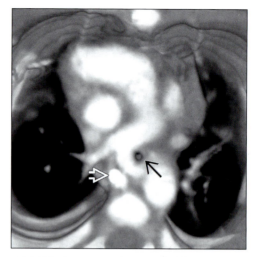

Axial CTA shows anomalous origin of left pulmonary artery, which courses between esophagus (identified by nasogastric tube, open arrow) and stenosed distal trachea (arrow).

TERMINOLOGY

Abbreviations and Synonyms
- Anomalous origin of the left pulmonary artery
- Aberrant left pulmonary artery

Definitions
- The left branch pulmonary artery originates from the proximal right branch pulmonary artery and forms a "sling" around the distal trachea as it passes leftward between trachea and esophagus

IMAGING FINDINGS

General Features
- Best diagnostic clue
  - Classic imaging appearance: Asymmetric lung inflation, narrowing of distal trachea which is displaced towards the left, anterior impression on mid-esophagus
  - It is the only vascular ring to course between the trachea and esophagus (compresses trachea from behind and esophagus from front)
- Morphology
  - Type I: Carina in normal location at T4-5 ⇒ predominant hyperinflation of right lung
    - With normal ("eparterial") right upper lobe bronchus
    - With tracheal bronchus (bronchus suis = "pig bronchus") to right upper lobe
  - Type II: Low carina at T6, with diffuse stenosis of intermediate left bronchus (ILB) by complete cartilaginous rings and absent membranous portion of trachea at multiple levels ("ring-sling" complex) ⇒ bilateral hyperinflation
    - Initial bifurcation at T4 into right upper lobe bronchus and ILB, which bifurcates at T6 into bridging right lower lobe bronchus and left mainstem bronchus
    - Lower ILB bifurcation is compressed by left pulmonary artery sling
    - Absent or abortive right upper lobe bronchus
    - Diffusely stenosed ILB (as in IIA) bifurcates at T6 into bridging right and left mainstem bronchus (low "inverted T" airway bifurcation)

Radiographic Findings
- Radiography
  - It is the only vascular ring associated with asymmetric lung inflation and aeration
  - Lateral view: Round soft tissue density between the distal trachea and esophagus
  - Posterior compression of the trachea, typically distally at the level of the distal trachea or carina

DDx: Other Causes Of Air Trapping, Masses And Tracheal Compression

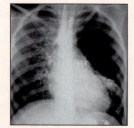

Lobar Emphysema

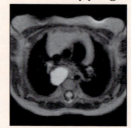

Bronchogenic Cyst

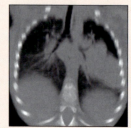

Lymphadenopathy

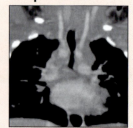

Double Aortic Arch

PULMONARY SLING

Key Facts

Terminology
- The left branch pulmonary artery originates from the proximal right branch pulmonary artery and forms a "sling" around the distal trachea as it passes leftward between trachea and esophagus

Imaging Findings
- It is the only vascular ring to course between the trachea and esophagus (compresses trachea from behind and esophagus from front)
- Type I: Carina in normal location at T4-5 ⇒ predominant hyperinflation of right lung
- Type II: Low carina at T6, with diffuse stenosis of intermediate left bronchus (ILB) by complete cartilaginous rings and absent membranous portion of trachea at multiple levels ("ring-sling" complex) ⇒ bilateral hyperinflation
- It is the only vascular ring associated with asymmetric lung inflation and aeration
- Lateral view: Round soft tissue density between the distal trachea and esophagus
- Barium swallow: It is the only vascular ring that leads to an anterior indentation on the esophagus
- The left pulmonary artery arises from the right, rather than the main, pulmonary artery
- Degree of tracheal compression typically severe
- When complete tracheal rings are present, the trachea will have a very round (rather than oval) appearance with an abnormally small diameter

Clinical Issues
- Most common signs/symptoms: Severe stridor, hypoxia, ventilator dependency

---

  - Distal trachea or right main bronchus may be bowed anteriorly
  - Low position of the left hilum

Fluoroscopic Findings
- Barium swallow: It is the only vascular ring that leads to an anterior indentation on the esophagus
- Trachea is compressed at same level from posteriorly

Echocardiographic Findings
- Echocardiogram
  - Absence of normal pulmonary artery bifurcation
  - Anomalous origin of left pulmonary artery from proximal right pulmonary artery
  - Associated other cardiac anomalies

Other Modality Findings
- CT and MR Features
  - Cross sectional imaging obtained to confirm diagnosis and delineate anatomy prior to surgery
  - Pulmonary sling and tracheal compression typically best demonstrated on axial CT or MR images
  - The left pulmonary artery arises from the right, rather than the main, pulmonary artery
  - The left pulmonary artery forms a "sling" around the trachea as it passes leftward between the trachea and esophagus
  - Degree of tracheal compression typically severe
  - Distal trachea and carina often displaced to the left
  - Often findings of coexisting congenital heart disease present
  - When complete tracheal rings are present, the trachea will have a very round (rather than oval) appearance with an abnormally small diameter

Imaging Recommendations
- Best imaging tool: Multidetector-row CTA is faster and logistically easier to perform than MRI in these critically ill infants on a ventilator
- Protocol advice
  - Thin axial slices are most helpful to depict sling anatomy
  - Coronal images or 3D reconstructions display effect of sling on tracheobronchial tree

DIFFERENTIAL DIAGNOSIS

Middle mediastinal mass
- Lymphadenopathy
- Bronchogenic cyst
- Esophageal duplication cyst

Primary bronchial malformation
- Congenital lobar emphysema/bronchial atresia
- Tracheobronchomalacia
- Complete cartilaginous ring

Midline descending aorta carina compression syndrome
- Descending aorta immediately anterior to spine, leading to "crowding" of mediastinum: Posterior compression on carina or left main stem bronchus
- May be isolated, or associated with right lung hypoplasia, arch anomalies

PATHOLOGY

General Features
- General path comments
  - Frequently associated with significant hypoplasia/dysplasia of distal trachea and main stem bronchi
  - Hemodynamics: Determined by associated cardiac anomaly
  - Pulmonary hypertension from severe hypoxia
- Genetics: No specific genetic defect identified
- Etiology
  - Embryology
    - Agenesis or obliteration of the left sixth aortic arch, which normally forms the left branch pulmonary artery
    - Arterial supply of left lung via persistent primitive artery originating from right pulmonary artery

PULMONARY SLING

- Pathophysiology: Severe stridor secondary to
  - Compression of distal trachea, carina, main stem bronchi: Uneven inflation of the lungs (obstructive emphysema > atelectasis)
  - Associated tracheobronchomalacia
  - Associated intrinsic airway narrowing (complete cartilaginous rings): Types IIA and IIB
- Associated abnormalities: Other congenital malformations (50%), lung hypoplasia, horseshoe lung

Gross Pathologic & Surgical Features
- The left pulmonary artery arises from the right, rather than the main, pulmonary artery
- The left pulmonary artery forms a "sling" around the trachea as it passes leftward between the trachea and esophagus
- It enters hilum of left lung posteriorly to left main stem bronchus
- Severe compression of distal trachea and right main stem bronchus
- Main stem bronchi have abnormal horizontal course ("inverted T"), with abnormal branching patterns to upper and lower lobes (types IIA and IIB)
- Often associated with with complete tracheal cartilaginous rings (50%)

CLINICAL ISSUES

Presentation
- Most common signs/symptoms: Severe stridor, hypoxia, ventilator dependency
- Other signs/symptoms: Noisy breathing, "seal bark" cough, apneic spells, recurrent pulmonary infections early in life

Demographics
- Age: Typically presents in neonatal period

Natural History & Prognosis
- Type II: Less favorable than other vascular rings, due to associated anomalies (60-80%)
  - Intrinsic tracheobronchial anomalies (complete rings, absent membranous portion of trachea), tracheomalacia
  - Congenital heart disease: Aortic arch anomalies, ventricular septal defect (10%), atrial septal defect (20%), patent ductus arteriosus (25%), single ventricle, tetralogy of Fallot, partial anomalous pulmonary venous return, persistent left superior vena cava (20%)
  - Pulmonary and systemic anomalies: Hypoplastic right lung, horseshoe lung, tracheo-esophageal fistula, imperforate anus, absence of gallbladder, Meckel diverticulum, biliary atresia, Hirschsprung disease

Treatment
- Surgical division of left pulmonary artery from its anomalous origin, with implantation to its normal location of origin, from main pulmonary artery
- Tracheobronchial reconstruction if there are complete cartilaginous rings or other associated tracheobronchial malformation (Types IIA and IIB)

DIAGNOSTIC CHECKLIST

Image Interpretation Pearls
- Anterior indentation on esophagus = left pulmonary artery (LPA) sling

SELECTED REFERENCES
1. Backer CL: Vascular rings and pulmonary artery sling. In: Mavroudis C, Backer CL ed. Pediatric cardiac surgery. 3rd ed. Philadelphia, Mosby. 234-50, 2003
2. Eichhorn J et al: Images in cardiovascular medicine. Time-resolved three-dimensional magnetic resonance angiography for assessing a pulmonary artery sling in a pediatric patient. Circulation. 106(14):e61-2, 2002
3. Hwang H-K et al: Horseshoe lung with pseudo-ring-sling complex. Pediatr Pulmonology. 34(5):402-4, 2002
4. Park SC et al: Vascular ring and pulmonary artery sling. In: Anderson RH et al, ed. Pediatric Cardiology. vol 2. 2nd ed. London, Churchill Livingstone.1559-75, 2002
5. Bove T et al: Tracheobronchial compression of vascular origin. Review of experience in infants and children. J Cardiovasc Surg (Torino). 42(5):663-6, 2001
6. Hodina M et al: Non-invasive imaging of the ring-sling complex in children. Pediatr Cardiol. 22(4):333-7, 2001
7. Lee KH et al: Use of imaging for assessing anatomical relationships of tracheobronchial anomalies associated with left pulmonary artery sling. Pediatr Radiol. 31(4):269-78, 2001
8. Woods RK et al: Vascular anomalies and tracheoesophageal compression: a single institution's 25-year experience. Ann Thorac Surg. 72(2):434-8; discussion 438-9, 2001
9. Berdon WE: Rings, slings, and other things: vascular compression of the infant trachea updated from the midcentury to the millennium--the legacy of Robert E. Gross, MD, and Edward B. D. Neuhauser, MD. Radiology. 216(3):624-32, 2000
10. Di Cesare E et al: Pulmonary artery sling diagnosed by magnetic resonance imaging. Magn Reson Imaging. 15(9):1107-9, 1997
11. Donnelly LF et al: The spectrum of extrinsic lower airway compression in children: MR imaging. AJR. 168:59-62, 1997
12. Siripornpitak S et al: Pulmonary artery sling: anatomical and functional evaluation by MRI. J Comput Assist Tomogr. 21(5):766-8, 1997
13. Pu WT et al: Diagnosis and management of agenesis of the right lung and left pulmonary artery sling. Am J Cardiol. 78(6):723-7, 1996
14. Newman B et al: Left pulmonary artery sling: diagnosis and delineation of associated tracheobronchial anomalies with MR. Pediatr Radiol. 26(9):661-8, 1996
15. Katz M et al: Spiral CT and 3D image reconstruction of vascular rings and associated tracheobronchial anomalies. J Comput Assist Tomogr. 19(4):564-8, 1995
16. Phillips RR et al: Pulmonary artery sling and hypoplastic right lung: diagnostic appearances using MRI. Pediatr Radiol. 23(2):117-9, 1993
17. Vogl TJ et al: MRI in pre- and postoperative assessment of tracheal stenosis due to pulmonary artery sling. J Comput Assist Tomogr. 17(6):878-86, 1993
18. Backer CL et al: Pulmonary artery sling. Results of surgical repair in infancy. J Thorac Cardiovasc Surg. 103(4):683-91, 1992
19. Sade RM et al: Pulmonary artery sling. J Thorac Cardiovasc Surg. 69(3):333-46, 1975
20. Berdon WE et al: Vascular anomalies and the infant lung: rings, slings, and other things. Semin Roentgenol. 7:39-63, 1972

PULMONARY SLING

IMAGE GALLERY

Typical

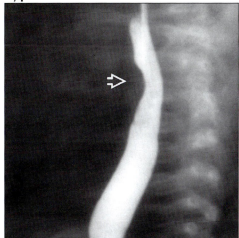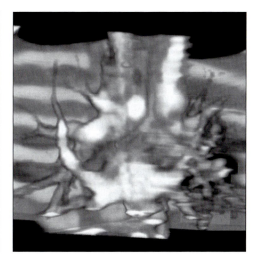

(Left) Lateral upper GI shows typical anterior indentation on esophagus *(arrow)* by type I LPA sling. *(Right)* Coronal CTA shows stenosis of distal trachea caused by right-sided compression by LPA sling vessel.

Variant

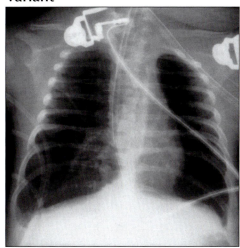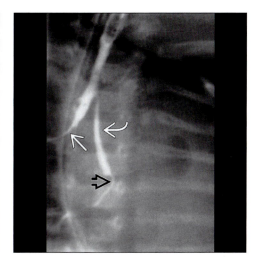

(Left) Anteroposterior radiograph of respirator-dependent infant with Down syndrome shows asymmetric hyperinflation of the lungs, right greater then left. *(Right)* Anteroposterior shows type IIA tracheobronchial anomaly, with high bifurcation into RUL *(arrow)* and diffusely narrowed intermediate left bronchus *(curved arrow)*, with low LPA sling indentation *(open arrow)* and bridging right bronchus.

Variant

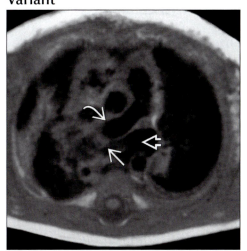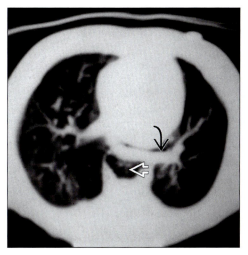

(Left) Axial T1WI MR shows proximal aspect of LPA sling *(curved arrow)*, and diffusely stenosed intermediate left bronchus *(arrow)*. Note horseshoe lung segment in posterior mediastinum *(open arrow)*. *(Right)* Axial NECT shows distal aspect of LPA sling, traveling to left lung *(curved arrow)*, and horseshoe lung segment in posterior mediastinum *(open arrow)*.

SUBGLOTTIC HEMANGIOMA

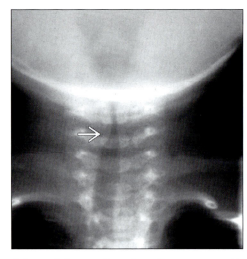

Anteroposterior radiograph shows asymmetric subglottic narrowing of initial portion of trachea (arrow) in a two week old infant with stridor.

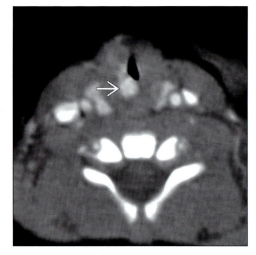

Axial CECT shows discrete localized mass posterior lateral wall of trachea (arrow). It densely enhances with contrast administration and causes focal tracheal compression.

TERMINOLOGY

Abbreviations and Synonyms
- Infantile hemangioma
- Subglottic hemangioma

Definitions
- Hemangioma located in the soft tissues of neck which affect subglottic airway
- May be isolated or associated with other hemangiomas of the trunk or particularly the face

IMAGING FINDINGS

General Features
- Best diagnostic clue
  - Asymmetrical subglottic narrowing in young child
  - Mass bulging into the airway on cross sectional imaging
  - Mass which enhances in subglottic space
  - Mass partially obstructing airway
  - Highly vascular mass in the neck
- Location
  - Subglottic space of the trachea
  - Lesion may be circumferential, bilateral, unilateral
  - Usually asymmetric affecting only one side, L > R
  - Posterior lateral position most common
  - Most common other site of hemangiomas is lower face with 8% having a beard type distribution which increases likelihood of symptomatic airway obstruction
  - With or without posterior extension to neck or mediastinum
- Size: Usually small
- Morphology: Well-defined highly vascular lesion

Radiographic Findings
- Radiography
  - Non rotated anteroposterior (AP) and lateral films of the airway
    - Asymmetric subglottic narrowing

CT Findings
- CECT
  - Enhancing, localized, usually solitary subglottic mass
  - Rarely calcify
  - Intense and uniform enhancement with contrast
  - Retains nodular contrast-enhancement
  - Involuting hemangiomas show decreased central flow

MR Findings
- T1WI
  - Smooth, lobulated, homogeneous, hyperintense lesions

DDx: Subglottic Airway Obstruction

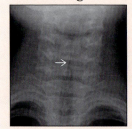

Viral Croup

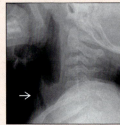

Viral Croup

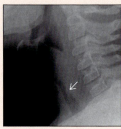

Membranous Croup

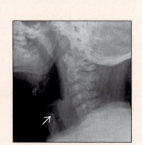

Tracheal Granuloma

SUBGLOTTIC HEMANGIOMA

Key Facts

Terminology
- Hemangioma located in the soft tissues of neck which affect subglottic airway
- May be isolated or associated with other hemangiomas of the trunk or particularly the face

Imaging Findings
- Asymmetrical subglottic narrowing in young child
- Lesion may be circumferential, bilateral, unilateral
- Enhancing, localized, usually solitary subglottic mass
- Smooth, lobulated, homogeneous, hyperintense lesions
- With large masses, either CT or MRI useful
- 3D reconstructions help define mass and degree of tracheal compression

Top Differential Diagnoses
- Subglottic stenosis
- Tracheal granuloma
- Viral croup
- Membranous croup

Clinical Issues
- Croup-like symptoms in infants less than 6 months
- Inspiratory stridor
- Associated with cutaneous hemangiomas in 50% of cases
- Majority of lesions have progressive airway obstruction during proliferative phase
- Diagnosis made at endoscopy
- Combinations of therapy used in 75% of children

  - Flow voids within or adjacent to mass
- T2WI: Spin-echo images show hyperintensity
- T1 C+: With gadolinium, lesions have peripheral nodular enhancement and progressive, prolonged contrast material in lesion
- MRI is useful if there is extensive involvement

Imaging Recommendations
- Best imaging tool
  - With large masses, either CT or MRI useful
    - 3D reconstructions help define mass and degree of tracheal compression
    - Images the airway compression and extent of mass
  - MRI most sensitive but sedation is usually needed
    - Imaging takes longer and infant has tracheal compression
  - CT with contrast utilized if severe airway obstruction present
- Protocol advice
  - Radiographs: High quality, non rotated AP and lateral
    - When abnormal, follow up with endoscopy
  - CT
    - Good contrast bolus technique
    - Adjust the radiation dose for pediatric patient

DIFFERENTIAL DIAGNOSIS

Subglottic stenosis
- Congenital stenosis
  - May be associated with other anomalies
- Acquired stenosis
  - Usually a history of prior intubation or injury

Tracheal granuloma
- History of prior intubation or tracheotomy

Viral croup
- Symmetric subglottic narrowing
- Occurs in children 8 months to three years

Membranous croup
- Intraluminal filling defects from inflammation
- Never occurs in young infants or children

Tracheal papillomatosis
- Affects entire trachea, bronchi, and lungs

PATHOLOGY

General Features
- Genetics
  - Likely genetic linkage of growth factors
  - Various protein makers such as glucose 1 protein deficiency
- Etiology: Hemangioma is a lesion that arises by endothelial hyperplasia whereas vascular malformations are lesions that arise by dysmorphogenesis and exhibit normal endothelial turnover
- Epidemiology: Subglottic hemangiomas account for 1.5% of all congenital anomalies of the larynx
- Associated abnormalities
  - Other hemangiomas most common in the face, extremity or trunk
    - Cutaneous hemangiomas in 50% of cases

Gross Pathologic & Surgical Features
- Submucosal mass with abnormal red color reflecting vascularity of lesion

Microscopic Features
- Stages of life cycle of hemangioma documented by light and electron microscopy and immunohistochemical techniques
- Proliferation phase has increased fibroblast growth factor and endothelial growth factor
- Involution phase has endothelial apoptosis and downregulation of angiogenesis with accumulation of mast cells
- Biological markers include glucose transporter protein which is seen in all stages

Staging, Grading or Classification Criteria
- Mulliken and Glowacki classification (1982), subsequently modified in 1996

SUBGLOTTIC HEMANGIOMA

○ Reflects the cellular kinetics and clinical behavior

CLINICAL ISSUES

Presentation
- Most common signs/symptoms
  ○ Croup-like symptoms in infants less than 6 months
  ○ Signs of airway obstruction maybe progressive
  ○ Inspiratory stridor
  ○ Hoarseness or abnormal cry
  ○ Typically stridor if less than 6 months of age
  ○ Age of presentation and degree of obstruction does not alter outcome
- Other signs/symptoms
  ○ Associated with cutaneous hemangiomas in 50% of cases
  ○ PHACE syndrome: Posterior fossa brain malformations, hemangiomas, arterial anomalies, coarctation of the aorta and cardiac defects, and eye abnormalities
    - 7% have subglottic hemangiomas
  ○ Kasabach-Merritt syndrome rarely associated with subglottic hemangiomas
    - May be life threatening
    - Associated with massive trapping of platelets, coagulopathy, and death
    - Large, extensive hemangiomas in the body with rapid growth and platelet trapping

Demographics
- Age
  ○ Presents during first year of life
    - May be present at birth
    - Average age is four months
  ○ Usually symptomatic prior to 6 months of age
- Gender: Females are affected twice as often as males

Natural History & Prognosis
- Unpredictable
  ○ Majority of lesions have progressive airway obstruction during proliferative phase
    - Lesions may grow rapidly
    - May need to be treated as airway obstruction may be progressive
  ○ Resolution of the symptoms during involutive phase
    - Natural history of lesions are that they involute spontaneously
- Benign condition but can have fatal outcome
  ○ With treatment, 30-70% mortality rate has been reported
  ○ Complications include bleeding, ulceration, airway obstruction
- Diagnosis made at endoscopy
  ○ Soft, slightly reddened, submucosal, compressible mass
  ○ Biopsy of mass not necessary as bleeding may occur

Treatment
- General principles
  ○ Combinations of therapy used in 75% of children
  ○ Complications are common with all treatments
  ○ A multitude of medical and surgical modalities have been proposed
- Conservative monitoring
  ○ Used in children with < 30% narrowing without respiratory or feeding difficulty
  ○ Need to have immediate access to care as lesions may grow quickly and obstruct
- Corticosteroids, systemic
  ○ Often used in association with other treatments
  ○ Positive response is seen in 30-60% of cases in first two weeks
  ○ Rebound growth may occur when steroids are tapered
  ○ Some hemangiomas do not respond
  ○ Side effects include infection, growth restriction, cushingoid features
- Corticosteroids, intralesional
  ○ After intralesional injection, children must be intubated
  ○ Repeated endoscopy and multiple injections with prolonged intubation times are a concern
- CO_2 laser therapy
  ○ Reported success rates are variable and may be operator dependent
  ○ Most patients also treated with other forms of therapy
  ○ Complications include thermal damage to cricoid
- Laryngotracheoplasty: Direct excision of small masses
- Tracheotomy to bypass the airway obstruction
  ○ Does not influence the natural history of hemangioma
  ○ Useful with multiple lesions of the glottis and trachea
  ○ Glottic and supraglottic involvement with airway obstruction
- Interferon
  ○ Used in life threatening hemangiomas of infancy
  ○ May cause low grade fever, neutropenia, anemia, and spastic diplegia in 5-20% of treated patients
- Vincristine therapy
  ○ Used as an alternative to Interferon when other therapies fail
- Direct excision of subglottic hemangiomas
  ○ Usually need tracheotomy
  ○ Usually had prior "failed" surgeries
  ○ Recommended for bilateral or circumferential lesions, and for patients who do not respond to other treatments

SELECTED REFERENCES

1. Pransky SM et al: Management of subglottic hemangioma. Curr Opin Otolaryngol Head Neck Surg. 12(6):509-512, 2004
2. Rahbar R et al: The Biology and Management of Subglottic Hemangioma: Past, Present, Future. Laryngoscope. 114(11):1880-1891, 2004
3. Re M et al: Role of endoscopic CO2 laser surgery in the treatment of congenital infantile subglottic hemangioma. Experience in the Department of Otolaryngology, "Sick Children Hospital", Toronto, Canada. Acta Otorhinolaryngol Ital. 23(3):175-9, 2003
4. Poetke M et al: PHACE syndrome: new views on diagnostic criteria. Eur J Pediatr Surg. 12(6):366-74, 2002

SUBGLOTTIC HEMANGIOMA

IMAGE GALLERY

Typical

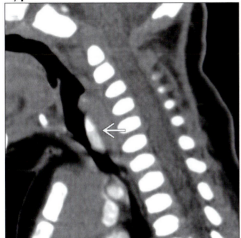
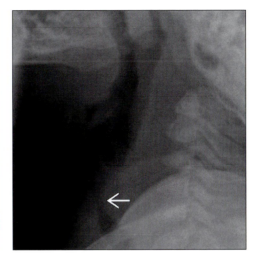

(Left) Sagittal CECT shows mass indenting the posterior wall of the trachea in the subglottic space *(arrow)*. It densely enhances with contrast administration. *(Right)* Lateral radiograph shows severe narrowing in subglottic space *(arrow)*. The narrowing appears circumferential and is below the vocal cords and above the thoracic inlet.

Typical

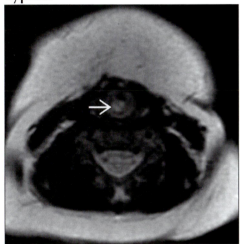
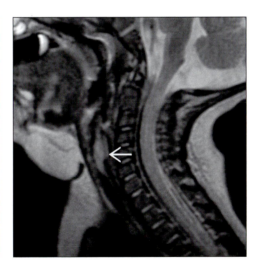

(Left) Axial T2WI MR shows an enhancing mass indenting posterolateral submucosa of the trachea *(arrow)*. The mass compromises the tracheal airway by narrowing the lumen. *(Right)* Sagittal T2WI MR shows well localized mass *(arrow)* posterior to the trachea in the immediate subglottic space.

Typical

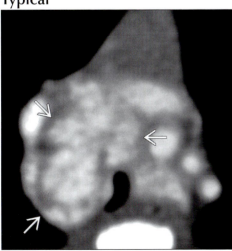
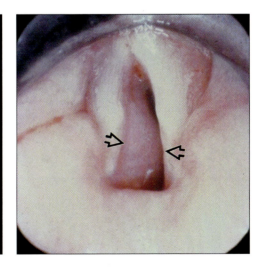

(Left) Axial CECT shows nodular enhancing mass *(arrows)* narrowing the tracheal airway. Mass is circumferential but affects right side greater than left and extends into the mediastinum. *(Right)* Endoscopic photograph demonstrating bulging red mass *(arrows)* protruding into the trachea at the level of the subglottic space with narrowing of the airway.

INNOMINATE ARTERY COMPRESSION SYNDROME

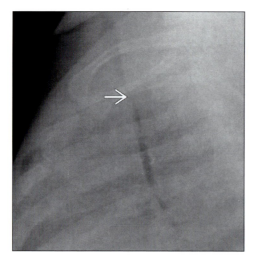

Lateral radiograph shows discrete narrowing of the anterior portion of the trachea (arrow) at the thoracic inlet in an infant that presented with stridor.

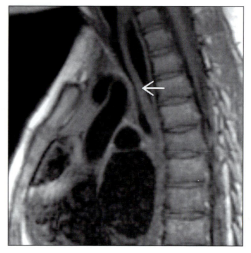

Sagittal T1WI MR shows the innominate artery immediately anterior to trachea and causing discrete anterior tracheal compression (arrow) as it ascends rightward and superiorly.

TERMINOLOGY

Abbreviations and Synonyms
- Tracheomalacia

Definitions
- Tracheal compression secondary to the innominate artery
  - Likely related to lack of rigidity of the infantile cartilage of trachea

IMAGING FINDINGS

General Features
- Best diagnostic clue
  - Narrowing of trachea from anterior compression secondary to the innominate artery on any imaging study
    - Narrowing and compression occurs at thoracic inlet
    - Tracheal narrowing can be seen in asymptomatic infants
- Location: Localized compression of the anterior trachea at thoracic inlet
- Size: Decrease in tracheal lumen
- Morphology: Infant trachea lacks rigidity and prone to vascular compression

Radiographic Findings
- Radiography
  - On lateral radiography, anterior aspect of trachea is compressed
  - Compression is just below thoracic inlet
  - Left-sided aortic arch identified
  - Lung aeration not affected

Fluoroscopic Findings
- Esophagram
  - On barium swallow, may see gastroesophageal reflux and dynamic airway changes
  - Airway fluoroscopy is not normally performed as children are endoscoped

CT Findings
- CECT
  - Tracheal narrowing confined to level at which innominate artery crosses anterior to trachea
  - Marked narrowing of the trachea in superior mediastinum
  - Innominate artery immediately abuts area of tracheal narrowing
  - Evaluates other structures in superior mediastinum
    - Excludes masses or malformations
- CTA
  - 3D reformatted images show relationship of vessels to trachea

DDx: Tracheal Compression

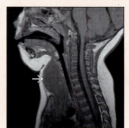

Lymphatic Mass

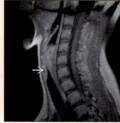

Polychondritis

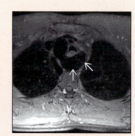

Vascular Ring

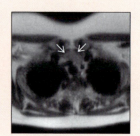

Aberrant Thymus

INNOMINATE ARTERY COMPRESSION SYNDROME

Key Facts

Terminology
- Tracheal compression secondary to the innominate artery
- Likely related to lack of rigidity of the infantile cartilage of trachea

Imaging Findings
- Location: Localized compression of the anterior trachea at thoracic inlet
- On lateral radiography, anterior aspect of trachea is compressed
- CT or MR defines degree of tracheal compression by the innominate artery

Top Differential Diagnoses
- Masses which compress the trachea
- Normal structures in an atypical position
- Vascular anomalies
- Lymphatic malformation compressing airway
- Pre- or post-operative congenital heart disease

Pathology
- Spectrum of severity from severe narrowing with symptoms to asymptomatic
- Infant's innominate artery arises from aortic arch more to left than it does in adults

Clinical Issues
- Presentation includes stridor, apnea, dyspnea
- Most children treated conservatively and outgrow disease
- Surgical therapy is controversial
- Reserved for those with severe symptoms and who fail conservative management

---

- Virtual airway endoscopy

MR Findings
- Anterior narrowing of the trachea as innominate artery crosses
- Allows evaluation of other vessels and structures
- 3D reformatted shows relationships

Echocardiographic Findings
- Echocardiogram: Normal study as tracheomalacia not usually associated with congenital heart disease

Other Modality Findings
- Endoscopy shows fixed, pulsatile compression from the anterior aspect of the trachea just below thoracic inlet

Imaging Recommendations
- Best imaging tool
  - Lateral chest radiograph shows anterior tracheal narrowing
  - CT or MR defines degree of tracheal compression by the innominate artery
  - Diagnosis confirmed at endoscopy
- Protocol advice
  - Positive pressure from intubation may stent the trachea and mask obstruction
  - CT
    - Needed only in moderate to severe cases or prior to consideration for surgery
    - Performed to evaluate vascular compression and relationship to the airway
    - Excludes other causes of compression
  - MR
    - Study can be done but if young child, usually sedation is necessary
    - Anatomy well seen on axial, sagittal and coronal imaging

DIFFERENTIAL DIAGNOSIS

Masses which compress the trachea
- Mass is characterized by CECT or MR
- Bronchogenic cysts can be superior mediastinal in location
- Duplication cyst
- Large neurofibroma or retropharyngeal masses
- Lymphoma in the anterior mediastinum
- Thymic cysts

Normal structures in an atypical position
- Aberrant thyroid or aberrant thymic tissue
  - Can be identified on tissue characterization on imaging

Vascular anomalies
- Compression of the trachea and the esophagus
- Most common is right aortic arch with aberrant left subclavian artery
- Double aortic arch

Lymphatic malformation compressing airway
- Lymphatic malformation can infiltrate the mediastinum and cause airway compression

Pre- or post-operative congenital heart disease
- May be associated with tracheal narrowing for a number of reasons

PATHOLOGY

General Features
- General path comments
  - Spectrum of severity from severe narrowing with symptoms to asymptomatic
  - Innominate may normally indent trachea in 30% of infants under age two
  - Infant's innominate artery arises from aortic arch more to left than it does in adults
  - Superior mediastinum "crowded" in infants secondary to thymus
  - Some speculate that large thymus contributes to the crowding

INNOMINATE ARTERY COMPRESSION SYNDROME

- ○ Combination of these factors in theory leads to innominate artery compressing trachea
- Genetics: No genetic predisposition
- Etiology
  - ○ Narrowing of trachea at thoracic inlet secondary to compression by innominate artery
    - Infantile trachea relatively flaccid, lacking rigidity
    - In infants, the innominate artery arises from the aortic arch left of trachea
    - As it crosses trachea, occasionally causes moderate tracheal compression
    - Leads to compression of trachea as the innominate artery crosses obliquely
    - Leads to compression of trachea as innominate ascends superiorly in neck
  - ○ Frequently associated with esophageal atresia
    - Dilated esophagus compresses posterior wall of the trachea
    - Displaces the trachea anteriorly which causes innominate to compress
    - May need aortopexy if symptomatic
- Associated abnormalities
  - ○ Esophageal atresia, post-repair
  - ○ Severe and persistent gastroesophageal reflux with failure to thrive
  - ○ Thoracic deformity with small superior mediastinum
  - ○ Laryngomalacia with severe reflux
  - ○ Large thymus

Gross Pathologic & Surgical Features
- Anterior wall of the trachea demonstrates abnormal cartilage related to vascular compression
- Cartilage compression causes a decrease in luminal size of the trachea in infants

Microscopic Features
- Infant trachea may have immature cartilage and not as rigid

CLINICAL ISSUES

Presentation
- Most common signs/symptoms
  - ○ Presentation includes stridor, apnea, dyspnea
    - Feeding accentuates the symptoms
    - Occasional bradycardia and reflex apnea
    - Symptoms will typically resolve as the child grows
  - ○ Many children will have mild anterior compression (normal variant) on lateral radiographs and they are asymptomatic
- Other signs/symptoms
  - ○ Failure to thrive due to feeding and airway problems
  - ○ Children with severe gastroesophageal reflux may have tracheomalacia

Demographics
- Age: Young infants
- Gender: More common in males

Natural History & Prognosis
- The compression and resultant symptoms typically decrease over time as child grows

Treatment
- Most children treated conservatively and outgrow disease
- Children with esophageal atresia may need aortopexy
- Surgical therapy is controversial
  - ○ Reserved for those with severe symptoms and who fail conservative management
  - ○ Aortopexy and re-implantation of innominate artery origin

DIAGNOSTIC CHECKLIST

Image Interpretation Pearls
- Always look at the trachea
- Walls should be parallel
- Tracheal narrowing
  - ○ Does not always indicate clinical abnormality in young children
  - ○ Usually related to a specific condition
  - ○ At thoracic inlet is caused by innominate artery compression
  - ○ By the innominate artery may occur in asymptomatic infants

SELECTED REFERENCES

1. Faust RA et al: Cine magnetic resonance imaging for evaluation of focal tracheomalacia: innominate artery compression syndrome. Int J Pediatr Otorhinolaryngol. 65(1):27-33, 2002
2. Weber TR et al: Aortic suspension (aortopexy) for severe tracheomalacia in infants and children. Am J Surg. 184(6):573-7; discussion 577, 2002
3. Simoneaux SF et al: MR imaging of the pediatric airway. Radiographics. 15(2):287-98; discussion 298-9, 1995
4. Mandell GA et al: Innominate artery compression of the trachea: relationship to cervical herniation of the normal thymus. Radiology. 190(1):131-5, 1994
5. Hawkins JA et al: Innominate artery compression of the trachea. Treatment by reimplantation of the innominate artery. J Thorac Cardiovasc Surg. 103(4):678-82, 1992
6. Guys JM et al: Esophageal atresia, tracheomalacia and arterial compression: role of aortopexy. Eur J Pediatr Surg. 1(5):261-5, 1991
7. Vogl T et al: MR imaging in pediatric airway obstruction. J Comput Assist Tomogr. 14(2):182-6, 1990
8. Strife JL et al: Tracheal compression by the innominate artery in infancy and childhood. Radiology. 139:73-5, 1981
9. Berdon WE et al: Vascular anomalies and the infant lung: rings, slings, and other things. Semin Roentgenol. 7:39-63, 1972
10. Berdon WE et al: Innominate artery compression of the trachea in infants with stridor and apnea. Radiology. 92:272-8, 1969

INNOMINATE ARTERY COMPRESSION SYNDROME

IMAGE GALLERY

Typical

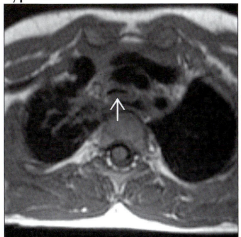
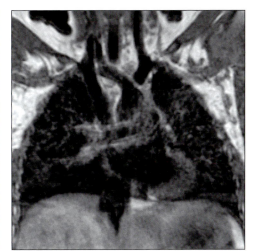

(Left) Axial T1WI MR shows anterior compression of trachea by the innominate artery as it crosses to the right (arrow). The normal innominate artery has an origin to the left of trachea. *(Right)* Coronal T1WI MR shows the origin of innominate artery from the aorta to left of trachea. It usually crosses the trachea and moves rightward before branching.

Typical

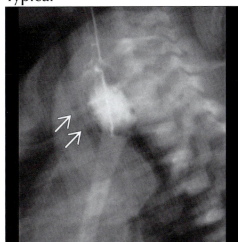
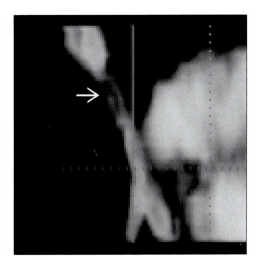

(Left) Lateral upper GI shows catheter in proximal pouch in a newborn with esophageal atresia. Note the long segment tracheal narrowing at thoracic inlet (arrows). *(Right)* 3D CECT reconstruction shows airway narrowing which affects the anterior portion of the trachea at the level of the thoracic inlet (arrow).

Typical

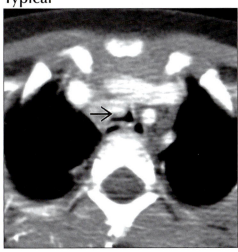
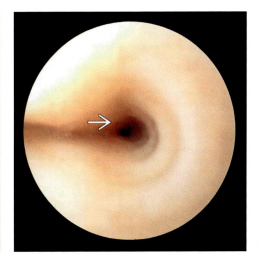

(Left) Axial CECT shows the indentation of the trachea by the innominate artery (arrow). Note the degree of trachea narrowing of the anterior wall. *(Right)* Endoscopic photograph shows narrowing of the anterior portion of trachea and tracheal collapse (arrow). Mass usually pulsates making evaluation easier. Image is oriented the same as prior axial CT.

RIGHT ARCH WITH ABERRANT LEFT SCA

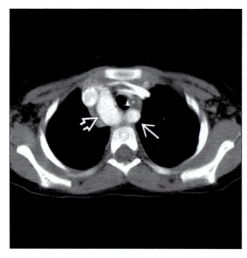

Axial CTA shows right aortic arch (open arrow) and aberrant left subclavian artery (arrow). Airway was compressed at more inferior image.

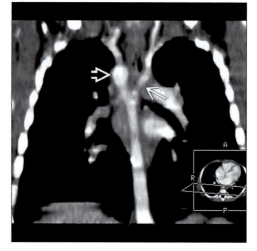

Coronal CTA shows right arch (open arrow) and aberrant left subclavian artery (arrow).

TERMINOLOGY

Definitions
- Aortic arch to right of trachea; left subclavian artery (LSA) takes off from proximal descending aorta, and it courses behind esophagus

IMAGING FINDINGS

General Features
- Best diagnostic clue
  - Aortic arch located to right of trachea, coursing over right main stem bronchus
  - Large vessel arising from the distal aorta and passing behind the esophagus with oblique course to the left
  - In 60% there is dilatation of the origin of the aberrant subclavian artery (aortic diverticulum of Kommerell)

Radiographic Findings
- Radiography
  - Chest radiography
    - Aortic arch indentation on right of trachea, which is deviated to the left
    - More soft tissue density over right vertebral pedicle than over left
    - Right-sided descending aorta line
    - Lateral view demonstrates indentation on the posterior aspect of the trachea
    - If aneurysmal dilatation of aortic diverticulum or subclavian, there may be prominence of the left mediastinum

Fluoroscopic Findings
- Barium swallow findings
  - Frontal view: Oblique filling defect coursing from right-inferior to left-superior
  - Lateral view: Posterior indentation
  - Large posterior indentation: Aortic diverticulum of Kommerell

CT Findings
- Axial images define patency of arch segments, branching patterns
- Axial and coronal reconstructions depict constricting effect on tracheal airway, if present

MR Findings
- Coronal thin-section images through the junction of the transverse and descending aorta demonstrate origin and proximal aspect of the aberrant vessel, as it passes posterior to the esophagus
- Axial and coronal images show effect on tracheobronchial tree

DDx: Right Aortic Arch

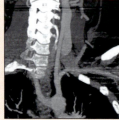
L Arch, Aberrant RSA

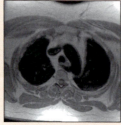
L Arch, Aberrant RSA

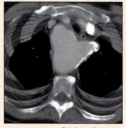
Aneurysmal LSA Origin

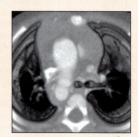
Mirror Image R Arch

RIGHT ARCH WITH ABERRANT LEFT SCA

Key Facts

Imaging Findings
- Aortic arch located to right of trachea, coursing over right main stem bronchus
- Large vessel arising from the distal aorta and passing behind the esophagus with oblique course to the left
- In 60% there is dilatation of the origin of the aberrant subclavian artery (aortic diverticulum of Kommerell)
- Frontal view: Oblique filling defect coursing from right-inferior to left-superior
- Lateral view: Posterior indentation

Pathology
- The left ductus persists as ligamentum arteriosum, which completes the vascular ring
- Left ligamentum arteriosum connects to subclavian artery ⇒ loose vascular ring
- Left ligamentum arteriosum connects to aortic diverticulum of Kommerell ⇒ tight vascular ring
- Most common congenital anomaly of aortic arch

Clinical Issues
- Right arch with aberrant LSA: Incidental finding, often asymptomatic (only symptoms in 5%)
- Right arch with aberrant LSA and constricting (symptomatic) left ligamentum arteriosum: Division of ligamentum via left thoracotomy

Diagnostic Checklist
- Right arch, no airway compression on radiograph, aberrant LSA on esophagram: No further work-up needed (non-constricting ring)
- Right arch with airway compression and aberrant LSA on esophagram: Perform cross-sectional imaging

Echocardiographic Findings
- Echocardiogram
  - Defines right arch, branching pattern
  - Origin of aberrant LSA is well seen, especially in the presence of an aortic diverticulum of Kommerell

Imaging Recommendations
- Best imaging tool
  - Multidetector-row CTA with 3D reconstruction
    - Advantages: Fast, generally no need for sedation/anesthesia, no need for intubation, and therefore better evaluation of airway compression
    - Disadvantage: Radiation dose
  - Multiplanar MRI
    - Advantage: No radiation dose
    - Disadvantage: Takes longer to perform than multidetector-row CT
- Protocol advice
  - Axial thin slices through tracheobronchial tree, proximal descending aorta to show aberrant LSA
  - Coronal imaging/reformats to depict airway compression

DIFFERENTIAL DIAGNOSIS

Right aortic arch with mirror image branching
- Associated with cyanotic congenital heart disease (CHD)
  - Tetralogy of Fallot, pulmonary atresia with ventricular septal defect: 25% incidence right arch
  - Truncus arteriosus: 30-40% incidence right arch

Double aortic arch with dominant right arch
- Left arch often not well seen, atretic segment and not left ligamentum arteriosum maintains fibrous continuity of vascular ring
- Characterized by tracheal narrowing, is nearly always symptomatic (stridor)

Left aortic arch with aberrant right subclavian artery
- Mirror image of right aortic arch with aberrant LSA
- Oblique posterior esophageal indentation from left-inferior to right-superior
- Isolated abnormality, incidentally found and usually without airway compression
- Rarely symptomatic from esophageal compression (dysphagia lusoria)

PATHOLOGY

General Features
- General path comments
  - All arch anomalies are a spectrum of the hypothetical double arch model of Edwards, with point of interruption:
    - Normal development: Distal to right subclavian artery (RSA)
    - Right arch, mirror image branching: Distal to left subclavian artery
    - Right arch, aberrant LSA: Between left common carotid and LSA
    - Left arch, aberrant RSA: Between right common carotid and RSA
  - Aberrant LSA rarely may lie anterior to the trachea (5%)
  - When associated with coarctation, aberrant subclavian artery can serve as a major collateral when it arises distally to coarctation
  - Embryology-anatomy
    - Related to embryological persistence of the right fourth aortic arch
    - Retroesophageal (Kommerell) diverticulum: Remnant of embryonic left fourth aortic arch and connects to left ductus ligament
    - LSA can arise directly from the descending aorta or can arise from an aortic diverticulum (Kommerell)

MIDLINE DESCENDING AORTA

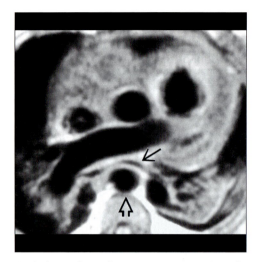

Axial shows descending aorta (open arrow) to be anterior to spine, instead of in left paraspinal location. Left main bronchus (arrow) is compressed between MDA and pulmonary artery.

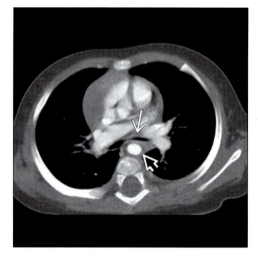

Axial CECT shows descending aorta (open arrow) to be anterior to spine, instead of in a left paraspinal location. Left main bronchus (arrow) is compressed between MDA and pulmonary artery.

TERMINOLOGY

Abbreviations and Synonyms
- Midline descending aorta - airway compression syndrome, MDA-ACS

Definitions
- Descending aorta positioned immediately anterior to vertebral bodies rather than in normal left paravertebral location
- Malposition leads to abnormal stacking of structures in the confined space between the spine and the anterior chest wall
- Can occur as an isolated lesion or in association with hypoplastic right lung and resultant mediastinal shift, right arch and left-sided descending aorta, double aortic arch, right aortic arch with left subclavian artery

IMAGING FINDINGS

General Features
- Best diagnostic clue
  o Classic imaging appearance: On cross-sectional imaging, aorta positioned immediately anterior to spine with associated airway compression
  o The distal airway, most typically the carina or main bronchi, is extrinsically compressed between the abnormally positioned descending aorta posteriorly and the pulmonary arteries anteriorly

Radiographic Findings
- Radiography
  o Radiographs often normal
  o Although radiography often able to depict compression of the trachea from vascular rings, radiographs insensitive to compression of the carina and proximal bronchi in children
  o Asymmetric air trapping usually not present on chest radiographs

CT Findings
- CECT
  o Imaging test of choice for work up of extrinsic airway compression
    ▪ Rapid multidetector CT depicts abnormalities
    ▪ Data can be displayed in multiple planes
    ▪ Most patients are infants and small children and sedation can often be avoided as compared to MRI
  o Aorta demonstrated anterior to vertebral bodies instead of in normal left paravertebral location
  o Carina or proximal main bronchus compressed between descending aorta posteriorly and pulmonary arteries anteriorly

DDx: Extrinsic Airway Compression

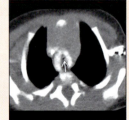
Double Aortic Arch

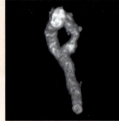
Double Aortic Arch

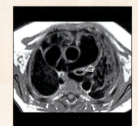
Pulmonary Sling

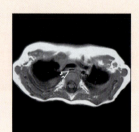
Thoracic Deformity

MIDLINE DESCENDING AORTA

Key Facts

Terminology
- Midline descending aorta - airway compression syndrome, MDA-ACS
- Descending aorta positioned immediately anterior to vertebral bodies rather than in normal left paravertebral location
- Malposition leads to abnormal stacking of structures in the confined space between the spine and the anterior chest wall
- Can occur as an isolated lesion or in association with hypoplastic right lung and resultant mediastinal shift, right arch and left-sided descending aorta, double aortic arch, right aortic arch with left subclavian artery

Imaging Findings
- Classic imaging appearance: On cross-sectional imaging, aorta positioned immediately anterior to spine with associated airway compression
- Radiographs often normal
- Although radiography often able to depict compression of the trachea from vascular rings, radiographs insensitive to compression of the carina and proximal bronchi in children
- Imaging test of choice for work up of extrinsic airway compression
- Aorta demonstrated anterior to vertebral bodies instead of in normal left paravertebral location

---

- ○ Associated findings such as arch anomalies or hypoplastic lung also well demonstrated
- ○ Typically do not see air trapping within lungs
- CTA: CECT performed as a CTA

MR Findings
- T1WI
  - ○ Aorta demonstrated anterior to vertebral bodies instead of in normal left paravertebral location
  - ○ Carina or proximal main bronchus compressed between descending aorta posteriorly and pulmonary arteries anteriorly
- MRA: Can be utilized to generate images that can better be used for communication purposes
- At most institutions MRI has been replaced with multidetector CT and CTA in the evaluation of children with suspected extrinsic airway compression
- MRI can well demonstrate findings
- Advantage is lack of ionizing radiation and non-dependence on IV contrast
- Most young children will need sedation to obtain an MRI and in a child with airway compression avoiding sedation is an important issue

Angiographic Findings
- Conventional: No longer performed in work-up of extrinsic airway compression and suspicion of vascular ring

DIFFERENTIAL DIAGNOSIS

Non-vascular mediastinal mass
- Small middle mediastinal masses such as duplication cyst, adenopathy

Double aortic arch
- Compression typically of upper trachea between aortic arches

Other arch anomalies
- Arch anomalies may have anatomy that compresses airway and leads to stridor

Anomalous origin of the pulmonary artery (pulmonary sling)
- Only vascular ring associated with asymmetric lung aeration
- Often associated with other congenital heart disease
- Associated with tracheal rings

Airway compression associated with thoracic deformity
- Typically occurs in children older than infancy
- Thoracic deformity present

Endobronchial obstruction such as from foreign body
- May be acute or chronic in presentation

PATHOLOGY

General Features
- General path comments
  - ○ Etiology of isolated position of midline descending aorta unknown
  - ○ Descending aorta positioned immediately anterior to vertebral bodies rather than in normal left paravertebral location
  - ○ Malposition leads to abnormal stacking of structures in the confined space between the spine and the anterior chest wall
  - ○ The distal airway, most typically the carina or main bronchi, is extrinsically compressed between the abnormally positioned descending aorta posteriorly and the pulmonary arteries anteriorly
- Associated abnormalities
  - ○ Abnormally positioned descending aorta can occur in isolation as a primary abnormality
  - ○ Even when occurs as a primary abnormality, it almost always is in association with other congenital heart disease or other congenital abnormalities or syndromes

MIDLINE DESCENDING AORTA

- Very uncommon to have an otherwise healthy child with an isolated midline descending aorta: Airway compression syndrome
- Midline descending aorta often occurs "secondary" in association with other arch anomalies
- Double aortic arch
  - Also often present in patients with double aortic arch
  - Patients following surgical repair for double aortic arch with persistent airway symptoms, midline descending aorta may be cause of persistent airway compression
- Right aortic arch with left aberrant subclavian artery
  - Most cases of right aortic arch with left aberrant subclavian artery not associated with airway symptoms
  - When airway compression is present in right aortic arch with aberrant subclavian artery, compression is often of the trachea at the level of the aberrant subclavian artery and associated Kommerell's diverticulum
  - Also midline descending aorta often a contributing anatomic factor to airway compression at lower portion of airway in region of carina and main bronchi
  - Surgical ligation of the ligamentum arteriosum will typically relieve airway symptoms regardless of the anatomic cause of the airway compression

CLINICAL ISSUES

Presentation
- Most common signs/symptoms: Stridor
- Recurrent pneumonia
- Chronic atelectasis
- Wheezing refractory to medical therapy
- Cor pulmonale
- Bronchoscopy demonstrates pulsatile, fixed compression of distal airway from posterior aspect
- Patients who have persistent respiratory symptoms after surgical therapy for double aortic arch may have airway compression secondary to midline descending aorta

Demographics
- Age
  - Typically present in infants
  - Most common vascular cause of extrinsic airway compression to present in infancy
- Gender: No predilection by gender

Natural History & Prognosis
- Surgery reserved for severe cases
- Children will often grow out of compression over time

Treatment
- In severe cases, aortopexy may relieve symptoms by causing a re-shifting of the abnormally stacked anatomic structures
- Descending aorta cannot be surgically moved because of origin of multiple intercostal arteries
- If in association with other abnormalities, surgical treatment of associated abnormality may relieve airway symptoms

SELECTED REFERENCES

1. Boiselle PM: Multislice helical CT of the central airways. Radiol Clin North Am. 41(3):561-74, 2003
2. Donnelly LF et al: Aberrant subclavian arteries: cross-sectional imaging findings in infants and children referred for evaluation of extrinsic airway compression. AJR Am J Roentgenol. 178(5):1269-74, 2002
3. Fleck RJ et al: Imaging findings in pediatric patients with persistent airway symptoms after surgery for double aortic arch. AJR Am J Roentgenol. 178(5):1275-9, 2002
4. Pacharn P et al: Low-tube-current multidetector CT for children with suspected extrinsic airway compression. AJR Am J Roentgenol. 179(6):1523-7, 2002
5. Donnelly LF: The aortic sling: malpositioned aortic arch surrounding and compressing the trachea in a patient with thoracic deformity. AJR Am J Roentgenol. 176(6):1606-7, 2001
6. Berdon WE: Rings, slings, and other things: vascular compression of the infant trachea updated from the midcentury to the millennium--the legacy of Robert E. Gross, MD, and Edward B. D. Neuhauser, MD. Radiology. 216(3):624-32, 2000
7. Walner DL et al: Utility of radiographs in the evaluation of pediatric upper airway obstruction. Ann Otol Rhinol Laryngol. 108(4):378-83, 1999
8. Donnelly LF et al: Airway compression in children with abnormal thoracic configuration. Radiology. 206(2):323-6, 1998
9. Hungate RG et al: Left mainstem bronchial narrowing: a vascular compression syndrome? Evaluation by magnetic resonance imaging. Pediatr Radiol. 28:527-32, 1998
10. Donnelly LF et al: The spectrum of extrinsic lower airway compression in children: MR imaging. AJR Am J Roentgenol. 168(1):59-62, 1997
11. Donnelly LF et al: Extrinsic airway compression secondary to pulmonary arterial conduits: MR findings. Pediatr Radiol. 27(3):268-70, 1997
12. Donnelly LF et al: The Spectrum of Extrinsic Lower Airway Compression In Children: MR Imaging. AJR. 168:59-62, 1997
13. Donnelly LF et al: Anomalous midline location of the descending aorta: a cause of compression of the carina and left mainstem bronchus in infants. AJR. 64:705-7, 1995

MIDLINE DESCENDING AORTA

IMAGE GALLERY

Typical

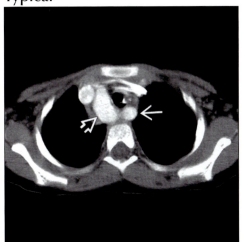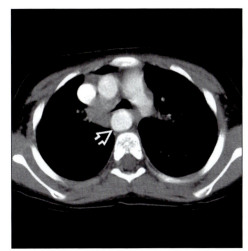

(Left) Axial CECT shows right aortic arch (open arrow) with aberrant left subclavian artery (arrow). This is same patient as in next 3 images. *(Right)* Axial CECT in same patient with right aortic arch as shown on left shows midline position of descending aorta (arrow).

Typical

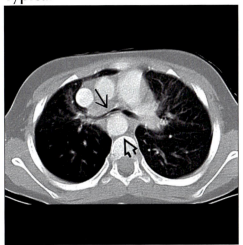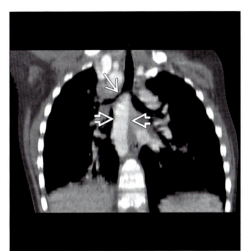

(Left) Axial CECT in same patient as shown above shows midline position of descending aorta (open arrow) causing compression of the right main bronchus (arrow). *(Right)* Coronal CECT in same patient as shown on left shows midline descending aorta (open arrows) anterior to spine with compression of right main bronchus (arrow).

Typical

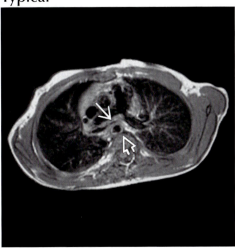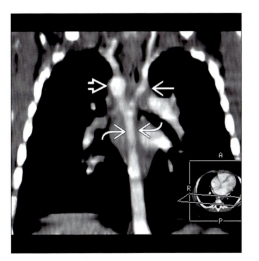

(Left) Axial T1WI MR in child with stridor & history of repaired double aortic arch shows midline descending aorta (open arrow) & associated compression of left main bronchus (arrow) against right pulmonary artery. *(Right)* Coronal CECT shows right aortic arch (open arrow) with anomalous left subclavian artery (arrow). Note midline course of descending aorta (curved arrows).

54

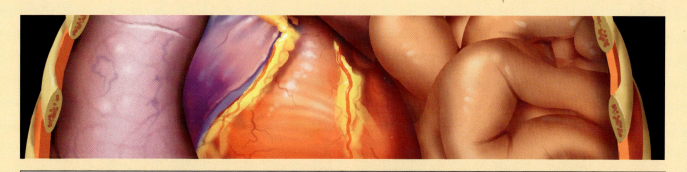

SECTION 2: Chest

Introduction and Overview
Chest	2-2

Congenital "Lung" Lesions
Cystic Adenomatoid Malformation	2-6
Pulmonary Sequestration	2-10
Bronchogenic Cyst	2-14
Congenital Lobar Emphysema	2-18
Congenital Diaphragmatic Hernia	2-22
Bronchial Atresia	2-26

Neonatal Chest Issues
Surfactant Deficient Disease	2-30
Neonatal Pneumonia	2-34
Meconium Aspiration Syndrome	2-38
Transient Tachypnea of the Newborn	2-42
Pulmonary Interstitial Emphysema	2-46
Bronchopulmonary Dysplasia	2-50
Umbilical Catheter Complications	2-54
Chylothorax	2-58

Chest Infection
Viral Lung Infection	2-62
Round Pneumonia	2-66
Parapneumonic Effusion and Empyema	2-70
Pneumonia with Cavitary Necrosis	2-74

Anterior Mediastinum
Normal Thymus	2-78
Lymphoma, Thoracic	2-82
Germ Cell Tumors, Mediastinum	2-86

Pulmonary Masses
Pleuropulmonary Blastoma	2-90
Pulmonary Inflammatory Pseudotumor	2-94

Miscellaneous
Child Abuse, Rib Fractures	2-98
Neuroblastoma, Thoracic	2-102
Discitis	2-106
Cystic Fibrosis, Lung	2-110
Sickle Cell, Acute Chest Syndrome	2-114
Pulmonary Arteriovenous Malformation	2-118
Lung Contusion and Laceration	2-122
Papillomatosis	2-126
Pectus Excavatum	2-130
Chronic Esophageal Foreign Body	2-134

CHEST

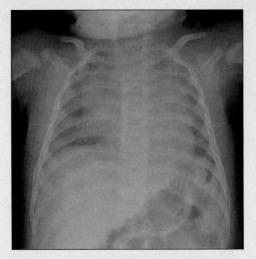 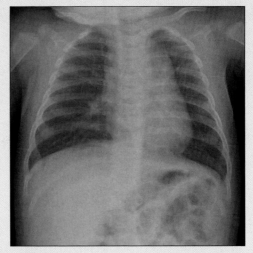

Anteroposterior radiograph shows prominent cardiothymic silhouette, low lung volumes, and increased lung density. Expiratory technique was suspected and radiograph repeated (see right image).

Anteroposterior radiograph repeated in same patient as on left shows normal sized heart and clear lungs. Previous findings were related to expiratory technique.

Neonatal Chest

Diffuse Pulmonary Disease Causing Respiratory Distress

- Respiratory distress in the newborn is most commonly related to diffuse pulmonary disease
- Causes of respiratory distress in children can be divided into two large categories
- Small babies with decreased lung volumes/granular opacities
  - Surfactant deficient disease
  - Beta-hemolytic Streptococcal pneumonia
- Large babies with increased lung volumes/streaky perihilar opacities
  - Meconium aspiration syndrome
  - Other neonatal pneumonias
  - Transient tachypnea of the newborn

Focal Causes Of Respiratory Distress

- Focal space occupying lesions in the thorax can compress functioning lung and lead to respiratory distress
- Differential diagnosis: Focal lesions
  - Abnormalities of the diaphragm
    - Congenital diaphragmatic hernia
    - Phrenic nerve palsy/paralyzed hemidiaphragm
  - Lung Masses: Containing air during neonatal period
    - Congenital cystic adenomatoid malformation
    - Congenital lobar emphysema
    - Persistent pulmonary interstitial emphysema
  - Lung masses: Typically not containing air during neonatal period
    - Sequestration
    - Bronchogenic cyst

Neonatal Intensive Care Unit (NICU) Issues

- Monitoring support apparatus
  - Umbilical arterial catheters
    - Route: Umbilical artery (inferiorly) to iliac artery (superiorly) to aorta
    - High lines: Positioned with tip in descending aorta (T8-T10)
    - Low lines: Tip positioned below level of L3
  - Umbilical venous catheters
    - Route: Umbilical vein to left portal vein to ductus venosus to hepatic vein to inferior vena cava
    - Tip left below right atrium
  - Esophageal intubation
    - Endotracheal tube over esophagus, air in esophagus, gas distended bowel in abdomen
  - Extracorporeal membrane oxygenation (ECMO)
    - Last resort therapy for respiratory failure
    - Prolonged form of circulatory bypass of the lungs
    - Arteriovenous ECMO: Right common carotid artery & internal jugular vein sacrificed & arterial catheter placed with tip in aortic arch & venous catheter tip placed in right atrium
    - Venovenous EMCO from right atrium also alternative
  - High frequency oscillator ventilation
    - Often used in contrast to conventional ventilators
    - Supraphysiologic rates of ventilation with very low tidal volumes
    - Air vibrated in and out of lung
    - Mean airway pressure of oscillator can be adjusted to move level of diaphragm to desired location, most often at 10 and a half posterior ribs
  - Pulmonary interstitial emphysema
    - Barotrauma results in air entering interstitial spaces/lymphatics
    - Bubbles and linear lucencies seen on radiographs
    - Warning sign of other air block complications such as pneumothorax
  - Bronchopulmonary dysplasia (BPD)
    - Injury to lungs through combination of mechanical ventilation and oxygen toxicity
    - Hazy density (second week of life)
    - Over next weeks to months, coarse lung markings, bubble-like lucencies, asymmetric aeration

Acute Diffuse Lung Consolidation In Neonates

- Differential diagnosis

CHEST

Key Issues

Normal Variants Mistaken For Disease
- Normal thymus
  - Commonly seen as prominent soft tissue mass in anterior mediastinum in children
  - Quite large up to 5 years of age, decreased by 10 years, should not be prominent mass during second decade of life
- Chest wall variants: May mimic palpable masses on physical exam

Abnormalities Commonly Overlooked
- Widened paravertebral soft tissues
  - Normally: Right paravererbral soft tissues not visualized and left less in diameter than adjacent pedicle
  - Abnormally widened: Neuroblastoma, discitis, extralobar sequestration, duplication cysts
- Airway compression
  - Abnormal tracheal compression or deviation (right arch) as in vascular rings
- Rib anomalies
  - Rib fractures in child abuse, rib erosions in neuroblastoma

CT Chest Protocols
- Because of low attenuation of lungs, chest CT in children and particularly small infants can be performed with low tube current (mA) without noise rendering images non-diagnostic
- Use size appropriate protocols for pediatric chest CT

- Edema (often related to development of patent ductus arteriosus)
- Diffuse pulmonary hemorrhage
- Worsening surfactant deficiency (typically only during first days of life)
- Superimposed pneumonia
- Artifact - diffuse micro - atelectasis
  - In infants, if the radiograph is obtained during expiration, the lungs may appear completely opacified artifactually
  - Repeat chest radiograph if indicated

Issues In Pediatric Community-Acquired Pneumonia

Confirmation And Exclusion Of Pneumonia
- Signs and symptoms of pneumonia often nonspecific in children
- Radiography findings affect diagnosis made in 21% of cases and management decisions in up to 34% of cases

Characterize Infectious Agent
- Primary decision in children is whether child has viral or bacterial disease: Does the child need to be on antibiotics?
- Viral disease: Radiographic findings
  - Bilateral, increased peribronchial opacities, hyperinflation, subsegmental atelectasis
- Bacterial disease: Radiographic findings
  - Unilateral, segmental to lobar, air space disease, air-bronchograms, often pleural effusions
- Radiographs have a negative predictive value for excluding bacterial infection of 92%
  - Valuable in minimizing children placed on antibiotics unnecessarily

Evaluation Of Failure To Clear
- In children, post obstructive pneumonia from bronchogenic carcinoma is not a concern and routine follow-up radiographs to ensure resolution of pneumonia are not indicated
- Reserved for persistent or recurrent symptoms and those children with underlying conditions
- Differential diagnosis for failure to clear
  - Infected developmental lesion
  - Bronchial obstruction (foreign body)
  - Gastroesophageal reflux and aspiration
  - Underlying systemic disorder (immunodeficiency, sickle cell anemia, cystic fibrosis)

Complications Related To Pneumonia
- Potential complications include
  - Parapneumonic effusions (empyema, transudative effusion, inadequate drainage), parenchymal complications (cavitary necrosis, abscess), purulent pericarditis
- Clinical issues
  - Primary evaluation of parapneumonic effusions
    - Imaging studies to help grade whether effusion is empyema vs. transudative effusion to help gage aggressiveness of therapy
    - Ultrasound grading fluid as complex (echogenic fronds, septae, and debris) vs. simple (anechoic fluid)
    - Complex effusions have decreased hospital stay if treated aggressively where as simple do not
    - CT and decubitus radiographs less helpful
  - Evaluation of the child with persistent or progressive symptoms
    - Child who is persistently septic despite antibiotics or pleural drainage, almost always has underlying purulent complication
    - CECT best imaging test of choice: Identifies and guides therapy to-loculated, persistent pleural collection, lung parenchymal complications (cavitary necrosis, lung abscess), or purulent pericarditis

Lung Mass In Children
- There are a number of other lung masses that can develop in children beyond the neonatal period

CHEST

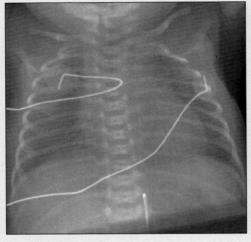

Anteroposterior radiograph in a pre-term neonate shows low lung volumes and diffuse lung granular opacities consistent with surfactant deficient disease. Contrast to radiograph on right.

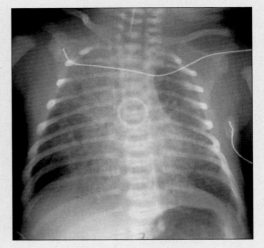

Anteroposterior radiograph in a term neonate shows ropy, perihilar markings and increased lung volumes consistent with meconium aspiration syndrome. Contrast to radiograph on left.

Differential Diagnosis
- Congenital lung masses (congenital cystic adenomatoid malformation, congenital lobar emphysema, sequestration, bronchogenic cyst)
- Pleuropulmonary blastoma
- Pulmonary inflammatory pseudotumor
- Pulmonary arteriovenous malformation
- Papillomatosis
- Granulomatous disease
- Metastatic disease

Mediastinal Lesions

Differential Diagnosis For Common Mediastinal Masses
- Anterior mediastinal masses
  - Normal thymus
  - Lymphoma
    - By far, the most common pathologic anterior mediastinal mass in children
    - Typically occurs during second decade of life
  - Germ cell tumors (teratoma)
  - Thymoma
- Middle mediastinal masses
  - Lymphadenopathy
  - Duplication cysts
- Posterior mediastinal masses
  - Neuroblastoma
    - In a young child, a posterior mediastinal mass is neuroblastoma until proven otherwise

Chest Wall Issues

Pectus Excavatum
- Haller index: Ratio of transverse left to right divided by anterior to posterior diameter of chest
  - > 3.2 considered candidate for non-invasive pectus repair
  - Measured on axial CT

Differential Diagnosis Of Malignant/Aggressive Chest Wall Lesions
- Osteomyelitis
- Langerhans cell histiocytosis
- Ewing sarcoma
- Primitive neuroectodermal tumor (Askin tumor)

Normal Variants
- Mild asymmetries in chest wall may cause protuberances to be palpated on physical exam and suspected to be aggressive malignancies
- Tilted sternum, asymmetric anterior convex ribs, asymmetric costal cartilages, cartilaginous rests

Common Chronic Or Recurrent Pulmonary Issues In Children

Acute Chest Syndrome In Sickle Cell Anemia
- Rib infarcts cause splinting and resultant collapse of lung

Cystic Fibrosis
- Most common lethal inherited disease in Caucasians

Immunodeficiency
- Both congenital and acquired immunodeficiencies may present during childhood
- Pulmonary infectious complications common

Related References
1. Donnelly LF: Fundamentals of Pediatric Radiology. Philadelphia: W.B. Saunders, 2001
2. Donnelly LF et al: Abnormalities of the chest wall in pediatric patients. AJR Am J Roentgenol. 173(6):1595-601, 1999
3. Donnelly LF et al: Localized radiolucent chest lesions in neonates: causes and differentiation. AJR Am J Roentgenol. 172(6):1651-8, 1999
4. Donnelly LF: Maximizing the usefulness of imaging in children with community-acquired pneumonia. AJR Am J Roentgenol. 172(2):505-12, 1999

CHEST

IMAGE GALLERY

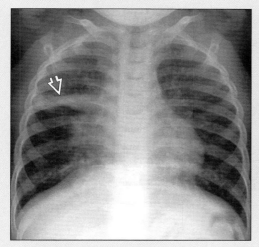
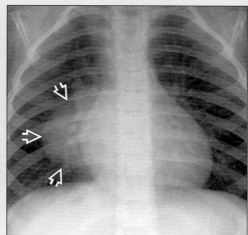

(Left) Anteroposterior radiograph shows increased perihilar markings, hyperinflation, and band of atelectasis *(arrow)* consistent with viral illness. Contrast to radiograph on right. *(Right)* Anteroposterior radiograph shows well-circumscribed opacity *(arrows)* in superior segment of right lower lobe consistent with focal, bacterial pneumonia. Contrast to radiograph on left.

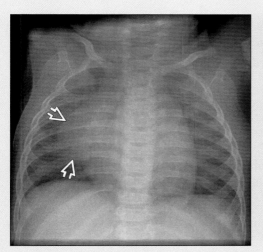
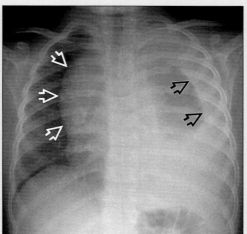

(Left) Anteroposterior radiograph in an infant shows prominent thymic shadow *(arrows)*, normal for age. Contrast to image on right. *(Right)* Anteroposterior radiograph in 6 year old child shows prominent thymic shadow *(white arrows)* with associated pleural effusion *(black arrows)*. Case proved to be lymphoma.

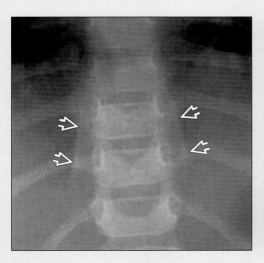
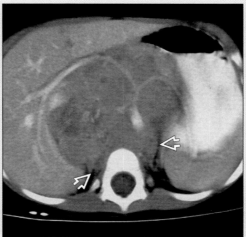

(Left) Anteroposterior radiograph shows widening of both right and left paravertebral soft tissues *(arrows)*. Right is visualized. Left is wider than adjacent pedicle and inferolaterally oriented. *(Right)* Axial CECT in same patient as on left shows large heterogeneous mass causing the widened paravertebral soft tissues *(arrows)*, consistent with neuroblastoma.

CYSTIC ADENOMATOID MALFORMATION

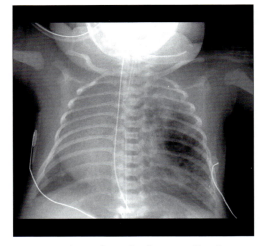

Anteroposterior radiograph shows multicystic mass containing air in left chest of a neonate. There is mediastinal shift to the right. NG tube is below diaphragm.

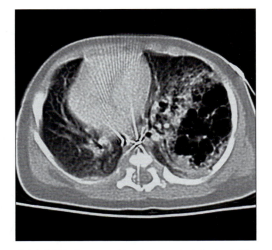

Axial CECT shows multicystic mass in left chest. The cysts contain air and cause mediastinal shift (same infant as shown on left).

TERMINOLOGY

Abbreviations and Synonyms
- Congenital cystic adenomatoid malformation (CCAM)

Definitions
- Congenital lung mass of adenomatoid proliferation

IMAGING FINDINGS

General Features
- Best diagnostic clue
  - Multicystic mass with air in cysts
  - Imaging appearance depends upon size of cysts and whether cysts fluid filled
  - Cysts communicate with bronchial tree at birth and fill with air early in life
- Location
  - Pulmonary
    - No lobar predilection, unlike congenital lobar emphysema
  - Most lesions confined to single lobe
  - Most lesions solitary
    - Multiple discontinuous CCAM reported
- Size
  - Three types based on size of cysts in lesion at imaging/pathology
    - CCAM type 1 (50%): 1 or more large (2-10 cm) cysts
    - CCAM type 2 (40%): Numerous small cysts of uniform size
    - CCAM type 3 (< 10%): Appears solid on gross inspection and imaging but have microcysts
- Morphology
  - Multicystic masses
    - Size of cysts variable
    - Content of cysts (air, fluid, air and fluid) variable

Radiographic Findings
- Radiography
  - Variable appearance
    - Dependent upon size and content of cysts
  - Solid to multicystic mass with variable amounts of air and fluid
  - Mass that appears solid
    - Type 3 CCAM
    - Mass with cysts that remain filled with fluid
  - May cause mass effect
  - If prenatal diagnosis, initial chest radiograph may appear normal or minimally abnormal
    - This does not mean that lesion has resolved
    - CT should be performed, lesion will be demonstrated
    - Most common with type 2 CCAM

DDx: Lung Masses In Young Children

| CDH | Sequestration | Cavitary Necrosis |

CYSTIC ADENOMATOID MALFORMATION

Key Facts

Imaging Findings
- Multicystic mass with air in cysts
- Imaging appearance depends upon size of cysts and whether cysts fluid filled
- Cysts communicate with bronchial tree at birth and fill with air early in life
- No lobar predilection, unlike congenital lobar emphysema
- Most lesions confined to single lobe
- Most lesions solitary
- Three types based on size of cysts in lesion at imaging/pathology
- If prenatal diagnosis, initial chest radiograph may appear normal or minimally abnormal
- CT should be performed, lesion will be demonstrated
- Most common with type 2 CCAM
- MR usually only used in prenatal diagnosis

Pathology
- Lesions are in communication with bronchial tree at birth
- Type 2 lesions associated with other congenital anomalies (50%)
- Epidemiology: Incidence: 1 per 100,000 births

Clinical Issues
- Symptomatic CCAM managed with surgical resection
- Management of asymptomatic CCAM controversial: Most advocate elective resection because of risks of infection and malignancy

CT Findings
- NECT
  - Solid mass to multicystic mass
    - Cysts of variable size
    - Cysts contain air and/or fluid
- CECT
  - No evidence of systemic arterial supply (presence suggests sequestration)
  - Cyst walls and solid components demonstrate variable enhancement
  - Mass effect demonstrated as mediastinal shift or adjacent lung compression
  - CCAM type 3 (< 10%): Appears solid on gross inspection and imaging but have microcysts

MR Findings
- T1WI
  - MR usually only used in prenatal diagnosis
  - Isointense lesion
- T2WI
  - Hyperintense mass
  - Often demonstrates mediastinal shift
  - Compression of adjacent lung
  - May be associated with fetal hydrops

Ultrasonographic Findings
- Grayscale Ultrasound
  - Ultrasound used primarily in prenatal diagnosis
  - Echogenic mass
  - Mass effect on adjacent lung
  - Compression of adjacent lung
- Color Doppler: No evidence of systemic arterial supply
- Prenatal sonography
  - Echogenic fetal lung mass
  - Mediastinal shift
  - Fetal hydrops may occur
  - Polyhydramnios may occur
  - CCAM type 2 may become less apparent on serial fetal ultrasound and may be subtle on chest radiography

Imaging Recommendations
- Best imaging tool
  - Radiography is the initial imaging study of choice in postnatal diagnosis
  - CT is utilized for further characterization of lesions for presurgical planning
  - CT is utilized to identify lesions diagnosed prenatally but not evident on radiographs
- Protocol advice
  - CT should be used with prenatal diagnosis and no findings shown by radiography
  - CT should be performed with IV contrast to exclude presence of systemic arterial blood supply

DIFFERENTIAL DIAGNOSIS

Sequestration
- Typically do not contain air during the neonatal period
- Systemic arterial supply to mass demonstrated
- Only become air-filled when infected
- Usually in left lower lobe

Congenital diaphragmatic hernia (CDH)
- Appears as multicystic, air-containing mass
- CCAM more likely to have air-fluid levels than CDH
- Appearance does not change in position with CCAM over serial films, can with CDH
- Position of support apparatus altered with CDH (i.e. nasogastric (NG) tube, umbilical venous catheter (UVC)) can help with diagnosis NG tube
- Lack of bowel gas in abdomen

Cavitary necrosis complicating pneumonia
- When patients with pneumonia have a cystic mass in the pneumonia, it may be secondary to developing cavitary necrosis or an underlying CCAM
- Both have similar CT and radiographic appearance
- Cavitary necrosis tends to be surrounded by consolidated lung (not always with CCAM)

CYSTIC ADENOMATOID MALFORMATION

- Children with cavitary necrosis tend to be more critically ill
- Temporal history most helpful
  - Does patient have previous normal chest X-ray (CXR)? (cavitary necrosis)
  - Has the lesion progressed during illness? (cavitary necrosis)
  - Is the lesion decreasing or resolving after acute illness? (cavitary necrosis)

PATHOLOGY

General Features
- General path comments
  - Congenital lung mass of adenomatoid proliferation
  - Lesions are in communication with bronchial tree at birth
  - Hamartomatous proliferation of terminal bronchioles
  - Mass proliferation causes arrest of adjacent alveolar development
  - Cysts lined by respiratory epithelium
- Genetics
  - Can be associated with deletions on chromosome 18
  - Type 2 lesions associated with other congenital anomalies (50%)
    - Renal, skeletal, intestinal, cardiac
- Etiology: Unknown
- Epidemiology: Incidence: 1 per 100,000 births
- Associated abnormalities: Type 2 lesions associated with other congenital anomalies (50%)

Gross Pathologic & Surgical Features
- Solid to multicystic mass

Microscopic Features
- Cysts lined with respiratory epithelium

Staging, Grading or Classification Criteria
- Types 1-3 as above

CLINICAL ISSUES

Presentation
- Most common signs/symptoms
  - Respiratory distress in newborn period
  - Recurrent lung infections
  - Asymptomatic, prenatal diagnosis

Demographics
- Age
  - Most commonly present during infancy or detected prenatally
  - Can present at any age
- Gender: M = F

Natural History & Prognosis
- Prenatal CCAM can regress and become smaller
- Prenatal CCAM can cause compression of adjacent structures and lead to hydrops
- Post-natal CCAM are at risk for becoming infected
- Small risk for malignant degeneration (rhabdomyosarcoma) reported

Treatment
- Prenatally detected lesions typically followed with ultrasound/MRI
  - If lesion does not progress in size and fetus does not develop hydrops, conservative prenatal management
  - If lesion associated with complication, fetal interventions considered
    - Aspiration of dominant cyst
    - Resection of lesion
- Symptomatic CCAM managed with surgical resection
- Management of asymptomatic CCAM controversial: Most advocate elective resection because of risks of infection and malignancy
  - Lesions easier to resect electively than after infection
  - Typically wait until child out of neonatal period for non-symptomatic lesions

DIAGNOSTIC CHECKLIST

Image Interpretation Pearls
- Most true multicystic pulmonary masses that contain air in neonatal period are CCAM

SELECTED REFERENCES

1. Achiron R et al: Fetal lung lesions: a spectrum of disease. New classification based on pathogenesis, two-dimensional and color Doppler ultrasound. Ultrasound Obstet Gynecol. 24(2):107-14, 2004
2. Berrocal T et al: Congenital anomalies of the tracheobronchial tree, lung, and mediastinum: embryology, radiology, and pathology. Radiographics. 24(1):e17, 2004
3. Davenport M et al: Current outcome of antenatally diagnosed cystic lung disease. J Pediatr Surg. 39(4):549-56, 2004
4. Johnson AM et al: Congenital anomalies of the fetal/neonatal chest. Semin Roentgenol. 39(2):197-214, 2004
5. Khosa JK et al: Congenital cystic adenomatoid malformation of the lung: indications and timing of surgery. Pediatr Surg Int. 20(7):505-8, 2004
6. Teoh L et al: Congenital cystic adenomatoid malformation: importance of postnatal chest computed tomography scans. J Paediatr Child Health. 40(11):654-5, 2004
7. Usui N et al: Outcome predictors for infants with cystic lung disease. J Pediatr Surg. 39(4):603-6, 2004
8. Gornall AS et al: Congenital cystic adenomatoid malformation: accuracy of prenatal diagnosis, prevalence and outcome in a general population. Prenat Diagn. 23(12):997-1002, 2003
9. Sauvat F et al: Management of asymptomatic neonatal cystic adenomatoid malformations. J Pediatr Surg. 38(4):548-52, 2003
10. Monni G et al: Prenatal ultrasound diagnosis of congenital cystic adenomatoid malformation of the lung: a report of 26 cases and review of the literature. Ultrasound Obstet Gynecol. 16(2):159-62, 2000
11. Donnelly LF et al: Localized radiolucent chest lesions in neonates: causes and differentiation. AJR Am J Roentgenol. 172(6):1651-8, 1999
12. Cleveland RH: A radiologic update on medical diseases of the newborn chest. Pediatr Radiol. 25:631-7, 1995

CYSTIC ADENOMATOID MALFORMATION

IMAGE GALLERY

Typical

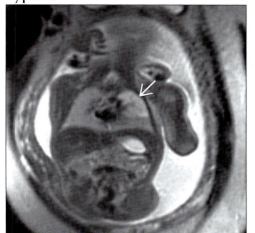
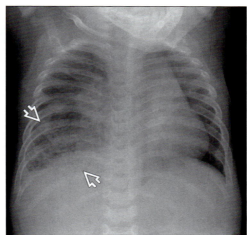

(Left) Coronal T2WI MR shows high signal mass *(arrow)* in left upper lobe of a fetus. *(Right)* Anteroposterior radiograph on day 3 of life shows heterogeneous lucency *(arrows)* in right lower lobe.

Typical

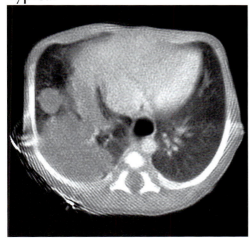
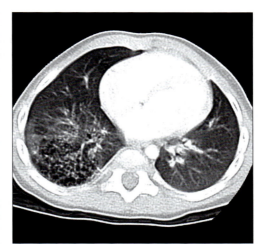

(Left) Axial CECT on day 1 of life in same patient as above right shows solid appearing mass related to retained fetal fluid within the cysts. *(Right)* Axial CECT on day three of life in same patient as on left shows mass with multiple small cysts containing air.

Typical

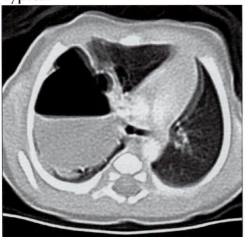
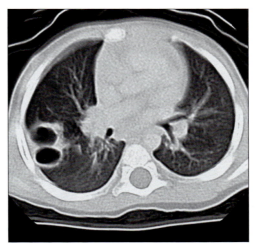

(Left) Axial CECT shows large, predominantly solitary cyst with air-fluid level. *(Right)* Axial CECT shows air-filled cystic mass with surrounding aerated lung.

PULMONARY SEQUESTRATION

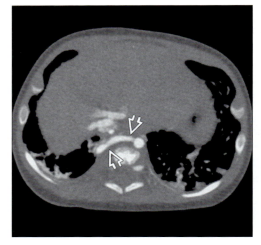

Axial CECT in patient with complex congenital heart disease shows left systemic artery (arrows) to right lower lobe from descending aorta.

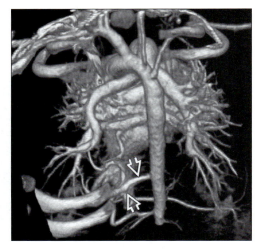

CTA in same patient as on left posterior view, shows systemic arterial supply (arrows) to right lower lobe opacity arising from descending aorta.

TERMINOLOGY

Abbreviations and Synonyms
- Sequestration

Definitions
- Congenital area of abnormal lung that does not connect to the bronchial tree or pulmonary arteries
- Involved lung is dysplastic and nonfunctioning
- Arterial supply is typically from systemic source arising from descending aorta
- Divided into intralobar and extralobar types
  - Intralobar type has venous drainage into inferior pulmonary vein
  - Extralobar type has venous drainage often systemic, however drainage variable
- May occur in conjunction with other congenital lung lesions such as congenital cystic adenomatoid malformation

IMAGING FINDINGS

General Features
- Best diagnostic clue
  - Persistent lung opacity over multiple presentations with pneumonia-like symptoms
    - Most common in left lower lobe
  - Identification of systemic arterial supply
- Location
  - Most common location is left lower lobe, followed by right lower lobe
  - Systemic arterial supply most commonly arises from descending aorta
    - May arise from below the hemidiaphragm in 20% of cases
- Diagnostic feature: Systemic artery arising from the aorta and feeding sequestration
- Identification of the supplying systemic artery is characteristic and documentation that surgeons are interested in
- Any imaging modality that can identify a systemic artery arising from the aorta and feeding sequestration has been advocated for diagnosis
  - CT/CTA
  - MRI/MRA
  - Ultrasound with color Doppler (particularly in neonates)
  - Arteriography (no longer utilized)
- Imaging differentiation between intralobar and extralobar sequestration
  - Difficult if not impossible with imaging
  - Extralobar have separate pleural covering
  - Different patterns of venous drainage emphasized but variable between intra and extralobar

DDx: Focal Pediatric Lung Mass

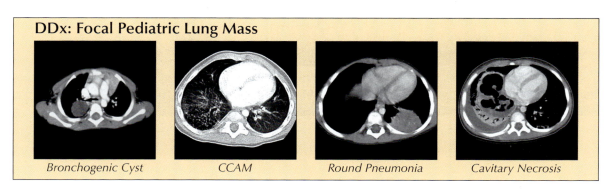

Bronchogenic Cyst | CCAM | Round Pneumonia | Cavitary Necrosis

PULMONARY SEQUESTRATION

Key Facts

Terminology
- Congenital area of abnormal lung that does not connect to the bronchial tree or pulmonary arteries
- Involved lung is dysplastic and nonfunctioning
- Arterial supply is typically from systemic source arising from descending aorta
- Divided into intralobar and extralobar types
- Intralobar type has venous drainage into inferior pulmonary vein
- Extralobar type has venous drainage often systemic, however drainage variable
- May occur in conjunction with other congenital lung lesions such as congenital cystic adenomatoid malformation

Imaging Findings
- Persistent lung opacity over multiple presentations with pneumonia-like symptoms
- Most common location is left lower lobe, followed by right lower lobe
- Systemic arterial supply most commonly arises from descending aorta
- May arise from below the hemidiaphragm in 20% of cases
- Diagnostic feature: Systemic artery arising from the aorta and feeding sequestration
- Identification of the supplying systemic artery is characteristic and documentation that surgeons are interested in

---

- Both may have drainage via pulmonary veins, azygous system, or inferior vena cava (IVC)
- Differentiation does not affect surgical management but demonstration of venous anatomy may be helpful for surgical planning

Radiographic Findings
- Radiography
  - Often seen as persistent lower lobe opacity that is unchanged over multiple radiographs
  - Most common in left lower lobe
  - Does not typically contain air unless infected
  - Does not appear as air-containing mass during neonatal period
  - If infected, may appear as multi-cystic air-containing mass
  - Extralobar sequestration may present as a paraspinal mass
    - Paraspinal lines displaced laterally
    - May have similar appearance to neuroblastoma

CT Findings
- NECT
  - Opacification of lower lobe lung parenchyma
  - May have cystic air-filled components if infected or if occurring in conjunction with congenital cystic adenomatoid malformation
- CECT
  - Systemic arterial supply demonstrated
  - Typically artery arises from descending aorta and extends into abnormal area of lung
  - Systemic artery may arise from other systemic sources as well
    - Reports have included areas such as coronary arteries
- CTA
  - In cases of suspected sequestration, CT should be set up as CTA in order to demonstrate systemic arterial supply
  - 3D reconstruction helpful in communicating anatomy for surgical planning

MR Findings
- MRI can be utilized to demonstrate systemic arterial supply
- Both high flow gradient echo sequences as well as gadolinium arteriography can demonstrate artery
- Has been replaced with CTA because of: Rapidity at which CT can be performed often eliminates need for sedation and better demonstration of lung by CT as compared to MRI
- Fetal MRI
  - Lesions may be seen prenatally as pulmonary mass
  - High T2W signal
  - Systemic arterial supply may be demonstrated

Ultrasonographic Findings
- Grayscale Ultrasound
  - Ultrasound may be used in newborns to demonstrate systemic arterial supply via Doppler
  - Abnormal lung is often opacified providing acoustic window
- Color Doppler: Demonstration of systemic arterial supply
- Fetal sonography
  - Echogenic lung mass
  - Doppler demonstration of systemic arterial supply

Angiographic Findings
- Conventional
  - Conventional angiography was historic mainstay of demonstrating systemic arterial supply
  - Has been replaced by CTA

Non-Vascular Interventions
- There are reports of utilizing embolization with infarction of abnormal lung as a treatment alternative to surgical excision

Imaging Recommendations
- If sequestration suspected on basis of chest radiography or fetal sonography: Contrast-enhanced helical CT of chest
  - CT can identify systemic arterial feeder
  - Further characterize lung opacity

BRONCHOGENIC CYST

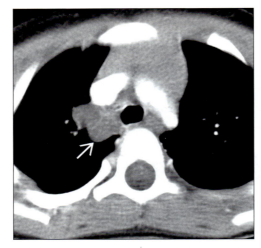

Axial CECT shows homogeneous, well-circumscribed, rounded fluid attenuation lesion in right paratracheal region (arrow) with no perceptible rim or internal enhancement.

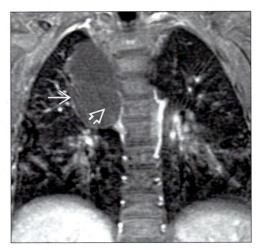

Coronal T1 C+ MR shows oblong, well-circumscribed, low signal lesion (open arrow) with barely perceptible enhancing thin rim (arrow) in the right paravertebral region.

TERMINOLOGY

Abbreviations and Synonyms
- Foregut duplication cyst

Definitions
- Bronchogenic cysts are part of the family of foregut duplication cysts: Bronchogenic cysts, enteric cysts, neurenteric cysts
- They are developmental lesions that result from abnormal ventral budding of the tracheobronchial tree between the 26th and 40th days of gestation

IMAGING FINDINGS

General Features
- Best diagnostic clue: Well-defined mass in the paratracheal or subcarinal region that is of homogeneously increased signal on a T2 weighted sequences
- Location
  o May be mediastinal or in the lung parenchyma
  o Mediastinal: More common than pulmonary
    ▪ Mediastinal 65-90%
    ▪ Majority in the middle mediastinum
    ▪ Typically paratracheal, carinal, or hilar
    ▪ Pericarinal most common
  o Pulmonary: Majority in the medial third of the lungs
    ▪ More frequent in the lower lobes
    ▪ Equal incidence in both lungs
  o Rare occurrence in thymus, diaphragm, neck, pericardium, and retroperitoneum
- Size: Variable sizes
- Well-defined ovoid or round mass with smooth borders
- Almost always solitary
- Rarely multilocular
- Typically do not communicate with airway and do not contain air
  o Air presence indicates infection
  o Parenchymal lesions more likely to communicate with airway than mediastinal lesions
- May have mass effect and cause airway compression or compress esophagus
  o Air-trapping (hyperinflation)
  o Lung collapse
  o Dysphagia and vomiting

Radiographic Findings
- Radiography
  o Nonspecific
  o Well-defined mass with smooth borders
  o Soft tissue density
  o Typically in the mediastinum or central lung

DDx: Bronchogenic Cyst

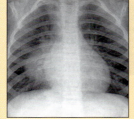

Round Pneumonia

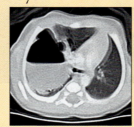

Infected CCAM

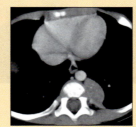

Neuroblastoma

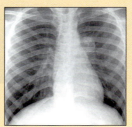

Lymphadenopathy

BRONCHOGENIC CYST

Key Facts

Terminology
- Bronchogenic cysts are part of the family of foregut duplication cysts: Bronchogenic cysts, enteric cysts, neurenteric cysts
- They are developmental lesions that result from abnormal ventral budding of the tracheobronchial tree between the 26th and 40th days of gestation

Imaging Findings
- Best diagnostic clue: Well-defined mass in the paratracheal or subcarinal region that is of homogeneously increased signal on a T2 weighted sequences
- Mediastinal: More common than pulmonary
- Typically paratracheal, carinal, or hilar
- Pulmonary: Majority in the medial third of the lungs
- May have mass effect and cause airway compression or compress esophagus

Top Differential Diagnoses
- Round pneumonia
- Congenital cystic adenomatoid malformation (CCAM)
- Neurogenic tumors
- Lymphadenopathy

Clinical Issues
- Infants: Respiratory distress or dysphagia
- Older children: Chest pain and dysphagia
- Symptoms more common in mediastinal lesions
- Younger children are more likely to present with symptoms

  - Usually need CT or MR for further evaluation

Fluoroscopic Findings
- May be incidentally noted on upper gastrointestinal (GI) studies, especially if the lesions are the cause of symptoms such as vomiting or dysphagia
- Can indent esophagus

CT Findings
- NECT
  - Homogeneous well circumscribed lesion
  - Cyst contents variable: Water to proteinaceous
  - Hence CT attenuation is variable
  - 50% water attenuation
- CECT
  - Well-defined, typically with nonenhancing or minimally enhancing thin wall
  - More prominent wall enhancement and wall thickening may be seen with infection
  - No central enhancement

MR Findings
- T1WI
  - Well-circumscribed lesion
  - Homogeneous signal intensity unless infected
  - Variable signal due to varying amounts of proteinaceous material, but usually water signal
  - Imperceptible wall
- T2WI: Signal is almost always equal to or greater than cerebrospinal fluid (CSF)
- STIR: Markedly increased signal, equal to or greater than CSF
- T1 C+
  - May have a thin rim of mild enhancement
  - Thicker enhancing wall implies infection
  - No central enhancement

Ultrasonographic Findings
- Grayscale Ultrasound
  - Increasingly being diagnosed on pre-natal imaging
  - Incidental finding on echocardiography
  - Retroperitoneal bronchogenic cysts more likely to be discovered by ultrasound than their intrathoracic counterparts
- Color Doppler: No associated abnormal flow
- M-mode: Well-circumscribed hypoechoic or anechoic lesion with posterior acoustic enhancement

Imaging Recommendations
- Best imaging tool
  - MR with T2 weighted and STIR imaging shows homogeneous signal as high or higher than CSF
  - Contrast-enhanced T1 weighted imaging shows no or minimal rim enhancement without central enhancement
- Protocol advice
  - T2 or STIR in planes to show anatomical relationships and homogeneously increased signal
  - Post-contrast fat-suppressed T1 to demonstrate no or a thin rim of enhancement without central enhancement

DIFFERENTIAL DIAGNOSIS

Round pneumonia
- Bronchogenic cysts may cause mass effect (airway) whereas round pneumonia will not
- Follow-up radiographs will show resolution of round pneumonia
- Patient usually has a fever and cough

Congenital cystic adenomatoid malformation (CCAM)
- More often not unilocular like bronchogenic cyst
- Most often contain air (shortly after birth) unlike bronchogenic cyst
- May contain fluid if infected (air-fluid level) or if images soon after birth (may be completely fluid-filled)

Neurogenic tumors
- Usually more solid appearing on cross sectional imaging

BRONCHOGENIC CYST

- May be calcified
- May have scalloping of ribs or vertebrae

Lymphadenopathy
- Differentiation by chest radiograph is difficult unless multiple nodal groups are enlarged
- Generally multilobular
- Necrotic nodes
  - Usually have associated pulmonary findings of infection (e.g. histoplasmosis or tuberculosis)
  - Thick rim of enhancement
  - Usually other nearby nodes are enlarged but not necrotic

Vascular malformations
- Tend to be more multilocular
- Invaginate around structures rather than displace with mass effect
- May contain phleboliths if there is a venous component
- More likely to extend into the neck

Primary pulmonary malignancies
- Pleuropulmonary blastoma
  - Rare
  - Solid components on CT and MRI
  - Heterogeneous appearance on CECT and MR
  - Pleural based and often peripheral in position
  - Pleural effusion common in pulmonary blastoma

Pulmonary sequestration
- Mass is more heterogeneous than bronchogenic cyst
- More ill-defined
- Supplying vessel arising from descending aorta is often visible

PATHOLOGY

General Features
- General path comments
  - Bronchogenic cysts do not communicate with the bronchial tree and do not contain air unless they become infected
  - Cysts are lined with ciliated epithelium
  - Walls may contain smooth muscle or cartilage
- Etiology
  - Bronchogenic cysts are developmental lesions that result from abnormal budding of the ventral foregut
    - Early budding results in mediastinal cysts
    - Later budding results in lung parenchymal cysts
- Epidemiology: Frequency unknown due to large asymptomatic population

Gross Pathologic & Surgical Features
- Well-circumscribed
- Contents usually thick or gelatinous fluid

Microscopic Features
- Lined by ciliated respiratory epithelium
- Occasionally may contain gastric mucosa or bronchial cartilage

CLINICAL ISSUES

Presentation
- Most common signs/symptoms
  - Infants: Respiratory distress or dysphagia
  - Older children: Chest pain and dysphagia
  - Symptoms more common in mediastinal lesions
- Other signs/symptoms
  - Younger children are more likely to present with symptoms
  - Cysts more likely to be incidentally discovered in older children
  - Consider in children with recurrent infection

Demographics
- Age: All ages
- Gender: No sex predilection

Natural History & Prognosis
- Propensity for infection
- Case reports of malignancy arising in lesions

Treatment
- Surgical resection recommended in children
- Morbidity increases when lesions are symptomatic

DIAGNOSTIC CHECKLIST

Image Interpretation Pearls
- T2 weighted or STIR imaging is most accurate, demonstrating homogeneous increased signal
- CT attenuation varies due to proteinaceous contents of fluid
- Middle mediastinum and central one third of lungs
- Thin rim on contrast enhanced imaging

SELECTED REFERENCES

1. Yoon YC et al: Intrapulmonary bronchogenic cyst: CT and pathologic findings in five adult patients. AJR Am J Roentgenol. 179(1):167-70, 2002
2. Ashizawa K et al: Anterior mediastinal bronchogenic cyst: demonstration of complicating malignancy by CT and MRI. Br J Radiol. 74(886):959-61, 2001
3. Donnelly LF et al: Fundamentals of Pediatric Radiology. Philadelphia; W.B. Saunders. 2001
4. McAdams HP et al: Bronchogenic cyst: imaging features with clinical and histopathologic correlation. Radiology. 217(2):441-6, 2000
5. Griscom NT et al: Diseases of the trachea, bronchi, and smaller airways. Radiol Clin N Amer. 31:605-15, 1993
6. Suen HC et al: Surgical management and radiological characteristics of bronchogenic cysts. Ann Thorac Surg. 55(2):476-81, 1993
7. Chapman KR et al: Spontaneous disappearance of a chronic mediastinal mass. Chest. 87(2):235-6, 1985
8. Mendelson DS et al: Bronchogenic cysts with high CT numbers. AJR. 140:463-5, 1983

BRONCHOGENIC CYST

IMAGE GALLERY

Typical

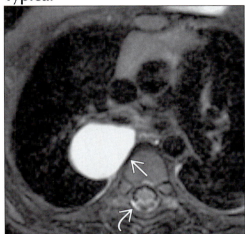
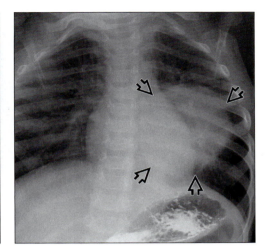

(Left) Axial T2WI MR shows homogeneous, well-circumscribed ovoid mass (arrow) with signal greater than CSF (curved arrow). (Right) Anteroposterior radiograph shows large, smooth, homogeneous, left retrocardiac parenchymal mass (arrows).

Variant

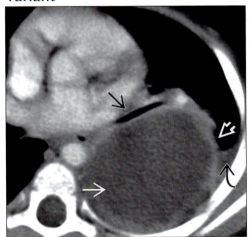
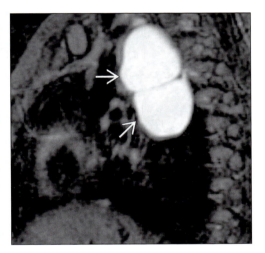

(Left) Axial CECT shows infected bronchogenic cyst (white arrow) adjacent to the left lower lobe bronchus (black arrow) with a thick rim (open white arrow), and reactive pleural effusion (curved arrow). (Right) Sagittal STIR MR shows a well-circumscribed homogeneously high signal mass which appear to have two separate lobules (arrows).

Typical

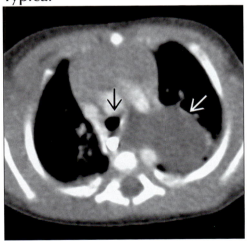
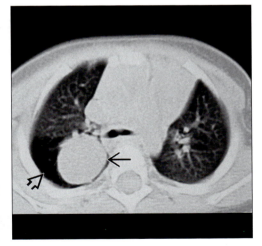

(Left) Axial CECT shows fluid attenuation mass in middle mediastinum (white arrow), with no perceptible rim. The lesion has mass effect, displacing the trachea (black arrow) to the right. (Right) Axial CECT shows mass in right upper lobe (arrow). There is compression of the right upper lobe bronchus with resultant hyperinflation of the right upper lobe (open arrow).

CONGENITAL LOBAR EMPHYSEMA

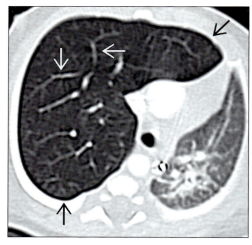

Axial CECT shows marked hyperinflation of the right upper lobe (black arrows) with associated deviation of the mediastinum to the left. Vessels in right lung are attenuated (white arrows).

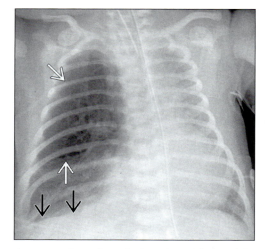

Anteroposterior radiograph shows hyperinflation of the right upper (white arrows) with flattening of the right hemidiaphragm (black arrows) and deviation of the mediastinum to the left.

TERMINOLOGY

Abbreviations and Synonyms
- Congenital lobar emphysema (CLE), congenital lobar pneumonia, infantile lobar emphysema, congenital lobar hyperinflation

Definitions
- Progressive over-distention of a pulmonary lobe due to obstruction
- Not a specific disease but a condition that may result from a variety of etiologies

IMAGING FINDINGS

General Features
- Best diagnostic clue: Radiodense lobe that progressively becomes hyperlucent and hyperexpanded
- Location
  - There is a lobar predilection
    - Left upper lobe: 42%
    - Right middle lobe: 35%
    - Right upper lobe: 21%
    - 1% in each lower lobe
  - Occasionally more than one lobe involved
  - Sometimes only a portion of a lobe involved
- Lucency and hyperexpansion caused by air in distended alveoli

Radiographic Findings
- Radiography
  - Initially after birth, lobe may be filled with fetal lung fluid and appear as radiodensity
  - May have a reticular pattern as fluid is cleared via distended lymphatics
  - Fluid eventually replaced by air
    - Hyperlucent, hyperexpanded lobe
  - Compression of ipsilateral lung
  - Deviation of mediastinum to contralateral side
  - Pulmonary vessels may appear attenuated and displaced
  - Occasionally ribs are separated and diaphragm is depressed
  - Increased retrosternal lucency on lateral view
  - No decompression of lung when patient is in ipsilateral decubitus position
  - Classic progression: Radiodense lobe that becomes progressively hyperlucent and hyperexpanded

Fluoroscopic Findings
- Esophagram
  - Being replaced by CT and MR to evaluate for anomalous origin of the pulmonary artery
    - Passes between trachea and esophagus

DDx: Lucent Hemithorax In A Neonate

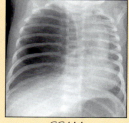

CCAM

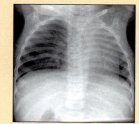

Lung Hypoplasia

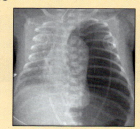

Pneumothorax

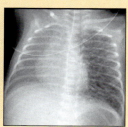

PIE

CONGENITAL LOBAR EMPHYSEMA

Key Facts

Terminology
- Progressive over-distention of a pulmonary lobe due to obstruction
- Not a specific disease but a condition that may result from a variety of etiologies

Imaging Findings
- Left upper lobe: 42%
- Lucency and hyperexpansion caused by air in distended alveoli
- Initially after birth, lobe may be filled with fetal lung fluid and appear as radiodensity
- No decompression of lung when patient is in ipsilateral decubitus position
- Hyperlucent lung
- Vessels attenuated: Smaller than those in adjacent lung
- Mediastinal and tracheal deviation
- Compression of remainder of ipsilateral lung

Top Differential Diagnoses
- Congenital cystic adenomatoid malformation (CCAM)
- Pulmonary artery hypoplasia
- Pulmonary hypoplasia

Pathology
- Dilated alveoli
- Alveolar walls are thinned but intact
- Defective cartilage in bronchial walls seen in less than 50%

Clinical Issues
- Majority symptomatic in neonatal period and infancy
- 50% present in first 4 weeks; 75% in first 6 months

CT Findings
- NECT
  - Detection of multiple abnormal areas and multilobar involvement becoming more common with increased use of CT
  - Lucency caused by air in distended alveoli
    - Hyperlucent lung
    - Vessels attenuated: Smaller than those in adjacent lung
  - Mediastinal and tracheal deviation
  - Compression of remainder of ipsilateral lung

MR Findings
- T1WI: May demonstrate anomalous pulmonary artery or other cause of extrinsic compression
- T2* GRE: Fetal MR demonstrates high signal expanded lobe with compression of ipsilateral remaining lung and mediastinal deviation

Ultrasonographic Findings
- Grayscale Ultrasound
  - Prenatal sonography
    - Distended, fluid-filled upper lobe mass
    - May cause mediastinal deviation

Angiographic Findings
- Conventional: Slow filling of attenuated pulmonary arteries

Nuclear Medicine Findings
- V/Q Scan
  - Ventilation-perfusion (V/Q) imaging
    - Ventilation initially diminished; then develop retention of isotope in affected lobe
    - Matching decreased perfusion in same distribution

Imaging Recommendations
- Best imaging tool
  - Diagnosis typically made by chest radiography
  - CT usually performed to
    - Confirm diagnosis
    - Exclude other causes of hyperlucent lung lesions in neonates
    - Evaluate for a causal lesion
    - Define extent of disease
- Protocol advice
  - Frontal and lateral chest radiograph
  - CECT

DIFFERENTIAL DIAGNOSIS

Congenital cystic adenomatoid malformation (CCAM)
- Air is contained in abnormal cystic structures of varying sizes

Pulmonary artery hypoplasia
- Affected lung is small
- Ipsilateral pulmonary artery is absent
- No air-trapping

Pulmonary hypoplasia
- Affected lung is small
- Ipsilateral bronchus is small or absent
- No air-trapping

Bronchial atresia
- Central tubular, rounded, or branching mass

Persistent pulmonary interstitial emphysema (PIE)
- In rare cases, PIE can persist and present as expanding hyperlucent mass
- Air is located in interstitium so pulmonary vessels are surrounded by air and seen as lines or dots within central portion of lucency

Congenital diaphragmatic hernia (CDH)
- Air within bowel loops, most commonly within left hemithorax
- Left diaphragm not seen
- Decreased or no bowel gas seen in upper abdomen

CONGENITAL LOBAR EMPHYSEMA

Pneumothorax
- In neonate, contralateral lung usually shows underlying lung disease

PATHOLOGY

General Features
- General path comments
  - CLE related to overdistention of alveoli
  - Two forms
    - Hypoalveolar → normal or fewer alveoli than expected
    - Polyalveolar → more alveoli than expected
  - Difference not clinically important
- Etiology
  - Cause found in approximately 50% of cases
  - Most likely related to bronchial obstruction with a ball valve phenomenon
    - Air enters involved region but has difficulty leaving → progressive hyperinflation
  - Wall
    - Deficient, immature, or dysplastic bronchial cartilage
    - Redundant bronchial mucosal folds
    - Stenotic or kinked bronchus
  - Lumen
    - Inspissated mucus plug
    - Mucosal web or fold
  - Extrinsic compression
    - Pulmonary arterial sling
    - Tetralogy of Fallot with absent pulmonary valve
    - Patent ductus arteriosus
    - Pulmonic stenosis
    - Dilated superior vena cava with anomalous pulmonary venous return
    - Foregut duplication cyst
- Associated abnormalities
  - Can be associated anomalies such as congenital heart disease in 14-50% of patients
    - PDA, ASD, VSD, TAPVR, tetralogy of Fallot

Gross Pathologic & Surgical Features
- Hyperexpanded lobe is rounded
- Sponge-like appearance
- Resected lobe does not deflate
- Compressed ipsilateral lobe will reinflate

Microscopic Features
- Dilated alveoli
- Alveolar walls are thinned but intact
- Defective cartilage in bronchial walls seen in less than 50%
- May see more alveoli than expected

Staging, Grading or Classification Criteria
- Polyalveolar: Increased number of alveoli than expected
- Hypoalveolar: Normal / < alveoli than expected

CLINICAL ISSUES

Presentation
- Most common signs/symptoms
  - Respiratory distress in neonatal period
  - May be progressive
- Other signs/symptoms
  - Asymmetry of movement of chest with respiration
  - Use of accessory muscles of respiration
  - Decreased breath sounds on affected side
  - Hyperresonant hemithorax

Demographics
- Age
  - May be diagnosed in utero
  - Majority symptomatic in neonatal period and infancy
    - 50% present in first 4 weeks; 75% in first 6 months
  - May present with symptoms later in childhood or may be an incidental finding
- Gender: M:F = 1.8:1
- Ethnicity: Most common in Caucasians

Natural History & Prognosis
- Fluid seen in neonatal period is removed by lymphatics and capillary reabsorption
- Lobe subsequently filled with air by collateral air drift
- May cause progressive respiratory distress as lobe continues to expand and cause lung compression and mediastinal shift → can be fatal if not resected
- Some patients have minor symptoms and can be observed
- Over time involved lobe becomes small with diminished markings
- No increased risk of malignancy or infection

Treatment
- Bronchoscopy to exclude endobronchial lesion
- Electively intubate opposite lung
- Place patient in ipsilateral decubitus position
- Surgical lobectomy
  - May need to be performed as an emergency if progressive hyperinflation occurs → can be life-threatening
- Conservative treatment has been advocated for patients with
  - Minimal symptoms
  - Incidental presentation

SELECTED REFERENCES

1. Berrocal T et al: Congenital anomalies of the tracheobronchial tree, lung, and mediastinum: embryology, radiology, and pathology. Radiographics. 24(1):e17, 2004
2. Daltro P et al: CT of congenital lung lesions in pediatric patients. AJR Am J Roentgenol. 183(5):1497-506, 2004
3. Tander B et al: Congenital lobar emphysema: a clinicopathologic evaluation of 14 cases. Eur J Pediatr Surg. 13(2):108-11, 2003
4. Donnelly LF et al: Localized lucent chest lesions in neonates. AJR. 212:837-40, 1999

CONGENITAL LOBAR EMPHYSEMA

IMAGE GALLERY

Typical

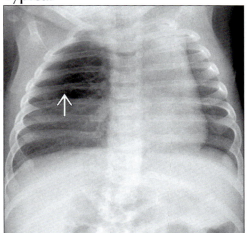
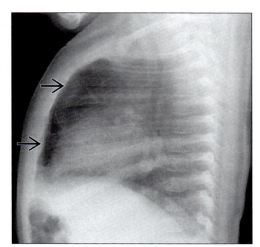

(Left) Anteroposterior radiograph shows hyperlucent right upper lobe (arrow) with mass effect causing deviation of the mediastinum towards the left hemithorax. (Right) Lateral radiograph shows an increase in the size of the retrosternal airspace (arrows) extending down to the diaphragm. The lung in this region is also hyperlucent.

Variant

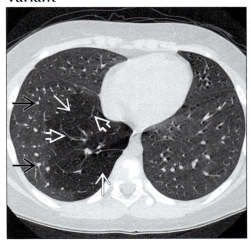
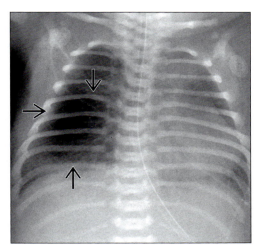

(Left) Axial HRCT shows involvement of the medial basal segment the right lower lobe which is hyperlucent (white arrows). The pulmonary vessels in this region are attenuated (open arrows), being appreciably smaller than those in the remainder of the right lower lobe (black arrows). (Right) Anteroposterior radiograph shows hyperinflation of the right lower lobe (arrows) with deviation of the mediastinum to the left.

Typical

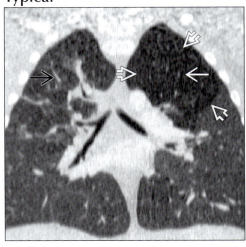
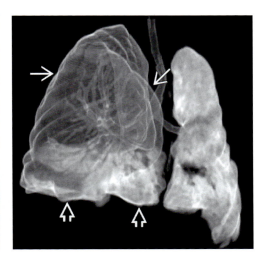

(Left) Coronal CECT shows hyperlucency of the left upper lobe (open arrows) with attenuation of vessels (white arrow). Compare with more normal size right upper lobe vessels (black arrow). (Right) appearance on a 3D surface-rendered CT demonstrating hyperinflation of the right upper lobe which is more rounded than usual (arrows). Note compression of the right lower lobe (open arrows).

CONGENITAL DIAPHRAGMATIC HERNIA

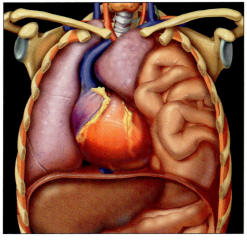

Graphic shows posterior defect in left hemidiaphragm with herniation of stomach & small bowel into left hemithorax. There is rightward mediastinal shift & compression of both ipsilateral and contralateral lung.

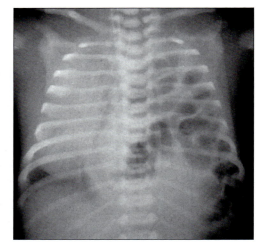

Anteroposterior radiograph shows aerated cystic mass in left hemithorax, mediastinal shift to left, and absence of gas in upper abdomen.

TERMINOLOGY

Abbreviations and Synonyms
- Congenital diaphragmatic hernia (CDH)
- Bochdalek hernia: Posterior hernia, most common type of CDH
- Morgagni hernia: Anterior, much less common in neonates

Definitions
- Herniation of abdominal contents into the chest typically via a posterior defect in the diaphragm

IMAGING FINDINGS

General Features
- Best diagnostic clue: Bubble-like lucencies that appear like bowel within chest
- Location
  o More common on left than right (5:1)
  o May contain variable abdominal contents: Stomach, small and large bowel, liver
- Size
  o Amount of herniated content variable
  o Large CDH causes compression of pulmonary tissue and resultant pulmonary hypoplasia
- Morphology: Herniated abdominal viscera potentially including stomach, bowel, liver

Radiographic Findings
- Radiography
  o Radiographic appearance depends on hernia contents and whether air present within herniated bowel
  o XR initially after birth may show hernia as radiodense (prior to air introduced into bowel)
    ▪ May inject air via nasogastric (NG) to make diagnosis of bowel in chest
  o Later when air introduced into bowel: Appears as air-containing cystic mass resembling bowel
  o Decreased bowel gas in abdomen
  o Right-sided hernia often contains liver and not bowel (soft tissue density)
  o Mediastinal shift away from hernia
  o Low volumes of ipsilateral or contralateral lung (from hypoplasia)
  o Abnormal position of support apparatus may be clue to diagnosis
    ▪ NG tube lodged with tip at esophagogastric junction
    ▪ NG tube above diaphragm documenting stomach in hernia
    ▪ Deviation of the intrathoracic descending portion of nasogastric tube away from side of hernia

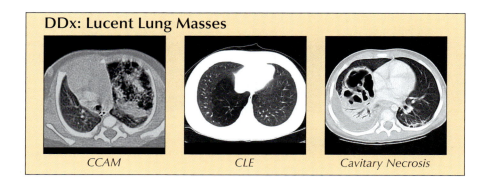

DDx: Lucent Lung Masses

CCAM | CLE | Cavitary Necrosis

CONGENITAL DIAPHRAGMATIC HERNIA

Key Facts

Terminology
- Congenital diaphragmatic hernia (CDH)
- Bochdalek hernia: Posterior hernia, most common type of CDH

Imaging Findings
- Best diagnostic clue: Bubble-like lucencies that appear like bowel within chest
- More common on left than right (5:1)
- Large CDH causes compression of pulmonary tissue and resultant pulmonary hypoplasia
- Radiographic appearance depends on hernia contents and whether air present within herniated bowel
- XR initially after birth may show hernia as radiodense (prior to air introduced into bowel)
- Later when air introduced into bowel: Appears as air-containing cystic mass resembling bowel
- Decreased bowel gas in abdomen
- Right-sided hernia often contains liver and not bowel (soft tissue density)
- Mediastinal shift away from hernia
- Abnormal position of support apparatus may be clue to diagnosis

Pathology
- Degree of lung hypoplasia: Major factor in determining prognosis
- Up to 1/3 have associated major malformations
- Congenital heart disease reported in up to 50%
- Approximately 8% have known syndromes

Clinical Issues
- Severe respiratory distress
- Most commonly presents at birth

- Apex convexity of umbilical venous catheter towards side of hernia
- Post-operative radiographic appearance
  - Resolution of herniated contents
  - ipsilateral hypoplastic lung may not fill space vacated by repaired hernia
  - Some of the gortex graft materials used to fix diaphragmatic defects can contain air post-operatively
    - Can mimic pneumothorax
- Fluoroscopy
  - Upper GI can be used to document that air containing structures in chest represent bowel and not cysts
  - Rarely necessary

CT Findings
- NECT
  - Shows multiple loops of bowel in chest
  - Oral contrast documents bowel-containing nature of hernia
  - Not typically used for diagnosis of CDH; may be obtained if other cystic chest mass suspected

MR Findings
- Fetal MRI
  - T2 weighted images
    - Multiple serpentine high signal structures seen in chest representing bowel loops
    - If liver herniated, appears as low signal structure
    - Mediastinal shift: Displacement of cardiac structures
    - Decreased lung volumes
    - Lack of normal bowel in abdomen
    - Can be associated with hydrops fetalis

Ultrasonographic Findings
- Grayscale Ultrasound
  - Prenatal ultrasound
    - Mixed echogenic mass seen in hemithorax
    - Displacement of cardiac structures
    - Absence of stomach bubble in normal position
  - Post-natal ultrasound
    - Not often utilized in evaluation of CDH
    - Can be utilized to evaluate for paralyzed diaphragm (paradoxical motion)
    - When question of elevated, paralyzed diaphragm vs. CDH

Imaging Recommendations
- Best imaging tool: Chest radiography
- Protocol advice: Look for diagnostic clues in position of support apparatus

DIFFERENTIAL DIAGNOSIS

Congenital cystic adenomatoid malformation (CCAM)
- Appears as multicystic, air-containing mass
- CCAM more likely to have air-fluid levels than CDH
- Appearance does not change in position with CCAM over serial films, can with CDH
- Position of support apparatus altered with CDH

Congenital lobar emphysema (CLE)
- Hyperlucent lung as compared to air filled bowel in CDH
- Often involves upper lobe vs. originating from below in CDH

Pneumonia complicated by cavitary necrosis
- Usually not in neonatal period
- Cysts surrounded by opacified lung

PATHOLOGY

General Features
- General path comments
  - Herniation of abdominal contents into the chest typically via a posterior defect in the diaphragm
  - Often via left pleuroperitoneal foramen
  - Herniated abdominal contents can compress ipsilateral and contralateral lung and prevent normal development of lung

BRONCHIAL ATRESIA

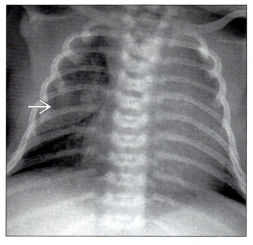

Anteroposterior radiograph shows relatively increased density in the right upper lobe (white arrow) in a neonate. This had been seen on prenatal imaging as a fluid-filled structure.

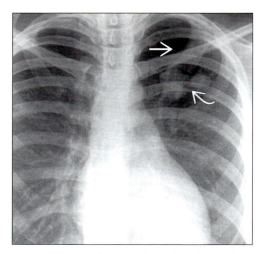

Anteroposterior radiograph shows branching tubular opacities in the left upper lobe (curved arrow) with hyperinflation distal to and surrounding the lesion (arrow).

TERMINOLOGY

Definitions
- Congenital atresia of a proximal segmental bronchus with normal distal architecture

IMAGING FINDINGS

General Features
- Best diagnostic clue: Hilar mass or tubular branching mass surrounded by hyperinflated lung
- Location
  - Most common location: Apicoposterior segment left upper lobe
  - Next most likely: Right upper lobe, right middle lobe; lower lobe bronchi rare
- Morphology
  - Round or branching tubular mass of dilated fluid-filled bronchi distal to an atretic proximal segmental bronchus
  - Occasionally the dilated bronchi may be partially or completely fluid-filled

Radiographic Findings
- Round or ovoid mass adjacent to the hilum (bronchocele)
- Branching tubular opacities (mucoid impaction of dilated bronchi) distal to segmental bronchus
- Distal lung hyperinflated
- Diminished vascularity
- Neonates; lobe or segment may be fluid filled, gradually replaced by air

CT Findings
- CECT
  - Central, low to intermediate attenuation, rounded or branching tubular mass
  - Hyperinflated distal lung with decreased vascularity
  - Distinguish bronchocele from other causes of a nodular mass
  - Multiplanar reconstructions help to demonstrate bronchial anatomy
- HRCT: Airtrapping confirmed in hyperlucent distal lung on expiratory images

MR Findings
- T1WI: Rounded or tubular branching mass is high signal due to proteinaceous content mucus
- T2WI: Central mass is high signal

Ultrasonographic Findings
- Obstetric ultrasound
  - Can be detected in utero
  - Fluid-filled upper lobe
    - Differential

DDx: Hyperlucent Lung

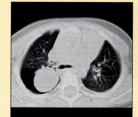
Bronchogenic Cyst

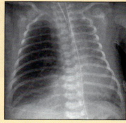
Lobar Emphysema

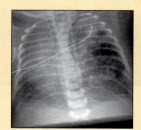
CCAM

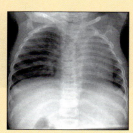
Pulm Hypoplasia

BRONCHIAL ATRESIA

Key Facts

Terminology
- Congenital atresia of a proximal segmental bronchus with normal distal architecture

Imaging Findings
- Best diagnostic clue: Hilar mass or tubular branching mass surrounded by hyperinflated lung
- Most common location: Apicoposterior segment left upper lobe
- Next most likely: Right upper lobe, right middle lobe; lower lobe bronchi rare
- Neonates; lobe or segment may be fluid filled, gradually replaced by air
- Can be detected in utero

Top Differential Diagnoses
- Congenital lobar emphysema
- Congenital cystic adenomatoid malformation (CCAM)
- Allergic bronchopulmonary aspergillosis (ABPA)

Pathology
- Aeration of distal lung through collateral air drift
- Focal atresia of proximal segmental bronchus
- Mucoid-filled dilated bronchi distal to atretic bronchus
- Distal lung hyperinflated but otherwise normal

Clinical Issues
- Most common signs/symptoms: Majority asymptomatic: Incidental discovery on a chest radiograph
- Recurrent respiratory tract infections
- Gender: F:M = 2:1

- Cystic adenomatoid malformation
- Congenital diaphragmatic hernia
- Bronchopulmonary foregut malformations
- Lobar emphysema

Nuclear Medicine Findings
- V/Q Scan: Ventilation/perfusion imaging demonstrates matched segmental ventilation and perfusion defects

Imaging Recommendations
- Best imaging tool: CT usually allows for more definite diagnosis
- Protocol advice: Contrast-enhanced axial images with multiplanar reconstructions

DIFFERENTIAL DIAGNOSIS

Congenital lobar emphysema
- No mass
- Usually involves entire lobe
- Often symptomatic in infancy
- Mass effect common
  - Compression of ipsilateral and/or contralateral lung
  - Mediastinal shift to opposite side

Bronchogenic cyst
- Can be similar with airtrapping and a central mass

Congenital cystic adenomatoid malformation (CCAM)
- Similar appearances in utero and neonatal period
- Most common congenital lung malformation (25% of all congenital pulmonary lesions)
- Often symptomatic in neonatal period
- No associated central mass
- No lobar predilection
- Multicystic types (types 2 and 3) more easy to differentiate than single cyst (type 1)

Allergic bronchopulmonary aspergillosis (ABPA)
- Associated bronchiectasis is usually widespread
- Often bilateral and multifocal
- Patients symptomatic
- Known underlying condition
  - Asthma
  - Cystic Fibrosis
- Nodular opacities come and go with exacerbations

Carcinoid tumor, slow growing endobronchial tumor
- Mass not as large as mucoid impaction
- Distal lung usually not hyperexpanded but atelectatic

Solitary pulmonary nodule (SPN)
- No hyperinflation distal to nodule

Pulmonary (lung) agenesis
- Complete absence of lung parenchyma, bronchus, and pulmonary artery
- Opaque hemithorax

Pulmonary aplasia
- Blind ending rudimentary bronchus
- No normal architecture distal
- Opaque hemithorax

Pulmonary hypoplasia
- Bronchus and lung present
- Decreased number and size of vessels, airways, and alveoli
- Mediastinal shift of the contralateral lung towards hypoplastic lung
- Commonly symptomatic with recurrent infections and respiratory distress

Pulmonary artery agenesis
- Complete absence of unilateral pulmonary artery
- Associated with other cardiac lesions
- Affected lung is smaller
- Ipsilateral hilum small on chest radiograph
- Lung may be hyperlucent
- No airtrapping

BRONCHIAL ATRESIA

Pulmonary vein atresia
- Usually presents in infancy/childhood with recurrent infection or hemoptysis
- Affected lung is small with resultant mediastinal shift
- Unilateral reticular opacities with septal lines
- Absent vein best seen in CT

Scimitar syndrome (hypogenetic lung syndrome)
- Hypoplastic lung
- Mediastinal deviation towards affected lung
- Partial anomalous pulmonary venous drainage via a systemic vein
- Usually right-sided
- Tubular opacity curves along right heart border

Pulmonary sequestration
- Recurrent infections
- Usually in left lower lobe
- Systemic arterial supply, usually from aorta
- Venous drainage may be systemic (extralobar) or via pulmonary veins (intralobar)

PATHOLOGY

General Features
- General path comments
  - Obliteration or severe narrowing of proximal lumen segmental bronchus
  - Aeration of distal lung through collateral air drift
  - Distal lung: Normal architecture
  - Embryology-anatomy
    - Thought to occur between 5th and 15th week of gestation
- Etiology
  - Uncertain
    - Possibly intrauterine interruption of arterial supply to bronchus → ischemia and scarring of primitive bronchus
- Associated abnormalities
  - Congenital lobar emphysema
  - Pulmonary sequestration
  - Congenital adenomatoid malformation
  - Bronchogenic cyst
  - Pericardial defects
  - Anomalous pulmonary venous return

Gross Pathologic & Surgical Features
- Focal atresia of proximal segmental bronchus
- Mucoid-filled dilated bronchi distal to atretic bronchus
- Distal lung hyperinflated but otherwise normal

Microscopic Features
- No specific features, nonspecific inflammation distal to atresia

CLINICAL ISSUES

Presentation
- Most common signs/symptoms: Majority asymptomatic: Incidental discovery on a chest radiograph
- Recurrent respiratory tract infections
- Chronic cough
- Dyspnea, wheezing

Demographics
- Gender: F:M = 2:1

Natural History & Prognosis
- Excellent

Treatment
- Surgical resection for repeated infections
- If asymptomatic, may not need any treatment

DIAGNOSTIC CHECKLIST

Image Interpretation Pearls
- Tubular or rounded mass centrally with hyperinflation of the distal lung in the distribution of a segmental bronchus
- Diminished vascularity in affected lung segment

SELECTED REFERENCES

1. Berrocal T et al: Congenital anomalies of the tracheobronchial tree, lung, and mediastinum: embryology, radiology, and pathology. Radiographics. 24(1):e17, 2004
2. Daltro P et al: CT of congenital lung lesions in pediatric patients. AJR Am J Roentgenol. 183(5):1497-506, 2004
3. Zylak CJ et al: Developmental lung anomalies in the adult: radiologic-pathologic correlation. Radiographics. 22 Spec No:S25-43, 2002
4. Donnelly LF et al: Localized radiolucent chest lesions in neonates: causes and differentiation. AJR Am J Roentgenol. 172(6):1651-8, 1999
5. Mori M et al: Bronchial atresia: report of a case and review of the literature. Surg Today. 23(5):449-54, 1993
6. Kinsella D et al: The radiological imaging of bronchial atresia. Br J Radiol. 65(776):681-5, 1992
7. Kuhn C et al: Coexistence of bronchial atresia and bronchogenic cyst: diagnostic criteria and embryologic considerations. Pediatr Radiol. 22(8):568-70, 1992
8. Keslar P et al: Radiographic manifestation of anomalies of the lung. Radiol Clin North Am. 29:255-70, 1991
9. Mata JM et al: CT of congenital malformations of the lung. Radiographics. 10(4):651-74, 1990
10. Cohen AM et al: Computed tomography in bronchial atresia. AJR Am J Roentgenol. 135(5):1097-9, 1980
11. Simon G et al: Atresia of an apical bronchus of the left upper lobe: Report of 3 cases. Br J Dis Chest. 57:126-32, 1963

BRONCHIAL ATRESIA

IMAGE GALLERY

Typical

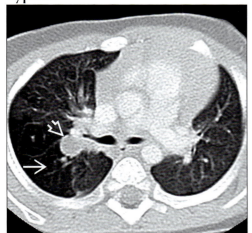
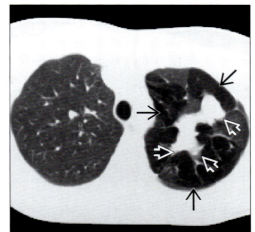

(Left) Axial CECT shows a rounded lesion centrally adjacent to the right upper lobe bronchus (open arrow). The distal lung is hyperlucent with decrease in pulmonary vascularity (arrow). (Right) Axial CECT shows branching tubular structure in the left upper lobe (open arrows). Distal to these dilated fluid bronchi is hyperlucent lung with decreased vascularity (arrows).

Typical

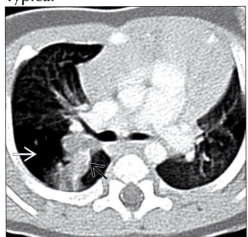
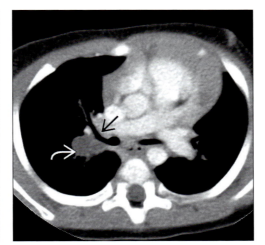

(Left) Axial CECT shows lobulated lesion centrally at the origin of the right upper lobe bronchus (black arrow). Distal to this lesion is hyperlucent lung with diminished vascularity (white arrow). (Right) Axial CECT shows a small rounded fluid attenuation nodule (curved arrow) posterior to the bronchus supplying the anterior segment of the right upper lobe (arrow).

Typical

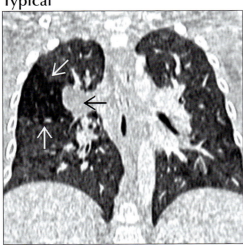
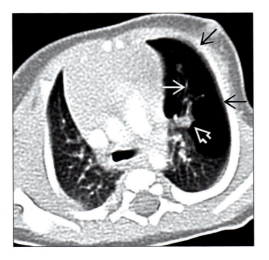

(Left) Coronal CECT shows diminished vascularity in a segmental distribution (white arrows) distal to a rounded, dilated, proximally obstructed bronchus = bronchocele (black arrow). (Right) Axial CECT shows hyperlucency in the anterior segment of the left upper lobe (black arrows), with decreased caliber of the vessels (white arrow). Central rounded opacity consistent with a bronchocele (open arrow).

SURFACTANT DEFICIENT DISEASE

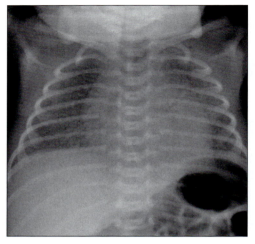

Anteroposterior radiograph shows pulmonary hypoventilation and reticulonodular densities bilaterally. The premature infant is 8 hours old, born at 28 weeks gestational age.

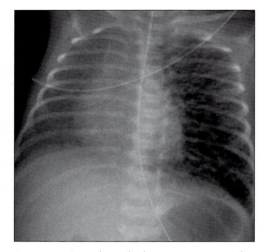

Anteroposterior radiograph shows a premature infant who has RDS and developed pulmonary interstitial emphysema of the left lung with mediastinal shift to the right.

TERMINOLOGY

Abbreviations and Synonyms
- Surfactant deficiency disease (SDD)
- Respiratory distress syndrome (RDS)
- Hyaline membrane disease
- Lung disease of prematurity

Definitions
- Common: Lung disease occurring in the premature infants due to lack of surfactant
  - Microatelectasis, abnormal pulmonary compliance are hallmarks of disease
- Very uncommon: Rare lung disease which is congenital or acquired due to lack of proteins to make surfactant
  - Protein B and C deficiencies
  - Can occur with meconium aspiration syndrome
  - Usually present later in infancy with interstitial lung disease

IMAGING FINDINGS

General Features
- Best diagnostic clue
  - Initial findings are low lung volumes and diffuse reticular granular opacities
  - Air bronchograms and poor lung expansion
  - Cardiac size is normal
  - Subsequent imaging shows significant bilateral lung disease
    - Localized areas of atelectasis
    - Focal hyperinflation
    - Air block issues with pneumothorax, pneumomediastinum
    - Complications of patent ductus arteriosus
    - Bronchopulmonary dysplasia or chronic lung disease of premature infant
- Size: Premature infants less than 32 weeks gestation
- Morphology: Small airways with hyaline membranes

Radiographic Findings
- Radiography
  - Initial Features
    - Low lung volumes secondary to micro-collapse
    - Diffuse granular opacities represent collapsed alveoli interspersed with open alveoli
    - Air bronchograms demonstrate patent bronchi in abnormal lung
    - Diffuse bilateral airspace disease
    - Pleural effusions very uncommon

DDx: Respiratory Distress

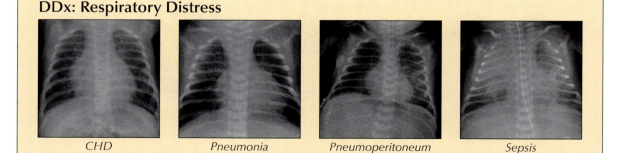

CHD | Pneumonia | Pneumoperitoneum | Sepsis

SURFACTANT DEFICIENT DISEASE

Key Facts

Terminology
- Respiratory distress syndrome (RDS)
- Hyaline membrane disease
- Common: Lung disease occurring in the premature infants due to lack of surfactant
- Very uncommon: Rare lung disease which is congenital or acquired due to lack of proteins to make surfactant

Imaging Findings
- Initial findings are low lung volumes and diffuse reticular granular opacities
- Subsequent imaging shows significant bilateral lung disease
- Low lung volumes secondary to micro-collapse
- Intubation and ventilatory support changes the imaging appearance
- High incidence of patent ductus arteriosus (PDA) which shows pulmonary edema (white out of lungs with cardiomegaly)
- Bronchopulmonary dysplasia in 17-55% of premature infants
- Best imaging tool: Chest radiograph with comparison to prior imaging

Pathology
- Immature type II pneumocytes cannot produce surfactant
- Deficiency of surfactant results in alveolar atelectasis
- Occurs in 40,000 infants each year in USA

Clinical Issues
- Disease of premature infants (< 36 weeks gestation, < 2.5 kg)

- Potential complications include: Pulmonary interstitial emphysema, pneumomediastinum, pneumothorax, superimposed pneumonia, pulmonary hemorrhage, bronchopulmonary dysphasia
  - Features after surfactant administration
    - Clearing of granular opacities and increased lung volumes
    - May have asymmetric or partial response
  - Findings after several days
    - Intubation and ventilatory support changes the imaging appearance
    - High incidence of patent ductus arteriosus (PDA) which shows pulmonary edema (white out of lungs with cardiomegaly)
  - Bronchopulmonary dysplasia in 17-55% of premature infants
    - Chronic lung disease characterized by focal areas of atelectasis, focal hyperinflation; pulmonary hyperinflation

CT Findings
- HRCT
  - Not typically used to make diagnosis of SDD
  - Bronchopulmonary dysplasia (BPD) demonstrates bilateral disease
    - Peribronchial thickening and prominent interlobular septum
    - Subpleural parenchymal bands
    - Hyperexpanded cyst-like areas, cobblestone appearance
    - Mosaic attenuation with airtrapping

Other Modality Findings
- Premature infants have many associated diseases
  - Intracranial ultrasound used to access for hemorrhage
  - Abdominal films for necrotizing enterocolitis

Imaging Recommendations
- Best imaging tool: Chest radiograph with comparison to prior imaging

DIFFERENTIAL DIAGNOSIS

Congenital heart disease (CHD)
- Echocardiography is gold standard for diagnosis
- Patent ductus arteriosus is common in infants less than 1000 gm
  - Usually closed with prostaglandin inhibitor
  - Surgical or thorascopic surgery done if contra-indication present

Group B streptococcal (GBS) pneumonia
- Most common type of pneumonia in neonates
- More common in premature infants
- Acquired during birth (25% of women colonized)
- Bilateral granular opacities and low lung volumes
- Pleural effusion common (67%): Only differentiating factor from SDD

Pneumoperitoneum
- Tachypnea may be secondary to a wide variety of causes
- Perforation likely secondary to necrotizing enterocolitis

Sepsis
- Streptococcus and gram negative organism are most common

Meconium aspiration syndrome
- Term infants
- High lung volumes
- Rope-like densities

PATHOLOGY

General Features
- General path comments: Hyaline membranes are proteinaceous exudates formed in alveoli
- Genetics: Mothers who deliver premature infants are more likely to have subsequent premature infants
- Etiology

SURFACTANT DEFICIENT DISEASE

- Immature type II pneumocytes cannot produce surfactant
- Surfactant normally coats alveoli and decreases surface tension allowing alveoli to stay open
- Deficiency of surfactant results in alveolar atelectasis
- Decreased lung compliance is associated with interstitial edema
- Secondary surfactant insufficiency occurs
  - Intrapartum asphyxia
  - Pulmonary infections
  - Meconium aspiration pneumonia
- Epidemiology
  - Males > females
  - Most common cause of death in live newborn infants
  - Occurs in 40,000 infants each year in USA
  - More common in infants of diabetic mothers
  - Common in all causes of premature labor and delivery
- Associated abnormalities
  - Premature infants have many associated abnormalities
    - Intracranial hemorrhage
    - Necrotizing enterocolitis
    - Patent ductus arteriosus
    - Metabolic problems of hypothermia, hypoglycemia
    - Delayed developmental milestones

CLINICAL ISSUES

Presentation
- Most common signs/symptoms
  - History of prematurity
  - Respiratory distress
- Other signs/symptoms
  - Metabolic acidosis
  - Cyanosis due to right to left shunting
  - Hypothermia

Demographics
- Age
  - Disease of premature infants (< 36 weeks gestation, < 2.5 kg)
  - Infants less than 27 weeks have a higher incidence of sequelae
  - One half of premature infants will have surfactant deficiency
- Gender: Equal
- Ethnicity: All races worldwide in premature infants

Natural History & Prognosis
- Acute complications
  - Alveolar rupture with pneumothorax, pneumomediastinum, pulmonary intersitial emphysema
  - Infections
  - Intracranial hemorrhage, periventricular leukomalacia
  - Patent ductus arteriosus with shunting and wide pulse pressure
  - Pulmonary hemorrhage
  - Necrotizing enterocolitis with or without perforation
  - Apnea
- Chronic complications
  - Bronchopulmonary dysplasia defined as
    - Abnormal chest radiograph at 30 days
    - Oxygen requirement at 36 weeks
  - Retinopathy of prematurity
  - Increased incidence of sudden death
  - Gastroesophageal reflux
  - Neurologic impairment in 10-70% depending on age
  - Family psychodynamic changes

Treatment
- Prenatal prevention with treatment of mother
  - Efforts to delay delivery allows fetus to mature
  - Maternal steroids will cross the placenta and increase surfactant
- Surfactant administration
  - Can be given in nebulized or aerosol forms
  - Injected into trachea via endotracheal tube or via catheter inserted into trachea
  - May be given prophylactically or after symptoms develop
  - Improves oxygenation and ventilator setting requirements, decreased air-block complications, decreased incidence of intracranial hemorrhage, decreased bronchopulmonary dysplasia, and decreased death rates
  - Increased risk of patent ductus arteriosus and pulmonary hemorrhage
- Mechanical ventilation with positive end-expiratory pressure (PEEP)
  - High frequency ventilation
- Meet special needs of premature patient
  - Respiratory support with endotracheal tube
  - Monitor temperature, prevent hypothermia
  - Treat metabolic acidosis
  - Intravenous access with fluid and caloric needs

SELECTED REFERENCES

1. Kuhn JP et al: Caffey's Pediatric Diagnostic Imaging. Tenth Edition, Volume I Philadelphia: Mosby. 78-88, 2004
2. Lemons JA et al: Very low birth weight outcomes of the National Institute of Child health and human development neonatal research network, January 1995 through December 1996. NICHD Neonatal Research Network. Pediatrics. 107(1):E1, 2001
3. Whitsett JA et al: Acute respiratory disorders in neonatology. In: Avery GB, Fletcher MA, MacDonald MG, eds. Pathophysiology and Management of the Newborn. 5th ed. JB Lippincot. 485, 1999
4. Kossel H et al: 25 years of respiratory support of newborn infants. J Perinat Med. 25(5):421-32, 1997
5. Swischuk KE et al: Immature lung problems: can our nomenclature be more specific? AJR. 166:917-8, 1996
6. Cleveland RH: A radiologic update on medical diseases of the newborn chest. Pediatr Radiol. 25:631-7, 1995
7. Merenstein GB et al: Surfactant replacement therapy for respiratory distress syndrome. Pediatrics. 87:946-7, 1991

SURFACTANT DEFICIENT DISEASE

IMAGE GALLERY

Typical

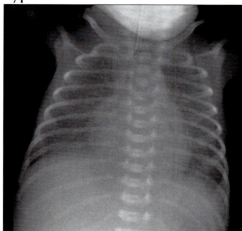 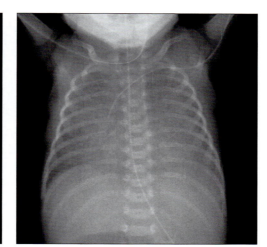

(Left) Anteroposterior radiograph shows intubated 27 week premature infant at 2 days of age with pulmonary hypoventilation and reticular and nodular densities bilaterally. *(Right)* Anteroposterior radiograph shows same patient at 5 days of age with diffuse increase in bilateral interstitial lung disease. This is typical for a functioning patent ductus arteriosus.

Typical

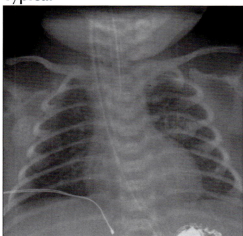 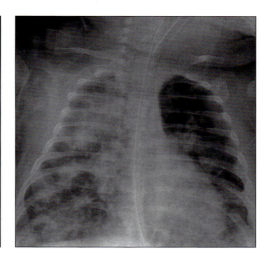

(Left) Anteroposterior radiograph shows initial exam on a 26 week premature infant who is intubated. The mechanical ventilation changes the radiographic appearance of RDS. *(Right)* Anteroposterior radiograph shows same patient at 18 days with residual significant lung disease characterized by focal areas of hyperinflation bilaterally and pulmonary parenchymal disease.

Typical

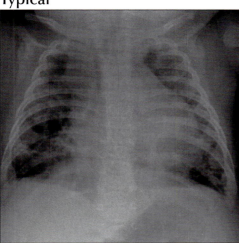 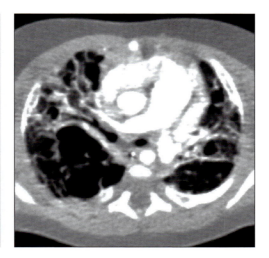

(Left) Anteroposterior radiograph of the chest demonstrates bilateral lung disease with focal areas of hyperinflation and coarse parenchymal bands which are more obvious at the base. Infant is 2 months of age and has BPD. *(Right)* Axial CECT shows focal areas of hyperinflation or cysts with dense parenchymal bands of lung disease. These findings are typical of bronchopulmonary dysplasia.

NEONATAL PNEUMONIA

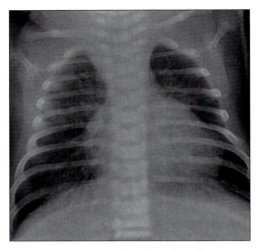

Anteroposterior radiograph at three days of age shows increased interstitial lung markings bilaterally which mimics other entities. Culture positive for group B streptococcus infection.

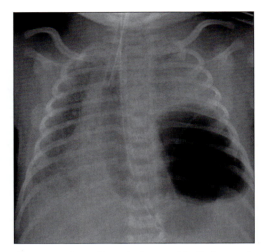

Anteroposterior radiograph shows a left diaphragmatic hernia in a 2 month old who had a prior history of streptococcal pneumonia. Diaphragmatic hernias have also been seen with history of chlamydia pneumonia.

TERMINOLOGY

Definitions
- Pneumonia occurring in neonate within the first 28 days of life
- Lung infection occurs in-utero, during delivery, or during the first 30 days of life

IMAGING FINDINGS

General Features
- Best diagnostic clue
  - Patchy asymmetric perihilar densities and hyperinflation
  - May be unilateral or bilateral
  - May or may not have effusions
    - Approximately 25% of group B infections have effusions
  - May be reticulonodular in appearance
  - May have pulmonary hypoventilation
  - May be interstitial
  - Complications include pneumothorax, pneumomediastinum, pneumatoceles
- Location
  - Chest
  - May have other systemic signs of infection
    - Sepsis, hypovolemia and shock
    - Neonatal meningitis
    - Intracranial calcifications with toxoplasmosis, rubella, cytomegalovirus, herpes simplex virus (HSV) (TORCH)
    - Bone lesions can be seen in syphilis
    - Premature infants may have systemic candidiasis
- Size
  - Usually bilateral
  - Can be unilateral

Radiographic Findings
- Radiography
  - Group B pneumonia
    - Most common neonatal pneumonia
    - Different appearance than other causes of neonatal pneumonia
    - Low lung volumes and granular opacities similar to surfactant deficiency
    - Pleural effusion in 25%: Only differentiating factor from surfactant deficiency
  - Other types of neonatal pneumonia
    - Bilateral hyperinflation
    - Rope-like perihilar markings
    - Areas of atelectasis
    - Pleural effusions not uncommon
    - May have pneumothorax and other air-block complications

DDx: Neonatal Lung Disease

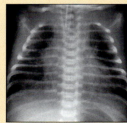
Meconium Aspiration

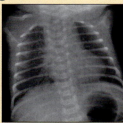
Transient Tachypnea

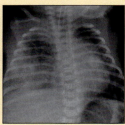
CCAM

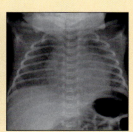
Surfactant Deficiency

NEONATAL PNEUMONIA

Key Facts

Terminology
- Pneumonia occurring in neonate within the first 28 days of life
- Lung infection occurs in-utero, during delivery, or during the first 30 days of life

Imaging Findings
- Group B pneumonia
- Most common neonatal pneumonia
- Different appearance than other causes of neonatal pneumonia
- Low lung volumes and granular opacities similar to surfactant deficiency
- Pleural effusion in 25%: Only differentiating factor from surfactant deficiency
- Other types of neonatal pneumonia
- Bilateral hyperinflation
- Rope-like perihilar markings
- Areas of atelectasis
- Pleural effusions not uncommon
- May have pneumothorax and other air-block complications

Top Differential Diagnoses
- Surfactant deficient disease
- Congenital cystic adenomatoid malformation (CCAM) of the chest
- Meconium aspiration syndrome
- Transient tachypnea of the newborn
- Congenital heart disease

Pathology
- Occurs in approximately 1% of term neonates and 10% of preterm neonates

CT Findings
- CECT: Usually not done
- HRCT: Occasionally done when infant is older to evaluate residual disease

Imaging Recommendations
- Best imaging tool
  - Chest radiography
  - Other imaging may aid in specific diagnosis
    - Cranial CT or ultrasound may show calcifications associated with TORCH infections
    - Extremity imaging may show osteitis associated with specific lesions
    - Ultrasound may demonstrate systemic signs of diseases

DIFFERENTIAL DIAGNOSIS

Surfactant deficient disease
- Premature infants less than 32 weeks gestation
- Reticulonodular densities in both lung
- Pulmonary hypoinflation
- Mimics group B streptococcus infections

Congenital cystic adenomatoid malformation (CCAM) of the chest
- Usually localized mass in one portion of lung
- Cystic and or solid component
- May have mass effect

Meconium aspiration syndrome
- Usually history of meconium staining or aspiration
- Coarse lung markings bilaterally
- Hyperinflation of the lungs
- Complications include pneumothorax, pneumomediastinum

Transient tachypnea of the newborn
- Occurs in term infants who have C-sections or abrupt deliveries
- Interstitial lung disease bilaterally
- Infants are usually well except for tachypnea
- Radiographs done to exclude other causes of tachypnea

Congenital heart disease
- Infants present with tachypnea
  - Usually afebrile
- Cyanosis or "gray" appearance
- Echocardiography is diagnostic

PATHOLOGY

General Features
- Etiology
  - Before delivery: Congenital or transplacental infection
    - Hematogenous spread from mother to fetus in utero
    - Severe pneumonia occurs with congenital rubella
    - TORCH
    - Other rare causes: Varicella zoster, adenovirus, enteroviruses, mycobacterium tuberculosis (< 200 reported cases), and listeria
    - Syphilis presents with systemic signs
  - During delivery: Infection occurs during vaginal delivery
    - Occurs during birth or as a result of maternal infection
    - Etiologic agents are those colonizing maternal birth canal
    - Group B hemolytic streptococcus (GBS) is the most common organism
    - 25% of woman are colonized by the organism
    - Organisms include GBS, E.coli, Klebsiella, Proteus, Chlamydia, Candida, Bacteroides, HSV, enteroviruses
    - HSV is most common cause of viral perinatal pneumonia worldwide
    - Chlamydia may have delayed appearance
  - Postnatal or after delivery
    - Viral: Respiratory syncytial virus influenza most common

NEONATAL PNEUMONIA

- Community acquired bacterial pneumonia (S. pneumoniae, H. influenza) may also occur
- Bacterial pneumonias are Pseudomonas, Klebsiella, Serratia, Enterobacter, Staphylococcus aureus (methicillin-sensitive and resistant)
- Fungal: Postnatal Candida pneumonia may occur in disseminated disease
○ Risk factors
- Neonates have immature pulmonary anatomy and immature host defense mechanisms
- Preterm infants more immature, therefore at increased risk
- Anatomical anomalies predispose or may cause pneumonia such as tracheoesophageal fistula, cleft palate
- Critically ill infants: Normal mucocutaneous barriers disrupted with invasive devices and procedures
- Maternal fever
- Maternal amniotitis, fever, sepsis
• Epidemiology
○ Occurs in approximately 1% of term neonates and 10% of preterm neonates
○ Mortality rate for perinatally acquired pneumonia: 20%
○ Mortality rate for postnatally acquired pneumonia: 50%
○ Bacteremia is present in as many as 46% of infants with perinatal pneumonia
○ Most common cause in the first week of life is GBS
- 57% of infants with pneumonia have GBS isolated from blood or tracheal secretions
- Vaginal colonization occurs in nearly 30% of pregnant women
- Without chemoprophylaxis, 50% of newborns born to colonized women will acquire colonization
• Associated abnormalities: Most frequent cause of septicemia in neonate

CLINICAL ISSUES

Presentation
• Most common signs/symptoms
○ Respiratory distress
- Nasal flaring, retractions, grunting, cyanosis
○ Symptoms usually begin within first 48 hours of life
- Chlamydia pneumonia may have delayed onset
- Most infants present with systemic signs not localized to chest
○ High risk
- Premature infants
- Infants with immunosuppression
- Infants with congenital heart disease
• Other signs/symptoms
○ Tachycardia, hypothermia
○ Irritability, lethargy, poor feeding
○ Chlamydia pneumonia: Has long incubation - acquired at birth, but presents at 2-12 weeks
- Presents with conjunctivitis and respiratory complaints

○ Candidal pneumonia: Infant often presents at birth with maculopapular rash
○ Herpes simplex pneumonia: Rapidly progressive and fatal
○ S. aureus may cause a severe necrotizing pneumonia with pneumatocele formation

Demographics
• Age: Neonates within first 28 days of life

Natural History & Prognosis
• Depends on organism and success of treatment: Early intervention and aggressive therapy are key
○ Usually associated with sepsis
○ May affect multiple organs
• Can be associated with intraventricular hemorrhage, neurological damage, and developmental delay

Treatment
• Perinatal screening and treatment prior to delivery
○ Maternal GBS vaccination to cause transplacental transfer of passive immunity
• GBS intrapartum chemoprophylaxis recommended
○ Positive perinatal screening culture
○ GBS during pregnancy
○ Maternal GBS vaccination to cause transplacental transfer of passive immunity
• Respiratory support, oxygen
• Broad spectrum antibiotics (a penicillin + an aminoglycoside) until organism identified
• Viral pneumonia: Acyclovir; adjunctive hyperimmune immunoglobulin may improve outcome
• Mechanical ventilation as needed
• Surfactant replacement may be of benefit
• ECMO used as last resort

DIAGNOSTIC CHECKLIST

Image Interpretation Pearls
• Usually bilateral diffuse disease
• Chest radiographs are nonspecific

SELECTED REFERENCES

1. Kuhn JP et al: Caffey's Pediatric Diagnostic Imaging. Tenth Edition, Volume I Philadelphia: Mosby, Chapter 3. p.88-89, 2004
2. Apisarnthanarak A et al: Ventilator-associated pneumonia in extremely preterm neonates in a neonatal intensive care unit: characteristics, risk factors, and outcomes. Pediatrics. 112(6 Pt 1):1283-9, 2003
3. Campbell JR: Neonatal pneumonia. Semin Respir Infect. 11(3):155-62, 1996
4. Potter B et al: Neonatal radiology. Acquired diaphragmatic hernia with group B streptococcal pneumonia. J Perinatol. 15(2):160-2, 1995
5. Ablow RC et al: The radiographic features of early onset Group B streptococcal neonatal sepsis. Radiology. 124(3):771-7, 1977
6. Ablow RC et al: A comparison of early-onset group B steptococcal neonatal infection and the respiratory-distress syndrome of the newborn. N Engl J Med. 294(2):65-70, 1976

NEONATAL PNEUMONIA

IMAGE GALLERY

Typical

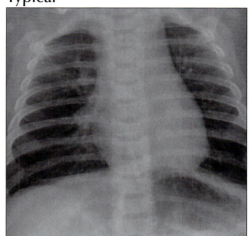
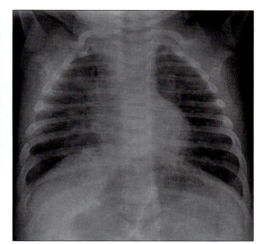

(Left) Anteroposterior radiograph shows marked hyperinflation of lungs in a 28 day old infant proven to have respiratory syncytial virus. The radiograph does not demonstrate significant interstitial disease. *(Right)* Anteroposterior radiograph shows coarse lung markings in a two week old infant who had conjunctivitis, and tachypnea. The findings are nonspecific but the infants cultures were positive for Chlamydia.

Typical

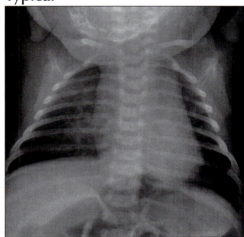
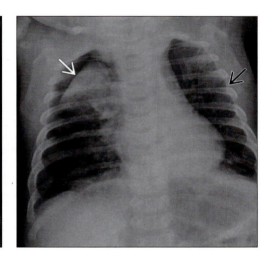

(Left) Anteroposterior radiograph in a two week only infant with herpes pneumonia. Prominent intersitial pattern in the lung is present. *(Right)* Anteroposterior radiograph shows one month old infant with respiratory syncytial virus complicated by apical right pneumothorax (white arrow). Radiograph demonstrates hyperinflation as the lung herniates between soft tissues of lateral chest wall (black arrow).

Typical

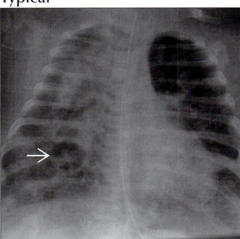
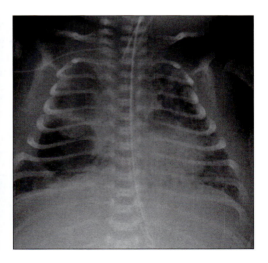

(Left) Anteroposterior radiograph shows neonate with Pseudomonas pneumonia superimposed on lung disease due to prematurity. A pneumatocele is identified in the right lower lung (arrow). *(Right)* Anteroposterior radiograph shows focal areas of hyperinflation in a neonate who had staphylococcal sepsis. Patient had several pneumatoceles which healed slowly.

MECONIUM ASPIRATION SYNDROME

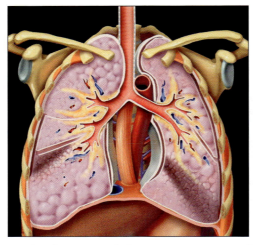

Graphic demonstrates findings: Asymmetric areas of hyperinflation and atelectasis as well as increased, rope-like perihilar densities.

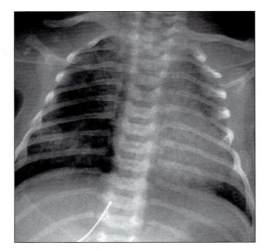

Anteroposterior radiograph shows hyperinflation of both lungs with coarse focal areas of increased density.

TERMINOLOGY

Abbreviations and Synonyms
- Meconium aspiration syndrome (MAS)

Definitions
- Respiratory distress that occurs secondary to intrapartum or intrauterine aspiration of meconium

IMAGING FINDINGS

General Features
- Best diagnostic clue
  - Coarse heterogeneous opacities associated with increased lung volumes bilaterally in a term infant
  - Hyperinflated lungs
  - Rope-like perihilar densities
- Location
  - Bilateral disease usually in middle two thirds of the lung
  - Frequently asymmetric
- Size: Variable
- Morphology
  - Hyperinflated segments
  - Focal areas of atelectasis

Radiographic Findings
- Radiography
  - High lung volumes, often asymmetric
  - Areas of asymmetric patchy hyperinflation and atelectasis
  - Rope-like perihilar densities
  - Pleural effusion uncommon
  - Chest radiograph useful to assess for complications
    - Endotracheal tube position
    - Pneumothorax occurs 20-40%
    - Pneumomediastinum
    - Pulmonary interstitial emphysema

CT Findings
- CECT
  - Not performed in acute disease
  - Occasionally done for chronic disease
    - Focal areas of lung involvement
    - Emphysematous bleb lesions
    - Bilateral residual disease

Ultrasonographic Findings
- Grayscale Ultrasound
  - In utero ultrasound done to monitor infant fluid and causes of fetal distress
  - Cranial ultrasound done as part of extracorporeal membrane oxygenation (ECMO) work-up

DDx: Term Infants With Lung Disease

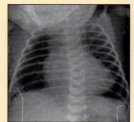

CHD

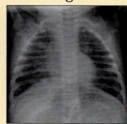

Chlamydia Pneumonia

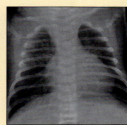

Pneumonia

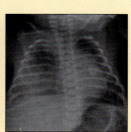

CCAM

MECONIUM ASPIRATION SYNDROME

Key Facts

Terminology
- Respiratory distress that occurs secondary to intrapartum or intrauterine aspiration of meconium

Imaging Findings
- Coarse heterogeneous opacities associated with increased lung volumes bilaterally in a term infant
- Pleural effusion uncommon
- Best imaging tool: Chest radiograph

Top Differential Diagnoses
- Congenital heart disease (CHD)
- Neonatal pneumonia
- Transient tachypnea of the newborn
- Congenital chest mass such as congenital cystic adenomatoid malformation (CCAM)

Pathology
- Meconium is a tenacious, thick and viscous material in neonatal bowel
- Occurs in term infants who have in-utero or intrapartum hypoxia or stress
- Meconium may be detected in amniotic fluid of 10-20% of newborns > 34 weeks gestation
- 25,000-30,000 cases of meconium aspiration yearly in USA

Clinical Issues
- Cyanosis, nasal flaring, intercostal retractions
- Airway obstruction
- Surfactant dysfunction
- Chemical pneumonitis
- Meconium injury contributes to high pulmonary vascular resistance

---

- Renal ultrasound occasionally done to exclude renal dysplasia associated pulmonary hypoplasia (Potters syndrome)

Imaging Recommendations
- Best imaging tool: Chest radiograph
- Protocol advice: Initial radiographs not predictive of outcome

DIFFERENTIAL DIAGNOSIS

Congenital heart disease (CHD)
- Clues to congenital heart disease may be present
  - Abnormal heart size or configuration
  - Aortic arch on right or abnormal abdominal situs
  - Decreased or increased pulmonary flow
- Echocardiography is gold standard for defining lesion

Neonatal pneumonia
- Patchy asymmetric perihilar densities and hyperinflation
- Usually no history or presence of meconium aspiration
- Chlamydia, herpes, streptococcal pneumonia the most common

Transient tachypnea of the newborn
- Occurs secondary to delayed clearance of fetal pulmonary fluid (often in cesarean section)
- Key feature is benign course
- Findings of normal heart size with prominent interstitial markings

Congenital chest mass such as congenital cystic adenomatoid malformation (CCAM)
- Focal areas of parenchymal lung abnormality
- Unilateral, may have mediastinal shift
- Pleural effusions may be present

PATHOLOGY

General Features
- General path comments
  - Meconium is a tenacious, thick and viscous material in neonatal bowel
    - Green-black substance of mucus, vernix, epithelial cells, lanugo, fatty acids, and bile
    - Normal passage of meconium occurs in first 24 hours after birth
- Genetics: No predisposition
- Etiology
  - Intrauterine aspiration
    - When fetus is hypoxic, there is passage of meconium into amniotic fluid which then enters the lung
    - Risk factors include placental insufficiency, maternal hypertension, preeclampsia, oligohydramnios, maternal drug use
  - Aspirated meconium causes injury by several mechanisms
    - Mechanical obstruction of small airways due to tenacious nature with resultant airtrapping and complications such as pneumothorax and pneumomediastinum
    - Chemical pneumonitis causes inflammation of airways and parenchyma
    - Surfactant inactivation strips surfactant from alveolar surface causing diffuse atelectasis
    - Pulmonary hypertension causes pulmonary vasoconstriction which leads to persistent pulmonary hypertension
    - Infection alters amniotic fluid, increasing risk of bacterial infection
- Epidemiology
  - Occurs in term infants who have in-utero or intrapartum hypoxia or stress
  - Meconium rarely found in amniotic fluid prior to 34 weeks gestation
  - Meconium may be detected in amniotic fluid of 10-20% of newborns > 34 weeks gestation
    - 5% will develop meconium aspiration syndrome

PULMONARY INTERSTITIAL EMPHYSEMA

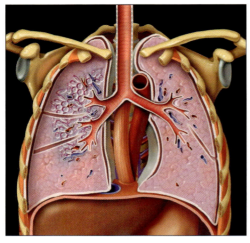

Graphic shows round and linear lucencies secondary to air escaping into the pulmonary interstitium.

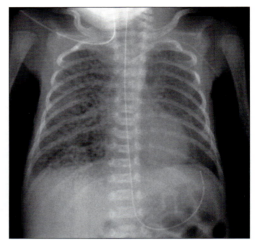

Anteroposterior radiograph shows right-sided bubble-like lucencies consistent with PIE.

TERMINOLOGY

Abbreviations and Synonyms
- Pulmonary interstitial emphysema (PIE)

Definitions
- Abnormal location of pulmonary air within the interstitium and lymphatics; usually secondary to barotrauma

IMAGING FINDINGS

General Features
- Best diagnostic clue: Bubble-like or linear lucencies within the lung

Radiographic Findings
- Radiography
  - Bubble-like or linear lucencies within the lung
  - Lucencies typically uniform in size
  - Often radiate from hilum
  - May be focal (one lobe) or diffuse and bilateral
  - Involved lung usually noncompliant: Static lung volume seen on multiple consecutive chest radiographs, even with change in volume of uninvolved lung from radiograph to radiograph
  - Serves as a warning sign for other pending air-block complications: Pneumothorax, pneumomediastinum
  - Finding is typically transient
  - Rarely, PIE may persist and form large air-filled cystic mass: Persistent pulmonary interstitial emphysema
    - May act as mass lesion and compress other thoracic structures and cause progressive respiratory distress
    - Initial management conservative: Decubitus positioning, selective intubation opposite lung
    - Usually affects single lobe
    - Most commonly left upper lobe
    - Sometimes requires surgical resection

CT Findings
- CT not obtained to evaluate routine typical PIE
  - PIE may be seen when CT obtained for other reasons
  - CT is often utilized to evaluate persistent PIE and differentiate from other neonatal causes of lucent lung masses
- CT findings: Air surrounds pulmonary arterial branches which are seen as soft tissue linear or dot-like densities surrounded by abnormal gas collections
  - This pattern of central linear and dot-like densities is characteristic for PIE

DDx: Lung Lucencies In Neonates

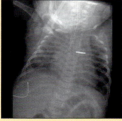
BPD

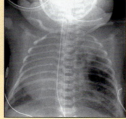
CCAM

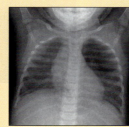
Lobar Emphysema

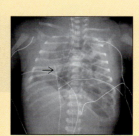
Diaphragmatic Hernia

PULMONARY INTERSTITIAL EMPHYSEMA

Key Facts

Terminology
- Abnormal location of pulmonary air within the interstitium and lymphatics; usually secondary to barotrauma

Imaging Findings
- Best diagnostic clue: Bubble-like or linear lucencies within the lung
- Lucencies typically uniform in size
- Often radiate from hilum
- May be focal (one lobe) or diffuse and bilateral
- Involved lung usually noncompliant: Static lung volume seen on multiple consecutive chest radiographs, even with change in volume of uninvolved lung from radiograph to radiograph
- Serves as a warning sign for other pending air-block complications: Pneumothorax, pneumomediastinum
- Finding is typically transient
- CT findings: Air surrounds pulmonary arterial branches which are seen as soft tissue linear or dot-like densities surrounded by abnormal gas collections

Clinical Issues
- Presence influences care givers to alter support: Switching from conventional to high-frequency ventilation
- Usually occurs during first several days of life
- Almost always during first week of life
- Almost always occurs only in infants on ventilator support

○ Characteristic pattern seen in 82% of patients with persistent PIE
○ Helps to differentiate persistent PIE from other hyperlucent lung masses in children such as congenital lobar emphysema, cystic adenomatoid malformation

DIFFERENTIAL DIAGNOSIS

Partially treated surfactant deficiency disease (SDD)
- With treatment of SDD with exogenous surfactant, there may be partial clearing of collapsed alveoli
- Pattern of alternating distended and collapsed acini may mimic pulmonary interstitial emphysema
- Important to know timing of surfactant therapy in relationship to time of radiograph

Developing bronchopulmonary dysplasia (chronic lung disease)
- Bubble-like lucencies that are seen with developing bronchopulmonary dysplasia (BPD) can appear similar to PIE
- Age is helpful: PIE typically occurs during first week of life, BPD later
- Acuteness of onset: PIE is abrupt, BPD changes are gradual

Congenital cystic adenomatoid malformation (CCAM)
- Typically present at birth
- Cysts often more variable in size and static
- PIE more transient and most typical bubble-like lucencies are small

Congenital lobar emphysema
- Typically seen at birth
- May present as fluid density on initial radiographs
- Generalized lucency of entire lobe rather than small focal lucencies seen with PIE

Congenital diaphragmatic hernia
- Not commonly confused with PIE
- Large lucencies with bowel-like appearance in chest
- Typically seen immediately after birth
- Position of support apparatus helpful
- Paucity of gas in abdomen

PATHOLOGY

General Features
- General path comments
  ○ Barotrauma results in increased alveolar pressure and alveolar rupture
  ○ Rupture of overdistended pulmonary alveoli leads to entry of air into the pulmonary interstitium
  ○ Air escape into adjacent lung interstitium and lymphatics is referred to as pulmonary interstitial emphysema
  ○ Air is distributed along bronchovascular structures and appears on radiography as radiolucent bubble-like and linear densities
  ○ Air may further dissect and lead to pneumothorax or pneumomediastinum

CLINICAL ISSUES

Presentation
- Most common signs/symptoms: Usually asymptomatic
- Other signs/symptoms: Difficulty with ventilation secondary to development of pneumothorax
- Typically presents on routine neonatal unit radiographs prior to symptoms
- Serves as a warning sign for other pending air block complications: Pneumothorax, pneumomediastinum
- Presence influences care givers to alter support: Switching from conventional to high-frequency ventilation
- Usually occurs during first several days of life
- Almost always during first week of life

PULMONARY INTERSTITIAL EMPHYSEMA

- Almost always occurs only in infants on ventilator support
- Usually is transient

Demographics
- Age
  - Premature infants
  - Usually during first days of life

Natural History & Prognosis
- Usually transient
- Can develop into persistent PIE

Treatment
- Often switching from conventional to high-frequency ventilation
- Increased frequency of clinical and radiographic monitoring for air-block complications such as pneumothorax
- For persistent pulmonary interstitial emphysema
  - Conservative management initial therapy
  - High frequency ventilation
  - Decubitus positioning with affected side down
  - Selective intubation of opposite lung
  - Surgery reserved for unmanageable respiratory distress
  - In one series, 53% of patients with persistent PIE required surgical resection

DIAGNOSTIC CHECKLIST

Consider
- Consider age of patient and rapidity of development to differentiate PIE from developing bronchopulmonary dysplasia

SELECTED REFERENCES

1. Corbett HJ et al: Pulmonary sequestration. Paediatr Respir Rev. 5(1):59-68, 2004
2. Johnson AM et al: Congenital anomalies of the fetal/neonatal chest. Semin Roentgenol. 39(2):197-214, 2004
3. Donnelly LF et al: CT findings and temporal course of persistent pulmonary interstitial emphysema in neonates: a multiinstitutional study. AJR Am J Roentgenol. 180(4):1129-33, 2003
4. Donnelly LF: Fundamentals of Pediatric Radiology. Philadelphia; W.B. Saunders, 2001
5. Frerking I et al: Pulmonary surfactant: functions, abnormalities and therapeutic options. Intensive Care Med. 27(11):1699-717, 2001
6. Suresh GK et al: Current surfactant use in premature infants. Clin Perinatol. 28(3):671-94, 2001
7. Khatua S et al: Advances in management of meconium aspiration syndrome. Indian J Pediatr. 67(11):837-41, 2000
8. Cohen MC et al: Solitary unilocular cyst of the lung with features of persistent interstitial pulmonary emphysema: report of four cases. Pediatr Dev Pathol. 2(6):531-6, 1999
9. Donnelly LF et al: Localized lucent chest lesions in neonates. AJR. 212:837-40, 1999
10. Newman B: Imaging of medical disease of the newborn lung. Radiol Clin North Am. 37(6):1049-65, 1999
11. Ogawa Y et al: Strategy for the prevention and treatment of chronic lung disease of the premature infant. Pediatr Pulmonol Suppl. 18:212-5, 1999
12. Agrons GA et al: Lung disease in premature neonates: impact of new treatments and technologies. Semin Roentgenol. 33(2):101-16, 1998
13. Breysem L et al: Bronchopulmonary dysplasia: correlation of radiographic and clinical findings. Pediatr Radiol. 27(8):642-6, 1997
14. Jabra AA et al: Localized persistent pulmonary interstitial emphysema: CT findings with radiographic-pathologic correlation. AJR Am J Roentgenol. 169(5):1381-4, 1997
15. Cleveland RH: A radiologic update on medical diseases of the newborn chest. Pediatr Radiol. 25:631-7, 1995
16. Wood BP: The newborn chest. Radiol Clin North Am. 31(3):667-76, 1993
17. Azizkhan RG et al: Acquired lobar emphysema (overinflation): clinical and pathological evaluation of infants requiring lobectomy. J Pediatr Surg. 27(8):1145-51; discussion 1151-2, 1992
18. Schneider JR et al: The changing spectrum of cystic pulmonary lesions requiring surgical resection in infants. J Thorac Cardiovasc Surg. 89(3):332-9, 1985

PULMONARY INTERSTITIAL EMPHYSEMA

IMAGE GALLERY

Typical

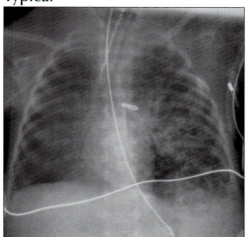
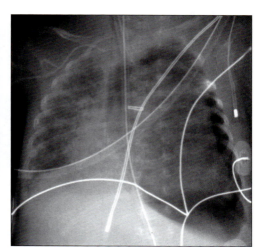

(Left) Anteroposterior radiograph in intubated premature infant shows bubble-like lucencies in left hemithorax. *(Right)* Same premature infant as on left obtained two days after previous chest radiograph shows development of left-sided pneumothorax.

Typical

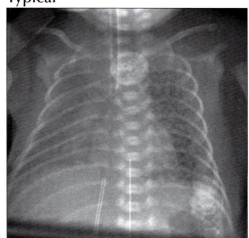
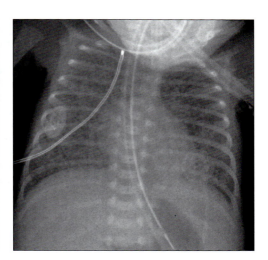

(Left) Anteroposterior radiograph shows there are bubble-like lucencies in the left lung consistent with PIE. *(Right)* Anteroposterior radiograph in premature infant shows bubble-like lucencies bilaterally, more so on left than right.

Typical

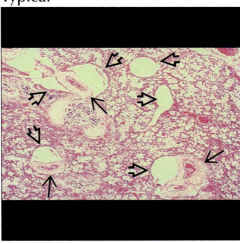
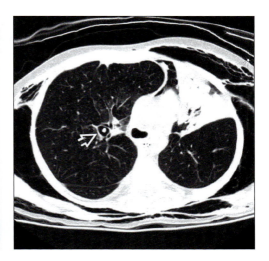

(Left) Micropathology shows gas collections (open arrows) in pulmonary interstitium and lymphatics. Gas surrounds bronchial arteries (arrows). *(Right)* Axial NECT shows round soft tissue density with surrounding air (arrow). This represents interstitial gas surrounding a vessel and is the typical appearance of PIE on CT.

BRONCHOPULMONARY DYSPLASIA

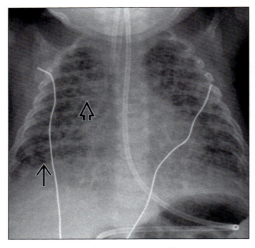

Anteroposterior radiograph shows diffusely distributed coarse reticular opacities (open arrow) with intervening lucencies (arrow) in hyperinflated lungs.

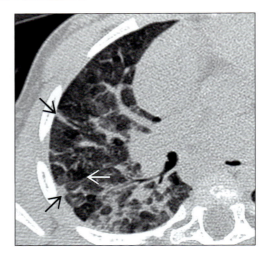

Axial HRCT shows airtrapping on this expiratory image (white arrow). Linear and triangular shaped subpleural opacities (black arrows) and mosaic attenuation are also present.

TERMINOLOGY

Abbreviations and Synonyms
- Bronchopulmonary dysplasia (BPD), chronic lung disease of infancy, chronic lung disease of prematurity (CLD)

Definitions
- Premature infants with oxygen dependency at 28 days of age and chest radiograph abnormalities
- Mechanical ventilation and supplemental oxygen needed to maintain an arterial oxygen > 50 mmHg in premature infants at 28 days with chest radiograph abnormalities
- Radiologically evident lung disease and a need for supplemental oxygen at 36 postconceptual weeks

IMAGING FINDINGS

General Features
- Best diagnostic clue: Ill-defined coarse reticular and band-like opacities with intervening small rounded lucencies
- Location: Diffuse throughout both lungs
- Size: Lungs are hyperinflated

Radiographic Findings
- Radiography
  - Early
    - Homogeneously increased opacities bilaterally primarily related to retained fluid and/or patent ductus arteriosus
  - Subsequently
    - Heterogeneous appearance with focal lucencies separated by coarse reticular and band-like opacities of fibrosis and atelectasis
    - More opacities in the upper lobes with hyperinflation at the bases
  - Overall hyperinflation of the lungs develops
  - Relatively decreased anteroposterior diameter of the chest in comparison to children with other causes of obstructive lung disease such as asthma
  - Surviving infants may subsequently develop normal radiographs in childhood
  - May be left with linear opacities with focal lucencies and hyperexpansion
  - Originally described 4 characteristic stages are rarely seen nowadays

CT Findings
- HRCT
  - Mosaic attenuation
  - Foci of air trapping on expiratory images
  - Subpleural triangular opacities

DDx: Bronchopulmonary Dysplasia

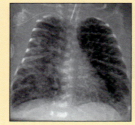
PIE

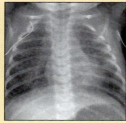
Neonatal Pneumonia

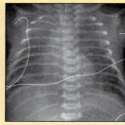
Meconium Aspiration

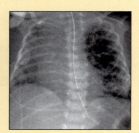
CCAM

BRONCHOPULMONARY DYSPLASIA

Key Facts

Terminology
- Radiologically evident lung disease and a need for supplemental oxygen at 36 postconceptual weeks

Imaging Findings
- Best diagnostic clue: Ill-defined coarse reticular and band-like opacities with intervening small rounded lucencies
- Overall hyperinflation of the lungs develops
- Surviving infants may subsequently develop normal radiographs in childhood
- Foci of air trapping on expiratory images
- Subpleural triangular opacities
- Architectural distortion

Top Differential Diagnoses
- Pulmonary interstitial emphysema (PIE)
- Meconium aspiration
- Neonatal pneumonia
- Congenital cystic adenomatoid malformation (CCAM)

Pathology
- Prematurity < 32 weeks gestational age
- Barotrauma: Prolonged ventilation support with large tidal volume
- High inspired oxygen concentrations
- Most common chronic pulmonary disease of infancy
- Incidence is growing due to improved survival of infants, both term and preterm, with surfactant deficiency disease and other diseases that require prolonged ventilation

---

- Linear and reticular opacities
- Reduced bronchial lumen: Pulmonary arterial ratio
- Architectural distortion
- Findings correlate with pulmonary function abnormalities

Nuclear Medicine Findings
- V/Q Scan: Ventilation/perfusion mismatch and reversed mismatch

Imaging Recommendations
- Best imaging tool: Chest radiograph
- Protocol advice
  - Anteroposterior radiograph
  - If CT is being considered, optimal results are obtained with a HRCT either under anesthesia or using controlled-ventilation

DIFFERENTIAL DIAGNOSIS

Pulmonary interstitial emphysema (PIE)
- Air in the interstitium
- Lucencies are more linear than in BPD
- More commonly occurs by day 3 of life in premature infants: BPD occurs later
- May be unilateral or focal unlike the diffuse rounded lucencies of BPD
- Usually rapid onset with no evidence of abnormal lucencies on preceding radiograph

Meconium aspiration
- Aspiration of meconium stained amniotic fluid leads to a toxic pneumonitis
- Usually post mature infants that are small for gestational age who have had distress in-utero
- Radiographic changes occur rapidly
- Marked hyperinflation and air block phenomena are more common: Pneumothorax and pneumomediastinum

Neonatal pneumonia
- May occur in full term infants
- Group B beta-hemolytic streptococcus is most common organism
- Early onset of symptoms can be associated with sepsis
- Often bilateral and diffuse, but may be unilateral
- Can be associated with an effusion unlike BPD

Congenital cystic adenomatoid malformation (CCAM)
- May be a term infant without history of ventilation or neonatal oxygen need
- May not present until older
- May appear as a fluid-filled mass in immediate neonatal period
- Communication with bronchi present at birth: Air-filled soon after birth
- Usually unilateral or involve portion of a lobe

Pulmonary lymphangiectasia
- Hyperplasia of lymphatic channels
- May be term infants
- Often associated with effusion which may be chylous
- Increased reticular markings: Kerley B lines
- Primary lymphangiectasia usually presents early and often is fatal

Congenital lobar emphysema
- May occur in full term infants
- May not be symptomatic
- Unilateral and usually unilobar
- Associated with mass effect: Compressive atelectasis of the adjacent lung and mediastinum

PATHOLOGY

General Features
- Genetics: Increased incidence if family history of asthma and atopy
- Etiology
  - Prematurity < 32 weeks gestational age
  - Barotrauma: Prolonged ventilation support with large tidal volume
  - High inspired oxygen concentrations

BRONCHOPULMONARY DYSPLASIA

- o Increased fluid retention
- o Lower respiratory tract infection with Ureaplasma urealyticum
- o Surfactant deficiency disease
- o Persistent pulmonary hypertension
- Epidemiology
  - o Most common chronic pulmonary disease of infancy
  - o Incidence is growing due to improved survival of infants, both term and preterm, with surfactant deficiency disease and other diseases that require prolonged ventilation
  - o Decreased mortality and less severe disease in survivors due to use of maternal steroids and exogenous surfactant
  - o Low (< 2,500g), very low (< 1,500g), and extremely low (< 1,000g) birth weight infants
  - o Incidence > 50% in infants with extremely low birth weight < 1000g
  - o Uncommon in infants > 32 weeks gestational age
- Associated abnormalities
  - o Surfactant deficiency disease
  - o Persistent pulmonary hypertension
  - o Patent ductus arteriosus
  - o Tracheobronchomalacia
  - o Gastroesophageal reflux

Gross Pathologic & Surgical Features
- Atelectasis
- Hyperinflated alveoli
- Thickened bronchial walls

Microscopic Features
- 4 Stages: Acute injury, exudative bronchiolitis, proliferative bronchiolitis, and obliterative fibroproliferative bronchiolitis
- Alveolar septal fibrosis
- Decreased number of alveoli
- Simple, abnormally formed alveoli
- Dilated alveoli
- Abnormal capillary configuration

CLINICAL ISSUES

Presentation
- Most common signs/symptoms
  - o Early: Tachypnea, tachycardia, increased work of breathing, ventilator and supplemental oxygen dependent
  - o Later
    - Increased susceptibility to respiratory tract infection in first two years of life in survivors
    - Hyperresponsiveness of respiratory tract
    - Symptoms improve as the patient ages
    - Abnormal pulmonary function and decreased exercise tolerance in late childhood and adulthood is not unusual

Demographics
- Age
  - o Premature infants, usually less than 32 weeks gestation at birth
  - o Nowadays uncommon when infants were equal to or greater than 34 weeks gestational age at birth
- Gender: Males tend to be more symptomatic and get more severe degrees of BPD

Natural History & Prognosis
- Increased risk for pulmonary infections in first 2 years of life with increased morbidity and mortality, especially with respiratory syncytial virus
- Slowly improving pulmonary function and fewer respiratory infections later in childhood
- Abnormal pulmonary function with increased airway hyperreactivity may persist into adulthood in severe bronchopulmonary dysplasia
- Reduced exercise tolerance
- Neurodevelopmental delay

Treatment
- Prevention
  - o Prenatal administration of steroids to mother
  - o Exogenous surfactant administration
- Low tidal volume ventilation and wean to continuous positive airway pressure (CPAP) as soon as possible
- Avoid high pressure ventilation
- Avoid high inspired oxygen concentrations
- Close patent ductus arteriosus and avoid fluid retention

DIAGNOSTIC CHECKLIST

Image Interpretation Pearls
- Coarse reticular opacities with ill-defined lucencies
- Subpleural triangular opacities on HRCT

SELECTED REFERENCES

1. Eber E et al: Long term sequelae of bronchopulmonary dysplasia (chronic lung disease of infancy). Thorax. 56(4):317-23, 2001
2. Howling SJ et al: Pulmonary sequelae of bronchopulmonary dysplasia survivors: high-resolution CT findings. AJR Am J Roentgenol. 174(5):1323-6, 2000
3. Aquino SL et al: High-resolution inspiratory and expiratory CT in older children and adults with bronchopulmonary dysplasia. AJR Am J Roentgenol. 173(4):963-7, 1999
4. Soler C et al: Pulmonary perfusion scintigraphy in the evaluation of the severity of bronchopulmonary dysplasia. Pediatr Radiol. 27(1):32-5, 1997
5. Oppenheim C et al: Bronchopulmonary dysplasia: value of CT in identifying pulmonary sequelae. AJR Am J Roentgenol. 163(1):169-72, 1994
6. Griscom NT et al: Bronchopulmonary dysplasia: radiographic appearance in middle childhood. Radiology. 171(3):811-4, 1989
7. Davis JM et al: Changes in pulmonary mechanics after the administration of surfactant to infants with respiratory distress syndrome. N Engl J Med. 319(8):476-9, 1988
8. Nickerson BG et al: Family history of asthma in infants with bronchopulmonary dysplasia. Pediatrics. 65(6):1140-4, 1980
9. Northway WH Jr et al: Pulmonary disease following respirator therapy of hyaline-membrane disease. Bronchopulmonary dysplasia. N Engl J Med. 16;276(7):357-68, 1967

BRONCHOPULMONARY DYSPLASIA

IMAGE GALLERY

Typical

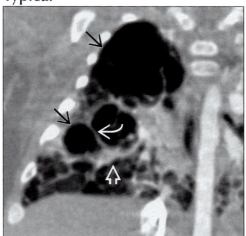
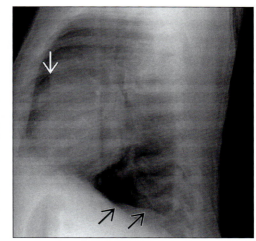

(Left) Coronal CECT shows rounded lucencies of airtrapping (black arrows) surrounded by coarse reticular (curved arrow) and band-like (open arrow) opacities. (Right) Lateral radiograph shows hyperinflation with flattened hemidiaphragms (black arrows). Note relatively normal/narrow anteroposterior (AP) diameter with no increased retrosternal air space (white arrow).

Typical

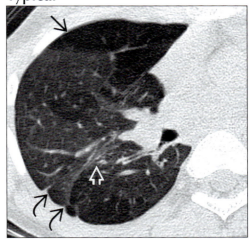
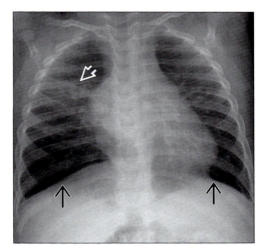

(Left) Axial HRCT shows mosaic attenuation and airtrapping on an expiratory HRCT image (black arrow), with subpleural triangular opacities (curved arrows) and architectural distortion (open arrow). (Right) Anteroposterior radiograph shows hyperinflation with flattened diaphragm (arrows) with lucent lower lungs zones and linear opacities in the upper lung zones (open arrow).

Typical

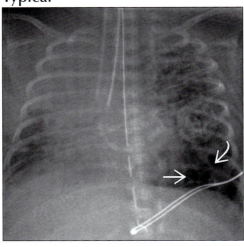
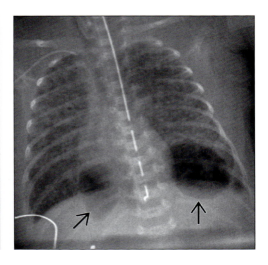

(Left) Anteroposterior radiograph shows hyperinflated left lung with rounded lucencies (arrow) and intervening coarse reticular opacities (curved arrow). Note endotracheal, the malposition and RVC collapse. (Right) Anteroposterior radiograph shows hyperinflated lungs with coarse reticular opacities and smaller rounded lucent areas. Note bilateral lower lobe pneumatoceles from an air leak (arrows).

UMBILICAL CATHETER COMPLICATIONS

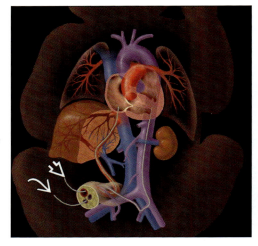

Graphic shows UVC (open arrow) passing through umbilical vein and ductus venosus to IVC/RA junction and UAC (curved arrow) passing through umbilical artery, IIA, CIA, and aorta.

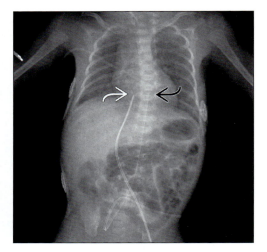

Anteroposterior radiograph shows good positioning of both UVC & UAC. UVC (white arrow) just above the diaphragm in RA (T8). UAC (black arrow) T7-8, which is below ductus arteriosus (DA) and above celiac axis.

TERMINOLOGY

Abbreviations and Synonyms
- Umbilical arterial catheter (UAC), umbilical venous catheter (UVC) aneurism

Definitions
- Umbilical venous catheter
  - UVC: Umbilical stump: Umbilical vein → left portal vein (LPV) → ductus venosus → middle or left hepatic vein → inferior vena cava (IVC)/right atrium (RA)
  - Indications
    - General access (85%)
    - Common for premature infants
    - Emergency vascular access for fluid and medication in newborn
    - Total parenteral nutrition (TPN)
    - Exchange transfusion
    - Central venous pressure monitoring
- Umbilical arterial catheter
  - UAC: Umbilical stump: Umbilical artery → internal iliac artery (IIA) → common iliac artery (CIA) → aorta
  - Indication
    - Frequent blood sampling
    - Continuous monitoring of arterial blood pressure
    - Angiography (cardiac)
    - Medication
    - Exchange transfusion

IMAGING FINDINGS

General Features
- Location
  - Ideal: UVC tip just above diaphragm (T8-T9)
  - Ideal "high line": UAC tip T6-T10 (T7-T9)
  - Acceptable "low line": UAC tip below L3

Radiographic Findings
- Radiography
  - UVC optimal location: Beyond liver at IVC/RA junction (approximately T8-T9)
    - UVC tip just above diaphragm on radiograph
  - UAC optimal location: (High line) between T6 and T10 to avoid major aortic branches
    - Ductus arteriosus (DA)
    - Celiac axis (T12)
    - Superior mesenteric artery (T12-L1)
    - Renal arteries (L1-L2)
    - Inferior mesenteric artery (L3)
    - Aortic bifurcation (L4)
  - UAC alternative location: (Low line) between L3 and L5
    - May be associated with higher risk of vascular complications (thrombosis, vasospasm)

DDx: Malpositioned Tubes And Catheters

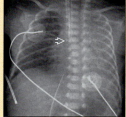

RMB Intubation

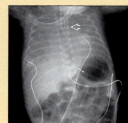

ETT In Esophagus

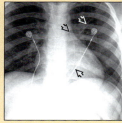

PICC In PA

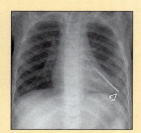

FT In Airway

UMBILICAL CATHETER COMPLICATIONS

Key Facts

Terminology
- UVC: Umbilical stump: Umbilical vein → left portal vein (LPV) → ductus venosus → middle or left hepatic vein → inferior vena cava (IVC)/right atrium (RA)
- UAC: Umbilical stump: Umbilical artery → internal iliac artery (IIA) → common iliac artery (CIA) → aorta

Imaging Findings
- Ideal: UVC tip just above diaphragm (T8-T9)
- Ideal "high line": UAC tip T6-T10 (T7-T9)
- Acceptable "low line": UAC tip below L3
- Anterior posterior chest/abdomen radiograph: Evaluate catheter position
- Ultrasound: Evaluate for thrombus or other complication

Pathology
- Complications of umbilical catheters may be due to
- Malpositioning
- Thrombus/thromboembolism
- Infection
- Epidemiology: True incidence of catheter complications unknown because of variability of reporting and monitoring

Clinical Issues
- In general, reposition or remove catheter
- Depending on extent and location, thrombus may be observed, treated medically, or surgically removed
- Other complications treated individually

Ultrasonographic Findings
- Grayscale Ultrasound
  - Catheter is well-defined, parallel, linear echogenic structure within the vascular lumen
  - Thrombus
    - Heterogeneous echogenic mass in lumen of vessel
    - May be located at catheter tip or may surround catheter
    - May occlude vessel lumen
    - May propagate into artery or vein branches
    - Evaluate perfusion of kidneys if thrombus in aorta
  - Calcification
    - Echogenic structure in vessel lumen with posterior shadowing
  - Pseudoaneurysm
    - Irregular outpouching of artery which contains turbulent high velocity flow on Doppler
    - Uncommon complication of UAC
  - Liver abscess (UVC)
    - Nonspecific mass
    - May have heterogeneous echotexture
    - No internal flow by Doppler
  - TPN ascites
    - Peritoneal fluid may be hypoechoic
    - May contain debris

Angiographic Findings
- Thrombus
  - Filling defect in vessel lumen or abrupt occlusion of vessel
  - May see collateral vessels
- Pseudoaneurysm
  - Focal outpouching of vessel
  - Usually artery
- Stricture

Imaging Recommendations
- Best imaging tool
  - Anterior posterior chest/abdomen radiograph: Evaluate catheter position
  - Ultrasound: Evaluate for thrombus or other complication

DIFFERENTIAL DIAGNOSIS

Malpositioned tubes and catheters
- Right mainstem bronchus (RMB) intubation
  - Tip beyond carina
  - May see left lung atelectasis due to obstruction of left mainstem bronchus by endotracheal tube (ETT)
- Esophageal intubation
  - May be difficult to appreciate by radiograph
  - Lungs may become opacified due to collapse
  - ETT may not project over tracheal air column
  - Frequently see gas-filled esophagus, stomach, and bowel due to inflation of ETT
- Peripherally inserted central venous catheter (PICC) fracture
  - Catheter may embolize to heart or lung
- Enteric tube malposition
  - Tube may perforate stomach or esophagus and extend into the retroperitoneum or peritoneum
- Feeding tube (FT) placement in airway
  - May perforate lung and cause bronchopleural fistula → pneumothorax
- PICC tip too low in RA
  - May cause arrhythmia
  - May perforate RA wall and cause cardiac tamponade

PATHOLOGY

General Features
- General path comments
  - Complications of umbilical catheters may be due to
    - Malpositioning
    - Thrombus/thromboembolism
    - Infection
  - UVC malposition in vascular structures
    - Portal vein (PV)
    - Superior mesenteric vein (SMV)
    - Splenic vein
    - Superior vena cava (SVC)
    - Internal jugular (IJ) vein

UMBILICAL CATHETER COMPLICATIONS

- May pass through patent foramen ovale (PFO) into left atrium (LA) and possibly into pulmonary vein
- Catheter may fracture and migrate to heart or pulmonary artery branch
○ UAC malposition in vascular structures
- Celiac trunk
- Superior mesenteric artery (SMA)
- Renal artery (RA)
- Internal iliac artery branches, such as the superior gluteal, inferior gluteal, and pudendal arteries
- May pass through ductus arteriosus into pulmonary arteries (PA)
- May pass into subclavian artery or other great vessels off aortic arch
○ UVC tip low within liver and instillation of hypertonic solution into portal system
- May cause thrombosis of PV
- Rarely leads to portal hypertension and cirrhosis
- May see calcification or thrombus in the PV, umbilical vein, or ductus venosus
- PV at higher risk of thrombosis because of slow flow
○ Sequela of UVC malposition in heart and lung
- Occlusion of pulmonary vein → focal pulmonary edema, hemorrhage, or infarction
- Arrhythmia, thrombotic endocarditis, atrial wall perforation, cardiac tamponade, hydrothorax
○ UVC extraluminal malposition
- May perforate LA wall and enter or perforate pericardium
- May perforate the lung via pulmonary vein
- May perforate the vein in liver
○ UVC erosion into hepatic parenchyma
- Instill medication/TPN into liver tissue
- Ultrasound may show liver mass and extraluminal position of catheter
- Parenchyma may calcify
- If parenchyma ruptures, may see ascites
○ UVC erosion into biliary system
- Biliary-venous fistula
○ UAC thrombus
- Majority are self-limiting
- May occlude artery and cause ischemia
- May become infected and cause septic emboli or mycotic aneurysm
- May become calcified
- May require surgical removal
○ UVC thrombus
- Majority are self-limiting
- May become infected and cause septic emboli
- May become calcified
○ Sepsis
- UVC is highest risk factor for sepsis in neonates
- More than half of catheter tips colonized with bacteria
○ Air embolism
○ Phlebitis
○ Septic osteoarthritis
○ Bowel perforation
- Epidemiology: True incidence of catheter complications unknown because of variability of reporting and monitoring

CLINICAL ISSUES

Presentation
- Most common signs/symptoms
  ○ UAC thrombosis or vasospasm
    - Skin blanching, lower extremity pallor, pulselessness, paralysis
    - Skin and muscle ischemia → ulceration and muscle necrosis
    - May rarely require amputation
  ○ UVC
    - Variable
- Other signs/symptoms
  ○ Symptoms depend on specific complication
  ○ Thrombosis may be asymptomatic
    - May form collaterals to compensate for occlusion
    - May be nonocclusive and found incidentally by ultrasound
  ○ Portal venous hypertension from portal venous thrombosis
    - May rarely lead to cirrhosis
  ○ Long term UAC thrombosis
    - Leg length discrepancy due to decreased arterial perfusion to involved leg

Demographics
- Age
  ○ Newborn
  ○ Often premature infant

Natural History & Prognosis
- Depends on complication
- Thrombi frequently resolve without treatment
- Thrombus may cause severe problems depending on location and extent
  ○ Arterial thrombus may cause ischemia or infarction of distal tissue (usually buttock or lower extremity)
  ○ Portal venous thrombus may rarely result in cirrhosis or abscess in liver
- Chronic arterial occlusion with collaterals to lower extremity
  ○ May result in chronic arterial insufficiency to lower extremity → claudication and slow growth
  ○ Leg length discrepancy

Treatment
- In general, reposition or remove catheter
- Depending on extent and location, thrombus may be observed, treated medically, or surgically removed
- Other complications treated individually

SELECTED REFERENCES

1. Kim JH et al: Does umbilical vein catheterization lead to portal venous thrombosis? Prospective US evaluation in 100 neonates. Radiology. 219(3):645-50, 2001
2. Hogan MJ: Neonatal vascular catheters and their complications. Radiol Clin North Am. 37(6):1109-25, 1999
3. Coley BD et al: Neonatal total parenteral nutrition ascites from liver erosion by umbilical vein catheters. Pediatr Radiol. 28(12):923-7, 1998
4. Narla LD et al: Evaluation of umbilical catheter and tube placement in premature infants. Radiographics. 11(5):849-63, 1991

UMBILICAL CATHETER COMPLICATIONS

IMAGE GALLERY

Typical

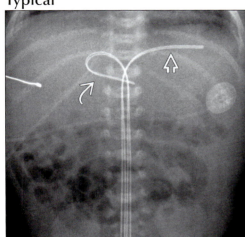
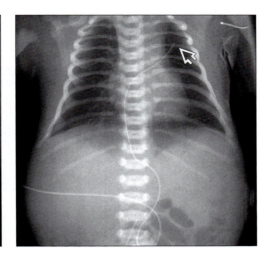

(Left) Anteroposterior radiograph shows two UVCs malpositioned in the liver. The *(open arrow)* points to a UVC likely in the left PV. The *(curved arrow)* points to a catheter likely in a right PV branch. *(Right)* Anteroposterior radiograph shows a malpositioned UVC with tip extending through PFO, through LA, and into a left upper lobe pulmonary vein branch *(arrow)*.

Typical

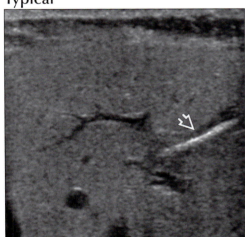
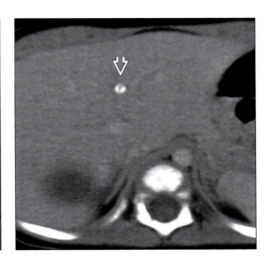

(Left) Ultrasound shows a linear echogenic calcification located in a branch of the portal vein *(arrow)*. *(Right)* Axial CECT shows a round calcification in the region of the obliterated ductus venosus *(arrow)*, likely the sequela of a prior thrombus. Likely no clinical significance.

Typical

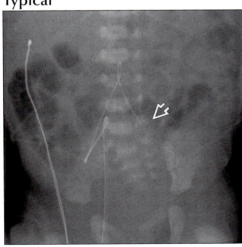
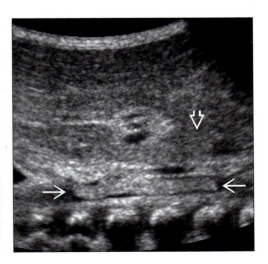

(Left) Anteroposterior radiograph shows a malpositioned UAC with tip likely in the SMA *(arrow)*. *(Right)* Sagittal ultrasound shows echogenic thrombus located in abdominal aorta *(arrows)* posterior to liver *(open arrow)*. Thrombus also impaired renal arterial flow, not seen on this image.

CHYLOTHORAX

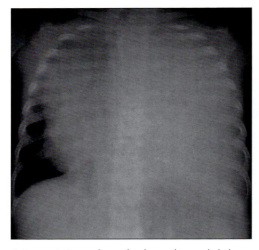

Anteroposterior radiograph shows large chylothorax secondary to lymphatic malformation in a 23 month old male. There is significant mediastinal shift to the right.

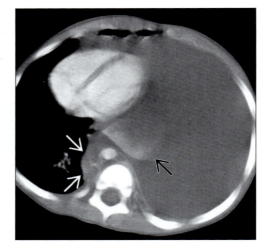

Axial CECT of same patient shows large pleural effusion, collapsed lung (black arrow), and abnormal soft tissue mass in the right paraspinal lymphatic malformation (white arrows).

TERMINOLOGY

Abbreviations and Synonyms
- Chylous fluid in pleural space

Definitions
- Lymphatic fluid in pleural space secondary to congenital or acquired conditions

IMAGING FINDINGS

General Features
- Best diagnostic clue
  - Increased density of a hemithorax secondary to an effusion
    - Mediastinal shift may also be present
  - Persistent pleural effusion following cardiac surgical repairs
    - Left thoracotomy procedures
    - Post-operative Glenn and Fontan procedures
    - Fluid accumulation occurs after oral intake is resumed
  - Lymphangiectasia presents with bilateral intersitial edema
    - Congenital lymphangiectasia
  - Newborn with congenital heart disease
    - Turner syndrome
    - Noonan syndrome
  - Newborn with congenital lymphedema or anasarca
  - Bone disease with chylothorax
    - Gorham syndrome or "vanishing" bone disease
- Location: Pleural space thoracic cavity
- Size: Variable
- Morphology
  - Pleural effusion which has fat microglobulins
  - Interstitial lung disease

Radiographic Findings
- Radiography
  - Chylothorax is nonspecific finding (persistent pleural effusion)
    - Post-operative cardiac or chest surgery
    - Left-sided fluid more common
    - Associated with variety of congenital and acquired lesions
  - Depends on the underlying etiology of chylothorax
    - Clinical history important
    - Other anomalies contribute to making correct diagnosis
  - Lymphangiectasia has normal heart with interstitial edema

CT Findings
- CECT
  - Neonates with mass in chest

DDx: Interstitial Edema

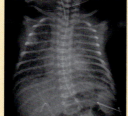
TAPVR

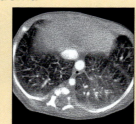
TAPVR

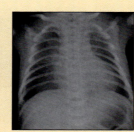
Transient Tachypnea

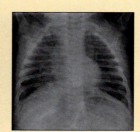
Neonatal Pneumonia

CHYLOTHORAX

Key Facts

Terminology
- Chylous fluid in pleural space
- Lymphatic fluid in pleural space secondary to congenital or acquired conditions

Imaging Findings
- Chylothorax is nonspecific finding (persistent pleural effusion)
- Depends on the underlying etiology of chylothorax
- Pleural effusion may be unilateral or bilateral
- Effusion usually without debris or septations

Top Differential Diagnoses
- Congenital heart disease with prominent venous pattern and effusions
- Pulmonary edema with effusions
- Pneumonia and effusions
- Interstitial pneumonia

Pathology
- Trauma to thoracic duct
- Congenital malformations or associations
- Congenital masses
- Obstruction to thoracic duct venous return
- Complication of increase in pulmonary artery pressure
- Malignant etiology
- Infectious etiology
- Diagnosis of chylothorax made by thoracentesis demonstrating chylomicrons

Clinical Issues
- Depends on etiology of chylous effusion
- Conservative or medical treatment

- Will help identify mass, congenital anomaly or lesions as cause of effusion
- Cystic adenomatoid malformation most common
- May occur in post-operative congenital heart disease
  - Older children
    - Helps define underlying abnormality
    - Large tumors may obstruct thoracic duct
    - Trauma to duct from surgery or accident
  - Pleural effusion may be unilateral or bilateral
    - Typically L > R
    - May look for complications including loculated fluid, lung disease and venous anatomy
  - Lymphangiectasia demonstrates diffuse interstitial thickening of interstitial spaces

Ultrasonographic Findings
- Grayscale Ultrasound
  - Effusion usually without debris or septations
  - Vascular evaluation of superior vena cava and brachiocephalic veins to exclude thrombosis

Imaging Recommendations
- Best imaging tool
  - No imaging needed if fat microglobulins are seen in pleural fluid
  - Imaging may be done to discover underlying cause of chylothorax such as mass
- Protocol advice
  - CT with contrast
    - Useful to evaluate for underlying cause
    - Useful in congenital heart disease

DIFFERENTIAL DIAGNOSIS

Congenital heart disease with prominent venous pattern and effusions
- In the newborn, total anomalous pulmonary venous return (TAPVR) simulates prominent interstitial pattern of lymphangiectasia
- Cardiac enlargement may or may not be present
- Abnormal cardiac contour
- Pleural fluid may or may not be present
- Post-operative coarctation repair in infants: 1%
- Post-operative surgery in Glenn and Fontan anastomosis

Pulmonary edema with effusions
- Non cardiac causes of pulmonary edema

Pneumonia and effusions
- Significant lung disease usually present plus pleural fluid
- Children usually febrile with cough

Hemothorax
- Secondary to trauma

Interstitial pneumonia
- Infants usually tachypnea with fever
- May simulate radiographic findings of lymphangiectasia

PATHOLOGY

General Features
- Genetics
  - Congenital heart patients may have genetic predisposition
  - Noonan syndrome is autosomal dominant or sporadic (Chromosome 12q)
  - Turner syndrome is the absence of one X chromosome (Karyotype 45,X)
- Etiology
  - Chylothorax
    - Thoracic duct is major lymphatic vessel
    - Begins near lower part of spine and collects lymph
    - Drains lymph from lower limbs, pelvis abdomen
    - Normally drains into the left brachiocephalic vessel
    - Drainage is variable in 30% of cases
    - Obstruction, anomaly, or trauma results in chylothorax
  - Trauma to thoracic duct
    - May occur during delivery

CHYLOTHORAX

- Post-operative congenital heart surgery most common
- Post-operative pneumonectomy or congenital diaphragmatic hernia
- Post-operative scoliosis surgery
  - Congenital malformations or associations
    - Congenital chylothorax is most common
    - Congenital lymphangiectasia, Turner syndrome, Noonan syndrome, Gorham syndrome, Lymphangiomatosis
  - Congenital masses
    - Large lymphatic malformations (cystic hygromas)
    - Cystic adenomatoid malformation of lung (CCAM)
    - Pulmonary sequestration
    - Diaphragmatic hernia
  - Obstruction to thoracic duct venous return
    - Left, right, or bilateral brachiocephalic vein clot
    - Superior vena cava clot
  - Complication of increase in pulmonary artery pressure
    - Cavopulmonary shunts (Glenn and Fontan procedures)
    - Severe pulmonary hypertension
  - Malignant etiology
    - Lymphoma is the most common
    - Large thoracic masses in the thorax may obstruct the duct
    - Metastatic disease to interstitial spaces of lung
  - Infectious etiology
    - Tuberculosis
    - Filariasis
- Epidemiology: Diverse depending on the underlying cause

Gross Pathologic & Surgical Features
- Depends on the underlying etiology
- Diagnosis of chylothorax made by thoracentesis demonstrating chylomicrons
  - Effusion milky white in appearance
  - A level of triglyceride greater than 110mg/dl reflects a 99% chance fluid is chyle
- Serum abnormal in lymphangiectasia
  - Lymphocyte depletion
  - Hypoalbuminemia

Microscopic Features
- Depends on the underlying cause
- Lymphangiectasia demonstrates dilated, ectatic lymph channels in the lung
- Gorham disease shows diffuse proliferation of dilated lymphatic channels in bone, soft tissue and lung

CLINICAL ISSUES

Presentation
- Most common signs/symptoms
  - Depends on etiology of chylous effusion
  - Tachypnea and dyspnea
  - Classic symptoms of pleural effusion
    - Decreased breath sounds usually with cough
  - Symptoms occur post-operative following resumption of feeding
  - Lymphangiectasia presents in infancy with tachypnea
- Other signs/symptoms
  - Children may have failure to gain weight and grow
  - Immunosuppression has been reported

Demographics
- Age: Variable depending on cause
- Gender: Depends on etiology

Natural History & Prognosis
- Depends on etiology
- Thoracic duct injury may resolve spontaneously in 50%
  - Other pathways of lymphatic drainage develop

Treatment
- Conservative or medical treatment
  - Treat underlying cause of chyle
  - Decrease chyle production
    - Fat restricted oral diet
    - Total parental nutrition (TPN)
- Surgical options
  - Indications for surgical intervention
    - Chyle leak greater than 1 L/d for five days
    - Persistent leak for more than two weeks
  - Thoracentesis or draining procedure of pleural space
  - Thoracic duct ligation
  - Pleuroperitoneal shunt difficult in children
  - Pleurodesis
- Treat underlying cause of chylothorax
  - Removal of chest masses
  - Gorham syndrome treated aggressively
  - Lymphatic malformations
    - Benign masses may grow and obstruct important structures
    - Some resolve spontaneously and decrease in size
    - Current therapy includes sclerotherapy, surgical removal

SELECTED REFERENCES

1. Young S et al: Severe congenital chylothorax treated with octreotide. J Perinatol. 24(3):200-2, 2004
2. Caspi J et al: Effects of controlled antegrade pulmonary blood flow on cardiac function after bidirectional cavopulmonary anastomosis. Ann Thorac Surg. 76(6):1917-21; discussion 1921-2, 2003
3. Miller GG. Related Articles et al: Treatment of chylothorax in Gorham's disease: case report and literature review. Can J Surg. 45(5):381-2, 2002
4. Pettitt TW et al: Treatment of persistent chylothorax after Norwood procedure with somatostatin. Ann Thorac Surg. 73(3):977-9, 2002
5. Chung CJ et al: The pediatric airway: a review of differential diagnosis by anatomy and pathology. Neuroimaging Clin N Am. 10(1):161-80, ix, 2000
6. Chung CJ et al: Children with congenital pulmonary lymphangiectasia: after infancy. AJR Am J Roentgenol. 173(6):1583-8, 1999
7. Browse NL et al: Management of chylothorax. Br J Surg. 84(12):1711-6, 1997

CHYLOTHORAX

IMAGE GALLERY

Typical

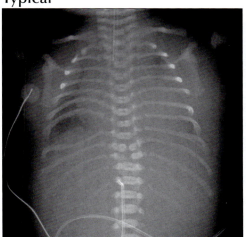
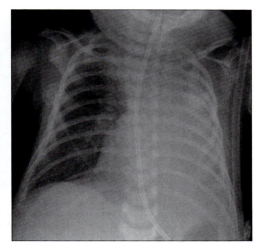

(Left) Anteroposterior radiograph shows massive soft tissue anasarca, left effusion, congenital anomalies in a newborn with hydrops. The fluid in the left chest was chylous. *(Right)* Anteroposterior radiograph shows opacification of the left hemithorax in an 8 day old infant following repair of coarctation. Chylothorax is a known complication of the procedure.

Typical

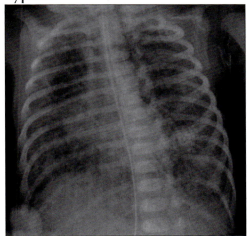
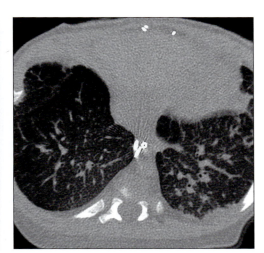

(Left) Anteroposterior radiograph shows bilateral symmetric increase in interstitial markings in infant with congenital lymphangiectasia. Prior to feeding the chest radiograph was normal. *(Right)* Axial CECT shows prominent interstitial lung markings and thickening of the interlobular septa in older patient with biopsy proven lymphangiectasia.

Typical

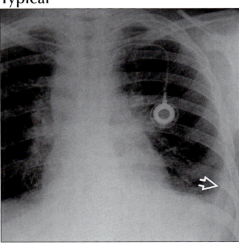
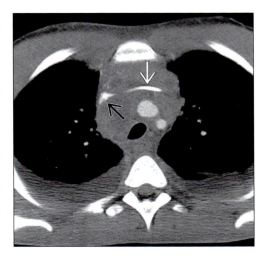

(Left) Anteroposterior radiograph shows mediastinal mass with left effusion (arrow) in patient with recurrent lymphoma. *(Right)* Anteroposterior CECT adolescent patient with recurrent lymphoma with bilateral effusion secondary to superior vena caval obstruction (black arrow). Patient has a compressed central line from left arm filled with contrast (white arrow). Fluid drained from both sides of hemithoraces was chylous.

VIRAL LUNG INFECTION

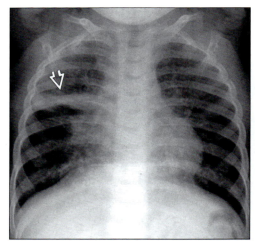

Anteroposterior radiograph in child with viral illness shows symmetric hyperinflation, increased peribronchial markings, and band of atelectasis (arrow) in right upper lobe.

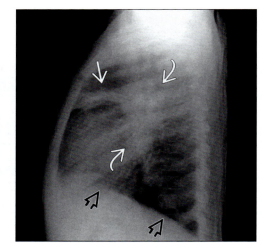

Lateral radiograph in same patient shows flatted hemidiaphragms (open arrows) and prominent/indistinct hila (curved arrows). Note atelectasis (arrow).

TERMINOLOGY

Abbreviations and Synonyms
- Bronchiolitis

Definitions
- Viral infection of the lower respiratory tract

IMAGING FINDINGS

General Features
- Best diagnostic clue: Increased peribronchial markings and hyperinflation
- Location: Bilateral and symmetric hyperinflation

Radiographic Findings
- Radiography
  - Major goal of imaging (chest radiography) is to differentiate viral from bacterial pneumonia
  - Best imaging clue for viral disease
    - Increased peribronchial markings
    - Hyperinflation
  - Lack of focal lung consolidation (hallmark for bacterial infection)
  - Increased peribronchial markings
    - Symmetric, coarse linear markings radiating from the hila into the lung
    - Central portions of the lungs may appear "dirty" or "busy"
    - Very subjective finding
    - Hila may appear prominent on lateral view
  - Hyperinflation
    - Hyperlucency
    - Depression of the diaphragm to more than 10 posterior ribs
    - Flattening of the diaphragms (best seen on lateral view)
    - Increased anteroposterior chest diameter (in infants chest wider than tall on lateral view)
    - Hyperinflation often much better appreciated on lateral view
  - Subsegmental atelectasis
    - Wedge-shaped or triangular areas of density most commonly seen in the mid or lower lung
    - Misinterpretation of subsegmental atelectasis as opacities suspicious for bacterial pneumonia is one of the most common errors in pediatric radiology
  - Hilar lymphadenopathy
    - Can be seen in lower respiratory tract infection in children
    - Does not have as alarming significance in this setting as when seen in adults

DDx: Lower Respiratory Track Symptoms

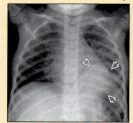
Bacterial Pneumonia

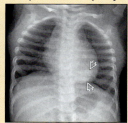
Sequestration

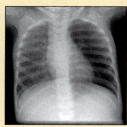
Bronchial Foreign Body

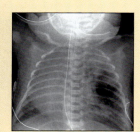
Infected CCAM

VIRAL LUNG INFECTION

Key Facts

Terminology
- Bronchiolitis

Imaging Findings
- Best diagnostic clue: Increased peribronchial markings and hyperinflation
- Lack of focal lung consolidation (hallmark for bacterial infection)
- Increased peribronchial markings
- Symmetric, coarse linear markings radiating from the hila into the lung
- Hyperinflation
- Hyperinflation often much better appreciated on lateral view
- Subsegmental atelectasis

Pathology
- Combination of narrowing of the lumen of small airways from edema and necrotic debris and mucus in the airway lumen leads to small airway occlusion
- Airway occlusion results in hyperinflation and areas of subsegmental atelectasis
- Anatomic consideration render small children more predisposed to air trapping and collapse
- < 2 years of age: 80% are viral
- > 2 years of age: 49% are viral

Clinical Issues
- Supportive
- Do not need antibiotics

CT Findings
- Not used to make diagnosis of viral disease but CT may be obtained in patient with viral disease
- Prominent and ill-defined hila with peribronchial markings radiating into the lung
- Ground-glass opacities
- Increased interstitial markings
- Mild hilar lymphadenopathy may be present

Imaging Recommendations
- Best imaging tool
  - Chest radiography is the best diagnostic tool to try to differentiate bacterial from viral lower respiratory tract infection
  - Performance of chest radiography in identifying and excluding bacterial pneumonia
    - Positive predictive value 30%
    - Negative predictive value 92%
  - Since the goal is to treat all children with possible bacterial pneumonia with antibiotics while minimizing the number of children unnecessarily treated with antibiotics, the high negative predictive value of chest radiography is helpful

DIFFERENTIAL DIAGNOSIS

Bacterial pneumonia
- Focal lung consolidation
- Lack of increased peribronchial markings
- Pleural effusions more common with bacterial infection

Asthma
- Increased peribronchial markings and hyperinflation
- Virtually identical appearance to viral lower respiratory tract infection
- Both asthma and viral disease are related to inflammation of the small airways

Left to right shunts
- In infants, left to right shunts may have similar appearance
- Increased pulmonary arterial flow may mimic increased peribronchial markings
- Shunts, like viral disease, typically have hyperinflation
- Shunts have associated cardiomegaly

Infected congenital lesions
- Infected congenital lesions such as congenital cystic adenomatoid malformations or sequestrations may present with respiratory symptoms
- Focal solid or cystic mass present rather than diffuse bilateral process

Aspirated bronchial foreign body
- May present with wheezing very similar to viral disease
- Asymmetric hyperinflation
- Static lung volume throughout respiratory cycle

PATHOLOGY

General Features
- General path comments
  - Viral infection involves the airways
  - Inflammation of the small airways results in peribronchial edema
  - Combination of narrowing of the lumen of small airways from edema and necrotic debris and mucus in the airway lumen leads to small airway occlusion
  - Airway occlusion results in hyperinflation and areas of subsegmental atelectasis
  - Anatomic consideration render small children more predisposed to air trapping and collapse
    - Small airway lumen diameter
    - Poorly developed collateral circulation of ventilation
    - More abundant production of mucus
- Etiology
  - Most common viral infections in one series of community acquired pneumonia (2000)
    - Respiratory syncytial virus 29%
    - Rhinovirus 58%
    - Parainfluenza virus (1, 2, 3) 25%

VIRAL LUNG INFECTION

- Adenovirus 7%
- Influenza A & B 4%
- Coronavirus 3%
- Human herpesvirus 3%
○ Most common bacterial
  - Streptococcus pneumoniae 37%
  - Haemophilus influenza 9%
  - Mycoplasma pneumoniae 7%
  - Chlamydia pneumoniae 3%
  - Staphylococcus pneumonia 0%
- Epidemiology
  ○ Respiratory tract infection is the most common cause of illness in children and continues to be a significant cause of morbidity and mortality
  ○ Evaluation of potential lower respiratory tract infection one of the most common indications for imaging in children
  ○ Etiology of lower respiratory tract infection varies with age
  ○ Preschool children (4 months to 5 years)
    - Viruses majority of lower respiratory tract infections
  ○ School age children (> 5 years)
    - Viruses still most common
    - Mycoplasma pneumoniae 30%
    - Streptococcus pneumoniae becomes more frequent
  ○ Another study of lower respiratory tract infections showed
    - < 2 years of age: 80% are viral
    - > 2 years of age: 49% are viral
    - For all ages: 47% viral, 38% bacterial, 15% mixed viral/bacterial
- Associated abnormalities: May lead to bronchiolitis obliterans

CLINICAL ISSUES

Presentation
- Most common signs/symptoms
  ○ Cough
  ○ Wheezing
- Other signs/symptoms
  ○ Often upper respiratory tract (sinus) symptoms
  ○ May have fever
  ○ Hypoxia/respiratory failure in severe cases
  ○ Difficult to differentiate bacterial from viral lower respiratory tract infection on basis of physical exam or any other available laboratory tests

Demographics
- Age: Typical and striking radiographic findings of viral disease more often seen in young children (< 5 years of age)

Natural History & Prognosis
- Resolution of symptoms over time

Treatment
- Supportive
- Do not need antibiotics

DIAGNOSTIC CHECKLIST

Consider
- If any question of asymmetry, consider aspirated foreign body

SELECTED REFERENCES

1. Copley SJ: Application of computed tomography in childhood respiratory infections. Br Med Bull. 61:263-79, 2002
2. Virkki R et al: Differentiation of bacterial and viral pneumonia in children. Thorax. 57(5):438-41, 2002
3. Donnelly LF: Practical issues concerning imaging of pulmonary infection in children. J Thorac Imaging. 16(4):238-50, 2001
4. Donnelly LF: Fundamentals of Pediatric Radiology. Philadelphia; W.B. Saunders, 2001
5. Juven T et al: Etiology of community-acquired pneumonia in 254 hospitalized children. Pediatr Infect Dis J. 19(4):293-8, 2000
6. Markowitz RI et al: The spectrum of pulmonary infection in the immunocompromised child. Semin Roentgenol. 35(2):171-80, 2000
7. Donnelly LF: Maximizing the usefulness of imaging in children with community-acquired pneumonia. AJR Am J Roentgenol. 172(2):505-12, 1999
8. Katz DS et al: Radiology of pneumonia. Clin Chest Med. 20(3):549-62, 1999
9. Brunelle F: [Radiologic approach to community-acquired pneumonia] Arch Pediatr. 5 Suppl 1:26s-27s, 1998
10. Donnelly LF et al: Cavitary necrosis complicating pneumonia in children: sequential findings on chest radiography. AJR Am J Roentgenol. 171(1):253-6, 1998
11. Donnelly LF et al: The yield of CT of children who have complicated pneumonia and noncontributory chest radiography. AJR Am J Roentgenol. 170(6):1627-31, 1998
12. Donnelly LF et al: Pneumonia in children: decreased parenchymal contrast enhancement--CT sign of intense illness and impending cavitary necrosis. Radiology. 205(3):817-20, 1997
13. Donnelly LF et al: CT appearance of parapneumonic effusions in children: findings are not specific for empyema. AJR Am J Roentgenol. 169(1):179-82, 1997
14. Wahlgren H et al: Radiographic patterns and viral studies in childhood pneumonia at various ages. Pediatr Radiol. 25(8):627-30, 1995
15. Korppi M et al: Comparison of radiological findings and microbial aetiology of childhood pneumonia. Acta Paediatr. 82(4):360-3, 1993
16. Condon VR: Pneumonia in children. J Thoracic Imaging. 6:31-44, 1991
17. Kirkpatrick JA: Pneumonia in children as it differs from adult pneumonia. Semin Roentgenol. 15(1):96-103, 1980

VIRAL LUNG INFECTION

IMAGE GALLERY

Typical

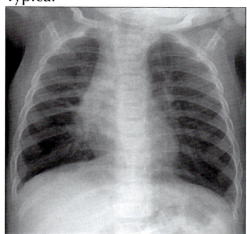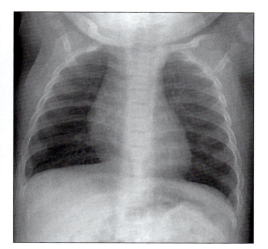

(Left) Anteroposterior radiograph in a patient while ill shows increased peribronchial markings as prominent and indistinct linear densities radiating from hilum. *(Right)* Anteroposterior radiograph in same child as to left shows normal appearance for contrast. Note absence of prominent and indistinct markings from hilum.

Typical

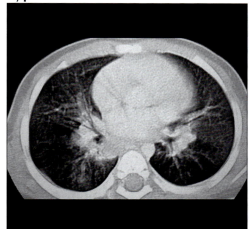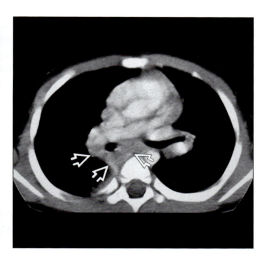

(Left) Axial CECT (lung windows) obtained for other reasons shows CT findings of viral disease for illustrative purposes: Increased prominence and indistinctness of interstitial and vascular markings and perihilar areas. *(Right)* Axial CECT (mediastinal windows) on same patient as on left shows increased soft tissue (arrows) surrounding right hilum not unexpected in viral disease.

Typical

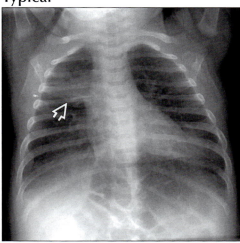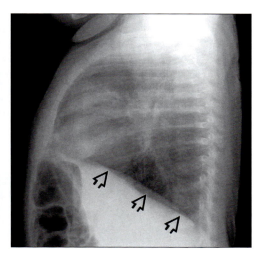

(Left) Anteroposterior radiograph shows increased perihilar markings. There is atelectasis (arrow) in a portion of the right upper lobe. There is hyperinflation. *(Right)* Lateral radiograph shows hyperinflation as increased anterior to posterior diameter and flattened hemidiaphragms (arrows). The hila are prominent supportive of the finding of increased perihilar markings.

ROUND PNEUMONIA

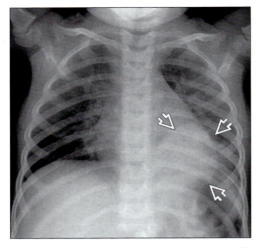

Anteroposterior radiograph in a 2 year old boy with fever and cough shows very round opacification (arrows) in left lower lobe consistent with round pneumonia.

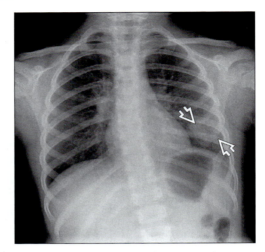

Anteroposterior radiograph shows round opacity (arrows) in left lower lobe consistent with round pneumonia.

TERMINOLOGY

Definitions
- Bacterial pneumonia with a very round, well-defined appearance on chest radiography, simulating a mass
- Should typically only be seen up to approximately 8 years of age
- Typically occurs with streptococcal pneumoniae infection

IMAGING FINDINGS

General Features
- Best diagnostic clue: Round lung opacity with well-defined borders in a child less than 8 years of age
- Location
  - More common in lower lobes
  - Most common in superior segment of lower lobes
  - No peripheral or central predisposition
- Size
  - May vary in size related to time of imaging diagnosis in relation to development of pneumonia
  - With growth, eventually may present as lobar pneumonia and no longer appear round
  - Reported size varies between 1-7 cm

Radiographic Findings
- Radiography
  - Round lung opacity
  - Supportive findings of air space disease
    - Air bronchograms
  - May progress to lobar pneumonia if child's illness progresses and serial films obtained
  - Respects lobar anatomy without crossing fissures

CT Findings
- NECT
  - CT not advocated in suspected cases of round pneumonia but may be obtained to evaluate for possibility of a mass
  - CT of abdomen obtained for pain may also show round pneumonia in lower lobes as cause of abdominal pain
  - CT shows round opacity
  - Air-bronchograms may be present
  - Respects lobar anatomy and does not cross fissures
  - No other specific CT findings
- CECT
  - May show normal pulmonary vessels coursing through lesion
  - There will be no enhancing rim or wall
  - No systemic arterial supply from descending aorta (seen with sequestration)

DDx: Focal Lung Masses In Children

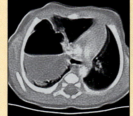
CCAM

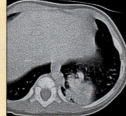
Sequestration

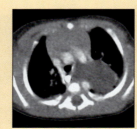
Bronchogenic Cyst

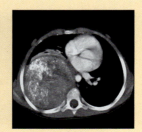
Neuroblastoma

ROUND PNEUMONIA

Key Facts

Terminology
- Bacterial pneumonia with a very round, well-defined appearance on chest radiography, simulating a mass

Imaging Findings
- More common in lower lobes
- Reported size varies between 1-7 cm
- Air bronchograms
- Respects lobar anatomy without crossing fissures
- If child has symptoms of pneumonia and "round" density on chest radiograph, additional imaging with modalities such as CT not necessary
- Follow-up radiograph several weeks after antibiotic therapy may be helpful to document resolution of the process
- This is one of the few indications concerning pneumonia in children where a follow-up chest radiograph may be indicated even if the child becomes asymptomatic in order to exclude underlying mass

Pathology
- In children, collateral pathways of air circulation are not well developed until approximately 8 years of age
- After 8 years of age, if round mass seen on chest radiograph, high suspicion for other pathology
- Etiology: Most commonly seen with streptococcal pneumoniae infection

Clinical Issues
- Cough and fever
- May present with abdominal pain

---

  o Presence of central cavity favors alternative diagnosis

MR Findings
- Not utilized in work-up of round pneumonia
- If MRI of chest performed because round mass suspected as neuroblastoma, findings may be encountered
- Round pneumonia will appear as high signal mass within pulmonary parenchyma

Imaging Recommendations
- If child has symptoms of pneumonia and "round" density on chest radiograph, additional imaging with modalities such as CT not necessary
- Follow-up radiograph several weeks after antibiotic therapy may be helpful to document resolution of the process
- This is one of the few indications concerning pneumonia in children where a follow-up chest radiograph may be indicated even if the child becomes asymptomatic in order to exclude underlying mass
- If greater than 8 years of age, increased suspicion for other causes of mass should be considered and CT obtained

DIFFERENTIAL DIAGNOSIS

Bronchogenic cyst
- May appear as round, well-defined soft tissue mass on chest radiography
- Very similar appearance to round pneumonia
- Only contains air or air fluid levels if infected
- Most common in perihilar areas
- CT: Well-defined mass that is water attenuated which may have an enhancing rim and no air bronchograms

Neuroblastoma
- If pneumonia is posterior, may simulate posterior mediastinal mass such as neuroblastoma
- Round pneumonia will have acute rather than obtuse borders with mediastinum
- Rib erosion/destruction seen with neuroblastoma
- Calcifications present in up to 85% of thoracic neuroblastoma
- Neuroblastoma may also appear as paraspinal mass with widening of paraspinal stripe on radiography

Congenital cystic adenomatoid malformation (CCAM)
- May appear as solid appearing lesion typically soon after birth
- Most CCAM are cystic and communicate with the bronchial tree at birth and as a result quickly fill with air
- "Solid" type 3 CCAM are exceedingly rare

Pulmonary sequestration
- Most common in the left lower lobe
- Present as recurrent pneumonia
- Round pneumonia almost never recurs in same location
- Systemic arterial supply to sequestration from descending aorta
- Sequestration typically do not appear as round

PATHOLOGY

General Features
- General path comments
  o In children, collateral pathways of air circulation are not well developed until approximately 8 years of age
    - Channels of Lambert
    - Pores of Kohn
  o Lack of well developed collateral circulation thought to hinder spread of bacterial infection and predispose to "round" appearance on radiography
  o After 8 years of age, if round mass seen on chest radiograph, high suspicion for other pathology
  o There are rarely reported cases in adults
- Etiology: Most commonly seen with streptococcal pneumoniae infection

NORMAL THYMUS

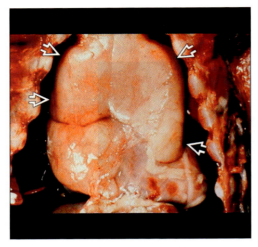

Gross pathology from autopsy of child who died of SIDS shows normal but prominently sized thymus (arrows). The anterior ribs have been removed.

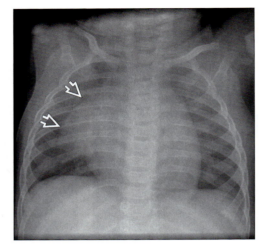

Anteroposterior radiograph shows prominent but normal thymus with rightward triangular projection (arrows) ("sail sign"). Lateral view (not shown) showed no displacement of airway.

TERMINOLOGY

Abbreviations and Synonyms
- Thymic sail sign

Definitions
- Normal organ in anterior superior mediastinum involved in production of T-cells
- "Thymos" is Greek for "warty excrescence"

IMAGING FINDINGS

General Features
- Best diagnostic clue: Patient age: Can be quite large up to 5 years of age
- Location: Anterior superior mediastinum
- Size
  ○ Variable
  ○ Upper limit of normal dependent upon patient age
- Morphology: Smooth contours, homogeneous attenuation

Radiographic Findings
- Radiography
  ○ Variability in size and appearance
  ○ Quite large on chest X-ray (CXR) up to 5 years of age
  ○ Decreases in relative size by end of first decade of life
  ○ Should not have a prominent mass during 2nd decade
  ○ More common in boys: 80% of prominent thymuses in boys
  ○ Contour: Convex, undulating with ribs
    ■ Abnormal contour: Irregular, lobulated, poorly defined
  ○ Shape: Variable
    ■ Sail sign: May have triangular extension out laterally that looks like a sail
    ■ Usually to right, but can be to left
    ■ Not to be confused with spinnaker sail sign: Lifted thymic shadow from pneumomediastinum
  ○ Consistency: Homogeneous, no calcification or low attenuation
  ○ Normal thymus does not displace or compress airway or vascular structures

Fluoroscopic Findings
- Fluoroscopy can be utilized to help differentiate normal, prominent thymus from mass
- Normal thymus is "soft" and changes contour with respirations
- Abnormal mass tends to be "harder" and less compliant with respirations
- Not often utilized currently

CT Findings
- Consistency: Homogeneous attenuation

DDx: Other Mediastinal Masses

Lymphoma | LCH | Thymic Cyst

NORMAL THYMUS

Key Facts

Imaging Findings
- Variability in size and appearance
- Quite large on chest X-ray (CXR) up to 5 years of age
- Decreases in relative size by end of first decade of life
- Should not have a prominent mass during 2nd decade
- More common in boys: 80% of prominent thymuses in boys
- Contour: Convex, undulating with ribs
- Shape: Variable
- Sail sign: May have triangular extension out laterally that looks like a sail
- Consistency: Homogeneous, no calcification or low attenuation
- Normal thymus does not displace or compress airway or vascular structures
- Shape on axial imaging
- Young children: Quadrilateral with convex borders
- Teenagers: Triangular
- Thymic volume can decrease/re-grow by > 40% volume with chemotherapy
- If chest radiograph demonstrates prominent thymus that is questionably normal for age, imaging options include
- Repeat chest radiograph in 6 weeks
- CT of chest with contrast
- Ultrasound to demonstrate normal architecture

Pathology
- Largest actual size of thymus occurs in teenage years
- But largest size relative to rest of chest occurs in infancy

---

  - No calcifications or areas of low attenuation
- Smooth borders, not irregular
- Shape on axial imaging
  - Young children: Quadrilateral with convex borders
  - Teenagers: Triangular
- Normal thymus does not displace or compress vascular structures or airway
- Associated findings such as pericardial effusion, pleural effusion, pulmonary disease favor pathology
- CT often utilized to differentiate between prominent but normal thymus and mediastinal mass
- Retrocaval thymus
  - Normal variant
  - Posterior extension of thymus between superior vena cava (SVC) and great arteries
  - Can mimic mediastinal mass or right upper lobe collapse
  - Only thymic variant that occasionally displaces structures (airway, vessels)
  - Retrocaval thymus is contiguous with anterior thymic tissue
  - Homogeneous attenuation, similar to rest of thymus
- Aberrant cervical thymus
  - Arrested migration along thymopharyngeal duct may result in aberrant cervical thymus
  - Cervical mass of normal thymic tissue
  - Mandibular angle to thoracic inlet
  - Homogeneous attenuation, similar to thymus
- Thymic rebound
  - Widened mediastinum when following up lymphoma suspicious for malignancy
  - Thymic volume can decrease/re-grow by > 40% volume with chemotherapy
  - Timing of CT in relationship to chemotherapy cycle important
  - Recurrent mass may represent normal thymic rebound after chemotherapy
  - Appearance and location of tissue in area of normal thymus

MR Findings
- Findings as on CT
- Homogeneous signal

Ultrasonographic Findings
- Historic description is that thymus is of homogeneous echogenicity, with low frequency transducers
- High frequency transducers now demonstrate normal thymic septa as echogenic linear or dot-like echogenicities
  - Considered characteristic for normal thymus
- Can be used to diagnose ectopic thymus or document normal but prominent thymus

Nuclear Medicine Findings
- PET
  - Normal thymus shows mild PET uptake
  - Typically much less intense uptake than seen in with lymphoma
  - Differentiation of recurrent lymphoma vs. normal thymus (thymic rebound) can be problematic at times

Imaging Recommendations
- If chest radiograph demonstrates prominent thymus that is questionably normal for age, imaging options include
  - Repeat chest radiograph in 6 weeks
  - CT of chest with contrast
  - Ultrasound to demonstrate normal architecture
- Features associated with normal thymus
  - Age
    - Can be quite large up to 5 years of age
  - Gender
    - 80% of prominent thymuses are in boys
  - Contour
    - Normal: Convex, undulating
    - Abnormal: Lobulated, poorly defined, irregular
  - Shape
    - Variable
    - Can drape over cardiac silhouette and make heart look prominent
    - Can have prominent triangular extension leftward or rightward called "sail sign"
  - Consistency
    - Homogeneous

NORMAL THYMUS

- No calcifications, areas of low attenuation
- Relationship to adjacent structures
  - Normal thymus "soft"
  - Does not compress adjacent structures: Airway and superior vena cava
- Associated findings that favor abnormal thymus
  - Pleural or pericardial effusion
  - Lung disease

DIFFERENTIAL DIAGNOSIS

Lymphoma
- By far most common cause of pathologic anterior mediastinal mass in children
- Prominent normal thymus occurs in infants
- Lymphoma typically occurs in older children/teenagers
- Irregular margins
- Compression of venous structures and airway
- Associated pleural effusion, pericardial effusion, lung involvement

Germ cell tumor (teratoma)
- Calcifications and fat attenuation

Thymic cyst
- Presence of cysts in region of thymus

Langerhans cell histiocytosis (LCH)
- Thymic involvement common in autopsy series of LCH
- Thymic mass with calcifications or low attenuation
- Lung cysts
- Hepatomegaly, periportal low attenuation, liver mass

Neuroblastoma
- Posterior mediastinal mass

PATHOLOGY

General Features
- General path comments
  - Normal thymus prominent in relationship to relative size of thorax at birth and during first 5 years of life
  - Begins to become smaller relative to chest by the end of 1st decade of life
  - Continues to decrease in size for remainder of adulthood
  - Largest actual size of thymus occurs in teenage years
    - But largest size relative to rest of chest occurs in infancy

Microscopic Features
- Normal thymus has connective tissue septa that show up on ultrasound as linear and dot-like foci of high echogenicity

CLINICAL ISSUES

Presentation
- Most common signs/symptoms: Prominent normal thymus not associated with symptoms
- History
  - Historically enlarged thymus blamed for multiple problems including thymic asthma, SIDS, anesthesia related death, status thymicolymphaticus
  - Advent of radiographs allowed for demonstration of prominent thymus on CXR
  - Thymic radiation utilized to reduce thymic size
    - First described in 1905
    - At time recommended as prophylactic treatment of all neonates
    - Continued in some regions until 1960s
    - Many credit these adverse events for rallying birth of 1st radiologic subspecialty: Pediatric radiology

SELECTED REFERENCES

1. Takahashi K et al: Characterization of the normal and hyperplastic thymus on chemical-shift MR imaging. AJR Am J Roentgenol. 180(5):1265-9, 2003
2. Frush DP et al: Imaging evaluation of the thymus and thymic disorders in children. In: Pediatric Chest Imaging, eds. Strife JL, Lucaya J. Berlin; Springer-Verlag, 187-208, 2001
3. Han BK et al: Thymic ultrasound. II. Diagnosis of aberrant cervical thymus. Pediatr Radiol. 31(7):480-7, 2001
4. Han BK et al: Thymic ultrasound. I. Intrathymic anatomy in infants. Pediatr Radiol. 31(7):474-9, 2001
5. Mendelson DS: Imaging of the thymus. Chest Surg Clin N Am. 11(2):269-93, x, 2001
6. Sklair-Levy M et al: Age-related changes in CT attenuation of the thymus in children. Pediatr Radiol. 30(8):566-9, 2000
7. Hasselbalch H et al: Thymus size in infants from birth until 24 months of age evaluated by ultrasound. A longitudinal prediction model for the thymic index. Acta Radiol. 40(1):41-4, 1999
8. Jacobs MT et al: The right place at the wrong time: historical perspective of the relation of the thymus gland and pediatric radiology. Radiology. 210:11-6, 1999
9. Hasselbalch H et al: Thymus size evaluated by sonography. A longitudinal study on infants during the first year of life. Acta Radiol. 38(2):222-7, 1997
10. Hasselbalch H et al: Sonographic measurement of thymic size in healthy neonates. Relation to clinical variables. Acta Radiol. 38(1):95-8, 1997
11. Molina PL et al: Thymic masses on MR imaging. AJR Am J Roentgenol. 155(3):495-500, 1990
12. Han BK et al: Normal thymus in infancy: sonographic characteristics. Radiology. 170(2):471-4, 1989
13. Siegel MJ et al: Normal and abnormal thymus in childhood: MR imaging. Radiology. 172(2):367-71, 1989
14. St Amour TE et al: CT appearances of the normal and abnormal thymus in childhood. J Comput Assist Tomogr. 11(4):645-50, 1987

NORMAL THYMUS

IMAGE GALLERY

Typical

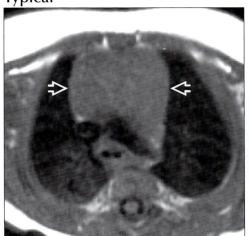 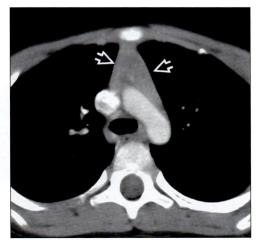

(Left) Axial T1WI MR shows normal thymus (arrows) in an infant. Note quadrilateral shape, smooth borders, and homogeneous signal, and nondisplacement of airway and vessels. *(Right)* Axial CECT in a teenager shows normal thymus (arrows) with triangular shape, homogeneous attenuation, smooth borders, and lack of compression of adjacent structures.

Typical

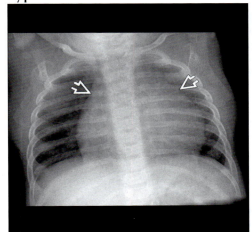 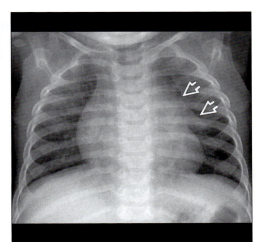

(Left) Anteroposterior radiograph in infant shows normal appearance with thymus (arrows) draped over cardiac silhouette. *(Right)* Anteroposterior radiograph in an infant shows normal thymus with triangular extension to left (arrows). Note smooth borders.

Variant

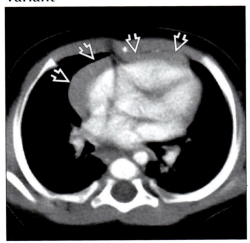 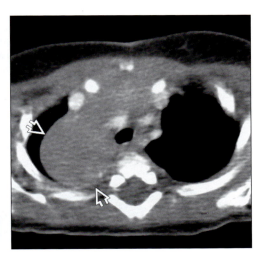

(Left) Axial CECT in a young child shows normal thymus (arrows) extending inferiorly, draped over anterior aspect of heart. This should not be confused with a pericardial effusion. *(Right)* Axial CECT in young child shows retrocaval thymus, a normal variant. The thymus extends posteriorly between great vessels and veins, simulating a mass (arrows).

LYMPHOMA, THORACIC

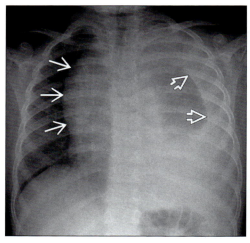

Anteroposterior radiograph shows mediastinal mass (arrows) and large left pleural effusion (open arrows).

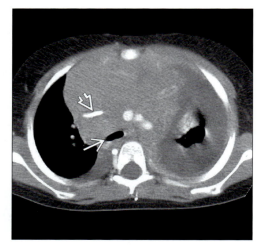

Axial CECT in same patient shows mediastinal mass, bilateral effusions, narrowing of the SVC (open arrow) and compression of the trachea (arrow) from round to oval in configuration.

TERMINOLOGY

Definitions
- Lymphoma: Malignant neoplasm that most commonly involves the lymph nodes of the mediastinum
- Categorized into Hodgkin, non-Hodgkin, and lymphoproliferative disorder

IMAGING FINDINGS

General Features
- Best diagnostic clue: Abnormal anterior mediastinal mass
- General imaging features: Lymphoma in general
  - Anterior superior mediastinal mass
  - Associated findings and complications
    - Superior vena cava obstruction
    - Central airway compression/obstruction
    - Pleural effusion
    - Pericardial effusion
  - Hodgkin lymphoma
    - 85% intrathoracic involvement at presentation
    - Most commonly involves anterior superior mediastinal nodes
    - Nodes rarely calcify before treatment: 5% post therapy
    - Lung: Near 0% at presentation, almost always in conjunction with nodes
    - Multiple pulmonary nodules or multifocal consolidation
    - Pleural effusion (15%)
  - Non-Hodgkin lymphoma
    - Initially, 50% intrathoracic involvement
    - Anterior and posterior nodes equally likely except lymphoblastic and large B-cell lymphoma primarily involve anterior mediastinum
    - Lung: Multiple pulmonary nodules may cavitate
    - Airspace mass (solitary or multiple, includes pseudolymphoma)
    - Diffuse reticular thickening (lymphocytic interstitial pneumonia)
    - Pleura: Effusions or focal pleural mass
  - Post transplant lymphoproliferative disorder (PTLD)
    - Nodules: Peripheral and basilar, no air-bronchograms, rarely cavitate
    - Focal consolidation: Bronchiolitis obliterans organizing pneumonia (BOOP) like
    - Hilar and mediastinal adenopathy
    - Mediastinal nodes more common with cardiac transplant
    - Lung nodules more common with immunodeficiency

DDx: Large Mediastinal Mass

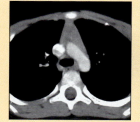

Normal Thymus Teen

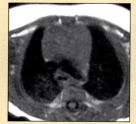

Normal Thymus Young

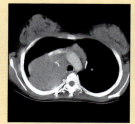

Pseudotumor

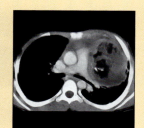

Teratoma

LYMPHOMA, THORACIC

Key Facts

Imaging Findings
- Anterior superior mediastinal mass
- Associated findings and complications
- Superior vena cava obstruction
- Central airway compression/obstruction
- Pleural effusion
- Pericardial effusion
- Hodgkin lymphoma
- 85% intrathoracic involvement at presentation
- Non-Hodgkin lymphoma
- Initially, 50% intrathoracic involvement
- 60% of children with mediastinal lymphoma have associated respiratory symptoms from airway compression
- CT showing greater than 50% reduction in area of trachea at level of obstruction associated with potential development of respiratory failure during induction of anesthesia
- Most mediastinal lymphomas are PET avid

Top Differential Diagnoses
- Normal thymus
- Pulmonary pseudotumor
- Germ cell tumor
- Thymoma

Clinical Issues
- Lymphoma uncommon in young children
- Hodgkin: Good, 90% cure
- Non-Hodgkin: Depends on bulk and histopathologic diagnosis

Radiographic Findings
- Radiography
  o Mediastinal mass
  o Look for evidence of complications listed above
  o Normal trachea should not be displaced posteriorly
    ▪ When displaced posteriorly or narrowed, evidence of airway compression
    ▪ Finding can be used to help differentiate mediastinal mass from normal thymus in young children

Fluoroscopic Findings
- Fluoroscopy during respiration quick way to tell normal thymus (soft and pliable during respiratory cycle) from mediastinal mass (hard, non-moving)

CT Findings
- Mediastinal mass
  o Irregular borders, heterogeneous attenuation and enhancement, compression of adjacent structures, irregular shape
    ▪ Normal thymus: Homogeneous attenuation and enhancement, no associated compression, smooth borders, quadrilateral shape in young children and triangular in teenagers
  o Lack of calcifications
    ▪ Calcifications in anterior mediastinal mass suggest pulmonary pseudotumor or germ cell tumor
- Airway compression
  o 60% of children with mediastinal lymphoma have associated respiratory symptoms from airway compression
  o Airway compression associated with increased chance of death during induction of anesthesia
  o CT showing greater than 50% reduction in area of trachea at level of obstruction associated with potential development of respiratory failure during induction of anesthesia
  o In addition, combination of both airway compression and superior vena cava (SVC) obstruction associated with even greater risk
- Other associated complications: Pleural or pericardial effusions, lung involvement

MR Findings
- MRI not typically utilized to evaluate mediastinal lymphoma

Nuclear Medicine Findings
- PET
  o Most mediastinal lymphomas are PET avid
  o In comparison with conventional imaging and PET, PET changed the initial staging and/or treatment in 10.5% of patients
  o There is slight uptake in normal thymus which can present a diagnostic dilemma

Other Modality Findings
- Galium often utilized to follow lymphoma with most lymphomas being gallium avid

Imaging Recommendations
- Best imaging tool
  o CT most commonly utilized for anatomic extent of disease
  o PET may also show promise in management

DIFFERENTIAL DIAGNOSIS

Normal thymus
- Large normal thymus typically occurs in young children, < 5 years of age
- Lymphoma uncommon in young patients, more common in teenagers
- Normal thymus: Homogeneous attenuation, smooth borders, does not compress adjacent structures

Pulmonary pseudotumor
- "Granulomatous disease gone wild"
- If you see a mediastinal mass or hilar lymphadenopathy that contains calcifications in a child, consider pulmonary pseudotumor
- Evidence of old granulomatous disease, such as calcified pulmonary nodules

Germ cell tumor
- May demonstrate fat or calcium

Demographics
- Age

GERM CELL TUMORS, MEDIASTINUM

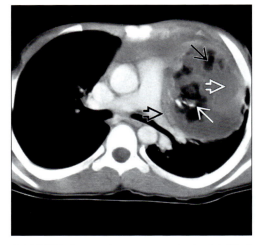

Axial CECT shows a large mass containing fat (black arrow), calcium (white arrow), and soft tissue (white open arrow) attenuation material with preservation of fat planes (black open arrow).

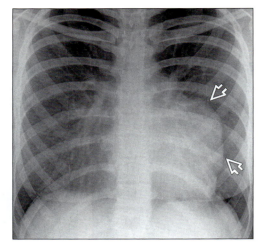

Anteroposterior radiograph shows a convex contour abnormality of the cardiomediastinal silhouette in the region of the left atrial appendage (arrows).

TERMINOLOGY

Abbreviations and Synonyms
- Germ cell tumors (GCT), mediastinal germ cell tumors (MGCT), teratoma, seminomas, nonseminomatous

Definitions
- Tumor derived from primordial germ cells that differentiate into embryonic and extraembryonic structures
- Teratoma: Majority are benign and mature = mature teratoma
  - Malignant or potentially malignant: Immature teratoma; malignant; teratoma with malignant components
- Malignant germ cell tumor = seminomas and non seminomatous germ cell tumors
- Seminoma: Germinoma and dysgerminoma
- Nonseminomatous germ cell tumor (NSGCT): Embryonal cell, endodermal sinus/yolk sac, choriocarcinoma, and mixed germ cell tumor

IMAGING FINDINGS

General Features
- Best diagnostic clue: Large anterior mediastinal mass arising within or adjacent to the thymus

- Location
  - Anterior mediastinum
  - Posterior mediastinum in 3-8%
- Morphology
  - Mature Teratoma: Classically demonstrates a combination of soft tissue, fat, calcium, and fluid signal/attenuation
  - Seminoma: Homogeneous, bulky soft tissue mass
  - NSGCT: Heterogeneous soft tissue masses

Radiographic Findings
- Radiography
  - Mature teratoma
    - Lopsided, round, sharply-marginated, anterior mediastinal mass
    - ≈ 25% calcify: Central or peripheral, curvilinear or solid; rarely may form teeth
  - Seminoma
    - Bulky, lobulated, anterior mediastinal mass
    - Calcification rare
  - NSGCT
    - Large, anterior mediastinal mass: Smooth or lobulated
    - Pleural or pericardial effusions may be present
    - May have signs of invasion of local structures
    - Pulmonary metastases not uncommon

CT Findings
- NECT

DDx: Anterior Mediastinal Mass

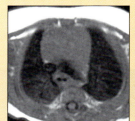
Normal Thymus

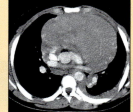
Lymphoma

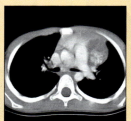
Vascular Malf

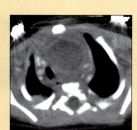
Thymic Cyst

GERM CELL TUMORS, MEDIASTINUM

Key Facts

Terminology
- Tumor derived from primordial germ cells that differentiate into embryonic and extraembryonic structures
- Teratoma: Majority are benign and mature = mature teratoma
- Seminoma: Germinoma and dysgerminoma
- Nonseminomatous germ cell tumor (NSGCT): Embryonal cell, endodermal sinus/yolk sac, choriocarcinoma, and mixed germ cell tumor

Imaging Findings
- Best diagnostic clue: Large anterior mediastinal mass arising within or adjacent to the thymus
- Mature Teratoma: Classically demonstrates a combination of soft tissue, fat, calcium, and fluid signal/attenuation
- CECT better defines extent of lesion and invasion into or erosion of structures
- Mature teratoma: Enhancement of rim of cyst and septations
- Seminoma: Mild enhancement
- NSGCT: Enhancement of peripheral soft tissue around central necrotic region

Top Differential Diagnoses
- Thymoma
- Lymphoma
- Vascular malformation

Pathology
- Etiology: Local transformation of primordial germ cells that are misplaced during embryogenesis

---

- Mature teratoma
  - Prevascular, extending predominantly into one side of the mediastinum
  - Closely applied to great vessels or pericardium
  - One or more cystic areas
  - May demonstrate complications such as endobronchial rupture, pleural or pericardial effusions
  - CT sensitive for detecting fat, fluid, and calcified components
- Seminoma
  - Large, lobulated mass of near homogeneous soft tissue attenuation
  - Less commonly heterogeneous with central areas of low attenuation (necrosis)
  - Often straddles midline
  - May extend into middle and posterior mediastinum
  - May infiltrate fat planes or invade structures
  - Calcification rare
  - May have lymphadenopathy
- NSGCT
  - Large, heterogeneous attenuation
  - Often have a prominent central area of low attenuation ($\approx$ 50%)
  - Irregular margins with obliterated fat planes
  - May invade lung, chest wall, and diaphragm
  - Lymphadenopathy and lung or liver metastases may be present
- CECT
  - CECT better defines extent of lesion and invasion into or erosion of structures
  - Mature teratoma: Enhancement of rim of cyst and septations
  - Seminoma: Mild enhancement
  - NSGCT: Enhancement of peripheral soft tissue around central necrotic region

MR Findings
- T1WI
  - Mature teratoma: Well-circumscribed lesions with regions of signal representing fat, soft tissue, calcium, and fluid depending on contents
    - Fluid varies in signal due to varying protein content
- T2WI
  - Mature teratoma: Well-circumscribed with signal dependent on tissue types in lesion
    - Fluid is of increased signal

Imaging Recommendations
- Best imaging tool: CECT demonstrates differing tissue components and demonstrates extent of disease and complications

DIFFERENTIAL DIAGNOSIS

Normal thymus
- Normal thymus appears as a large quadrilateral shaped, homogeneous mass in young children

Thymoma
- Thymoma associated with paraneoplastic syndromes
- Usually older (> 40 years)

Lymphoma
- Lymphoma rarely calcifies before treatment

Vascular malformation
- May have fluid and calcium components, but not fat
- May have soft tissue attenuation following bleed or infection

Thymic cyst
- Congenital or acquired
- Asymptomatic, calcification rare

Thymolipoma
- Predominantly fat; often has a whorled appearance

PATHOLOGY

General Features
- General path comments: Derived from all 3 cell lines or embryologic cell rests

GERM CELL TUMORS, MEDIASTINUM

- Etiology: Local transformation of primordial germ cells that are misplaced during embryogenesis
- Epidemiology: Mature teratoma: 24% of anterior mediastinal tumors in children → 10% in adults
- Associated abnormalities
  - NSGCT
    - 20% Klinefelter syndrome (gynecomastia, testicular atrophy, increased Follicle stimulating hormone)
    - Associated with hematologic malignancies which usually occur at same time

Gross Pathologic & Surgical Features
- Mature teratoma: Well-encapsulated tumor that usually have a prominent cyst → multilocular > unilocular
  - Most have a solid component, but rarely entirely solid
  - May be adherent to mediastinal structures
- Seminoma: Unencapsulated, well-circumscribed, large, usually solid mass
  - Central hemorrhage, necrosis, and cyst formation are rare
  - May adhere to or invade mediastinal structures
- NSGCT: Unencapsulated, irregularly marginated, heterogeneous large masses
  - Large areas of necrosis, hemorrhage, and cyst formation
  - Invade local structures

Microscopic Features
- Mature teratoma
  - Multiple tissues representing one or more of the germinal layers: Ectoderm, mesoderm, and endoderm
- Seminoma
  - Uniform sheets of round cells admixed with lymphocytes
- Nonseminomatous
  - Embryonal: Large malignant cells arranged in sheets or tubular/acinar patterns
  - Endodermal sinus: Glandular cords of neoplastic cells
  - Choriocarcinoma: Large, round, multinucleated cells (syncytiotrophoblastic) arranged in sheets; hemorrhage

CLINICAL ISSUES

Presentation
- Most common signs/symptoms
  - Mediastinum is the most common site of extragonadal germ cell tumors (50-70%)
  - Mature teratoma: 60% of germ cell tumors
    - Usually asymptomatic; large tumors may present with dyspnea or chest pain
    - Infants may present with respiratory distress
    - Gastric/pancreatic juices may cause erosion into tracheobronchial tree, pericardium, pleural space, and lung
  - Seminoma: 30% of germ cell tumors
    - Usually symptomatic (70-80%)
    - Most common malignant germ cell tumor of mediastinum
    - Symptoms related to tumor size and location, and compression or invasion of adjacent structures
    - Chest pain, shortness of breath, hoarseness, dysphagia are most common
    - Less commonly: Fever, weight loss, superior vena cava obstruction (10%), aortic or pulmonary artery compression
    - Elevated beta-human chorionic gonadotropin (β-HCG) in ≈ 10%; normal alpha fetoprotein (AFP)
  - Nonseminomatous: 10% of germ cell tumors
    - Usually symptomatic (90-100%)
    - Related to invasion or compression of adjacent mediastinal structures; proportional to tumor size
    - Chest pain, dyspnea, cough, fever, weight loss
    - ↑ AFP in ≈ 80%, ↑ β-HCG in ≈ 60%, ↑ lactose dehydrogenase (LDH) in ≈ 30%

Demographics
- Age: Most common under 40 years
- Gender
  - Mature teratoma: M = F
  - Seminoma and nonseminomatous germ cell tumor
    - Children: M = F
    - Teenagers and adults: M > F

Natural History & Prognosis
- Mature Teratoma: Excellent prognosis with complete excision
- Seminoma: Majority (90%) have good prognosis with a 5 year survival rate of 88%
- Nonseminomatous GCT: Variable depending on AFP, beta-hCG, and LDH levels, and presence of nonpulmonary metastases (poor prognosis)

Treatment
- Mature teratoma: Surgery
- Seminoma: Chemotherapy followed by radiation for bulky tumors and surgery for residual disease
- Nonseminomatous: Chemotherapy and surgery

SELECTED REFERENCES

1. Strollo DC et al: Primary mediastinal malignant germ cell neoplasms: imaging features. Chest Surg Clin N Am. 12(4):645-58, 2002
2. Choi SJ et al: Mediastinal teratoma: CT differentiation of ruptured and unruptured tumors. AJR. 171:591-4, 1998
3. Moran CA et al: Primary germ cell tumors of the mediastinum: I. Analysis of 322 cases with special emphasis on teratomatous lesions and a proposal for histopathologic classification and clinical staging. Cancer. 80(4):681-90, 1997
4. Strollo DC et al: Primary mediastinal tumors: Part I. Tumors of the anterior mediastinum. Chest. 112:511-22, 1997
5. Rosado-de-Christenson ML et al: From the archives of the AFIP. Mediastinal germ cell tumors: Radiologic and pathologic correlation. Radiographics. 12:1013-30, 1992

GERM CELL TUMORS, MEDIASTINUM

IMAGE GALLERY

Typical

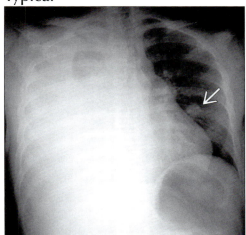
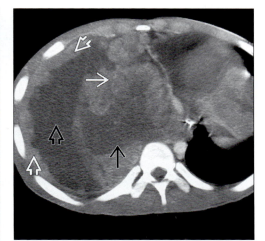

(Left) Anteroposterior radiograph in patient with seminoma shows complete opacification of right hemithorax with deviation of mediastinum to left. Rounded lesion adjacent to left heart border *(arrow)* was solitary metastasis. *(Right)* Axial CECT in same patient shows heterogeneous mass with solid *(white arrow)* and necrotic *(black arrow)* regions. Note pleural thickening *(white open arrows)* and effusion *(black open arrow)*.

Typical

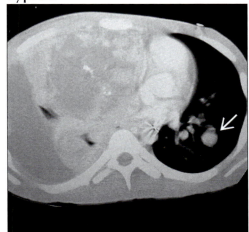
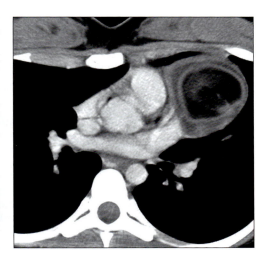

(Left) Axial CECT in same patient shows a well-circumscribed metastatic nodule in the left lower lobe *(arrow)* with complete opacification of the right hemithorax. *(Right)* Axial CECT shows a well-circumscribed mass containing fat, fluid, and soft tissue attenuation material, adherent to the pulmonary artery.

Typical

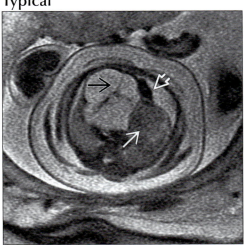
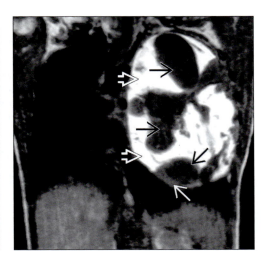

(Left) Axial T2* GRE MR shows a fetal MR demonstrating a cystic mass *(black arrow)* with soft tissue *(white arrow)* and calcific signal regions *(white open arrow)*. Necropsy confirmed teratoma. *(Right)* Coronal STIR MR shows a well-circumscribed mass containing soft tissue *(white arrow)*, fat *(black arrows)* and fluid *(white open arrows)* signal material in a mature teratoma.

PLEUROPULMONARY BLASTOMA

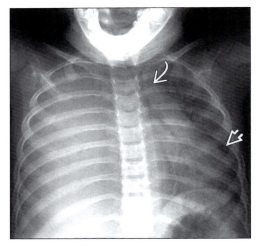

Anteroposterior radiograph shows opacification of the right hemithorax with leftward shift of the trachea (curved arrow), mediastinum and heart (open arrow). No rib erosions are seen.

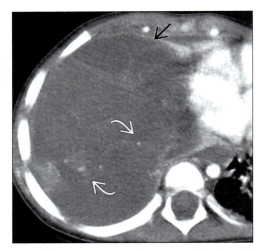

Axial CECT shows a large soft tissue mass filling the right chest, pushing the heart leftward. A pleural effusion is anterior to mass (arrow). Vessels traverse the mass (curved arrows).

TERMINOLOGY

Abbreviations and Synonyms
- Pleuropulmonary blastoma (PPB)

Definitions
- Rare aggressive malignant primary neoplasm of the pleuropulmonary mesenchyme occurring in early childhood associated with poor prognosis

IMAGING FINDINGS

General Features
- Best diagnostic clue
  ○ Large thoracic soft tissue mass (type II and III)
    ▪ Heterogeneous low attenuation
    ▪ May have associated pleural effusion
    ▪ Contralateral mediastinal shift
    ▪ Typically no chest wall invasion
  ○ Lung cyst (type I)
  ○ Child less than 5 years old
- Location
  ○ Intrathoracic (100%)
  ○ Pleural-based or intraparenchymal
  ○ My invade or arise in mediastinum and diaphragm
  ○ May arise in lung cysts: Congenital cystic adenomatoid malformation (CCAM), bronchogenic cyst, cystic mesenchymal hamartoma, pulmonary sequestration cysts
- Size: Large
- Morphology: Heterogeneous soft tissue mass and/or cysts

Radiographic Findings
- Radiography
  ○ Frequently presents late as opacified hemithorax with contralateral mediastinal shift
  ○ May present as a mediastinal mass
  ○ Diaphragmatic masses have been reported
  ○ Incidental finding of a pulmonary cyst (type I)
  ○ Pneumothorax
  ○ Hemothorax

CT Findings
- CECT
  ○ Type I PPB
    ▪ Benign-appearing air-filled lung cysts
  ○ Type II and III PPB
    ▪ Usually large heterogeneous solid mass originating from pulmonary pleura or parenchyma
    ▪ May also arise in mediastinum and diaphragm
    ▪ Can invade mediastinum, vessels, and diaphragm
    ▪ Rarely invades chest wall
    ▪ Metastases: CNS, bone, liver

DDx: Pediatric Chest Mass

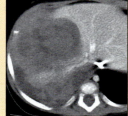
Undiff Sarcoma

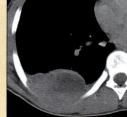
Ewing Sarcoma

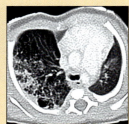
CCAM

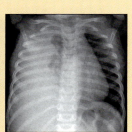
Empyema

PLEUROPULMONARY BLASTOMA

Key Facts

Terminology
- Pleuropulmonary blastoma (PPB)
- Rare aggressive malignant primary neoplasm of the pleuropulmonary mesenchyme occurring in early childhood associated with poor prognosis

Imaging Findings
- Large thoracic soft tissue mass (type II and III)
- Typically no chest wall invasion
- Lung cyst (type I)
- Frequently presents late as opacified hemithorax with contralateral mediastinal shift

Top Differential Diagnoses
- Rhabdomyosarcoma
- Undifferentiated sarcoma
- Ewing sarcoma
- Primitive neuroectodermal tumor (PNET)
- Parapneumonic effusion/empyema
- Other lung cysts (type I)

Clinical Issues
- Respiratory distress
- Gender: M = F
- High association (25%) with close relatives with childhood cancers: Should screen family

Diagnostic Checklist
- Consider PPB when see large chest mass in young child
- Type I PPB is radiographically indistinguishable from benign lung cysts
- Argument for surgical excision of all lung cysts found in children

---

- Rarely involves lymph nodes
- Frequently associated with pleural effusion
- Typically unilateral

Ultrasonographic Findings
- Grayscale Ultrasound
  - Solid heterogeneous mass (types II and III)
  - Pleural fluid

Imaging Recommendations
- Best imaging tool
  - CECT
    - Typically used to evaluate initial extent of disease and follow after resection and treatment
- Protocol advice: Routine CECT generally adequate

DIFFERENTIAL DIAGNOSIS

Rhabdomyosarcoma
- Solid mass
- May be indistinguishable
- May invade chest wall

Undifferentiated sarcoma
- May be indistinguishable
- May be more likely to invade chest wall

Ewing sarcoma
- Frequently associated with rib destruction
- More likely extrapleural, not associated with pleural effusion

Primitive neuroectodermal tumor (PNET)
- Frequently invades chest wall (Askin tumor)
- May have similar appearance

Pulmonary inflammatory pseudotumor
- Often contains calcifications
- Typically smaller than PPB

Parapneumonic effusion/empyema
- Similar chest radiograph: Opacified hemithorax with contralateral mediastinal shift
- Evaluate pleural fluid
  - Culture
  - Cytology
- Resolves with antibiotics and pleural fluid drainage

Other lung cysts (type I)
- Congential lung cysts
  - CCAM
  - Bronchogenic cyst
  - Pulmonary sequestration
- Radiographically indistinguishable from type I PPB

Neuroblastoma
- Posterior mediastinum
- Extension into widened neural foramen and spinal canal
- Rib erosion
- May contain coarse calcifications

PATHOLOGY

General Features
- General path comments
  - Primitive pulmonary tumor analogous to Wilms tumor in the kidney, neuroblastoma in the adrenal gland, and hepatoblastoma in the liver
  - Histologically distinct from the adult pulmonary blastoma, which has malignant epithelial and mesenchymal components
    - PPB has no malignant epithelial component
- Genetics: Cytogenetic analysis: Polysomy of chromosome 8 (present in all mesenchymal elements, but not in epithelial cells)
- Etiology: Unknown
- Epidemiology
  - Very uncommon tumor
  - High incidence of childhood cancers in close family members (25%)

Gross Pathologic & Surgical Features
- Soft, fleshy, friable, vascular tumor (types II and III)
- Cystic (type I)

PLEUROPULMONARY BLASTOMA

Microscopic Features
- Primitive blastema and a malignant mesenchymal stroma that often demonstrates heterologous elements such as cartilage differentiation
- Myxoid components resemble embryonal rhabdomyosarcoma
- Blastema components may show numerous mitoses (20/HPF) and foci of necrosis
- Cystic component lined by benign respiratory-type epithelium

Staging, Grading or Classification Criteria
- Type I: Purely cystic
- Type II: Cystic and solid
- Type III: Solid

CLINICAL ISSUES

Presentation
- Most common signs/symptoms
  - Respiratory distress
    - Often present at late stage with symptoms from airway compression
  - +/- Fever
- Other signs/symptoms: Occasionally cystic lung lesion found incidentally on chest radiograph (type I)

Demographics
- Age
  - Type I: 10 months
  - Type II: 34 months
  - Type III: 44 months
- Gender: M = F
- Familial childhood cancer
  - High association (25%) with close relatives with childhood cancers: Should screen family
  - Patient at higher risk of developing other childhood cancer

Natural History & Prognosis
- Type I
  - Presents at younger age
  - Better prognosis than types II and III
  - Complete surgical resection may be curative
  - Recurrent type I disease frequently progresses to more malignant type (II or III)
- Type II and III
  - Present at slightly older age
  - Worse prognosis
- Overall, aggressive tumor with poor prognosis

Treatment
- Type I: Complete surgical resection +/- chemotherapy
- Type II: Surgical resection + chemotherapy
  - Benefit of local radiation controversial
- Type III: Surgical resection + chemotherapy, consider neoadjuvant chemotherapy
  - Benefit of local radiation controversial

DIAGNOSTIC CHECKLIST

Consider
- Consider PPB when see large chest mass in young child
- Type I PPB is radiographically indistinguishable from benign lung cysts
  - Argument for surgical excision of all lung cysts found in children

Image Interpretation Pearls
- Consider solid tumor such as PPB when presented with a chest radiograph with an opacified hemithorax and cardiomediastinal shift
- PPB rarely invades the chest wall, unlike other solid pediatric chest tumors

SELECTED REFERENCES

1. Naffaa LN et al: Imaging findings in pleuropulmonary blastoma. Pediatr Radiol. 2005
2. Dosios T et al: Pleuropulmonary blastoma in childhood. A malignant degeneration of pulmonary cysts. Pediatr Surg Int. 20(11-12):863-5, 2004
3. Hasiotou M et al: Pleuropulmonary blastoma in the area of a previously diagnosed congenital lung cyst: report of two cases. Acta Radiol. 45(3):289-92, 2004
4. MacSweeney F et al: An assessment of the expanded classification of congenital cystic adenomatoid malformations and their relationship to malignant transformation. Am J Surg Pathol. 27(8):1139-46, 2003
5. Sebire NJ et al: Gains of chromosome 8 in pleuropulmonary blastomas of childhood. Pediatr Dev Pathol. 5(2):221-2, 2002
6. Granata C et al: Pleuropulmonary blastoma. Eur J Pediatr Surg. 11(4):271-3, 2001
7. Papagiannopoulos KA et al: Pleuropulmonary blastoma: is prophylactic resection of congenital lung cysts effective? Ann Thorac Surg. 72(2):604-5, 2001
8. Parsons SK et al: Aggressive multimodal treatment of pleuropulmonary blastoma. Ann Thorac Surg. 72(3):939-42, 2001
9. Perdikogianni C et al: Pleuropulmonary blastoma: an aggressive intrathoracic neoplasm of childhood. Pediatr Hematol Oncol. 18(4):259-66, 2001
10. Indolfi P et al: Pleuropulmonary blastoma: management and prognosis of 11 cases. Cancer. 89(6):1396-401, 2000
11. Kukkady A et al: Pleuropulmonary blastoma: four cases. Pediatr Surg Int. 16(8):595-8, 2000
12. Nicol KK et al: The cytomorphology of pleuropulmonary blastoma. Arch Pathol Lab Med. 124(3):416-8, 2000
13. Wright JR Jr: Pleuropulmonary blastoma: A case report documenting transition from type I (cystic) to type III (solid). Cancer. 88(12):2853-8, 2000
14. Priest JR et al: Pleuropulmonary blastoma: a clinicopathologic study of 50 cases. Cancer. 80(1):147-61, 1997
15. Priest JR et al: Pleuropulmonary blastoma: a marker for familial disease. J Pediatr. 128(2):220-4, 1996
16. Dehner LP: Pleuropulmonary blastoma is THE pulmonary blastoma of childhood. Semin Diagn Pathol. 11(2):144-51, 1994

PLEUROPULMONARY BLASTOMA

IMAGE GALLERY

Typical

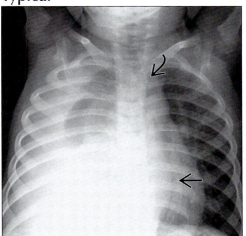
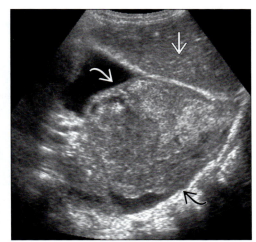

(Left) Anteroposterior radiograph shows near complete opacification of the right chest with leftward shift of the trachea *(curved arrow)*. There is shift of the left paraspinal line *(arrow)*. *(Right)* Sagittal ultrasound shows a solid mass *(curved arrows)* at the right posterior costophrenic angle, above the liver *(arrow)*. It is surrounded by pleural fluid (black around mass).

Typical

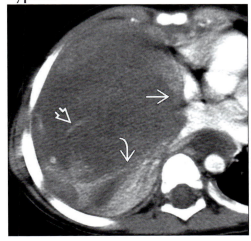
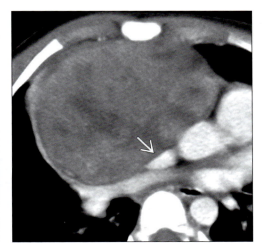

(Left) Axial CECT shows a large solid PPB filling the right chest and pushing the lung posteriorly *(curved arrow)* and the heart leftward *(arrow)*. Large vessel courses through tumor *(open arrow)*. *(Right)* Axial CECT shows a large heterogeneous anterior mediastinal PPB that pushes the mediastinal vascular structures to the left and posteriorly. Note the effacement of the SVC *(arrow)*.

Other

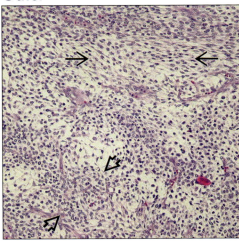
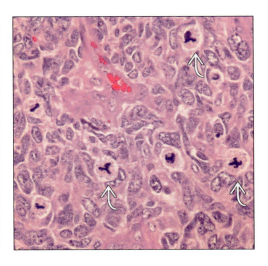

(Left) Micropathology, low power shows a biphasic cell pattern, with a myxoid pattern *(arrows)* and spindle cells *(open arrows)*. Pattern resembles embryonal rhabdomyosarcoma, common in PPB. *(Right)* Micropathology, high power shows dense cellularity, nuclear anaplasia, and frequent atypical mitoses *(arrows)* which are characteristic of PPB.

PULMONARY INFLAMMATORY PSEUDOTUMOR

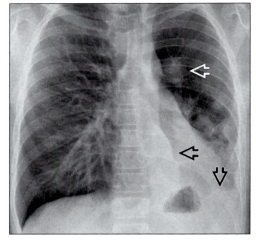

Anteroposterior radiograph shows a lobulated well-circumscribed mass abutting pleura and obscuring descending aorta (black arrows). White arrow points to a separate pleural mass, rare.

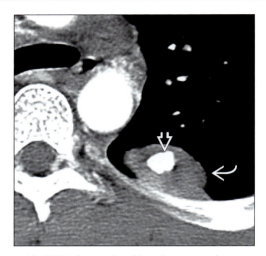

Axial CECT shows pleural-based mass in the same patient (curved arrow). The open arrow points to a calcification in the mass, seen in 25% of cases, but more common in children.

TERMINOLOGY

Abbreviations and Synonyms
- Inflammatory myofibroblastic tumor, inflammatory myofibrohistiocytic proliferation, histiocytoma, fibrous histiocytoma, plasma cell-histiocytoma complex, plasma cell granuloma, plasma cell tumor, xanthoma, fibroxanthoma, xanthogranuloma

Definitions
- Most common primary lung mass in children
  - 50% of benign pediatric intrapulmonary tumors
- Mass consists of inflammatory cells and myofibroblastic spindle cells

IMAGING FINDINGS

General Features
- Best diagnostic clue
  - Solid, sharply circumscribed chest mass
  - No pathognomonic features
- Location
  - May be anywhere in chest
    - Pleura
    - Lung parenchyma
    - Mediastinum
    - Endobronchial
    - Intravascular/intracardiac
    - Esophagus
- Size
  - Variable
    - Average 4-5 cm
    - May fill the hemithorax
- Morphology: Solid, sharply circumscribed, and lobulated, but wide range of appearances

Radiographic Findings
- Radiography
  - Wide range of appearances
    - Most common: Solitary, peripheral, sharply circumscribed, lobulated mass most commonly located in the lower lobes
    - May originate as an infiltrating mass in mediastinum
    - May mimic progressive atelectasis
    - Endobronchial lesions may cause air-trapping, post-obstructive atelectasis, or pneumonia
    - Often calcifies

Fluoroscopic Findings
- Esophagram
  - Esophageal narrowing
    - When mass invades or arises in esophagus

CT Findings
- CECT

DDx: Pediatric Solid Pulmonary Mass

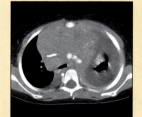
Lymphoma

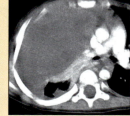
PPB

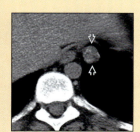
Osteosarcoma Met

PULMONARY INFLAMMATORY PSEUDOTUMOR

Key Facts

Terminology
- Most common primary lung mass in children
- Mass consists of inflammatory cells and myofibroblastic spindle cells

Imaging Findings
- Nonspecific sharply circumscribed solid mass
- 25% have calcifications, but more frequent in children
- Adenopathy rare

Top Differential Diagnoses
- Sarcoma
- Metastatic pulmonary mass
- Lymphoma
- Granulomatous disease

Pathology
- Etiology: Likely unregulated inflammatory reparative response to injured tissue

Clinical Issues
- Age: Most common second decade, but may occur at any age
- Controversial relationship between inflammatory pseudotumor and tumor
- Most consider pediatric inflammatory pseudotumors to have no malignant potential
- Progression to sarcoma has been reported

Diagnostic Checklist
- Definitive diagnosis by imaging alone difficult
- Biopsy or excision usually required for exclusion of malignancy

---

- Nonspecific sharply circumscribed solid mass
  - May be found virtually anywhere in chest
- Heterogeneous attenuation and enhancement
- 25% have calcifications, but more frequent in children
  - Amorphous, mixed, fleck-like, or heavy
- Adenopathy rare
- Sometimes associated with atelectasis and pleural effusion
- 5% multiple
- 10% endobronchial
- Mediastinal mass
  - Encase and sometimes narrow bronchi
  - Compress mediastinal vessels

MR Findings
- T1WI: Intermediate heterogeneous signal intensity mass
- T2WI
  - High signal intensity
  - Best for evaluating cardiac involvement or vascular lesion

Imaging Recommendations
- Best imaging tool
  - Depends on location
    - CECT: Lung parenchyma, pleura, mediastinum
    - MRI: Cardiac or vascular involvement
    - Esophagram: Evaluate esophageal involvement when mass abuts esophagus
- Protocol advice: Routine protocols generally adequate

DIFFERENTIAL DIAGNOSIS

Sarcoma
- More likely to be large and invade adjacent structures
- Histologic similarities (spindle cells) with fine needle aspirations and frozen sections, often requiring more tissue for exclusion of malignancy
- May be radiographically indistinguishable

Other aggressive primary neoplasm
- Pleuropulmonary blastoma (PPB), Ewing sarcoma, etc.
- Biopsy typically required for exclusion

Metastatic pulmonary mass
- More likely multiple
- Less likely calcified, except for osteosarcoma

Lymphoma
- Usually associated with more extensive adenopathy
- May be radiographically indistinguishable
- Untreated lymphoma does not typically calcify

Granulomatous disease
- Nodules tend to be smaller, multiple, and frequently calcified
- Frequently have associated calcified hilar and mediastinal lymph nodes
- May be radiographically indistinguishable

Pulmonary sequestration
- Solid well-circumscribed mass with occasional cystic areas
- Systemic arterial supply
- Most commonly located at left posteromedial lung base

Hamartoma
- Round or oval sharply defined pulmonary mass
- Congenital tumor composed of lung's normal elements in abnormal proportions
- Seen in older children or adults
- Occasionally calcify

Chondroma
- Carney's triad: Pulmonary chondroma, gastric smooth muscle tumor (leiomyoma/leiomyosarcoma), and extra-adrenal paraganglioma: Usually young, mostly female patients
- No lung lobe predilection
- 45% calcify
- Considered by some as a hamartoma

PULMONARY INFLAMMATORY PSEUDOTUMOR

Hemangioma
- Rare, usually solitary
- Histology: Sclerosing hemangioma of the lung

Other endobronchial masses (if endobronchial mass)
- Foreign body
- Carcinoid
- Mucoepidermoid tumor

PATHOLOGY

General Features
- Etiology: Likely unregulated inflammatory reparative response to injured tissue
- Epidemiology: Frequently occurs in children with prior pneumonia (20%), but no definite link

Gross Pathologic & Surgical Features
- Firm, gray, well-defined, lobulated parenchymal masses with a whorled and heterogeneous appearance

Microscopic Features
- Proliferation of spindle-shaped fibroblasts and permeation of collagen with lymphocytes, fibrosis, granulomatous inflammation, lymphoid hyperplasia, and intraalveolar fibrosis at the edge of the tumor
- 3 histologic subtypes
  - Fibrous histiocytic pattern
    - Most common
    - Spindle-shaped myofibroblasts arranged in whorls
  - Organizing pneumonia pattern
    - Airways filled with plump fibroblasts
    - Foamy histiocytes and parenchyma replaced with a mixture of histiocytes, mononuclear cells, and fibroblasts
  - Lymphohistiocytic pattern
    - Least common
    - Mixture of lymphocytes and plasma cells with only minimal fibrous connective tissue
- Fine needle aspiration (FNA)
  - Cytomorphology
    - Nonspecific mixed inflammatory infiltrate
    - Spindle cell component, typically fibroblasts
    - Some cells have reactive cytological changes and atypia, making it difficult to differentiate from a malignant neoplastic process

CLINICAL ISSUES

Presentation
- Most common signs/symptoms
  - Nonspecific
    - Cough
    - Chest pain
    - Fever
    - Dyspnea
    - Hemoptysis
- Other signs/symptoms
  - Asthma exacerbation (endobronchial lesion)
  - Malaise
  - Weight loss
  - SVC syndrome (mediastinal mass)

Demographics
- Age: Most common second decade, but may occur at any age
- Gender: M ≥ F

Natural History & Prognosis
- Unpredictable natural history
  - Majority slowly increase in size, rarely spontaneously regress
- Controversial relationship between inflammatory pseudotumor and tumor
  - Most consider pediatric inflammatory pseudotumors to have no malignant potential
  - Progression to sarcoma has been reported
- 5% behave aggressively
  - May invade chest wall, mediastinum, diaphragm, pericardium
- Delayed diagnosis and treatment may result in encroachment on hilar and mediastinal structures
  - Rarely, may result in sclerosing mediastinitis
- Prognosis excellent with complete surgical excision

Treatment
- Treatment of choice: Surgical resection
- Locally aggressive lesions may require more radical surgery such as pneumonectomy
- Steroids and possibly nonsteroidal antiinflammatory drugs in cases that are incompletely resectable
- Radiation therapy controversial
- Chemotherapy controversial

DIAGNOSTIC CHECKLIST

Image Interpretation Pearls
- Often nonspecific mass with malignant tumor high in differential diagnosis
- Definitive diagnosis by imaging alone difficult
  - Biopsy or excision usually required for exclusion of malignancy

SELECTED REFERENCES

1. Hosler GA et al: Inflammatory pseudotumor: a diagnostic dilemma in cytopathology. Diagn Cytopathol. 31(4):267-70, 2004
2. Narla LD et al: Inflammatory pseudotumor. Radiographics. 23(3):719-29, 2003
3. Kim JH et al: Pulmonary inflammatory pseudotumor--a report of 28 cases. Korean J Intern Med. 17(4):252-8, 2002
4. Dahabreh J et al: Inflammatory pseudotumor: a controversial entity. Eur J Cardiothorac Surg. 16(6):670-3, 1999
5. Hedlund GL et al: Aggressive manifestations of inflammatory pulmonary pseudotumor in children. Pediatr Radiol. 29(2):112-6, 1999
6. Verbeke JI et al: Inflammatory myofibroblastic tumour of the lung manifesting as progressive atelectasis. Pediatr Radiol. 29(11):816-9, 1999
7. Agrons GA et al: Pulmonary inflammatory pseudotumor: radiologic features. Radiology. 206(2):511-8, 1998
8. Jayne D et al: Endobronchial inflammatory pseudotumour exacerbating asthma. Postgrad Med J. 73(856):98-9, 1997

PULMONARY INFLAMMATORY PSEUDOTUMOR

IMAGE GALLERY

Variant

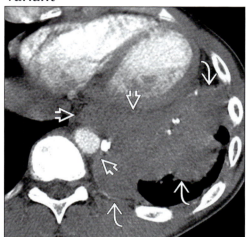
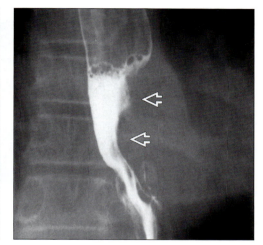

(Left) Axial CECT shows a large lobulated solid mass (curved arrows) containing calcifications. It shows aggressive features of encasing aorta, esophagus, and pericardium (open arrows). (Right) Anteroposterior upper GI shows narrowing and distortion of distal esophagus (arrows) in the same patient caused by invasion by mass. This caused dysphagia.

Variant

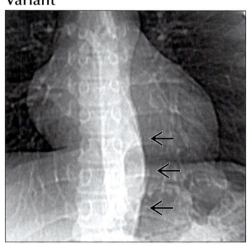
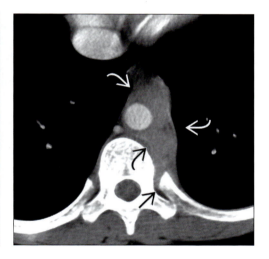

(Left) Anteroposterior radiograph shows an abnormally wide posterior mediastinum (arrows), due to a mass which is better delineated on the CT to the right. (Right) Axial CECT shows an infiltrating solid posterior mediastinal mass which partially encases the descending aorta (curved arrows) and extends between the rib and vertebral body (arrow).

Variant

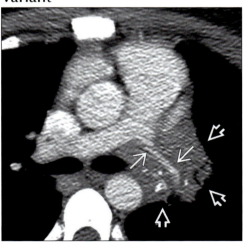
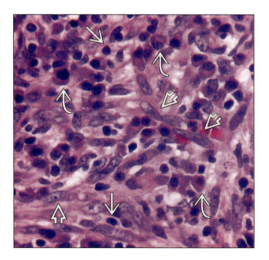

(Left) Axial CECT shows a mediastinal mass containing calcifications (open arrows) which encases and narrows the left pulmonary artery (arrows). (Right) Micropathology, high power shows mixture of spindle cells (open arrows), lymphocytes (arrows), and plasma cells (curved arrows), characteristic of inflammatory pseudotumor.

CHILD ABUSE, RIB FRACTURES

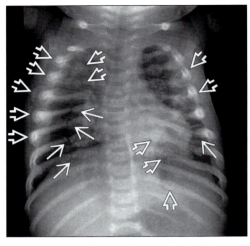

Anteroposterior radiograph shows multiple rib fractures of various ages including acute (arrows) and subacute (open arrows).

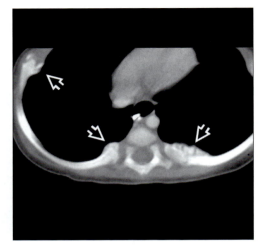

Axial CECT on child with suspected abdominal abuse shows callus formation involving rib fractures (arrows) of the bilateral posterior medial ribs and right anterior lateral rib.

TERMINOLOGY

Abbreviations and Synonyms
- Nonaccidental trauma (the more politically correct and less graphic term), battered child syndrome, child abuse, Kempe-Silverman syndrome

Definitions
- Child abuse is the intentional infliction of pain and suffering on a child
  - May be both physical and/or emotional
  - Harm by caretakers may be neglect (63%), physical abuse (19%), sexual abuse (10%), psychological abuse (8%)
- Rib fractures secondary to trauma other than child abuse are rare in infants

IMAGING FINDINGS

General Features
- Best diagnostic clue: Posterior rib fractures, adjacent to transverse process, in an infant or young child
- Location: Posterior ribs

Radiographic Findings
- Radiography
  - Rib fractures secondary to trauma such as falls or motor vehicle accidents are common in older children and adults
    - Young children's ribs are cartilaginous and pliable and rarely fracture from direct blow
  - Rib fractures in infants are almost always secondary to abuse
  - Rib fractures in children < 1 year of age
    - 82% Secondary to abuse
    - 7.7% Accidental injuries
    - 2.6% Birth trauma
    - 7.7% Underlying metabolic disease (prematurity, osteogenesis imperfecta, rickets)
  - Positive predictive value of a rib fracture for abuse in children < 3 years of age = 95%
  - Rib fracture only radiographic manifestation of child abuse in up to 29% of cases
  - Rib fractures represented 48% of bony injuries from abuse in another study
  - Rib Fractures: Radiographic appearance
    - Acute rib fractures appear as linear lucencies
    - Rib fractures may occur anterior, lateral, or posterior in abuse
    - Posterior rib fractures most common and most specific for abuse
    - Posterior ribs fracture over adjacent transverse spinous process

DDx: Rib Fractures In Infants

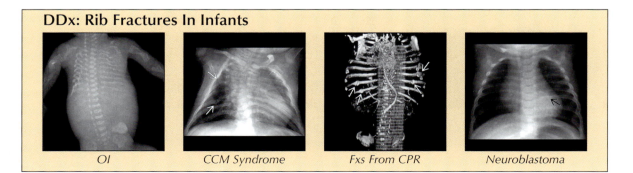

OI | CCM Syndrome | Fxs From CPR | Neuroblastoma

CHILD ABUSE, RIB FRACTURES

Key Facts

Terminology
- Child abuse is the intentional infliction of pain and suffering on a child
- Rib fractures secondary to trauma other than child abuse are rare in infants

Imaging Findings
- Positive predictive value of a rib fracture for abuse in children < 3 years of age = 95%
- Rib fracture only radiographic manifestation of child abuse in up to 29% of cases
- Rib fractures represented 48% of bony injuries from abuse in another study
- Radiography often insensitive to acute fractures as they may be nondisplaced, incomplete, or superimposed with multiple other bony structures

- Other tests that may be used to document findings of abuse
- Repeat skeletal survey in 2 weeks
- Skeletal scintigraphy
- Abdominal CT
- MRI of the brain

Pathology
- 1 out of every 100 children abused
- Parents are 77% of perpetrators

Clinical Issues
- Physical abuse much more common in young children
- Children < 1 year of age represent 44% of all abuse related deaths

---

- Radiography often insensitive to acute fractures as they may be nondisplaced, incomplete, or superimposed with multiple other bony structures
- Oblique images of chest may be helpful
- Fractures much easier to identify after callus formation becomes radiographically evident
- Callus formation becomes radiographically evident in 10-14 days following injury
○ Follow-up skeletal surveys
- Follow-up radiographic skeletal survey after 2 weeks often advocated to document extent of injuries and identify previous occult injuries after callus formation present
- Additional information regarding skeletal trauma identified in 61% of cases
- Definitive fractures increased by 27%
- Most common fractures identified on follow-up radiographic surveys include rib fractures and metaphyseal corner fractures
○ Other radiographic findings
- Metaphyseal corner fracture (highly specific)
- Scapulae fractures (specific)
- Spiral fracture of long bone in nonambulatory infant (highly suspicious)
- Multiple fractures of different ages (highly specific)
- Spinous process fracture (specific)
- Sternal fractures (specific)
- Extraskeletal manifestations

CT Findings
- CT of chest not advocated for identifying rib fractures but CT of abdomen often performed to evaluate for intraabdominal injuries or CT of chest rarely performed to evaluate for mediastinal trauma
- On such studies, important to search for and identify rib fractures
- CT Findings
  ○ Posterior rib fractures in the region of the costovertebral joints
  ○ Lung contusion: Crescentic shaped opacities, posterior location, subpleural sparing of opacified lung
  ○ Duodenal hematoma
  ○ Solid abdominal organ laceration
  ○ Pancreatitis

Nuclear Medicine Findings
- Bone Scan
  ○ Skeletal scintigraphy advocated as useful adjunct to radiographic surveys in documenting skeletal trauma or further investigating possible injuries seen on radiographs
  ○ In one study of cases which underwent both bone scan and radiography
    - 33% had injuries seen on both studies
    - 44% seen on radiography only
    - 25% seen on bone scan alone
    - Metaphyseal lesions harder to demonstrate on bone scan (65% not apparent)

Imaging Recommendations
- When abuse suspected, skeletal survey obtained to document the presence of findings of abuse for legal reasons so that the child can be removed from the abuser
- Identification and reporting of radiographic findings of abuse is important task
  ○ False-positive findings may result in removal of a non-abused child from their family
  ○ False-negative findings may result in returning a child to potentially life-threatening environment
- Other tests that may be used to document findings of abuse
  ○ Repeat skeletal survey in 2 weeks
  ○ Skeletal scintigraphy
  ○ Abdominal CT
  ○ MRI of the brain

DIFFERENTIAL DIAGNOSIS

Entities associated with multiple fractures
- Osteogenesis imperfecta (OI) and Menkes syndrome
  ○ Excessive Wormian bone formation (along cranial sutures)

CHILD ABUSE, RIB FRACTURES

○ Osteopenia

Birth trauma
- Rarely results in rib fractures
- Rib fractures only occur with large babies and difficult deliveries
- In one study of 34,946 births, no rib fractures were identified

Trauma from cardiopulmonary resuscitation (CPR)
- Fractures as a result of CPR are very rare in children
- One study showed incidence of fractures from CPR in children was 0.6%
- Most fractures involve anterior ribs
- Posterior rib fractures very rare and normally do not occur immediately adjacent to transverse process as seen in abuse

Neuroblastoma
- Can lead to rib erosion
- Should not be confused with rib fractures seen in abuse

Cerebrocostomandibular syndrome (CCM)
- Rare genetic syndrome
- Characteristic congenital gaps in ossified portions of posterior ribs
- Should not be mistaken for rib fractures

PATHOLOGY

General Features
- General path comments
  ○ Tight hold of an infants chest by adult sized hands and substantial squeezing results in potential fractures of the anterior, lateral, and posterior ribs
  ○ Posterior ribs most common location and most specific for abuse
  ○ Posterior medial rib fractures result from levering of posterior rib on transverse process
  ○ Squeezing mechanism results in fulcrum-type injury and fracture of posterior medial rib over costovertebral joint
- Epidemiology
  ○ Unfortunately common
  ○ Three million cases of suspected abuse reported in 2000 with close to one million substantiated, in USA alone
  ○ 1 out of every 100 children abused
  ○ Parents are 77% of perpetrators
  ○ 30% of fractures in infants are secondary to abuse
  ○ Fracture present in up to 55% of abused children
  ○ Up to 48% of bony injuries in infants are rib fractures

Gross Pathologic & Surgical Features
- Disruption of the cortex and adjacent bony trabeculae
- Hemorrhage and potential disruption of periosteum
- Four states: Inflammation, soft callus formation, hard callus, remodeling

CLINICAL ISSUES

Presentation
- Most common signs/symptoms
  ○ Varies depending on sites of injury and type of abuse
  ○ Lethargy not uncommon secondary to central nervous system injury
- Other signs/symptoms: Refusal to use extremity, seizures, unexplained bruising

Demographics
- Age
  ○ Physical abuse much more common in young children
  ○ Children < 1 year of age represent 44% of all abuse related deaths
- Gender
  ○ Girls abused slightly more often then boys
  ○ Sexual abuse: Girls are four times as likely to be abused then boys

Treatment
- Identification of abuse
- Documentation of abuse
- Removal of child from hostile environment

SELECTED REFERENCES

1. Barsness KA et al: The positive predictive value of rib fractures as an indicator of nonaccidental trauma in children. J Trauma. 54(6):1107-10, 2003
2. Lonergan GJ et al: From the archives of the AFIP. Child abuse: radiologic-pathologic correlation. Radiographics. 23(4):811-45, 2003
3. Mandelstam SA et al: Complementary use of radiological skeletal survey and bone scintigraphy in detection of bony injuries in suspected child abuse. Arch Dis Child. 88(5):387-90; discussion 387-90, 2003
4. Carty H et al: Non-accidental injury: a retrospective analysis of a large cohort. Eur Radiol. 12(12):2919-25, 2002
5. Bulloch B et al: Cause and clinical characteristics of rib fractures in infants. Pediatrics. 105(4):E48, 2000
6. Kleinman PK et al: Mechanical factors associated with posterior rib fractures: laboratory and case studies. Pediatr Radiol. 27(1):87-91, 1997
7. Kleinman PK et al: Follow-up skeletal surveys in suspected child abuse. AJR Am J Roentgenol. 167(4):893-6, 1996
8. Conway JJ et al: The role of bone scintigraphy in detecting child abuse. Semin Nucl Med. 23(4):321-33, 1993
9. Kleinman PK: Diagnostic imaging in infant abuse. AJR. 155:703-12, 1990
10. Silverman FN: Child abuse: the conflict of underdetection and overreporting. Pediatrics. 80(3):441-3, 1987
11. Silverman FN: Unrecognized trauma in infants, the battered child syndrome, and the syndrome of Ambroise Tardieu. Rigler Lecture. Radiology. 104(2):337-53, 1972
12. Silverman FN: The battered child. Manit Med Rev. 45(8):473-7, 1965
13. Kempe CH et al: The battered-child syndrome. By C. Henry Kempe, Frederic N. Silverman, Brandt F. Steele, William Droegemueller, and Henry K. Silver. Landmark article July 7, 1962

CHILD ABUSE, RIB FRACTURES

IMAGE GALLERY

Typical

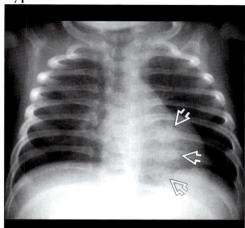
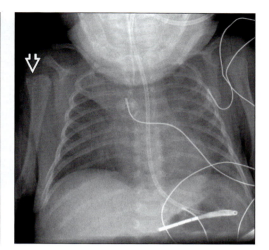

(Left) Anteroposterior radiograph shows multiple rib fractures (arrows) of the left posterior ribs with surrounding callus formation. (Right) Anteroposterior radiograph shows corner fracture (arrow) of proximal metaphysis of right humerus. There is also right upper lobe collapse.

Typical

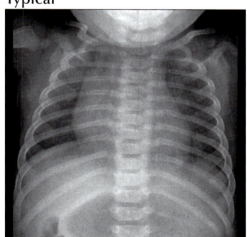
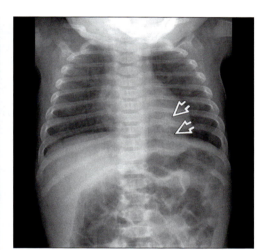

(Left) Anteroposterior radiograph obtained at presentation in an infant suspected of abuse shows no definitive fractures. Next two images on same patient. (Right) Anteroposterior radiograph obtained two weeks later shows at least two healing rib fractures (arrows) in left posterior chest.

Typical

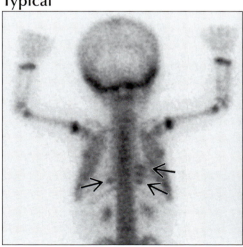
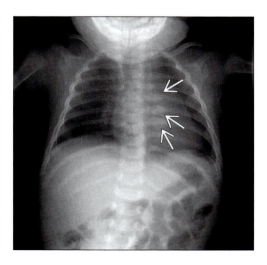

(Left) Anteroposterior bone scan in same patient as directly above shows posterior rib fractures (arrows) with three adjacent fractures on left and one on right. (Right) Anteroposterior radiograph (different patient) shows multiple, left posterior rib fractures (arrows) as thickened areas of rib from callus. The patient had other fractures elsewhere of varying ages.

NEUROBLASTOMA, THORACIC

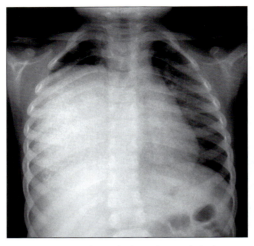

Anteroposterior radiograph shows large calcified mass in right hemithorax with rib erosion.

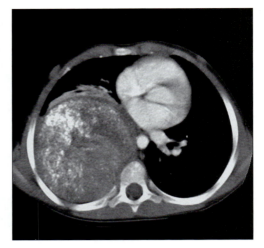

Axial CECT on same patient as on left shows large calcified mass in right hemithorax displacing right lung anteriorly and causing leftward mediastinal shift.

TERMINOLOGY

Abbreviations and Synonyms
- Neuroblastoma, thoracic (NBT)

Definitions
- Malignant thoracic tumor of primitive neural crest cells
- Invasive mass that tends to surround and encase vessels and invade neuroforamina into spinal canal
- Tendency to invade into spinal canal via neuroforamina
  - Important to recognize for presurgical planning
- Metastasizes most commonly to liver and bone
  - Low attenuation focal liver lesions or diffuse heterogeneous liver
  - Destructive bony lesions (marrow mets in up to 60% at diagnosis)
  - Lung metastasis less common but can occur
- Prognosis and patterns of disease dependent on age
  - < 1 year of age: Better prognosis, mets to liver and skin
  - > 1 year of age: Worse prognosis, mets to bone

IMAGING FINDINGS

General Features
- Best diagnostic clue: Posterior mediastinal (paraspinal) mass with calcifications
- Location: Posterior mediastinum

Radiographic Findings
- Radiography
  - Soft tissue mass in posterior mediastinum
  - Rib involvement
    - Widening of intercostal spaces
    - Erosion/destruction of ribs
  - Calcifications: Common (up to 30% by radiography)
  - Paravertebral soft tissue widening
    - May be present prior to rib erosion
    - Normally the right inferior paravertebral soft tissues are not visualized in children: Any visualization is abnormal
    - Normally the left inferior paravertebral soft tissues are seen
    - Should not exceed width of ipsi-level spinal pedicle
    - Normally are inferomedial in orientation
    - Inferolateral orientation is abnormal
  - Bone metastasis
    - Lucent or sclerotic lesions
  - Pedicle erosion from intraspinal extension

DDx: Solid Chest Mass In A Child

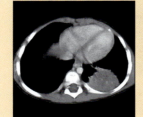
Pneumonia

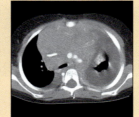
Lymphoma

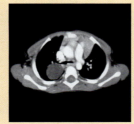
Bronchogenic Cyst

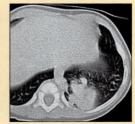
Sequestration

NEUROBLASTOMA, THORACIC

Key Facts

Terminology
- Malignant thoracic tumor of primitive neural crest cells
- Tendency to invade into spinal canal via neuroforamina

Imaging Findings
- Soft tissue mass in posterior mediastinum
- Rib involvement
- Calcifications: Common (up to 30% by radiography)
- Paravertebral soft tissue widening
- Bone metastasis
- Calcification seen on CT in up to 85%

Pathology
- Most commonly arises from the adrenal gland but can arise anywhere along sympathetic chain, including posterior mediastinum
- Third most common pediatric malignancy behind leukemia and central nervous system tumors

Clinical Issues
- Mean age at presentation 22 Months
- Features associated with a better prognosis
- Thoracic primary
- Age at diagnosis < 1 year, histological grade (Shimada system), decreased n-myc amplification (copies of gene), anatomic staging, stage 4S: Near 100% survival

CT Findings
- Posterior mediastinal mass, more commonly in inferior mediastinum but can occur in superior mediastinum/cervical region
- Mass often heterogeneous from necrosis, hemorrhage
- Calcification seen on CT in up to 85%

MR Findings
- Heterogeneous in signal and contrast-enhancement
- Tends to be high in signal on T2WI/low in signal on T1WI
- Excellent for detecting extension of tumor into spinal canal and organ of origin (abdominal lesions)

Ultrasonographic Findings
- Grayscale Ultrasound
  - Heterogeneously echogenic mass
  - More often used with abdominal than chest masses

Nuclear Medicine Findings
- PET: Role of PET not defined in NBT, many tumors are PET positive
- Bone scintigraphy (Technetium-99m MDP)
  - Uptake seen in bony metastasis (both cortical and marrow)
  - Calcified primary mass often also demonstrates uptake (up to 74% of cases)
- Metaiodobenzylguanidine (MIBG)
  - Avid uptake related to catecholamine production
  - Excellent for following extent of disease in MIBG avid tumors
  - Approximately 30% of NBT are not MIBG avid

Imaging Recommendations
- CT or MRI (controversial as to which one) for defining local extent of disease
- MIBG and bone scan for determining distal extent of disease

DIFFERENTIAL DIAGNOSIS

Widening of inferior paravertebral soft tissues
- Normal paravertebral soft tissues
  - May be more prominent in obese patients
  - May be more prominent on recumbent films: Upright films
  - If in question, obtain
  - Should not exceed adjacent pedicle in thickness or be inferolaterally oriented
- Thoracic discitis
  - Similar widening of paravertebral soft tissues
  - Narrowing of disc space, loss of definition of vertebral endplates

Mediastinal mass in child less than 3 years of age
- Neuroblastoma until proven otherwise
- Pneumonia: Posterior located
  - No evidence of rib erosion or intraspinal extension
  - Air bronchograms, parapneumonic effusion
- Bronchogenic cyst
  - Fluid density, homogeneous attenuation
  - May occasionally be paraspinal
- Extralobar sequestration
  - May appear very similar to NBT as paraspinal mass
- Lymphoma
  - Anterior mediastinal mass

PATHOLOGY

General Features
- General path comments
  - Malignant tumor of primitive neural crest cells
  - Most commonly arises from the adrenal gland but can arise anywhere along sympathetic chain, including posterior mediastinum

NEUROBLASTOMA, THORACIC

- Continuous spectrum with more benign counterparts: Ganglioneuroma and ganglioneuroblastoma (determined by degree of cellular maturation)
- Genetics
  - Increased copies of n-myc proto oncogene associated with poor prognosis (n-myc amplification)
  - CD44, glycoprotein on cell surface, increased levels = better prognosis
- Epidemiology
  - Third most common pediatric malignancy behind leukemia and central nervous system tumors
  - 8-10% of childhood cancer
  - 15% of childhood cancer deaths
  - Most common abdominal malignancy in children
  - Posterior mediastinum 20% of NBT cases
- Associated abnormalities
  - Von Recklinghausen disease, Beckwith-Wiedemann syndrome, Hirschsprung disease,
  - Most cases of NBT occur in children without associations

Gross Pathologic & Surgical Features
- Often areas of necrosis or hemorrhage

Microscopic Features
- Immature, undifferentiated sympathetic cells: Small, round blue cells
- Homer Wright rosettes: Circular orientation of groups of cells
- Shimada classification: Combines histologic features and age of patient to separate into unfavorable and favorable histology categories for prognosis

Staging, Grading or Classification Criteria
- Evans anatomic staging (prognosis - % survival)
  - 1: Confined to organ of interest (90%)
  - 2: Extension beyond organ but not crossing midline (75%)
  - 3: Extension crossing midline (vertebral column) (30%)
  - 4: Distal metastasis (10%)
  - 4S: Age < 1 year, metastatic disease confined to skin, liver, and bone marrow (near 100%)

CLINICAL ISSUES

Presentation
- Most common signs/symptoms: Pain
- Other signs/symptoms
  - Malaise, irritability, weight loss, neurologic symptoms, opsoclonus-myoclonus (movement of eyes and extremities), cerebellar ataxia (more common with chest NBT)
  - Skin mets: "Blueberry muffin syndrome"
  - Skull base mets: "Raccoon eyes"
  - Massive hepatomegaly from mets - Pepper syndrome
- Approximately 95% of patients with neuroblastoma have elevated levels of catecholamines (vanillylmandelic acid, VMA) in urine

Demographics
- Age
  - Mean age at presentation 22 Months
  - Younger age of presentation associated with better prognosis
  - May be diagnosed prenatally
  - NBT most common malignancy of first week of life

Natural History & Prognosis
- Features associated with a better prognosis
  - Thoracic primary
  - Age at diagnosis < 1 year, histological grade (Shimada system), decreased n-myc amplification (copies of gene), anatomic staging, stage 4S: Near 100% survival
- Some lesions may spontaneously regress and mature into less malignant tumors (ganglioneuroma)

Treatment
- Options: Chemotherapy, surgical resection, bone marrow transplantation, radiation
- Based upon anatomic stage, age, and histologic features
- Less aggressive lesions may be treated with surgical resection alone
- For stage 4S: Many institutions no treatment with spontaneous resolution

DIAGNOSTIC CHECKLIST

Consider
- Always remember to look for rib erosions when a focal chest mass is seen in children
- Look for subtle widening of paraspinal stripe

SELECTED REFERENCES

1. Kushner BH: Neuroblastoma: a disease requiring a multitude of imaging studies. J Nucl Med. 45(7):1172-88, 2004
2. Matthay KK et al: Central nervous system metastases in neuroblastoma: radiologic, clinical, and biologic features in 23 patients. Cancer. 98(1):155-65, 2003
3. Mehta K et al: Imaging neuroblastoma in children. Crit Rev Comput Tomogr. 44(1):47-61, 2003
4. Pfluger T et al: Integrated imaging using MRI and 123I metaiodobenzylguanidine scintigraphy to improve sensitivity and specificity in the diagnosis of pediatric neuroblastoma. AJR Am J Roentgenol. 181(4):1115-24, 2003
5. Lonergan GJ et al: Neuroblastoma, ganglioneuroblastoma, and ganglioneuroma: radiologic-pathologic correlation. Radiographics. 22(4):911-34, 2002
6. Meyer JS et al: Imaging of neuroblastoma and Wilms' tumor. Magn Reson Imaging Clin N Am. 10(2):275-302, 2002
7. Donnelly LF et al: Differentiating normal from abnormal inferior thoracic paravertebral soft tissues on chest radiography in children. Radiology. 175:489-93, 2000
8. Brodeur GM et al: Neuroblastoma. In: Pizzo PA, Poplack DG, eds. Principles and practice of pediatric oncology. 3rd ed. Philadelphia: Lippincott-Raven. 761-97, 1997
9. Suc A et al: Metastatic neuroblastoma in children older than one year: prognostic significance of the initial metaiodobenzylguanidine scan and proposal for a scoring system. Cancer. 77(4):805-11, 1996

NEUROBLASTOMA, THORACIC

IMAGE GALLERY

Typical

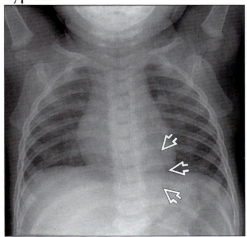
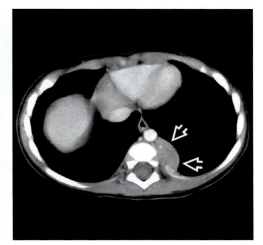

(Left) Anteroposterior radiograph in a young child shows left paraspinal mass *(arrows)*. There is no evidence of rib erosions. CT to right same patient. *(Right)* Axial CECT on same patient as on left shows left paraspinal mass *(arrows)*. There is no intraspinal extension.

Typical

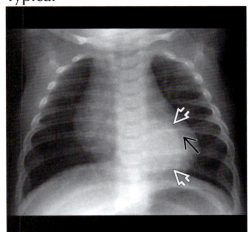
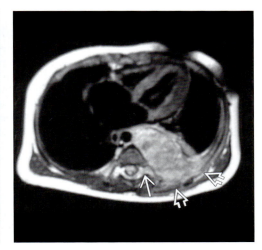

(Left) Anteroposterior radiograph shows left retrocardiac density *(open arrows)*. There is also widening of the right 7-8th intercostal distance and rib erosion *(arrow)*. *(Right)* Axial T1 C+ MR on same patient as on left shows findings paraspinal mass with evidence of posterior chest wall invasion *(open arrows)* and intraspinal extension *(arrow)*.

Typical

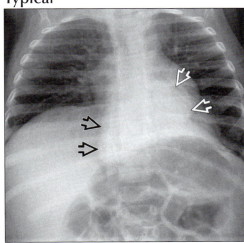
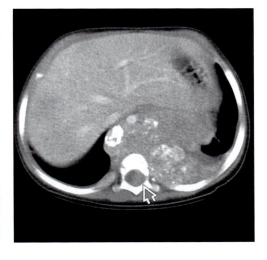

(Left) Anteroposterior radiograph shows widening of the right paraspinal stripe *(black arrows)* and retrocardiac mass *(white arrows)*. CT to right from same patient. *(Right)* Axial NECT on same patient as on left shows large paravertebral mass with calcifications and intraspinal extension *(arrow)*.

DISCITIS

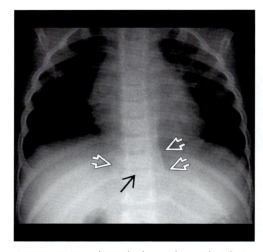

Anteroposterior radiograph shows abnormal widening of the right and left paraspinal soft tissues (open arrows) and loss of height of the disc space at the level (arrow).

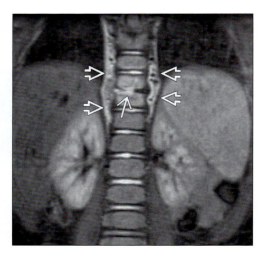

Coronal T2WI MR in same patient as on left shows edema and widening of paraspinal soft tissues (open arrows), narrowing of the disc (arrow), and high signal of adjacent vertebral bodies.

TERMINOLOGY

Abbreviations and Synonyms
- Infectious spondylitis

Definitions
- Inflammatory process of the intervertebral disc space often with unknown etiology

IMAGING FINDINGS

General Features
- Best diagnostic clue: Disc space narrowing and end plate irregularity
- Location
  - Single disc involved
  - Lumbar spine most commonly effected
    - Particularly in younger children
    - Most common sites are L3-4 and L2-3
    - Followed by L4-5, L1-2, L5-S1
  - Lower thoracic spine can also be involved
    - More common in teenagers and older children
- Imaging sensitivity: One study showed that the following imaging parameters were positive in the evaluation of discitis
  - Radiography 82% of patients
  - Bone scan 72%
  - MRI 100%

Radiographic Findings
- Radiography
  - Radiographic changes often lag behind development of symptoms
    - Initial radiographs often normal
    - Estimated that radiographic findings do not develop often until at least 12 days of symptoms
  - Radiographic findings in lumbar discitis
    - Irregularity or poor definition of adjacent vertebral endplates
    - Sclerosis of adjacent vertebral bodies
    - Narrowing of the intervertebral disc space
  - Radiographic findings in thoracic discitis
    - Paravertebral soft tissue widening
    - May be present prior to disc space narrowing
    - Normally the right inferior paravertebral soft tissues are not visualized in children: Any visualization is abnormal
    - Normally the left inferior paravertebral soft tissues are seen
    - Should not exceed width of ipsi-level spinal pedicle (abnormal)
    - Normally are inferomedial in orientation
    - Inferolateral orientation: Abnormal
    - Irregularity or poor definition of adjacent vertebral endplates

DDx: Lower Back Pain In Children

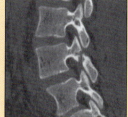
Spondylolysis

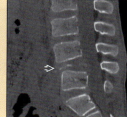
LCH

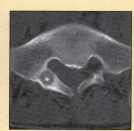
Osteoid Osteoma

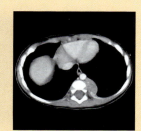
Neuroblastoma

DISCITIS

Key Facts

Terminology
- Infectious spondylitis
- Inflammatory process of the intervertebral disc space often with unknown etiology

Imaging Findings
- Lumbar spine most commonly effected
- Most common sites are L3-4 and L2-3
- Lower thoracic spine can also be involved
- Radiographic changes often lag behind development of symptoms
- Radiographic findings in lumbar discitis
- Irregularity or poor definition of adjacent vertebral endplates
- Sclerosis of adjacent vertebral bodies
- Narrowing of the intervertebral disc space
- Radiographic findings in thoracic discitis
- Paravertebral soft tissue widening
- May be present prior to disc space narrowing

Pathology
- Blood cultures or cultures from tissue sampling of disc area yield positive results in only 1/3 of cases
- When identified, Staphylococcus aureus is most common etiologic agent

Clinical Issues
- Diagnosis is often delayed because of nonspecific presentation
- Most common in children 6 months to 4 years
- Lumbar location most common in this age group
- Second peak during 10-14 years of age
- Thoracic location most common in this age group

- Sclerosis of adjacent vertebral bodies
- Narrowing of the intervertebral disc space

CT Findings
- CT may be performed to evaluate for cause of abdominal pain
- CT may show excessive soft tissues at level of discitis
- Easy to overlook when evaluating for abdominal pain
- Disc space narrowing difficult to determine on axial images
- Sagittal and coronal reconstructions of spine and specific attention to bone windows can be helpful

MR Findings
- T1WI
  - Disc space narrowing
  - Loss of low signal normally seen along cortical margin of adjacent vertebral bodies
  - Low marrow signal in adjacent vertebral bodies
- T2WI
  - Widening of the paravertebral soft tissues with edema (high T2) signal
  - Loss of high T2 signal of affected disc space and disc space narrowing
  - High T2 signal in adjacent vertebral bodies
- STIR
  - High T2 signal seen in adjacent vertebral bodies as on T2W sequences
  - May be helpful if having problems with homogeneous fat saturation related to anatomic location of disc affected
- T1 C+
  - Enhancement may be present in disc space and adjacent vertebral bodies
  - Enhancement may also be seen in adjacent soft tissues
  - Focal nonenhancing area surrounded by enhancing tissue may represent abscess

Non-Vascular Interventions
- Imaging guided needle aspiration or core biopsy of affected disc space and adjacent vertebral body bone is advocated by some to evaluate for etiologic agent prior to placing patient on antibiotics
- CT guidance most commonly utilized

Nuclear Medicine Findings
- Bone Scintigraphy
  - Increased uptake in the vertebral bodies on each side of the involved disc
  - Usually positive within 1-2 days of onset of symptoms
  - Therefore often positive much sooner than radiographs

Imaging Recommendations
- Protocol advice
  - Persistent back pain is not normal in children
  - If persistent back pain and normal radiography, other imaging such as bone scan or lumbar MRI should be obtained

DIFFERENTIAL DIAGNOSIS

Lower back pain in children
- Muscle strain
  - Probably most common cause lower back pain in children
  - Particularly in athletes
  - Typically, no imaging findings
  - Improves with time/rest
- Spondylolysis
  - Defects in pars interarticularis
  - Occur in 5% of children, many asymptomatic
  - Most common diagnosis seen by imaging
  - Most common at L5-S1 followed by L4-5
  - Can be secondary to acute or chronic stress injuries
  - Lucent defect seen through pars on lateral view

DISCITIS

- Discontinuity of neck of "Scotty dog" seen on oblique lumbar view: Often cause more confusion than help in making diagnosis
- Scheuermann disease
  - End plate irregularity, disc space narrowing, limbus vertebrae
  - Greater than 3 vertebral bodies > 5 degrees of anterior wedging
  - More common in thoracic than lumbar spine
  - Differentiated from discitis by multi-level involvement
- Focal masses of the spine: Sclerotic or lucent
  - Osteoblastoma
  - Osteoid osteoma
  - Aneurysmal bone cyst
  - Neuroblastoma metastatic disease
  - Leukemia
  - Langerhans cell histiocytosis (LCH) - vertebral plana

Widening of lower thoracic paraspinal soft tissues

- Normal variation
  - Soft tissues wider in obese patients
  - Recumbent technique can make paravertebral soft tissues wider: Repeat film upright
- Neuroblastoma
  - Rib erosion
  - Intraspinal extension
  - Calcifications in mass
  - Typically younger age
- Extralobar sequestration
  - May present as paraspinal mass
  - Look for systemic arterial supply
- Bronchogenic cyst
  - May occasionally present as paraspinal mass
  - Homogeneous water attenuation on CT

PATHOLOGY

General Features

- General path comments: Infectious or non-infectious inflammation of disc
- Etiology
  - Exact etiology unknown
  - Most commonly no infectious agent identified
    - Blood cultures or cultures from tissue sampling of disc area yield positive results in only 1/3 of cases
    - When identified, Staphylococcus aureus is most common etiologic agent
    - 55% of identified causes were Staphylococcus aureus in one study
- Associated abnormalities: May lead to disc fibrosis and less commonly vertebral body fusion

CLINICAL ISSUES

Presentation

- Most common signs/symptoms
  - Presentation variable and often nonspecific
  - Diagnosis is often delayed because of nonspecific presentation
  - In one study, the diagnosis was often delayed with a mean of 42 days between presentation and diagnosis
- Other signs/symptoms
  - Pain may not be localized to area of discitis
    - Pain may be abdominal, hip, knee
  - Fever, irritability, malaise: Particularly in infants
  - Refusal to walk or sit up, limping
  - Elevated sedimentation rate and white cell count

Demographics

- Age
  - Most common in children 6 months to 4 years
    - Lumbar location most common in this age group
  - Age is younger than mean age for presentation of osteomyelitis
    - Mean age of presentation for discitis 3 years
    - Mean age of presentation for osteomyelitis 7.5 years
  - Second peak during 10-14 years of age
    - Thoracic location most common in this age group

Natural History & Prognosis

- Typically process resolves
- Symptoms typically decrease within several days after onset of antibiotics
- Most patients eventually become asymptomatic despite methods of treatment chosen

Treatment

- Controversial
- Most treat with bed rest and antibiotics
  - Some advocate percutaneous needle biopsy (or open biopsy) when blood cultures negative prior to placing on antibiotics
  - Others advocate no antibiotic therapy
  - Most cases improve rapidly with antibiotic therapy and are treated for 4-6 week course
- Immobilization sometimes necessary in those who do not respond to antibiotics
  - Shown to decrease symptoms
- In one study, the following treatments utilized with all patients recovering
  - Bed rest 100%
  - Plaster cast immobilization 50%
  - Antibiotics 40%
  - Traction 23%

SELECTED REFERENCES

1. Early SD et al: Childhood diskitis. J Am Acad Orthop Surg. 11(6):413-20, 2003
2. Garron E et al: Nontuberculous spondylodiscitis in children. J Pediatr Orthop. 22(3):321-8, 2002
3. Brown R et al: Discitis in young children. J Bone Joint Surg Br. 83(1):106-11, 2001
4. Donnelly LF et al: Differentiating normal from abnormal inferior thoracic paravertebral soft tissues on chest radiography in children. Radiology. 175:489-93, 2000
5. Fernandez M et al: Discitis and vertebral osteomyelitis in children: an 18-year review. Pediatrics. 105(6):1299-304, 2000
6. Garcia FF et al: Diagnostic imaging of childhood spinal infection. Orthop Rev. 22(3):321-7, 1993
7. Crawford AH et al: Diskitis in children. Clin Orthop. (266):70-9, 1991

DISCITIS

IMAGE GALLERY

Typical

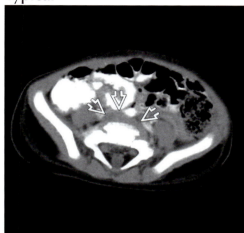
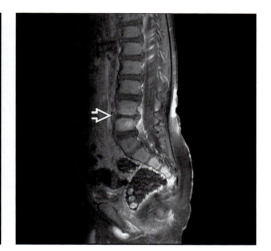

(Left) Axial CECT obtained in a young child with abdominal pain shows increased soft tissues (arrows) anterior to vertebral bodies, not noted prospectively. (Right) Sagittal T1 C+ MR of lumbar spine obtained later in same patient shows disc space narrowing and posterior protrusion at L4-5 (arrow) and enhancement of adjacent vertebral bodies and soft tissues.

Typical

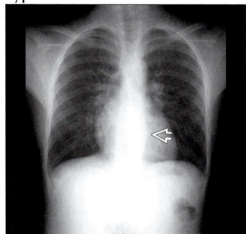
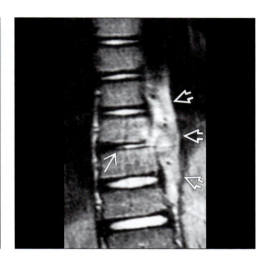

(Left) Anteroposterior radiograph shows left paraspinal widening (arrow). Next image same patient. (Right) Coronal T2WI MR shows disc space narrowing and loss of signal (arrow), increased signal in adjacent vertebral bodies, and increased paraspinal soft tissues (open arrows).

Typical

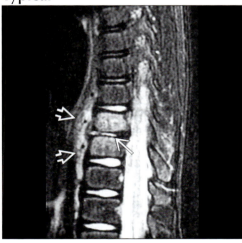
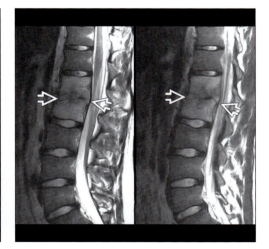

(Left) Sagittal T2WI MR in same patient as above shows disc space narrowing (arrow), increased signal in adjacent vertebral bodies, and increased paraspinal soft tissues (open arrows). (Right) Sagittal T2WI MR images show increased T2W signal in vertebral bodies and decreased disk space width at T12-L1 (arrows). Note loss of definition of adjacent vertebral endplates.

CYSTIC FIBROSIS, LUNG

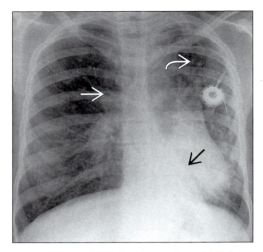

Posteranterior radiograph shows collapsed left lower lobe (black arrow) with hyperinflation and reticulonodular opacities (curved white arrow), and bronchiectasis (white arrow).

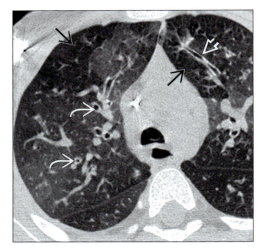

Axial HRCT shows mosaic attenuation with air-trapping (arrows), bronchial wall thickening (curved arrows) and bronchiectasis with a non-tapering bronchus (open arrow).

TERMINOLOGY

Abbreviations and Synonyms
- Cystic fibrosis (CF), mucovicidosis

Definitions
- Autosomal recessive multisystem disorder of exocrine gland function characterized in the respiratory tract by recurrent infection, chronic obstruction and chronic sinusitis with nasal polyps

IMAGING FINDINGS

General Features
- Best diagnostic clue: Predominately upper lobe bronchiectasis and mucous plugging in hyperinflated lungs
- Location: Lungs, sinuses, gastrointestinal tract, genitourinary tract, sweat glands

Radiographic Findings
- Radiography
  o Early: Hyperinflation and/or lobar atelectasis
    ▪ Increased perihilar markings
  o Later: Upper lobe predominant bronchiectasis
  o Multiple small, ill-defined opacities in lung periphery from small airways mucoid impaction
  o Persistent atelectasis → subsegmental, segmental, or lobar
  o Pneumonia (recurrent): Pseudomonas aeruginosa, Staph. aureus, Haemophilus influenzae
  o Pulmonary arterial enlargement
  o Adenopathy from chronic inflammation: Hilar > mediastinal
  o Cor pulmonale
  o Apical cystic airspaces
    ▪ Cystic bronchiectasis, bullae, or sequela of prior abscesses
  o Predisposed to spontaneous pneumothorax
  o 10% develop allergic bronchopulmonary aspergillosis (ABPA)
  o Brasfield scoring system demonstrates good correlation between radiographs and pulmonary function
    ▪ Scored on extent of air-trapping, nodular and cystic lesions, linear markings, large opacities (atelectasis or consolidation), and general severity
    ▪ Similar grading systems for high resolution chest CT findings

CT Findings
- More sensitive than radiographs for detecting mild disease
- Best imaging modality for detection of bronchial wall thickening and dilatation

DDx: Recurrent Respiratory Symptoms And Bronchiectasis

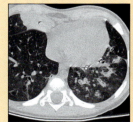

Rec Aspiration

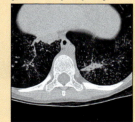

Immotile Cilia

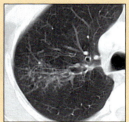

Asthma And ABPA

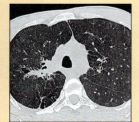

CGD

CYSTIC FIBROSIS, LUNG

Key Facts

Terminology
- Autosomal recessive multisystem disorder of exocrine gland function characterized in the respiratory tract by recurrent infection, chronic obstruction and chronic sinusitis with nasal polyps

Imaging Findings
- Best diagnostic clue: Predominately upper lobe bronchiectasis and mucous plugging in hyperinflated lungs
- Predisposed to spontaneous pneumothorax
- "Signet ring sign" on CT: Dilated bronchus in association with adjacent artery on axial images
- Secretions within peripheral small centrilobular bronchioles can give V- or Y-shaped opacities: "Tree-in-bud"
- HRCT will detect subtle disease and will better demonstrate extent of changes of CF and complications
- Consider controlled ventilation technique for HRCT in infants and young children

Top Differential Diagnoses
- Recurrent aspiration
- Asthma
- Bronchopulmonary dysplasia
- Immotile cilia syndrome

Clinical Issues
- Highest prevalence in Caucasians of Northern European origin: 1:3,200
- Most fatalities due to progressive lung disease but also liver failure and massive hemoptysis

---

- Cylindrical, varicose and saccular bronchiectasis (in order of severity)
  - "Signet ring sign" on CT: Dilated bronchus in association with adjacent artery on axial images
- Secretions within peripheral small centrilobular bronchioles can give V- or Y-shaped opacities: "Tree-in-bud"
- Expiration HRCT will show associated small airway disease indicated by air trapping and a more pronounced "mosaic pattern"

Angiographic Findings
- DSA: May have extensive systemic collaterals to lungs

Nuclear Medicine Findings
- V/Q Scan: Matched ventilation and perfusion defects

Imaging Recommendations
- Best imaging tool
  - Chest radiographs usually sufficient for long-term follow-up and most acute exacerbations
  - HRCT will detect subtle disease and will better demonstrate extent of changes of CF and complications
- Protocol advice
  - HRCT most sensitive for detecting bronchiectasis with expiratory images to determine airtrapping
  - Consider controlled ventilation technique for HRCT in infants and young children

DIFFERENTIAL DIAGNOSIS

Recurrent aspiration
- Often have predisposing neuromuscular abnormalities
- Bronchiectasis in lower lobes and posterior segments i.e. the dependent portions of lungs
- Pneumonia can sometimes be related to a preceding episode of choking or gagging with feeds

Asthma
- Especially when complicated by ABPA and bronchiectasis
- May be seasonal
- History of allergies

Bronchopulmonary dysplasia
- Improves as the patient ages
- Recurrent aspiration
- History of prematurity

Immotile cilia syndrome
- Dysfunction of cilia in respiratory and auditory epithelium
- Lower lobe predominant
- May have situs inversus
- May have associated cardiac anomalies

Immunodeficiency states such as chronic granulomatous disease (CGD)
- CGD
  - Recurrent lungs abscesses
  - Staphylococcal abscesses in other organs also

PATHOLOGY

General Features
- General path comments
  - Lungs normal at birth
  - Airways colonized with pseudomonas
- Genetics
  - Autosomal recessive
  - Abnormality of a gene located on long arm of chromosome 7
  - Genetic heterogeneity with over 900 known mutations
  - Correlation between phenotype and genotype is being recognized
- Etiology
  - Pathologic changes acquired from abnormal chloride transport
  - Abnormal chloride transport produces thick, viscous mucus → not expectorated, becomes secondarily infected
  - Repeated infections eventually destroy airways
- Epidemiology

CYSTIC FIBROSIS, LUNG

- Most common lethal inherited disease in Caucasians
- Highest prevalence in Caucasians of Northern European origin: 1:3,200
- Associated abnormalities: Pancreatic, gastrointestinal, hepatobiliary, and genitourinary abnormalities

Gross Pathologic & Surgical Features

- Bronchial walls thickened and chronically inflamed with granulation tissue and fibrosis
- Bronchial artery hypertrophy
- Leads to bronchial wall weakness, recurrent infections, parenchymal volume loss and distortion
- Colonization with pseudomonas

Microscopic Features

- No specific features, chronic inflammation of both airway wall and lung

CLINICAL ISSUES

Presentation

- Most common signs/symptoms: Recurrent respiratory tract infections
- Other signs/symptoms
  - With mild disease, may be asymptomatic
  - Chest
    - Wheezing, chronic cough, hemoptysis, progressive respiratory failure, cor pulmonale
    - Digital clubbing
    - Pansinusitis and nasal polyps
  - Intestinal tract
    - Meconium peritonitis, meconium ileus (10-15% of newborns with CF), distal intestinal obstruction syndrome = meconium ileus equivalent, intussusception, rectal prolapse
  - Hepatobiliary
    - Cirrhosis, portal hypertension, hypersplenism, esophageal varices that may bleed, cholelithiasis
  - Pancreas
    - Steatorrhea: Frequent, bulky, greasy, large, foul-smelling stools that float in water
    - 8% develop diabetes mellitus
    - Occasional deficiency of vitamins A, D, E, and K → fat-soluble vitamins
  - Urogenital
    - Delayed sexual development, azoospermia due to failure of vas deferens to develop, undescended testes, hydrocele, secondary amenorrhea
  - Dry skin, salty taste to skin
  - Failure to thrive
- Clinical Profile
  - Diagnosis: Positive sweat test > 60 mEq/L
    - May be difficult to get enough sweat in infants
  - Genotyping important but cannot establish diagnosis without other supporting laboratory and clinical findings or a positive family history
  - Pulmonary function tests: Unreliable until 4-6 years of age
    - Obstructive pattern at all ages
    - May develop a restrictive pattern as disease advances
  - Bronchoalveolar lavage: Airway inflammation with increased neutrophils even in absence of infection
    - Pseudomonas aeruginosa
  - Semen analysis
    - Azoospermia should be confirmed with testicular biopsy

Demographics

- Age: Fetus (meconium peritonitis) to young adult (recurrent respiratory tract infection) at presentation
- Gender
  - M:F = 1:1
  - More severe manifestations in females
- Ethnicity
  - Highest prevalence in Caucasians of Northern European origin: 1:3,200
  - African Americans: 1:17,000
  - Hispanics: 1:9,200
  - Asian Americans: 1:31,000
  - Clinical manifestations similar between races

Natural History & Prognosis

- Improving life expectancy, but life span shortened
- Most fatalities due to progressive lung disease but also liver failure and massive hemoptysis

Treatment

- Pancreatic enzymes
- Respiratory therapy
  - Postural drainage
  - Bronchodilators
  - Prophylactic antibiotics
  - Aerosolized rhDNase
  - Lung transplants for endstage disease
  - Hemoptysis may require bronchial artery embolization
- Gene therapy promising

DIAGNOSTIC CHECKLIST

Image Interpretation Pearls

- Hyperinflation with upper lobe predominant bronchiectasis and mucous plugging

SELECTED REFERENCES

1. Brody AS et al: High-resolution computed tomography in young patients with cystic fibrosis: distribution of abnormalities and correlation with pulmonary function tests. J Pediatr. 145(1):32-8, 2004
2. McGuinness G et al: CT of airways disease and bronchiectasis. Radiol Clin North Am. 40(1):1-19, 2002
3. Long FR et al: Technique and clinical applications of full-inflation and end-exhalation controlled-ventilation chest CT in infants and young children. Pediatr Radiol. 31(6):413-22, 2001
4. Helbich TH et al: Cystic fibrosis: CT assessment of lung involvement in children and adults. Radiology. 213(2):537-44, 1999
5. Stern RC: The diagnosis of cystic fibrosis. N Engl J Med. 336(7):487-91, 1997
6. Wood BP: Cystic fibrosis. Radiology 204:1-10, 1997
7. Davis PB et al: Cystic fibrosis. Am J Respir Crit Care Med. 154(5):1229-56, 1996
8. Bhalla M et al: Cystic fibrosis: scoring system with thin-section CT. Radiology. 179(3):783-8, 1991

CYSTIC FIBROSIS, LUNG

IMAGE GALLERY

Typical

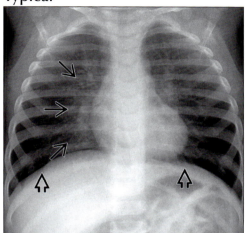
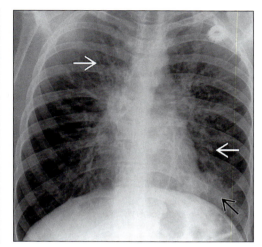

(Left) Anteroposterior radiograph shows typical changes of early cystic fibrosis with hyperinflation (open arrows on flattened hemidiaphragms) and increased perihilar markings (arrows). *(Right)* Posteroanterior radiograph shows coarse reticulonodular (white arrows) opacities of peribronchial thickening and mucous plugging. Also note exacerbating lingular consolidation (black arrow).

Variant

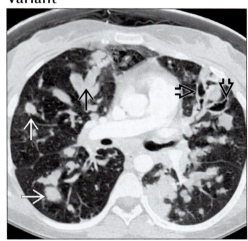
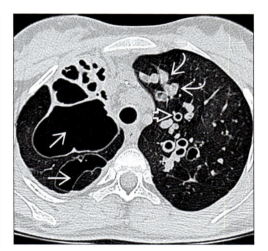

(Left) Axial CECT shows dilated bronchi with thickened walls (open arrows), most filled with large mucous plugs (white arrows) giving the appearance of gloved fingers (black arrow). *(Right)* Axial HRCT shows large cystic spaces (arrows) and mucous plugging (curved arrows) with bronchiectasis. Note signet ring appearance (open arrow) and mosaic attenuation.

Typical

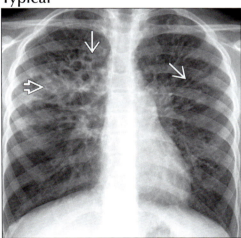
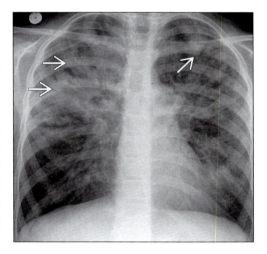

(Left) Posteroanterior radiograph shows hyperinflation with bilateral upper lobe predominant bronchiectasis (arrows), with a more confluent opacity in the right upper lobe (open arrow). *(Right)* Posteroanterior radiograph shows subsequent development of extensive mucous plugging in these ectatic, thick-walled bronchi (arrows). Note the marked upper lobe predominance.

SICKLE CELL, ACUTE CHEST SYNDROME

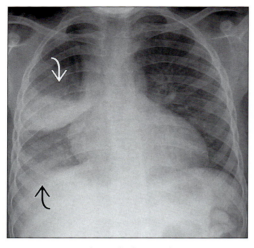

Anteroposterior radiograph shows right upper lobe and right lower lobe opacities (arrows) in Hb SS patient with respiratory distress and fever, consistent with ACS. Note cardiomegaly.

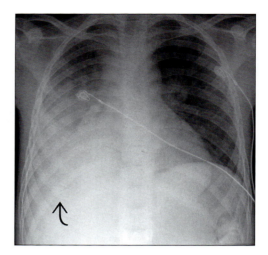

Anteroposterior radiograph shows recurrent extensive right lung opacification in same Hb SS patient 11 months later (arrow). ACS is recurrent in 80% of patients.

TERMINOLOGY

Abbreviations and Synonyms
- Acute chest syndrome (ACS)
- Sickle cell disease (Hb SS)

Definitions
- Appearance of new pulmonary opacity on chest radiograph accompanied by fever and respiratory symptoms (cough, tachypnea, and chest pain) in patient with Hb SS

IMAGING FINDINGS

General Features
- Best diagnostic clue: Pulmonary opacity in patient with Hb SS who has fever and respiratory symptoms
- Location: Lower lobes predominate, but may be in any lobe
- Size: Variable
- Morphology: Ill-defined air space disease

Radiographic Findings
- Radiography
  o Lung parenchyma
    - Initial chest radiograph may be normal (46%)
    - Lobar, segmental, subsegmental opacity due to pneumonia, atelectasis or infarct
    - Lower lobes predominate
    - Interstitial thickening due to scarring from prior episodes
    - Pulmonary edema
  o Pleura
    - Pleural effusion due to pneumonia or infarcts
    - Pleural effusion due to left heart failure
  o Heart
    - Cardiomegaly due to chronic anemia and high output heart failure
  o Skeletal
    - Avascular necrosis (AVN) humeral heads
    - H-shaped vertebrae
    - Enlarged ribs due to marrow expansion
    - Bone sclerosis due to bone infarcts
  o Upper abdomen
    - Small spleen, may be calcified (autosplenectomy)

CT Findings
- NECT
  o Limited clinical use for ACS
  o Findings consistent with lobar pneumonia, pulmonary edema or atelectasis
  o Pleural effusion common
  o May see healed bone infarcts

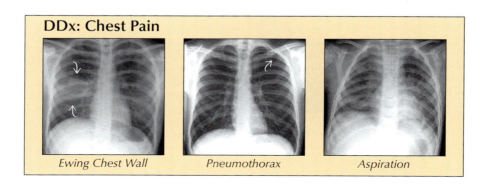

DDx: Chest Pain — Ewing Chest Wall, Pneumothorax, Aspiration

SICKLE CELL, ACUTE CHEST SYNDROME

Key Facts

Terminology
- Acute chest syndrome (ACS)
- Appearance of new pulmonary opacity on chest radiograph accompanied by fever and respiratory symptoms (cough, tachypnea, and chest pain) in patient with Hb SS

Imaging Findings
- Lobar, segmental, subsegmental opacity due to pneumonia, atelectasis or infarct
- Lower lobes predominate
- Cardiomegaly due to chronic anemia and high output heart failure
- Avascular necrosis (AVN) humeral heads
- H-shaped vertebrae

Pathology
- General path comments: Red blood cells sickle when deoxygenated
- Multifactorial, exact cause rarely determined
- Fat embolism causing pulmonary infarction
- Pneumonia
- Rib infarction with hypoinflation from splinting, leading to atelectasis
- ACS occurs in up to 50% with Hb SS
- Recurrent episodes in 80%
- Much more common in young children than adults

Clinical Issues
- ACS: Leading cause of death in Hb SS
- Second most common cause of hospitalization in Hb SS patients

---

- Intravenous iodinated contrast historically avoided to prevent potential sickling
  - Little data
- HRCT
  - Limited clinical use for ACS
  - Mosaic perfusion due to microvascular occlusion
    - Paucity of small vessels in periphery of lung
    - Ground glass attenuation, possibly due to hemorrhagic edema
  - Acute chest syndrome sequelae
    - Parenchymal bands
    - Septal thickening
    - Peripheral wedge-shaped opacities
    - Architectural distortion
    - Traction bronchiectasis

Nuclear Medicine Findings
- Bone Scan
  - Often see foci of abnormal radiotracer uptake in ribs
    - Decreased or increased uptake: Acute or subacute bone infarcts
  - Often find other bone infarcts vs. osteomyelitis
  - Commonly see increased skull uptake
  - Increased spleen uptake due to calcification
  - Delayed renal uptake
- Pulmonary Perfusion Scintigraphy
  - Limited clinical use in ACS
  - Etiology may be sickling erythrocytes vs. pneumonia vs. fat emboli
  - Defects often resolve quickly with supportive therapy
  - May mimic pulmonary embolism

Imaging Recommendations
- Best imaging tool
  - Chest radiograph for evaluation of cardiopulmonary disease
  - Bone scan to evaluate for bone infarcts as cause of pain and ACS
- Protocol advice
  - Routine frontal and lateral chest radiograph
  - Bone scan: Oblique spot images of ribs may increase sensitivity for rib infarcts

DIFFERENTIAL DIAGNOSIS

Chest pain
- Pneumothorax
  - See visceral pleural line with lucency lateral to line
- Pulmonary edema related to high output heart failure
  - Opacities may be more diffuse and bilateral
  - May be radiographically indistinguishable
- Aspiration
  - Lower lobe opacities, similar to ACS
  - May resolve quickly, similar to ACS
- Primary or metastatic lung mass
  - Rare
  - Opacity may appear more well-circumscribed

PATHOLOGY

General Features
- General path comments: Red blood cells sickle when deoxygenated
- Genetics
  - Valine substitution for glutamic acid in hemoglobin beta subunit (Hb S)
    - Hb S has some protection from malaria
    - Normal hemoglobin (Hb A)
  - Sickle cell anemia (Hb SS)
    - Exposure to low oxygen tension → HbS becomes less soluble and forms large polymers
    - Results in a distorted erythrocyte (sickle cell) → vaso-occlusion and hemolysis
  - May also occur in Hb SC, Hb SB°, Hb SB+
- Etiology
  - ACS: Not fully understood and frequently difficult to definitively determine exact cause
    - Multifactorial, exact cause rarely determined
    - Fat embolism causing pulmonary infarction
    - Pneumonia
    - Rib infarction with hypoinflation from splinting, leading to atelectasis
  - Infection
    - Documented in 30% of cases

SICKLE CELL, ACUTE CHEST SYNDROME

- More common cause of ACS in children
- Most common pathogens: Chlamydia pneumoniae, Mycoplasma pneumoniae, respiratory syncytial virus
- Pulmonary opacity persists longer than cases where infection not documented
○ Pulmonary fat embolism
- Emboli with fat and necrotic bone marrow in 9%
- Frequently have bone pain, decreased hemoglobin and platelet count, increased plasma free fatty acids and phospholipase A2
- Diagnosis supported by lipid-laden macrophages in bronchoalveolar lavage fluid
○ Rib infarction with hypoventilation from pain and/or analgesics
- High correlation between rib infarction and pulmonary opacity
- Pain may result in splinting, leading to atelectasis
- Incentive spirometry may decrease atelectasis and prevent pulmonary complications of ACS
- Analgesics may decrease splinting, but may cause hypoventilation
○ Pulmonary thrombus
- Potential cause, but rarely documented
○ Iatrogenic pulmonary edema
- Over-hydration with intravenous fluids may exacerbate
- Epidemiology
○ Hb SS most prevalent inherited disorder among African-Americans
- Hb SS occurs in 0.14% African-American population
- Hb SA in 8% African-American population
○ Average life expectancy 42 years for men and 48 years for women
○ Lung is one of the major organs affected by Hb SS
- Acute: ACS
- Chronic: Sickle cell chronic lung disease
○ ACS occurs in up to 50% with Hb SS
- Recurrent episodes in 80%
- Much more common in young children than adults

CLINICAL ISSUES

Presentation
- Most common signs/symptoms
○ Wheezing, cough, and fever most common in patients less than 10 years of age
- Milder and more likely due to infection
- Chest pain rare in this age group
- Upper lobe disease more common in children
○ Dyspnea, arm and leg pain more common in adults
- More frequently afebrile

Natural History & Prognosis
- ACS: Leading cause of death in Hb SS
○ Responsible for up to 25% of deaths
- The opacification may rapidly appear and resolve
○ Resolution often delayed in cases with documented bacterial pneumonia

- Second most common cause of hospitalization in Hb SS patients
- More common in young children
○ Highest incidence 2-4 years of age
- More severe in patients over 20 years old
- Complications
○ Respiratory failure
- Pulmonary emboli (bone marrow, fat, thrombus)
- Bronchopneumonia
- Chronic lung disease from repeat episodes of ACS
- Pulmonary hemorrhage
- Cor pulmonale
- May lead to multiorgan system failure
○ Strong correlation with neurologic events
- Altered mental status, seizures, neuromuscular abnormalities, anoxic brain injury, intracranial hemorrhage
○ Sepsis
○ Hypovolemic shock from splenic sequestration

Treatment
- Supportive, because the cause remains largely unknown
○ Oxygen and adequate hydration
- Overhydration may lead to pulmonary edema
○ Pain control
○ Incentive spirometry
○ Antibiotics for presumed pneumonia
○ Bronchodilators
○ Blood transfusions
- Prevention
○ Pneumococcal vaccination
- At higher risk for pneumonia from encapsulated organisms because of poor or absent splenic function
○ Haemophilus influenza vaccination
○ Hydroxyurea
- Reduces sickling by ↑ fetal hemoglobin level
- Reduces incidence in patients with recurrent ACS

DIAGNOSTIC CHECKLIST

Consider
- ACS in patient with Hb SS and pulmonary opacity

SELECTED REFERENCES

1. Siddiqui AK et al: Pulmonary manifestations of sickle cell disease. Postgrad Med J. 79(933):384-90, 2003
2. Vinchinsky EP et al: Causes and outcomes of the acute chest syndrome in sickle cell disease. National Acute Chest Syndrome Study Group. N Engl J Med. 342(25):1855-65, 2000
3. Crowley JJ et al: Imaging of sickle cell disease. Pediatr Radiol. 29(9):646-61, 1999
4. Martin L et al: Acute chest syndrome of sickle cell disease: radiographic and clinical analysis of 70 cases. Pediatr Radiol. 27(8):637-41, 1997
5. Bhalla M et al: Acute chest syndrome in sickle cell disease: CT evidence of microvascular occlusion. Radiology. 187(1):45-9, 1993
6. Gelfand MJ et al: Simultaneous occurrence of rib infarction and pulmonary infiltrates in sickle cell disease patients with acute chest syndrome. J Nucl Med. 34(4):614-8, 1993

SICKLE CELL, ACUTE CHEST SYNDROME

IMAGE GALLERY

Typical

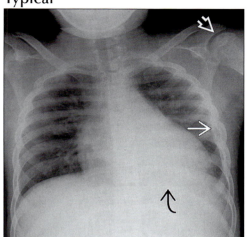
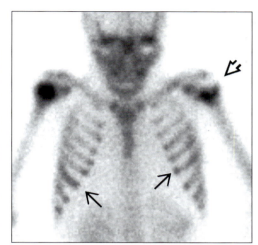

(Left) Anteroposterior radiograph shows common findings in ACS: Cardiomegaly, left lower lobe opacity (curved arrow), pleural effusion (arrow). Note AVN in left humeral head (open arrow). (Right) Anteroposterior bone scan shows absent uptake in left humeral head in same patient, which corresponds to AVN (open arrow). Heterogeneous rib uptake likely due to infarcts (arrows).

Typical

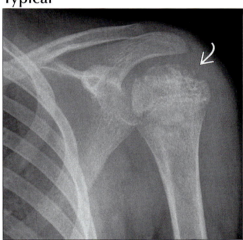
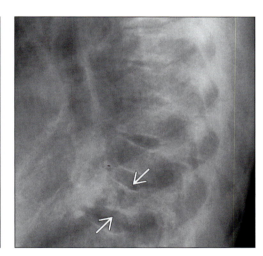

(Left) Anteroposterior radiograph shows irregularity and flattening of humeral head (arrow) of Hb SS patient, consistent with AVN. Hb SS patients with bone infarcts more commonly develop ACS. (Right) Lateral radiograph shows multiple vertebral endplate compression deformities (arrows) of vertebral bodies, sometimes called "H-shaped vertebrae" seen in Hb SS.

Typical

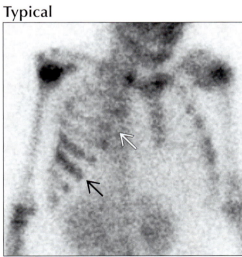
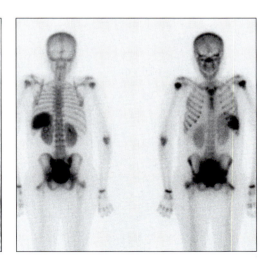

(Left) Oblique bone scan shows areas of abnormal increased (black arrow) and decreased (white arrow) uptake in ribs, consistent with rib infarcts in patient with Hb SS and chest pain. (Right) Bone scan shows typical findings in Hb SS including abnormal uptake in spleen, delayed renal uptake, and abnormal uptake in calvaria.

PULMONARY ARTERIOVENOUS MALFORMATION

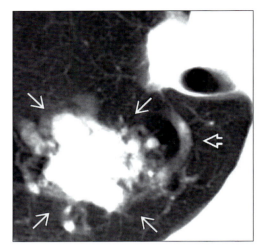

Axial CECT shows a lobulated lung nodule (arrows) with prominent feeding artery (open arrow). On soft tissue windows, enhancement of the nodule was similar to other vascular structures.

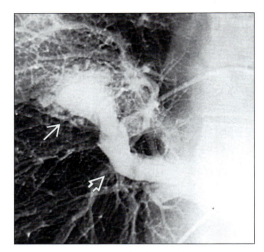

Anteroposterior angiography shows a large vein (open arrow) draining the nidus (arrow) of an arteriovenous malformation in the right medial lung.

TERMINOLOGY

Abbreviations and Synonyms
- Pulmonary arteriovenous malformation (PAVM)
- Pulmonary arteriovenous fistula (PAVF)

Definitions
- Abnormal direct communication between pulmonary artery and vein
  - Most are congenital
  - Problems mainly due to right to left shunt

IMAGING FINDINGS

General Features
- Best diagnostic clue: CECT: Smoothly marginated brightly enhancing nodule with enlarged feeding artery and draining vein
- Location
  - 50-70% located in the lower lobes
  - 70% unilateral
  - 36% multiple lesions
- Size: Typically 1-5 cm, but may be larger than 10 cm
- Morphology
  - 3 typical appearances
    - Large single sac
    - Plexiform mass of dilated vascular channels
    - Dilated and often tortuous direct connection between artery and vein

Radiographic Findings
- Radiography
  - Sharply defined pulmonary nodule, which may have lobulated borders
  - Uniform density
  - Curvilinear opacities medial to nodule
    - Represent feeding arteries and draining veins

CT Findings
- CECT
  - Best imaging modality for diagnosis of PAVM (98% sensitivity)
    - More sensitive than conventional angiography
    - Provides better anatomic detail than angiography
  - Enhancement of nodule similar to enhancement of other vascular structures
  - Large feeding artery and draining vein
  - Multidetector-row CT (MDCT)
    - Recent development which increases sensitivity for finding small PAVMs
    - Allows for retrospective decrease in image slice thickness, below 1mm collimation
    - 3-Dimensional (3D) reconstructions, Maximum intensity projections (MIPs) allow for creation of angiographic images noninvasively

DDx: Pediatric Pulmonary Nodule Or Pulmonary Vascular Lesion

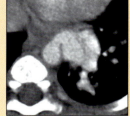
Aorta-Pulm Shunt

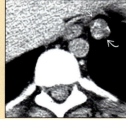
Osteosarcoma Met

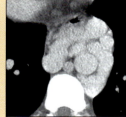
Varices

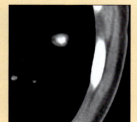
Granuloma

PULMONARY ARTERIOVENOUS MALFORMATION

Key Facts

Terminology
- Abnormal direct communication between pulmonary artery and vein
- Problems mainly due to right to left shunt

Imaging Findings
- Best diagnostic clue: CECT: Smoothly marginated brightly enhancing nodule with enlarged feeding artery and draining vein
- 50-70% located in the lower lobes

Top Differential Diagnoses
- Pulmonary varix
- Pulmonary metastasis
- Granuloma
- Pulmonary pseudotumor

Pathology
- Hereditary hemorrhagic telangiectasia (HHT), aka Rendu-Osler-Weber syndrome
- HHT accounts for 70% of patients with PAVMs
- 15-35% of patients with HHT have PAVM
- Should screen family members of patient with HHT and PAVM, because 35% incidence of PAVM found

Clinical Issues
- Mucocutaneous telangiectasia or epistaxis (suspect HHT)
- Incidental solitary pulmonary nodule on chest radiograph
- Physical signs of right to left shunt or complications of PAVM
- Most are congenital
- Other causes: Trauma, surgery, infection

MR Findings
- 3D MR angiography may be alternative to CT in characterizing PAVMs
- In general, MR has been less sensitive and specific than CT, with lower resolution
  - T2: Flow void may be indistinguishable from surrounding air in lung or calcification
  - GRE: May help to confirm nodule contains high flow (high flow = high signal)

Ultrasonographic Findings
- Contrast-enhanced echocardiography
  - May be helpful in distinguishing between intracardiac and intrapulmonary shunts

Angiographic Findings
- DSA
  - Selective pulmonary angiography
    - Large feeding artery
    - Nidus
    - Large early draining vein
  - Less sensitive, but may be more specific than CT
    - Some vascular lung lesions, such as a pulmonary varix, may be difficult to distinguish by CT

Nuclear Medicine Findings
- Lung perfusion scan
  - Confirms right to left shunt, especially if contrast-enhanced echocardiography or the 100% oxygen method is not available
  - Method: Peripheral IV injection of macroaggregated albumin labeled with technetium Tc-99m
    - Normally, particles trapped in pulmonary capillaries
    - In right to left shunt, the particles pass through the lungs and trapped in the brain and kidneys
    - Calculate shunt fraction

Imaging Recommendations
- Best imaging tool
  - CECT
    - Increasingly sensitive in detecting smaller lesions with the development of MDCT
    - Clearly depicts anatomy for pre-transcatheter embolization planning
    - 3D reconstructions and MIPs allow for creation of angiographic images noninvasively
    - Invasive angiography typically reserved for therapeutic intervention
- Protocol advice: CECT, using MDCT if possible, for superior detection of PAVMs and presurgical/transcatheter embolization planning

DIFFERENTIAL DIAGNOSIS

Pulmonary varix
- Enlarged pulmonary vein
- No large feeding artery or nidus
- Angiography may be needed for diagnosis, as appearance by CT may be similar to PAVM

Systemic artery to pulmonary vein shunt
- Vessel arises from systemic artery rather than pulmonary artery
- Most commonly seen following surgery for cyanotic congenital cardiac disease

Retroperitoneal varices
- Tubular vessels located in esophageal hiatus
- Usually history of end stage liver disease and other collateral veins in abdomen
- No arterial component

Pulmonary metastasis
- E.g., osteosarcoma, testicular carcinoma, renal cell carcinoma, rhabdomyosarcoma, lymphoma, etc.
- Frequently multiple and seen in the setting of known primary malignant tumor
- Typically not associated with large vessels

Granuloma
- Frequently smoothly marginated
- Frequently densely calcified or central calcification
- Often associated with calcified hilar and mediastinal lymph nodes
- Less enhancement than PAVM

PULMONARY ARTERIOVENOUS MALFORMATION

- Not associated with large vessels

Pulmonary pseudotumor
- Most common primary lung mass in children
- Typically less enhancement than PAVM
- May contain coarse calcifications
- No large vessels

PATHOLOGY

General Features
- Genetics
  - HHT 1: Gene locus 9q3
  - HHT 2: Gene locus 12q
- Etiology
  - Congenital (most common)
    - One theory is incomplete resorption of the vascular septa during embryogenesis
  - Acquired
    - Surgery for congenital cyanotic heart disease: Late complication of Glenn and Fontan procedures
    - Hepatopulmonary syndrome: 47% with end stage liver disease acquire abnormal arterial venous communications
    - Rarely discrete PAVMs on chest radiograph
    - Infection: tuberculosis, actinomycosis, schistosomiasis
- Associated abnormalities
  - Hereditary hemorrhagic telangiectasia (HHT), aka Rendu-Osler-Weber syndrome
    - HHT accounts for 70% of patients with PAVMs
    - 15-35% of patients with HHT have PAVM
    - Autosomal dominant, variable penetrance
    - Clinical triad of epistaxis, telangiectasias, family history of syndrome
    - Should screen family members of patient with HHT and PAVM, because 35% incidence of PAVM found
  - Congenital cyanotic heart disease
  - End stage liver disease
  - Prior infection with tuberculosis, actinomycosis, schistosomiasis

Microscopic Features
- Thin-walled vascular channels lined with endothelium
- Scant connective tissue stroma

Staging, Grading or Classification Criteria
- Simple PAVM = 80%
  - Single feeding segmental artery leading to single draining pulmonary vein
  - Associated with nonsepte aneurysms
- Complex PAVM = 20%
  - Two or more feeding arteries and veins
  - Often in lingula and right middle lobe

CLINICAL ISSUES

Presentation
- Most common signs/symptoms
  - Mucocutaneous telangiectasia or epistaxis (suspect HHT)
  - Incidental solitary pulmonary nodule on chest radiograph
  - Physical signs of right to left shunt or complications of PAVM
- Other signs/symptoms
  - Right to left shunt
    - Dyspnea, cyanosis, clubbing
    - Congestive heart failure
  - Neurologic (paradoxical emboli)
    - Brain abscess
    - Embolic stroke, transient ischemic attack
  - Hemoptysis
    - May be massive
  - Murmurs or bruits with auscultation over PAVM

Demographics
- Age
  - Most are congenital
  - 10% detected in infancy or childhood
  - Incidence gradually increases through the fifth and sixth decades of life
  - Other causes: Trauma, surgery, infection
- Gender
  - M:F = 1:2
  - Male predominance in newborns

Natural History & Prognosis
- Not carefully studied
- Lesions larger than 2 cm usually treated to avoid neurologic complications and heart failure

Treatment
- Options, risks, complications
  - Endovascular coil or balloon occlusion
    - High success rate, permanent occlusion in > 90%
    - Low morbidity and mortality
    - Systemic embolization of balloon, coil, or air rare
    - Postembolization syndrome: Transient fever, pleuritic chest pain
  - Rarely requires open surgery

SELECTED REFERENCES

1. Abujudeh H: Pulmonary varix: blood flow is essential in the diagnosis. Pediatr Radiol. 34(7):567-9, 2004
2. Faughnan ME et al: Pulmonary arteriovenous malformations in children: outcomes of transcatheter embolotherapy. J Pediatr. 145(6):826-31, 2004
3. Miyabe H et al: Paradoxical brain embolism caused by pulmonary arteriovenous fistula and coincident pulmonary embolism--a case report. Angiology. 55(5):577-81, 2004
4. Goyen M et al: Pulmonary arteriovenous malformation: Characterization with time-resolved ultrafast 3D MR angiography. J Magn Reson Imaging. 13(3):458-60, 2001
5. Rubin GD: Techniques for performing multidetector-row computed tomographic angiography. Tech Vasc Interv Radiol. 4(1):2-14, 2001
6. Pick A et al: Pulmonary arteriovenous fistula: presentation, diagnosis, and treatment. World J Surg. 23(11):1118-22, 1999
7. Gossage JR et al: Pulmonary arteriovenous malformations. A state of the art review. Am J Respir Crit Care Med. 158(2):643-61, 1998
8. Mitchell RO et al: Pulmonary arteriovenous malformation in the neonate. J Pediatr Surg. 28(12):1536-8, 1993

PULMONARY ARTERIOVENOUS MALFORMATION

IMAGE GALLERY

Typical

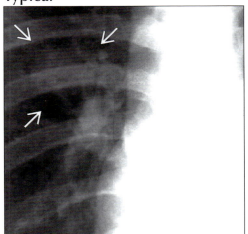
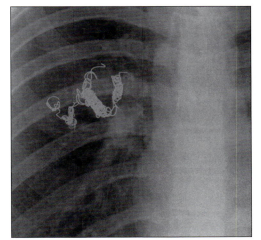

(Left) Anteroposterior radiograph shows a faint opacity near the superior right hilum *(arrows)*. *(Right)* Anteroposterior radiograph shows placement of coils to occlude the arteriovenous malformation (AVM) seen on the left radiograph. Images below show the CT and angiographic appearance of the AVM.

Typical

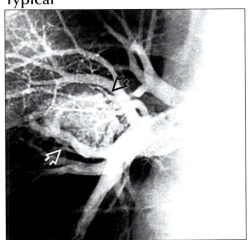
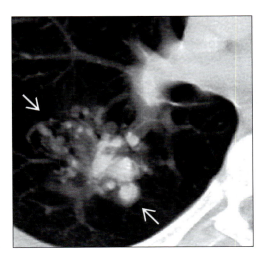

(Left) Anteroposterior catheter angiography shows early images of a selective right lower lobe pulmonary angiogram, with filling of the nidus of a PAVM in the right lower lobe *(arrows)*. *(Right)* Axial CECT shows a lobulated lung nodule *(arrows)*. On soft tissue windows, enhancement of the nodule was similar to other vascular structures.

Typical

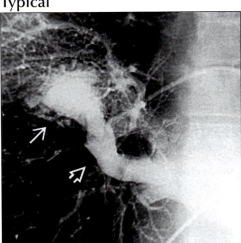
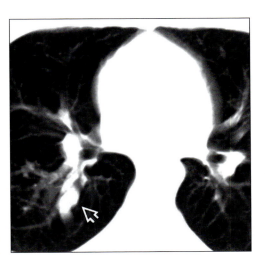

(Left) Anteroposterior catheter angiography shows a large vein *(open arrow)* draining the nidus *(arrow)* of a pulmonary arteriovenous malformation in the medial right lower lobe. *(Right)* Axial CECT shows portions of the large draining vein *(open arrow)* arising from the pulmonary arteriovenous malformation see in the pulmonary angiogram in the left image.

LUNG CONTUSION AND LACERATION

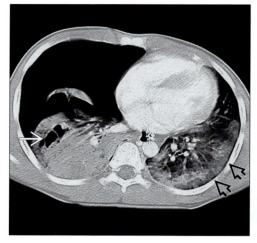

Axial CECT shows left posterior, crescentic contusion with subpleural sparing (open arrows). Large pneumothorax, collapsed lung, and cavity consistent with laceration (arrow).

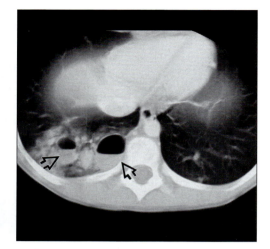

Axial CECT on 10 year old girl in motor vehicle accident shows multiple cavities (arrows) with surrounding lung opacity consistent with lung laceration.

TERMINOLOGY

Definitions
- Lung contusion: Hemorrhage and edema formation in the alveoli and interstitium as a result of alveolar capillary damage secondary to blunt chest trauma
- Lung laceration: Frank tear within the lung parenchyma as a result of chest trauma
- Identification of lung contusions and differentiation from other causes of lung opacity in presence of blunt chest trauma has relevance to child's prognosis

IMAGING FINDINGS

General Features
- Best diagnostic clue
  - Lung opacity that is posterior in location, non-segmental in distribution, crescentic in shape, amorphous, and mixed confluent and nodular quality
  - Subpleural sparing of peripheral lung
- Location: Posterior most common

Radiographic Findings
- Radiography
  - Radiography is insensitive diagnostic test for detecting lung contusions
  - 69% of lung contusions are either underestimated (24%) or not identified (45%) on initial chest radiography in patients with contusions shown by CT
  - Contusions
    - Opacities appear soon after trauma, < 6 hours
    - Adjacent to ribs and vertebral bodies
    - Located at impaction or contrecoup lung injury
    - Irregular patchy areas of airspace consolidation (mild)
    - Hemorrhage and edema in peribronchovascular interstitium
    - Diffuse extensive homogeneous consolidation (severe)
    - Improvement within 24-48 hours
    - Complete clearing within 10 days unless develops ARDS or other cause of airway opacification
  - Lacerations
    - May appear hours or days after trauma
    - At point of maximum impact or contrecoup location
    - Thin-walled air-filled cysts (pneumatoceles)
    - With or without air-fluid levels
    - May fill with blood (hematoma), rarely hematomas expand
    - Single or multiple
    - Oval or spherical
    - Unilocular, multilocular

DDx: Lung Consolidation After Trauma

Pre-Existing Pneumonia | Atelectasis | Aspiration

LUNG CONTUSION AND LACERATION

Key Facts

Terminology
- Lung contusion: Hemorrhage and edema formation in the alveoli and interstitium as a result of alveolar capillary damage secondary to blunt chest trauma
- Lung laceration: Frank tear within the lung parenchyma as a result of chest trauma
- Identification of lung contusions and differentiation from other causes of lung opacity in presence of blunt chest trauma has relevance to child's prognosis

Imaging Findings
- Radiography is insensitive diagnostic test for detecting lung contusions
- 69% of lung contusions are either underestimated (24%) or not identified (45%) on initial chest radiography in patients with contusions shown by CT
- CT findings of lung contusion
- Posterior location most common (75%)
- Crescentic (50%) or amorphous (45%) shape
- Mixed areas of both confluent lung opacification and nodular quality (70%) typical
- Subpleural sparing
- 1-2 mm region of uniformly non-opacified subpleural lung, separating the area of lung consolidation from the adjacent chest wall

Pathology
- Blunt trauma most common cause of death in children
- 80% of chest injuries are secondary to blunt trauma
- Lung contusion most common type of chest injury in children

---

- 2-14 cm diameter
- Persist for up to 4 months
- Gradual decrease in size, 1-2 cm/week
- Weeks to months to resolve
  - Bronchial injury
    - Very rare
    - Persistent pneumothorax despite chest tube placement
    - Lung falls away from hilum

CT Findings
- CT for blunt pulmonary trauma
  - CT uncommonly performed for the primary evaluation purpose of evaluating for blunt pulmonary trauma
  - Inferior lung is often visualized when CT is performed to evaluate for traumatic injury to the contents of the abdomen and pelvis
  - CT of chest (CTA) may be performed to evaluate for suspected aortic trauma
  - Important to recognize pulmonary contusions because of relevance to prognoses in blunt trauma patients
- CT findings of lung contusion
  - Posterior location most common (75%)
  - Crescentic (50%) or amorphous (45%) shape
  - Mixed areas of both confluent lung opacification and nodular quality (70%) typical
  - More common in lower lobes
  - Subpleural sparing
    - 1-2 mm region of uniformly non-opacified subpleural lung, separating the area of lung consolidation from the adjacent chest wall
    - Seen with many lung contusions and not with other causes of lung opacity such as atelectasis or pneumonia
    - Larger the lung contusion, the less likely subpleural sparing is to be present
- CT findings of lung laceration
  - Presence of air or fluid-filled cavity within region of findings of lung contusion
  - The cavity indicates that a frank tear of the lung parenchyma has occurred and is considered a more severe injury

Imaging Recommendations
- Chest radiographs usually sufficient to follow course of blunt trauma

DIFFERENTIAL DIAGNOSIS

Aspiration
- Radiographic findings may be similar to contusion
- Posterior location, lower lobes more common
- Absence of subpleural sparing
- Aspiration can occur in head trauma

Pneumonia
- A child in blunt trauma may have a lung contusion
- If acquired in hospital, occurs later in hospital course
- If contusion worsens after 48 hours, consider superinfection

Atelectasis
- Triangular shape
- Segmental distribution
- Obvious signs of volume loss
- Lack of subpleural sparing

PATHOLOGY

General Features
- General path comments
  - Rapid deceleration mechanism encountered in most motor vehicle accidents and relative increase plasticity of anterior chest wall in children as compared to adults determine the CT appearance of lung contusions
  - Rib fractures occur much more often in adults than in children related to the increased pliability of the anterior chest wall in children

LUNG CONTUSION AND LACERATION

- Increased pliability of chest wall in children in combination with contra-coup forces of rapid deceleration injury compresses the relatively fixed posterior lung against the immediately adjacent, less compliant posterior ribs and vertebral column
- Distribution of the disruptive forces along the least mobile regions of lung explains both posterior location and crescentic shape of most contusions
- Also explains the non-segmental distribution
- Subpleural sparing
  - Lung contusion result of alveolar capillary damage with extravasation of edema and hemorrhage into alveoli and interstitial spaces
  - Terminal arterial branches terminate prior to subpleural region of lung
  - Resultant sparse vascularity of this region may protect subpleural lung from hemorrhage
  - Subpleural lung also compressed against adjacent chest wall during injury, "squeezing" the extravasated blood and edema into more central lung
  - Larger contusions may have tendency to hemorrhage into subpleural lung secondary to persistent bleeding following trauma - may explain why sign is less common in larger contusions
- Lung laceration
  - Frank tear of lung parenchyma results in formation of disrupted cavity that fills with hemorrhage and/or air
- Etiology
  - Most lung contusions secondary to blunt chest trauma
  - Most commonly related to motor vehicle accidents
  - Other causes include child struck by car, fall from height
  - Penetrating chest trauma less common in children: Stabbing, gun shot, rib fracture puncturing lung
  - Child abuse
    - Lung contusions not uncommon in child abuse
    - Documentation of presence of lung contusion and differentiation from other causes of lung opacity may facilitate evidence in criminal proceedings and help with decisions regarding removal of child from a high risk environment
- Epidemiology
  - Blunt trauma most common cause of death in children
    - 80% of chest injuries are secondary to blunt trauma
  - Presence of lung contusion in pediatric trauma patient increases morbidity from 1.3% without contusion to 10.8% with contusion
  - Chest trauma secondary to only brain injuries as cause of death from blunt trauma
- Associated abnormalities
  - Lung contusion most common type of chest injury in children
  - Injuries to bronchi, great vessels, esophagus, and diaphragm are all much less common

Gross Pathologic & Surgical Features
- Air spaces filled with blood

CLINICAL ISSUES

Presentation
- Most common signs/symptoms: Usually no specific symptoms from contusions, pneumatoceles, or hematomas
- Other signs/symptoms: May present with respiratory failure in large contusions

Natural History & Prognosis
- Variable, usually related to other injures

Treatment
- Supportive therapy, surveillance for other major organ injuries, observation for complications
- Complications: Infection, hemopneumothorax, or hemoptysis

SELECTED REFERENCES

1. Sartorelli KH et al: The diagnosis and management of children with blunt injury of the chest. Semin Pediatr Surg. 13(2):98-105, 2004
2. Hall A et al: The imaging of paediatric thoracic trauma. Paediatr Respir Rev. 3(3):241-7, 2002
3. Sivit CS: Pediatric thoracic trauma: imaging considerations. Emerg Radiol. 9(1):21-5, 2002
4. Rashid MA: Contre-coup lung injury: evidence of existence. J Trauma. 48(3):530-2, 2000
5. Allen GS et al: Pulmonary contusion in children: diagnosis and management. South Med J. 91(12):1099-106, 1998
6. Lowe LH et al: Traumatic aortic injuries in children: radiologic evaluation. AJR Am J Roentgenol. 170(1):39-42, 1998
7. Donnelly LF et al: Subpleural sparing: a CT finding of lung contusion in children. Radiology. 204(2):385-7, 1997
8. Karaaslan T et al: Traumatic chest lesions in patients with severe head trauma: a comparative study with computed tomography and conventional chest roentgenograms. J Trauma. 39(6):1081-6, 1995
9. Taylor GA et al: Active hemorrhage in children after thoracoabdominal trauma: clinical and CT features. AJR Am J Roentgenol. 162(2):401-4, 1994
10. Mirvis SE et al: Imaging in acute thoracic trauma. Semin Roentgenol 27:184-210, 1992
11. Bonadio WA et al: Post-traumatic pulmonary contusion in children. Ann Emerg Med. 18(10):1050-2, 1989
12. Schild HH et al: Pulmonary contusion: CT vs plain radiograms. J Comput Assist Tomogr. 13(3):417-20, 1989
13. Sivit CJ et al: Chest injury in children with blunt abdominal trauma: evaluation with CT. Radiology. 171(3):815-8, 1989
14. Wagner RB et al: Pulmonary contusion. Evaluation and classification by computed tomography. Surg Clin North Am. 69(1):31-40, 1989
15. Wagner RB et al: Classification of parenchymal injuries of the lung. Radiology. 167(1):77-82, 1988
16. Wagner RB et al: Quantitation and pattern of parenchymal lung injury in blunt chest trauma. Diagnostic and therapeutic implications. J Comput Tomogr. 12(4):270-81, 1988

LUNG CONTUSION AND LACERATION

IMAGE GALLERY

Typical

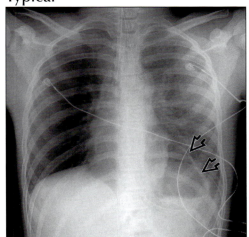
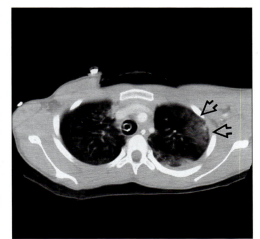

(Left) Anteroposterior radiograph shows 14 year old boy in motor vehicle accident with traumatic diaphragmatic hernia *(arrows)*. There is a large left lung contusion which is poorly visualized. *(Right)* Axial CECT in same patient shows peripheral lung contusion in left upper lobe with subpleural sparing *(arrows)*.

Typical

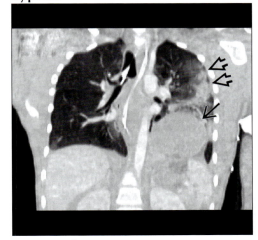
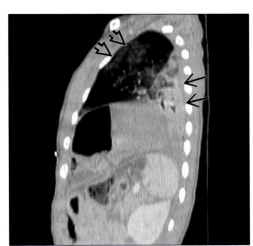

(Left) Coronal CECT in same patient as above shows traumatic diaphragmatic hernia *(arrow)* and left upper lobe lung contusion with subpleural sparing *(open arrows)*. Note Right bronchial intubation. *(Right)* Sagittal CECT in same patient as on left shows anterior left upper lobe lung contusion with subpleural sparing *(open arrows)* and left lower lobe collapse without subpleural sparing *(arrows)*.

Typical

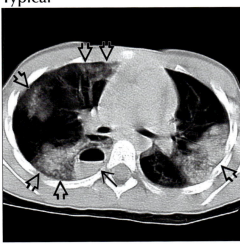
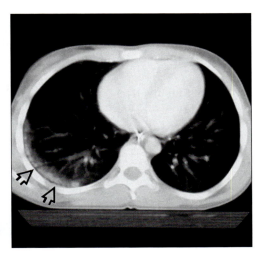

(Left) Axial CECT shows bilateral areas of air space opacification some of which show subpleural sparing *(open arrows)*. Note cystic structure *(arrow)* consistent with a lung laceration. *(Right)* Axial CECT shows crescentic, posterior, non-segmental opacity with subpleural sparing *(arrows)* classic for lung contusion.

PAPILLOMATOSIS

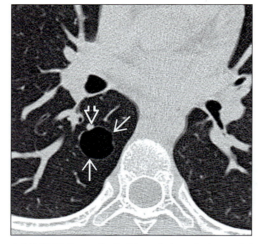

Axial HRCT shows classic thin walled cyst in the medial basal segment of the right lower lobe (arrows). The adjacent nodular density (open arrow) is a pulmonary arterial branch.

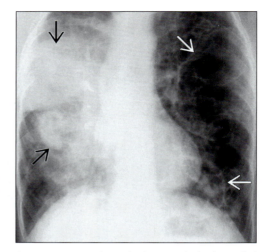

Anteroposterior radiograph shows multiple thin-walled cysts predominantly in the left lung (white arrows) with nodules and masses predominantly in the right lung (black arrows).

TERMINOLOGY

Abbreviations and Synonyms
- Recurrent respiratory papillomatosis (RRP)
- Juvenile-onset recurrent respiratory papillomatosis (JORRP)
- Laryngeal/laryngotracheal/tracheal papillomatosis
- Juvenile laryngeal papillomatosis

Definitions
- Benign tumors of the aerodigestive tract due to infection with human papilloma virus (HPV)

IMAGING FINDINGS

General Features
- Best diagnostic clue: Cauliflower-like growth in larynx
- Location
  - Larynx involved in 95% of cases
  - Tracheobronchial tree and lung parenchyma less common
  - Nasopharynx, oropharynx, esophagus are rarer sites
- Size: 1-2 mm to several centimeters
- Morphology
  - Warty lesions of larynx and tracheobronchial tree
  - Endobronchial spread leads to round nodules that may cavitate
  - Thin > thick walled cavities

Radiographic Findings
- Radiography
  - Larynx, trachea, and main bronchi: Multifocal nodular irregularity of the wall
  - Lung: Multiple solid or cavitated nodules
    - As nodules enlarge more likely to cavitate
    - Cavities may be thick or thin walled
    - Slow growth (years)
    - Air-fluid level suggests superinfection
    - Atelectasis and postobstructive pneumonia uncommon
    - Large mass suggests malignant degeneration

Fluoroscopic Findings
- Confirms that tracheal irregularity is not related to adherent secretions

CT Findings
- Useful to evaluate trachea and airways for papillomas
- Parenchymal nodules are well circumscribed and have mild homogeneous enhancement
- Dorsal distribution, may be related to gravity and dependent seeding of the lung
- Nodules communicate with adjacent airways
- Heterogeneous enhancement and irregular nodules or large growing mass suggest malignant degeneration

DDx: Cysts And Nodules

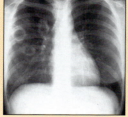

Wegener

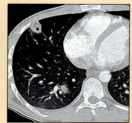

Septic Emboli

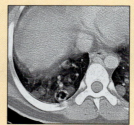

Metastases

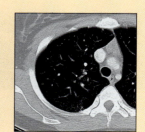

Tuberous Sclerosis

PAPILLOMATOSIS

Key Facts

Terminology
- Benign tumors of the aerodigestive tract due to infection with human papilloma virus (HPV)

Imaging Findings
- Larynx involved in 95% of cases
- Endobronchial spread leads to round nodules that may cavitate
- Lateral airway radiographs best for laryngotracheal disease
- CT useful to determine extent of disease and to identify complications

Top Differential Diagnoses
- Wegener granulomatosis
- Langerhans cell histiocytosis
- Invasive fungal disease

Pathology
- Perinatal transmission of human papilloma virus from infected mother to child
- Increased risk with: Vaginal delivery; firstborn child; and mother < 20 years of age

Clinical Issues
- Most common signs/symptoms: Hoarseness/voice change
- Frequent recurrences and disease exacerbations are the norm
- Malignant degeneration more common in longstanding disease with history of prior irradiation and smoking
- Need for repeated debulking is typical

- Lymphadenopathy suspicious for malignant degeneration

Imaging Recommendations
- Best imaging tool
  - Lateral airway radiographs best for laryngotracheal disease
  - Radiographs for uncomplicated pulmonary disease
  - CT useful to determine extent of disease and to identify complications
- Protocol advice: CT in prone position may identify small peripheral nodules in dorsal dependent regions

DIFFERENTIAL DIAGNOSIS

Metastases
- Variable size sharply defined
- Cavitation usually seen in squamous cell histology or sarcomas

Wegener granulomatosis
- Trachea: Circumferential wall thickening in subglottic region
- Paranasal sinus or renal disease
- Pulmonary nodules that may form thick-walled cavities

Septic emboli
- Endocarditis
- Lemierre syndrome: Thrombophlebitis of a neck vein from an upper respiratory tract infection, with septic emboli
- Trachea normal

Pneumatoceles
- Transient and usually follow known insult (trauma, infection, hydrocarbon ingestion)
- Trachea normal

Tuberous sclerosis
- Women, cysts randomly distributed
- May have nodules (multifocal micronodular pneumocyte hyperplasia)
- Trachea normal

Langerhans cell histiocytosis
- Nodules and/or cysts, primarily in upper lung zones
- Trachea normal

Sjögren
- History of sicca syndrome
- 1/3 have thin-walled cysts
- Trachea normal

Invasive fungal disease
- Aspergillus most common
- Immunocompromised host
- Commonly have ground-glass halo
- Trachea usually normal

Septic emboli
- Patient usually acutely ill
- Trachea normal

Subglottic hemangioma
- Usually presents in infancy with stridor
- Strongly enhancing nodule on CT

PATHOLOGY

General Features
- General path comments
  - Projections of keratinized stratified squamous epithelium overlying a fibrovascular core
  - Most commonly occur at junctions between squamous and ciliated respiratory epithelium
    - True and false vocal cords
    - Subglottis and epiglottis
  - Repeated trauma to ciliated epithelium induces squamous metaplasia and facilitates spread to new areas
- Etiology
  - Perinatal transmission of human papilloma virus from infected mother to child
    - Increased risk with: Vaginal delivery; firstborn child; and mother < 20 years of age

PAPILLOMATOSIS

- Elective cesarian section is not recommended as it is not protective
- Rarely occurs in non-twin sibling pairs
- Multiple strains of HPV can cause disease, but vast majority from HPV-6 and HPV-11
- HPV-11 more common and causes more severe disease
- HPV-16 and HPV-18 have greatest risk of malignant degeneration
- Tracheal or central bronchial involvement in ≈ 5%
- Peripheral airway or alveolar involvement in < 1%
  - Surgical manipulation of laryngeal papillomas increases risk of dissemination
  - More common in chronic infection with large papillomata
- Second peak in adults of same lesion = adult-onset recurrent respiratory papillomatosis (AORRP)
  - Etiology most likely sexual transmission of HPV
  - M:F = 4:1
- Epidemiology
  - U.S.: 4.3 cases per 100,000 children
  - Commonest cause of a laryngeal tumor in children

Gross Pathologic & Surgical Features
- Sessile or papillary lesions with vascular core covered by squamous epithelium

Microscopic Features
- Lung and laryngeal lesions composed of squamous cells, cavities lined with squamous epithelium
- Squamous atypia common even in benign lesions
- Distinction between benign and malignant disease may be difficult

CLINICAL ISSUES

Presentation
- Most common signs/symptoms: Hoarseness/voice change
- Other signs/symptoms
  - Weak cry, wheezing, stridor, choking, complete airway obstruction, failure to thrive
  - Laryngoscopy/bronchoscopy: Warty laryngeal growth
  - Polymerase chain reaction on tissue for viral typing: Helps to determine prognosis as most severe disease with HPV-11
  - Pulmonary functions tests: Pattern of upper airway obstruction

Demographics
- Age
  - Mean age at diagnosis is 3.8 years
  - First presentation after 5 years of age raises possibility of sexual abuse
- Gender: Male = female
- Ethnicity: Caucasian (63%) > African-American (28%) > Asian-American or Native-American (2%)

Natural History & Prognosis
- Frequent recurrences and disease exacerbations are the norm
- Occasionally may be a self limiting infection
  - Variable and unpredictable
- Tracheal involvement in 2-17% of patients without tracheostomies
- Tracheostomies have significant morbidity
  - ≈ 50% develop peristomal and tracheal lesions
- Lung nodules grow very slowly, usually measured in decades
- May cavitate
  - Can become secondarily infected
- May get postobstructive atelectasis and pneumonia
- 2% incidence of squamous cell carcinoma degeneration
  - High suspicion needs to be maintained
    - Any change in nodule should be investigated for malignant transformation
  - Malignant degeneration more common in longstanding disease with history of prior irradiation and smoking
    - Adults: Larynx
    - Pediatric patients: Tracheobronchial tree
- Disseminated disease: Death due to respiratory failure

Treatment
- Laser ablation of laryngeal or airway lesion for debulking
  - Virus may be aerosolized during ablation
    - Increased risk of transbronchial spread to lungs
    - Risk to operating room personnel
- Need for repeated debulking is typical
- Interferon and antiviral agents (cidofovir and acyclovir) may slow growth, but are not curative
- 3-Carbinol, retinoic acid, and photodynamic therapy have variable effect
- Tracheostomy needed in 10-15% → increase risk of spread to trachea

SELECTED REFERENCES

1. Prince JS et al: Nonneoplastic lesions of the tracheobronchial wall: radiologic findings with bronchoscopic correlation. Radiographics. 22 Spec No:S215-30, 2002
2. Shah KV et al: Risk factors for juvenile onset recurrent respiratory papillomatosis. Pediatr Infect Dis J. 17(5):372-6, 1998
3. Bauman NM et al: Recurrent respiratory papillomatosis. Pediatr Clin North Am. 43(6):1385-401, 1996
4. Kashima HK et al: A comparison of risk factors in juvenile-onset and adult-onset recurrent respiratory papillomatosis. Laryngoscope. 102(1):9-13, 1992
5. Kawanami T et al: Juvenile laryngeal papillomatosis with pulmonary parenchymal spread. Case report and review of the literature. Pediatr Radiol. 15:102-4, 1985
6. Kramer SS et al: Pulmonary manifestations of juvenile laryngotracheal papillomatosis. AJR. 144:687-94, 1985
7. Mounts P et al: Association of human papillomavirus subtype and clinical course in respiratory papillomatosis. Laryngoscope. 94(1):28-33, 1984

PAPILLOMATOSIS

IMAGE GALLERY

Typical

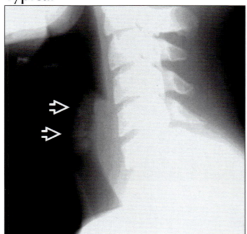 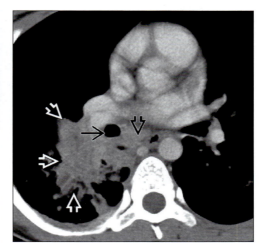

(Left) Lateral radiograph shows a cauliflower-like growth in the glottis and subglottic airway (arrows). (Right) Axial CECT shows heterogeneously enhancing mass (white open arrows), extending into the azygoesophageal recess (black open arrow), surrounding the left lower lobe bronchus (arrow). This was found to be a squamous cell carcinoma at biopsy.

Typical

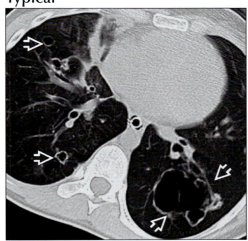 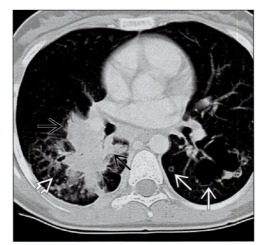

(Left) Axial NECT shows predominantly thin-walled cysts in the bilateral lower lobes, of varying sizes (arrows). (Right) Axial CECT shows ill-defined mass in the right lower lobe (black arrows) with postobstructive pneumonia (open arrow). Note predominantly thin-walled cysts in the dependent portions of the left lower lobe (white arrows).

Typical

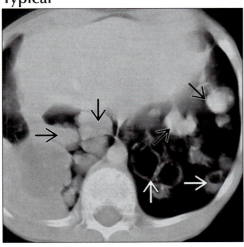 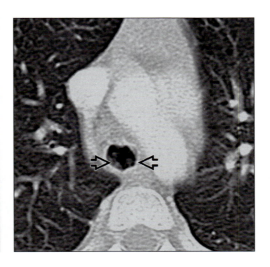

(Left) Axial CECT shows multiple nodular densities in both lower lobes (black arrows). Some of these are at differing stages of cavitation (white arrows). (Right) Axial CECT shows nodularity of the distal trachea (arrows). The patient had recurrent papillomatosis at this site.

PECTUS EXCAVATUM

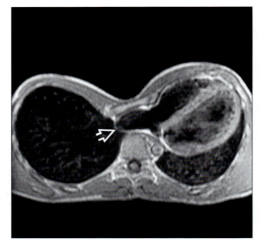

Axial T1WI MR in child with Marfan syndrome shows severe pectus deformity with right atrium (arrow) immediately behind sternum. Atrial laceration could occur at Nuss procedure

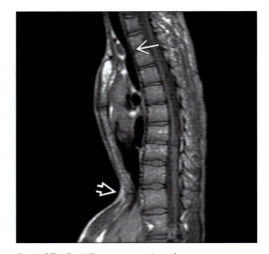

Sagittal T1 C+ MR on same patient shows severe pectus deformity. Xyphoid (open arrow) almost rests on spinal column. Trachea is narrowed (arrow) at thoracic inlet.

TERMINOLOGY

Abbreviations and Synonyms
- Funnel chest

Definitions
- Pectus excavatum represents a depression of the sternum and anterior ribs posteriorly resulting in a sunken appearance of the anterior inferior chest wall
- Pectus carinatum by contrast represents a prominent anterior convexity (pigeon chest)
- Most often pectus excavatum is asymptomatic except for cosmetic concerns
- However, it may be associated with exercise intolerance, restrictive lung disease, central airway compression, mitral valve prolapse, and Wolff-Parkinson-White syndrome
- Currently, in severe cases, pectus excavatum is most commonly treated by means of minimally invasive repair (Nuss procedure)
  - A transverse, curved metal bar is surgically inserted internal to the sternum and rib cage and then "inverted" popping the chest into a more normal configuration
  - In "long" superior to inferior deformities, two bars may be utilized
  - Bar(s) remain in place for up to several years
  - Most of the imaging done for pectus excavatum is done for pre-operative planning and follow-up of the Nuss procedure

IMAGING FINDINGS

Radiographic Findings
- Radiography
  - Pectus excavatum on chest radiography
    - Right heart border is frequently obliterated because the depressed thoracic wall replaces aerated lung at the right heart border
    - Heart is displaced to the left and rotated (mitral configuration) may mimic cardiomegaly
    - Degree of depression best seen on lateral chest radiograph, sternum seen more posterior than most anterior position of anterior ribs
    - Central airway compression from thoracic deformity often difficult to visualize on radiographs, better see on CT
  - Post-Nuss Procedure
    - Nuss bar appears as transverse metal bar with "T" shaped stabilizer at one end
    - Chest radiography often utilized to follow-up for potential complications following Nuss procedure
    - Bar displacement or rotation 9.2%
    - Pneumothorax 4.8%

DDx: Chest Wall Deformity or Mass

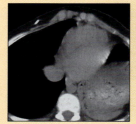
Pectus Carinatum

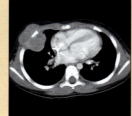
Askin Tumor

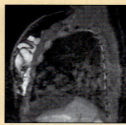
Lymphatic Malfor.

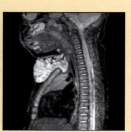
Hemangioma

PECTUS EXCAVATUM

Key Facts

Terminology
- Pectus excavatum represents a depression of the sternum and anterior ribs posteriorly resulting in a sunken appearance of the anterior inferior chest wall
- Pectus carinatum by contrast represents a prominent anterior convexity (pigeon chest)
- Currently, in severe cases, pectus excavatum is most commonly treated by means of minimally invasive repair (Nuss procedure)
- A transverse, curved metal bar is surgically inserted internal to the sternum and rib cage and then "inverted" popping the chest into a more normal configuration

Imaging Findings
- Right heart border is frequently obliterated because the depressed thoracic wall replaces aerated lung at the right heart border
- Nuss bar appears as transverse metal bar with "T" shaped stabilizer at one end
- Bar displacement or rotation 9.2%
- Pre-Nuss procedure evaluation with CT
- Haller index > 3.2 considered great enough deformity for surgical candidacy
- Right atrium may be anomalously positioned immediately posterior to deep side of sternum and may predispose to potential laceration of atrium during placement of bar
- Central airway compression

- Pleural effusion 2.0%
- Thoracic outlet obstruction 0.8%
- Cardiac injury during placement of bar 0.4%
  - Lateral radiograph is best view to evaluate for migration of fixation bar
    - Best to obtain baseline study including lateral several days after bar placed for baseline position
    - Most commonly the bar will rotate with anterior portion moving superior or inferior
    - May occur after trauma
    - Rotation also less commonly found in axial plane

CT Findings
- Pre-Nuss procedure evaluation with CT
  - Technical features
    - Noncontrast, low mA images obtained through chest
    - Sagittal and 3D reconstruction may be helpful for communication purposes
  - Haller index
    - Calculation used to determine severity of pectus deformity and serves as indicator for Nuss procedure candidacy
    - Measured in axial plane at level of the most severe anterior to posterior chest narrowing
    - Ratio of transverse, left-to-right diameter of the chest divided by sagittal, anterior-to-posterior diameter of the chest
    - Measurements are made "internally" from inner aspect of bony chest wall to inner aspect of bony chest wall
    - Haller index > 3.2 considered great enough deformity for surgical candidacy
  - Characterization of superior-to-inferior extent of pectus excavatum deformity
    - May be focal depression vs. more diffusely depressed from superior to inferior
    - Length of depression determines if one or two transverse bars are needed
    - Best shown on sagittal reconstructed images
  - Heart position
    - Evaluation for compression, displacement, or distortion of cardiac structures
    - Pectus excavatum may cause distortion of cardiac structures
    - Right atrium may be anomalously positioned immediately posterior to deep side of sternum and may predispose to potential laceration of atrium during placement of bar
    - Information critical to surgical planning
  - Central airway compression
    - Thoracic deformities such as pectus excavatum may distort mediastinal anatomy and result in compression of the thoracic airway
    - Most common sites of compression: Carina/proximal main bronchi, trachea at thoracic inlet
  - Associated rib or vertebral anomalies
    - May be present in association with pectus excavatum
- CT evaluation for palpable anterior chest wall mass
  - Mild pectus deformities may be associated with a tilted sternum, prominent asymmetric anterior convex ribs, or prominent asymmetric costal cartilages that may be palpated and suspected to represent a chest wall mass
  - Such subjects are often referred to cross-sectional imaging to evaluate for mass
  - Important to state the reason for the palpable abnormality in addition to stating that no aggressive masses are present as referring physician can palpate abnormality
  - 3D reconstruction often helpful for communication and occasionally diagnostic aids

MR Findings
- May be used to evaluate for central airway compression in patients with thoracic deformity
- May be used to evaluate for palpable anterior chest wall masses

Echocardiographic Findings
- Echocardiogram: May show findings of mitral valve prolapse

PECTUS EXCAVATUM

Imaging Recommendations
- Best imaging tool
  - CT for pre-Nuss procedure, evaluation for central airway compression
  - Lateral chest radiography to evaluate for migration of bar in Nuss procedure (base-line view recommended)
- Protocol advice: Pre-Nuss chest CT does not require contrast and may be done at low mA

DIFFERENTIAL DIAGNOSIS

Pectus carinatum
- Opposite of pectus excavatum
- Anterior chest convex outward: Pigeon chest

Chest wall aggressive lesions
- Palpable bony asymmetry associated with mild pectus deformity may be mistaken for soft tissue mass

Chest wall vascular malformation or hemangioma
- Lymphatic malformation, venous malformations, and hemangiomas commonly involve chest wall

PATHOLOGY

General Features
- Etiology: Poorly understood
- Epidemiology: 1% of population affected
- Associated abnormalities: Pectus excavatum: Frequently associated with Marfan's syndrome, Poland syndrome, scoliosis, and Pierre Robin syndrome

CLINICAL ISSUES

Presentation
- Most common signs/symptoms
  - Most common isolated cosmetic problem
  - Exercise intolerance not uncommon
- Other signs/symptoms
  - Cardiac (pulmonic murmur, mitral valve prolapse, syncope, Wolff-Parkinson-White syndrome) and respiratory (severe restriction) symptoms
  - Central airway compression resulting in stridor
  - Restrictive lung disease is the result of decreased compliance of both the lung and chest wall
  - Restriction results in hypoventilation, hypoxic vasoconstriction, pulmonary artery hypertension, cor pulmonale, hypercapnia and respiratory failure

Demographics
- Age: Any

Natural History & Prognosis
- May lead to restrictive lung disease or central airway compression

Treatment
- Conservative management for mild cases
- Non-invasive pectus repair (Nuss procedure)
  - Excellent results > 85% of patients
  - Relatively safe procedure with minimal morbidity
- Ravitch pectus excavatum repair
  - More traditional surgical repair
  - One article has shown similar success rates and hospitalization length to Nuss procedure

SELECTED REFERENCES

1. Daunt SW et al: Age-related normal ranges for the Haller index in children. Pediatr Radiol. 34(4):326-30, 2004
2. Haecker FM et al: Minimally invasive repair of pectus excavatum (MIRPE)--the Basel experience. Swiss Surg. 9(6):289-95, 2003
3. Fonkalsrud EW et al: Comparison of minimally invasive and modified Ravitch pectus excavatum repair. J Pediatr Surg. 37(3):413-7, 2002
4. Croitoru DP et al: Experience and modification update for the minimally invasive Nuss technique for pectus excavatum repair in 303 patients. J Pediatr Surg. 37(3):437-45, 2002
5. Donnelly LF: Use of three-dimensional reconstructed helical CT images in recognition and communication of chest wall anomalies in children. AJR Am J Roentgenol. 177(2):441-5, 2001
6. Raichura N et al: Breath-hold MRI in evaluating patients with pectus excavatum. Br J Radiol. 74(884):701-8, 2001
7. Sidden CR et al: Radiologic considerations in patients undergoing the Nuss procedure for correction of pectus excavatum. Pediatr Radiol. 31(6):429-34, 2001
8. Hebra A et al: Outcome analysis of minimally invasive repair of pectus excavatum: review of 251 cases. J Pediatr Surg. 35(2):252-7; discussion 257-8, 2000
9. Donnelly LF et al: Abnormalities of the chest wall in pediatric patients. AJR Am J Roentgenol. 173(6):1595-601, 1999
10. Donnelly LF et al: Anterior chest wall: frequency of anatomic variations in children. Radiology. 212(3):837-40, 1999
11. Haje SA et al: Growth disturbance of the sternum and pectus deformities: imaging studies and clinical correlation. Pediatr Radiol. 29(5):334-41, 1999
12. Donnelly LF et al: Airway compression in children with abnormal thoracic configuration. Radiology. 206(2):323-6, 1998
13. Grissom LE et al: Thoracic deformities and the growing lung. Semin Roentgenol. 33(2):199-208, 1998
14. Nuss D et al: A 10-year review of a minimally invasive technique for the correction of pectus excavatum. J Pediatr Surg. 33(4):545-52, 1998
15. Donnelly LF et al: The spectrum of extrinsic lower airway compression in children: MR imaging. AJR Am J Roentgenol. 168(1):59-62, 1997
16. Donnelly LF et al: Asymptomatic, palpable, anterior chest wall lesions in children: is cross-sectional imaging necessary? Radiology. 202(3):829-31, 1997

PECTUS EXCAVATUM

IMAGE GALLERY

Typical

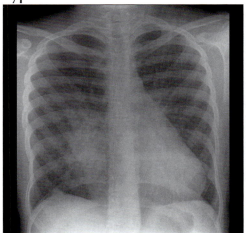
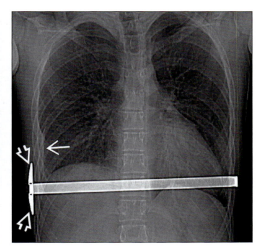

(Left) Anteroposterior radiograph shows pectus deformity with loss of right heart border seen on frontal view mimicking right middle lobe opacity. (Right) Anteroposterior radiograph after Nuss procedure shows transverse metal bar with "T" shaped stabilization device (open arrows) at one end. Note small right pleural effusion (arrow).

Typical

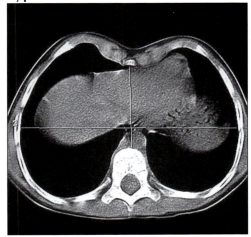
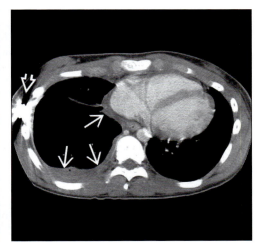

(Left) Axial NECT shows pectus excavatum with lines measuring "Haller index". Lines begin and end at internal aspect of bony chest wall. (Right) Axial CECT after Nuss procedure shows edge of stabilization bar (open arrow), small pleural effusion (arrows), and resolution of pectus deformity.

Typical

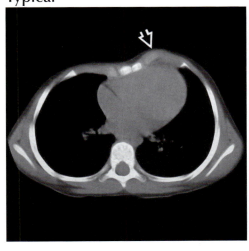
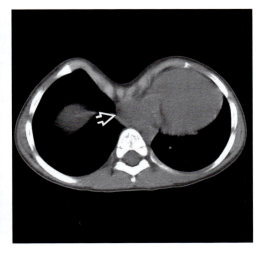

(Left) Axial CECT shows mild pectus deformity causing asymmetric convex left anterior rib which was palpated and suspected of being a rib mass (arrow). (Right) Axial NECT shows pectus with right atrium (arrow) immediately posterior to xiphoid and potentially at risk for laceration during placement of transverse bar. Heart is shifted to left.

CHRONIC ESOPHAGEAL FOREIGN BODY

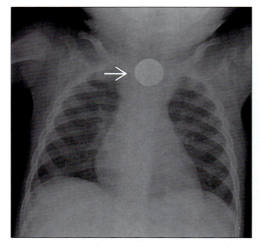

Anteroposterior radiograph shows coin in esophagus (arrow) in this eight month old infant who was wheezing for the last week and recently had decreased oral intake.

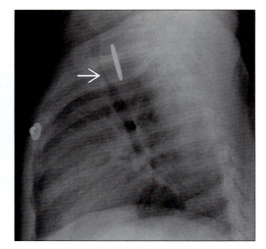

Lateral radiograph shows coin in esophagus with tracheal narrowing anteriorly (arrow) and increase in distance between esophagus and trachea secondary to inflammatory reaction.

TERMINOLOGY

Definitions
- Foreign body in the esophagus which has been there for a prolonged period of time
- Usually causes airway or feeding symptoms in infants and toddlers

IMAGING FINDINGS

General Features
- Best diagnostic clue
  - Radiopaque object in region of esophagus
  - High suspicion when airway is narrowed
    - Airway displaced anteriorly
    - Proximal esophagus may be dilated
  - May present with complications
    - Abscess
    - Pneumomediastinum/mediastinitus
    - Pneumothorax
- Location
  - Most common site is upper esophagus at thoracic inlet
  - Second most common site is level of carina and aortic arch
    - Normal physiologic narrowing is present at this level
  - Third most common site is distal esophagus slightly above gastroesophageal junction
  - Obstruction at other sites suggest underlying abnormality
    - Anastomotic stricture after repair of esophageal atresia
    - Vascular ring
- Size: Variable
- Morphology
  - Variable depending on foreign body
  - Coins are the most commonly swallowed foreign body
    - Coins in esophagus will appear in coronal plane (en face) on anteroposterior (AP) view
    - Coins in trachea will appear in sagittal plane (on end) on AP view
  - Button batteries show a characteristic double-density (2-layer) shadow
    - Laterally, their edges are rounded with a step-off junction at the positive and negative terminal
    - Important to identify since they may cause caustic burn injury to esophagus
  - Non-radiopaque foreign body
    - Hot dog is most common
    - Plastic toys are also commonly ingested

Radiographic Findings
- Radiography

DDx: Esophageal Narrowing

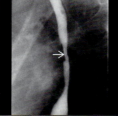
Epidermolysis Bullosa

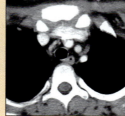
Candida Esophagitis

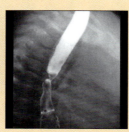
Esophageal Stenosis

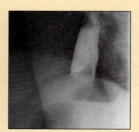
Achalasia

CHRONIC ESOPHAGEAL FOREIGN BODY

Key Facts

Terminology
- Foreign body in the esophagus which has been there for a prolonged period of time

Imaging Findings
- Radiopaque object in region of esophagus
- High suspicion when airway is narrowed
- May present with complications
- Most common site is upper esophagus at thoracic inlet
- Obstruction at other sites suggest underlying abnormality
- Coins are the most commonly swallowed foreign body
- Button batteries show a characteristic double-density (2-layer) shadow
- AP and lateral chest radiograph best initial study
- Esophagram for nonradiopaque foreign bodies
- CECT to diagnose complications such as abscess or mediastinitis

Top Differential Diagnoses
- Airway obstruction
- Achalasia
- Tracheal stenosis
- Esophagitis

Pathology
- Retained foreign body may cause perforation, inflammatory reaction, and strictures of esophagus

Clinical Issues
- Respiratory or airway problems most common
- Cough, stridor, fever, wheezing
- Dysphagia, drooling, vomiting, gagging

- Radiopaque foreign body in esophagus
  - Entire or portion of foreign body may be radiolucent
- Tracheal narrowing and/or anterior tracheal bowing
- Mediastinal mass
  - Secondary to abscess
- Lateral radiograph
  - Increased distance between trachea and esophagus
  - Dilatation of esophagus
  - Tracheal narrowing and anterior displacement
- Complications may be evident
  - Pneumomediastinum
  - Abscess

Fluoroscopic Findings
- Esophagram
  - Useful for evaluating nonradiopaque foreign bodies
  - May diagnose strictures or underlying cause
  - Identify fistula or perforation

CT Findings
- CECT
  - Radiopaque foreign body may be isodense to bone
  - Mediastinitis and abscess
  - Maybe useful following removal of chronic foreign body
    - Esophageal leak
    - Mediastinitis
    - Esophageal diverticulum

Imaging Recommendations
- Best imaging tool
  - AP and lateral chest radiograph best initial study
  - Esophagram for nonradiopaque foreign bodies
  - CECT to diagnose complications such as abscess or mediastinitis
- Protocol advice
  - Initial survey includes chest, lateral neck, and supine abdominal radiographs
  - Barium swallow for nonradiopaque foreign bodies
    - Use water soluble contrast if occult perforation is suspected
  - CECT indications for complications
    - Plain radiography is negative
    - High suspicion of esophageal foreign body
    - Used to evaluate for esophageal perforation
    - Complications of foreign body such as abscess or pneumothorax

DIFFERENTIAL DIAGNOSIS

Airway obstruction
- May simulate foreign bodies in the esophagus
- Retropharyngeal abscess
- Croup
- Asthma

Achalasia
- Failure of normal relaxation of lower esophageal sphincter
- Dilatation of esophagus

Tracheal stenosis
- Presents with airway problems especially when feeding
- Congenital lesion often associated with other anomalies

Esophagitis
- Inflammatory reaction which alters peristalsis
- Gastroesophageal reflux

Epidermolysis bullosa
- Multiple esophageal strictures
- Skin changes

Strictures of the esophagus
- Many foreign bodies wedge proximal to esophageal strictures
  - Nonradiopaque the most common (meat)
- Esophageal atresia repair is the most common
- Need esophagram to diagnose stricture with or without foreign body

CHRONIC ESOPHAGEAL FOREIGN BODY

PATHOLOGY

General Features
- Etiology: Ingestion of foreign body
- Epidemiology
  - Thousands of cases in the US each year
  - Common for toddlers to explore their environment and place objects in mouth
- Associated abnormalities
  - Complications
    - Respiratory symptoms due to migration of foreign body into mediastinum or soft tissues
    - Mediastinitis
    - Abscess
    - Esophageal perforation following removal of chronic foreign bodies
    - Esophageal diverticula
    - Granulomas: Can lead to tracheal stenosis, lobar atelectasis, and bronchoesophageal fistulas
    - Retained foreign body may cause perforation, inflammatory reaction, and strictures of esophagus

Gross Pathologic & Surgical Features
- Localized inflammation and possible perforation of the esophagus

CLINICAL ISSUES

Presentation
- Most common signs/symptoms
  - Respiratory or airway problems most common
    - Cough, stridor, fever, wheezing
    - Chronic upper respiratory infection (URI)
    - Pneumonia
    - Hemoptysis, choking, cyanosis
  - Gastrointestinal symptoms
    - Dysphagia, drooling, vomiting, gagging
  - Chest pain when swallowing
  - Fever of unknown origin
  - Failure to thrive
  - Commonly ingested items
    - Chicken or fish bones
    - Coins
    - Batteries
    - Buttons
    - Plastic toys

Demographics
- Age
  - Most are younger than 5 years
  - Typically 8 months to 2 years of age
  - Can occur at any age
- Gender: Males slightly higher incidence

Natural History & Prognosis
- Foreign bodies present for > 24 hours have increased risk of esophageal perforation
- Vast majority of ingested objects pass through gastrointestinal tract without problems

Treatment
- Success rate is 95-100% regardless of technique
- Strategy depends on three things
  - Type and location of foreign body
  - Amount of time foreign body present in esophagus
  - Degree of removal experience at facility
- General complications prior to or without treatment
  - Most common complication is perforation and subsequent mediastinitis
  - Rare complications include tracheoesophageal fistula and aortoesophageal fistula
- Endoscopy or surgery
  - Use immediately for sharp objects and irregular or unknown foreign bodies
  - Use immediately for batteries in esophagus
    - Cause damage by pressure against wall of esophagus, from leakage of caustic alkali, and electrical current they generate
    - Injury can occur in as short a time as 1 hour
    - Full-thickness burns can occur in 4 hours
    - Lodging in the esophagus occurs in less than 1% of cases
    - Check battery type as most batteries do not cause injury
  - Batteries in stomach may be observed initially
    - Repeat radiography 24 hours after presentation with removal if still in stomach
- Esophagoscopy
  - Rigid esophagoscopy most successful for retrieval of foreign body
    - Requires general anesthesia
    - Requires intubation: Protected airway
  - Flexible esophagoscopy
    - Requires sedation
    - Intubation not necessary
- Foley catheter extraction under fluoroscopy
  - Relatively contraindicated in patients with known esophageal abnormalities
  - Rarely used in chronic foreign bodies
- Increased soft tissues between foreign body (FB) and trachea indicative of chronic inflammation and predictive of more difficult removal of FB

SELECTED REFERENCES

1. Miller RS et al: Chronic esophageal foreign bodies in pediatric patients: a retrospective review. Int J Pediatr Otorhinolaryngol. 68(3):265-72, 2004
2. Naidoo RR et al: Chronic retained foreign bodies in the esophagus. Ann Thorac Surg. 77(6):2218-20, 2004
3. Soprano JV et al: Four strategies for the management of esophageal coins in children. Pediatrics. 105(1):e5, 2000
4. Castellote A et al: Cervicothoracic lesions in infants and children. Radiographics. 19(3):583-600, 1999
5. Gilchrist BF et al: Pearls and perils in the management of prolonged, peculiar, penetrating esophageal foreign bodies in children. J Pediatr Surg. 32(10):1429-31, 1997
6. Macpherson RI et al: Esophageal foreign bodies in children: diagnosis, treatment, and complications. AJR Am J Roentgenol. 166(4):919-24, 1996
7. Campbell JB et al: Catheter removal of blunt esophageal foreign bodies in children. Survey of the Society for Pediatric Radiology. Pediatr Radiol. 19(6-7):361-5, 1989
8. Nandi P et al: Foreign body in the oesophagus: review of 2394 cases. Br J Surg. 65(1):5-9, 1978

CHRONIC ESOPHAGEAL FOREIGN BODY

IMAGE GALLERY

Typical

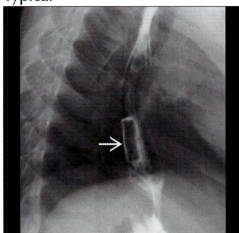
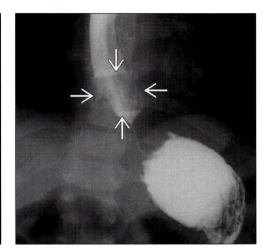

(Left) Lateral esophagram shows scrabble piece (arrow) outlined by barium in an eleven year old who had symptoms of esophagitis for past week. He denied swallowing anything which means you can not trust the history in kids! (Right) Anteroposterior esophagram shows scrabble piece (arrows) at gastroesophageal junction. The patient had no underlying abnormality of the esophagus except mild esophagitis from presence of the foreign body.

Typical

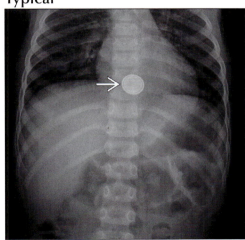
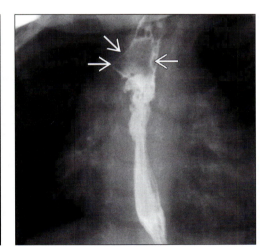

(Left) Anteroposterior radiograph shows button battery (arrow) in esophagus with characteristic double-density (2-layer) shadow. Laterally, their edges are rounded with a step-off junction at the positive and negative terminal. (Right) Anteroposterior esophagram shows large, nonradiopaque foreign body (arrows) proximal to anastomotic stricture in a patient who is post-operative tracheoesophageal fistula repair.

Typical

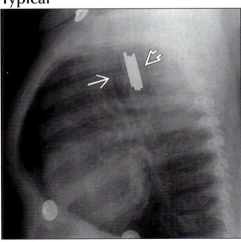
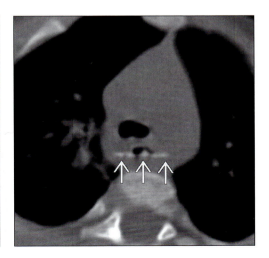

(Left) Lateral radiograph shows four coins in the esophagus (open arrow) with anterior displacement of airway and significant airway narrowing (arrow) indicating inflammation. (Right) Axial NECT after contrast esophagram demonstrates localized leak (arrows) into the mediastinum secondary to esophageal perforation which occurred during removal of the coins in the esophagus.

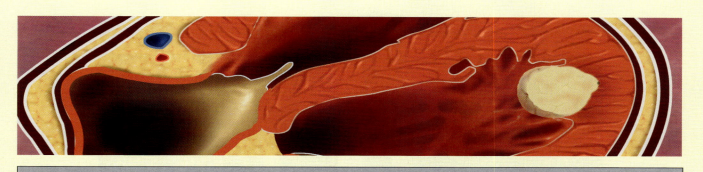

SECTION 3: Cardiac

Introduction and Overview
Cardiac   3-2

Left to Right Shunts (Non-Cyanotic, Increased Pulmonary Arterial Flow)
Ventricular Septal Defect (VSD)   3-6
Atrial Septal Defect (ASD)   3-10
Atrioventricular Septal Defect (AVSD)   3-14
Patent Ductus Arteriosus (PDA)   3-18

Cyanotic, Decreased Pulmonary Arterial Flow
Tetralogy of Fallot   3-22
Pulmonary Atresia   3-26
Ebstein Anomaly   3-30
D-Transposition of the Great Arteries   3-34
Tricuspid Atresia   3-38

Cyanotic, Increased Pulmonary Arterial Flow
Truncus Arteriosus   3-42
Total Anomalous Pulmonary Venous Return   3-46

Congestive Heart Failure (Increased Venous Flow)
Hypoplastic Left Heart Syndrome   3-50
Left Coronary Artery Anomalous Origin   3-54
Myocarditis   3-58
Cardiomyopathy   3-62

Abnormalities Often Associated with Complex Congenital Heart Disease
Double Outlet Right Ventricle   3-66
L-Transposition of the Great Arteries   3-70
Heterotaxia Syndromes   3-74

Obstructive Lesions of the Aorta and Pulmonary Arteries
Aortic Coarctation   3-78
Aortic Stenosis   3-82
Pulmonary Artery Stenosis   3-86

Miscellaneous
Operative CHD Procedures   3-90
Right Ventricular Dysplasia   3-94
Scimitar Syndrome   3-98
Rhabdomyoma   3-102
Kawasaki Disease   3-104
Rheumatic Heart Disease   3-108

CARDIAC

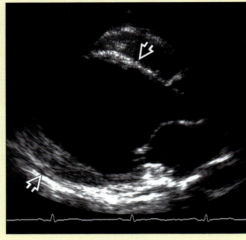

Echocardiogram shows marked dilatation of the left ventricle (arrows) in a child with dilated cardiomyopathy.

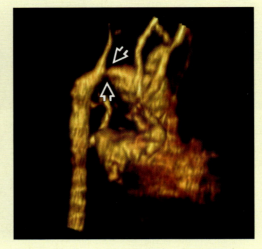

Surface 3D image created from data from CTA shows coarctation of the aorta (arrows) with dilatation of ascending aorta.

Imaging Modalities In Congenital Heart Disease (CHD)

- Days in which CHD was characterized by chest radiography and defined by angiography are gone
  - Certainly both still play some role in the diagnosis and management of CHD
- Modalities are utilized to define the morphology, connections, and function in CHD

Echocardiography (Ultrasound)

- Mainstay of diagnosing CHD especially during the fetal and neonatal periods
- Can demonstrate highly detailed anatomic information
- Functional information also able to be provided
- Color Doppler can be utilized to identify areas of stenosis and regurgitation
- Echocardiography more limited in older children, adults, and post surgical patients due to decreased acoustic window

CT Arteriography (CTA)

- With the advent of multidetector CT technology, CTA has rapidly become a useful tool in the evaluation of patients with CHD
- It is often utilized to complement those areas where echocardiography has difficulty
- CT is useful in depicting those anatomic structures which do not have a good acoustic window on echocardiography such as the pulmonary arteries, aorta, pulmonary veins, and conduits
  - Depicting the anatomic relationships of complex CHD
  - Post-operative complications such as stenoses, occlusions, and pseudoaneurysm
- CT vs. MRI
  - Benefits of CT include rapid acquisition time, avoidance of need for sedation in many cases, greater access to critically ill infants, lung visualization
  - Disadvantages of CT include use of ionizing radiation, dependence on IV contrast bolus, and relative lack of functional information

MRI

- MRI offers both anatomic and functional information
- MRI can be obtained without ionizing radiation
- Key imaging sequences
  - "Black blood" imaging with cardiac-gated spin echo or double inversion recovery imaging
    - Demonstrates anatomic detail and spacial relationships between adjacent structures
    - Allows for precise measurements of anatomic structures
  - "Bright blood" imaging with cardiac-gated cine MR with
    - T2* GRE steady state sequence (FLASH, SPGR); older sequences good for flow abnormalities
    - Steady state free precession (FIESTA, TRUFISP, balanced fast field echo); newer sequences with shows better contrast between myocardium and lumen
    - Can demonstrate dynamic findings such as turbulent flow related to stenosis and regurgitation
    - Data can be processed for functional information such as ventricular ejection fraction
  - MR angiography
    - Post-gadolinium MR arteriography with maximum intensity projection (MIP) or shaded surface 3D reconstructions can demonstrate complex anatomic relationships

CARDIAC

Key Information

Imaging In CHD
- Imaging modalities used to evaluate CHD define morphology, connections, and function
- Days in which CHD characterized by chest radiography and defined by angiography are gone

Echocardiography
- Mainstay of diagnosing and characterizing CDH especially during fetal and neonatal periods
- Demonstrates both anatomy and function
- Can be technically limited in older children, adults, and postoperative patients from lack of adequate acoustic window

CT
- Excellent at depicting anatomic relationships of complex CHD, structures sometimes not seen well by echo (pulmonary arteries, conduits, aorta), post-operative complications such as stenoses, occlusion, and pseudoaneurysms
- Easily obtainable in critically ill patients

MRI
- Offers both anatomic and functional information
- No ionizing radiation
- Demonstrates anatomic detail, spacial relationships, evidence of turbulent flow related to stenosis and regurgitation, functional measurements such as ventricular ejection fractions

Angiography

- The use of diagnostic angiography in cases where a percutaneous intervention is not being performed has dramatically decreased with improvements in non-invasive imaging tools such as echocardiography, MRI, and CT
- Percutaneous interventional procedures such as atrial septal defect and ventricular septal defect closures and balloon dilatations have increased in number
  - Diagnostic angiography is often performed as part of these interventional procedures for anatomic definition and procedure guidance

Radiography

Current Role Of Radiography In Imaging CHD
- The exact diagnosis of a specific CHD by radiography is often difficult and sometimes impossible, particularly in complex CHD
  - Ability has been overemphasized in radiology educational efforts
  - Many of the classically described radiographic findings of specific CHD do not manifest until after the neonatal period
    - Now that most CHD is diagnosed and often surgically treated in neonatal period, value of these classic imaging findings is decreased
  - However, in some cases the radiologist may be the first person to recognize that radiographic findings in a newborn suggest a cardiac rather than pulmonary cause of respiratory distress

Approach To The Chest Radiograph
- Pulmonary vascularity
  - Most important radiographic finding needed to generate appropriate category of CHD
    - It is also most difficult to evaluate
  - Normal pulmonary flow
    - Normal state of pulmonary flow - just right
  - Increased pulmonary arterial flow
    - Pulmonary arterial branches appear too prominent in both size and number
    - Pulmonary arterial structures appear "crisp" and well-defined
    - Guideline: If diameter of interlobar pulmonary artery is larger than diameter of the trachea, increased pulmonary arterial flow is present
    - Such findings are indicative of a left-to-right shunt or admixture lesion
    - In large left-to-right shunts in infants, marked hyperinflation will often be present
    - Sometimes appearance of left-to-right shunt may be easily confused with findings of viral lung disease; look for cardiomegaly
  - Increased pulmonary venous flow
    - Pulmonary structures are prominent in size and distribution but borders are indistinct and poorly defined
    - Indicative of pulmonary venous congestion, such as seen with pulmonary edema
    - With large left-to-right shunts, there is often both components of increased pulmonary arterial and venous flow
    - If you can make out any distinct pulmonary arterial structures, a component of increased pulmonary arterial flow is most likely present
  - Decreased pulmonary arterial flow
    - Lack of visualized arterial structures throughout lung
    - All patients with decreased pulmonary arterial flow will be cyanotic
- Heart size
  - Size of cardiac silhouette may be normal or enlarged
  - In older children and adults, there are often findings that suggest a specific chamber that is enlarged
  - In neonates and young children, you are doing well if you can determine between cardiomegaly and normal
  - Rule in adults that cardiac silhouette should not be wider than half of chest does not work well in young children

CARDIAC

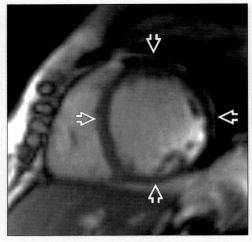

T2* GRE MR shows markedly dilated left ventricle (arrows) in patient with dilated cardiomyopathy.

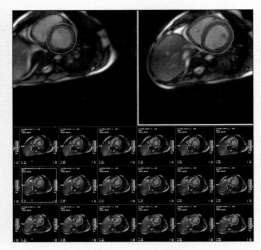

T2* GRE MR data processed to calculate ejection fraction in same patient with dilated cardiomyopathy. Regions of interest calculate volume of left ventricle at end diastole and end systole.

- Lateral view much more helpful in determining presence of cardiomegaly
- If heart projects posterior to oblique line drawn down tracheal air column or projects over vertebral bodies, cardiomegaly should be considered to be present
- Situs
  - Determination of "sidedness" of patient
  - Anatomic determinations to be made to determine situs
    - Cardiac apex, stomach bubble, liver
  - When there is dis-concordance between the position of the cardiac apex and stomach bubble (they are on opposite sides), there is a very high incidence (near 100%) of congenital heart disease
  - Bilateral right sidedness (asplenia)
    - Associated with complex cyanotic CHD
    - Other: Malrotation, microgastria, midline gallbladder, azygous continuation of the inferior vena cava
  - Bilateral left sidedness (polysplenia)
    - Less associated with complex CHD, more commonly associated with left-to-right shunts
    - Other: Malrotation, azygous continuation of the inferior vena cava, lack of a gallbladder
- Aortic arch
  - Identification of a right aortic arch raises possibility of CHD
  - Imaging findings of right aortic arch
    - Aortic knob on right (difficult in infants)
    - Descending aorta seen on right
    - Trachea indented on right side
    - Trachea gradually oriented left inferiorly (normally oriented right inferiorly)

Categorization Of CHD

Cyanosis
- Decreased flow
  - Tetrology of Fallot
  - Ebstein anomaly (giant heart)
  - Pulmonary atresia with intact ventricular septum (giant heart)
- Increased flow
  - Truncus arteriosis
  - Total anomalous pulmonary venous return
- Variable flow
  - D-transposition of the great arteries
  - Tricuspid atresia

Acyanosis
- Increased pulmonary arterial flow (left-to-right shunts)
  - Ventricular septal defect, atrial septal defect, arteriovenous canal, patent ductus arteriosis
- Increased pulmonary venous flow (congestive heart failure in the newborn)
  - Left sided anatomic obstruction
    - Coarctation of the aorta, aortic stenosis, left ventricular dysfunction [anomalous origin of the left coronary artery, myocarditis, shock myocardium (birth asphyxia), glycogen storage disease, infant of diabetic mother], hypoplastic left heart, mitral stenosis, cor triatriatum, pulmonary venous atresia/stenosis
  - Systemic "badness"
    - Anemia, polycythemia, hypoglycemia, hyperglycemia, hypothyroidism, hyperthyroidism, sepsis, peripheral arteriovenous malformations (hepatic hemangioendothelioma, vein of Galen malformation)
- Normal pulmonary flow
  - Obstructive lesions
    - Coarctation of the aorta, aortic stenosis, pulmonary artery stenosis
  - Post surgical issues

Related References

1. Boxt LM: Magnetic resonance and computed tomographic evaluation of congenital heart disease. J Magn Reson Imaging. 19(6):827-47, 2004
2. Higgins CB: Cardiac imaging. Radiology. 217(1):4-10, 2000

CARDIAC

IMAGE GALLERY

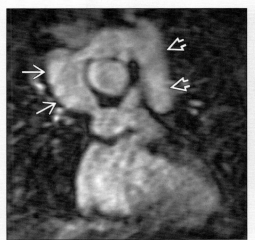
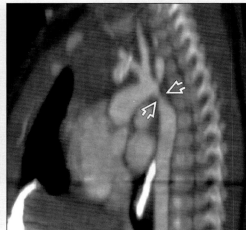

(Left) Coronal T2* GRE MR shows total anomalous pulmonary venous return with vertical vein *(open arrows)* traversing rightward and contiguous with superior vena cava *(arrows)*, making "snowman" appearance. *(Right)* Sagittal reconstructed image from CTA data shows coarctation of the aorta *(arrows)*.

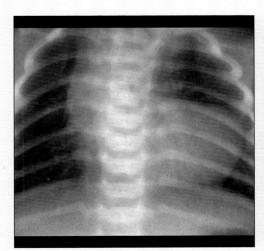
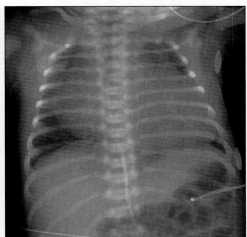

(Left) Radiograph shows decreased pulmonary arterial flow, deficient main pulmonary artery, cardiomegaly with upturned cardiac apex, and right-sided aortic arch in patient with tetrology of Fallot. *(Right)* Radiograph shows decreased pulmonary arterial flow and massive cardiomegaly in patient with Ebstein abnormality.

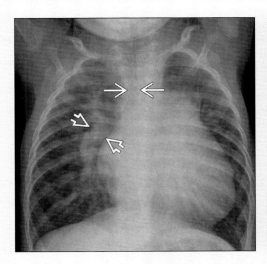
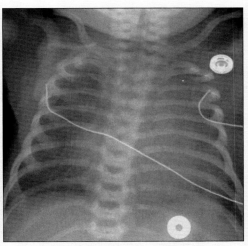

(Left) Radiograph shows cardiomegaly and increased, distinct pulmonary arterial flow in left-to-right shunt (VSD). Note interlobar artery *(open arrows)* is > in diameter than trachea *(arrows)*. *(Right)* Radiograph shows cardiomegaly and increased, indistinct vessels consistent with increased pulmonary venous flow in interrupted aortic arch. No distinct pulmonary vessels can be identified.

VENTRICULAR SEPTAL DEFECT (VSD)

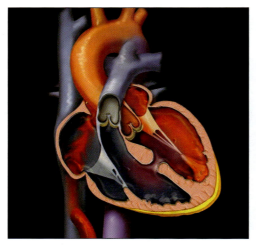

Graphic shows defect in the muscular portion of the interventricular septum, leading to left-to-right shunting, with associated right ventricular volume overload and enlargement.

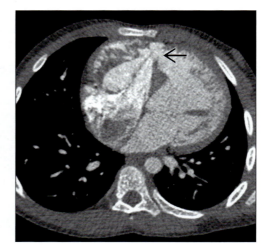

Axial CTA shows muscular ventricular septal defect (arrow) in the apical portion of the ventricular septum. Usually, muscular septal defects are multiple and some close spontaneously.

TERMINOLOGY

Definitions
- Cardiac anomalies characterized by defect(s) in the ventricular septum
  - Perimembranous septal defect
  - Muscular or trabecular septal defect
  - Inlet which is associated with atrioventricular septal defect (AVSD)
  - Outlet septal defect or supracristal VSD
- Cardiac anomalies with VSD associated with other congenital lesions
  - Intrinsic part of congenital heart lesion: Tetralogy of Fallot, truncus arteriosus, double outlet right ventricle
  - Associated with other congenital lesions: Coarctation, tricuspid atresia

IMAGING FINDINGS

General Features
- Best diagnostic clue
  - Chest radiograph with cardiomegaly and increased pulmonary artery flow, left atrial enlargement in a small child
  - Defect in the ventricular septum on any imaging modality
- Location
  - Membranous or perimembranous defects occurs in 80%
    - Defects lie in the outflow tract of the left ventricle immediately beneath the aortic valve
  - Inlet VSD occurs in 8-10%
    - Posterior and inferior defects, beneath the septal leaflet of the tricuspid valve
    - Associated atrioventricular septal defects with usual involvement of atrioventricular valves
  - Outlet septum occurs in 5%
    - Conal, subpulmonary, subaortic, supracristal, or infundibular
    - Malalignment defects associated with truncus arteriosus, tetralogy of Fallot, and double outlet right ventricle
    - Supracristal defect located about the crista muscle high in ventricular outlet portion which may cause prolapse of aortic coronary cusp with development of aortic insufficiency and injury to aortic valve
  - Muscular or trabecular VSD occurs in 5-10%
    - Confined to the muscular portion of the interventricular septum
    - Central muscular, apical muscular, marginal or have multiple defects described as "swiss cheese" muscular septum

DDx: CHD With Left-To-Right Shunts

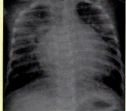
Large AVSD

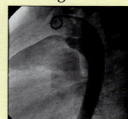
Patent Ductus

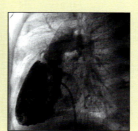
Double Outlet

VENTRICULAR SEPTAL DEFECT (VSD)

Key Facts

Terminology
- Cardiac anomalies characterized by defect(s) in the ventricular septum
- Perimembranous septal defect
- Muscular or trabecular septal defect
- Inlet which is associated with atrioventricular septal defect (AVSD)
- Outlet septal defect or supracristal VSD
- Cardiac anomalies with VSD associated with other congenital lesions

Imaging Findings
- Chest radiograph with cardiomegaly and increased pulmonary artery flow, left atrial enlargement in a small child
- Defect in the ventricular septum on any imaging modality
- Primary diagnosis with echocardiography

Top Differential Diagnoses
- Atrioventricular canal defects
- Patent ductus arteriosus
- Double outlet right ventricle

Clinical Issues
- Small VSD: Children are asymptomatic but have a heart murmur
- Moderate or large VSD: Children have tachypnea, tachycardia, and diaphoresis, failure to thrive
- Small defects may close spontaneously
- Moderate and large defects treated medically and followed by surgical approach
- Surgical treatment depends on the site of VSD

- Size: Defects can be small, moderate or large and involve adjacent structures

Radiographic Findings
- Radiography
  - Small VSD
    - Normal chest radiograph does not exclude a small shunt
  - Moderate to large VSD
    - Cardiomegaly with increased size of main pulmonary artery, increased pulmonary artery flow, left atrial enlargement and usually small aorta
    - Main pulmonary artery is high in position in infants and frequently confused with aortic knob
    - Heart failure may occur with venous edema
    - Hyperinflation is seen in large shunts due to abnormal lung compliance and possibly bronchial compression by dilated pulmonary arteries
  - Supracristal VSD
    - Left-to-right shunt is usually small as the anterior leaflet of aortic valve prolapses and may partially cover defect
    - May have evidence of dilated ascending aorta if aortic insufficiency is present
    - Difficult to diagnosis on chest radiographs

CT Findings
- CECT: Not usually done for diagnosis but occasionally performed to evaluate tracheal-bronchial compression

MR Findings
- Delineates cardiac anatomy and quantification of physiologic function
- Morphologic information provided by electrocardiography (ECG) gated spin-echo and cine MR imaging
- Shunt volume can be estimated by using volumetric cine MR imaging or velocity encoded cine MR imaging
- High-resolution three dimensional examination of vessels

Echocardiographic Findings
- Echocardiography findings
  - Characterizes type, location and number of septal defect(s), function and hemodynamic assessment
  - Echocardiography is utilized as main diagnostic modality in infants and young children

Angiographic Findings
- Cardiac catheterization and angiography findings
  - Catheterization utilized in complex lesions to obtain hemodynamic information and delineate anatomy
  - Left anterior oblique view profiles the ventricular septum
  - Aortogram done to assess for aortic insufficiency in supracristal VSD

Imaging Recommendations
- Primary diagnosis with echocardiography

DIFFERENTIAL DIAGNOSIS

Atrioventricular canal defects
- Chest radiograph demonstrates cardiomegaly and increased flow
- Congenital defect involving the atrial and ventricular septum and associated atrioventricular valves
- Presents early with clinical symptoms of large shunt
- High association with trisomy 21

Patent ductus arteriosus
- When shunt is large, chest radiograph demonstrates cardiomegaly and increased flow
- Persistent flow through the ductus from high pressure aorta to the main pulmonary artery
- Presents early and has loud continuous murmur during both systole and diastole

Double outlet right ventricle
- Both great vessels have their origin from the right ventricle; aortic mitral discontinuity is present and valves are at similar level

VENTRICULAR SEPTAL DEFECT (VSD)

- Pulmonary artery pressure is lower than systemic, and there is significant flow into the pulmonary arteries which simulates clinically and radiographically a large left-to-right shunt
- Considered a complex lesion and there are many variants and classifications

PATHOLOGY

General Features
- General path comments
  - Location of VSD important for surgical repair
  - Multiple defects occur, especially in the trabecular septum
  - Embryology
    - Complex, dependent on location of defect and associated anomalies
  - Pathophysiology
    - The determinants of left-to-right shunt are defect size, and relative resistance or pressure in the ventricular chambers which may reflect systemic or pulmonary artery pressure
    - Small defects have high resistance to flow across the defect, and have small shunts
    - Moderate size VSD have moderate shunts and moderate flow
    - Large sized VSDs are defined as a defect that approximates the size of the aorta (which may have large flow)
    - The increased flow increases the work of the right ventricle and increases the volume of venous return to the left atrium and ventricle
    - Marked volume overload occurs and child develops tachycardia and congestive heart failure
    - Long term increase in flow to pulmonary arteries is associated with vessel injury
    - Pulmonary hypertension occurs although the complex interaction between vascular endothelium and smooth muscle reaction is incompletely understood
    - Pulmonary hypertension may be reversible and those with early hypertension may need early surgical closure
- Genetics: No specific genetic defect in majority
- Epidemiology
  - Accounts for 20% of all congenital heart lesions
  - Most common congenital lesion
  - Most common congenital lesion associated with other heart lesions

CLINICAL ISSUES

Presentation
- Most common signs/symptoms
  - Small VSD: Children are asymptomatic but have a heart murmur
  - Moderate or large VSD: Children have tachypnea, tachycardia, and diaphoresis, failure to thrive
    - Congestive heart failure may occur
  - Dependent on size of shunt, associated lesion, and pulmonary vascular pressure
- Other signs/symptoms: Loud systolic murmur near the left heart border

Demographics
- Age
  - Although defect is present at birth, children not symptomatic immediately due to high pulmonary vascular resistance of the newborn
  - Moderate or large shunts usually are symptomatic in the first few months of life
- Gender: M = F

Natural History & Prognosis
- Most small muscular VSD close spontaneously
- Untreated large shunt will develop pulmonary vascular disease
- Reversal of shunt from right to left with late onset cyanosis
- Associated cardiac anomalies determine final outcome
- Lifetime risk of bacterial endocarditis

Treatment
- Small defects may close spontaneously
  - Many small muscular defects close spontaneously
  - Aneurysm of the ventricular septum may be part of spontaneous closure
- Moderate and large defects treated medically and followed by surgical approach
  - Medical therapy with diuretics and afterload reduction
  - Many infants improve and will grow
  - Poor growth, congestive heart failure may be indication for early surgery
- Surgical treatment depends on the site of VSD
- Perimembranous VSD: Surgical closure of shunt lesion usually performed with right atrial approach, on bypass during first or second year if shunt is moderate or large
- Outlet defects such as supracristal VSD are closed earlier to prevent aortic sinus prolapse, injury to the valve leaflet and subsequent aortic regurgitation
- Muscular lesions require more difficult surgical approach; recent catheter closure devices being utilized

SELECTED REFERENCES
1. Wang ZJ et al: Cardiovascular shunts: MR imaging evaluation. Radiographics. 23 Spec No:S181-94, 2003
2. Varaprasathan GA et al: Quantification of flow dynamics in congenital heart disease: applications of velocity-encoded cine MR imaging. Radiographics. 22(4):895-905; discussion 905-6, 2002
3. McDaniel NL et al: Ventricular Septal Defects. In:Allen HD, Gutgesell HP, (eds) Ventricular Septal Defects in Moss and Adams, Heart Disease in Infants, Children, and Adolescents; Lippincott williams&Wilkins, Philadelphia. Vol 1, pages 636-651, 2001
4. Parsons JM et al: Morphological evaluation of atrioventricular septal defects by magnetic resonance imaging. Br Heart J 64:138-45, 1990
5. Baker EJ et al: Magnetic resonance imaging at a high field strength of ventricular septal defects in infants. Br Heart J 62:305-10, 1989

VENTRICULAR SEPTAL DEFECT (VSD)

IMAGE GALLERY

Typical

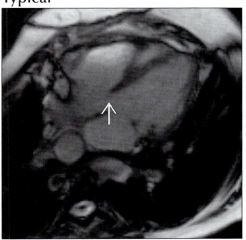 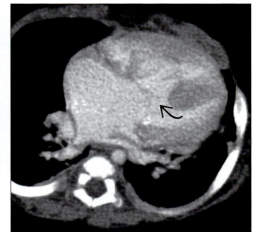

(Left) STIR MR four chamber view demonstrating high membranous ventricular septal defect *(arrow)* in this adolescent patient. *(Right)* Axial CTA shows marked atrial enlargement in young patient with a VSD. Ventricular septal defect *(curved arrow)* occurring within the septum is identified.

Typical

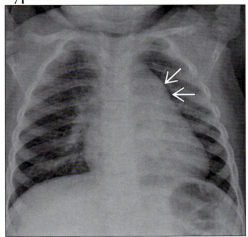 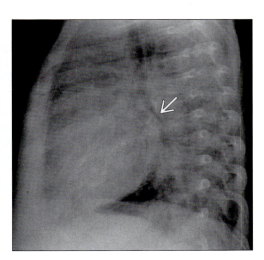

(Left) Anteroposterior radiograph shows enlargement of main pulmonary artery *(arrows)* and increase in pulmonary arterial flow in small child with perimembranous ventricular septal defect. *(Right)* Lateral radiograph shows displacement of left main stem bronchus posteriorly *(arrow)*. This is attributed to left atrial enlargement which is frequently seen in large ventricular septal defects.

Variant

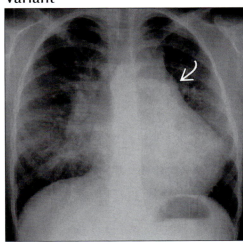 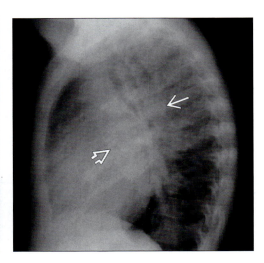

(Left) Anteroposterior radiograph shows elevated apex of heart, convex pulmonary artery segment *(arrow)* with pruning of vessels in a patient who had unoperated large VSD and pulmonary hypertension. *(Right)* Lateral radiograph shows right ventricular enlargement with central dilatation of right *(open arrow)* and left *(arrow)* pulmonary arteries.

ATRIAL SEPTAL DEFECT (ASD)

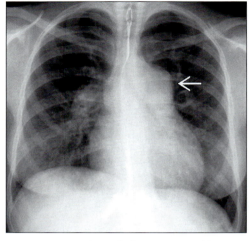

Anteroposterior radiograph shows 26 year old woman with Eisenmenger secondary to untreated ASD. Marked enlargement of the main (arrow), right and left pulmonary arteries is seen.

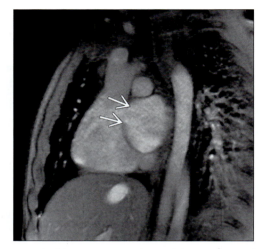

Sagittal oblique MR cine shows defect in interatrial septum (arrows). MR was used for sizing of this defect for possible Amplatz device occlusion.

TERMINOLOGY

Abbreviations and Synonyms
- Atrial septal defect (ASD)

Definitions
- Defect(s) in the atrial septum of the heart which can be isolated anomaly or associated with other congenital heart lesions
- 10% of congenital heart lesions in children yet 30% congenital lesions in adults

IMAGING FINDINGS

General Features
- Best diagnostic clue
  - Defect in the atrial septum seen on any imaging modality
    - Patent foramen ovale
    - Secundum atrial septal defect
    - Ostium primum defect/atrioventricular septal defect (AVSD)
    - Sinus venosus defect
- Location
  - Foramen ovale is a normal interatrial communication that in utero allows flow from inferior vena cava to freely enter the left atrium
  - Secundum atrial septal defect is oval defect bordered by the fossa ovalis
  - Ostium primum defect occurs in anterior and inferior portion of septum
  - Atrioventricular canal defect involves atrial and ventricular portions of septum
  - Sinus venosus defect occurs superiorly in atrial septum near superior vena cava
- Size: Variable
- Morphology
  - Patent foramen ovale
    - Interatrial communication
    - The limbus is a thick muscular ridge which borders on the foramen ovale
    - After birth, left atrial pressure is higher and thin tissue flap on the left atrial side forced against the limbus, achieving physiologic closure usually during first few weeks
    - Persistence of foramen ovale with right to left shunt occurs in congenital lesions with elevated right atrial pressures such as tricuspid atresia, Ebstein anomaly, hypoplastic right ventricle, and others
    - Persistence of foramen ovale with left-to-right shunt is important in lesions such as hypoplastic left heart, mitral atresia
  - Ostium primum defect

DDx: Prominent Main Pulmonary Artery

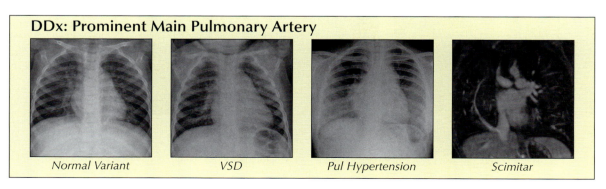

Normal Variant   VSD   Pul Hypertension   Scimitar

ATRIAL SEPTAL DEFECT (ASD)

Key Facts

Terminology
- Defect(s) in the atrial septum of the heart which can be isolated anomaly or associated with other congenital heart lesions
- 10% of congenital heart lesions in children yet 30% congenital lesions in adults

Imaging Findings
- Defect in the atrial septum seen on any imaging modality
- Patent foramen ovale
- Secundum atrial septal defect
- Ostium primum defect/atrioventricular septal defect (AVSD)
- Sinus venosus defect
- Primary diagnosis made by echocardiography in infants and children
- MR is emerging as accurate alternative for depiction of function, flow, and anatomy in older patients

Top Differential Diagnoses
- Normal chest
- Ventricular septal defect
- Pulmonary hypertension
- Scimitar syndrome

Clinical Issues
- Secundum ASD: Majority of patients are asymptomatic
- Spontaneous closure occurs in many children
- Transcatheter percutaneous closure device is current treatment
- Adults may have pulmonary hypertension from unrecognized ASD

  - Located in the most anterior and inferior aspect of the atrial septum
  - Simplest form AVSD
  - May exist in isolation but commonly exists with a cleft in anterior leaflet of mitral valve
 - Secundum defect
  - Bordered by the edge of the fossa ovalis and the exposed circumference of the ostium secundum
 - Sinus venosus defect
  - Upper atrial septum and is contiguous with the superior vena cava
  - Lesion is posterior to the fossa ovalis
  - Almost always associated with anomalous connection of the right upper pulmonary vein into superior vena cava

Radiographic Findings
- Radiography
 - Chest radiograph in secundum ASD
  - Small and moderate defects have normal chest radiographs
  - Large defects show mild cardiomegaly with main pulmonary artery normal or increased in size, shunt vascularity
 - Chest radiograph in primum ASD or AVSD
  - Young child with cardiomegaly and increased pulmonary vascularity
  - Volume overload of the right atrium, right ventricle, and pulmonary arteries
 - Chest radiograph in sinus venosus defect
  - Horizontal position of the right upper pulmonary vein as it enters the superior vena cava
 - Chest radiograph in adults with pulmonary hypertension
  - Classic enlarged, convex main pulmonary artery with peripheral decrease in size of vessels
  - Right ventricular enlargement on lateral film

CT Findings
- CTA: Defect in the atrial septum, enlargement of the right atrium, right ventricular enlargement and increase in size of pulmonary arteries and veins

MR Findings
- Morphologic information by ECG gated spin echo and cine MR imaging
- MR is emerging as an accurate and noninvasive alternative for depiction of function, flow, and anatomy
 - Can evaluate shunt severity by quantitating the ratio of pulmonary flow to systemic flow
 - MR angiography permits high-resolution three dimensional evaluation of the vessels
 - Shunt volume can be estimated by using volumetric cine MR imaging or velocity encoded cine MR imaging
- Useful to look at size and position of the defect and/or associated other congenital heart lesions
 - Sinus venosus defects and venous anatomy depicted well
- Used to evaluate the atrial septal occluder position and relationships with pulmonary venous return, coronary sinus, and mitral valve

Echocardiographic Findings
- Echocardiogram
 - Demonstrates "drop out" in atrial septum best seen on apical four chamber view and subcostal imaging
 - Transesophageal echo utilized in older patients and during placement of closure device

Angiographic Findings
- Cardiac catheterization and angiography findings
 - Utilized for transcatheter percutaneous treatment with closure device
 - In AVSD, can be used to hemodynamically evaluate pulmonary artery pressure and anatomy

Imaging Recommendations
- Best imaging tool
 - Primary diagnosis made by echocardiography in infants and children
 - Catheterization done for percutaneous treatment with closure devices

ATRIAL SEPTAL DEFECT (ASD)

- MR is emerging as accurate alternative for depiction of function, flow, and anatomy in older patients

DIFFERENTIAL DIAGNOSIS

Normal chest
- Main pulmonary artery can be prominent normally particularly between ages of 8 and 12
- Not associated with any heart disease

Ventricular septal defect
- Small shunts have normal radiographs
- Moderate or large shunts have cardiomegaly and increased arterial and venous flow

Pulmonary hypertension
- In adults or children there are many other causes of pulmonary hypertension
- Most commonly, it is secondary to chronic lung disease

Scimitar syndrome
- Associated with anomalous venous return to the right atrium
- Usually can visualize the anomalous "scimitar" vein

PATHOLOGY

General Features
- General path comments
  - Embryology
    - Defect occurs during the fifth week of gestation in AVSD
  - Pathophysiology; volume overload
    - ASD: Low pressure shunt
    - VSD, AVSD: High pressure shunts
    - Eventually all lead to pulmonary hypertension if untreated
- Genetics
  - No specific genetic defect in majority of children
  - Holt Oram syndrome has ASD with upper extremity anomalies which occurs in families
  - Ostium primum and AVSD associated with trisomy 21 in 65% of children
- Epidemiology: 10% of all congenital heart lesions but true incidence is much higher as many close spontaneously

CLINICAL ISSUES

Presentation
- Most common signs/symptoms
  - Secundum ASD: Majority of patients are asymptomatic
    - Eisenmenger or pulmonary hypertension is rare because ASD usually recognized and treated
    - Occasionally, there are neurologic symptoms from paradoxical emboli or atrial dysrhythmias
  - Atrioventricular canal defects or ostium primum defects
    - Feeding difficulties with dyspnea, diaphoresis, increased work of breathing, failure to thrive
    - Infants with mitral regurgitation may have marked tachypnea and failure to thrive
  - Sinus venosus defect
    - Usually asymptomatic in children or symptoms related to hemodynamics of left-to-right shunt
- Other signs/symptoms: Heart murmur is usually systolic ejection murmur, with widely split second heart sound

Demographics
- Age
  - Atrioventricular canal defect patients may present in the first week of life
  - Secundum defects present with asymptomatic heart murmurs
- Gender: Secundum defects: F:M = 1:2

Natural History & Prognosis
- Patent foramen ovale usually closes during first months of life
  - May persist if there is associated heart disease
- Untreated large shunt may develop pulmonary vascular disease or paradoxical embolus, or atrial arrhythmias due to atrial dilation or pulmonary hypertension

Treatment
- Secundum ASD
  - Spontaneous closure occurs in many children
  - Transcatheter percutaneous closure device is current treatment
  - Adults may have pulmonary hypertension from unrecognized ASD
  - Large defects may need Dacron patch or direct suture closure
    - 100% closure achieved with no mortality
- Ostium primum defects not amenable to device closure due to proximity of the atrioventricular valve tissue
  - Usually operated at 3-5 years of age
- Atrioventricular canal
  - Surgical repair done in first year of life for symptomatic patients
- Sinus venosus defect
  - More complex surgical repair as right superior pulmonary vein needs to be redirected to left atrium
  - Surgical repair associated with normal life expectancy

SELECTED REFERENCES

1. Beerbaum P et al: Atrial septal defects in pediatric patients: noninvasive sizing with cardiovascular MR imaging. Radiology. 228(2):361-9, 2003
2. Lapierre C et al: Evaluation of a large atrial septal occluder with cardiac MR imaging. Radiographics. 23 Spec No:S51-8, 2003
3. Wang ZJ et al: Cardiovascular shunts: MR imaging evaluation. Radiographics. 23 Spec No:S181-94, 2003
4. Porter C et al: Atrial Septal Defects, In: Allen HD, Gugesell HP. Moss and Adams, Heart Disease in Infants, Children, and Adolescents, Lippincott Williams&Wilkins, Philadelphia. 603-617, 2001

ATRIAL SEPTAL DEFECT (ASD)

IMAGE GALLERY

Typical

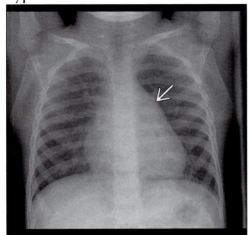
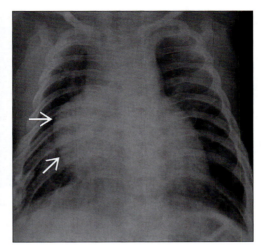

(Left) Anteroposterior radiograph shows mild cardiomegaly with prominent pulmonary artery (arrow) in this asymptomatic 6 year old child with secundum atrial septal defect. *(Right)* Anteroposterior radiograph shows 3 month child with an enlarged right atrium (arrows) and known ostium primum defect. Radiograph demonstrates 11 paired ribs which suggests trisomy 21.

Typical

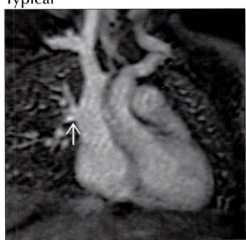
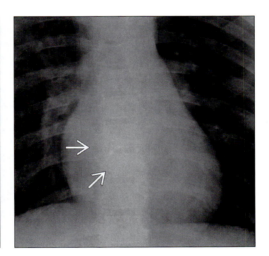

(Left) Coronal MRA Depicts anomalous venous return of right upper pulmonary vein (arrow) in a patient with sinus venosus defect. This creates a left-to-right shunt. *(Right)* Anteroposterior radiograph Shows position deployed Amplatz device utilized to close atrial septal defect (arrows). It has a circular rim on both sides of the atrium best seen on lateral.

Other

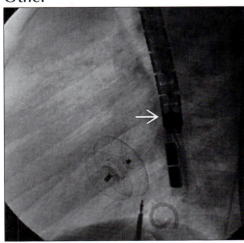
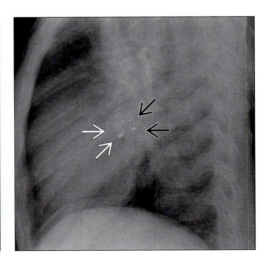

(Left) Lateral radiograph Shows the deployment of Amplatz device which was monitored by transesophageal echo (arrow). Transvenous delivery device is seen with the tip in inferior vena cava. *(Right)* Lateral radiograph After percutaneous placement of an Amplatz device. The white arrows are on the device in the right atrium and the black arrows are on device in the left atrium.

ATRIOVENTRICULAR SEPTAL DEFECT (AVSD)

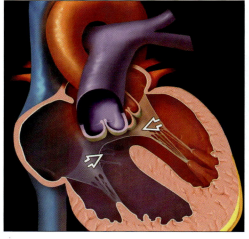

Graphic shows defect (arrows) in atrio and ventricular septum connecting right atrium (RA) and ventricle to left atrium and ventricle.

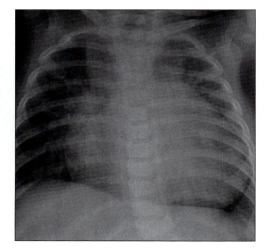

Anteroposterior radiograph Shows cardiomegaly in a one month infant. There is enlargement of all chambers and increase in pulmonary artery flow secondary to left-to-right shunting.

TERMINOLOGY

Abbreviations and Synonyms
- Atrioventricular septal defect (AVSD)
  - Atrioventricular canal defect (AVC)
  - Endocardial cushion defect
  - Complete atrioventricular canal defect (CAVC)
- Ostium primum defect
  - Partial atrioventricular canal defect (PAVC)
  - Partial atrioventricular septal defect
  - Incomplete endocardial cushion defect

Definitions
- Broad spectrum of defects characterized by involvement in atrial septum, ventricular septum and one or both of the atrioventricular-ventricular (AV) valves
  - A complete AVSD indicates the presence of both atrial and ventricular septal defects with a common AV valve
  - A partial AVSD defect indicates atrial septal involvement with separate mitral and tricuspid valve orifices
  - Unbalanced AVSD indicates that one ventricular chamber is hypoplastic compared with the other depending on direction of AV valve flow
- 42-48% of patients have Down syndrome or trisomy 21 have an AVC

IMAGING FINDINGS

General Features
- Best diagnostic clue
  - Chest radiograph
    - Large heart with large main pulmonary artery and increased pulmonary artery flow
    - Serial radiographs to evaluate for pulmonary hypertension
    - Mitral insufficiency may occur both pre and post-operative
    - When mitral insufficiency is severe, the left atrium can be large and cause left lower lobe collapse
    - Children with large shunts have increased incidence of upper respiratory infections and pneumonia
    - Pulmonary hypertension patients have abnormal lung compliance and lungs are hyperinflated with eversion of the diaphragms: Does not necessarily imply infection
- Location
  - Complete atriventricular canal
    - Large defect in the anterior inferior portion of the atrial septum
    - Large defect in the ventricular septum
    - Common atrioventricular valve orifice

DDx: Common Left-To-right Shunts

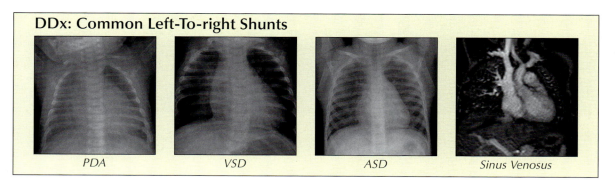

PDA   VSD   ASD   Sinus Venosus

ATRIOVENTRICULAR SEPTAL DEFECT (AVSD)

Key Facts

Terminology
- Atrioventricular septal defect (AVSD)
- Endocardial cushion defect
- Ostium primum defect
- Broad spectrum of defects characterized by involvement in atrial septum, ventricular septum and one or both of the atrioventricular-ventricular (AV) valves

Imaging Findings
- Large heart with large main pulmonary artery and increased pulmonary artery flow
- Echocardiography in infants and young children defines the lesion
- Demonstration of left-to-right shunt, severity of mitral regurgitation, tricuspid regurgitation

Top Differential Diagnoses
- Ventricular septal defect (VSD)
- Atrial septal defect (ASD)
- Patent ductus arteriosus (PDA)
- Sinus venosus atrial septal defect

Clinical Issues
- Large shunts present early with tachypnea, tachycardia, and failure to thrive
- Small shunts may be well tolerated through first decade and children may be asymptomatic
- Medical management until surgery depending on lesion and severity
- Elective repair in children 2-5 years, unless mitral regurgitation is present
- Single ventricle physiology may necessitate a staged procedure such as Glenn and then Fontan

---

- When AV valve opens towards one ventricle, an unbalanced canal defect is present
- Right ventricular or left ventricular dominance can occur
- Results in single ventricle physiology
- Unbalanced canal defect refers to hypoplasia of one ventricle
- Hypoplasia of the inlet and outlet septum, resulting in hypoplasia of the chamber with malalignment of the ventricular septum
  - Ostium primum defect
    - Defect in the anterior inferior aspect of the atrial septum
    - May be isolated defect in atrial septum but coexistent cleft in the anterior leaflet of the mitral valve is frequently present
    - 5 leaflet AV valve is present with separate valve orifices to right and left ventricle
    - Tricuspid and mitral valve leaflets adhere to the crest of the interventricular septum and a mitral valve cleft is present
- Size: Broad spectrum of size of defects in atrioventricular septum and respective sizes of the ventricles
- Morphology
  - Complete atrioventricular canal
    - Defect in anterior inferior aspect of atrial septum
    - Defect in ventricular septum
    - Abnormal mitral valve attachments
  - Ostium primum defect: Defect in anterior inferior aspect of atrial septum

CT Findings
- CECT
  - Not done for diagnosis but may identify the atrial and ventricular defects
  - Large heart with increased size of pulmonary arteries
  - Large right-sided structures such as right atrium right ventricle, pulmonary artery

Echocardiographic Findings
- Echocardiogram
  - Echocardiography in infants and young children defines the lesion
    - Primum defects have echo dropout in lower portion of the septum, cleft in mitral valve
    - Anterior and superior displacement of the aorta with elongation and narrowing of left ventricular outflow tract
- Color Doppler
  - Demonstration of left-to-right shunt, severity of mitral regurgitation, tricuspid regurgitation
    - Left ventricular outflow tract obstruction can be quantified

Angiographic Findings
- Conventional
  - Cardiac catheterization is not usually done for anatomy but done to measure pulmonary vascular resistance
    - Left ventriculogram shows cleft in mitral valve, shunts, respective size of the ventricles and also left ventricular outflow tract obstruction

Imaging Recommendations
- Best imaging tool
  - Echocardiography in infants and young children defines the lesion
    - Primum defects have echo dropout in lower portion of the septum, mitral valve cleft
    - Complete AVSD demonstrate varying degree of absence of septum, size of defect and relative size of the ventricles

DIFFERENTIAL DIAGNOSIS

Ventricular septal defect (VSD)
- Most common congenital heart disease (CHD) with left-to-right shunt
- Most common CHD associated with other lesions
- Cardiac enlargement with increased pulmonary flow

Atrial septal defect (ASD)
- Defect is in the superior portion of the atrial septum

ATRIOVENTRICULAR SEPTAL DEFECT (AVSD)

- Presents in older children and children usually asymptomatic from shunt
- Left-to-right shunt usually not large but it can cause Eisenmenger physiology in adult if unrecognized

Patent ductus arteriosus (PDA)
- Communication between the high pressure aorta with the lower pressure pulmonary artery
- Left-to-right shunt usually presents in infancy
- Closed by percutaneous occlusion devices

Sinus venosus atrial septal defect
- Defect high in the right atrial septum
- Usually associated with anomalous venous drainage of the right upper lobe vein
- Volume overloads the right atrium, the right ventricle and the pulmonary arteries

PATHOLOGY

General Features
- Genetics: Associated with trisomy 21 in 44-48%
- Etiology
  - Malformation occurring during the 5th week of gestation
  - Abnormal or inadequate fusion of the superior and inferior endocardial cushion
  - Abnormal fusion of the ventricular (trabecular) portion of the septum
- Epidemiology
  - 4-8 out of 1,000 live births have congenital heart defects
  - 5-8% have AVSD
- Associated abnormalities
  - Trisomy 21 children have constellation of clinical and radiographic findings
    - Chest radiograph may show 11 ribs, double manubrial ossification center in 80%
    - Many skeletal malformations, spectrum of retardation

CLINICAL ISSUES

Presentation
- Most common signs/symptoms
  - Complete atrial ventricular defect
    - Large shunts present early with tachypnea, tachycardia, and failure to thrive
    - Mitral insufficiency adds complexity and earlier symptoms
  - Partial atrial ventricular defect
    - Small shunts may be well tolerated through first decade and children may be asymptomatic
    - Mitral insufficiency adds complexity and earlier symptoms
- Other signs/symptoms
  - Pathophysiology of lesions
    - Degree of left-to-right shunting is determined by the size of defect and the relative compliance of atria and ventricles
    - Right ventricular compliance reflects pulmonary vascular resistance
    - Infants have high pulmonary vascular resistance and therefore rarely have shunts
    - As pulmonary vascular resistance decreases, left-to-right shunting increases with age
    - Subsequent enlargement of right atrium, right ventricular enlargement and increase in pulmonary vascularity
    - Degree of regurgitation through mitral vale cleft depends on its size and also whether there are left-sided lesions such as coarctation
    - Cleft directs regurgitant blood through atrial defect

Demographics
- Age: Infants and children
- Gender: Both male and female

Natural History & Prognosis
- Complete atrioventricular canal presents in infancy with symptoms
- Children assessed for surgical repair
  - Post-operative course may be complicated by mitral insufficiency
  - Pulmonary hypertension occurs in unoperated children

Treatment
- Medical management until surgery depending on lesion and severity
- Surgical management: Partial AVSD
  - Closed by pericardial patch via right atrial approach
  - Percutaneous closure devices not usually done as the inferior attachment may injure AV valves
- Surgical management: Complete AVSD, mortality rate is 3%
  - Elective repair in children 2-5 years, unless mitral regurgitation is present
  - Complications include mitral insufficiency which may require reoperation, valvuloplasty or replacement
  - Arrhythmias such as sinus node dysfunction or heart block
- Surgical management: Complete unbalanced AVSD
  - Single ventricle physiology may necessitate a staged procedure such as Glenn and then Fontan

SELECTED REFERENCES

1. Ten Harkel AD et al: Development of left atrioventricular valve regurgitation after correction of atrioventricular septal defect. Ann Thorac Surg. 79(2):607-12, 2005
2. Formigari R et al: Better surgical prognosis for patients with complete atrioventricular septal defect and Down's syndrome. Ann Thorac Surg. 78(2):666-72; discussion 672, 2004
3. Freeman SB et al: Population-based study of congenital heart defects in Down syndrome. Am J Med Genet. 80(3):213-7, 1998
4. van Son JA et al: Predicting feasibility of biventricular repair of right-dominant unbalanced atrioventricular canal. Ann Thorac Surg. 63(6):1657-63, 1997
5. Tweddell JS et al: Twenty-year experience with repair of complete atrioventricular septal defects. Ann Thorac Surg. 62(2):419-24, 1996

ATRIOVENTRICULAR SEPTAL DEFECT (AVSD)

IMAGE GALLERY

Typical

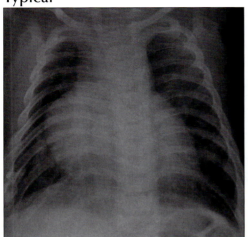
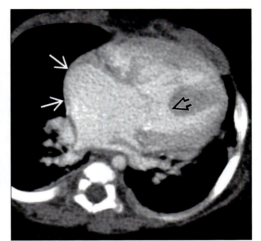

(Left) Anteroposterior radiograph shows and enlarged heart in a young patient. The right atrium is prominent and there were eleven paired ribs indicating likely trisomy 21. Infant had large AVSD. *(Right)* Axial CECT shows infant with complete atrioventricular septal defect. The right atrium is marked enlarged (arrows) and there is communication (open arrow) at atrial and ventricular level.

Typical

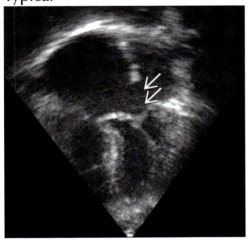
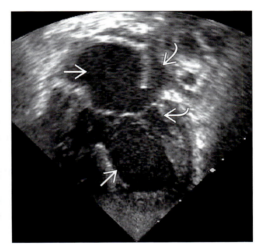

(Left) Four chamber view echocardiogram shows echo drop out in the inferior portion of the atrial septum (arrows) which is characteristic of a primum atrial septal defect. *(Right)* Four chamber view echocardiogram shows striking asymmetry of ventricular size in infant with unbalanced AVSD. The RA and right ventricle (RV) (arrows) are much larger than left atrium (LA) and left ventricle (LV) (curved arrows).

Typical

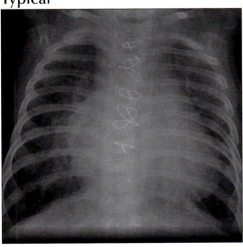
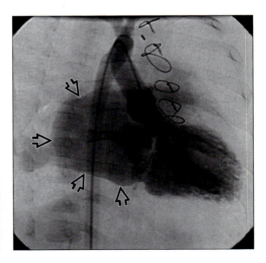

(Left) Anteroposterior radiograph shows post-operative chest following AVSD repair in a child with tachypnea and loud diastolic murmur. Asymmetry of pulmonary edema due to mitral insufficiency. *(Right)* Right anterior oblique left ventricular angiogram shows significant mitral regurgitation with contrast filling enlarged left atrium (arrows), following AVSD repair.

PATENT DUCTUS ARTERIOSUS (PDA)

CLINICAL ISSUES

Presentation
- Most common signs/symptoms
  - Characteristic machinery-like murmur
  - Bounding peripheral pulses
  - Congestive heart failure
  - Special situation: Premature infant recovering from surfactant deficiency disease
    - Decrease in hypoxia
    - Drop in pulmonary vascular resistance
    - Shunt flow through ductus arteriosus increases
    - Clinical and radiographic signs of congestive heart failure (cardiomegaly, pulmonary edema)
- Other signs/symptoms
  - Subacute bacterial endocarditis
    - Need for treatment of clinically "silent" PDA (incidentally detected with echocardiography) is controversial
  - Ductal aneurysm
    - Can result from premature narrowing of ductus on pulmonary side

Natural History & Prognosis
- Irreversible pulmonary hypertension (Eisenmenger physiology) resulting in shunt reversal, development of cyanosis
- Isolated PDA: Excellent prognosis with early closure
- When associated with complex heart disease: Prognosis determined by underlying disorder
- Persistent fetal circulation, pulmonary hypertension: Treatment with extracorporeal membrane oxygenation (ECMO) is often necessary to disrupt vicious circle
  - Hypoxia → pulmonary vasoconstriction → decreased pulmonary flow → more severe hypoxia

Treatment
- To close ductus in premature infants: Indomethacin
  - Side effects: Renal failure, intestinal perforation, intracranial hemorrhage
- To keep ductus open (cyanotic heart disease): Prostaglandin E1
- Term infants, older children: Surgical clipping or ligation
  - Can be performed at bedside under video-assisted thoracoscopic and/or robotic guidance
  - Complications: Inadvertent ligation of aortic isthmus, pulmonary artery, recurrent laryngeal nerve injury
- Endovascular closure with duct occluder devices and/or coils
  - Small ductus (< 4 mm): Gianturco coils
  - Large ductus (> 4 mm): Ivalon plug, Rashkind and Amplatz duct occluders
  - Complications: Protrusion of occluder device into left pulmonary artery orifice (→ decreased left lung perfusion), peripheral embolization
  - Incomplete closure in 10-20%

SELECTED REFERENCES

1. Cannon JW et al: Application of robotics in congenital cardiac surgery. Semin Thorac Cardiovasc Surg Pediatr Card Surg Annu. 6:72-83, 2003
2. Hillman ND et al: Patent ductus arteriosus. In: Mavroudis C, Backer CL, ed. Pediatric cardiac surgery. 3rd ed. Philadelphia, Mosby. 223-33, 2003
3. Morgan-Hughes GJ et al: Morphologic assessment of patent ductus arteriosus in adults using retrospectively ECG-gated multidetector CT. AJR Am J Roentgenol. 181(3):749-54, 2003
4. Anil SR et al: Coil occlusion of the small patent arterial duct without arterial access. Cardiol Young. 12(1):51-6, 2002
5. Jan SL et al: Isolated neonatal ductus arteriosus aneurysm. J Am Coll Cardiol. 39(2):342-7, 2002
6. Thanopoulos BD et al: Patent ductus arteriosus equipment and technique. Amplatzer duct occluder: intermediate-term follow-up and technical considerations. J Interv Cardiol. 14(2):247-54, 2001
7. Day JR et al: A spontaneous ductal aneurysm presenting with left recurrent laryngeal nerve palsy. Ann Thorac Surg. 72(2):608-9, 2001
8. Davies MW et al: A preliminary study of the application of the transductal velocity ratio for assessing persistent ductus arteriosus. Arch Dis Child Fetal Neonatal Ed. 82(3):F195-9, 2000
9. Gersony WN, Apfel HD: Patent ductus arteriosus and other aortopulmonary anomalies. In: Moller JH, Hoffman JIE, ed. Pediatric cardiovascular medicine, 1st ed. Philadelphia, Churchill Livingstone. 323-34, 2000
10. Alva C et al: Aneurysm of the pulmonary trunk with patent arterial duct. Cardiol Young. 9(1):70-2, 1999
11. Sandstede J et al: [Magnetic resonance imaging in persistent ductus arteriosus of Botalli] Rofo. 171(5):405-6, 1999
12. Schmidt M et al: Magnetic resonance imaging of ductus arteriosus Botalli apertus in adulthood. Int J Cardiol. 68(2):225-9, 1999
13. Acherman RJ et al: Aneurysm of the ductus arteriosus: a congenital lesion. Am J Perinatol. 15(12):653-9, 1998
14. Evangelista JK et al: Effect of multiple coil closure of patent ductus arteriosus on blood flow to the left lung as determined by lung perfusion scans. Am J Cardiol. 80(2):242-4, 1997
15. Arora R et al: Transcatheter coil occlusion of persistent ductus arteriosus using detachable steel coils: short-term results. Indian Heart J. 49(1):60-4, 1997
16. Dessy H et al: Echocardiographic and radionuclide pulmonary blood flow patterns after transcatheter closure of patent ductus arteriosus. Circulation. 94(2):126-9, 1996
17. Sharma S et al: Computed tomography and magnetic resonance findings in long-standing patent ductus. Case reports. Angiology. 47(4):393-8, 1996
18. Strouse PJ et al: Magnetic deflection forces from atrial septal defect and patent ductus arteriosus-occluding devices, stents, and coils used in pediatric-aged patients. Am J Cardiol. 78(4):490-1, 1996
19. Chien CT et al: Potential diagnosis of hemodynamic abnormalities in patent ductus arteriosus by cine magnetic resonance imaging. Am Heart J 122:1065-73, 1991

ATRIOVENTRICULAR SEPTAL DEFECT (AVSD)

IMAGE GALLERY

Typical

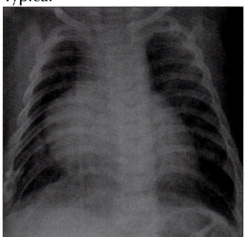
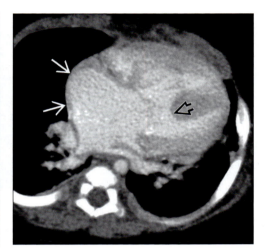

(Left) Anteroposterior radiograph shows and enlarged heart in a young patient. The right atrium is prominent and there were eleven paired ribs indicating likely trisomy 21. Infant had large AVSD. *(Right)* Axial CECT shows infant with complete atrioventricular septal defect. The right atrium is marked enlarged (arrows) and there is communication (open arrow) at atrial and ventricular level.

Typical

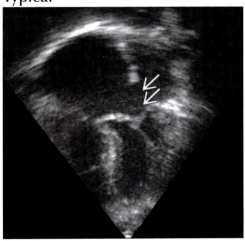
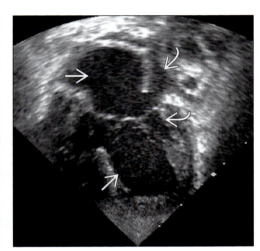

(Left) Four chamber view echocardiogram shows echo drop out in the inferior portion of the atrial septum (arrows) which is characteristic of a primum atrial septal defect. *(Right)* Four chamber view echocardiogram shows striking asymmetry of ventricular size in infant with unbalanced AVSD. The RA and right ventricle (RV) (arrows) are much larger than left atrium (LA) and left ventricle (LV) (curved arrows).

Typical

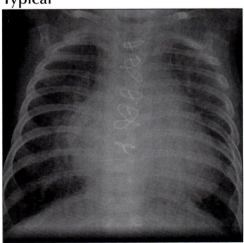
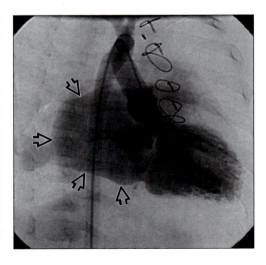

(Left) Anteroposterior radiograph shows post-operative chest following AVSD repair in a child with tachypnea and loud diastolic murmur. Asymmetry of pulmonary edema due to mitral insufficiency. *(Right)* Right anterior oblique left ventricular angiogram shows significant mitral regurgitation with contrast filling enlarged left atrium (arrows), following AVSD repair.

PATENT DUCTUS ARTERIOSUS (PDA)

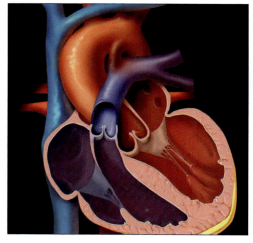

Graphic shows dilated left ventricle and enlargement of ascending aorta compared to pulmonary artery, indicative of volume overload of left heart from aortic to pulmonary (left-to-right) shunt through PDA.

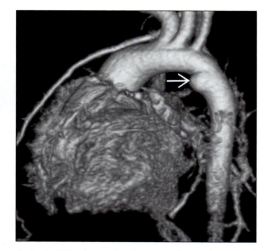

Sagittal CTA shows focal outpouching of proximal descending aorta (arrow), consistent with remnant of ductus arteriosus ("ductus bump"), which is a normal variant and not to be confused with an aneurysm.

TERMINOLOGY

Abbreviations and Synonyms
- Patent ductus arteriosus (PDA), persistent arterial duct, patent ductus Botalli

Definitions
- Persistent postnatal patency of the normal prenatal connection from the pulmonary artery to the proximal descending aorta
- Category: Acyanotic, increased pulmonary blood flow
- Hemodynamics: L → R shunt between aorta and pulmonary artery
- PDA is frequently an essential part of complex congenital heart disease
  - Hypoplastic left heart syndrome, preductal coarctation, interrupted aortic arch: Conduit for systemic perfusion (R → L flow)
  - D-Transposition: Necessary for admixture between systemic and pulmonary circuits (L → R flow)
  - Pulmonary atresia and other severe cyanotic heart disease with right-sided obstruction: Conduit for pulmonary perfusion (L → R flow)
- PDA is part of persistent fetal circulation syndrome: R → L flow
  - Severe lung disease (meconium aspiration, surfactant deficiency disease, neonatal pneumonia)
  - Primary pulmonary hypertension of neonate

IMAGING FINDINGS

General Features
- Best diagnostic clue: Ductus bump

Radiographic Findings
- Radiography
  - Cardiomegaly (left atrium and left ventricle)
  - Increased pulmonary vascularity
  - Wide vascular pedicle (large aortic arch with "ductus bump")

CT Findings
- CTA
  - Volume renditions of aortic arch depict ductus arteriosus
  - Excellent modality for sizing of ductus prior to cardiac catheterization for placement of occluder device

MR Findings
- Cardiac-gated T1 weighted (black blood) imaging
  - Sagittal oblique plane through aortic arch depicts ductus
- Gradient echo steady-state free precession cine MRI for right ventricular function in cases with Eisenmenger pulmonary hypertension
- 3D gadolinium MRA with volume rendition

DDx: Ductus Arteriosus Associated With Other Heart Lesions

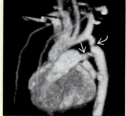

Preductal Coarctation

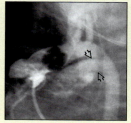

D-Transposition

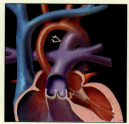

Hypoplastic Left Heart

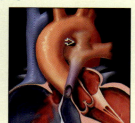

Pulmonary Atresia

PATENT DUCTUS ARTERIOSUS (PDA)

Key Facts

Terminology
- Persistent postnatal patency of the normal prenatal connection from the pulmonary artery to the proximal descending aorta
- Category: Acyanotic, increased pulmonary blood flow
- Hemodynamics: L → R shunt between aorta and pulmonary artery
- PDA is frequently an essential part of complex congenital heart disease
- PDA is part of persistent fetal circulation syndrome: R → L flow

Pathology
- With pulmonary hypertension pressure overload of right ventricle, reversal of shunt (R → L), leading to cyanosis (Eisenmenger physiology)
- When closed: Forms ligamentum arteriosum, which may calcify (incidental calcification in aortopulmonary window on chest radiograph or CT)

Clinical Issues
- Irreversible pulmonary hypertension (Eisenmenger physiology) resulting in shunt reversal, development of cyanosis
- To close ductus in premature infants: Indomethacin
- To keep ductus open (cyanotic heart disease): Prostaglandin E1
- Term infants, older children: Surgical clipping or ligation
- Endovascular closure with duct occluder devices and/or coils

Echocardiographic Findings
- Echocardiogram: Suprasternal notch view: Direct visualization of ductus
- M-mode: Increased left-atrium-to-aorta ratio (> 1.2:1)
- Pulsed Doppler
  - Diastolic flow reversal in descending and abdominal aorta (ductus steal)
  - Flow acceleration across a constricting ductus: Transductal velocity ratio (TVR)
- Color Doppler: For flow direction through ductus

Angiographic Findings
- Conventional
  - Cardiac catheterization only needed for associated complex cyanotic heart disease, and to determine reversibility of pulmonary hypertension
  - Placement of PDA closure device

Imaging Recommendations
- Protocol advice: Treatment decisions based on echocardiographic findings only in majority of cases

DIFFERENTIAL DIAGNOSIS

Other causes of L → R shunting
- Septal defects, atrioventricular canal

Persistent fetal circulation syndrome
- Pulmonary hypertension (primary or secondary to severe lung disease)
- Patent foramen ovale, PDA secondary to profound irreversible hypoxia

PATHOLOGY

General Features
- General path comments
  - In normal neonate ductus arteriosus closes functionally 18-24 hours after birth, anatomically at 1 month of age
  - PDA is persistence of normal prenatal structure after birth
  - Embryology
    - Ductus originates from primitive sixth aortic arch
  - Pathophysiology (for simple PDA)
    - L → R shunt to pulmonary artery
    - Volume overload of left-sided cardiac cambers
    - With pulmonary hypertension pressure overload of right ventricle, reversal of shunt (R → L), leading to cyanosis (Eisenmenger physiology)
    - Diastolic flow reversal in aorta can lead to renal and intestinal hypoperfusion: Renal dysfunction, necrotizing enterocolitis
- Genetics: No specific genetic defect identified in most cases of isolated PDA
- Etiology
  - Prematurity: Persistent postnatal hypoxia → failure of contraction of ductus
  - Term infant: Associated with maternal rubella
- Epidemiology
  - 10-12% of congenital heart disease
  - 1 per 2,500-5,000 live births
  - Slightly more common in females
  - Associated with prematurity (21-35%)

Gross Pathologic & Surgical Features
- Patent arterial duct, most often wider on aortic side
  - Length: 2-8 mm; diameter 4-12 mm
  - Makes an acute angle with aorta in simple PDA; blunt angle with associated congenital heart disease
- Contractile tissue mainly on pulmonary side, spirally arranged muscle bundles in media
  - Prostaglandin E1 present in fetal life maintains relaxation
  - Increased oxygen pressure causes constriction
- Thickening of intima with mucoid degeneration
- When closed: Forms ligamentum arteriosum, which may calcify (incidental calcification in aortopulmonary window on chest radiograph or CT)
- Can be right-sided

PATENT DUCTUS ARTERIOSUS (PDA)

CLINICAL ISSUES

Presentation
- Most common signs/symptoms
  - Characteristic machinery-like murmur
  - Bounding peripheral pulses
  - Congestive heart failure
  - Special situation: Premature infant recovering from surfactant deficiency disease
    - Decrease in hypoxia
    - Drop in pulmonary vascular resistance
    - Shunt flow through ductus arteriosus increases
    - Clinical and radiographic signs of congestive heart failure (cardiomegaly, pulmonary edema)
- Other signs/symptoms
  - Subacute bacterial endocarditis
    - Need for treatment of clinically "silent" PDA (incidentally detected with echocardiography) is controversial
  - Ductal aneurysm
    - Can result from premature narrowing of ductus on pulmonary side

Natural History & Prognosis
- Irreversible pulmonary hypertension (Eisenmenger physiology) resulting in shunt reversal, development of cyanosis
- Isolated PDA: Excellent prognosis with early closure
- When associated with complex heart disease: Prognosis determined by underlying disorder
- Persistent fetal circulation, pulmonary hypertension: Treatment with extracorporeal membrane oxygenation (ECMO) is often necessary to disrupt vicious circle
  - Hypoxia → pulmonary vasoconstriction → decreased pulmonary flow → more severe hypoxia

Treatment
- To close ductus in premature infants: Indomethacin
  - Side effects: Renal failure, intestinal perforation, intracranial hemorrhage
- To keep ductus open (cyanotic heart disease): Prostaglandin E1
- Term infants, older children: Surgical clipping or ligation
  - Can be performed at bedside under video-assisted thorascopic and/or robotic guidance
  - Complications: Inadvertent ligation of aortic isthmus, pulmonary artery, recurrent laryngeal nerve injury
- Endovascular closure with duct occluder devices and/or coils
  - Small ductus (< 4 mm): Gianturco coils
  - Large ductus (> 4 mm): Ivalon plug, Rashkind and Amplatz duct occluders
  - Complications: Protrusion of occluder device into left pulmonary artery orifice (→ decreased left lung perfusion), peripheral embolization
  - Incomplete closure in 10-20%

SELECTED REFERENCES

1. Cannon JW et al: Application of robotics in congenital cardiac surgery. Semin Thorac Cardiovasc Surg Pediatr Card Surg Annu. 6:72-83, 2003
2. Hillman ND et al: Patent ductus arteriosus. In: Mavroudis C, Backer CL, ed. Pediatric cardiac surgery. 3rd ed. Philadelphia, Mosby. 223-33, 2003
3. Morgan-Hughes GJ et al: Morphologic assessment of patent ductus arteriosus in adults using retrospectively ECG-gated multidetector CT. AJR Am J Roentgenol. 181(3):749-54, 2003
4. Anil SR et al: Coil occlusion of the small patent arterial duct without arterial access. Cardiol Young. 12(1):51-6, 2002
5. Jan SL et al: Isolated neonatal ductus arteriosus aneurysm. J Am Coll Cardiol. 39(2):342-7, 2002
6. Thanopoulos BD et al: Patent ductus arteriosus equipment and technique. Amplatzer duct occluder: intermediate-term follow-up and technical considerations. J Interv Cardiol. 14(2):247-54, 2001
7. Day JR et al: A spontaneous ductal aneurysm presenting with left recurrent laryngeal nerve palsy. Ann Thorac Surg. 72(2):608-9, 2001
8. Davies MW et al: A preliminary study of the application of the transductal velocity ratio for assessing persistent ductus arteriosus. Arch Dis Child Fetal Neonatal Ed. 82(3):F195-9, 2000
9. Gersony WN, Apfel HD: Patent ductus arteriosus and other aortopulmonary anomalies. In: Moller JH, Hoffman JIE, ed. Pediatric cardiovascular medicine, 1st ed. Philadelphia, Churchill Livingstone. 323-34, 2000
10. Alva C et al: Aneurysm of the pulmonary trunk with patent arterial duct. Cardiol Young. 9(1):70-2, 1999
11. Sandstede J et al: [Magnetic resonance imaging in persistent ductus arteriosus of Botalli] Rofo. 171(5):405-6, 1999
12. Schmidt M et al: Magnetic resonance imaging of ductus arteriosus Botalli apertus in adulthood. Int J Cardiol. 68(2):225-9, 1999
13. Acherman RJ et al: Aneurysm of the ductus arteriosus: a congenital lesion. Am J Perinatol. 15(12):653-9, 1998
14. Evangelista JK et al: Effect of multiple coil closure of patent ductus arteriosus on blood flow to the left lung as determined by lung perfusion scans. Am J Cardiol. 80(2):242-4, 1997
15. Arora R et al: Transcatheter coil occlusion of persistent ductus arteriosus using detachable steel coils: short-term results. Indian Heart J. 49(1):60-4, 1997
16. Dessy H et al: Echocardiographic and radionuclide pulmonary blood flow patterns after transcatheter closure of patent ductus arteriosus. Circulation. 94(2):126-9, 1996
17. Sharma S et al: Computed tomography and magnetic resonance findings in long-standing patent ductus. Case reports. Angiology. 47(4):393-8, 1996
18. Strouse PJ et al: Magnetic deflection forces from atrial septal defect and patent ductus arteriosus-occluding devices, stents, and coils used in pediatric-aged patients. Am J Cardiol. 78(4):490-1, 1996
19. Chien CT et al: Potential diagnosis of hemodynamic abnormalities in patent ductus arteriosus by cine magnetic resonance imaging. Am Heart J 122:1065-73, 1991

PATENT DUCTUS ARTERIOSUS (PDA)

IMAGE GALLERY

Typical

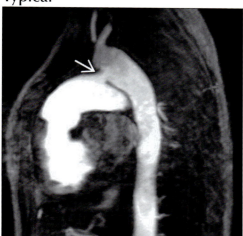
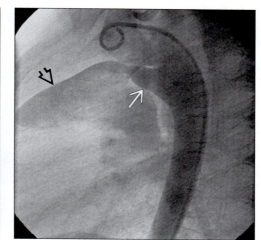

(Left) Sagittal oblique MRA shows PDA *(arrow)*, connecting dilated main pulmonary artery with proximal descending aorta, in adolescent with pulmonary arterial hypertension (Courtesy L. Sena, MD). *(Right)* Lateral angiography, aortic arch injection, shows filling of main pulmonary artery *(open arrow)* via a large PDA *(arrow)*, which has a broad insertion onto the proximal descending aorta.

Variant

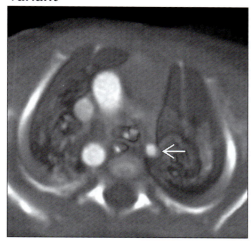
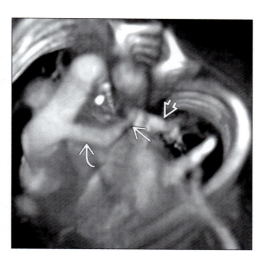

(Left) Axial CTA in infant with complex cyanotic lesion with absent central left pulmonary artery shows right aortic arch and left PDA *(arrow)*. *(Right)* CTA, superior view of volume rendition, shows PDA *(arrow)* supplying hilar portion of left pulmonary artery *(open arrow)* from left brachiocephalic artery *(curved arrow)*.

Typical

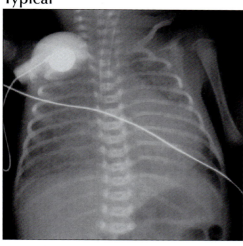
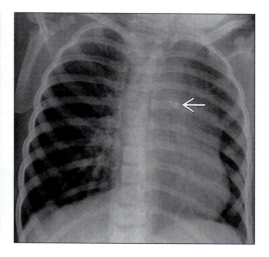

(Left) Anteroposterior radiograph in premature infant recovering from surfactant deficiency disease shows pulmonary edema and cardiomegaly from shunting PDA. *(Right)* Anteroposterior radiograph following endovascular occlusion of PDA shows Amplatz ductus closure device in situ *(arrow)*.

TETRALOGY OF FALLOT

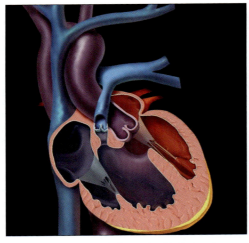

Graphic shows subvalvular (infundibular) pulmonary stenosis, small pulmonary valve, large aortic valve overriding high ventricular septal defect, right ventricular hypertrophy, and right-sided aortic arch.

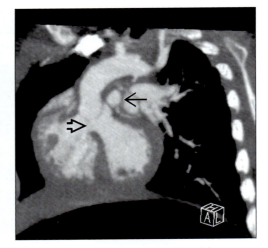

Coronal oblique CTA shows hypoplastic main pulmonary artery (arrow) and high (membranous) ventricular septal defect (open arrow) with overriding aorta.

TERMINOLOGY

Abbreviations and Synonyms
- Tetralogy of Fallot (TOF), 4 Fallot

Definitions
- Infundibular right ventricular outflow tract (RVOT) stenosis, subaortic ventricular septal defect (VSD), overriding aorta and right ventricle (RV) hypertrophy
- Category: Cyanotic, normal heart size, ↓ vascularity
- Hemodynamics: Outflow obstruction of RV
- Spectrum: Pink Fallot - classic Fallot - pulmonary atresia, VSD, multiple collaterals

IMAGING FINDINGS

General Features
- Best diagnostic clue: Infundibular stenosis of RVOT

Radiographic Findings
- Radiography
  - RV hypertrophy, concave pulmonary artery (PA) segment: "Boot-shaped heart" = "coeur en sabot"
  - Decreased pulmonary vascularity (oligemia)
  - Normal heart size at birth
  - Right-sided aortic arch in 25%
    - TOF is the most common lesion with right arch

CT Findings
- CTA
  - Pre-operative: Multidetector row CT can diagnose coronary anomalies, obviating need for angiography
  - Post-operative: Cardiac-gated cine CT can perform assessment of RV function in patients with contra-indication for MRI
    - CTA is less affected by metal artifact than MRI, to assess results of interventions (stents, coils)

MR Findings
- T1WI
  - Cardiac-gated axial images for pre-operative definition of PA anatomy, PA stenosis
  - Post-operative PA anatomy, patency of Blalock-Taussig shunts
- T2* GRE
  - Short-axis steady-state free precession (SSFP) cine MRI for right and left ventricular volumes, function, ejection fraction, regurgitation fraction
    - Functional MRI: Bi-ventricular response to exercise and recovery
    - Presence of RVOT outflow tract akinesia/aneurysm and wide annulus correlates with need for pulmonary valve replacement
- MRA
  - Gadolinium-enhanced MRA: For depiction of PA anatomy and aortopulmonary collaterals

DDx: Cyanosis, Decreased Pulmonary Vascularity

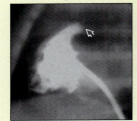
Pulmonary Atresia

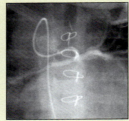
Hypoplastic PAs

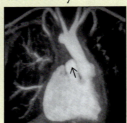
Double Outlet RV

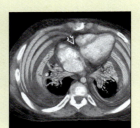
Tricuspid Atresia

TETRALOGY OF FALLOT

Key Facts

Terminology
- Infundibular right ventricular outflow tract (RVOT) stenosis, subaortic ventricular septal defect (VSD), overriding aorta and right ventricle (RV) hypertrophy
- Category: Cyanotic, normal heart size, ↓ vascularity
- Hemodynamics: Outflow obstruction of RV
- Spectrum: Pink Fallot - classic Fallot - pulmonary atresia, VSD, multiple collaterals

Imaging Findings
- Best diagnostic clue: Infundibular stenosis of RVOT
- RV hypertrophy, concave pulmonary artery (PA) segment: "Boot-shaped heart" = "coeur en sabot"
- Short-axis steady-state free precession (SSFP) cine MRI for right and left ventricular volumes, function, ejection fraction, regurgitation fraction
- Gadolinium-enhanced MRA: For depiction of PA anatomy and aortopulmonary collaterals
- Phase-contrast MRA for estimate of RV function (ejection fraction) and pulmonary regurgitation

Clinical Issues
- Modified Blalock-Taussig shunt: Interposition of Gore-Tex graft
- Complete repair: Enlargement of RVOT, VSD closure
- Pulmonary valve or conduit replacement in adult life after early complete repair
- Pulmonary regurgitation: RV volume overload, diastolic and systolic dysfunction, reciprocal LV systolic dysfunction, arrhythmias
- Percutaneous balloon dilatation of residual pulmonary valve stenosis and/or peripheral PA stenosis (with stent placement)

- Phase-contrast MRA for estimate of RV function (ejection fraction) and pulmonary regurgitation

Echocardiographic Findings
- Echocardiogram
  - Location VSD, additional muscular VSDs
  - Degree of aortic override, position of arch
  - RVOT obstruction, function of pulmonary valve
  - Anatomy of branch PAs

Angiographic Findings
- Conventional
  - Coronary anatomy
  - PA stenosis: Balloon angioplasty with stenting
  - Anatomy/distribution of aortopulmonary collaterals

Imaging Recommendations
- Best imaging tool: Initial diagnosis with echocardiography
- Protocol advice
  - MRI or CTA for detailed PA anatomy
  - Cardiac catheterization for coronary anatomy, percutaneous interventions
  - MRI in older child/young adult with poor acoustic window; is becoming gold standard for functional assessment of post-operative regurgitation and ventricular dysfunction

DIFFERENTIAL DIAGNOSIS

Pulmonary atresia with VSD and multiple aortopulmonary collaterals
- Extreme end of TOF spectrum

Pulmonary atresia with intact ventricular septum
- Massive cardiomegaly with right atrial enlargement at birth

Double outlet right ventricle with pulmonary stenosis
- Characterized by discontinuity between mitral and aortic valve, with subaortic conus

Tricuspid atresia
- Large right atrium

PATHOLOGY

General Features
- General path comments
  - Pathophysiology: Balance between RVOT obstruction and VSD determines shunt direction
    - Classic TOF: Right-to-left shunting, decreased pulmonary flow, cyanosis
    - "Pink" TOF: Left to right shunting, normal to increased pulmonary flow, congestive heart failure
  - Embryology
    - Abnormal bulbotruncal rotation and septation
    - Primary hypoplasia of infundibular septum
- Genetics
  - Chromosomal anomalies in 11% (chromosome 22)
  - Other congenital anomalies in 16%; 8% syndromal
- Epidemiology
  - Incidence: 3-5 per 10,000 live births
  - Fourth most common congenital heart anomaly
  - Most common cyanotic heart lesion
- Associated abnormalities
  - PA branch stenosis or hypoplasia
  - Absence of pulmonary valve: Severe pulmonary regurgitation → aneurysmal dilatation of PAs → tracheobronchial compression
  - Patent foramen ovale
  - Right aortic arch, mirror image branching (25%)
  - Coronary anomalies: Left anterior descending arising from right coronary and crossing RVOT (4%), with implications for surgical repair

TETRALOGY OF FALLOT

Gross Pathologic & Surgical Features
- Anterior/cephalad deviation of infundibular septum, hypertrophic outlet septum and anterior muscle bands
- Hypoplastic pulmonary valve annulus with deformed and stenosed, often bicuspid, pulmonary valve
- Large perimembranous subaortic VSD, with aortic override of 15-95%

CLINICAL ISSUES

Presentation
- Most common signs/symptoms
  - Varying degrees of cyanosis at birth (most often apparent by 3 month)
  - Older child: Cyanotic spells, relieved by squatting
  - Congestive heart failure (large VSD)
- Other signs/symptoms
  - Clubbing of fingers and toes
  - After repair: Decreased exercise tolerance, RV dysfunction
  - Severe arrhythmias, which may be fatal
    - RV dilatation from pulmonary regurgitation
    - Damage to conduction system during VSD closure
    - Scar from right ventriculotomy → ectopy focus
  - Bacterial endocarditis
  - Stroke due to paradoxical embolus to brain
  - Hyperviscosity syndrome due to polycythemia

Natural History & Prognosis
- 10% of untreated patients live more than 20 years
- Short term: Excellent results after early complete repair
- Long term: Determined by right ventricular diastolic and systolic dysfunction, chronic regurgitation leading to dilatation, arrhythmias, risk of sudden death
  - Timing of pulmonary valve replacement determined by results of functional MRI

Treatment
- Palliative shunt
  - Classic Blalock-Taussig shunt: End-to-side subclavian artery to PA (opposite from aortic arch)
  - Modified Blalock-Taussig shunt: Interposition of Gore-Tex graft
  - Central shunt: Ductus-like connection between aorta and PA
- Complete repair: Enlargement of RVOT, VSD closure
  - With transannular and/or RV patch: Post-operative pulmonary regurgitation, RV dysfunction, arrhythmias
  - Rastelli shunt: Valved conduit between RV and pulmonary arteries in case of severe RVOT stenosis or pulmonary valve atresia
- Pulmonary valve or conduit replacement in adult life after early complete repair
  - Conduit stenosis: RV pressure overload, systolic dysfunction
  - Pulmonary regurgitation: RV volume overload, diastolic and systolic dysfunction, reciprocal LV systolic dysfunction, arrhythmias
  - Timely surgery decreases RV size, increases ejection fraction, improves exercise capacity
- Percutaneous balloon dilatation of residual pulmonary valve stenosis and/or peripheral PA stenosis (with stent placement)

SELECTED REFERENCES

1. van Straten A et al: Right ventricular function late after total repair of tetralogy of Fallot. Eur Radiol. 2005
2. Raman SV et al: Usefulness of multidetector row computed tomography to quantify right ventricular size and function in adults with either tetralogy of Fallot or transposition of the great arteries. Am J Cardiol. 95(5):683-6, 2005
3. Geva T et al: Factors associated with impaired clinical status in long-term survivors of tetralogy of Fallot repair evaluated by magnetic resonance imaging. J Am Coll Cardiol. 43(6):1068-74, 2004
4. van Straten A et al: Right ventricular function after pulmonary valve replacement in patients with tetralogy of Fallot. Radiology. 233(3):824-9, 2004
5. Kang IS et al: Differential regurgitation in branch pulmonary arteries after repair of tetralogy of Fallot: a phase-contrast cine magnetic resonance study. Circulation. 107(23):2938-43, 2003
6. Nieman K et al: Coronary anomaly imaging by multislice computed tomography in corrected tetralogy of Fallot. Heart. 89(6):664, 2003
7. Roest AA et al: Tetralogy of Fallot: postoperative delayed recovery of left ventricular stroke volume after physical exercise assessment with fast MR imaging. Radiology. 226(1):278-84, 2003
8. Davlouros PA et al: Right ventricular function in adults with repaired tetralogy of Fallot assessed with cardiovascular magnetic resonance imaging: detrimental role of right ventricular outflow aneurysms or akinesia and adverse right-to-left ventricular interaction. J Am Coll Cardiol. 40(11):2044-52, 2002
9. Helbing WA et al: ECG predictors of ventricular arrhythmias and biventricular size and wall mass in tetralogy of Fallot with pulmonary regurgitation. Heart. 88(5):515-9, 2002
10. Roest AA et al: Exercise MR imaging in the assessment of pulmonary regurgitation and biventricular function in patients after tetralogy of fallot repair. Radiology. 223(1):204-11, 2002
11. Uebing A et al: Influence of the pulmonary annulus diameter on pulmonary regurgitation and right ventricular pressure load after repair of tetralogy of Fallot. Heart. 88(5):510-4, 2002
12. Vliegen HW et al: Magnetic resonance imaging to assess the hemodynamic effects of pulmonary valve replacement in adults late after repair of tetralogy of fallot. Circulation. 106(13):1703-7, 2002
13. Holmqvist C et al: Pre-operative evaluation with MR in tetralogy of fallot and pulmonary atresia with ventricular septal defect. Acta Radiol. 42(1):63-9, 2001
14. Doyle TP et al: Tetralogy of Fallot and pulmonary atresia with ventricular septal defect. In: Moller JH, Hoffman JIE ed. Pediatric cardiovascular medicine, 1st ed. Philadelphia, Churchill Livingstone. 391-408, 2000
15. Helbing WA et al: Clinical applications of cardiac magnetic resonance imaging after repair of tetralogy of Fallot. Pediatr Cardiol. 21(1):70-9, 2000
16. Beekman RP et al: Usefulness of MRI for the pre-operative evaluation of the pulmonary arteries in Tetralogy of Fallot. Magn Reson Imaging. 15(9):1005-15, 1997
17. Greenberg SB et al: Tetralogy of Fallot: diagnostic imaging after palliative and corrective surgery. J Thorac Imaging. 10(1):26-35, 1995

TETRALOGY OF FALLOT

IMAGE GALLERY

Typical

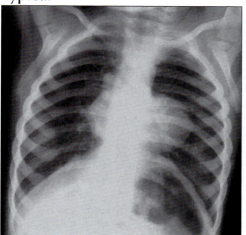 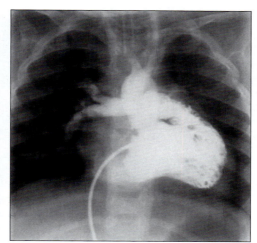

(Left) Anteroposterior radiograph shows classic "boot"-shaped heart due to right ventricular enlargement and concave pulmonary artery segment, with pulmonary oligemia *(Right)* Anteroposterior angiography with right ventricular injection: Simultaneous filling of aorta and normal caliber of pulmonary arteries. Note heavy trabeculation in right ventricular outflow tract, leading to minor subpulmonary stenosis.

Typical

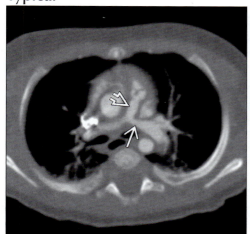 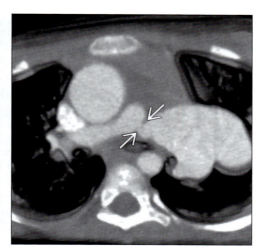

(Left) Axial CTA shows small dysplastic pulmonic valve, hypoplastic main pulmonary artery (open arrow) and origin stenosis left branch pulmonary artery (arrow). *(Right)* Axial CTA shows origin stenosis (arrows) with aneurysmal post-stenotic dilatation of left branch pulmonary artery.

Variant

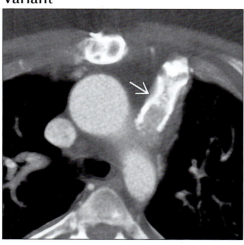 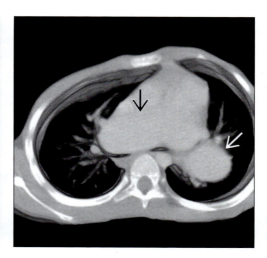

(Left) Axial CTA shows calcified stenotic conduit (arrow) in 26 year old man who underwent repair for tetralogy of Fallot in infancy. *(Right)* Axial CTA shows massively dilated pulmonary arteries (right, black arrow; left, white arrow), compressing the tracheobronchial tree. Child presented with stridor, and was diagnosed with tetralogy of Fallot with absent pulmonary valve.

PULMONARY ATRESIA

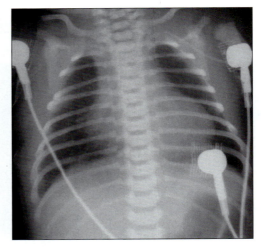

Graphic shows pulmonary atresia with intact ventricular septum. Note patent foramen ovale, dilatation of right atrium and right ventricular hypertrophy. Pulmonary arteries are perfused by patent ductus arteriosus.

Anteroposterior radiograph in patient with pulmonary atresia and intact ventricular septum after right Blalock-Taussig shunt placement (note rib splaying) reveals right cardiomegaly and pulmonary oligemia.

TERMINOLOGY

Abbreviations and Synonyms
- Pulmonary atresia (PAt) with ventricular septal defect (VSD) and multiple aortopulmonary collateral arteries (MAPCAs)
  - Also sometimes referred to as "Truncus arteriosus type 4" or "Pseudotruncus" (misnomers)
- PAt, intact VS: Pulmonary atresia with intact ventricular septum

Definitions
- Two distinct entities, differentiated by presence or absence of a VSD
  - PAt, VSD, MAPCAs: Hypoplastic/absent pulmonary arteries (PAs), MAPCAs supply one or both lungs
  - PAt, intact VS: Normal sized PAs supplied by ductus arteriosus, patent foramen ovale (PFO)
- Both are characterized by underdevelopment of right ventricular outflow tract (RVOT) and pulmonary valve
  - PAt, VSD, MAPCAs: At extreme end of the spectrum of RVOT-obstructive (Fallot-type) heart lesions, with complex and highly variable PA anatomy
- Category: Cyanotic, cardiomegaly, decreased and/or irregular pulmonary vasculature
- Hemodynamics: Extreme outflow obstruction of right ventricle (RV), (almost) entire cardiac output goes into dilated overriding ascending aorta

IMAGING FINDINGS

General Features
- Best diagnostic clue: Atresia of RVOT and/or pulmonary valve

Radiographic Findings
- Radiography
  - Extreme "boot-shaped" appearance of heart
  - Right-sided aortic arch common
  - Diminutive hilar shadows
  - Irregular branching patterns of MAPCAs
  - PAt, intact VS: Severe cardiomegaly from massive right atrial dilatation

CT Findings
- CTA
  - Better than echocardiography for PA anatomy
  - CTA best used to provide anatomic road-map for subsequent catheterization
    - Saves overall radiation, contrast, procedure time
  - CTA is excellent modality for unstable post-operative patients

MR Findings
- T1WI: PAt, VSD, MAPCAs: Cardiac-gated axial images for pre-operative definition of PA anatomy

DDx: Cyanosis, Decreased Pulmonary Vascularity

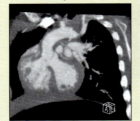
Tetralogy Of Fallot

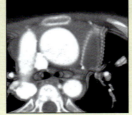
Conduit Thrombosis

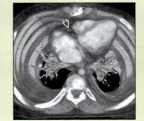
Tricuspid Atresia

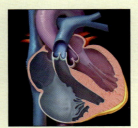
Ebstein Anomaly

PULMONARY ATRESIA

Key Facts

Terminology
- Two distinct entities, differentiated by presence or absence of a VSD
- Both are characterized by underdevelopment of right ventricular outflow tract (RVOT) and pulmonary valve
- Category: Cyanotic, cardiomegaly, decreased and/or irregular pulmonary vasculature
- Hemodynamics: Extreme outflow obstruction of right ventricle (RV), (almost) entire cardiac output goes into dilated overriding ascending aorta

Imaging Findings
- Best diagnostic clue: Atresia of RVOT and/or pulmonary valve
- CTA best used to provide anatomic road-map for subsequent catheterization

Pathology
- Pathophysiology of PAt, VSD, MAPCAs: Balance between flow though PAs and MAPCAs determines pulmonary perfusion
- Pathophysiology of PAt, intact VS: Obligatory right → left shunt through PFO
- Hilar arteries = true PAs
- Presence and confluence of central portions of true PAs important for surgical repair

Clinical Issues
- Progressive cyanosis after birth with closure of ductus arteriosus
- Prognosis is guarded, depends on feasibility of surgery
- PAt, VSD, MAPCAs: Staged complete repair
- PAt, intact VS: Type of repair dependent on RV size and RV-dependency on coronary circulation

---

- T2* GRE: Short- and long-axis steady-state free precession (SSFP) cine MRI for functional assessment, tricuspid regurgitation
- MRA: Coronal gadolinium-enhanced MRA for detailed analysis of PA anatomy and MAPCAs

Echocardiographic Findings
- Echocardiogram
  - PAt, VSD, MAPCAs
    - Characterizes intracardiac anatomy, position and size of VSD, aortic root override
    - Development of branch PAs, their confluence
  - PAt, intact VS
    - Morphology of interatrial septum: Is there any restriction to flow across PFO?
    - Size of RV and tricuspid annulus (expressed as a "z-score"), degree of tricuspid regurgitation: Important for planning of surgical repair

Angiographic Findings
- Conventional
  - PAt, VSD, MAPCAs
    - Selective injection with pressure recordings of all MAPCAs, imaging of true PAs
    - Pulmonary venous wedge injections for retrograde filling of diminutive PAs
  - PAt, intact VS
    - Suprasystemic pressure recordings in RV
    - Detailed imaging of coronary anatomy through RV and aortic root injections: RV to coronary communications, stenoses, interruptions

Imaging Recommendations
- Protocol advice
  - PAt, VSD, MAPCAs
    - Initial diagnosis with echocardiography
    - CT or MR for assessment of PA anatomy, post-operatively for shunt/conduit patency
    - Cardiac catheterization for hemodynamic assessment, selective injection studies and catheter-based interventions

DIFFERENTIAL DIAGNOSIS

Tetralogy of Fallot
- At least partial patency of RVOT

Complex cyanotic heart lesions with component of (sub)pulmonary stenosis
- Double outlet right ventricle
- Transposition of great arteries with VSD
- Single ventricle
- Tricuspid atresia

Ebstein anomaly
- May mimic PAt, intact VS with large tricuspid annulus and massive tricuspid regurgitation

PATHOLOGY

General Features
- General path comments
  - Embryology (PAt, VSD, MAPCAs)
    - RVOT obstruction → hypoplasia of PAs
    - Persistence or hypertrophy of primitive arterial connections to lungs
    - Hypertrophy of bronchial arteries
  - Pathophysiology of PAt, VSD, MAPCAs: Balance between flow though PAs and MAPCAs determines pulmonary perfusion
    - PA flow at sub-systemic pressures, restricted by narrow caliber and eventual closure of ductus arteriosus
    - MAPCA flow leads to increased lung perfusion at systemic pressures (unless restricted by stenosis)
    - Degree of cyanosis determined by intracardiac admixture and amount of pulmonary flow
    - Large amount of pulmonary blood flow through unrestricted MAPCAs → congestive heart failure
  - Pathophysiology of PAt, intact VS: Obligatory right → left shunt through PFO
    - Pulmonary arteries supplied by PDA

PULMONARY ATRESIA

- Small heavily trabeculated right ventricle with suprasystemic pressures
- Depending on size of tricuspid valve annulus: Severe tricuspid regurgitation, leading to massive right atrial dilatation (comparable to Ebstein anomaly)
- Transmyocardial sinusoids connecting right ventricular cavity with coronary artery system cause coronary flow reversal during diastole, leading to myocardial ischemia and infarction
- Epidemiology: Rare congenital cyanotic heart lesions, often classified together with tetralogy of Fallot

Gross Pathologic & Surgical Features
- Hilar arteries = true PAs
- Presence and confluence of central portions of true PAs important for surgical repair
- MAPCAs originating from
  - Ascending aorta
  - Brachiocephalic or intercostal arteries
  - Ductus arteriosus
  - Descending aorta (most common)

Microscopic Features
- Pulmonary vascular disease develops in vascular bed of high-flow MAPCAs → increase in cyanosis

CLINICAL ISSUES

Presentation
- Most common signs/symptoms
  - Progressive cyanosis after birth with closure of ductus arteriosus
  - Congestive heart failure with large unobstructed high-flow MAPCAs
- Other signs/symptoms: Failure to thrive, polycythemia, finger clubbing

Natural History & Prognosis
- Progressive cyanosis due to development of pulmonary vascular disease → irreversible pulmonary hypertension
- Life expectancy when untreated less than 10 years
- Survival into adulthood now possible: "Adult congenital heart disease"
  - Need for lifelong follow-up with multiple imaging tests
- Prognosis is guarded, depends on feasibility of surgery

Treatment
- Prostaglandin E1 to keep ductus arteriosus open
- Palliative: Systemic-to-PA shunt (Blalock-Taussig, central), initial banding of high-flow MAPCAs
- PAt, VSD, MAPCAs: Staged complete repair
  - Unifocalization of MAPCAs and true PAs (if existent, to allow for PA growth)
  - Early one-stage repair in infancy, with incorporation of all MAPCAs in PA conduit, may be feasible
  - Complete repair with incorporation of MAPCAs and PAs in conduit, connected to reconstructed RVOT, closure of VSD (may not be possible due to high pressure in pulmonary system from residual stenosis/hypoplasia and pulmonary vascular disease)
  - Catheter-based interventions (balloon angioplasty with stenting of stenoses, coil embolization of small superfluous and/or bleeding MAPCAs)
- PAt, intact VS: Type of repair dependent on RV size and RV-dependency on coronary circulation
  - Restriction in flow across PFO: Balloon atrial septostomy
  - Catheter-based or surgical pulmonary valvotomy
  - Sudden decompression of RV through valvotomy, RVOT repair or transannular patch may lead to myocardial ischemia/infarction
  - When RV is too hypoplastic for bi-ventricular repair: Cavopulmonary (Glenn) shunt, staged completion of univentricular repair (Fontan)

SELECTED REFERENCES

1. Roche KJ et al: Assessment of vasculature using combined MRI and MR angiography. AJR Am J Roentgenol. 182(4):861-6, 2004
2. Baque J et al: Evaluation of pulmonary atresia with magnetic resonance imaging. Heart. 87(2):159, 2002
3. Okada M et al: Modified Blalock-Taussig shunt patency for pulmonary atresia: assessment with electron beam CT. J Comput Assist Tomogr. 26(3):368-72, 2002
4. Holmqvist C et al: Pre-operative evaluation with MR in tetralogy of fallot and pulmonary atresia with ventricular septal defect. Acta Radiol. 42(1):63-9, 2001
5. Doyle TP et al: Tetralogy of Fallot and pulmonary atresia with ventricular septal defect. In: Moller JH, Hoffman JIE ed. Pediatric cardiovascular medicine, 1st ed. Philadelphia, Churchill Livingstone. 391-408, 2000
6. Freedom RM: Pulmonary atresia and intact ventricular septum. In: Moller JH, Hoffman JIE ed. Pediatric cardiovascular medicine. 1st ed. Philadelphia, Churchill Livingstone. 442-460, 2000
7. Powell AJ et al: Accuracy of MRI evaluation of pulmonary blood supply in patients with complex pulmonary stenosis or atresia. Int J Card Imaging. 16(3):169-74, 2000
8. Ichida F et al: Evaluation of pulmonary blood supply by multiplanar cine magnetic resonance imaging in patients with pulmonary atresia and severe pulmonary stenosis. Int J Card Imaging. 15(6):473-81, 1999
9. Westra SJ et al: Cardiac electron-beam CT in children undergoing surgical repair for pulmonary atresia. Radiology 213(2):502-12, 1999
10. Choe YH et al: MR imaging of non-visualized pulmonary arteries at angiography in patients with congenital heart disease. J Korean Med Sci. 13(6):597-602, 1998
11. Frank H et al: Magnetic resonance imaging of absent pulmonary valve syndrome. Pediatr Cardiol. 17(1):35-9, 1996
12. Taneja K et al: Comparison of computed tomography and cineangiography in the demonstration of central pulmonary arteries in cyanotic congenital heart disease. Cardiovasc Intervent Radiol. 19(2):97-100, 1996
13. Kersting-Sommerhoff BA et al: Evaluation of pulmonary blood supply by nuclear magnetic resonance imaging in patients with pulmonary atresia. J Am Coll Cardiol. 11(1):166-71, 1988
14. Rees RS et al: Magnetic resonance imaging of the pulmonary arteries and their systemic connections in pulmonary atresia: comparison with angiographic and surgical findings. Br Heart J. 58(6):621-6, 1987

PULMONARY ATRESIA

IMAGE GALLERY

Typical

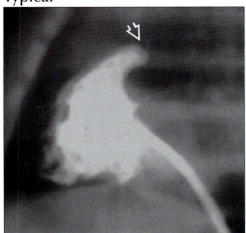
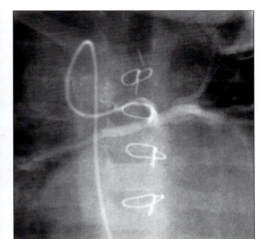

(Left) Lateral angiography shows occlusion at the pulmonary valve (arrow). The right ventricle is small, but there is a normally developed right ventricular outflow tract. *(Right)* Anteroposterior angiography shows selective injection of confluent hypoplastic branch pulmonary arteries in patient with pulmonary atresia with VSD.

Typical

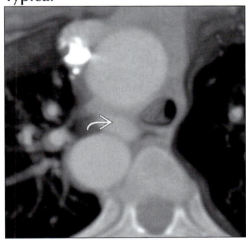
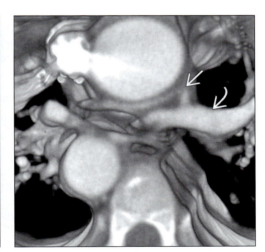

(Left) Axial CTA shows right aortic arch and large aortopulmonary collateral (arrow) originating from descending aorta. Note asymmetry and irregularity of pulmonary vasculature. *(Right)* Axial CTA, same patient as previous image, shows right aortic arch, aortopulmonary collateral (curved arrow) and confluence (arrow) of hypoplastic true branch pulmonary arteries.

Typical

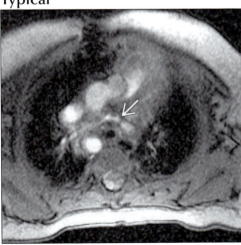
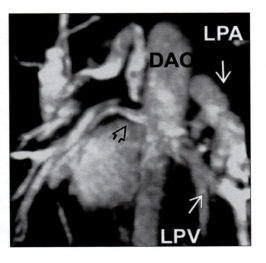

(Left) Axial MR cine shows hypoplastic confluent branch pulmonary arteries (arrow). Note right-sided aortic arch. *(Right)* Coronal MRA shows well-developed left pulmonary artery (LPA, arrows), whereas right lung is mainly supplied by aortopulmonary collaterals (open arrow). (LPV: Left pulmonary vein; DAO: Descending aorta). (Courtesy L. Sena, MD).

EBSTEIN ANOMALY

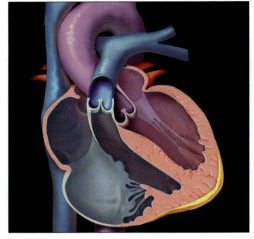

Graphic depicts downward displacement of the posterior valve leaflet, which has become incorporated into the right ventricular (RV) wall, leading to "atrialization" of the inflow portion of the RV.

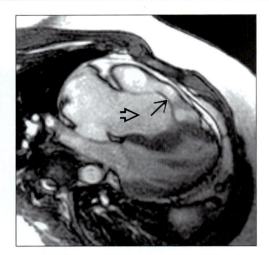

Four chamber view MR cine shows dilated right atrium, low placement of septal leaflet of tricuspid valve (arrow), atrialized portion of right ventricle (open arrow).

TERMINOLOGY

Definitions
- Downward displacement of the septal and posterior leaflets of the tricuspid valve
- Classic plain film appearance: Massive right-sided cardiomegaly ("box-shaped" heart)
- Category: Cyanotic, (severe) cardiomegaly, normal or decreased pulmonary vascularity
- Hemodynamics: Determined by severe tricuspid valve regurgitation
  - Volume overload to right heart
  - Right-to-left shunting through patent foramen ovale (PFO) → cyanosis

IMAGING FINDINGS

General Features
- Best diagnostic clue: Downward displacement of septal tricuspid leaflet (≥ 8 mm/m² body surface area)
- Location: Tricuspid valve

Radiographic Findings
- Radiography
  - Severe right-sided cardiomegaly
    - Heart size can be near normal in newborn period but also can be massively enlarged at birth
    - Heart increases gradually in size over time, reaching massive proportions in untreated cases during adulthood
    - Cardiothoracic ratio used as a parameter for follow up
  - Small vascular pedicle
  - May mimic large pericardial effusion

CT Findings
- Electron beam cine CT has been used for functional analysis of ventricular contraction

MR Findings
- T1WI: Right chamber best seen on long axis imaging
- T2* GRE
  - Cardiac-gated steady-state free precession cine-MRI
    - Ventricular volumes, ejection fraction of each ventricle, tricuspid regurgitation fraction
    - Left ventricular function affected by right ventricular dilatation, bowing of septum, mitral valve prolapse

Echocardiographic Findings
- Echocardiogram
  - Right chamber enlargement, "atrialized" portion of right ventricle
  - Enlarged tricuspid annulus (expressed in z-score)
  - Apical displacement of septal tricuspid leaflet (> 15 mm in children < 14 year; > 20 mm in adults)

DDx: Right-Sided Obstructive Cyanotic Heart Lesions

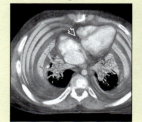
Tricuspid Atresia

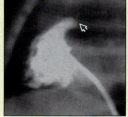
Pulmonary Atresia

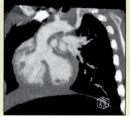
Tetralogy Of Fallot

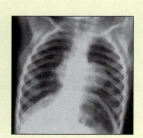
TGA, Pulm Stenosis

EBSTEIN ANOMALY

Key Facts

Terminology
- Downward displacement of the septal and posterior leaflets of the tricuspid valve
- Classic plain film appearance: Massive right-sided cardiomegaly ("box-shaped" heart)
- Category: Cyanotic, (severe) cardiomegaly, normal or decreased pulmonary vascularity
- Hemodynamics: Determined by severe tricuspid valve regurgitation
- Volume overload to right heart
- Right-to-left shunting through patent foramen ovale (PFO) → cyanosis

Imaging Findings
- Best diagnostic clue: Downward displacement of septal tricuspid leaflet (≥ 8 mm/m² body surface area)
- Severe right-sided cardiomegaly
- Cardiac-gated steady-state free precession cine-MRI
- Ventricular volumes, ejection fraction of each ventricle, tricuspid regurgitation fraction

Clinical Issues
- Wide spectrum of findings and ages at first presentation; some patients are asymptomatic
- Chronic right heart failure
- Presence of cyanosis depends on balance between right and left atrial pressure
- Prognosis is highly variable, dependent on hemodynamic significance of tricuspid regurgitation, presence of cyanosis
- Tricuspid valve replacement and/or reconstruction (valvuloplasty) is the definitive repair procedure

---

- Color Doppler
  - Tricuspid regurgitation
  - PFO with right-to-left shunting

Angiographic Findings
- Conventional
  - Characteristic notch at inferior right ventricular border at insertion of displaced anterior tricuspid leaflet
  - Seldom required for primary diagnosis

Nuclear Medicine Findings
- Radionuclide imaging
  - Decreased left ventricular ejection fraction in 50%

Imaging Recommendations
- Protocol advice
  - Anatomic and functional assessment with echocardiography in infants
  - Cine MRI in (young) adults

DIFFERENTIAL DIAGNOSIS

Large atrial septal defect (ASD)
- Acyanotic
- Increased pulmonary vascularity
- Left-to-right flow through ASD

Pericardial effusion
- Acyanotic
- Easy differentiation with echocardiography

Tricuspid insufficiency
- Primary, due to dysplastic valve
- Often secondary to pulmonary atresia with intact ventricular septum

Uhl anomaly and arrhythmogenic right ventricular dysplasia (ARVD)
- Similar but distinct entities with congenital absence (Uhl) or fatty infiltration (ARVD) of right ventricular myocardium
- May be differentiated from Ebstein anomaly with spin-echo and cine MRI

Right-sided obstructive cyanotic heart lesions with decreased pulmonary vascularity
- Tetralogy of Fallot
- Pulmonary atresia
  - With ventricular septal defect and aortopulmonary collaterals
  - With intact ventricular septum
    - Ebstein anomaly and pulmonary atresia with intact ventricular septum are the two lesions that cause the most severe cardiomegaly
- Tricuspid atresia
- Transposition of the great arteries (TGA) with pulmonary stenosis
- Double outlet right ventricle with pulmonary stenosis

PATHOLOGY

General Features
- General path comments
  - Massive right-sided chamber enlargement
  - Three compartments: Right atrium, atrialized non-contracting inlet portion and functional outlet portion of right ventricle
  - Ebstein anomaly frequently involves the left-sided tricuspid valve in congenitally corrected (L) transposition of the great arteries
  - Embryology
    - Insufficient separation of tricuspid valve leaflets and chordae tendineae from right ventricular endocardium
  - Pathophysiology
    - Massive tricuspid regurgitation
    - Volume overload to right side of heart
    - Right-to-left shunt through PFO → cyanosis
    - Left ventricular diastolic dysfunction may result from massive right-sided cardiac enlargement

EBSTEIN ANOMALY

- Arrhythmias due to conduction abnormalities are common
- Genetics: Most often sporadic
- Epidemiology
  - < 1% of congenital cardiac anomalies, incidence 1/210,000 live births
  - M:F = 1:1
- Associated abnormalities: PFO, secundum ASD in 90%

Gross Pathologic & Surgical Features
- Thickened valve leaflets, adherent to underlying myocardium
- Downward displacement of septal and posterior tricuspid leaflets
- Normally placed, redundant "sail-like" anterior tricuspid leaflet
- May occur on left side of the heart with congenitally corrected (L) transposition

CLINICAL ISSUES

Presentation
- Most common signs/symptoms
  - Wide spectrum of findings and ages at first presentation; some patients are asymptomatic
  - Chronic right heart failure
    - Decreased exercise tolerance (classified as New York Heart Association class I-IV)
  - Presence of cyanosis depends on balance between right and left atrial pressure
    - Physiological drop in pulmonary vascular resistance in neonatal period → decrease in right-to-left shunting through PFO → gradual improvement in cyanosis in first weeks of life
    - Polycythemia
- Other signs/symptoms
  - Hydrops fetalis in neonatal cases
  - Severe cardiomegaly in fetal life → pulmonary hypoplasia
  - Thrombosis, paradoxical embolus
  - Arrhythmias
    - Atrial fibrillation, atrial flutter → irregular heartbeat
    - Accessory atrioventricular conduction pathways (pre-excitation) → tachy-arrhythmias, which can be unexpected and fatal

Demographics
- Age: First presentation can range from newborn period through old age (average: 14 years)

Natural History & Prognosis
- Sudden death due to fatal atrial arrhythmias
- Uncomplicated pregnancies possible in women with hemodynamically well-balanced lesions
- Prognosis is highly variable, dependent on hemodynamic significance of tricuspid regurgitation, presence of cyanosis

Treatment
- Supportive treatment in cyanotic neonate: Oxygen, nitric oxide ventilation to lower pulmonary vascular resistance
- Systemic to pulmonary (Blalock-Taussig and central) shunts are ineffective
- Some patients benefit from total right-sided heart bypass procedures (Glenn → Fontan surgical treatment pathway)
- Tricuspid valve replacement and/or reconstruction (valvuloplasty) is the definitive repair procedure
  - Valvuloplasty and bioprosthesis placement are preferable to mechanical valve (allow growth; no need for life-long anticoagulation)
  - Valvuloplasty uses tissues from the existing valve (redundant anterior tricuspid leaflet)
  - Bioprosthesis: Homograft or xenograft (porcine valve)
- Indications for valve repair
  - NYHA Class III and IV
  - NYHA Class I and II with cardiothoracic ratio > 0.65
  - Significant cyanosis (arterial saturation < 80%) and/or polycythemia (Hb > 16 g/dl)
  - History of paradoxical embolus
  - Arrhythmia due to accessory atrioventricular pathway
- Arrhythmia treatments
  - Anti-arrhythmic drugs
  - Permanent pacemaker implantation
  - Radiofrequency ablation

SELECTED REFERENCES
1. Beerepoot JP et al: Case 71: Ebstein anomaly. Radiology. 231(3):747-51, 2004
2. Chauvaud S et al: Ebstein's anomaly: repair based on functional analysis. Eur J Cardiothorac Surg. 23(4):525-31, 2003
3. Dearani JA et al: Ebstein's anomaly of the tricuspid valve, In: Mavroudis C, Backer CL ed. Pediatric cardiac surgery. 3rd ed. Philadelphia, Mosby. 524-36, 2003
4. MacLellan-Tobert SG et al: Ebstein anomaly of the tricuspid valve. In: Moller JH, Hoffman JIE ed. Pediatric cardiovascular medicine, 1st ed. Philadelphia, Churchill Livingstone. 461-8, 2000
5. Ammash NM et al: Mimics of Ebstein's anomaly. Am Heart J. 134(3):508-13, 1997
6. Choi YH at al: MR imaging of Ebstein's anomaly of the tricuspid valve. Am J Roentgenol. 163:539-43, 1994
7. Eustace S et al: Ebstein's anomaly presenting in adulthood: the role of cine magnetic resonance imaging in diagnosis. Clin Radiol. 49(10):690-2, 1994
8. Farb A et al: Anatomy and pathology of the right ventricle (including acquired tricuspid and pulmonic valve disease). Cardiol Clin. 10(1):1-21, 1992
9. Lau MK et al: Magnetic resonance imaging of Ebstein's anomaly: report of two cases. J Formos Med Assoc. 91(12):1205-8, 1992
10. Saxena A et al: Late noninvasive evaluation of cardiac performance in mildly symptomatic older patients with Ebstein's anomaly of tricuspid valve: role of radionuclide imaging. J Am Coll Cardiol. 17(1):182-6, 1991
11. Kastler B et al: Potential role of MR imaging in the diagnostic management of Ebstein anomaly in a newborn. J Comput Assist Tomogr. 14(5):825-7, 1990
12. Link KM et al: MR imaging of Ebstein anomaly: results in four cases. AJR Am J Roentgenol. 150(2):363-7, 1988

EBSTEIN ANOMALY

IMAGE GALLERY

Typical

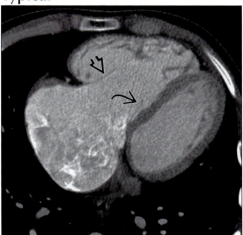 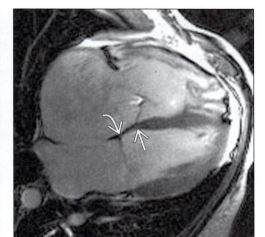

(Left) Axial CECT shows right atrial dilatation and apical displacement *(curved arrow)* of septal tricuspid leaflet. Note "sail-like" deformity of redundant anterior valve leaflet *(open arrow)*. *(Right)* Axial MR cine shows 16 mm distance between the septal leaflets of the mitral *(curved arrow)* and the tricuspid valve *(arrow)*, which is diagnostic of Ebstein anomaly.

Typical

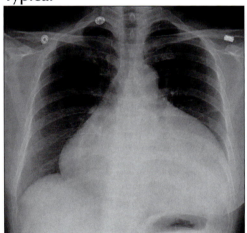 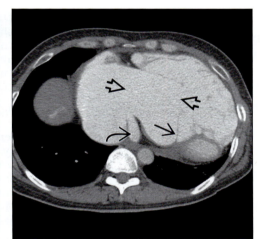

(Left) Anteroposterior radiograph of 48 year old woman with Ebstein anomaly shows massive right-sided cardiomegaly. *(Right)* Axial CECT shows apical displacement of septal tricuspid valve leaflet *(arrow)*, with atrialized portion of right ventricle *(between open arrows)*. Note dilatation of coronary sinus *(curved arrow)*.

Typical

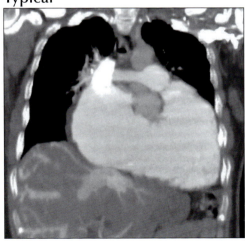 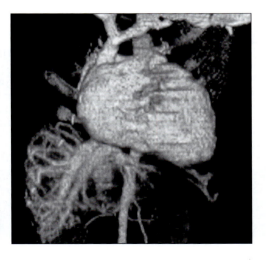

(Left) Coronal CTA depicts massive dilatation of right-sided cardiac chambers. Note reflux of contrast material into congested right hepatic veins, due to tricuspid regurgitation. *(Right)* CTA with shaded surface rendition also displays severe right-sided cardiomegaly and reflux into hepatic veins.

D-TRANSPOSITION OF THE GREAT ARTERIES

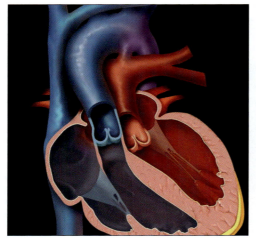

Graphic shows anteriorly-placed aorta, connected via infundibulum to right ventricle, and posteriorly-placed pulmonary artery, directly connected to left ventricle.

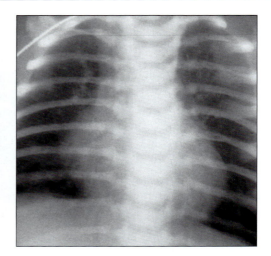

Anteroposterior radiograph shows classic "egg"-shaped heart, increased pulmonary vascularity and narrow mediastinum (due to abnormal anteroposterior relationship of great vessels and thymic involution).

TERMINOLOGY

Abbreviations and Synonyms
- Ventriculoarterial discordance with atrioventricular concordance

Definitions
- Aorta arises from right ventricle (RV) and pulmonary artery from left ventricle (LV)
- Category: Cyanotic, cardiomegaly, increased pulmonary vascularity
- Hemodynamics
  o RV connected with systemic circulation: Pressure overload
  o LV connected with pulmonary circulation: Volume overload
  o Incompatible with life without flow admixture: Patent foramen ovale (PFO), ventricular septal defect (VSD), patent ductus arteriosus (PDA)

IMAGING FINDINGS

General Features
- Best diagnostic clue: Great vessels lie parallel and almost in the same sagittal plane, with aortic valve in anterior position and slightly to the right (D-loop) of pulmonary valve

Radiographic Findings
- Radiography
  o May be normal in neonates
  o Cardiomegaly
  o Narrow mediastinum ("egg-on-side" heart)
  o Increased pulmonary vascularity

CT Findings
- CTA
  o Post-operative CTA shows altered great vessel anatomy, with anteriorly-positioned pulmonary artery (PA) and posterior aorta in same sagittal plane
    ▪ Traction on both branch PAs may lead to stenosis
    ▪ Anterior tracheal or left mainstem bronchus compression by ascending aorta, which is tethered by PAs in front of it
    ▪ Cardiac-gated multi-detector cine CT for ventricular function in patients with contra-indication for MRI
  o CTA is preferred modality after placement of metallic stents for branch pulmonary artery stenosis

MR Findings
- T1WI
  o Cardiac-gated axial images for segmental cardiac analysis: Atrioventricular concordance and ventriculoarterial discordance
    ▪ Presence of PFO, VSD, (sub-) pulmonary stenosis

DDx: Cyanosis With Increased Pulmonary Vascularity

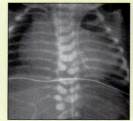
Truncus Arteriosus

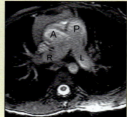
AP Window

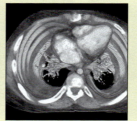
Tricuspid Atresia

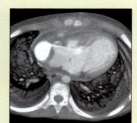
Single Ventricle

D-TRANSPOSITION OF THE GREAT ARTERIES

Key Facts

Terminology
- Ventriculoarterial discordance with atrioventricular concordance
- Aorta arises from right ventricle (RV) and pulmonary artery from left ventricle (LV)
- Category: Cyanotic, cardiomegaly, increased pulmonary vascularity
- Incompatible with life without flow admixture: Patent foramen ovale (PFO), ventricular septal defect (VSD), patent ductus arteriosus (PDA)

Imaging Findings
- Best diagnostic clue: Great vessels lie parallel and almost in the same sagittal plane, with aortic valve in anterior position and slightly to the right (D-loop) of pulmonary valve
- Narrow mediastinum ("egg-on-side" heart)
- Multiplanar steady-state free precession cine is the gold standard for cardiac function evaluation, ventricular volume measurements
- Conventional: Cardiac catheterization only needed for Rashkind procedure (emergency balloon atrial septostomy)

Pathology
- Coronary anomalies are frequent

Clinical Issues
- Complication of arterial switch: Traction on branch PAs by anteriorly transposed main PA, leading to branch origin stenosis
- Mustard/Senning procedures: RV failure, atrial thrombosis, arrhythmias

---

- Post-operative assessment of PA stenosis
- If metal artifact from stents: Double inversion sequence
- T2* GRE
  - Multiplanar steady-state free precession cine is the gold standard for cardiac function evaluation, ventricular volume measurements
    - RV dysfunction following atrial switch procedures, not able to sustain systemic circulation
    - Baffle obstruction after Mustard/Senning
- T1 C+: Delayed-enhancement myocardial MRI to detect ischemia complicating coronary transposition
- MRA
  - Gadolinium-enhanced MRA for post-operative PA stenosis
  - MR coronary angiography with navigator-echo respiratory gating to study patency of origins of transposed coronary arteries
  - Velocity-encoded phase contrast MRA with flow velocity measurements, allowing calculations of gradients across stenoses (PAs, atrial baffles)

Echocardiographic Findings
- Segmental cardiac analysis: Identification of atria, ventricles, great arteries and their connections
- Identification of PFO, VSD, PDA
- Proximal coronary artery anatomy

Angiographic Findings
- Conventional: Cardiac catheterization only needed for Rashkind procedure (emergency balloon atrial septostomy)

Imaging Recommendations
- Echocardiography allows for complete pre-operative diagnosis in majority
- CT or MRI for post-operative complications of pulmonary arteries, atrial baffle

DIFFERENTIAL DIAGNOSIS

Complex transposition
- Associated (sub-) pulmonary stenosis, VSD

Associated (pre-ductal) coarctation with PDA
- Small RV and aorta; large LV and pulmonary artery

Truncus arteriosus, aortopulmonary (AP) window, tricuspid atresia, single ventricle with unobstructed pulmonary flow
- All have cardiomegaly with increased vascularity

PATHOLOGY

General Features
- General path comments
  - Atria and ventricles are morphologic normal
  - Coronary anomalies are frequent
    - Right coronary artery dominance
    - Circumflex branch originates from right coronary
    - Single coronary ostium
  - Embryology
    - Single embryological error: Faulty separation of aorta and pulmonary artery from primitive bulbus cordis (cono-truncus)
    - Heart is otherwise structurally normal
  - Pathophysiology
    - Complete separation of pulmonary and systemic circulations
    - Survival dependent on admixture: PFO, VSD, PDA
- Genetics
  - No genetic factors identified
  - Not associated with extracardiac malformations or chromosomal abnormalities
- Epidemiology
  - Incidence: 1 in 3,000 live births
  - 5% of congenital heart disease
  - Males > females

D-TRANSPOSITION OF THE GREAT ARTERIES

Gross Pathologic & Surgical Features
- Infundibulum of RV connected to aortic valve, anterior and slightly to right of midline (D-loop)
- LV connected without infundibulum to pulmonary valve, posterior and slightly to left of aortic valve

CLINICAL ISSUES

Presentation
- Severe cyanosis not improving with oxygen, with little respiratory distress

Natural History & Prognosis
- Early death without communicating shunt
- Large VSD: Congestive heart failure in neonatal period
- Patients with large VSD and (sub-) pulmonic stenosis have mild symptoms and may survive for years without treatment
- Simple transposition: Good prognosis with early switch
- Complication of arterial switch: Traction on branch PAs by anteriorly transposed main PA, leading to branch origin stenosis
- Long-term prognosis determined by potential coronary abnormalities
- Complex transposition: Dependent on associated anomalies
- Mustard/Senning procedures: RV failure, atrial thrombosis, arrhythmias

Treatment
- Prostaglandin E1 to keep ductus arteriosus open
- Emergency balloon atrial septostomy (Rashkind)
- Surgical early: Arterial switch with transposition of coronaries (Jatene)
  - Late arterial switch not possible (pressure drops after birth in LV connected to pulmonary circulation, which is then no longer able to sustain systemic arterial pressures)
- Surgical late: Re-routing of venous flow in atria with pericardial baffle (Mustard) or reorientation of the atrial septum (Senning)

SELECTED REFERENCES

1. Raman SV et al: Usefulness of multidetector row computed tomography to quantify right ventricular size and function in adults with either tetralogy of Fallot or transposition of the great arteries. Am J Cardiol. 95(5):683-6, 2005
2. Taylor AM et al: MR coronary angiography and late-enhancement myocardial MR in children who underwent arterial switch surgery for transposition of great arteries. Radiology. 234(2):542-7, 2005
3. Lissin LW et al: Comparison of transthoracic echocardiography versus cardiovascular magnetic resonance imaging for the assessment of ventricular function in adults after atrial switch procedures for complete transposition of the great arteries. Am J Cardiol. 93(5):654-7, 2004
4. Roest AA et al: Cardiovascular response to physical exercise in adult patients after atrial correction for transposition of the great arteries assessed with magnetic resonance imaging. Heart. 90(6):678-84, 2004
5. Sorensen TS et al: Operator-independent isotropic three-dimensional magnetic resonance imaging for morphology in congenital heart disease: a validation study. Circulation. 110(2):163-9, 2004
6. Fogel MA et al: Mid-term follow-up of patients with transposition of the great arteries after atrial inversion operation using two- and three-dimensional magnetic resonance imaging. Pediatr Radiol. 32(6):440-6, 2002
7. McMahon CJ et al: Preoperative identification of coronary arterial anatomy in complete transposition, and outcome after the arterial switch operation. Cardiol Young. 12(3):240-7, 2002
8. Tulevski II et al: Usefulness of magnetic resonance imaging dobutamine stress in asymptomatic and minimally symptomatic patients with decreased cardiac reserve from congenital heart disease (complete and corrected transposition of the great arteries and subpulmonic obstruction). Am J Cardiol. 89(9):1077-81, 2002
9. Lidegran M et al: Magnetic resonance imaging and echocardiography in assessment of ventricular function in atrially corrected transposition of the great arteries. Scand Cardiovasc J. 34(4):384-9, 2000
10. Sidi D. Complete transposition of the great arteries. In: Moller JH, Hoffman JIE ed. Pediatric cardiovascular medicine, 1st ed. Philadelphia, Churchill Livingstone. 351-262, 2000
11. Tulevski II et al: Dobutamine-induced increase of right ventricular contractility without increased stroke volume in adolescent patients with transposition of the great arteries: evaluation with magnetic resonance imaging. Int J Card Imaging. 16(6):471-8, 2000
12. Gutberlet M et al: Arterial switch procedure for D-transposition of the great arteries: quantitative midterm evaluation of hemodynamic changes with cine MR imaging and phase-shift velocity mapping-initial experience. Radiology. 214(2):467-75, 2000
13. Chen SJ et al: Three-dimensional reconstruction of abnormal ventriculoarterial relationship by electron beam CT. J Comput Assist Tomogr. 22(4):560-8, 1998
14. Lorenz CH et al: Right ventricular performance and mass by use of cine MRI late after atrial repair of transposition of the great arteries. Circulation. 92(9 Suppl):II233-9, 1995
15. Blakenberg F et al: MRI vs echocardiography in the evaluation of the Jatene procedure. J Comput Assist Tomogr. 18(5):749-54, 1994
16. Hardy CE et al: Usefulness of magnetic resonance imaging for evaluating great-vessel anatomy after arterial switch operation for D-transposition of the great arteries. Am Heart J. 128(2):326-32, 1994
17. Beek FJ et al: MRI of the pulmonary artery after arterial switch operation for transposition of the great arteries. Pediatr Radiol 23:335-40, 1993
18. Theissen P et al: Magnetic resonance imaging of cardiac function and morphology in patients with transposition of the great arteries following Mustard procedure. Thorac Cardiovasc Surg. 39 Suppl 3:221-4, 1991
19. Chung KJ et al: Cine magnetic resonance imaging after surgical repair in patients with transposition of the great arteries. Circulation. 77(1):104-9, 1988
20. Rees S et al: Comparison of magnetic resonance imaging with echocardiography and radionuclide angiography in assessing cardiac function and anatomy following Mustard's operation for transposition of the great arteries. Am J Cardiol. 61(15):1316-22, 1988
21. Campbell RM et al: Detection of caval obstruction by magnetic resonance imaging after intraatrial repair of transposition of the great arteries. Am J Cardiol. 60(8):688-91, 1987
22. Matherne GP et al: Cine computed tomography for diagnosis of superior vena cava obstruction following the Mustard operation. Pediatr Radiol. 17(3):246-7, 1987

D-TRANSPOSITION OF THE GREAT ARTERIES

IMAGE GALLERY

Typical

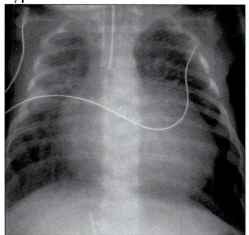
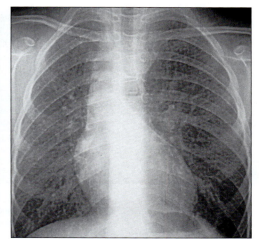

(Left) Anteroposterior radiograph shows "egg"-shaped heart, narrow mediastinum. *(Right)* Anteroposterior radiograph in older child who underwent Mustard repair for transposition shows abnormal contour of great vessels in upper mediastinum.

Typical

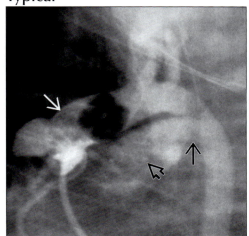
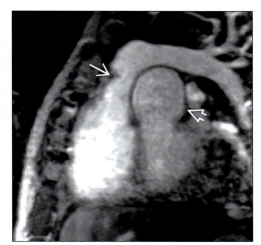

(Left) Lateral angiography shows reversed relationship between anteriorly placed aorta (white arrow) and posteriorly placed pulmonary artery (open arrow); patent ductus arteriosus (black arrow). *(Right)* Sagittal oblique MR cine shows typical post-operative anatomy after arterial switch operation. Note anastomotic stenosis in pulmonary artery (arrow), which is now located anteriorly to aortic root (open arrow).

Other

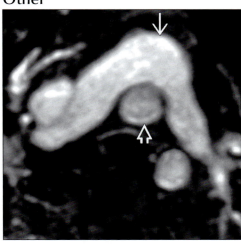
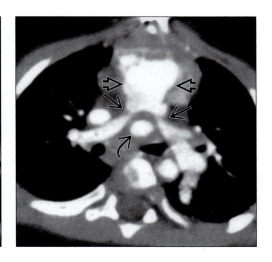

(Left) Axial MR cine, same patient as previous panel, shows pulmonary artery bifurcation (arrow) positioned anteriorly to ascending aorta (open arrow), with normal branch pulmonary arteries. (Both images courtesy of L. Sena, MD). *(Right)* Axial CTA shows anterior position of pulmonary outflow tract (open arrows) with respect to ascending aorta (curved arrow). Stenoses of origins of bilateral branch pulmonary arteries (arrows).

TRICUSPID ATRESIA

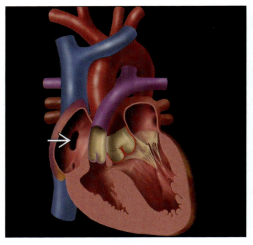

Graphic of tricuspid atresia where there is no forward flow into right ventricle. Graphic depicts atrial septal defect (arrow), ventricular septal defect, and hypoplastic right ventricle.

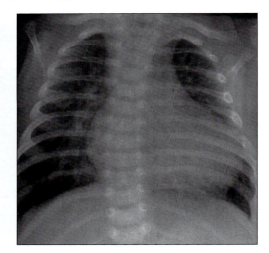

Anteroposterior radiograph shows marked cardiomegaly and increased pulmonary flow in this infant with tricuspid atresia, large VSD and no pulmonary valve stenosis.

TERMINOLOGY

Abbreviations and Synonyms
- Tricuspid atresia (TA)

Definitions
- Congenital absence or agenesis of the tricuspid valve and inlet portion of the right ventricle

IMAGING FINDINGS

General Features
- Best diagnostic clue
  - Absence of an inflow portion of the right ventricle with atretic tricuspid valve
  - Outlet portion of the right ventricle depends on the size of the ventricular septal defect (VSD)
- Location: Tricuspid valve is absent, fused or stenotic and size of VSD and right ventricle is variable
- Morphology
  - Type I: Normally related great arteries occurs in 70-80%
  - Type II: D-transposition of the great arteries occurs in 12-25%
  - Type III: L-transposition of the great vessels or malposition occurs in 3-6%
  - Ventricular septal defect can occur with atresia, stenosis or normal pulmonary valve

Radiographic Findings
- Radiography
  - Neonate chest is variable depending on size of VSD
    - Small VSD: Heart is usually normal in size and RV is hypoplastic and pulmonary flow is diminished
    - Large VSD: Heart is usually large with increased flow or transposition of the great arteries
    - Right aortic arch is present in 8% of patients
  - Surgery depends on defining the anatomy although many children require more than one surgical procedure
  - Post-operative chest imaging depends on anatomy and surgical repair
    - Aortopulmonary shunt such as a modified Blalock-Taussig shunt may demonstrate asymmetry of pulmonary flow
    - Bidirectional Glenn anastomosis may have asymmetry of blood flow
    - Pleural effusions related to elevation of pulmonary artery pressure, in part due to abnormal lymphatic drainage are common after surgery

CT Findings
- CECT

DDx: Cyanotic Congenital Heart Disease In First Week Of Life

Transposition | Tetralogy | Ebstein | TAPVR

TRICUSPID ATRESIA

Key Facts

Terminology
- Congenital absence or agenesis of the tricuspid valve and inlet portion of the right ventricle

Imaging Findings
- Neonate chest is variable depending on size of VSD
- Demonstrates post-operative anastomosis, relative size of pulmonary arteries, and presence of collateral venous anatomy
- Excellent for post-operative left ventricular functional assessment and anatomy of cavo-pulmonary artery anastomosis
- Protocol advice: Prior to imaging studies, knowledge of previous surgical procedure is critical to interpreting imaging particularity in Glenn anastomosis and Fontan procedures

Top Differential Diagnoses
- Transposition of the great arteries
- Tetralogy of Fallot
- Ebstein anomaly
- Total anomalous pulmonary venous return

Clinical Issues
- 50% of neonates present with cyanosis first 24 hours
- 30% present with signs of congestive heart failure
- Surgery usually involves a staged approach similar to single ventricle morphology
- Modified Blalock-Taussig shunt with systemic artery to pulmonary flow
- Bidirectional Glenn anastomosis with superior vena cava to pulmonary artery
- Modified Fontan procedure with inferior vena cava conduit to pulmonary artery

---

- o Demonstrates post-operative anastomosis, relative size of pulmonary arteries, and presence of collateral venous anatomy
- o Must know underlying anatomy and type of surgical repair to interpret contrast studies
- o Useful to assess for pulmonary artery embolus, collateral vessels, in children who have increasing cyanosis

MR Findings
- MR Cine
  - o Useful in older children or adults who can hold their breath and in whom the acoustical window is suboptimal
  - o Spin-echo or gradient-echo MR techniques used for anatomic imaging
  - o Gadolinium-enhanced imaging can be useful for functional and anatomic assessment
  - o Excellent for post-operative left ventricular functional assessment and anatomy of cavo-pulmonary artery anastomosis
  - o 3D contrast-enhanced MRA or spin-echo imaging can be used to assess connections and relations as well as the size of the proximal pulmonary arteries
  - o Can assess pulmonary artery branch stenosis

Echocardiographic Findings
- Echocardiogram
  - o In-utero and after birth modality of choice for specific cardiac anomalies
  - o Defines size and position of the VSD, the size of right ventricle and associated abnormalities

Angiographic Findings
- Cardiac catheterization prior to staged cardiac surgery repairs or complications
  - o Coiling of collateral arteries and veins to reduce work load of left ventricle

Other Modality Findings
- Newborn pattern of left axis deviation on electrocardiography (EKG) is usually diagnostic

Imaging Recommendations
- Best imaging tool
  - o Hallmark on any imaging modality is the lack of direct anatomic continuity between the right atrium and ventricle
  - o Ventricular anatomy, type and size of the ventricular septal defect and the relationship of the great vessels, ventriculoarterial connections, sources of pulmonary artery flow need to be accessed
- Protocol advice: Prior to imaging studies, knowledge of previous surgical procedure is critical to interpreting imaging particularity in Glenn anastomosis and Fontan procedures

DIFFERENTIAL DIAGNOSIS

Transposition of the great arteries
- Chest radiograph can be normal or have classic "egg" appearance
- Usually cyanotic within first 24 hours of birth

Tetralogy of Fallot
- Large aorta which is right sided in 25%, concave left hilum, and decreased peripheral flow

Ebstein anomaly
- Newborn chest may show massive cardiac heart
- Spectrum of disease which involves downward displacement of the septal and posterior leaflets of the tricuspid valve

Total anomalous pulmonary venous return
- Normal size heart, pulmonary edema, and effusion when obstructed

PATHOLOGY

General Features
- Genetics
  - o No genetic predisposition, multifactorial
  - o Associated with asplenia syndromes

TRICUSPID ATRESIA

- Etiology: Early embryologic insult with fusion of valve leaflet resulting in stenosis (partial fusion) or atresia (complete fusion) of the valves
- Epidemiology: 3% of congenital heart lesions

Microscopic Features
- Atretic valve is represented by a dimple in the floor of the right atrium

CLINICAL ISSUES

Presentation
- Most common signs/symptoms
  - 50% of neonates present with cyanosis first 24 hours
  - 30% present with signs of congestive heart failure
- Other signs/symptoms: Extracardiac anomalies may occur in 20% of patients

Demographics
- Age: Diagnosed in-utero, at birth
- Gender: M = F

Natural History & Prognosis
- Prenatal circulation
  - Blood from superior vena cava and inferior vena cava crosses foramen ovale into left atrium, left ventricle and aorta
  - Blood supply to lung is entirely through ductus arteriosus in fetus
- Postnatal circulation
  - All systemic flow is shunted across interatrial septal communication into left atrium
  - Admixture of systemic venous and pulmonary venous return
  - Left ventricular volume overload occurs as entire systemic, coronary, and pulmonary outputs are ejected by left ventricle
  - Degree of volume overloading increases if there is mild or no pulmonary outflow obstruction or if a systemic to pulmonary shunt has been performed
  - Patency of interatrial communication is essential for survival and obstruction may necessitate an atrial septectomy
  - Closure of the duct arteriosus in a neonate may result in severe hypoxemia requiring administration of prostaglandin E1 or surgical creation of systemic to pulmonary artery shunt
  - Patency of VSD is also essential to maintain intracardiac shunting for patient survival and oxygenation
    - Spontaneous closure may occur in 30-48% with a median age of 1.3 years
  - Blood enters the left atrium and in type I, a VSD may be present which permits left-to-right shunting and lung perfusion, usually blood flow to the lungs is decreased
  - In D-transposition of the great arteries and TA, lungs receive the blood flow from left ventricle and in general, there is over circulation
  - Children may be at risk for stroke, brain abscess, polycythemia, bacterial endocarditis
  - Atrial arrhythmias occur commonly in older children

Treatment
- Neonatal care depends on anatomy and pulmonary artery flow
  - Some infants need prostaglandin to maintain ductal patency with subsequent surgery
- Initial atrial septostomy if right to left atrial shunt is restrictive
- Surgery usually involves a staged approach similar to single ventricle morphology
  - Initial atrial septostomy if right to left atrial shunt is restrictive
  - Modified Blalock-Taussig shunt with systemic artery to pulmonary flow
    - Transient pulmonary edema may occur if shunt is large
    - May distort the pulmonary arteries at anastomosis
  - Bidirectional Glenn anastomosis with superior vena cava to pulmonary artery
    - Many have transient pulmonary edema and serous or chylous effusions
    - Develop collateral venous pathways if pulmonary artery pressure is increased
  - Modified Fontan procedure with inferior vena cava conduit to pulmonary artery
    - Techniques continue to be revised but current therapy is an extracardiac conduit connection from the inferior vena cava to the pulmonary circuit
    - Venous collaterals develop from elevated PA pressures and empty in various sites however increasing cyanosis occurs as this is unoxygenated blood entering the left side of the heart
    - Systemic arterial collaterals develop and there is left-to-right shunting which increases the pressure in pulmonary arteries and increases the work of left ventricle
    - Occasional complication of protein losing enteropathy, ascites
  - Cardiac transplantation is an option for failed Fontan

SELECTED REFERENCES

1. Lilje C et al: Magnetic resonance imaging follow up of total cavopulmonary connection. Heart. 91(3):395, 2005
2. Sittiwangkul R et al: Outcomes of tricuspid atresia in the Fontan era. Ann Thorac Surg. 77(3):889-94, 2004
3. Epstein, M: Tricuspid Atresia: In: Allen HD and Gutgesell HP (eds). Heart Disease in Infants and Children, and Adolescents. Lippincott Williams & Wilkins. Philadelphia. 1197-1215, 2001
4. Hess J: Long-term problems after cavopulmonary anastomosis: diagnosis and management. Thorac Cardiovasc Surg. 49(2):98-100, 2001
5. Freedom RM et al: The Fontan procedure: analysis of cohorts and late complications. Cardiol Young. 10(4):307-31, 2000
6. Rao PS: Tricuspid atresia: anatomy, imaging, and natural history. In: Braunwald E, Freedom R, eds. Atlas of Heart Disease: Congenital Heart Disease. Vol 12. Philadelphia, Pa: Current Medicine, 1997

TRICUSPID ATRESIA

IMAGE GALLERY

Typical

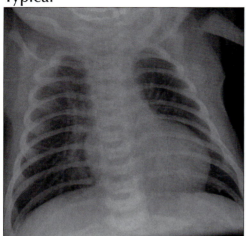
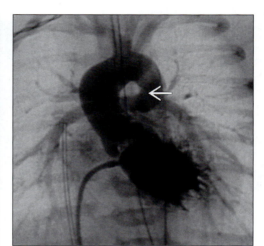

(Left) Anteroposterior radiograph shows a newborn with tricuspid atresia and normally related great vessels. Chest radiograph shows normal heart size, and normal pulmonary blood flow. *(Right)* Anteroposterior angiography shows catheter in the left ventricle with contrast in ascending aorta and a large patent ductus arteriosis (arrow) with significant flow to lung.

Typical

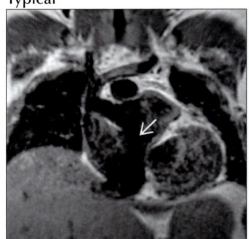
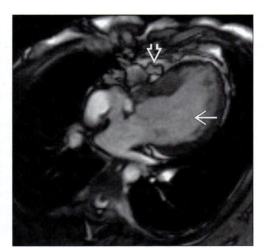

(Left) Coronal T1WI MR shows an absence of the tricuspid valve, no inlet portion of the right ventricle and a large patent foramen ovale (arrow) which connects the right and left atrium. *(Right)* Four chamber view MR shows enlarged left ventricular chamber (arrow) and absence of right ventricle (open arrow) in patient with tricuspid atresia and post-operative Fontan.

Other

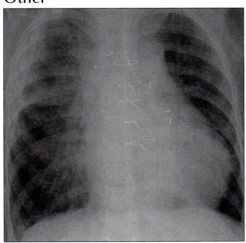
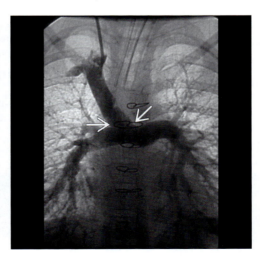

(Left) Anteroposterior radiograph shows right pleural effusion in patient who has tricuspid atresia, post-operative bidirectional Glenn anastomosis. Effusions are commonly seen in the immediate post-operative period. *(Right)* Anteroposterior angiography demonstrates a bidirectional Glenn anastamosis. The superior vena cava is anastomosed to pulmonary artery (arrows) and transient bilateral effusions are common.

TRUNCUS ARTERIOSUS

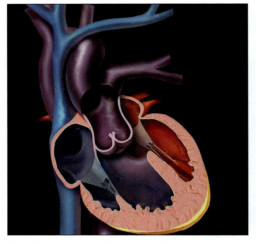

Graphic shows type 1 truncus with common truncal valve, overriding high VSD, giving rise to aorta (note right aortic arch) and main pulmonary artery. Cyanosis is due to flow admixture within ventricles and truncus.

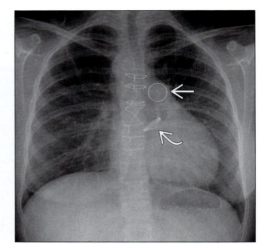

Anteroposterior radiograph in 15 year old girl who underwent repair for truncus arteriosus in infancy shows pulmonary conduit (arrow) and aortic (curved arrow) valve prostheses in place. Note right-sided aortic arch.

TERMINOLOGY

Abbreviations and Synonyms
- Common arterial trunk

Definitions
- Common arterial vessel arising from the heart, giving rise to aorta, pulmonary arteries (PAs) and coronaries
- Classic plain film appearance: Cardiomegaly, increased pulmonary vascularity, narrow mediastinum, right aortic arch
- Category: Cyanotic, cardiomegaly, increased pulmonary vascularity
- Hemodynamics
  o Both ventricles connected with pulmonary and systemic circulation
  o Flow admixture across ventricular septal defect (VSD) and within truncus → cyanosis
  o Postnatal drop in pulmonary vascular resistance → relative increase in pulmonary blood flow → volume overload of pulmonary circulation
- Truncus arteriosus is the heart lesion most commonly associated with right aortic arch (30-40%)
- Frequently associated with absent thymus and parathyroid glands: DiGeorge syndrome

IMAGING FINDINGS

General Features
- Best diagnostic clue: Common arterial trunk arising from both ventricles

Radiographic Findings
- Radiography
  o Cardiomegaly
  o Active pulmonary vascular congestion (shunt vascularity)
  o Right aortic arch common
  o Narrow mediastinum due to thymic agenesis
  o Dilated pulmonary arteries may compress neighboring bronchi → atelectasis

CT Findings
- CTA
  o Relationship of branch PAs with truncus
  o Coronary anatomy
  o Post-operative: Patency and size of conduit, calcification and stenosis
  o CTA is best technique to evaluate stent placement

MR Findings
- T1WI
  o Cardiac-gated axial images for pre-operative definition of PA anatomy

DDx: Cyanosis, Increased Pulmonary Vascularity

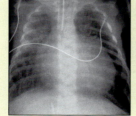
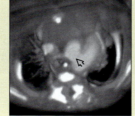
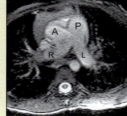
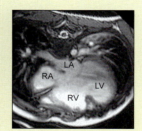

Transposition   *AP Window*   *AP Window*   *Unbalanced AV Canal*

TRUNCUS ARTERIOSUS

Key Facts

Terminology
- Common arterial vessel arising from the heart, giving rise to aorta, pulmonary arteries (PAs) and coronaries
- Classic plain film appearance: Cardiomegaly, increased pulmonary vascularity, narrow mediastinum, right aortic arch
- Category: Cyanotic, cardiomegaly, increased pulmonary vascularity
- Both ventricles connected with pulmonary and systemic circulation
- Flow admixture across ventricular septal defect (VSD) and within truncus → cyanosis
- Truncus arteriosus is the heart lesion most commonly associated with right aortic arch (30-40%)
- Frequently associated with absent thymus and parathyroid glands: DiGeorge syndrome

Imaging Findings
- Best diagnostic clue: Common arterial trunk arising from both ventricles
- MRI/CTA for post-operative assessment of conduit stenosis, stent placement

Clinical Issues
- Progressive congestive heart failure with drop in pulmonary vascular resistance in young infant
- Increasing cyanosis due to shunt reversal with development of pulmonary hypertension
- Surgical repair, with placement of conduit between right ventricle and PA, and closure of VSD
- Conduit revisions are frequently necessary throughout patient's life time

---

  - Post-operative: Conduit stenosis, anastomotic pseudoaneurysm
- T2* GRE: Steady-state free precession cine MRI: Truncal valve regurgitation, ventricular function
- MRA: Gadolinium-enhanced MRA for global anatomy, patency of PA conduit

Echocardiographic Findings
- Echocardiogram
  - Common arterial trunk originating from both ventricles
  - High (outlet) VSD immediately below truncal valve
  - Common truncal valve with 2 (5%), 3 (60%) or 4 (25%) cusps
- Color Doppler
  - Bidirectional flow across VSD
  - Truncal valve regurgitation

Angiographic Findings
- Conventional
  - Cardiac catheterization with angiography
    - To define the exact type of truncal anatomy
    - Truncal valve insufficiency
    - Hemodynamic study is gold standard for calculation of pulmonary vascular resistance

Imaging Recommendations
- Protocol advice
  - Primary diagnosis made with echocardiography
  - MRI/CTA for pre-operative delineation of PA anatomy
  - MRI/CTA for post-operative assessment of conduit stenosis, stent placement

DIFFERENTIAL DIAGNOSIS

Transposition of the great arteries
- Presents earlier in life with more severe cyanosis, ductus-dependent

Aortopulmonary window
- Congenital fenestration between separate ascending aorta and PA, with separate aortic and pulmonary valves

Common atrioventricular (AV) canal
- When unbalanced (right or left dominant): Cyanosis frequently occurs due to admixture

PATHOLOGY

General Features
- General path comments
  - Common outflow tract of both ventricles, over non-restrictive VSD
  - No separate outflow portion (infundibulum) of right ventricle
  - Right-sided aortic arch with mirror-image branching (30-40%)
  - Embryology
    - Lack of separation of primitive bulbus cordis into aorta and main PA
    - Associated persistence of primitive aortic arches
  - Pathophysiology: Congestive heart failure versus cyanosis (degree of cyanosis is determined by balance between pulmonary and systemic vascular resistance)
    - Marked increase in pulmonary blood flow in early neonatal period, due to drop in pulmonary vascular resistance → slight improvement in cyanosis but worsening congestive heart failure
    - Development of pulmonary vascular obstructive disease leads to improvement in congestive heart failure but worsening in cyanosis
- Genetics
  - Strong association with deletion on the long arm of chromosome 22 (22q11 syndrome)
  - CATCH-22: Conofacial anomaly, absent thymus, hypocalcemia, heart defect
  - Velocardiofacial (Shprintzen) syndrome

TRUNCUS ARTERIOSUS

- Theory: Abnormal migration of neural crest tissue that interferes with development of cardiac tube
- Epidemiology: 2% of congenital cardiac anomalies
- Associated abnormalities
  - Absent thymus and parathyroid glands
  - Persistence of primitive aortic arches

Gross Pathologic & Surgical Features
- Many variations exist, involving interruption of the aortic arch (11-14%), absence of a branch PA (hemitruncus) and patent ductus arteriosus
- Position of common trunk with respect to VSD
  - Predominantly positioned over right ventricle (42%)
  - Predominantly positioned over left ventricle (16%)
  - Equally shared (42%)

Staging, Grading or Classification Criteria
- Classification of Collett and Edwards
  - Type 1: Separation of common trunk into ascending aorta and main PA
  - Type 2: Common take-off of branch PAs from trunk, with no main PA
  - Type 3: Both branch PAs originate separately from posterolateral aspect of ascending aorta
  - Type 4: "Pseudotruncus", pulmonary arterial supply from major aortopulmonary collateral arteries (MAPCAs), arising from descending aorta; controversial entity, misnomer for pulmonary atresia with VSD and MAPCAs
- Classification of Van Praagh
  - Type A1: Same as Collett and Edwards type 1
  - Type A2: Collet and Edwards types 2 and 3 combined
  - Type A3: Unilateral pulmonary artery with collateral supply to contralateral lung
  - Type A4: Truncus with interrupted aortic arch

CLINICAL ISSUES

Presentation
- Most common signs/symptoms
  - Progressive congestive heart failure with drop in pulmonary vascular resistance in young infant
  - Increasing cyanosis due to shunt reversal with development of pulmonary hypertension
- Other signs/symptoms
  - T-cell immunodeficiency (thymic agenesis - DiGeorge syndrome)
  - Neonatal tetany (absent parathyroid glands)

Natural History & Prognosis
- Untreated: 65% 6 month and 75% 1 year mortality
- Intractable congestive heart failure
  - Marked increase in pulmonary flow after drop in pulmonary vascular resistance
  - Aggravated by presence of truncal valve regurgitation (in 50% of cases)
- Eventual shunt reversal with progressive cyanosis and sudden death
  - Pulmonary vascular obstructive disease with Eisenmenger physiology can develop as early as 6 months of age
- Post-operative course determined by function of PA conduit and morbidity of conduit replacement

Treatment
- Palliative: Banding of main PA
  - Initial palliation with PA banding is often unsatisfactory, with early development of pulmonary vascular disease → pulmonary hypertension
  - Early complete repair (at 2-6 weeks of life) is favored by most surgeons
- Surgical repair, with placement of conduit between right ventricle and PA, and closure of VSD
  - Conduit revisions are frequently necessary throughout patient's life time
    - Patient outgrows fixed conduit size
    - Calcification
    - Stenosis, neointimal hyperplasia
    - Anastomotic pseudoaneurysm
    - Conduit valve dysfunction (regurgitation)
  - Truncal valve dysfunction (regurgitation) is common → need for valvuloplasty, prosthesis

SELECTED REFERENCES

1. Muhler MR et al: Truncus arteriosus communis in a midtrimester fetus: comparison of prenatal ultrasound and MRI with postmortem MRI and autopsy. Eur Radiol. 14(11):2120-4, 2004
2. Razavi R et al: Diagnosis of hemi-truncus arteriosis by three-dimensional magnetic resonance angiography. Circulation. 109(3):E15-6, 2004
3. Mavroudis C, Backer CL: Truncus arteriosus. In: Mavroudis C, Backer CL ed. Pediatric cardiac surgery. 3rd ed. Philadelphia, Mosby. 339-52, 2003
4. Lim C et al: Truncus arteriosus with coarctation of persistent fifth aortic arch. Ann Thorac Surg. 74(5):1702-4, 2002
5. Murashita T et al: Giant pseudoaneurysm of the right ventricular outflow tract after repair of truncus arteriosus: evaluation by MR imaging and surgical approach. Eur J Cardiothorac Surg. 22(5):849-51, 2002
6. Taylor JFN: Persistent truncus arteriosus. In: Moller JH, Hoffman JIE ed. Pediatric cardiovascular medicine. 1st ed. Philadelphia, Churchill Livingstone. 499-510, 2000
7. Rajasinghe HA et al: Long-term follow-up of truncus arteriosus repaired in infancy: a twenty-year experience. J Thorac Cardiovasc Surg 113:869-78, 1997
8. Donnelly LF et al: MR imaging of conotruncal abnormalities. AJR Am J Roentgenol. 166(4):925-8, 1996
9. Levine JC et al: Anastomotic pseudoaneurysm of the ventricle after homograft placement in children. Ann Thorac Surg. 59(1):60-6, 1995
10. Engle MA et al: Endocarditis with aneurysm involving an aortic homograft used to correct a truncus arteriosus: medical-surgical salvage. Br Heart J. 67(5):409-11, 1992
11. Chrispin A et al: Echo planar imaging of normal and abnormal connections of the heart and great arteries. Pediatr Radiol. 16(4):289-92, 1986
12. Chrispin A et al: Transectional echo planar imaging of the heart in cyanotic congenital heart disease. Pediatr Radiol. 16(4):293-7, 1986

TRUNCUS ARTERIOSUS

IMAGE GALLERY

Typical

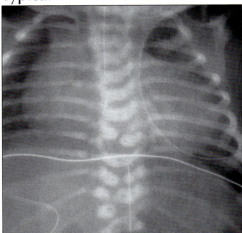
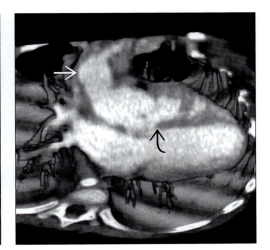

(Left) Anteroposterior radiograph shows cardiomegaly and multiple vertebral anomalies in cyanotic infant diagnosed with truncus on echocardiography. *(Right)* Coronal CTA shows large truncus overriding high ventricular septal defect (curved arrow). Note right aortic arch (arrow).

Typical

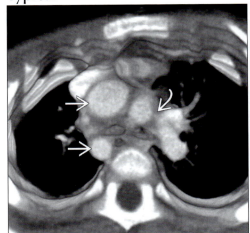
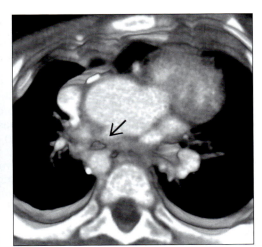

(Left) Axial CTA shows right aortic arch (arrows) and prominent left branch pulmonary artery, which was constricted in its mid-portion (curved arrow) by a surgically placed pulmonary artery band. *(Right)* Axial CTA shows small right pulmonary artery, originating from posterior aspect of large common trunk (arrow).

Typical

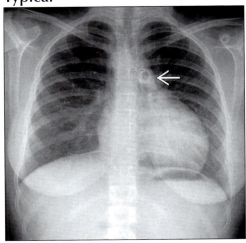
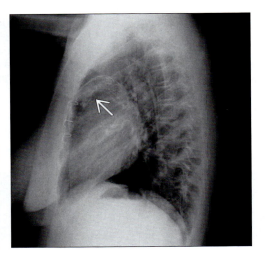

(Left) Anteroposterior radiograph shows stents in stenosed pulmonary artery homograft (arrow), which was placed in infancy as part of complete repair for truncus arteriosus. *(Right)* Lateral radiograph confirms stents in pulmonary artery homograft (arrow). This graft eventually had to be exchanged for a valved conduit, and aortic valve replacement was also required (see post-op film on first page of this dx).

TOTAL ANOMALOUS PULMONARY VENOUS RETURN

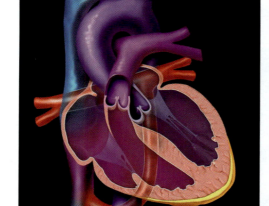

Graphic shows infradiaphragmatic TAPVR (type III) to inferior vena cava, constituting obligatory extracardiac left to right shunt. Mixed blood flows to left atrium through patent foramen ovale.

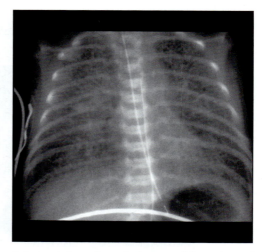

Anteroposterior radiograph shows small heart size and severe interstitial pulmonary edema in infant with obstructed infradiaphragmatic TAPVR (type III).

TERMINOLOGY

Abbreviations and Synonyms
- TAPVR = total anomalous pulmonary venous return (or "drainage")
  - Refers to hemodynamics: Where does pulmonary venous (PV) flow return (drain) to? (= right atrium)
- Total anomalous pulmonary venous connection
  - Refers to anatomy: Where do PVs connect to?

Definitions
- Failure of connection between PVs and left atrium
- Category: Cyanotic; heart size and pulmonary vascularity depend on type
- Hemodynamics
  - All pulmonary venous return goes to right heart (extracardiac left to right shunt)
  - Intracardiac right-to-left shunt through patent foramen ovale (PFO)
  - All types are admixture lesions
- Three types
  - Supracardiac TAPVR (type I, 40-50%): "Vertical" common pulmonary vein joins left innominate vein
  - Cardiac TAPVR (type II, 20-30%): Common pulmonary vein joins coronary sinus
  - Infracardiac TAPVR (type III, 10-30%): Common pulmonary vein joins portal vein, ductus venosus or inferior vena cava

IMAGING FINDINGS

General Features
- Best diagnostic clue: No PVs connecting to left atrium

Radiographic Findings
- Radiography
  - Cardiomegaly (types I, II), small heart (type III)
  - Shunt vascularity (types I, II), pulmonary edema (type III)
  - Wide mediastinum (type I, "snowman heart"), narrow mediastinum (types II, III; thymic atrophy)
  - Left vertical vein often visible in type I
  - Classic plain film appearance
    - Type I: "Snowman" heart
    - Type II: Indistinguishable from atrial septal defect (ASD)
    - Type III: Small heart, reticular pattern in the lungs: Edema

CT Findings
- 3D CT angiography: For post-operative evaluation of PV caliber and anastomoses
- Thickened interlobular septa, peribronchial cuffing and ground-glass opacities suggest anastomotic PV stenosis

DDx: Severe Cyanosis, Heart Failure In Newborn

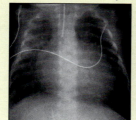

Transposition

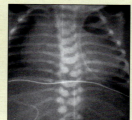

Truncus Arteriosus

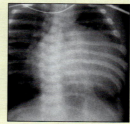

Hypoplastic L Heart

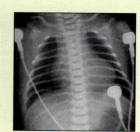

Pulmonary Atresia

TOTAL ANOMALOUS PULMONARY VENOUS RETURN

Key Facts

Terminology
- Failure of connection between PVs and left atrium
- Category: Cyanotic; heart size and pulmonary vascularity depend on type
- All pulmonary venous return goes to right heart (extracardiac left to right shunt)
- Intracardiac right-to-left shunt through patent foramen ovale (PFO)
- All types are admixture lesions

Imaging Findings
- Type I: "Snowman" heart
- Type II: Indistinguishable from atrial septal defect (ASD)
- Type III: Small heart, reticular pattern in the lungs: Edema

Pathology
- Lack of normal incorporation of primitive common PV into posterior wall of left atrium
- All types have PFO to allow for obligatory right-to-left flow, leading to varying degrees of cyanosis (less severe in types I, II: Pulmonary hypercirculation)
- Non-obstructive TAPVR (types I, II): ASD physiology, pulmonary plethora, congestive heart failure
- Obstructive TAPVR (type III): Common PV is obstructed by diaphragmatic hiatus → pulmonary venous congestion and edema
- Occasionally associated with other complex cyanotic heart disease, asplenia syndrome (type III), atrioventricular canal

MR Findings
- T1WI: Cardiac-gated black blood imaging: Anomalous connections best seen in axial plane
- T2* GRE: Steady-state free precession cine MRI for functional assessment, flow jets, regurgitation
- MRA
  - Velocity-encoded phase contrast MRA: For detection of PV anastomotic stenosis (flow velocities > 100 cm/sec are diagnostic)
  - Dynamic time-resolved Gadolinium-enhanced 3D MRA: for detailed depiction of PV anatomy

Echocardiographic Findings
- Echocardiogram
  - Lack of connection of PVs to left atrium
  - Right-sided chamber enlargement in types I, II
  - Patent foramen ovale (PFO)
  - Associated cardiac and abdominal situs abnormalities
  - Limited assessment for post-operative anastomotic PV obstruction

Angiographic Findings
- Conventional
  - Seldom required for primary diagnosis
  - Balloon atrial septostomy when flow across ASD is restricted
  - After repair: For diagnosis and treatment of anastomotic PV stenosis

Imaging Recommendations
- Protocol advice
  - Primary diagnosis with echocardiography
  - CT, MRI for post-operative PV anastomotic stenosis

DIFFERENTIAL DIAGNOSIS

Cor triatriatum
- Pulmonary venous connection occurred but remains stenotic, with lack of incorporation of common PV into left atrial wall

Hypoplastic left heart syndrome
- PVs insert normally into left atrium, left-to-right shunting through PFO

Persistent fetal circulation syndrome, primary pulmonary hypertension
- Associated with severe surfactant deficiency disease, meconium aspiration

PATHOLOGY

General Features
- General path comments
  - All pulmonary venous drainage eventually flows into right atrium
  - Embryology
    - Lack of normal incorporation of primitive common PV into posterior wall of left atrium
    - Persistence and enlargement of embryological pathways for pulmonary venous return via umbilicovitelline and cardinal veins
  - Pathophysiology
    - All types have PFO to allow for obligatory right-to-left flow, leading to varying degrees of cyanosis (less severe in types I, II: Pulmonary hypercirculation)
    - Non-obstructive TAPVR (types I, II): ASD physiology, pulmonary plethora, congestive heart failure
    - Obstructive TAPVR (type III): Common PV is obstructed by diaphragmatic hiatus → pulmonary venous congestion and edema
    - Left-sided cardiac chambers may be underdeveloped, especially in TAPVR type III, due to prenatal decrease in systemic blood flow
- Genetics
  - No specific genetic defect found
  - Occasionally associated with other complex cyanotic heart disease, asplenia syndrome (type III), atrioventricular canal
- Epidemiology

TOTAL ANOMALOUS PULMONARY VENOUS RETURN

- 1-3% of congenital heart disease
- More frequent in neonatal period
• Associated abnormalities
  - Single ventricle, atrioventricular septal defect, truncus arteriosus, tetralogy of Fallot, anomalous systemic venous connection
  - Asplenia (or rarely: Polysplenia) syndrome, biliary atresia

Gross Pathologic & Surgical Features

• Common PV is anastomosed via window with left atrium, and all other abnormal pulmonary venous connections are ligated

CLINICAL ISSUES

Presentation

• Most common signs/symptoms
  - Types I, II: Congestive heart failure
  - Type III: Severe cyanosis at birth
  - Patent ductus arteriosus: Persistent fetal circulation

Natural History & Prognosis

• No patients survive without surgical treatment
• Natural history is highly variable
  - Type I, II: Initially asymptomatic, with gradual development of congestive heart failure, when pulmonary vascular resistance drops (ASD physiology)
  - Type III, obstructive forms: Death within a month
• After surgical repair: Prognosis is determined by associated cardiac anomalies and development of PV anastomotic stenosis

Treatment

• Prostaglandin E1 to improve systemic perfusion in pulmonary hypertension
• Pre-operative extracorporeal membrane oxygenation (ECMO) is occasionally necessary to improve oxygenation and systemic perfusion
• Early surgical anastomosis of pulmonary venous confluence to left atrium
  - Anastomotic PV stenosis may occur in up to 18% of TAPVR repairs
  - Long-standing PV stenosis leads to irreversible pulmonary hypertension (arterial pulmonary vascular disease)
  - Reoperation is performed using sutureless technique, with pericardial patch augmentation of anastomotic stenoses

SELECTED REFERENCES

1. Roman KS et al: How is pulmonary arterial blood flow affected by pulmonary venous obstruction in children? A phase-contrast magnetic resonance study. Pediatr Radiol. 2005
2. Damry N et al: Non-invasive diagnosis of infracardiac total anomalous pulmonary venous return. JBR-BTR. 87(2):97, 2004
3. Dieter RS et al: Transseptal stent treatment of anastomotic stricture after repair of partial anomalous pulmonary venous return. J Endovasc Ther. 10(4):838-42, 2003
4. Kirshbom PM et al: Total anomalous pulmonary venous connection. In: Mavroudis C. Backer CL ed. Pediatric cardiac surgery. 3rd ed. Philadelphia, Mosby. 612-24, 2003
5. Valsangiacomo ER et al: Contrast-enhanced MR angiography of pulmonary venous abnormalities in children. Pediatr Radiol. 33(2):92-8, 2003
6. Valsangiacomo ER et al: Phase-contrast MR assessment of pulmonary venous blood flow in children with surgically repaired pulmonary veins. Pediatr Radiol. 33(9):607-13, 2003
7. Sridhar PG et al: Total anomalous pulmonary venous connection: helical computed tomography as an alternative to angiography. Indian Heart J. 55(6):624-7, 2003
8. Wang ZJ et al: Cardiovascular shunts: MR imaging evaluation. Radiographics. 23 Spec No:S181-94, 2003
9. Chen SJ et al: Validation of pulmonary venous obstruction by electron beam tomography in children with congenital heart disease. Ann Thor Surg 71:1690-2, 2001
10. Videlefsky N et al: Magnetic resonance phase-shift velocity mapping in pediatric patients with pulmonary venous obstruction. Am J Cardiol 87:589-93, 2001
11. Eimbeck F et al: Total anomalous pulmonary venous connection. In: Moller JH, Hoffman JIE ed. Pediatric cardiovascular medicine. 1st ed. Philadelphia, Churchill Livingstone. 409-20, 2000
12. Hong YK et al: Efficacy of MRI in complicated congenital heart disease with visceral heterotaxy syndrome. J Comput Assist Tomogr. 24(5):671-82, 2000
13. Kim TH et al: Helical CT angiography and three-dimensional reconstruction of total anomalous pulmonary venous connections in neonates and infants. AJR Am J Roentgenol. 175(5):1381-6, 2000
14. Masui T et al: Gadolinium-enhanced MR angiography in the evaluation of congenital cardiovascular disease pre- and postoperative states in infants and children. J Magn Reson Imaging. 12(6):1034-42, 2000
15. Choe YH et al: MRI of total anomalous pulmonary venous connections. J Comput Assist Tomogr. 18(2):243-9, 1994
16. Kim WS et al: Radiological evaluation of pulmonary vein obstruction including two examinations by magnetic resonance imaging. Pediatr Radiol. 23(1):6-11, 1993
17. Wang JK et al: Delineation of obstruction in total anomalous pulmonary venous connection utilizing magnetic resonance imaging. Am Heart J. 124(3):807-9, 1992
18. Livolsi A et al: MR diagnosis of subdiaphragmatic anomalous pulmonary venous drainage in a newborn. J Comput Assist Tomogr. 15(6):1051-3, 1991
19. Masui T et al: Abnormalities of the pulmonary veins: evaluation with MR imaging and comparison with cardiac angiography and echocardiography. Radiology. 181(3):645-9, 1991
20. Ross RD et al: Magnetic resonance imaging for diagnosis of pulmonary vein stenosis after "correction" of total anomalous pulmonary venous connection. Am J Cardiol. 60(14):1199-201, 1987

TOTAL ANOMALOUS PULMONARY VENOUS RETURN

IMAGE GALLERY

Typical

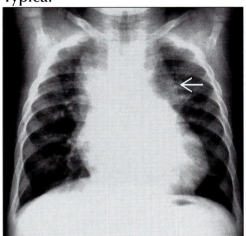
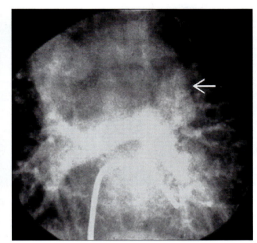

(Left) Anteroposterior radiograph shows "snowman" heart of TAPVR type I, with wide mediastinum and vertical vein *(arrow)*. *(Right)* Angiography shows flow from pulmonary venous confluence via vertical vein *(arrow)* into distended left brachiocephalic vein.

Variant

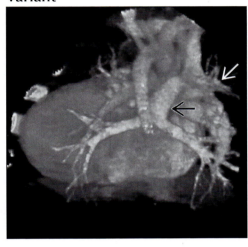
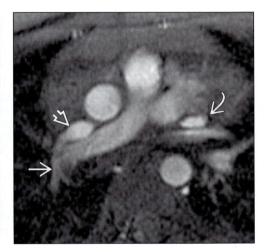

(Left) CTA, posterior view of volume rendition, shows anomalous connection of common pulmonary vein *(black arrow)* to posterior aspect of superior vena cava (SVC). Right upper pulmonary vein *(white arrow)* has separate insertion into SVC. *(Right)* Axial MR cine shows partial anomalous pulmonary venous drainage of right upper lobe vein *(arrow)* into right superior vena cava (SVC, *open arrow*). Note persistent left SVC *(curved arrow)*.

Other

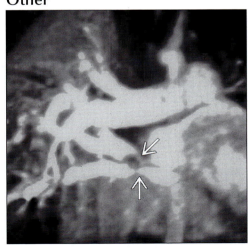
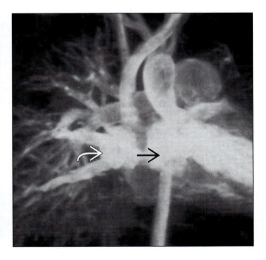

(Left) Coronal MRA shows anastomotic stenoses *(arrows)* of right-sided pulmonary veins in patient following TAPVR repair. *(Right)* Coronal MRA shows pericardial patch *(curved arrow)* to left atrium *(arrow)* conduit. Note asymmetric pulmonary vascular congestion in right lung.

HYPOPLASTIC LEFT HEART SYNDROME

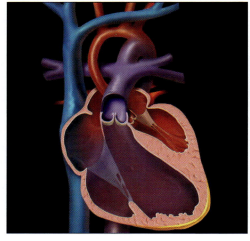

Graphic shows hypoplasia of LA, LV, aortic valve and ascending aorta. Systemic flow depends on patency of ductus arteriosus.

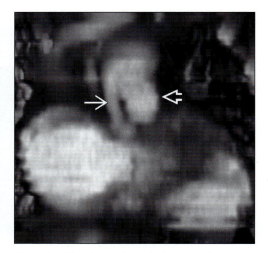

Coronal CTA shows hypoplastic ascending aorta (arrow), large main pulmonary artery (open arrow), which served as the main cardiac output conduit. Note dilatation of right atrium.

TERMINOLOGY

Abbreviations and Synonyms
- Hypoplastic left heart syndrome (HLHS)
- Aortic atresia

Definitions
- Hypoplasia/atresia of the ascending aorta, aortic valve, left ventricle (LV) and mitral valve
  - Secondary findings: Patent ductus arteriosus (PDA), juxtaductal coarctation
- Most severe congenital heart lesion presenting in neonatal period with congestive heart failure, cardiogenic shock and cyanosis
- Category: Cyanotic, cardiomegaly, increased pulmonary vascularity
- Hemodynamics
  - Severe obstruction to flow to systemic circulation = ductus-dependent
  - Retrograde flow in hypoplastic aortic arch and ascending aorta for cranial and coronary perfusion
  - Volume overload in pulmonary circulation
  - Left-to-right shunting through patent foramen ovale (PFO)
  - Flow admixture in right atrium → severe cyanosis

IMAGING FINDINGS

General Features
- Best diagnostic clue: Hypoplasia of ascending aorta, LV

Radiographic Findings
- Radiography
  - Cardiomegaly
  - Pulmonary venous congestion with interstitial fluid
  - Hyperinflation
  - Narrow mediastinum due to thymic atrophy

CT Findings
- CTA
  - Patency of aortopulmonary (Blalock-Taussig) and cavopulmonary (Glenn) shunts
  - Seroma associated with Blalock-Taussig shunt
  - Airway compression by dilated neo-aortic arch following Norwood repair

MR Findings
- T2* GRE
  - Short-axis steady-state free precession (SSFP) cine MRI for functional assessment of univentricular heart, to determine suitability for Fontan operation
  - SSFP cine MRI for ventricular volume measurements in marginally hypoplastic left heart, to determine feasibility of bi-ventricular repair

DDx: Left Heart Obstructive Lesions

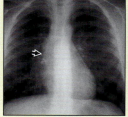

Valvular Aortic Stenosis

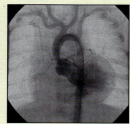

Willam Syndrome

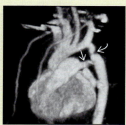

Preductal Coarctation

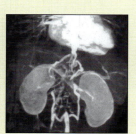

Mid Aortic Syndrome

HYPOPLASTIC LEFT HEART SYNDROME

Key Facts

Terminology
- Hypoplasia/atresia of the ascending aorta, aortic valve, left ventricle (LV) and mitral valve
- Most severe congenital heart lesion presenting in neonatal period with congestive heart failure, cardiogenic shock and cyanosis
- Category: Cyanotic, cardiomegaly, increased pulmonary vascularity
- Severe obstruction to flow to systemic circulation = ductus-dependent
- Retrograde flow in hypoplastic aortic arch and ascending aorta for cranial and coronary perfusion
- Flow admixture in right atrium → severe cyanosis

Imaging Findings
- Primary diagnosis made with echocardiography in majority of cases
- Post-operative: Functional MRI and interventional catheterizations for residua/sequelae of Fontan operation

Clinical Issues
- Medical: Prostaglandin E1 to keep PDA open
- Norwood: Atrial septectomy, construction of neo-aorta from pulmonary artery, Blalock-Taussig shunt for pulmonary perfusion (3 weeks)
- Conversion to hemi-Fontan (Glenn shunt between superior vena cava and right PA, 4-6 months)
- Fontan: Fenestrated venous conduit through right atrium of inferior caval flow to right PA (1.5-2 years)
- In some centers: Cardiac transplantation

- MRA: Velocity-encoded phase contrast (PC-) MRA for measurements of flow through aortic isthmus, PDA and PFO: Can predict response to intra-operative test closure of ASD and PDA to determine feasibility of bi-ventricular repair

Echocardiographic Findings
- Echocardiogram
  - HLHS increasingly diagnosed prenatally
    - Retrograde flow in diminutive ascending aorta
    - LV growth arrest only becomes manifest between 18-22 weeks of gestation
  - Postnatal diagnosis with echo sufficient for treatment planning
    - Diminutive ascending aorta < 5 mm
    - Small, thick-walled LV
    - Mitral valve size is expressed as a Z-score: Important parameter to decide whether a bi-ventricular repair is possible in marginally hypoplastic LVs
    - Dilatation of right-sided cardiac chambers and pulmonary artery (PA)
    - Size and location of ductus arteriosus
    - Patency of foramen ovale or presence of atrial septal defect
    - Abnormal ventricular wall motion (ischemic damage, fibroelastosis)
- Color Doppler
  - Hemodynamics of aortic root
  - Left-to-right shunting through PFO
  - Tricuspid regurgitation

Angiographic Findings
- Conventional
  - Cardiac catheterization with angiography
    - Can be done via umbilical artery catheter
    - Retrograde flow in hypoplastic ascending aorta
    - Filling of pulmonary arteries via ductus arteriosus

Other Modality Findings
- CTA, MRI: Occasionally performed after staged Norwood or Stanzel procedures
  - Residual stenosis of neo-aortic arch, coarctation
  - Functional assessment of marginally hypoplastic left heart with cine MRI and velocity-encoded phase contrast MRA, prior to Fontan operation

Imaging Recommendations
- Primary diagnosis made with echocardiography in majority of cases
- Post-operative: Functional MRI and interventional catheterizations for residua/sequelae of Fontan operation

DIFFERENTIAL DIAGNOSIS

Critical aortic stenosis, infantile coarctation, interrupted aortic arch
- Pressure overload of normally-developed left ventricle

Cranial (vein of Galen) or hepatic arteriovenous malformation
- Structurally normal heart with volume overload of all chambers

Cardiomyopathy, endocardial fibroelastosis
- Globally enlarged, structurally normal heart, myocardial dysfunction

Coronary arteriovenous fistula
- Left coronary originates from PA, myocardial infarction

Severe arrhythmias: Paroxysmal supraventricular tachycardia
- Characteristic electrocardiogram

PATHOLOGY

General Features
- General path comments
  - Underdevelopment of left-sided cardiac structures
    - Hypoplasia or atresia of aortic and mitral valves
    - Hypoplasia of LV and ascending aorta

HYPOPLASTIC LEFT HEART SYNDROME

- Compatible with normal fetal hemodynamics → no fetal compromise
- Embryology
  - Abnormal partitioning of primitive conotruncus into left and right ventricular outflow tracts → hypoplasia/atresia of aortic valve
  - Diminished prenatal antegrade flow through aorta → underdevelopment of LV and ascending aorta
- Pathophysiology
  - Severe obstruction to outflow of LV, which is diminutive
  - Pulmonary venous flow shunts through PFO into right atrium
  - Dilated right-sided cardiac chambers and PA
  - Systemic perfusion via PDA
- Genetics
  - No clear genetic defect demonstrated in majority
  - Not commonly associated with extracardiac malformations
- Epidemiology
  - 1-3 per 10,000 live births, M:F = 2:1
  - Fourth most common congenital heart lesion presenting under 1 year (7-9%)

Gross Pathologic & Surgical Features
- Severe hypoplasia of left-sided cardiac chambers and ascending aorta
- Large main pulmonary artery, ductus arteriosus
- Localized aortic coarctation (80%)
- Endocardial fibro-elastosis in small, thick-walled left ventricle

CLINICAL ISSUES

Presentation
- Most common signs/symptoms
  - No circulatory symptoms immediately at birth but rapid deterioration
    - Congestive heart failure (volume overload pulmonary circulation)
    - Cardiogenic shock after closure of PDA
    - Cyanosis (flow admixture in right heart)
    - Hypoxia → pulmonary hypertension, persistent fetal circulation
- Other signs/symptoms
  - Poor systemic perfusion, metabolic acidosis
    - Acute tubular necrosis, renal failure
    - Necrotizing enterocolitis

Natural History & Prognosis
- Death within days/weeks when untreated
- Poor prognosis without treatment; has improved substantially in recent years
- Determined by complications, residua and sequelae of staged Norwood repair and Fontan operation (right ventricular dysfunction, venous hypertension)
- Significant tricuspid regurgitation after surgical palliation correlates with poor outcome

Treatment
- Medical: Prostaglandin E1 to keep PDA open
- Prenatal: US-guided balloon dilatation of aortic valve in mid/late fetal period is now possible in a few centers
  - Change in fetal hemodynamics may enhance prenatal growth of left-sided cardiac structures
- Rashkind balloon atrial septostomy (in case of flow restriction across PFO)
- Palliative repair
  - Norwood: Atrial septectomy, construction of neo-aorta from pulmonary artery, Blalock-Taussig shunt for pulmonary perfusion (3 weeks)
  - Damus-Kaye-Stanzel anastomosis: Variation of Norwood with side-to-side anastomosis between PA and hypoplastic ascending aorta
  - Conversion to hemi-Fontan (Glenn shunt between superior vena cava and right PA, 4-6 months)
  - Fontan: Fenestrated venous conduit through right atrium of inferior caval flow to right PA (1.5-2 years)
- Marginally hypoplastic LV: Bi-ventricular repair may be feasible
  - LV volume is commonly underestimated with echocardiography
  - Functional MRI (SSPE-cine: Ventricular volumes, mass and function; PC-MRA: Flow volumes) is more reliable
- In some centers: Cardiac transplantation

SELECTED REFERENCES
1. Oye RG et al. Hypoplastic left heart syndrome. In: Mavroudis C, Backer CL ed. Pediatric cardiac surgery. 3rd ed. Philadelphia, Mosby. 560-574, 2003
2. Cheatham JP: Intervention in the critically ill neonate and infant with hypoplastic left heart syndrome and intact atrial septum. J Interv Cardiol. 14(3):357-66, 2001
3. Herman TE et al: Special imaging casebook. Hypoplastic left heart, prostaglandin therapy gastric focal foveolar hyperplasia and brown-fat necrosis. J Perinatol. 21(4):263-5, 2001
4. Bardo DM et al: Hypoplastic left heart syndrome. Radiographics. 21(3):705-17, 2001
5. Moadel-Sernick RM et al: Lymphoscintigraphy demonstrating thoracic duct injury in an infant with hypoplastic left heart syndrome. Clin Nucl Med. 25(5):335-6, 2000
6. Rosenthal A et al: Hypoplastic left heart syndrome. In: Moller JH, Hoffman JIE ed. Pediatric cardiovascular medicine, 1st ed. Philadelphia, Churchill Livingstone. 594-605, 2000
7. Fellows KE et al: MR imaging and heart function in patients pre- and post-Fontan surgery. Acta Paediatr Suppl. 410:57-9, 1995
8. Fogel MA et al: A study in ventricular-ventricular interaction. Single right ventricles compared with systemic right ventricles in a dual-chamber circulation. Circulation. 92(2):219-30, 1995
9. Kondo C et al: Nuclear magnetic resonance imaging of the palliative operation for hypoplastic left heart syndrome. J Am Coll Cardiol. 18(3):817-23, 1991
10. Norwood WI et al: Hypoplastic left heart syndrome. Ann Thorac Surg 1991:688-95, 1991

HYPOPLASTIC LEFT HEART SYNDROME

IMAGE GALLERY

Typical

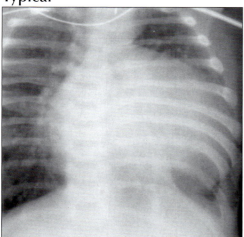
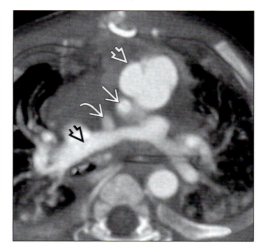

(Left) Anteroposterior radiograph shows right-sided cardiomegaly, pulmonary vascular congestion and narrow mediastinum due thymic atrophy. *(Right)* Axial CTA shows large main pulmonary artery (white open arrow), hypoplastic ascending aorta (arrow), and right-sided Blalock-Taussig (curved arrow) and cavopulmonary (Glenn, black open arrow) shunts.

Typical

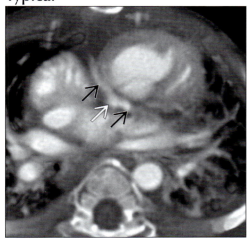
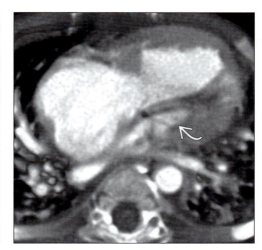

(Left) Axial CTA shows hypoplastic ascending aorta (white arrow) retrograde perfusion of the coronary arteries (black arrows). *(Right)* Axial CTA shows relative hypoplasia of left ventricle (curved arrow) and severe dilatation of right atrium and ventricle.

Variant

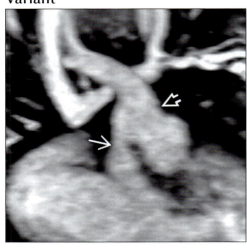
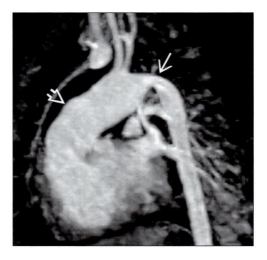

(Left) Coronal MRA shows Stanzel anastomosis between main pulmonary artery (open arrow) and hypoplastic ascending aorta (arrow). (Courtesy L. Sena, MD). *(Right)* Sagittal oblique MRA shows dilated main pulmonary artery (open arrow), serving as main cardiac outflow channel after Norwood repair. Note focal narrowing leading to obstruction in transverse aortic arch (arrow). (Courtesy L. Sena, MD).

LEFT CORONARY ARTERY ANOMALOUS ORIGIN

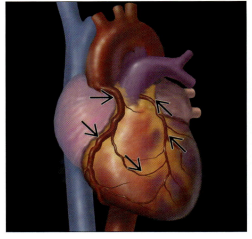

Graphic shows anomalous origin of left coronary artery from main pulmonary artery. Collateral flow develops from the right coronary artery which retrograde flows to pulmonary artery (arrows).

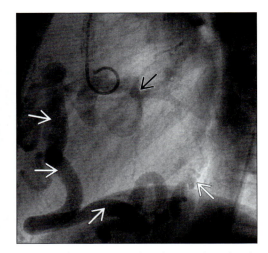

Lateral catheter angiography shows enlarged right coronary artery (white arrows), and retrograde filling of anomalous left coronary artery with flow into pulmonary artery (black arrow).

TERMINOLOGY

Abbreviations and Synonyms
- Bland-Garland-White syndrome
- Anomalous left coronary artery (ALCA)

Definitions
- Coronary artery origin anomaly which causes cardiac ischemia and leads to infarction, poor left ventricular function, and mitral valve regurgitation
  - Anomalous origin of left coronary artery from pulmonary artery is most common

IMAGING FINDINGS

General Features
- Best diagnostic clue
  - Chest radiograph, CT, MR that demonstrates poor left ventricular function, anomalous origin of a coronary artery, large tortuous collateral coronary vessels, and enlarged left atrium due to mitral regurgitation
  - Electrocardiogram demonstrating anterior lateral wall left ventricular infarct
  - Diagnosis usually made by cardiac echocardiography demonstrating anomalous coronary artery in child with poor left ventricular function
- Location
  - Right or left coronary artery origin anomaly which is usually isolated anomaly
    - Can be associated with other congenital heart lesions
    - Rarely associated with other syndromes or anomalies

Radiographic Findings
- Radiography: Marked left ventricular, left atrial enlargement with or without pulmonary edema

CT Findings
- CTA
  - Multi-detector CT angiography can demonstrate coronary artery anatomy
    - Volume rendered 3D depiction from contrast-enhanced imaging
    - Gating is difficult in infants partially related to fast heart rates

MR Findings
- MRA
  - MR cine gradient echo images can define anatomy and function and may be done for follow-up studies
    - Large coronary artery is clue to anomaly and significant collateral vessels are apparent

DDx: Causes Of Decreased Left Ventricular Function In Children

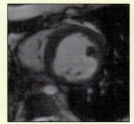
Cardiomyopathy

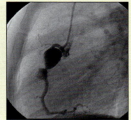
Kawasaki Disease

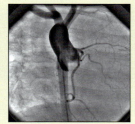
Single Coronary

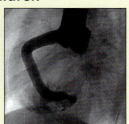
Coronary Fistula

LEFT CORONARY ARTERY ANOMALOUS ORIGIN

Key Facts

Terminology
- Coronary artery origin anomaly which causes cardiac ischemia and leads to infarction, poor left ventricular function, and mitral valve regurgitation
- Anomalous origin of left coronary artery from pulmonary artery is most common

Imaging Findings
- Chest radiograph, CT, MR that demonstrates poor left ventricular function, anomalous origin of a coronary artery, large tortuous collateral coronary vessels, and enlarged left atrium due to mitral regurgitation
- Electrocardiogram demonstrating anterior lateral wall left ventricular infarct
- Diagnosis usually made by cardiac echocardiography demonstrating anomalous coronary artery in child with poor left ventricular function

Top Differential Diagnoses
- Dilated cardiomyopathy
- Kawasaki disease
- Coronary artery fistula
- Single coronary artery origin

Clinical Issues
- 87% present in infancy with nonspecific symptoms of irritability, wheezing, failure to thrive
- Surgical therapy: Prognosis relates to left ventricular function
- Direct transfer of the left coronary artery to the aorta

Diagnostic Checklist
- This is a rare anomaly and an unusual cause of poor left ventricular function yet readily diagnosed by imaging

---

- Ventricular function quantitatively assessed on four chamber view and qualitatively assessed on stack of short axis views
  - Assess wall motion, thickness of ventricular wall, chamber size and degree of wall thickening
  - End diastolic volume is increased, abnormal shortening fraction is common

Echocardiographic Findings
- Echocardiogram
  - Abnormal origin of the coronary artery is recognized by color flow assessment demonstrating multiple collateral vessels, retrograde flow from left coronary artery to the pulmonary artery
  - Echocardiography demonstrates decreased left ventricular function, regional left wall functional abnormalities which typically represents an anterolateral infarct, mitral regurgitation

Angiographic Findings
- Conventional
  - Cardiac catheterization done only when echo or other imaging is not diagnostic
    - Information obtained on anatomy, pressures, and valve insufficiency
  - Selective injection: Right coronary angiography demonstrates
    - Enlarged right coronary artery, tortuous collateral vessels, retrograde filling of left coronary artery
    - Diminished left ventricular wall flow
  - Selective injections help define the anatomy and other anomalies
    - Coronary artery fistulas demonstrate enlargement of the coronary arteries and the exact site of entry into the atrium or ventricle

Other Modality Findings
- Myocardial perfusion with thallium and technetium permits evaluation of perfusion
- Exercise testing with perfusion techniques

Imaging Recommendations
- Best imaging tool

- Electrocardiograms in infants demonstrate an infarct pattern with loss of normal R-wave progression, abnormal Q-waves, and S-T segment depression
- Diagnosis is usually made at bedside by echocardiogram demonstrating decreased left ventricular function, anomalous origin of the coronary artery, collateral vessels

DIFFERENTIAL DIAGNOSIS

Dilated cardiomyopathy
- Most common cause of poor left ventricular function in an infant
- Similar clinical presentation with irritability, failure to thrive, wheezing

Kawasaki disease
- Multisystem disease that may develop coronary artery aneurysms
- Myocarditis is common and aneurysms occur in < 2% of children
- May develop stenosis associated with aneurysm and have clot with infarction

Coronary artery fistula
- May produce cardiac ischemia if there is a "steal" phenomena away from the ventricular wall

Single coronary artery origin
- 40% are associated with other anomalies including transposition, tetralogy
- Usually asymptomatic but occasional sudden deaths

PATHOLOGY

General Features
- General path comments
  - Embryology
    - Abnormalities in signaling pathways or alterations in local factors that direct coronary development
- Associated abnormalities

LEFT CORONARY ARTERY ANOMALOUS ORIGIN

- Coronary artery anomalies can be isolated anomalies or associated with other diseases
  - Important to identify for surgical purposes and planning
- Tetralogy of Fallot
  - 40% have an abnormally long, large conus artery
  - 5% have a left anterior descending coronary arising from the right coronary artery
- Transposition of the great arteries has coronary anomalies due to malposition of aorta
  - Left circumflex arises from the right coronary in 20%

Microscopic Features
- Signs of left ventricular ischemia, varying degrees of reparative changes in children who die or need transplant
  - Anterolateral papillary muscle is atrophic and scarred
  - Thinning and scarring of the anterolateral left ventricular wall and apex due to infarction

CLINICAL ISSUES

Presentation
- Most common signs/symptoms
  - Nonspecific symptoms with irritability, fussiness, wheezing, or failure to thrive
  - 87% present in infancy with nonspecific symptoms of irritability, wheezing, failure to thrive
- Other signs/symptoms: Diaphoresis, gray or poor color in association with symptoms
- Older child or adolescent
  - Usually asymptomatic until sudden catastrophic event with syncope, dysrhythmic event, occasional death
  - Chest pain or syncope associated with exercise suggesting coronary artery or heart disease

Demographics
- Age: 85-90% in infancy
- Gender: M:F ratio is similar

Natural History & Prognosis
- Fetal life: No harmful effects with normal myocardial perfusion
- Stage 1: Newborn with high pulmonary vascular resistance
  - Flow from main pulmonary artery into the anomalous coronary artery
  - No ischemia or symptoms as myocardium is perfused
- Stage 2: Pulmonary vascular resistance decreases
  - Drop in pulmonary artery pressure is inadequate to provide forward flow to the anomalous coronary artery
  - Low pulmonary artery pressure cannot perfuse adequately the left ventricular myocardium
  - Collateral vessels from the normal right coronary artery develop and the right coronary enlarges
  - Flow from right coronary artery system meets the high resistance of left ventricular myocardial bed, and preferential flow occurs into the low resistance pulmonary artery
  - Retrograde flow of fully oxygenated blood into the pulmonary artery creates a small left-to-right shunt
- Later stages: Cardiac symptoms or ischemia occurs
  - Myocardial steal occurs with increase in collateral vessels
  - Ischemia and infarct occur in anterolateral distribution, global ventricular dilation and dysfunction
  - Mitral valve regurgitation is common secondary to papillary muscle infarction

Treatment
- Medical therapy
  - Initial therapy stabilized the patient
    - Mechanical ventilation with oxygen to prevent hypoxia, treatment of shock and cardiac failure
    - Sedation to minimize activity and demands on failing myocardium
- Surgical therapy: Prognosis relates to left ventricular function
  - Direct transfer of the left coronary artery to the aorta
    - Button of tissue around the ostium of the coronary artery is transferred posteriorly to the aortic root
  - Bypass grafting
    - Proximal anomalous coronary is ligated, and bypass grafting used to reestablish perfusion
  - Surgical mortality is 5-10% and usually related to poor left ventricular function
    - Complications include bleeding, cardiac arrest, failure, stroke

DIAGNOSTIC CHECKLIST

Consider
- This is a rare anomaly and an unusual cause of poor left ventricular function yet readily diagnosed by imaging

SELECTED REFERENCES

1. Deibler AR et al: Imaging of congenital coronary anomalies with multislice computed tomography. Mayo Clin Proc. 79(8):1017-23, 2004
2. Frommelt PC et al: Congenital coronary artery anomalies. Pediatr Clin North Am. 51(5):1273-88, 2004
3. Schoenhagen P et al: Noninvasive imaging of coronary arteries: current and future role of multi-detector row CT. Radiology. 232(1):7-17, 2004
4. Matherne, GP et al: Congenital Abnormalities of the Coronary Vessels and the Aortic Root. In: Allen HD and Gutgesell HP (eds). Heart Disease in Infants and Children, and Adolescents. Lippincott Williams & Wilkins. Philadelphia. 675-688, 2001
5. Didier D et al: Detection and quantification of valvular heart disease with dynamic cardiac MR imaging. Radiographics. 20(5):1279-99; discussion 1299-301, 2000
6. Higgins CB: Cardiac imaging. Radiology. 217(1):4-10, 2000

LEFT CORONARY ARTERY ANOMALOUS ORIGIN

IMAGE GALLERY

Typical

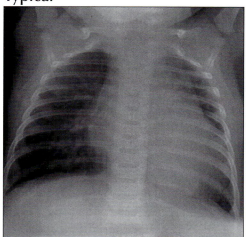
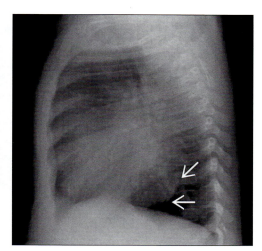

(Left) Anteroposterior radiograph shows a markedly enlarged transverse diameter with left ventricular enlargement secondary to infarct of left ventricle from an anomalous left coronary artery. *(Right)* Lateral radiograph shows an enlarged left ventricle (arrows) posterior to inferior vena cava in same infant who presented with irritability at four months of age. EKG showed infarct.

Other

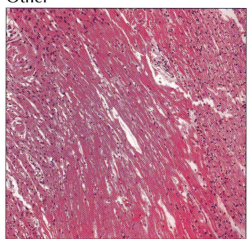
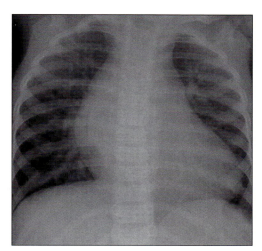

(Left) Micropathology, high power depicts ischemic necrosis with loss of nuclear material, increase in cellular debris from myocardial infarct secondary to anomalous origin of the coronary artery. *(Right)* Anteroposterior radiograph shows an enlarged heart with increase in pulmonary artery flow, secondary to left coronary artery fistula to the right atrium. Perfusion of myocardium may be bypassed.

Typical

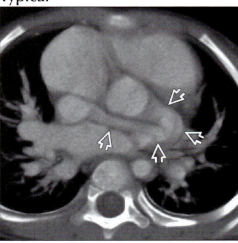
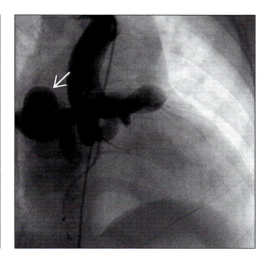

(Left) Axial CECT shows an example of left coronary artery to right atrial fistula. Marked enlargement of left coronary artery (arrows) can create a "steal" phenomenon and bypass myocardial perfusion. *(Right)* Anteroposterior catheter angiography shows a markedly enlarged left coronary artery with filling of the atrial appendage and right atrium (arrow) in three year old child.

MYOCARDITIS

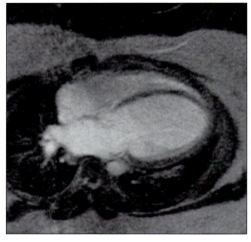

Four chamber view T2* GRE MR demonstrates an enlarged left ventricle. Ejection fraction compared to normal standards was calculated as 10% in this adolescent with myocarditis.

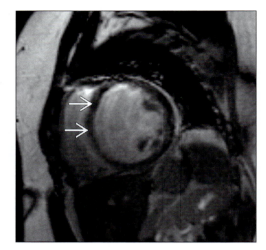

MR cine in the short axis plane shows increased left ventricle end diastolic volume with bowing of the septum (arrows). Multiple images in short axis are used to access functional imaging.

TERMINOLOGY

Definitions
- Process characterized by inflammatory infiltration of the myocardium with necrosis and/or degeneration of adjacent myocytes not typical of ischemic changes, which lead to myocardial dysfunction and heart failure
- Underlying etiology is not found in 50% of cases

IMAGING FINDINGS

General Features
- Best diagnostic clue
  - Echocardiography is gold standard in infants and children for assessing cardiac function and anatomy
  - Cardiac enlargement with left ventricular and left atrial enlargement, Kerly B lines, effusions
  - Endomyocardial biopsy may detect specific cause utilizing genetic markers, histologic and immunologic techniques
- Location: Cardiac muscle

Radiographic Findings
- Radiography
  - Cardiac enlargement with left ventricular and left atrial enlargement
  - Pleural effusions, R > L

CT Findings
- CTA: Occasionally done to access airway compression secondary to cardiac enlargement

MR Findings
- MR Cine
  - Ventricular function qualitatively assessed on four chamber view and quantitatively assessed on stack of short axis views
  - Assess wall motion, thickness of ventricular wall, chamber size and degree of wall thickening
  - End diastolic volume is increased, abnormal shortening fraction is common
  - Velocity encoded cine (VEC) MR
    - Valvular regurgitation can be quantified
- Gadolinium-enhanced MRI
  - Enhancement ratio calculated by dividing the enhancement of myocardium by the enhancement of skeletal muscle
  - Normal myocardial enhancement ratio < 2.5
  - Myocarditis enhancement ratio > 4.0

Echocardiographic Findings
- Echocardiogram

DDx: Systemic Diseases With Cardiac Involvement

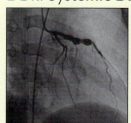

Kawasaki Disease

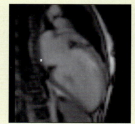

Duchenne

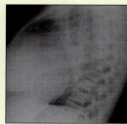

Sickle Cell Disease

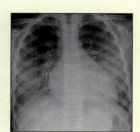

Rheumatic Heart

MYOCARDITIS

Key Facts

Terminology
- Process characterized by inflammatory infiltration of the myocardium with necrosis and/or degeneration of adjacent myocytes not typical of ischemic changes, which lead to myocardial dysfunction and heart failure

Imaging Findings
- Echocardiography is gold standard in infants and children for assessing cardiac function and anatomy
- Cardiac enlargement with left ventricular and left atrial enlargement, Kerly B lines, effusions
- Endomyocardial biopsy may detect specific cause utilizing genetic markers, histologic and immunologic techniques

Top Differential Diagnoses
- Cardiomyopathy
- Anomalous coronary artery (ACA)
- Kawasaki disease
- Cardiogenic shock

Pathology
- Cell types: Lymphocytic, eosinophilic, neutrophilic, giant cell, granulomatous, or mixed
- Distribution: Focal (outside vessel lumen), confluent, diffuse, or reparative (in fibrotic areas)

Clinical Issues
- Acute or fulminant cases need intensive care
- Cardiac transplantation may be necessary

- Echocardiography is performed to exclude other causes of heart failure (valvular, congenital) and to evaluate degree of cardiac dysfunction (usually diffuse hypokinesis and diastolic dysfunction)
- Left ventricular (LV) shortening fraction, end diastolic dimension, end systolic dimension, LV volume and LV posterior wall and septal thickness measurements related to mean values for age
- Echocardiography shows increased left ventricular end diastolic dimension and fractional shortening

Angiographic Findings
- Conventional: Endomyocardial biopsy performed in attempt to make specific diagnosis

Nuclear Medicine Findings
- Gallium-67 Scan: Antimyosin scintigraphy can identify myocardial inflammation with high sensitivity (91-100%) and negative predictive power (93-100%) but has low specificity (31-44%) and low positive predictive power (28-33%)

Other Modality Findings
- Leukocystosis, elevated sedimentation rates, and negative rheumatolic screening
- Elevated cardiac enzymes (creatine kinase or cardiac troponin)

Imaging Recommendations
- Best imaging tool
  - Echocardiography is gold standard particularity in young infants and children
  - Endomyocardial biopsies may establish specific underlying cause utilizing histologic, immunologic, and immunochemical criteria

DIFFERENTIAL DIAGNOSIS

Cardiomyopathy
- Broad categories of disease which include familial or specific genetic causes, myocardial protein mutations, metabolic, immunologic, ischemic, toxic induced, or inflammatory causes
- Myocarditis accounts for 3-30% of cardiomyopathies
- Idiopathic causes range from 57-68% of cases
- World Health Organization (WHO) classification includes dilated, hypertrophic and restrictive cardiomyopathy

Anomalous coronary artery (ACA)
- Congenital anomaly of the right or left coronary artery origin which may cause left ventricular ischemia, dysfunction, and shock
- Alternatively, may present with irritability, poor appetite and unrecognized cardiac symptoms
- Abnormal electrocardiogram (ECG) suggestive of ischemia or infarction
- Cardiac enzymes are elevated if infarct is present

Kawasaki disease
- Systemic disease of unknown etiology with fever, skin rash, lymphadenopathy, vasculitis
  - Transient myocarditis is common
  - Left ventricular dysfunction related to infarct in left ventricular wall secondary to aneurysm of coronary arteries

Cardiogenic shock
- Sepsis and other causes may present with cardiac shock

PATHOLOGY

General Features
- General path comments
  - Myocardial damage has 2 main phases
    - Acute phase (first 2 weeks): Myocyte destruction is a direct consequence of the offending agent
    - Chronic phase: Continuing myocyte destruction is autoimmune in nature
  - Molecular diagnostics may provides specific analysis and match with protein products
- Etiology

MYOCARDITIS

- Myocarditis likely is caused by a wide variety of infectious organisms, autoimmune disorders, and exogenous agents, with genetic and environmental predisposition
- Underlying etiology is not found in 50% of cases
- Most common viral infections include adenovirus, enterovirus, coxsackie, echovirus, poliovirus, influenza, cytomegalovirus, herpes simplex, rubella, mumps, human immunodeficiency (HIV)
- Children with AIDS may have myocarditis and have enterovirus engtomes detected on biopsy
- Non viral causes include rickettsia, bacteria, protozoa, other parasites, fungi and yeast
- Drug causes include antimicrobial medication
- Autoimmune or collagen-vascular disease such as systemic lupus, scleroderma
- Epidemiology: Incidence is estimated at 1-10 per 100,000 persons

Gross Pathologic & Surgical Features
- Active myocarditis is characterized by abundant inflammatory cells and myocardial necrosis
- Borderline myocarditis is characterized by an inflammatory response that is too sparse

Microscopic Features
- Eosin methylene blue (EMB) should reveal the simultaneous findings of lymphocyte infiltration and myocyte necrosis

Staging, Grading or Classification Criteria
- WHO Marburg classification (1996)
  - Cell types: Lymphocytic, eosinophilic, neutrophilic, giant cell, granulomatous, or mixed
  - Distribution: Focal (outside vessel lumen), confluent, diffuse, or reparative (in fibrotic areas)
  - Amount: None (grade 0), mild (grade 1), moderate (grade 2), or severe (grade 3)

CLINICAL ISSUES

Presentation
- Most common signs/symptoms
  - Clinical presentation varies from asymptomatic to acute cardiac decompensation
  - Chest pain is common in adolescents
  - Arrhythmia such as sinus tachycardia, atrioventricular disturbances
- Other signs/symptoms: In infants, irritability, lethargy, fever, wheezing, and failure to thrive

Demographics
- Age: Newborns and infants have increased susceptibility to myocarditis particularity of viral etiology
- Ethnicity
  - World Health Organization notes cardiovascular involvement after enteroviral infection is 1-4%
  - Differs in various populations and genetic patterns

Natural History & Prognosis
- Majority of cases of acute myocarditis have a benign course: Many of are not detected clinically
  - 2/3 with mild symptoms recover completely without any residual cardiac dysfunction
- Some patients develop heart failure, serious arrhythmias, circulatory collapse, and sudden death
  - 17% of children who died of sudden infant death syndrome (SIDS) had histopathologic evidence of myocarditis
  - 1/3 subsequently developing dilated cardiomyopathy
  - Mortality rate with Coxsackie virus B in newborns is 75%
  - Prognosis depends on organisim and patient

Treatment
- Acute or fulminant cases need intensive care
  - Treatment of congestive heart failure
  - Severe circulatory compromise may need extracorporeal membrane oxygenation (ECMO)
  - Ventricular assist device as a bridge to transplant
- Nonsteroidal antiinflammatory drugs are not effective and may actually enhance the myocarditis and increase mortality
- Continuous monitoring and assessment
- Immunosuppressive therapy may be appropriate
- Cyclosporine and steroids may be indicated if biopsy is positive
- Cardiac transplantation may be necessary
  - Donors for pediatric patients are limited
  - Survival rates following transplant 90% one year, 83% five year
- Recovery of left ventricular function occurs 36-60% of cases
- Research may provide ways to induce regeneration of cardiac muscle such as stem cells or utilizing angiogenesis techniques

SELECTED REFERENCES

1. Robinson J et al: Intravenous immunoglobulin for presumed viral myocarditis in children and adults. Cochrane Database Syst Rev. (1):CD004370, 2005
2. English RF et al: Outcomes for children with acute myocarditis. Cardiol Young. 14(5):488-93, 2004
3. Harmon WG et al: Myocardial and Pericardial Disease in HIV. Curr Treat Options Cardiovasc Med. 4(6):497-509, 2002
4. Towbin JA: Myocarditis. In: Allen HD and Gutgesell HP (eds). Heart Disease in Infants and Children, and Adolescents. Lippincott Williams & Wilkins. Philadelphia. 1197-1215, 2001
5. Friedrich MD et al: Contrast media-enhanced magnetic resonance imaging visualizes myocardial changes in the course of viral myocarditis. Circulation. 97:1802-9, 1998
6. Alpert JS et al: Update in cardiology: Myocarditis. Ann Intern Med. 125:40-6, 1996

MYOCARDITIS

IMAGE GALLERY

Typical

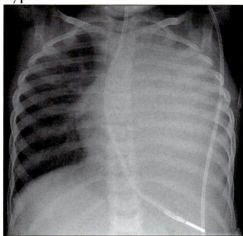
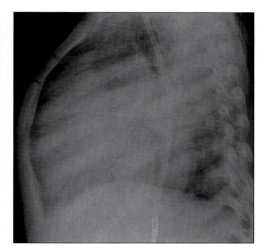

(Left) Anteroposterior radiograph shows collapse of the left lung related to left atrial enlargement in infant with myocarditis. Nasogastric tube is displaced due to left atrial enlargement. *(Right)* Lateral radiograph shows marked cardiomegaly with left atrial and left ventricular enlargement in patient who presented with wheezing. Volume loss in left lower lobe also seen.

Typical

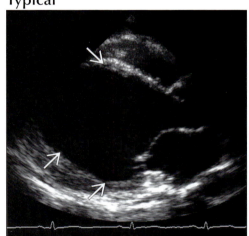
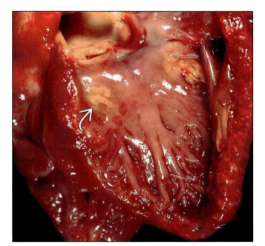

(Left) Echocardiogram shows marked left ventricular dilation (arrows) and bowing of the interventricular septum in child with dilated cardiomyopathy secondary to myocarditis. *(Right)* Gross pathology depicts mottled appearance of left ventricle from inflammatory myocarditis. Pale areas represent focal areas of necrosis (arrow) beneath the endocardial surface.

Typical

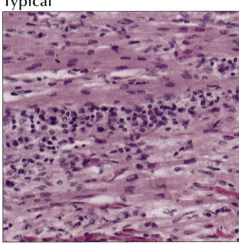
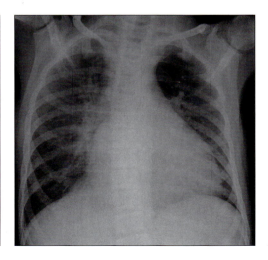

(Left) Micropathology, high power obtained from endomyocardial biopsy of the right ventricle demonstrating characteristic extensive cellular infiltrate with mixture of lymphocytes and neutrophils. *(Right)* Anteroposterior radiograph shows moderate cardiomegaly with pulmonary edema more prominent on the right than the left. Note left atrial enlargement.

CARDIOMYOPATHY

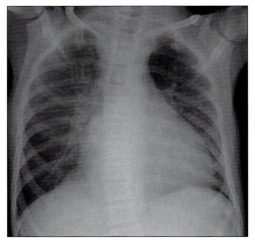

Anteroposterior radiograph shows cardiomegaly, left atrial enlargement with widening of the tracheal bifurcation. Asymmetry of pulmonary edema likely secondary to mitral regurgitation.

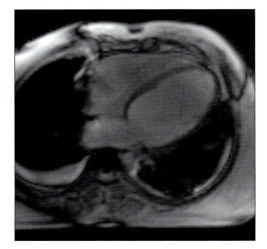

Axial MR imaging shows left ventricular chamber enlargement, thinning of the ventricular wall, and abnormal end diastolic volume. Patient had "idiopathic" dilated cardiomyopathy.

TERMINOLOGY

Abbreviations and Synonyms
- Dilated cardiomyopathy (DCM)
  - Congestive cardiomyopathy
- Hypertrophic cardiomyopathy (HCM)
  - Idiopathic hypertrophic subaortic stenosis, hypertrophic obstructive cardiomyopathy, asymmetric hypertrophic cardiomyopathy, and others

Definitions
- Cardiomyopathies are diffuse diseases of the myocardium which alter function
  - DCM has cardiac dilatation and decreased systolic function
    - Final common pathway of diverse diseases that lead to heart failure
    - Due to many etiologic factors
  - HCM has thickened septum and left ventricular free wall which maybe diffuse or focal

IMAGING FINDINGS

General Features
- Best diagnostic clue
  - DCM has dilated, thin-walled, poorly contracting ventricle with increased end-diastolic volume
  - HCM has thickened septum and left ventricle wall with decreased end-diastolic volume
- Location: Myocytes of the heart muscle particularly the ventricles
- Size
  - DCM shows diffuse changes of ventricular chambers
  - HCM demonstrates thickened interventricular septum extending into the free wall of the left ventricle

Radiographic Findings
- Radiography
  - Chest radiography in DCM is abnormal in 85%
    - Large left ventricle, large left atrium, pulmonary edema, right pleural effusions during acute presentation
    - Left lower lobe collapse from left main stem bronchus compression
  - Chest radiograph in HCM is normal in 85%

CT Findings
- CECT: Not used very much in children except for defining anomalies of coronary arteries

MR Findings
- T2* GRE

DDx: Diverse Causes Cardiomyopathy

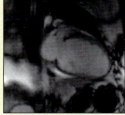
DCM: Duchenne

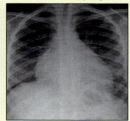
Rheumatic Heart

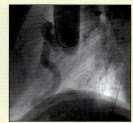
Ischemic

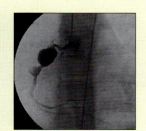
Kawasaki Disease

CARDIOMYOPATHY

Key Facts

Terminology
- Dilated cardiomyopathy (DCM)
- Hypertrophic cardiomyopathy (HCM)

Imaging Findings
- DCM has dilated, thin-walled, poorly contracting ventricle with increased end-diastolic volume
- HCM has thickened septum and left ventricle wall with decreased end-diastolic volume
- Chest radiography in DCM is abnormal in 85%
- Chest radiograph in HCM is normal in 85%
- MR imaging is used to evaluate the anatomy, function, perfusion and tissue characterization in children with cardiomyopathy
- Myocardial cell injury can be studied by injection of gadolinium and timing the appearance in myocardial cells
- Infants: Chest radiography, echocardiography, cardiac biopsy

Top Differential Diagnoses
- Many etiologies of cardiomyopathies: Duchenne muscular dystrophy
- Anomalous origin of left coronary artery
- Acute infectious myocarditis
- Kawasaki disease
- Idiopathic

Clinical Issues
- Infants present with tachycardia, diaphoresis and grunting respiratory effort
- HCM: Symptomatic patients have exercise intolerance, fatigue, chest pain, syncope
- Most common cause of sudden death

- ○ MR imaging is used to evaluate the anatomy, function, perfusion and tissue characterization in children with cardiomyopathy
- ○ Dynamic MR imaging allows accurate assessment of ventricular function
- ○ VEC MR combines measures of flow volume and velocity, and is good for serial measurements
- Myocardial cell injury can be studied by injection of gadolinium and timing the appearance in myocardial cells
  - ○ Acute enhancement can occur in myocarditis
  - ○ The degree of late myocardial enhancement may predict the extent of infarct and likelihood of recovery of function
  - ○ Intracardiac thrombi in 23%
- Wall thickness and myocardial tagging studies are helpful in DCM and also HCM
  - ○ Myocardial contrast agents being developed with potential interventional strategies

Echocardiographic Findings
- Echocardiogram
  - ○ DCM: Chamber dilatation, myocardial wall thinning, abnormal ejection fraction and increased end-diastolic volume
    - ▪ Intracardiac thrombi in 23%
  - ○ HCM: Thickening of interventricular septum and ventricular wall, dynamic outflow tract obstruction, systolic anterior motion of the mitral valve
- Power Doppler: Mitral regurgitation, subaortic obstruction during left ventricular systole

Angiographic Findings
- Cardiac catheterization
  - ○ Elevated ventricular filling pressures and pulmonary venous wedge pressure
  - ○ Diminished cardiac output, mitral regurgitation, normal coronary arteries
  - ○ Allows for myocardial biopsy to determine treatable causes (myocarditis)

Nuclear Medicine Findings
- Radionuclide Imaging
  - ○ PET scanning may show changes in perfusion
  - ○ Gallium uptake correlates with myocardial inflammation in DCM

Imaging Recommendations
- Best imaging tool
  - ○ Infants: Chest radiography, echocardiography, cardiac biopsy
  - ○ Older children: Cardiac MR with functional assessment
  - ○ Hypertrophic cardiomyopathy: PET and functional MR imaging

DIFFERENTIAL DIAGNOSIS

Many etiologies of cardiomyopathies: Duchenne muscular dystrophy
- Muscle biopsy demonstrates abnormal myocytes

Anomalous origin of left coronary artery
- Myocardial ischemia and infarction may occur with coronary anomalies

Acute infectious myocarditis
- Viral disease is the most common

Kawasaki disease
- May have myocarditis and occasional infarcts related to aneurysms

Idiopathic
- Most common

PATHOLOGY

General Features
- General path comments
  - ○ Physiology: HCM
    - ▪ Left ventricular hypertrophy is anatomic marker, small left ventricular cavity, increased left ventricular mass due to wall thickness

CARDIOMYOPATHY

- Diffuse and involves portions of ventricular septum and left ventricular free wall
- Abnormal mitral valve with alterations in size, shape
- Spectrum of severity and distribution of fibrous tissue formation within the myocardium
- Intramural coronary artery abnormalities occurs in 80% with increase in number yet decrease in luminal size
- Small vessel disease that may produce myocardial ischemia and necrosis
- Dynamic subaortic obstruction occurs with systolic anterior motion of the mitral valve contacts the ventricular septum and
  - Physiology: DCM
    - Diminished ventricular pump function, pooling of blood in atria
    - Increased wall tension, muscle hypertrophy, increased oxygen consumption and decreased myocardial efficiency
    - Decreased renal perfusion, activation of renin-angiotensin system with fluid retention, pulmonary edema and congestive heart failure
- Genetics
  - Hereditary: DCM (20-30%): Autosomal dominant, age dependent with variable expression
    - Gene mapping has provided many insights into multiple sarcomere proteins abnormalities
    - Duchenne muscular dystrophy is X-linked, chromosome band 21
  - HCM; genetically transmitted cardiovascular disease
- Etiology
  - Unknown in up to 85% of cases
  - Systemic diseases such as juvenile rheumatoid arthritis, systemic lupus, Kawasaki disease, polyarteritis nodosa, muscular dystrophy
  - Infectious: Bacterial (rheumatic), viral (Coxsackie), parasites (Chagas)
  - Toxic: Sulfonamides, chloramphenicol, alcohol, hemochromatosis
  - Metabolic: Hypo-/hyperthyroidism, maternal diabetes, hypocalcemia
  - Glycogen storage diseases, mucopolysaccharidoses, sphingolipidoses
  - Nutritional: Kwashiorkor, beriberi, carnitine or other trace element deficiencies
- Epidemiology
  - Incidence cardiomyopathy is 2-8/100,000
  - HCM occurs in 0.2% of population

Microscopic Features

- DCM: Molecular and histologic characteristics of specific diseases
  - Cascade of molecular and cellular events that lead to congestive heart failure
  - Lymphocytic infiltrate correlates with myocarditis

Staging, Grading or Classification Criteria

- Major types of cardiomyopathy
  - DCM: Biventricular dilatation, depressed systolic function
  - HCM: Left ventricular hypertrophy, left ventricular outflow tract obstruction
  - Restrictive cardiomyopathy
- Classifications are changing due to enhanced knowledge based on endomyocardial biopsy, mutant mouse models of disease, molecular diagnostics, and immunopathogenesis of diseases

CLINICAL ISSUES

Presentation
- Most common signs/symptoms
  - DCM: Symptomatic children have gradual onset of shortness of breath, exercise intolerance
    - Infants present with tachycardia, diaphoresis and grunting respiratory effort
  - HCM: Symptomatic patients have exercise intolerance, fatigue, chest pain, syncope
    - Difficult to screen for disease as many patients are asymptomatic
- Other signs/symptoms
  - Symptoms usually attributed to other causes such as upper respiratory infection
  - Most common cause of sudden death

Demographics
- Age: All ages
- Ethnicity: Worldwide disease with multiple different causes

Natural History & Prognosis
- 1/3 die, 1/3 improve with residual dysfunction, 1/3 recover completely
- Risks of pediatric cardiac transplantation include life-long immunosuppression, infections, growth disturbance, lymphoproliferative disease, malignancies

Treatment
- Cardiomyopathy: Supportive medical therapy
- DCM: Reduce the work of the heart, improve function
- HCM: Medical, surgical and interventional therapy
  - Implantable cardiac defibrillators when high risk
  - Alcohol septal ablation done percutaneously with infusion into septal perforating branches

SELECTED REFERENCES

1. Pujadas S et al: MR imaging assessment of cardiac function. J Magn Reson Imaging. 19(6):789-99, 2004
2. Tsirka AE et al: Improved outcomes of pediatric dilated cardiomyopathy with utilization of heart transplantation. J Am Coll Cardiol. 44(2):391-7, 2004
3. Cecchi F et al: Coronary microvascular dysfunction and prognosis in hypertrophic cardiomyopathy. N Engl J Med. 349(11):1027-35, 2003
4. Krombach, GA et al: Myocardial and Pericardial Diseases Chapter 7 in Higgins, Charles and DeRoos, Alberts, ed(s) Cardiovascular MRI & MRA Lippincot Williams & Wilkins, Philadelphia. 103-121, 2003
5. Strauss A et al: Pediatric cardiomyopathy--a long way to go. N Engl J Med. 348(17):1703-5, 2003
6. Varaprasathan GA et al: Quantification of flow dynamics in congenital heart disease: applications of velocity-encoded cine MR imaging. Radiographics. 22(4):895-905; discussion 905-6, 2002

CARDIOMYOPATHY

IMAGE GALLERY

Typical

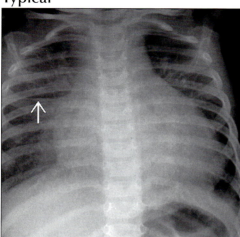
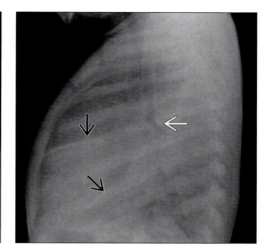

(Left) Anteroposterior radiograph shows cardiomegaly, indistinct vascularity, thickening of minor fissure *(arrow)*. Interstitial pulmonary edema. *(Right)* Lateral radiograph shows thickening of fissures *(black arrows)* and interstitial pulmonary edema. Left main stem bronchus *(white arrow)* is displaced posteriorly secondary to left atrial enlargement.

Typical

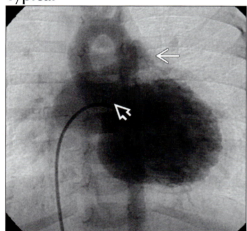
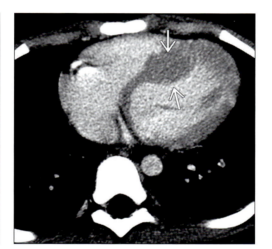

(Left) Anteroposterior left ventriculogram, shows dilatation of left ventricle, mitral regurgitation *(open arrow)* into dilated left atrium and enlarged left atrial appendage *(arrow)*. *(Right)* Axial CECT shows thickening of the interventricular septum *(arrows)* with thickening also of free wall and apex of left ventricle. The patient has hypertrophic cardiomyopathy.

Typical

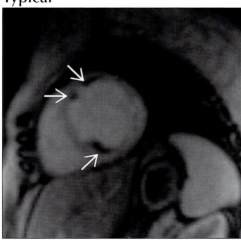
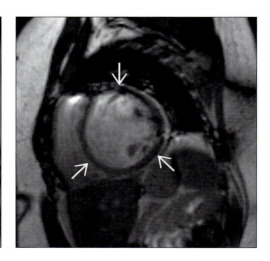

(Left) First pass perfusion image of a cardiac MR study in short axis plane demonstrates enhancement of the myocardium with nonenhancement of intraventricular thrombi *(arrows)*. *(Right)* MR cine short axis gradient echo sequence in a patient with a dilated cardiomyopathy demonstrates increased end diastolic volume. Ejection fraction was 10%. Note thinned left ventricular wall *(arrows)*.

DOUBLE OUTLET RIGHT VENTRICLE

- VSDs can be large and present early with significant shunting
- DORV without pulmonic stenosis radiographically simulates a large left-to-right shunt
- Distinguishing feature is that in VSD there is normal fibrous continuity between the posterior leaflet of the aortic valve and the anterior leaflet of the mitral valve

Tetralogy of Fallot (TOF)
- With severe outflow tract obstruction and VSD, the aorta over-rides the ventricular septum and simulates DORV with pulmonic stenosis
- Physiology may be similar but in TOF, there is aortic mitral continuity despite the anterior position of aorta and overriding of the right ventricle
- DORV and TOF both have increased incidence of right aortic arch

Transposition of the great arteries (TGA)
- Cyanosis occurs in first 24 hours of birth
- D-transposition of the great vessels (D-TGA), there is atrial-ventricular concordance and ventricular great vessel discordance; the RV gives origin to the aorta, and the pulmonary artery has an LV origin
  - The RV gives origin to the aorta, and the pulmonary artery has an LV origin

Truncus arteriosus
- Single arterial trunk with truncal valve arising from the ventricles and gives origin to the aorta, the coronary arteries, and the pulmonary arteries
- Distinguishing feature is that there is normal continuity between the posterior leaflet of the truncal valve and the anterior leaflet of the mitral valve

PATHOLOGY

General Features
- Genetics
  - Chromosomal abnormalities such as trisomy 13 or trisomy 18
  - DiGeorge syndrome, velocardiofacial syndrome and chromosome band 22q11 deletion is known as the CATCH-22 association
- Etiology
  - Conotruncal heart defect which may be of neural crest origin
  - Neural crest involved in the development of the cardiac septum
  - Occurs during the looping of the bulboventricular tube

CLINICAL ISSUES

Presentation
- Most common signs/symptoms
  - May be diagnosed in utero and usually has clinical symptoms at birth or in the first month of life
  - Failure to thrive, tachypnea
  - DORV with subaortic VSD without pulmonic stenosis present with symptoms of a large left-to-right shunt and early evidence of pulmonary hypertension
  - DORV with pulmonic stenosis presents with cyanosis, failure to thrive

Demographics
- Age: DORV accounts for 1-1.5% of all congenital heart disease, with an incidence of 1 per 10,000 live births
- Gender: No race or sex predilection

Treatment
- DORV with two developed ventricles
  - Closure of the VSD and placement of a right ventricle to pulmonary artery conduit
- Surgery depends on anatomy
  - Usually biventricular approach in transposition with placement of an intraventricular baffle
  - Norwood/Fontan procedure if there is hypoplasia of ventricle
  - Some children need palliation such as banding of pulmonary arteries to prevent pulmonary vascular resistance abnormalities
- Statistics depend on the specific type of DORV
  - Mortality rate after operation is higher for complex lesions
  - Fifteen year survival rate for non-complex lesions ranges from 85-90%
  - Children may have multiple other anomalies which affect outcome
  - Reoperation may be required and related to right ventricular outflow obstruction

SELECTED REFERENCES

1. Wyttenbach R et al: Cardiovascular magnetic Resonance of complete Congenital heart Disease in the Adult. In: Manning, Pennell (eds). Cardiovascular magnetic Resonance. Churchill Livingstone Philadelphia. 311-323, 2002
2. Brown JW et al: Surgical results in patients with double outlet right ventricle: a 20-year experience. Ann Thorac Surg. 72(5):1630-5, 2001
3. Hagler DJ. Double-Outlet Right Ventricle In Allen HD, Gutgesell HP (eds). Heart Disease in Infants, Children, and Adolescents. Lippincott Williams & Wilkins. Philadelphia. 1102-1128, 2001
4. Niezen RA et al: Double outlet right ventricle assessed with magnetic resonance imaging. Int J Card Imaging. 15(4):323-9, 1999
5. Yoo SJ et al: Magnetic resonance imaging of complex congenital heart disease. Int J Card Imaging. 15(2):151-60, 1999
6. Goldmuntz E et al: Frequency of 22q11 deletions in patients with conotruncal defects. J Am Coll Cardiol. 32(2):492-8, 1998

DOUBLE OUTLET RIGHT VENTRICLE

IMAGE GALLERY

Typical

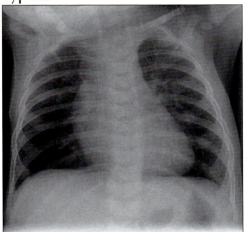
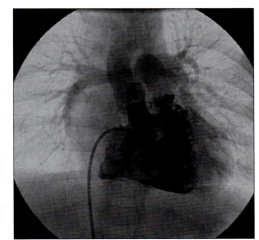

(Left) Anteroposterior radiograph shows a one year old patient who has DORV. Patient has a normal sized heart and normal pulmonary artery flow as there was mild pulmonic stenosis. *(Right)* Catheterization with right ventricular injection shows flow into both pulmonary artery and also ascending aorta. Child has DORV, normally related great vessels and mild pulmonic stenosis.

Typical

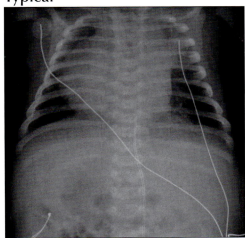
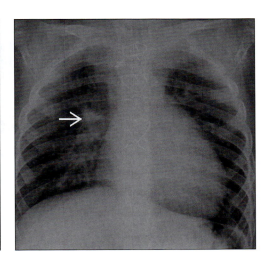

(Left) Radiograph of chest shows dextrocardia, malposition of stomach, and left-sided umbilical venous catheter due to midline liver. Suggests complex heart disease with asplenia or polysplenia. *(Right)* Anteroposterior radiograph shows child with complex heart disease, DORV with PS, total anomalous pulmonary venous return, post-operative shunt creating asymmetry of pulmonary flow (arrow).

Typical

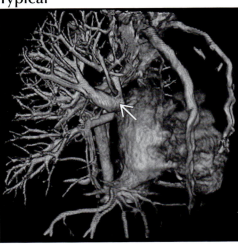
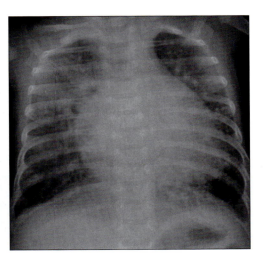

(Left) Oblique CECT in same patient as above shows asymmetry of pulmonary artery flow (arrow) in a patient with DORV, repaired total anomalous pulmonary venous return, and azygous continuation of inferior vena cava. *(Right)* Anteroposterior radiograph shows cardiomegaly with significant increase in pulmonary artery flow, and signs of venous edema. Infant had DORV with no pulmonic stenosis which explains the increased flow to lungs.

L-TRANSPOSITION OF THE GREAT ARTERIES

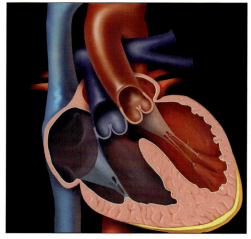

Graphic depicts left-sided ascending aorta, connected to left-sided trabeculated right ventricle. Right-sided pulmonary artery is connected to right-sided smooth-walled left ventricle. Note high VSD.

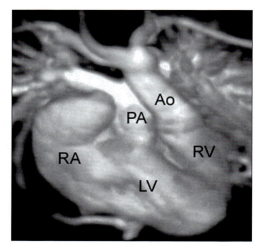

Oblique MRA shows abnormal side-to-side orientation of main pulmonary artery (PA) and ascending aorta (AO). LV = left ventricle; RV = right ventricle; RA = right atrium. (Courtesy Shi-Joon Yoo, MD).

TERMINOLOGY

Abbreviations and Synonyms
- "Congenitally corrected transposition" (misnomer)
- Discordant transposition

Definitions
- Inversion of ventricles and great arteries: Atrioventricular discordance and ventriculoarterial discordance
- Category: Dependent on associated anomalies
  - Ventricular septal defect (VSD, 60-70%): Acyanotic, increased pulmonary vascularity
  - Left ventricular outflow tract (subpulmonary) obstruction (30-50%): Cyanotic
  - Dysplasia (Ebstein anomaly) with regurgitation of left-sided atrioventricular (AV) valve: Pulmonary venous congestion/hypertension
  - Conduction abnormalities, heart block
  - Only 1% have no associated anomalies: True congenitally corrected transposition
- Hemodynamics
  - Right atrium connects via mitral valve to right-sided morphologic left ventricle (LV), which connects to pulmonary circulation
  - Left atrium connects via tricuspid valve to left-sided morphologic right ventricle (RV), which connects to systemic circulation
  - Hemodynamic sequelae dependent on associated anomalies
- Segmental analysis of atrial, ventricular and great vessel morphology, relationship and connections is required for complete description of this complex disorder

IMAGING FINDINGS

General Features
- Best diagnostic clue: Great vessels lie parallel and almost in the same coronal plane, with aortic valve in anterior position and slightly to the left (L-loop) of pulmonary valve
- Morphology
  - {S, L, L} heart: Atrial situs solitus, L-loop, L-transposed great arteries
    - Right-sided morphologic LV characterized by associated mitral valve, smooth wall and absent outflow chamber to pulmonary valve
    - Left-sided morphologic RV characterized by associated tricuspid valve, trabeculated wall with moderator band and infundibulum below aortic valve
  - {I, D, D} heart: Atrial situs inversus, D-loop, D-transposed great arteries
    - Mirror image of {S, L, L} heart

DDx: L-Transposition: Differentials & Associated Anomalies

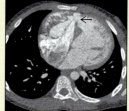
VSD

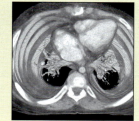
Tricuspid Atresia

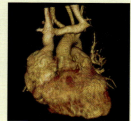
DORV

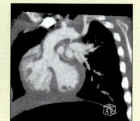
Tetralogy Of Fallot

L-TRANSPOSITION OF THE GREAT ARTERIES

Key Facts

Terminology
- Inversion of ventricles and great arteries: Atrioventricular discordance and ventriculoarterial discordance
- Category: Dependent on associated anomalies
- Ventricular septal defect (VSD, 60-70%): Acyanotic, increased pulmonary vascularity
- Left ventricular outflow tract (subpulmonary) obstruction (30-50%): Cyanotic
- Dysplasia (Ebstein anomaly) with regurgitation of left-sided atrioventricular (AV) valve: Pulmonary venous congestion/hypertension
- Only 1% have no associated anomalies: True congenitally corrected transposition

- Segmental analysis of atrial, ventricular and great vessel morphology, relationship and connections is required for complete description of this complex disorder

Imaging Findings
- Best diagnostic clue: Great vessels lie parallel and almost in the same coronal plane, with aortic valve in anterior position and slightly to the left (L-loop) of pulmonary valve
- T1WI: Multiplanar cardiac-gated T1WI and 3D gadolinium MRA for segmental cardiac analysis and anatomic evaluation

Clinical Issues
- Double switch operation to prevent late systemic ventricular (RV) failure

---

- Almost always associated with cardiac malposition: Mesocardia, dextroversion, true dextrocardia (25%)

Radiographic Findings
- Radiography
  - Classic plain film appearance: Straight upper left heart border
  - Other findings are determined by associated anomalies

CT Findings
- 3D CT angiography can depict abnormal atrioventricular and ventriculoarterial relationships

MR Findings
- T1WI: Multiplanar cardiac-gated T1WI and 3D gadolinium MRA for segmental cardiac analysis and anatomic evaluation
- T2* GRE: Dobutamine stress short-axis steady-state free precession cine MRI for functional evaluation of RV: Can it sustain the systemic circulation?

Echocardiographic Findings
- Echocardiogram
  - Segmental cardiac analysis: Identification of atria, ventricles, great arteries and their connections
  - Continuity between right-sided mitral and pulmonary valve annulus
  - Discontinuity between left-sided tricuspid and aortic valve annulus
  - Abnormally straight, vertical course of interventricular septum

Angiographic Findings
- Conventional: Cardiac catheterization with angiography defines ventricular inversion, abnormal ventriculoarterial connections, VSD, pulmonary outflow tract obstruction, left-sided tricuspid valve regurgitation

Imaging Recommendations
- Protocol advice
  - Echocardiography allows for complete pre-operative diagnosis in majority of cases
  - CT or MR as complementary noninvasive cross-sectional tests for more complex abnormalities

DIFFERENTIAL DIAGNOSIS

Congestive heart failure, increased pulmonary blood flow
- Isolated VSD
- Double inlet ventricle
- Tricuspid atresia with increased pulmonary blood flow
- Double outlet right ventricle (DORV) with subaortic VSD

Cyanosis, decreased pulmonary blood flow
- Tetralogy of Fallot

Atrioventricular discordance with ventriculoarterial concordance
- Isolated ventricular inversion, with each ventricle connected to its appropriate great artery, and physiology resembling D-Transposition

PATHOLOGY

General Features
- General path comments
  - Ventricular arrangement is not simply the mirror image of normal
  - Ventricles and great arteries form an L-loop (D-loop is normal)
  - Interventricular septum is more vertical in orientation than normal
  - Coronary distribution is mirror image of normal (right-sided coronary bifurcates into circumflex and anterior descending arteries)
  - Embryology: Primitive cardiac tube loops to the left (L-loop), leading to ventricular inversion and left-sided position of ascending aorta

L-TRANSPOSITION OF THE GREAT ARTERIES

- Pathophysiology
  - Determined by associated anomalies: VSD, subpulmonary stenosis, AV valve dysfunction
  - Late sequel: left-sided RV is not able to sustain systemic circulation
- Genetics
  - No genetic factors or chromosomal abnormalities identified
  - Not commonly associated with extracardiac malformations
- Epidemiology: Incidence: 1 in 13,000 live births, 1% of congenital heart disease, males > females
- Associated abnormalities
  - VSD: 80%
  - LV outflow tract (subpulmonary) obstruction: 30%
  - Left-sided tricuspid valve dysplasia, Ebstein anomaly, regurgitation: 30%
  - Can be associated with atrial situs inversus: Dextrocardia {I, D, D}
  - Rare: Ventricular hypoplasia, atrioventricular canal, straddling AV valves, aortic atresia, coarctation or interruption

Gross Pathologic & Surgical Features

- Right-sided morphologic LV connected without infundibulum to pulmonary valve, which is slightly posterior and to right of aortic valve
- Infundibulum of left-sided morphologic RV connected to aortic valve, which is slightly anterior and to left of pulmonary valve (L-loop)
- Pulmonary artery and ascending aorta lie nearly parallel in same coronal plane
- Interruption of conduction system of heart due to malalignment between atrial and ventricular septa: Disconnection between atrioventricular node and bundle of His → third degree heart block

CLINICAL ISSUES

Presentation

- Most common signs/symptoms
  - Congestive heart failure (VSD, systemic AV valve dysfunction)
  - Cyanosis (subpulmonary stenosis)
  - Rarely completely asymptomatic, presenting as incidental finding on chest radiograph (straight upper left heart border)
- Other signs/symptoms
  - Conduction disturbances: Bradycardia (heart block) and tachydysrhythmia
  - Decreased exercise tolerance due to dysfunction of systemic ventricle (RV)

Natural History & Prognosis

- Determined by presence of AV valve dysfunction
- Guarded prognosis due to progressive systemic AV valve and RV dysfunction after corrective surgery: 50% mortality after 15 years
- Patients with true congenitally corrected transposition may have a normal life expectancy

Treatment

- Surgical treatment focused on associated abnormalities
  - Congestive heart failure from VSD shunt: PA banding or VSD closure
  - Cyanosis from subpulmonary stenosis: Systemic to PA shunt (Blalock-Taussig) or LV to PA conduit (Rastelli)
  - Pulmonary venous hypertension from tricuspid valve dysfunction: Tricuspid valvuloplasty
- Double switch operation to prevent late systemic ventricular (RV) failure
  - Venous switch (Senning) re-routes the atrial blood into the appropriate ventricles
  - Ventricular (Rastelli) or arterial switch: Morphologic LV becomes systemic ventricle
- Pacemaker insertion

SELECTED REFERENCES

1. Sorensen TS et al: Operator-independent isotropic three-dimensional magnetic resonance imaging for morphology in congenital heart disease: a validation study. Circulation. 110(2):163-9, 2004
2. Tulevski II et al: Regional and global right ventricular dysfunction in asymptomatic or minimally symptomatic patients with congenitally corrected transposition. Cardiol Young. 14(2):168-73, 2004
3. Karl TR et al: Congenitally corrected transposition of the great arteries. In: Mavroudis C, Backer CL, ed. Pediatric cardiac surgery. 3rd ed. Philadelphia, Mosby. 476-495, 2003
4. Dodge-Khatami A et al: Comparable systemic ventricular function in healthy adults and patients with unoperated congenitally corrected transposition using MRI dobutamine stress testing. Ann Thorac Surg. 73(6):1759-64, 2002
5. Tulevski II et al: Usefulness of magnetic resonance imaging dobutamine stress in asymptomatic and minimally symptomatic patients with decreased cardiac reserve from congenital heart disease (complete and corrected transposition of the great arteries and subpulmonic obstruction). Am J Cardiol. 89(9):1077-81, 2002
6. Schmidt M et al: Tc-99m MIBI SPECT correlated with magnetic resonance imaging for cardiac evaluation of a patient with congenitally corrected transposition of the great arteries (L-TGA). Clin Nucl Med. 26(8):714-5, 2001
7. Freedom RM. Congenitally corrected transposition of the great arteries. In: Moller JH, Hoffman JIE ed. Pediatric cardiovascular medicine, 1st ed. Philadelphia, Churchill Livingstone. 391-408, 2000
8. Schmidt M et al: Congenitally corrected transposition of the great arteries (L-TGA) with situs inversus totalis in adulthood: findings with magnetic resonance imaging. Magn Reson Imaging. 18(4):417-22, 2000
9. Reddy GP et al: Case 15: Congenitally corrected transposition of the great arteries. Radiology 213:102-6, 1999
10. Chen SJ et al: Three-dimensional reconstruction of abnormal ventriculoarterial relationship by electron beam CT. J Comput Assist Tomogr. 22(4):560-8, 1998
11. Formanek AG: MR imaging of congenitally corrected transposition of the great vessels in adults. AJR Am J Roentgenol. 154(4):898-9, 1990
12. Park JH et al: MR imaging of congenitally corrected transposition of the great vessels in adults. AJR Am J Roentgenol. 153(3):491-4, 1989

L-TRANSPOSITION OF THE GREAT ARTERIES

IMAGE GALLERY

Typical

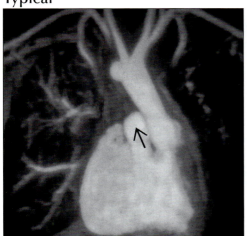
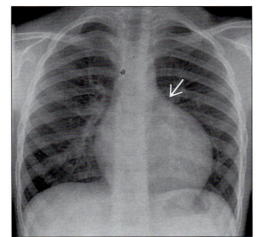

(Left) Coronal MRA shows L-loop of aortic arch, located to left of pulmonary outflow tract *(arrow)*. *(Right)* Anteroposterior radiograph in 8 year old girl with L-transposition and Ebstein anomaly of left-sided tricuspid valve shows typical abnormal contour of upper left heart border *(arrow)*. (Courtesy Shi-Joon Yoo, MD).

Typical

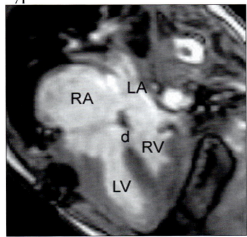
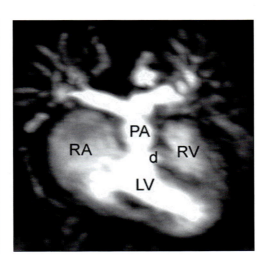

(Left) Four chamber view MR cine shows smooth-walled left ventricle (LV) connecting with right atrium (RA); trabeculated right ventricle (RV) connecting with left atrium (LA); d = high ventricular septal defect. *(Right)* Coronal oblique MIP shows pulmonary artery (PA) connecting with smooth-walled left ventricle (LV). (Courtesy Shi-Joon Yoo, MD).

Typical

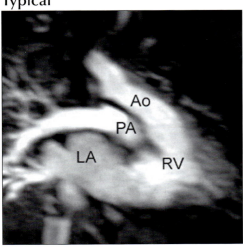
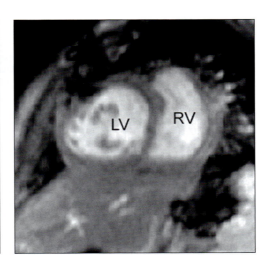

(Left) Sagittal oblique MIP shows aorta (Ao) connecting with trabeculated right ventricle (RV) *(Right)* Coronal oblique MR cine Shows ventricular inversion: Morphologic left ventricle (LV) is anatomically positioned on the right, and morphologic right ventricle (RV) on the left. (Courtesy Shi-Joon Yoo, MD).

HETEROTAXIA SYNDROMES

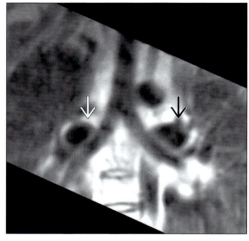

Coronal T1WI MR shows bilaterally symmetric hyparterial bronchi in polysplenia syndrome: Both pulmonary arteries arch over the mainstem bronchi (arrows). (Courtesy R. Krishnamurthy, MD).

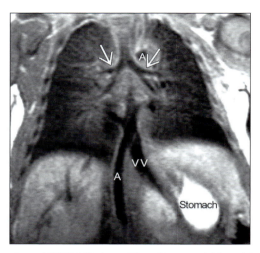

Coronal T1WI MR shows bilaterally eparterial bronchi (arrows), infradiaphragmatic pulmonary venous return (VV) and right aorta (A) in aspienia syndrome. (Courtesy Shi-Joon Yoo, MD).

TERMINOLOGY

Abbreviations and Synonyms
- Situs ambiguous, right/left isomerism, cardiosplenic syndromes, Ivemark syndrome

Definitions
- Disturbance of the normal left-right asymmetry in the position of thoracic and abdominal organs

IMAGING FINDINGS

General Features
- Best diagnostic clue: Abnormal symmetry in chest and abdomen

Radiographic Findings
- Radiography
  o Classic plain film appearance: Transverse midline liver, discrepancy between position of cardiac apex and stomach, bilateral left- or right-sidedness in the chest, findings of congenital heart disease (CHD)
  o Asplenia syndrome
    ▪ Bilateral minor fissures
    ▪ Symmetrical short mainstem bronchi with right-sided morphology (narrow carinal angle, early take-off of upper lobe bronchus)
    ▪ Pulmonary artery courses anterior to mainstem bronchus (eparterial bronchus)
    ▪ Cardiomegaly, pulmonary edema
  o Polysplenia syndrome
    ▪ No minor fissure on either side
    ▪ Symmetrical long mainstem bronchi with left-sided morphology (wide carinal angle)
    ▪ Pulmonary artery courses over and behind mainstem bronchus (hyparterial bronchus)
    ▪ Absent IVC shadow on lateral film, prominent azygous shadow on AP
  o Both syndromes
    ▪ Cardiac malposition (40%: Mesocardia, dextrocardia)
    ▪ Transverse liver
    ▪ Right-sided stomach bubble with levocardia, left-sided stomach bubble with dextrocardia, or midline stomach

CT Findings
- CTA
  o Rapid examination of chest and abdomen: Situs abnormalities, systemic and pulmonary venous connections, tracheobronchial anatomy
  o Best for post-operative patients with metallic coils, stents and clips
  o Can replace and often provide more anatomic information than diagnostic angiocardiography

DDx: Situs Abnormalities

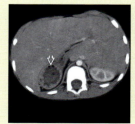 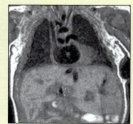 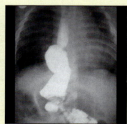 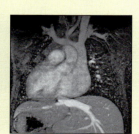

Situs Ambiguous | Common Atrium | Midline Stomach | Dextrocardia

HETEROTAXIA SYNDROMES

Key Facts

Terminology
- Disturbance of the normal left-right asymmetry in the position of thoracic and abdominal organs

Imaging Findings
- Best diagnostic clue: Abnormal symmetry in chest and abdomen
- Classic plain film appearance: Transverse midline liver, discrepancy between position of cardiac apex and stomach, bilateral left- or right-sidedness in the chest, findings of congenital heart disease (CHD)
- Rapid examination of chest and abdomen: Situs abnormalities, systemic and pulmonary venous connections, tracheobronchial anatomy
- T1WI: Multiplanar imaging (coronal, axial) for segmental analysis of intracardiac connections and defects
- T2* GRE: Cine MRI for ventricular volumes and function, to determine suitability for biventricular versus univentricular (Fontan) repair
- Gadolinium-enhanced 3D MRA: Comparable to CTA, better spatial resolution in coronal plane

Pathology
- Segmental approach to analysis of complex cardiac anomalies with cardiac malposition
- Any arrangement other than situs solitus or inversus is termed situs ambiguous (heterotaxia)

Clinical Issues
- Asplenia: Male neonate with severe cyanosis, susceptibility for infections
- Polysplenia: More variable, often presents later

MR Findings
- T1WI: Multiplanar imaging (coronal, axial) for segmental analysis of intracardiac connections and defects
- T2* GRE: Cine MRI for ventricular volumes and function, to determine suitability for biventricular versus univentricular (Fontan) repair
- MRA
  - Gadolinium-enhanced 3D MRA: Comparable to CTA, better spatial resolution in coronal plane
  - Ultrafast time-resolved Gd-MRA with repeated acquisitions allows for dynamic circulation study
  - Velocity-encoded phase contrast MRA for flow quantification

Echocardiographic Findings
- Echocardiogram: Often definitive test for characterization of intracardiac anomalies, abnormal systemic and/or pulmonary venous connections

Other Modality Findings
- Upper GI study: Malrotation is frequently associated

Imaging Recommendations
- Protocol advice
  - Echocardiography, followed by MRI
  - CTA for anatomic study in postoperative patients

DIFFERENTIAL DIAGNOSIS

Situs inversus totalis {I, L, L}
- Mirror image of normal
- Low association with CHD (3-5%); may be associated with immotile cilia syndrome (Kartagener): Sinusitis, bronchiectasis, infertility

True dextrocardia, abdominal situs solitus and levocardia, abdominal situs inversus
- Both have a high association with CHD (95-100%)

Dextroversion of the heart
- Heart is positioned in right chest with apex and stomach still directed toward the left
- In right pulmonary hypoplasia (scimitar syndrome), left-sided mass lesions (diaphragmatic hernia, cystic adenomatoid malformation of lung)

PATHOLOGY

General Features
- General path comments
  - Heterotaxy syndrome represents a spectrum, with overlap between classic asplenia and polysplenia manifestations, and other anomalies
  - Embryology
    - Early embryological disturbance (5th week of gestation), leading to complex anomalies
  - Pathophysiology
    - Determined by complexity of associated CHD
    - Asplenia syndrome with anomalous pulmonary venous connections: Findings of pulmonary venous outflow obstruction may be masked when there is restriction to pulmonary arterial inflow at the same time (pulmonary atresia)
- Genetics: No specific genetic defect in majority (usually sporadic)
- Epidemiology
  - Prevalence 1 per 22,000 to 24,000; 1-3% of CHD
  - Asplenia is more common in boys; equal sex ratio for polysplenia

Staging, Grading or Classification Criteria
- Segmental approach to analysis of complex cardiac anomalies with cardiac malposition
  - Viscero-atrial situs designated by S (solitus = normal) or I (inversus = mirror image of normal)
  - Always associated on same side are
    - Major lobe of liver, Inferior vena cava (IVC), anatomic right atrium, tri-lobed lung, eparterial bronchus

HETEROTAXIA SYNDROMES

- Spleen, stomach, descending aorta, anatomic left atrium, bi-lobed lung, hyparterial bronchus
  - Any arrangement other than situs solitus or inversus is termed situs ambiguous (heterotaxia)
  - Ventricular loop: D (normal) or L (inverted)
  - Orientation of great arteries (presence of transposition) also designated by D or L
  - Segmental analysis summarized by 3-letter code: {S, D, D}, {I, L, L}, {S, D, L}
  - Connections: Concordant or discordant
  - Associated abnormalities: Transposition of great arteries (TGA), double outlet right ventricle (DORV), total anomalous pulmonary venous return (TAPVR)
- Two major subtypes
  - Asplenia syndrome = double right-sidedness
    - Absence of a spleen
    - IVC and aorta on same side
    - Bilateral superior vena cavae (SVC, 36%), absent coronary sinus
    - Right isomerism of atrial appendages
    - Common atrium with band-like remnant of septum crossing atria in anteroposterior direction
    - Bilateral tri-lobed lungs
    - Bilateral eparterial bronchi
    - Associated with severe cyanotic CHD (atrioventricular septal defect, common atrioventricular valve, DORV, TGA, pulmonary stenosis/atresia)
    - Abnormalities of pulmonary venous connections: TAPVR (> 80%); often obstructed, below diaphragm (type III)
  - Polysplenia syndrome = double left-sidedness
    - Multiple spleens, anisosplenia, multilobed spleen
    - Abnormalities of systemic venous connections: Azygous continuation of IVC (>70%), hepatic veins drain separately into common atrium
    - Bilateral SVC (41%), one or both may connect to coronary sinus
    - Left isomerism of atrial appendages
    - Common atrium or large ostium primum ASD
    - Bilateral bi-lobed lungs
    - Bilateral hyparterial bronchi
    - Associated with less severe CHD [common atrium, ventricular septal defect (VSD)]

CLINICAL ISSUES

Presentation
- Most common signs/symptoms
  - Asplenia: Male neonate with severe cyanosis, susceptibility for infections
  - Polysplenia: More variable, often presents later
- Other signs/symptoms: Malrotation, volvulus, preduodenal portal vein, absent gallbladder, extrahepatic biliary atresia, short pancreas

Natural History & Prognosis
- First year mortality: 85% asplenia, 65% polysplenia

Treatment
- Supportive, prostaglandins, antibiotic prophylaxis
- Asplenia/polysplenia with pulmonary overcirculation: Pulmonary artery banding
- Asplenia with obstructed pulmonary flow and TAPVR: Delicate balance between pulmonary arterial inflow and venous outflow
  - Placement of palliative systemic to pulmonary artery (Blalock-Taussig or central) shunt increases inflow
  - TAPVR repair needs to be done at the same time, to reduce outflow obstruction
- Early biventricular repair, if possible
- Univentricular repair, step 1: Glenn or hemi-Fontan
- Polysplenia: Incorporation of azygous vein to cavopulmonary anastomosis (Kawashima operation)
  - Post-operative: Development of pulmonary to systemic venous collaterals, arteriovenous malformations, pulmonary vein stenosis
- Completion of modified Fontan operation, if possible
  - One or more hepatic veins may have to be excluded from Fontan shunt → veno-venous collaterals
  - CTA or MRA prior to catheterization as road map for coil embolization of collaterals

DIAGNOSTIC CHECKLIST

Image Interpretation Pearls
- Rigorous application of segmental analysis on cross-sectional study will resolve any complex case

SELECTED REFERENCES

1. Fulcher AS et al: Abdominal manifestations of situs anomalies in adults. Radiographics. 22(6):1439-56, 2002
2. Hong YK et al: Efficacy of MRI in complicated congenital heart disease with visceral heterotaxy syndrome. J Comput Assist Tomogr. 24:671-82, 2000
3. Marino B et al: Malposition of the heart. In: Moller JH, Hoffman JIE, ed. Pediatric cardiovascular medicine, 1st ed. Philadelphia, Churchill Livingstone. 621-41, 2000
4. Applegate KE et al: Situs revisited: Imaging of heterotaxy syndrome. RadioGraphics. 19:837-52, 1999
5. Gayer G et al: Polysplenia syndrome detected in adulthood: report of eight cases and review of the literature. Abdom Imaging. 24(2):178-84, 1999
6. Chen SJ et al: Usefulness of electron beam computed tomography in children with heterotaxy syndrome. Am J Cardiol. 81(2):188-94, 1998
7. Oleszczuk-Raschke K et al: Abdominal sonography in the evaluation of heterotaxy in children. Pediatr Radiol. 25 Suppl 1:S150-6, 1995
8. Winer-Muram HT: Adult presentation of heterotaxic syndromes and related complexes. J Thorac Imaging. 10(1):43-57, 1995
9. Bakir M et al: The value of radionuclide splenic scanning in the evaluation of asplenia in patients with heterotaxy. Pediatr Radiol. 24(1):25-8, 1994
10. Geva T et al: Role of spin echo and cine magnetic resonance imaging in presurgical planning of heterotaxy syndrome. Circulation 90:348-56, 1994
11. Niwa K et al: Magnetic resonance imaging of heterotaxia in infants. J Am Coll Cardiol. 23(1):177-83, 1994
12. Wang JK et al: Usefulness of magnetic resonance imaging in the assessment of venoatrial connections, atrial morphology, bronchial situs, and other anomalies in right atrial isomerism. Am J Cardiol. 74(7):701-4, 1994
13. Jelinek JS et al: MRI of polysplenia syndrome. Magn Reson Imaging. 7(6):681-6, 1989
14. Winer-Muram HT et al: The spectrum of heterotaxic syndromes. Radiol Clin North Am. 27(6):1147-70, 1989

HETEROTAXIA SYNDROMES

IMAGE GALLERY

Typical

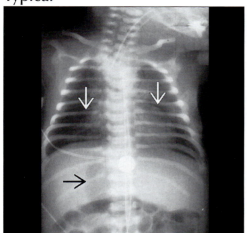
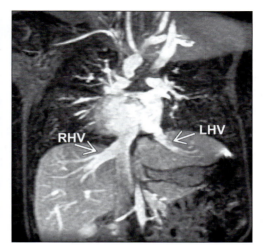

(Left) Anteroposterior radiograph shows transverse symmetrical liver shadow, gastric malposition *(black arrow)* and bilateral minor fissures *(white arrows)*, consistent with right isomerism (asplenia syndrome). *(Right)* Coronal MRA shows asplenia, with separate drainage of left (LHV) and right hepatic veins (RHV) into common atrium. *(Courtesy R. Krishnamurthy, MD).*

Typical

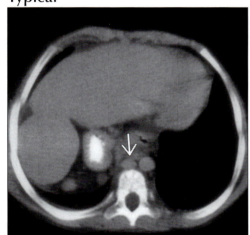
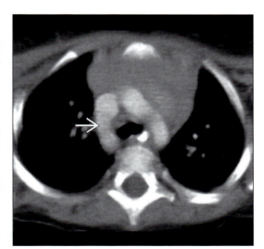

(Left) Axial NECT shows levocardia, right-sided stomach, multiple right-sided spleens, prominent azygous vein *(arrow)* to right of aorta. *(Right)* Axial CECT shows prominent azygous arch *(arrow)* in polysplenia patient with azygous continuation of inferior vena cava. *(Courtesy R. Krishnamurthy, MD).*

Typical

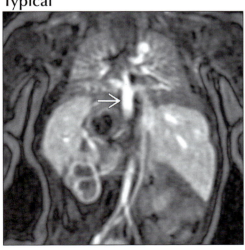
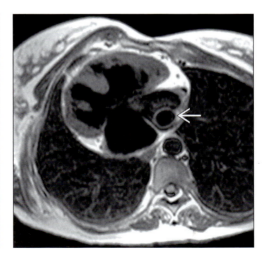

(Left) Coronal MRA shows infradiaphragmatic total anomalous pulmonary venous return *(arrow)* in asplenia syndrome. *(Courtesy R. Krishnamurthy, MD).* *(Right)* Axial T1WI MR shows balanced atrioventricular canal, dextrocardia and intra-atrial Fontan conduit *(arrow)* in asplenia syndrome. *(Courtesy R. Krishnamurthy, MD).*

AORTIC COARCTATION

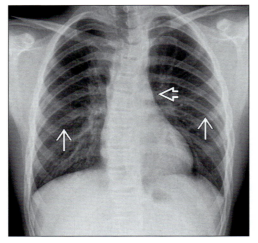

Anteroposterior radiograph shows rib notching (arrows) and post-stenotic dilatation in descending aorta ("3" sign, open arrow).

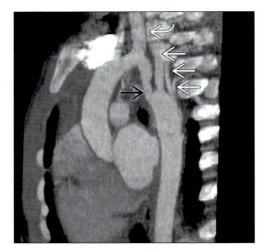

Sagittal oblique CTA shows severe postductal coarctation (black arrow) distal to take-off of left subclavian artery (curved arrow), with large collaterals (white arrows) feeding into descending aorta.

TERMINOLOGY

Definitions
- Narrowing of the aortic lumen with obstruction to blood flow
- Category: Acyanotic, normal heart size and pulmonary vascularity
- Hemodynamics: Left ventricular (LV) pressure overload

IMAGING FINDINGS

General Features
- Best diagnostic clue: Focal aortic narrowing, presence of collaterals
- Location
  - Preductal (infantile)
  - Juxtaductal or postductal (adult)
  - Abdominal: Middle aortic syndrome
- Morphology: Simple (isolated coarctation in adult) or complex (associated with other cardiac anomalies, presenting in infancy)

Radiographic Findings
- Radiography
  - Classic sign: Rib notching (above age 5 years)
  - Post-stenotic dilatation of proximal descending aorta: Figure 3 sign
  - LV hypertrophy: Rounded cardiac apex

Fluoroscopic Findings
- Esophagram: Impression by dilated descending aorta (reversed figure 3 or "ε" sign)

CT Findings
- CTA
  - Depicts coarctation site, percentage of stenosis and presence and location of collaterals
  - Multidetector row CT increasingly used in diagnosis
    - Advantage: Speed of exam
    - Disadvantage: Radiation dose, no hemodynamic data

MR Findings
- T1WI
  - "Black blood" imaging (cardiac-gated spin echo or double inversion recovery)
    - Sagittal oblique ("candy-cane") plane through aortic arch shows location of coarctation
    - Perpendicular views for cross-sectional diameter measurements
- T2* GRE
  - "White blood" imaging (cardiac-gated steady state free precession cine MR)

DDx: Coarctation, Left Ventricular Pressure Overload

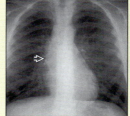
Aortic Valve Stenosis

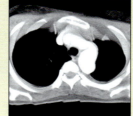
Pseudocoarctation

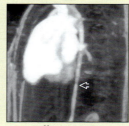
Diffuse Aortitis

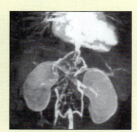
Abdominal Coarctation

AORTIC COARCTATION

Key Facts

Terminology
- Category: Acyanotic, normal heart size and pulmonary vascularity
- Hemodynamics: Left ventricular (LV) pressure overload

Imaging Findings
- Preductal (infantile)
- Juxtaductal or postductal (adult)
- Morphology: Simple (isolated coarctation in adult) or complex (associated with other cardiac anomalies, presenting in infancy)
- Echocardiography for primary diagnosis in infancy
- Older child: MR for pre-operative work-up and post-operative surveillance for re-coarctation, aneurysms
- Cardiac catheterization reserved for gradient measurement and intervention

Pathology
- In 50% associated with bicuspid aortic valve
- Focal shelf or waist lesion
- Diffuse narrowing of aortic isthmus

Clinical Issues
- Re-coarctation (< 3%, higher when operated in infancy)
- Post-operative aneurysms (24% after patch angioplasty)

Diagnostic Checklist
- Rib notching in asymptomatic individuals can be first clue to hemodynamically significant coarctation

---

- In sagittal oblique plane for anatomy, more reliable for diameters than black blood imaging
- Length of systolic (dark) flow jet correlates with hemodynamic significance
- Aortic regurgitation (bicuspid aortic valve)
- MRA
  - Velocity encoded phase-contrast MRA: For estimate of gradient, collateral flow and aortic valve regurgitation fraction
  - 3D Gadolinium-enhanced MRA: For anatomy and depiction of collaterals

Echocardiographic Findings
- Echocardiogram
  - Imaging of aortic arch and branches in suprasternal long axis view
  - Relationship of coarctation with patent ductus arteriosus (PDA)
- Pulsed Doppler: Estimate of gradient across coarctation

Angiographic Findings
- Conventional
  - Cardiac catheterization: Direct measurement of gradient
  - Intervention: Balloon angioplasty

Imaging Recommendations
- Protocol advice
  - Echocardiography for primary diagnosis in infancy
  - Older child: MR for pre-operative work-up and post-operative surveillance for re-coarctation, aneurysms
  - Cardiac catheterization reserved for gradient measurement and intervention

DIFFERENTIAL DIAGNOSIS

Hypoplastic left heart syndrome
- Congestive heart failure in newborn
- Hypoplastic LV
- Ductus-dependent systemic perfusion
- Retrograde flow in hypoplastic ascending aorta

Interrupted aortic arch
- Flow to descending aorta via PDA

Pseudocoarctation
- Elongation with kinking of aorta without obstruction

Takayasu arteritis
- Acquired inflammatory condition
- Acute phase: Aortic wall enhancement
- Chronic phase: Narrowing/occlusion of aorta and branch vessels

PATHOLOGY

General Features
- General path comments
  - In 50% associated with bicuspid aortic valve
  - Other associations: Ventricular septal defect (VSD, 33%), PDA (66%), transposition, subaortic and mitral stenosis ("parachute" deformity: Shone's syndrome), Taussig-Bing anomaly, endocardial fibro-elastosis
  - Embryology
    - Abnormal fetal hemodynamics (cardiac lesions that reduce left ventricular output and flow through aortic isthmus, e.g., VSD, hypoplastic left heart) can lead to preductal coarctation and diffuse hypoplasia of isthmus
  - Pathophysiology
    - Increase in systemic vascular resistance (LV afterload)
    - Hypertension due to renal hypoperfusion
    - Congestive heart failure (newborn, associated complex heart disease)
    - LV hypertrophy
    - Collaterals develop that bypass the stenosis (internal mammary, intercostal, epigastric)
- Genetics
  - Usually sporadic
  - Associated with Turner syndrome (20-36% have coarctation)

AORTIC COARCTATION

- Etiology
  - Two theories
    - Abnormal fetal hemodynamics (when associated with hypoplastic left heart or large VSD)
    - Postnatal contraction of fibrous ductal tissue in aortic wall at time of closure PDA
- Epidemiology
  - Incidence: 2-6 per 10,000 live births
  - More common in males (2:1), Caucasians
- Associated abnormalities
  - Berry aneurysms of circle of Willis
  - Scoliosis (in boys)

Gross Pathologic & Surgical Features
- Focal shelf or waist lesion
- Diffuse narrowing of aortic isthmus
- Post-stenotic dilatation of descending aorta

CLINICAL ISSUES

Presentation
- Most common signs/symptoms
  - Frequently asymptomatic, incidentally found
  - Infancy: Congestive heart failure (due to aortic arch interruption, associated anomalies)
  - Older child, adult: Hypertension, diminished femoral pulses, differential blood pressure between upper and lower extremities (arm-leg gradient)
- Other signs/symptoms: Bacterial endocarditis

Natural History & Prognosis
- Re-coarctation (< 3%, higher when operated in infancy)
- Post-operative aneurysms (24% after patch angioplasty)
- Long term survival decreased (late hypertension, coronary artery disease)

Treatment
- Resection and end-to-end anastomosis
- Interposition graft
- Prosthetic patch, subclavian flap aortoplasty
- Balloon angioplasty

DIAGNOSTIC CHECKLIST

Consider
- Diffuse hypoplasia of aortic isthmus, in addition to focal coarctation (important for surgical planning)

Image Interpretation Pearls
- Rib notching in asymptomatic individuals can be first clue to hemodynamically significant coarctation

SELECTED REFERENCES

1. Baum U et al: Multi-slice spiral CT imaging after surgical treatment of aortic coarctation. Eur Radiol. 15(2):353-5, 2005
2. Hager A et al: Follow-up of adults with coarctation of the aorta: comparison of helical CT and MRI, and impact on assessing diameter changes. Chest. 126(4):1169-76, 2004
3. Kinsara A et al: Noninvasive imaging modalities in coarctation of the aorta. Chest. 126(4):1016-8, 2004
4. Konen E et al: Coarctation of the aorta before and after correction: the role of cardiovascular MRI. AJR Am J Roentgenol. 182(5):1333-9, 2004
5. Smith Maia MM et al: Evolutional aspects of children and adolescents with surgically corrected aortic coarctation: clinical, echocardiographic, and magnetic resonance image analysis of 113 patients. J Thorac Cardiovasc Surg. 127(3):712-20, 2004
6. Araoz PA et al: MR findings of collateral circulation are more accurate measures of hemodynamic significance than arm-leg blood pressure gradient after repair of coarctation of the aorta. J Magn Reson Imaging. 17(2):177-83, 2003
7. Sebastia C et al: Aortic stenosis: spectrum of diseases depicted at multisection CT. Radiographics. 23 Spec No:S79-91, 2003
8. Godart F et al: Coarctation of the aorta: comparison of aortic dimensions between conventional MR imaging, 3D MR angiography, and conventional angiography. Eur Radiol. 12(8):2034-9, 2002
9. Haramati LB et al: MR imaging and CT of vascular anomalies and connections in patients with congenital heart disease: significance in surgical planning. Radiographics. 22(2):337-47; discussion 348-9, 2002
10. Holmqvist C et al: Collateral flow in coarctation of the aorta with magnetic resonance velocity mapping: correlation to morphological imaging of collateral vessels. J Magn Reson Imaging. 15(1):39-46, 2002
11. Rupprecht T et al: Determination of the pressure gradient in children with coarctation of the aorta by low-field magnetic resonance imaging. Pediatr Cardiol. 23(2):127-31, 2002
12. Gutberlet M et al: Quantification of morphologic and hemodynamic severity of coarctation of the aorta by magnetic resonance imaging. Cardiol Young. 11(5):512-20, 2001
13. Scholz TD et al: Aortic aneurysm following subclavian flap repair: diagnosis by magnetic resonance imaging. Pediatr Cardiol. 22(2):153-5, 2001
14. Bogaert J et al: Follow-up of patients with previous treatment for coarctation of the aorta: comparison between contrast-enhanced MR angiography and fast spin-echo MR imaging. Eur Radiol. 10:1847-54, 2000
15. Rocchini AP et al: Coarctation of the aorta and interrupted aortic arch. In: Moller JH, Hoffman JIE ed. Pediatric cardiovascular medicine, 1st ed. Philadelphia, Churchill Livingstone. 567-93, 2000
16. Riquelme C et al: MR imaging of coarctation of the aorta and its postoperative complications in adults: assessment with spin-echo and cine-MR imaging. Magn Reson Imaging. 17(1):37-46, 1999
17. Ho VB et al: Thoracic MR aortography: imaging techniques and strategies. Radiographics. 18(2):287-309, 1998
18. Julsrud PR et al: Coarctation of the aorta: collateral flow assessment with phase-contrast MR angiography. AJR Am J Roentgenol. 169(6):1735-42, 1997
19. Krinsky GA et al: Thoracic aorta: comparison of gadolinium-enhanced three-dimensional MR angiography with conventional MR imaging. Radiology. 202(1):183-93, 1997
20. Moresco KP et al: Abdominal aortic coarctation: CT, MRI, and angiographic correlation. Comput Med Imaging Graph. 19(5):427-30, 1995
21. Muhler EG et al: Evaluation of aortic coarctation after surgical repair: role of magnetic resonance imaging and Doppler ultrasound. Br Heart J. 70:285-90, 1993

AORTIC COARCTATION

IMAGE GALLERY

Typical

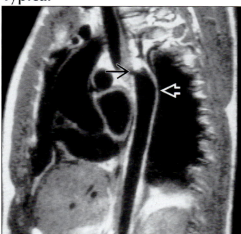
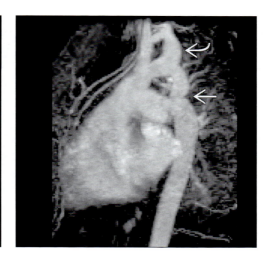

(Left) Sagittal oblique T1WI MR shows focal coarctation (arrow) distal to take-off of left subclavian artery (not shown) with post-stenotic dilatation of proximal descending aorta (open arrow). *(Right)* Sagittal oblique MRA shows shelf-like stenosis (arrow) at coarctation site, poststenotic dilatation of descending aorta, large caliber of subclavian artery (curved arrow), due to significant collateral flow.

Variant

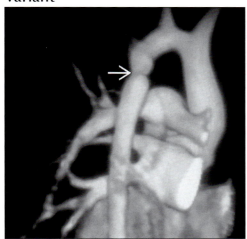
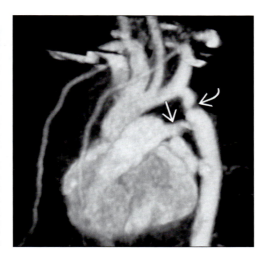

(Left) MRA, posterior oblique view of 3D volume rendition, shows diffuse hypoplasia of transverse aortic arch, with focal coarctation (arrow). *(Right)* Sagittal oblique CTA shows severe preductal coarctation (curved arrow). Note patent ductus arteriosus (arrow).

Variant

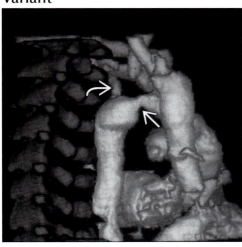
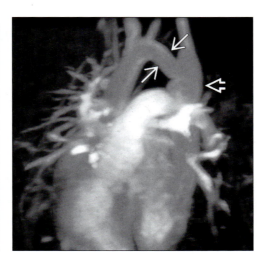

(Left) CTA, right lateral view of 3D surface rendition, shows focal narrowing (arrow) in transverse aortic arch, proximal to take-off of carotid arteries (curved arrow), indicative of pre-ductal coarctation in infant with complex cyanotic heart disease. *(Right)* Coronal oblique MRA in child with persistent hypertension after coarctation repair shows diffuse hypoplasia of aortic isthmus (arrows). Coarctation repair site (open arrow) is widely open.

AORTIC STENOSIS

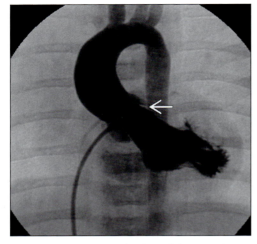

Anteroposterior angiography shows left ventriculogram in infant. Findings include thickened aortic valve leaflets (arrow), narrowed orifice, and post-stenotic dilatation of aorta.

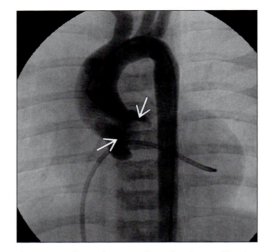

Anteroposterior catheter angiography shows dilatation of the ascending aorta, doming with restricted motion of aortic valve leaflets (arrows), and systolic ejection jet of unopacified blood.

TERMINOLOGY

Abbreviations and Synonyms
- Aortic stenosis (AS); aortic valvar stenosis; aortic valvular stenosis

Definitions
- Spectrum of aortic valve abnormalities which includes asymptomatic bicuspid aortic valve, or thickened and obstructing aortic valve stenosis, to severe neonatal aortic atresia and hypoplastic left heart
- Valvar stenosis is most common occurring in 80%

IMAGING FINDINGS

General Features
- Best diagnostic clue
  - Thickening valve leaflets with fusion
    - Bicuspid aortic valve is seen in 80%
    - Unicuspid aortic valve is seen in hypoplastic left heart, endocardial fibroelastosis
    - Quadracuspid is seen in truncal valves which may become stenotic or insufficient
  - High velocity jet of blood ejected into left ventricular outflow during systole
  - Post-stenotic dilation of the ascending aorta
  - Concentric left ventricular hypertrophy
- Location: Stenosis may be subvalvar, valvar (most common) or supravalvar
- Size: Valve annulus may be small for age, valve leaflets are thickened, commissures may be fused
- Morphology: Normal valve is tricuspid and mobile: Stenotic valve is usually thickened with restricted systolic motion

Radiographic Findings
- Radiography
  - Neonatal: Infants have normal chest or have mild cardiomegaly and edema
  - Childhood and adolescent: May have normal heart size even in severe AS
    - Dilatation of the ascending aorta due to jet phenomenon related to stenotic aortic valve
    - Following balloon valvotomy for treatment, the left ventricle may enlarge secondary to aortic regurgitation
    - Calcification of the valve is rare in childhood

CT Findings
- CTA
  - Rarely done for diagnosis as echocardiography is gold standard
  - Supravalvar stenosis (Williams syndrome) demonstrates concentric narrowing of ascending aorta

DDx: Dilatation Of Aorta

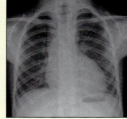
Hypertension

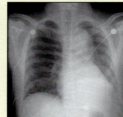
Marfan Disease

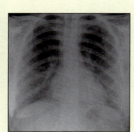
Coarctation

AORTIC STENOSIS

Key Facts

Terminology
- Aortic stenosis (AS); aortic valvar stenosis; aortic valvular stenosis
- Spectrum of aortic valve abnormalities which includes asymptomatic bicuspid aortic valve, or thickened and obstructing aortic valve stenosis, to severe neonatal aortic atresia and hypoplastic left heart
- Valvar stenosis is most common occurring in 80%

Imaging Findings
- Thickening valve leaflets with fusion
- Post-stenotic dilation of the ascending aorta
- Concentric left ventricular hypertrophy
- Location: Stenosis may be subvalvar, valvar (most common) or supravalvar
- Ventricular function can be qualitatively assessed on four chamber view and quantitatively assessed on a stack of short axis views
- Severity of stenosis and regurgitation can be evaluated
- 2D echocardiography is gold standard for making diagnosis in infants

Top Differential Diagnoses
- Rheumatic heart disease
- Marfan disease
- Systemic hypertension
- Ehlers-Danlos syndrome

Clinical Issues
- Severe stenosis > 55 mm usually treated with percutaneous balloon valvotomy

---

- May also have evidence of coarctation or pulmonary artery stenosis

MR Findings
- MR Cine
  - Ventricular function can be qualitatively assessed on four chamber view and quantitatively assessed on a stack of short axis views
  - Severity of stenosis and regurgitation can be evaluated
    - Evaluation of the flow jet: Signal loss caused by high velocity flow and turbulence
    - Assess valve motion: Abnormal motion of stenotic valve evaluated in a plane parallel to annulus
    - Evaluate thickening and bulging of valve leaflets
    - Secondary changes in chamber size and degree of wall thickening can be measured
    - Ventricular volumetric measurements can be made on several short-axis views of the ventricles and one can calculate the regurgitant fraction
    - Valvar regurgitation can be quantified by measuring the area or volume and the maximum length of the signal void in the receiving cavity, and the ratio of the area of the signal void to the area of the chamber receiving the regurgitant jet
  - Velocity encoded cine (VEC) MR imaging
    - Allows quantification of the transvalvar pressure gradient and valve area
    - Can quantify regurgitant fraction
    - Flow velocity maps across the valve can be generated
  - Calculation of regurgitant fraction and ventricular function can be followed on serial exams

Echocardiographic Findings
- 2D echocardiography is gold standard for making diagnosis in infants
  - In infants, important technique to assess the left ventricular function, aortic valve, gradient, and also for associated anomalies such as mitral insufficiency
- Doppler echocardiography
  - Systolic high velocity flow jet in the left ventricle outflow tract

Angiographic Findings
- Conventional
  - Cardiac catheterization is done for the purpose of interventional treatment with balloon valvotomy
  - Findings include: Thickened aortic valve, systolic flow jet into ascending aorta, enlarged ascending aorta and thickened left ventricle

DIFFERENTIAL DIAGNOSIS

Rheumatic heart disease
- Multisystem disease with fever, rash, carditis and valvular disease

Marfan disease
- Connective tissue disorder associated with aneurysmal dilation of the ascending aorta

Coarctation of the aorta
- May have dilation of aorta proximal to narrowing
- In infants, 75% may have associated bicuspid valve

Systemic hypertension
- Left ventricular hypertrophy and prominent ascending aorta

Ehlers-Danlos syndrome
- Connective tissue disease which is associated with aneurysmal dilation of large vessels

PATHOLOGY

General Features
- General path comments: Thickening of the aortic valve leaflets
- Genetics
  - Bicuspid aortic valve is one of most common congenital malformations
  - Williams syndrome is chromosomal abnormality of 7q11.2 and is autosomal dominant

AORTIC STENOSIS

- Epidemiology: Occurs in 3-6% of children with congenital cardiac defects
- Associated abnormalities
  - Endocarditis occurs in 4%
  - Williams syndrome: Associated with supravalvar aortic stenosis and pulmonary artery stenosis
  - Coarctation of the aorta: Associated with bicuspid aortic valve and aortic stenosis

Staging, Grading or Classification Criteria
- Grading of aortic stenosis
  - Mild has gradient of 25 mmHg or less
  - Moderate has gradient between 25-55 mmHg
  - Severe has gradient > than 55 mmHg
- Classification of aortic stenosis
  - Subvalvar is a membrane which partially obstructs left ventricular outflow
  - Valvar is the most common and occurs in 90% of cases
  - Supravalvar which is concentric narrowing in the ascending aorta

CLINICAL ISSUES

Presentation
- Most common signs/symptoms
  - Neonatal: Signs of poor or low cardiac output with tachypnea and feeding problems
  - Childhood: Usually asymptomatic but may have systolic murmur or suprasternal thrill
    - If prior valvotomy, there will be dilation of ascending aorta and large left ventricle secondary to aortic regurgitation (AR)
    - Sudden death which usually occurs during exercise
    - Children with Williams syndrome recognized due to multiple manifestations of disease

Demographics
- Age: 10-20% in the first year of life
- Gender: M: F = 4:1

Natural History & Prognosis
- Infants with critical aortic stenosis may be diagnosed in utero
  - Mortality relates to degree of stenosis, symptomatic less than 30 days and lower birth weights
    - Hypoplastic left heart has highest mortality
    - Endocardial fibroelastosis with decreased left ventricular outflow
    - Coronary blood flow to subendocardium reduced and ischemia may occur
- Children with aortic stenosis constitute 3-5% of all congenital heart defects
  - Usually stenosis progresses and 20% have associated lesions
  - 1% of sudden death is thought to be related to undetected AS
  - Once balloon valvotomy occurs, children will have both residual AS and AR

Treatment
- In infants, aortic stenosis may be part of the spectrum of hypoplastic left heart syndrome (HLHS)
  - Treatment with prostaglandin to maintain ductal patency
  - May need balloon atrial septostomy or Rashkind procedure with Staged Norwood procedure
  - Occasionally treated with heart transplant
- In infants, with "critical" aortic stenosis
  - Percutaneous balloon valvotomy is urgent treatment but infant may have aortic regurgitation
  - Surgical procedure called the Ross procedure is also done when valvotomy not adequate or regurgitation is moderate
    - Native pulmonary valve placed in aortic position and homograph placed for pulmonary valve
- In children, depends on degree of obstruction and progression
  - Mild stenosis is 25 mmHg and can be monitored with echocardiogram, EKG
  - Moderate stenosis 25-55 mmHg and 40% will require valvotomy
  - Severe stenosis > 55 mm usually treated with percutaneous balloon valvotomy
- Surgical aortic valvotomy
  - Performed for supravalvar aortic stenosis, resection of subaortic membrane, enlargement of aortic annulus
  - Mechanical valves usually need anticoagulation which is an issue in normal children
- Replacement of the aortic valve with the pulmonary valve (autograph) or Ross procedure
  - Pulmonary valve replaced with homograft or reconstruction with conduit
  - Indicated in peak to peak gradients > 70 mm and where valvotomy has failed
- All children need prophylaxis to prevent bacterial endocarditis

SELECTED REFERENCES

1. Alphonso N: Midterm results of the Ross procedure. Eur J Cardiothorac Surg. 25(6):925-30, 2004
2. Brown JW et al: Surgery for aortic stenosis in children: a 40-year experience. Ann Thorac Surg. 76(5):1398-411, 2003
3. Glockner JF et al: Evaluation of cardiac valvular disease with MR imaging: qualitative and quantitative techniques. Radiographics. 23(1):e9, 2003
4. Lupinetti FM et al: Comparison of autograft and allograft aortic valve replacement in children. J Thorac Cardiovasc Surg. 126(1):240-6, 2003
5. Al-Halees Z et al: The Ross procedure is the procedure of choice for congenital aortic valve disease. J Thorac Cardiovasc Surg. 123(3):437-41; discussion 441-2, 2002
6. Didier D et al: Detection and quantification of valvular heart disease with dynamic cardiac MR imaging. Radiographics. 20(5):1279-99; discussion 1299-301, 2000
7. Egito ES et al: Transvascular balloon dilation for neonatal critical aortic stenosis: early and midterm results. J Am Coll Cardiol. 29(2):442-7, 1997

AORTIC STENOSIS

IMAGE GALLERY

Typical

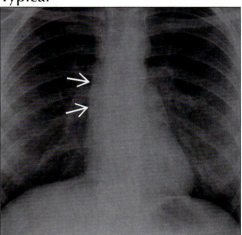
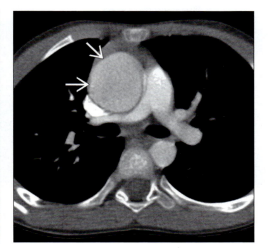

(Left) Anteroposterior radiograph of chest demonstrates convex appearance to right mediastinum which suggests dilation of ascending aorta *(arrows)* secondary to aortic valvar stenosis. *(Right)* Axial CECT shows post-stenotic dilation of ascending aorta *(arrows)* in this adolescent with aortic valvar stenosis. Note discrepancy in size of main pulmonary artery and ascending aorta.

Typical

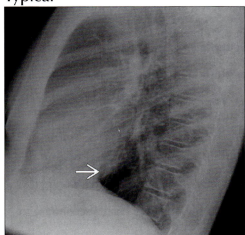
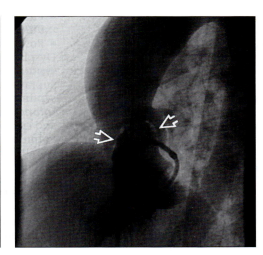

(Left) Lateral radiograph of chest demonstrating cardiac enlargement posterior to inferior vena cava *(arrow)* which is suggestive in children of left ventricular enlargement or hypertrophy. *(Right)* Angiography shows catheter in left ventricular injection via foramen ovale with thickened aortic valve leaflets *(arrows)*, doming of aortic valve, and post-stenotic dilation of ascending aorta.

Typical

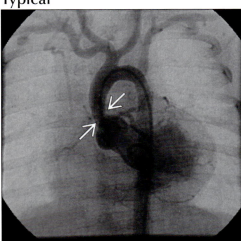
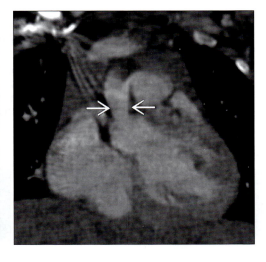

(Left) Anteroposterior angiography shows thickened left ventricular wall, normal AV, and concentric narrowing of the initial portion of ascending aorta *(arrows)*. Child has Williams syndrome. *(Right)* Coronal CTA shows supravalvar narrowing of ascending aorta *(arrows)* in six year old child with Williams syndrome. Note that narrowing is not discrete and involves origin of coronary arteries.

PULMONARY ARTERY STENOSIS

- Alagille syndrome is autosomal dominant related to mutations on chromosome 20p12
  - Pulmonic valve and peripheral stenosis associated with cholestatic jaundice in infancy
  - Butterfly vertebrae, abnormal facies, mental retardation, eye, renal anomalies
- Etiology
  - Pulmonary valvar stenosis is congenital anomaly
    - Maldevelopment of the pulmonary valve tissue and distal portion of the bulbus cordis
- Associated abnormalities
  - Most children are normal without any other lesions
  - Can be associated with other common congenital lesions in 10%
    - Infundibular stenosis and ventricular septal defect (VSD) in tetralogy of Fallot
    - Atrial septal defect, patent ductus arteriosus
    - Complex cardiac lesions
  - Williams syndrome
    - Supravalvar aortic stenosis, supravalvar PS, peripheral stenosis, coarctation
  - Noonan syndrome
    - Dysplastic pulmonary valve
  - Alagille syndrome
    - Pulmonary stenosis with multiple peripheral artery stenosis

Gross Pathologic & Surgical Features
- Valve thickened with fused commissure

Microscopic Features
- Valve thickened with fibrous, myxomatous, and collagenous tissue
- Noonan patients have excess tissue associated with the valve

Staging, Grading or Classification Criteria
- Pulmonary valvar stenosis; mild, moderate, severe
- Noonan syndrome has dysplastic pulmonary valve
- Alagille syndrome has PS and peripheral pulmonary artery stenosis
- Williams syndrome has supravalvar stenosis

CLINICAL ISSUES

Presentation
- Most common signs/symptoms
  - Mild stenosis: Usually asymptomatic with systolic ejection murmur
  - Moderate stenosis: Exertional dyspnea, easy fatigability
  - Infants may present with severe cyanosis
    - Decreased pulmonary flow, increased right ventricular pressure, tricuspid regurgitation and shunting from right atrium to left atrium
- Other signs/symptoms: Loud systolic ejection murmur and click at left upper heart border

Demographics
- Age
  - Critical pulmonic stenosis occurs in newborns
  - PS diagnosed 2-6 years during routine physical exam
- Gender: M = F

Natural History & Prognosis
- Critical pulmonic stenosis in infancy will progress and can be fatal if not treated
- Pulmonary valvar stenosis with mild gradient does not usually progress
  - Children have normal life expectancy
- Pulmonary valvar stenosis which is moderate will progress
  - Clinically well tolerated
  - After valvotomy, may have pulmonary insufficiency which is usually tolerated
- Mortality depends on the severity of lesions but mild to moderate have normal life expectancy

Treatment
- Observation medical management for mild valvar stenosis gradients less than 25 mmHg
- Balloon valvuloplasty is treatment of choice for moderate to severe gradients > 50 mmHg
  - Balloon catheter placed over wire
  - Balloon dilated greater than estimated pulmonary valve annulus while straddling valve
  - Long term decrease in right ventricular pressure and estimated gradient
  - Hemodynamically insignificant pulmonary insufficiency may occur in 80%
  - Recurrence of PS happens in 15% at ten years
  - Excellent outcome with survival similar to general population
  - Balloon valvotomy not as effective in dysplastic valves which may need surgery
- Angioplasty is done for branch stenosis
- Newborns with severe or critical pulmonic stenosis
  - May need immediate valvotomy
  - Prostaglandin for ductus arteriosus flow
  - Surgical valvotomy or palliative Blalock-Taussig shunt
  - Lesion may be associated with hypoplasia of right ventricle needing univentricular repair

DIAGNOSTIC CHECKLIST

Image Interpretation Pearls
- Normal adolescent has a prominent pulmonary artery

SELECTED REFERENCES

1. Braundwald E: Valvular Heart Disease. In: Braundwald E. Heart Disease: A Textbook of Cardiovascular Medicine. 6th ed W.B. Saunders Company, Philadelphia. 2001
2. Latson LA et al: Heart Disease in Infants, Children and Adolescents. Sixth edition, Lippincott Williams & Wilkins, Philadelphia. 820-43, 2001
3. Rao PS: Pulmonary Valve Disease. In: Alpert JS, Dalen JE and Rahimtoola SH (eds): Valvular Heart Disease. 3rd ed. Lippincott William and Wilkins, Philadelphia. 2000
4. Anand R et al: Natural history of asymptomatic valvar pulmonary stenosis diagnosed in infancy. Clin Cardiol. 20(4):377-80, 1997
5. Hayes CJ et al: Second natural history study of congenital heart defects. Results of treatment of patients with pulmonary valvar stenosis. Circulation. 87(2 Suppl):I28-37, 1993

PULMONARY ARTERY STENOSIS

IMAGE GALLERY

Typical

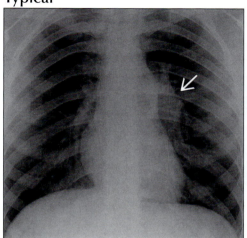
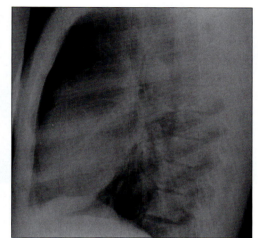

(Left) Anteroposterior radiograph shows post-stenotic dilatation of main pulmonary artery secondary to valvar pulmonic stenosis. The left pulmonary artery (arrow) is larger than the right due to direction of jet. *(Right)* Lateral radiograph shows nonprominence of pulmonary hila.

Typical

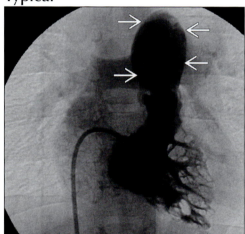
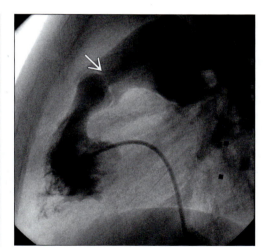

(Left) Anteroposterior angiography with contrast injection into trabeculated right ventricle demonstrates thickened valved leaflets and prominent post-stenotic dilatation of main pulmonary artery (arrows). *(Right)* Lateral angiography demonstrates doming of valve, thickening of leaflets, and narrowing of the orifice (arrow), and post-stenotic dilation of main pulmonary artery.

Variant

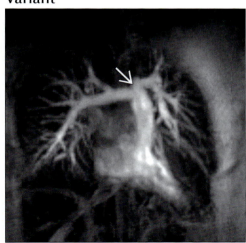
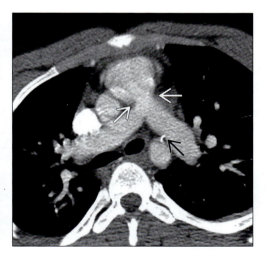

(Left) Coronal MRA in child with Alagille syndrome who had stenosis at the origin of the left pulmonary artery (arrow) and mild left peripheral stenosis. *(Right)* Axial CECT shows supravalvar narrowing (white arrows) of main pulmonary artery in 9 year old child with Williams syndrome. Incidental calcification of ligamentum arteriosum is seen (black arrow).

OPERATIVE CHD PROCEDURES

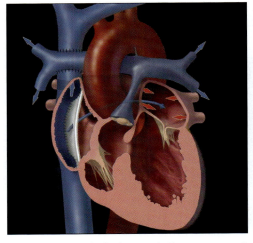

Graphic shows right bi-directional Glenn anastomosis and intra-atrial tunnel Fontan conduit with fenestration, placed in functionally univentricular heart (tricuspid atresia with ventricular septal defect).

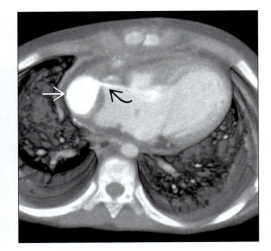

Axial CTA shows dense opacification of lateral tunnel Fontan conduit (arrow) with fenestration (curved arrow) toward common atrium, allowing decompression of elevated central venous pressure.

TERMINOLOGY

Definitions
- Pulmonary artery (PA) banding: Palliative procedure to decrease pulmonary perfusion in left → right shunt lesions, when definitive repair is not yet feasible
- Blalock-Taussig (BT) shunt: For initial palliation of cyanotic lesions with decreased pulmonary flow
  - Aortopulmonary shunt (high → low pressure): Size and length determine pressure drop
  - Performed via lateral thoracotomy
  - Classic BT shunt: Subclavian artery is ligated and connected end-to-side to ipsilateral PA
    - On side opposite aortic arch, to avoid kinking
    - Collaterals develop to ipsilateral upper extremity → unilateral rib notching
  - Modified BT shunt: Gore-Tex tube is interposed between subclavian and ipsilateral PA
    - Can be performed on either side
    - No compromise of upper extremity perfusion
  - Central shunt: Aorta to PA conduit, alternative to BT
- Glenn shunt: In complex cyanotic heart disease, as initial stage of Fontan operation
  - Cavopulmonary anastomosis (low pressure), performed via median sternotomy
    - Decreases volume load on single ventricle
    - Can be unilateral or bilateral [in case of bilateral superior vena cava (SVC)]
    - Can be unidirectional or (most often) bidirectional (i.e., perfuses both PAs)
  - Hemi-Fontan: Variation of Glenn, with temporary occlusion patch between right atrium and right PA
  - Kawashima operation: For azygos continuation Inferior vena cava (IVC)
    - (Hemi-)azygos vein is incorporated in cavopulmonary anastomosis
- Fontan: In complex heart disease, not suitable for bi-ventricular repair (single ventricle physiology)
  - IVC → right PA shunt
  - Classic Fontan: Anastomosis between right atrial appendage and right PA (for tricuspid atresia)
  - Intra-atrial lateral tunnel Fontan: Gore-Tex shunt
    - With fenestration, which serves as pop-off valve for elevated central venous pressures
    - Can be closed later with occluder device
  - Extra-cardiac conduit from IVC to right PA
- Mustard/Senning: Venous switch for L-transposition of the great arteries (TGA)
  - Mustard: Intra-atrial pericardial baffle redirects blood from right atrium to left ventricle (LV) and from left atrium to right ventricle (RV)
  - Senning: Flap fashioned from atrial septum redirects systemic and pulmonary venous blood to LV and RV
- Jatene: Arterial switch for L-TGA
  - Coronary arteries are also transposed

DDx: Systemic To Pulmonary Artery Shunts

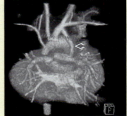
BT Shunt

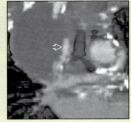
BT Shunt, Seroma

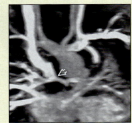
Glenn Shunt

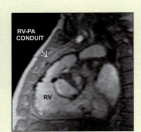
Rastelli Conduit

OPERATIVE CHD PROCEDURES

Key Facts

Terminology
- Blalock-Taussig (BT) shunt: For initial palliation of cyanotic lesions with decreased pulmonary flow
- Glenn shunt: In complex cyanotic heart disease, as initial stage of Fontan operation
- Fontan: In complex heart disease, not suitable for bi-ventricular repair (single ventricle physiology)
- Mustard/Senning: Venous switch for L-transposition of the great arteries (TGA)
- Jatene: Arterial switch for L-TGA
- Norwood: For hypoplastic left heart syndrome (HLHS)
- Rastelli: RV to PA conduit

Imaging Findings
- CTA is most versatile modality for post-op patients
- Short-axis cine MRI for calculation of ventricular volumes, ejection fraction, regurgitation fractions
- To determine suitability for biventricular versus univentricular (Fontan) repair
- For RV function after repair for tetralogy of Fallot, L-TGA, venous switch for D-TGA, Ebstein
- To study hemodynamic (in-)efficiency and thrombosis after Fontan or atrial baffle procedures
- PA anastomotic/conduit stenosis: Balloon dilatation, stent placement
- Image-guided percutaneous drainage of post-operative seromas after BT shunt placement

Pathology
- Adult congenital heart disease (ACHD) represents an increasing category of patients

---

  - Complication: Stretching of pulmonary artery branches, major airway compression
- LeCompte: For TGA with ventricular septal defect (VSD) and pulmonary stenosis
  - Tunnel connecting LV to aorta, closure VSD, connection PA to RV using pericardial patch
  - Avoids complications of Rastelli conduit
- Norwood: For hypoplastic left heart syndrome (HLHS)
  - Stage 1: Connection of main PA to descending aorta, side-to-side anastomosis of PA to hypoplastic aorta
    - BT shunt for PA perfusion
    - Sano shunt: RV → PA confluence (less PA overcirculation and better coronary flow than BT)
  - Stage 2: Take-down of BT shunt; creation of cavopulmonary (Glenn or hemi-Fontan) shunt
  - Stage 3: Completion of Fontan operation
- Damus-Kay-Stansel: Side-to-side anastomosis between ascending aorta and main PA, in selected cases of TGA and single ventricle with LV outflow tract obstruction
- Ross-Konno: In selected cases of aortic stenosis
  - Aortic valve replaced by patient's pulmonary valve
  - Pulmonary valve is substituted by valved conduit
- Rastelli: RV to PA conduit
  - For right ventricular outflow tract obstructive lesions
    - Pulmonary atresia, VSD, aortopulmonary collaterals
    - Tetralogy of Fallot
    - TGA with VSD and pulmonary stenosis
- Cardiac transplantation: For HLHS, end-stage CHD
  - More complicated in CHD patients: Abnormal situs, transposition, scarring from prior surgeries
  - Need for life-long immunosuppression
  - When pulmonary hypertension: Prognosis guarded

IMAGING FINDINGS

CT Findings
- CTA
  - CTA is most versatile modality for post-op patients
    - Generally no need for sedation
    - Fast, can be done on unstable post-op patients
    - Unlike MRI, patient monitoring equipment does not interfere with imaging procedure
    - Less affected by metal artifact (stents, coils, surgical clips and wires) than MRI
    - Depicts pulmonary and pleural disease, tracheobronchial compression by dilated vessels
    - 3D renditions very helpful to convey complex post-op findings to referring clinicians
- Specific indications
  - Patency of vascular conduits (BT, Glenn shunts)
  - Fontan patients: Flow admixture from upper/lower flow, may simulate thrombosis
    - Simultaneous upper and lower extremity injection

MR Findings
- T1WI
  - Double inversion recovery sequences are most helpful to minimize metal artifacts
  - Multiplanar imaging to demonstrate course of vascular conduits (BT shunts)
  - Evaluation for branch PA stenosis following Jatene
- T2* GRE
  - Short-axis cine MRI for calculation of ventricular volumes, ejection fraction, regurgitation fractions
    - To determine suitability for biventricular versus univentricular (Fontan) repair
    - For RV function after repair for tetralogy of Fallot, L-TGA, venous switch for D-TGA, Ebstein
    - To study hemodynamic (in-)efficiency and thrombosis after Fontan or atrial baffle procedures
    - Exercise and/or Dobutamine stress testing
- MRA
  - Flow measurements with phase contrast MRA to characterize Fontan hemodynamics
    - Inefficient "seesaw" pattern of flow in lateral tunnel Fontans, not in extracardiac conduits

Angiographic Findings
- Cardiovascular interventions
  - PA anastomotic/conduit stenosis: Balloon dilatation, stent placement
    - Common location: Adjacent to insertion BT shunt
    - Stenotic unifocalized aortopulmonary collaterals

OPERATIVE CHD PROCEDURES

- Stenosis of Rastelli conduits
- Transcatheter occlusion of modified BT shunts

Non-Vascular Interventions
- Image-guided percutaneous drainage of post-operative seromas after BT shunt placement
  - Progressive mediastinal widening
  - Airway and vascular/conduit compression
  - Can be diagnosed with ultrasound or CT

Nuclear Medicine Findings
- Lung perfusion scan: Differential lung uptake after Glenn and/or Fontan operations
  - Systemic uptake: Pulmonary arteriovenous fistulae

PATHOLOGY

General Features
- Epidemiology
  - Adult congenital heart disease (ACHD) represents an increasing category of patients
    - Increased survival in many congenital lesions
    - Need for repeated imaging procedures, catheterizations, re-operations, life-time follow-up
    - With new developments in cross-sectional cardiac imaging (CTA, MRI), radiologists should become more involved in multidisciplinary ACHD care

Staging, Grading or Classification Criteria
- Three ACHD patient groups with different prognoses
  - Those who have undergone complete repair
  - Those with uncorrected defects, presenting late
  - Those who underwent palliative procedures

CLINICAL ISSUES

Presentation
- Most common signs/symptoms
  - Sequelae of CHD: Arrhythmias, polycythemia, subacute bacterial endocarditis, conduit stenosis/infection, heart failure, pulmonary hypertension, stroke, hemoptysis, RV dysfunction
  - Residuals of CHD: Persistent VSD, valvular leaks, (re-)coarctation, aneurysms, collaterals, complications of Fontan and venous switch (baffle obstruction, systemic venous hypertension, thrombosis, protein losing enteropathy)
- Other signs/symptoms: Pregnancy-related complications, renal dysfunction, side effects of anticoagulation and immune suppression (post-transplant lymphoproliferative disease)

Natural History & Prognosis
- 70-75% of patients with CHD now reach adulthood

SELECTED REFERENCES
1. Garg R et al: Effects of metallic implants on magnetic resonance imaging evaluation of Fontan palliation. Am J Cardiol. 95(5):688-91, 2005
2. Greenberg SB et al: Magnetic resonance flow analysis of classic and extracardiac Fontan procedures: the seesaw sign. Int J Cardiovasc Imaging. 20(5):397-405; discussion 407-8, 2004
3. Laffon E et al: Quantitative MRI comparison of systemic hemodynamics in Mustard/Senning repaired patients and healthy volunteers at rest. Eur Radiol. 14(5):875-80, 2004
4. Connolly BL et al: Early mediastinal seroma secondary to modified Blalock-Taussig shunts--successful management by percutaneous drainage. Pediatr Radiol. 33(7):495-8, 2003
5. Eicken A et al: Hearts late after fontan operation have normal mass, normal volume, and reduced systolic function: a magnetic resonance imaging study. J Am Coll Cardiol. 42(6):1061-5, 2003
6. Hillman ND et al: Adult congenital heart disease. In: Mavroudis C, Backer CL ed. Pediatric cardiac surgery. 3rd ed. Philadelphia, Mosby. 818-47, 2003
7. Hjortdal VE et al: Effects of exercise and respiration on blood flow in total cavopulmonary connection: a real-time magnetic resonance flow study. Circulation. 108(10):1227-31, 2003
8. Hornung TS et al: Comparison of equilibrium radionuclide ventriculography with cardiovascular magnetic resonance for assessing the systemic right ventricle after Mustard or Senning procedures for complete transposition of the great arteries. Am J Cardiol. 92(5):640-3, 2003
9. Jacobs ML et al: The functional single ventricle and Fontan's operation. In: Mavroudis C, Backer CL ed. Pediatric cardiac surgery. 3rd ed. Philadelphia, Mosby. 496-523, 2003
10. Okada M et al: Modified Blalock-Taussig shunt patency for pulmonary atresia: assessment with electron beam CT. J Comput Assist Tomogr. 26(3):368-72, 2002
11. Tulevski II et al: Usefulness of magnetic resonance imaging dobutamine stress in asymptomatic and minimally symptomatic patients with decreased cardiac reserve from congenital heart disease (complete and corrected transposition of the great arteries and subpulmonic obstruction). Am J Cardiol. 89(9):1077-81, 2002
12. van Rijn RR et al: Development of a perigraft seroma around modified Blalock-Taussig shunts: imaging evaluation. AJR Am J Roentgenol. 178(3):629-33, 2002
13. Fogel MA et al: A simplified approach for assessment of intracardiac baffles and extracardiac conduits in congenital heart surgery with two- and three-dimensional magnetic resonance imaging. Am Heart J. 142(6):1028-36, 2001
14. Wang JK et al: Balloon angioplasty for obstructed modified systemic-pulmonary artery shunts and pulmonary artery stenoses. J Am Coll Cardiol. 37(3):940-7, 2001
15. Somerville J et al: Cardiac problems of adults with congenital heart disease. In: Moller JH, Hoffman JIE ed. Pediatric cardiovascular medicine, 1st ed. Philadelphia, Churchill Livingstone. 687-705, 2000
16. Fogel MA et al: Caval contribution to flow in the branch pulmonary arteries of Fontan patients with a novel application of magnetic resonance presaturation pulse. Circulation. 99(9):1215-21, 1999
17. Be'eri E et al: In vivo evaluation of Fontan pathway flow dynamics by multidimensional phase-velocity magnetic resonance imaging. Circulation. 98(25):2873-82, 1998
18. Seliem MA et al: Lung perfusion patterns after bidirectional cavopulmonary anastomosis (Hemi-Fontan procedure). Pediatr Cardiol. 18(3):191-6, 1997
19. Fogel MA et al: Late ventricular geometry and performance changes of functional single ventricle throughout staged Fontan reconstruction assessed by magnetic resonance imaging. J Am Coll Cardiol. 28(1):212-21, 1996
20. Rebergen SA et al: MR velocity mapping of tricuspid flow in healthy children and in patients who have undergone Mustard or Senning repair. Radiology. 194(2):505-12, 1995
21. Blakenberg F et al: MRI vs echocardiography in the evaluation of the Jatene procedure. J Comput Assist Tomogr. 18(5):749-54, 1994

OPERATIVE CHD PROCEDURES

IMAGE GALLERY

Typical

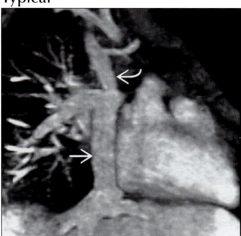
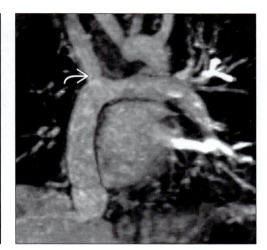

(Left) Coronal MRA shows extracardiac Fontan conduit (arrow), connecting inferior vena cava to right pulmonary artery. A cavopulmonary (Glenn) shunt is also noted (curved arrow). *(Right)* Coronal MRA shows connection of Fontan conduit to left pulmonary artery, and right-sided Glenn shunt (curved arrow). (Courtesy L. Sena, MD).

Typical

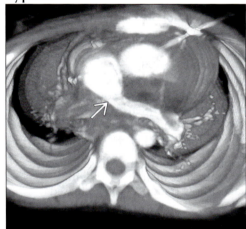
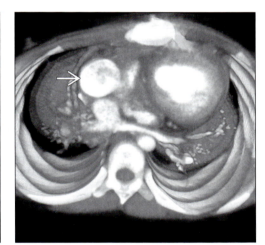

(Left) Axial CTA shows connection between Fontan conduit and left pulmonary artery (arrow). *(Right)* Axial CTA at a slightly lower level demonstrates artifact from flow admixture and turbulence within Fontan conduit (arrow), simulating thrombus.

Typical

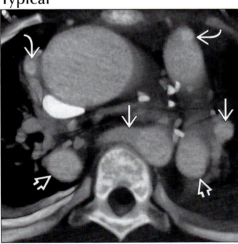
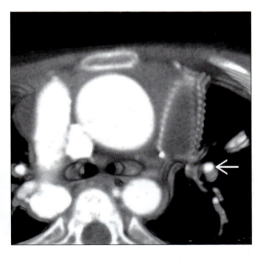

(Left) Axial CTA shows bilateral pericardial tube unifocalizations (open arrows) of aortopulmonary collaterals (arrows). Note Blalock-Taussig shunts (curved arrows) perfusing neo-pulmonary artery conduits. *(Right)* Axial CTA shows thrombosed Gore-Tex graft of left unifocalization conduit, with normal enhancement of intrapulmonary branches (arrow). Right-sided conduit is normally patent. Thrombosed conduit was successfully repaired.

RIGHT VENTRICULAR DYSPLASIA

- Typical EKG abnormalities
  - Epsilon waves: Small depolarizations at the beginning of the ST segment
  - T-wave inversions in early precordial leads V1-V3
- Biopsy showing fibrofatty infiltration
  - Sampling errors are common, since biopsies taken from thinned anterior wall are risky, and are therefore taken from septum, which is infrequently involved
- Gold standard: Autopsy

CLINICAL ISSUES

Presentation
- Most common signs/symptoms
  - Ventricular arrhythmias: Ventricular tachycardia with left bundle branch block morphology
  - Syncope
  - Sudden death
    - 3-4% of sudden deaths in young athletes in U.S.
    - Most common cause of sudden death in young athletes in Italy
- Other signs/symptoms: Heart failure: Isolated RV or biventricular

Demographics
- Age: Up to 5% of sudden deaths in young individuals < 45 years in the U.S.
- Gender: M:F = 2.7:1

Treatment
- Avoid vigorous athletics
- In the absence of arrhythmias, beta blocker therapy
- Catheter ablation
- Implantable cardioverter defibrillator
  - In patients with a history of ventricular tachyarrhythmia, cardiac arrest, or syncope
  - Antiarrhythmics may be needed for repeated discharges

SELECTED REFERENCES

1. Tandri H et al: Noninvasive detection of myocardial fibrosis in arrhythmogenic right ventricular cardiomyopathy using delayed-enhancement magnetic resonance imaging. J Am Coll Cardiol. 45(1):98-103, 2005
2. Abbara S et al: Value of fat suppression in the MRI evaluation of suspected arrhythmogenic right ventricular dysplasia. AJR Am J Roentgenol. 182(3):587-91, 2004
3. Bomma C et al: Misdiagnosis of arrhythmogenic right ventricular dysplasia/cardiomyopathy. J Cardiovasc Electrophysiol. 15(3):300-6, 2004
4. Castillo E et al: Arrhythmogenic right ventricular dysplasia: ex vivo and in vivo fat detection with black-blood MR imaging. Radiology. 232(1):38-48, 2004
5. Stevenson I et al: Magnetic resonance imaging in the diagnosis of arrhythmogenic right ventricular cardiomyopathy: the gold standard or just another imaging modality? J Interv Card Electrophysiol. 10(1):27-9, 2004
6. Tandri H et al: Magnetic resonance and computed tomography imaging of arrhythmogenic right ventricular dysplasia. J Magn Reson Imaging. 19(6):848-58, 2004
7. Tandri H et al: MRI of arrhythmogenic right ventricular cardiomyopathy/dysplasia. J Cardiovasc Magn Reson. 6(2):557-63, 2004
8. White JB et al: Relative utility of magnetic resonance imaging and right ventricular angiography to diagnose arrhythmogenic right ventricular cardiomyopathy. J Interv Card Electrophysiol. 10(1):19-26, 2004
9. Aviram G et al: MR evaluation of arrhythmogenic right ventricular cardiomyopathy in pediatric patients. AJR Am J Roentgenol. 180(4):1135-41, 2003
10. Bluemke DA et al: MR Imaging of arrhythmogenic right ventricular cardiomyopathy: morphologic findings and interobserver reliability. Cardiology. 99(3):153-62, 2003
11. Boxt LM et al: MR imaging of arrhythmogenic right ventricular dysplasia. Magn Reson Imaging Clin N Am. 11(1):163-71, 2003
12. Harper KW et al: Prediction rule for diagnosis of arrhythmogenic right ventricular dysplasia based on wall thickness measured on MR imaging. Comput Med Imaging Graph. 27(5):363-71, 2003
13. Kayser HW et al: Usefulness of magnetic resonance imaging in diagnosis of arrhythmogenic right ventricular dysplasia and agreement with electrocardiographic criteria. Am J Cardiol. 91(3):365-7, 2003
14. Keller DI et al: Arrhythmogenic right ventricular cardiomyopathy: diagnostic and prognostic value of the cardiac MRI in relation to arrhythmia-free survival. Int J Cardiovasc Imaging. 19(6):537-43; discussion 545-7, 2003
15. Tandri H et al: Controversial role of magnetic resonance imaging in the diagnosis of arrhythmogenic right ventricular dysplasia. Am J Cardiol. 92(5):649, 2003
16. Tandri H et al: Magnetic resonance imaging findings in patients meeting task force criteria for arrhythmogenic right ventricular dysplasia. J Cardiovasc Electrophysiol. 14(5):476-82, 2003
17. van der Wall EE et al: MR imaging in arrhythmogenic right ventricular dysplasia/cardiomyopathy. Int J Cardiovasc Imaging. 19(6):549-52, 2003
18. Kayser HWM et al: Diagnosis of arrhythmogenic right ventricular dysplasia: a review. Radiographics. May-Jun;22(3):639-48, 2002
19. McCaffrey F: Around pediheart: right ventricular dysplasia. Pediatr Cardiol. 22(4):320, 2001
20. Midiri M et al: MR imaging of arrhythmogenic right ventricular dysplasia. Int J Cardiovasc Imaging. 17(4):297-304, 2001
21. Immer FF et al: Images in cardiology. Visualising fatty deposits in familial arrhythmogenic right ventricular cardiomyopathy by magnetic resonance imaging. Heart. 84(1):52, 2000
22. Schick F et al: Fat- and water-selective MR cine imaging of the human heart: assessment of right ventricular dysplasia. Invest Radiol. 35(5):311-8, 2000
23. White RD et al: Right ventricular arrhythmia in the absence of arrhythmogenic dysplasia: MR imaging of myocardial abnormalities. Radiology. 207(3):743-51, 1998
24. Blake LM et al: MR features of arrhythmogenic right ventricular dysplasia. AJR Am J Roentgenol. 162(4):809-12, 1994
25. McKenna WJ et al: Diagnosis of arrhythmogenic right ventricular dysplasia/cardiomyopathy. Task Force of the Working Group Myocardial and Pericardial Disease of the European Society of Cardiology and of the Scientific Council on Cardiomyopathies of the International Society and Federation of Cardiology. Br Heart J. 71(3):215-8, 1994
26. Hamada S et al: Arrhythmogenic right ventricular dysplasia: evaluation with electron-beam CT. Radiology. 187(3):723-7, 1993
27. Dery R et al: Cine-computed tomography of arrhythmogenic right ventricular dysplasia. J Comput Assist Tomogr. 10(1):120-3, 1986

RIGHT VENTRICULAR DYSPLASIA

IMAGE GALLERY

Typical

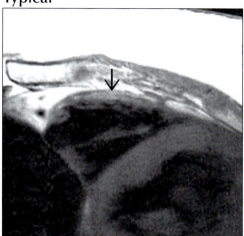
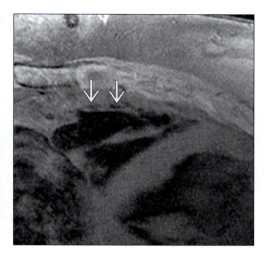

(Left) Axial T1WI MR shows diffuse fatty infiltration and thinning of right ventricular free wall (arrow). *(Right)* Axial T1WI MR shows decrease in signal intensity of some but not all areas on corresponding fat suppressed image (arrows), due to mixture of fibrous and fatty myocardial infiltration. (Courtesy F. Holmvang, MD).

Typical

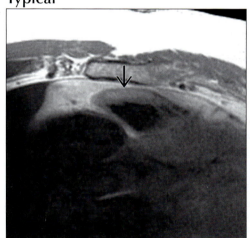
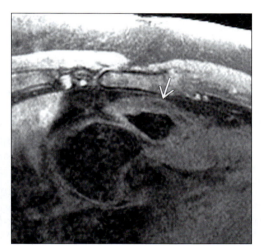

(Left) Axial T1WI MR shows extensive fatty deposits in the anterior wall of the right ventricular outflow tract (arrow). *(Right)* Axial T1WI MR with fat suppression shows low signal intensity in the same lesion (arrow), confirms that it represents a fatty deposit. (Courtesy F. Holmvang, MD).

Typical

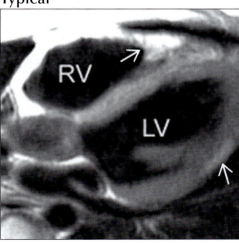
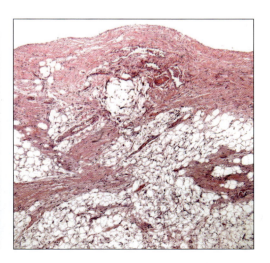

(Left) Axial T1WI MR shows diffuse fatty infiltration in the anterior right ventricular wall (RV, arrow), and small focal fatty deposit in posterior left ventricular wall (LV, arrow) as well. (Courtesy Shi-Joon Yoo, MD). *(Right)* Micropathology, low power, H&E shows multiple areas of extensive fatty infiltration of the myocardium. (Courtesy J. Stone, MD).

SCIMITAR SYNDROME

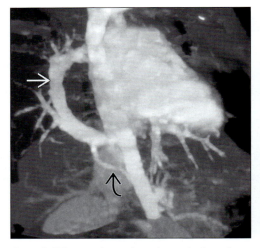

Coronal CTA, maximum intensity projection, shows total venous drainage of right lung via scimitar (arrow) vein to inferior vena cava, and systemic artery (curved arrow) from celiac axis to right lung base.

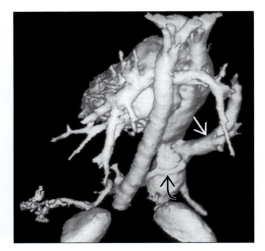

CTA, posterior view of shaded surface rendition, shows total venous drainage of right lung via scimitar (arrow) vein to inferior vena cava, and systemic artery (curved arrow) from celiac axis to right lung base.

TERMINOLOGY

Abbreviations and Synonyms
- Hypogenetic lung syndrome, congenital pulmonary venolobar syndrome

Definitions
- Right lung hypoplasia, anomalous right pulmonary venous connection to inferior vena cava (IVC)
- Often associated: Anomalous systemic arterial supply to right lung base
- Category: Acyanotic, right-sided cardiac chamber enlargement, increased pulmonary vascularity (partial anomalous pulmonary venous return)
- Hemodynamics: Venous flow from right lung returns to right atrium ⇒ volume overload of right heart [atrial septal defect (ASD) physiology]

IMAGING FINDINGS

General Features
- Best diagnostic clue: Scimitar sign = curved anomalous venous trunk, resembling a Turkish sword, in right medial costophrenic sulcus near right heart border, that increases in caliber in a caudad direction

Radiographic Findings
- Radiography
  ○ Right lung hypoplasia
  ○ Dextroversion of heart (no dextrocardia: Apex is still directed towards the left)
  ○ Prominent right atrium, active pulmonary vascular congestion: Shunt vascularity
  ○ Scimitar vein in right medial costophrenic sulcus

Fluoroscopic Findings
- Normal excursions of both hemidiaphragms, no air trapping

CT Findings
- Axial images show scimitar vein joining IVC
- CT angiography with 3D reconstruction most helpful to demonstrate anomalous systemic arterial supply, right pulmonary and mainstem bronchus hypoplasia

MR Findings
- Cardiac-gated T1WI: Anomalous pulmonary venous connection best seen in axial and coronal planes
- Phase-contrast MRA for shunt flow calculation
- Gadolinium-enhanced MRA, coronal acquisition with 3D reconstruction for anomalous right pulmonary venous and arterial development

Echocardiographic Findings
- Echocardiogram

DDx: Anomalous Pulmonary Venous Return (APVR), Right Lung Hypoplasia

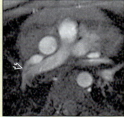

Partial APVR

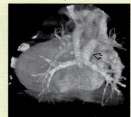

Total APVR Type 1

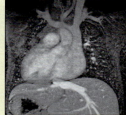

True Dextrocardia

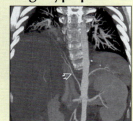

Sequestration

SCIMITAR SYNDROME

Key Facts

Terminology
- Right lung hypoplasia, anomalous right pulmonary venous connection to inferior vena cava (IVC)
- Category: Acyanotic, right-sided cardiac chamber enlargement, increased pulmonary vascularity (partial anomalous pulmonary venous return)
- Hemodynamics: Venous flow from right lung returns to right atrium ⇒ volume overload of right heart [atrial septal defect (ASD) physiology]

Imaging Findings
- Best diagnostic clue: Scimitar sign = curved anomalous venous trunk, resembling a Turkish sword, in right medial costophrenic sulcus near right heart border, that increases in caliber in a caudad direction
- CT angiography with 3D reconstruction most helpful to demonstrate anomalous systemic arterial supply, right pulmonary and mainstem bronchus hypoplasia
- CTA or MRA are better than echocardiography for complete assessment, and can replace diagnostic angiocardiography
- Angiography reserved for coil embolization

Clinical Issues
- Depending on age at presentation and size of left to right shunt
- Newborn: Congestive heart failure, right heart volume overload, pulmonary hypertension
- Young child: Recurrent infections in right lung base
- Older child and adult: Often asymptomatic (incidental finding on chest radiograph)

- No right pulmonary veins entering left atrium
- Scimitar vein connecting to IVC

Angiographic Findings
- Conventional
  - Scimitar vein opacifies during venous phase of pulmonary artery injection
  - Injection of abdominal aorta: Anomalous systemic arterial supply to right lung base (originating from celiac axis, right phrenic artery, descending aorta)
  - Used as road-map for coil embolization of systemic artery

Imaging Recommendations
- CTA or MRA are better than echocardiography for complete assessment, and can replace diagnostic angiocardiography
- Angiography reserved for coil embolization

DIFFERENTIAL DIAGNOSIS

Other forms of partial anomalous pulmonary venous connection
- Right pulmonary vein(s) to azygous vein, superior vena cava, right atrium (with sinus venosus atrial septal defect)

True dextrocardia with abdominal situs solitus
- Other complex cardiac anomalies

Isolated right pulmonary hypoplasia
- Normal right pulmonary venous connection to left atrium

Pulmonary sequestration
- Mass in right lung base not connected to bronchial tree, with systemic arterial supply and venous drainage to pulmonary (intralobar) or systemic (extralobar) veins

PATHOLOGY

General Features
- General path comments
  - Associated in 25% with other anomalies
    - Sinus venosus atrial septal defect most common
    - Ventricular septal defect, tetralogy of Fallot, patent ductus arteriosus
    - Diaphragmatic abnormalities: Accessory hemidiaphragm, hernia
    - Horseshoe lung (lung segment crossing over midline in posterior mediastinum)
  - Embryology
    - Primary abnormality in development of right lung, with secondary anomalous pulmonary venous connection
  - Pathophysiology
    - Obligatory left to right shunt to right atrium: ASD physiology
- Genetics: No specific genetic defect identified
- Associated abnormalities
  - Major
    - Absence of right pulmonary artery
    - Accessory diaphragm (duplication of diaphragm)
    - Absence or interruption of inferior vena cava
  - Minor: Tracheal trifurcation, diaphragmatic eventration or (partial) absence, phrenic cyst, horseshoe lung, esophageal or gastric lung, anomalous superior vena cava, absent left pericardium
  - Cardiac and spinal abnormalities

Gross Pathologic & Surgical Features
- Right lung (including pulmonary artery and bronchus) hypoplasia or agenesis
  - Right upper and middle lobes most commonly a/or hypogenetic
- Anomalous right pulmonary venous drainage to IVC (most frequent) or right atrium, superior vena cava, azygous vein, portal vein, hepatic vein
- Systemic arterialization of right lung base (without sequestration)

SCIMITAR SYNDROME

Microscopic Features
- Normal parenchyma in right lung base (as opposed to sequestration)
- Systemic artery branches anastomose with right pulmonary artery vascular bed in right lung base
- Long-standing shunt: Pulmonary vascular disease, leading to irreversible pulmonary hypertension (Eisenmenger physiology)

CLINICAL ISSUES

Presentation
- Most common signs/symptoms
  - Depending on age at presentation and size of left to right shunt
    - Newborn: Congestive heart failure, right heart volume overload, pulmonary hypertension
    - Young child: Recurrent infections in right lung base
    - Older child and adult: Often asymptomatic (incidental finding on chest radiograph)

Natural History & Prognosis
- Large shunt: Development of irreversible pulmonary hypertension
- Moderate to poor prognosis with neonatal presentation
- May be asymptomatic for many years with small shunt

Treatment
- Embolization of systemic arterial supply
- Baffling of common right pulmonary vein onto left atrium
- Surgical repair indicated when L - R shunt > 2:1

DIAGNOSTIC CHECKLIST

Consider
- Pre-operative identification of systemic arterial supply followed by embolization is important to avoid bleeding complications

Image Interpretation Pearls
- Recognize anomalous vessel in medial costophrenic sulcus
  - Runs perpendicular to expected course of right inferior pulmonary vein
  - Increases in caliber in caudad direction (as opposed to normal pulmonary vein)

SELECTED REFERENCES

1. Berrocal T et al: Congenital anomalies of the tracheobronchial tree, lung, and mediastinum: embryology, radiology, and pathology. Radiographics. 24(1):e17, 2004
2. Sinha R et al: Scimitar syndrome: imaging by magnetic resonance angiography and Doppler echocardiography. Indian J Chest Dis Allied Sci. 46(4):283-6, 2004
3. Konen E et al: Congenital pulmonary venolobar syndrome: spectrum of helical CT findings with emphasis on computerized reformatting. Radiographics. 23(5):1175-84, 2003
4. Kramer U et al: Scimitar syndrome: morphological diagnosis and assessment of hemodynamic significance by magnetic resonance imaging. Eur Radiol. 13 Suppl 4:L147-50, 2003
5. Marco de Lucas E et al: Scimitar syndrome: complete anatomical and functional diagnosis with gadolinium-enhanced and velocity-encoded cine MRI. Pediatr Radiol. 33(10):716-8, 2003
6. Vanderheyden M et al: Partial anomalous pulmonary venous connection or scimitar syndrome. Heart. 89(7):761, 2003
7. Reddy R et al: Scimitar syndrome: a rare cause of haemoptysis. Eur J Cardiothorac Surg. 22(5):821, 2002
8. Vaes MF et al: Scimitar syndrome. JBR-BTR. 85(3):160-1, 2002
9. Zylak CJ et al: Developmental lung anomalies in the adult: radiologic-pathologic correlation. Radiographics. 22 Spec No:S25-43, 2002
10. Do KH et al: Systemic arterial supply to the lungs in adults: spiral CT findings. Radiographics. 21(2):387-402, 2001
11. Gilkeson RC et al: Gadolinium-enhanced magnetic resonance angiography in scimitar syndrome: diagnosis and postoperative evaluation. Tex Heart Inst J. 27(3):309-11, 2000
12. Huddleston CB et al: Scimitar syndrome presenting in infancy. Ann Thor Surg. 67:154-60, 1999
13. Henk CB et al: Scimitar syndrome: MR assessment of hemodynamic significance. J Comput Assist Tomogr. 21(4):628-30, 1997
14. Baran R et al: Scimitar syndrome: confirmation of diagnosis by a noninvasive technique (MRI). Eur Radiol. 6(1):92-4, 1996
15. Ramseyer L et al: The scimitar syndrome: demonstration with magnetic resonance imaging. J Okla State Med Assoc. 89(9):324-5, 1996
16. Vrachliotis TG et al: Hypogenetic lung syndrome: functional and anatomic evaluation with magnetic resonance imaging and magnetic resonance angiography. J Magn Reson Imaging. 6(5):798-800, 1996
17. Boothroyd AE et al: Shoe, scimitar or sequestration: a shifting spectrum. Pediatr Radiol. 25(8):652-3, 1995
18. Woodring JH et al: Congenital pulmonary venolobar syndrome revisited. Radiographics. 14(2):349-69, 1994
19. Figa FH et al: Horseshoe lung--a case report with unusual bronchial and pleural anomalies and a proposed new classification. Pediatr Radiol. 23(1):44-7, 1993
20. Gao YA et al: Scimitar syndrome in infancy. J Am Coll Cardiol. 22(3):873-82, 1993
21. Baxter R et al: Scimitar syndrome: cine magnetic resonance imaging demonstration of anomalous pulmonary venous drainage. Ann Thorac Surg. 50(1):121-3, 1990
22. Partridge JB et al: Scimitar etcetera--the dysmorphic right lung. Clin Radiol. 39(1):11-9, 1988

SCIMITAR SYNDROME

IMAGE GALLERY

Typical

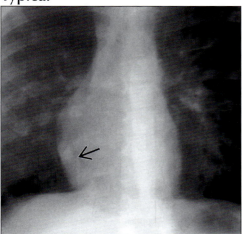
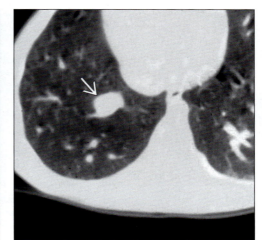

(Left) Anteroposterior radiograph shows shift of heart to right due to right lung hypoplasia, and characteristic shadow from scimitar vein in right medial lung base (arrow). *(Right)* Axial CECT shows tubular round shadow from scimitar vein in right lung base (arrow), which could be traced down to inferior vena cava.

Variant

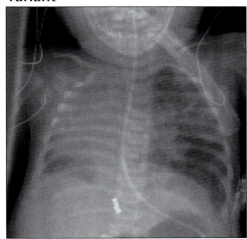
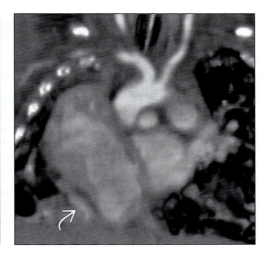

(Left) Anteroposterior radiograph shows dextroversion of heart due to right lung hypoplasia. Note embolization coil which was placed in systemic artery to right lung base. *(Right)* Coronal CTA demonstrates right heart dilatation and scimitar vein (curved arrow) to inferior vena cava.

Variant

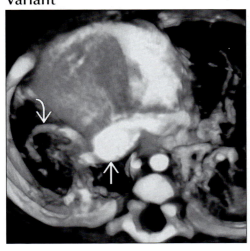
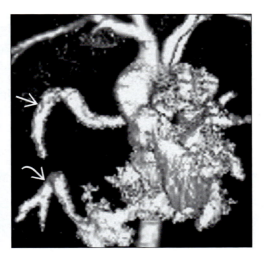

(Left) Axial CTA shows typical curved course of scimitar vein (curved arrow) to distended inferior vena cava (arrow). *(Right)* Coronal CTA, shaded surface rendition, shows prominent right pulmonary artery (arrow), despite ipsilateral lung hypoplasia, indicative of pulmonary hypertension. Also note scimitar vein (curved arrow).

RHABDOMYOMA

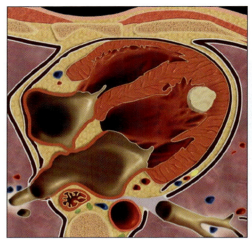

Graphic shows exophytic and partially intramural rhabdomyoma in apex of left ventricle.

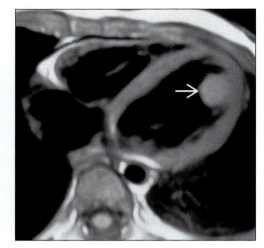

Axial T1WI MR shows round, well-demarcated intraluminal mass (arrow), originating from the free wall of the left ventricle, slightly hyperintense to myocardium.

TERMINOLOGY

Definitions
- Congenital myocardial mass (hamartoma)
- Classic imaging appearance: Intramural or exophytic
- Most common pediatric cardiac tumor
- Associated in up to 86% with tuberous sclerosis

IMAGING FINDINGS

General Features
- Best diagnostic clue: Cardiac mass within or contiguous with myocardium
- Location: Left or right ventricle, ventricular septum
- Size: < 1 mm to 8 cm
- Morphology
  - Well-circumscribed non-encapsulated intramyocardial nodules
  - Multiple in up to 90% of cases

Radiographic Findings
- Radiography
  - Normal chest radiograph in small masses
  - Cardiomegaly and signs of congestive heart failure (CHF) in large masses

CT Findings
- NECT: Masses are often hypodense compared with myocardium
- CECT: Intraluminal component may be assessed with contrast-enhanced studies

MR Findings
- T1WI, T2WI: Variable increased signal intensity compared with myocardium
- Cine MRI: Hemodynamic effect of mass, valvular leak
- Myocardial tagging study can differentiate tumor from contractile tissue

Echocardiographic Findings
- Echocardiogram
  - One or more hyperechoic masses
  - Focal impairment of myocardial wall motion
  - Intraluminal portion of mass may move across adjacent valve during parts of cardiac cycle
- Color Doppler: For obstructive masses, assessment of valvular dysfunction

Imaging Recommendations
- Protocol advice
  - Primary diagnosis with echocardiography
  - MRI helpful in large masses for surgical planning

DDx: Cardiac Tumors

Hemangioendothelioma

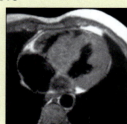
Cardiac Fibroma

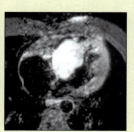
Cardiac Fibroma

RHABDOMYOMA

Key Facts

Terminology
- Congenital myocardial mass (hamartoma)
- Classic imaging appearance: Intramural or exophytic
- Most common pediatric cardiac tumor
- Associated in up to 86% with tuberous sclerosis

Imaging Findings
- Best diagnostic clue: Cardiac mass within or contiguous with myocardium
- Well-circumscribed non-encapsulated intramyocardial nodules
- Multiple in up to 90% of cases
- Primary diagnosis with echocardiography
- MRI helpful in large masses for surgical planning

Clinical Issues
- Obstruction to blood flow → congestive heart failure
- Arrhythmias
- Most regress spontaneously over time

DIFFERENTIAL DIAGNOSIS

Other benign connective tissue tumors
- Fibroma, myxoma, hemangioma

Teratoma
- Is a pericardial (not myocardial) tumor
- Contains all three germ cell layers: Cystic components, fat, calcium

Malignant cardiac tumors
- Rhabdomyosarcoma, angiosarcoma, malignant fibrous histiocytoma
- Metastases of Wilms tumor, neuroblastoma, lymphoma, osteosarcoma

PATHOLOGY

General Features
- General path comments
  - Embryology
    - All are congenital hamartomatous tumors
  - Pathophysiology
    - Mass may interfere with myocardial contraction
    - Exophytic masses frequently obstruct blood flow, or lead to valvular insufficiency
- Genetics
  - > 50% of children with tuberous sclerosis have rhabdomyomas, frequently multiple
  - Most rhabdomyomas occur in patients with tuberous sclerosis
- Epidemiology: Pediatric cardiac tumors are rare (1:100,000-1:30,000)

Gross Pathologic & Surgical Features
- Encapsulated intramyocardial or exophytic mass(es)

Microscopic Features
- Large vacuolated myocytes
- Glycogen-rich vacuoles stretch the perinuclear cytoplasm (spider cells)

CLINICAL ISSUES

Presentation
- Most common signs/symptoms
  - Obstruction to blood flow → congestive heart failure
  - Arrhythmias
  - Tumor embolization and thrombus formation (rare)
  - Large intracavitary tumors causing turbulent flow → hemolytic anemia and thrombocytopenia

Natural History & Prognosis
- Most regress spontaneously over time
- Poor prognosis for untreated large masses interfering with cardiac hemodynamics
- Excellent with complete or partial resection

Treatment
- Surgical excision is curative
- Partial resection of intraluminal component of large exophytic masses may be necessary
- Small intramural masses with no hemodynamic effect need no treatment

SELECTED REFERENCES

1. Cope JT et al: Cardiac tumors. In: Mavroudis C, Backer CL ed. Pediatric cardiac surgery. 3rd ed. Philadelphia, Mosby. 689-700, 2003
2. Kiaffas MG et al: Magnetic resonance imaging evaluation of cardiac tumor characteristics in infants and children. Am J Cardiol. 89(10):1229-33, 2002
3. Grebenc ML et al: Primary cardiac and pericardial neoplasms: radiologic-pathological correlation. Radiographics. 20:1073-103, 2000
4. Titus JL et al: Cardiac tumors. In: Moller JH, Hoffman JIE ed. Pediatric cardiovascular medicine, 1st ed. Philadelphia, Churchill Livingstone. 913-8, 2000

IMAGE GALLERY

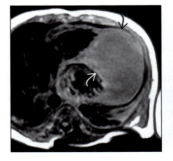 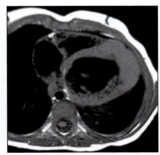

(Left) Axial T1WI MR shows mass (arrows), compressing left ventricular lumen. (Right) Axial T1WI MR at 2 years follow-up shows marked involution of mass.

KAWASAKI DISEASE

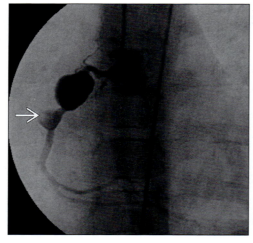

Anteroposterior angiography with catheter tip in the right coronary artery demonstrates fusiform aneurysms of the right coronary artery. Note the second aneurysm has clot within it (arrow).

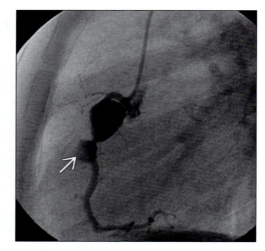

Lateral angiography during same injection demonstrates aneurysms and filling defect associated with clot (arrow). Kawasaki patients are at risk for thrombosis due to increase in platelets.

TERMINOLOGY

Abbreviations and Synonyms
- Mucocutaneous lymph node syndrome

Definitions
- Kawasaki disease (KD) is an acute self limited vasculitis of childhood that is characterized by multisystem disease that occurs in a characteristic progression
- Fever, nonexudative conjunctivitis, erythema of lips and oral mucosa, skin rash, and cervical lymphadenopathy
- Cardiac manifestations include myocarditis (50%), coronary artery aneurysms (3-15%), arrhythmias, and cardiac functional abnormalities related to ischemia

IMAGING FINDINGS

General Features
- Best diagnostic clue: Multiple fusiform and saccular coronary aneurysms
- Location: Multisystem disease affecting the skin, lymph nodes, mucous membranes, conjunctiva, myocardium, pericardium, coronary arteries, joints, bowel, gall gladder, kidney, urethra, and other systems

Radiographic Findings
- Radiography: Chest radiography is usually normal

CT Findings
- CTA
  - Can be utilized to demonstrate aneurysms and stenosis of coronary or other arteries
  - Reformatted images depict aneurysms and focal stenosis

MR Findings
- T2* GRE
  - MRI stress imaging with quantification of regional perfusion
  - Gradient-echo (GRE) cine MRI shows regional wall motion abnormality
  - Can measure cardiac function with end diastolic volumes, systolic ejection, and ejection fraction
- MRA
  - Accurately images coronary artery aneurysms, coronary occlusions, coronary stenosis and provides flow profiles
  - Cardiac-gated T1WI: Myocardial wall thinning, recently infarcted myocardium enhances with gadolinium
  - Used to depict and follow other aneurysms of thorax and abdomen or peripheral involvement

DDx: Multisystem Diseases With Vasculitis

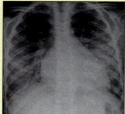
Rheumatic Fever

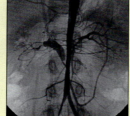
Takayasu Arteritis

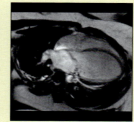
Viral Myocarditis

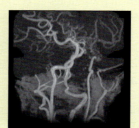
Moya Moya Disease

KAWASAKI DISEASE

Key Facts

Terminology
- Mucocutaneous lymph node syndrome
- Kawasaki disease (KD) is an acute self limited vasculitis of childhood that is characterized by multisystem disease that occurs in a characteristic progression
- Fever, nonexudative conjunctivitis, erythema of lips and oral mucosa, skin rash, and cervical lymphadenopathy
- Cardiac manifestations include myocarditis (50%), coronary artery aneurysms (3-15%), arrhythmias, and cardiac functional abnormalities related to ischemia

Imaging Findings
- Echocardiography is ideal technique with high specificity and sensitivity for detecting proximal aneurysms of coronary arteries
- Size, number and distribution of aneurysms
- Intravascular coronary ultrasound demonstrates findings in the wall of the vessels
- Coronary angiography demonstrates the aneurysms, size and extent of stenosis
- Cardiac MR in older children and adults for assessing function and aneurysms

Top Differential Diagnoses
- Exanthematous infections: Viral or bacterial
- Allergies or hypersensitivity reactions
- Vasculitides

Pathology
- Etiology: Remains elusive but clinical and epidemiologic features suggest infectious cause with abnormal immune response to toxin or infection

Ultrasonographic Findings
- Grayscale Ultrasound
  - Lymphadenopathy is usually non suppurative, unilateral, and in anterior triangle
  - Gall bladder may be hydropic
  - Kidneys have been reported to be enlarged
  - Aneurysms may be identified

Echocardiographic Findings
- Echocardiogram
  - Echocardiography is ideal technique with high specificity and sensitivity for detecting proximal aneurysms of coronary arteries
    - Aneurysms usually occur in first few centimeters of coronary arteries or at bifurcating vessels
    - Can assess internal vessel diameter, whether there is dilatation, ectasia or aneurysm
    - Size, number and distribution of aneurysms
  - Intravascular coronary ultrasound demonstrates findings in the wall of the vessels
- M-mode: Left ventricular function assessment with measurement of volumes, ejection fraction, and regional wall motion

Angiographic Findings
- Conventional
  - Coronary angiography demonstrates the aneurysms, size and extent of stenosis
    - Aneurysms occur at bifurcating sites
    - Acute thrombotic occlusion of a coronary may occur and thrombolytic therapy may be useful
  - Intravascular coronary ultrasound can be done to assess the wall of the vessels

Nuclear Medicine Findings
- Thallium myocardial perfusion imaging (SPECT)
  - Pharmacological stress testing with dipyridamole can demonstrate myocardial ischemia

Imaging Recommendations
- Best imaging tool
  - Echocardiography for initial and sequential studies
  - Cardiac MR in older children and adults for assessing function and aneurysms

DIFFERENTIAL DIAGNOSIS

Exanthematous infections: Viral or bacterial
- Septic shock syndrome has high fever, desquamation of hands and feet
- Rheumatic fever has skin rash, fever, arthritis, myocarditis, pericarditis, and multi-organ involvement
- Mononucleosis has fever, lymphadenopathy, splenomegaly, and liver disease

Allergies or hypersensitivity reactions
- Drug reactions, Stevens-Johnson syndrome, erythema multiforme have systemic signs, rash, fever yet usually do not have cardiac involvement

Vasculitides
- Systemic lupus erythematosus, polyarteritis nodosa, Takayasu have medium to large vessel disease and may have thrombocytosis, Moya Moya

PATHOLOGY

General Features
- General path comments
  - Laboratory evidence
    - C-reactive protein (CRP) elevated and returns to normal by 6 to 10 weeks
    - White blood cell count: 50% of children have < 15,000
    - Thrombocytosis with marked elevation of platelet counts appears second and third weeks
- Etiology: Remains elusive but clinical and epidemiologic features suggest infectious cause with abnormal immune response to toxin or infection
- Epidemiology
  - Japan: Incidence 50/100,000 children < 4 year (10x incidence in USA)

GASTROINTESTINAL

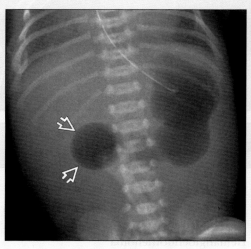

Radiograph of neonate shows proximal obstruction with dilated duodenal bulb (arrows) and stomach (double bubble) = duodenal atresia. Dilated duodenum indicative of long-standing obstruction.

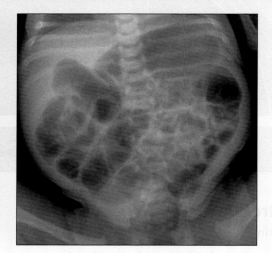

Radiograph of neonate with failure to pass meconium shows distal obstruction with multiple dilated loops of bowel. Contrast enema would be next imaging test of choice.

Neonates

High Intestinal Obstruction
- Differential diagnosis
  - Midgut volvulus: Malrotation
  - Duodenal atresia: Stenosis
  - Duodenal web
  - Annular pancreas
  - Jejunal atresia
- Duodenal atresia, stenosis, web, annular pancreas all part of same spectrum of anomalies and can occur in combination
- Double bubble: Air-filled and dilated duodenal bulb and stomach
  - Classic for duodenal atresia
  - Dilatation of duodenal bulb indicates chronic obstruction and presence of dilatation makes acute volvulus a very unlikely diagnostic consideration

Low Intestinal Obstruction
- Differential diagnosis
  - Hirschsprung disease
  - Meconium plug syndrome/small left colon syndrome
  - Ileal atresia (microcolon on enema)
  - Meconium ileus (microcolon on enema)

Vomiting Infant
- The primary anatomic concerns in the vomiting infants are hypertrophic pyloric stenosis (HPS) and malrotation
- Ultrasound is an ideal test for HPS and is typically the first test of choice in cases where the history and age of patient are highly suspicious for HPS
  - If HPS is not identified, US findings of malrotation such as a fluid-filled proximal duodenum and inversion of the normal relationship between superior mesenteric vein and artery should be evaluated
- If history is not classic for HPS, upper gastrointestinal (UGI) is suggest to evaluate for both HPS and other potential diagnoses such as malrotation

Common Abdominal Processes That May Cause Bowel Obstruction

Differential Diagnosis
- Appendicitis
  - Differential diagnosis for right lower quadrant (RLQ) pain
    - Ovarian pathology (torsion, cyst), mesenteric adenitis, pyelonephritis, segmental omental infarction, renal calculi, appendagitis
- Adhesions
- Intussusception
- Incarcerated inguinal hernia
- Meckel diverticulum
- Malrotation with midgut volvulus

Liver Masses

Differential For Patients < 5 Years
- Hepatoblastoma (+ alpha fetal protein)
- Hemangioendothelioma
- Mesenchymal hamartoma
- Metastatic disease (neuroblastoma)

Differential For Patients > 5 Years
- Hepatocellular carcinoma (+ alpha fetal protein)
- Undifferentiated embryonal sarcoma
- Hepatic adenoma
- Metastatic disease
- Lymphoma

Differential For Immunocompromised Patients
- Lymphoproliferative disorder
- Fungal infection

GASTROINTESTINAL

Key Information

Neonatal Bowel Obstruction
- Can be separated into high and low causes of obstruction
- Differentiation into high or low obstruction helpful in deciding on whether to do UGI or enema as next test of choice

Malrotation, Malrotation, Malrotation!
- Always consider malrotation/midgut volvulus when entertaining GI pathology in children
- A missed midgut volvulus can lead to bowel infarction and death

UGI In Infants And Children
- Multiple images of stomach and duodenal bulb not necessary
- Most important goal is documenting position of duodenojejunal junction and excluding malrotation

Consider Most Common Abdominal Problems First
- Appendicitis, intussusception, malrotation/volvulus

Radiosensitivity
- Infants 10x more radiosensitive than adults
- Optimize use of abdominal CT

Radiographic Bowel Appearances In Children
- Sigmoid in right lower quadrant 43%
- Difficult to differentiate small and large bowel

Technical Issues

Radiographic Studies Of The Abdomen
- For most indications in children, 2 views
  - Frontal supine view
  - "Free air view"
    - Upright view
    - Left lateral decubitus view
    - Cross table lateral view in neonates in NICU
  - In neonates and young children in which it is difficult to differentiate small and large bowel, an additional prone view may be helpful
    - On the prone view, gas moves into posterior structure such as rectum and ascending and descending colon
    - Combination of findings on prone and supine view can be helpful in differentiating air-filled colon from disproportionately dilated small bowel
- Exception to 2 view rule: Children being evaluated for possibility of/suspected constipation
  - Only requires a single frontal supine view
  - Constipation is a common cause of abdominal pain in children: Presents with pain, not with history of not using bathroom

How To Perform An UGI In Infants
- Technique
  - Child may be placed in immobilization device (octagon board) or held in position by parent at head of table and technologist at feet end
    - Immobilization device allows radiologist to concentrate on exam rather than child's moving and safety, rapidly position child for imaging, and minimize radiation dose for child and staff
    - Downside of immobilization is infants become irritated and less cooperative with drinking, can be anxiety producing for parents
  - Contrast can be administered by bottle in infants who will drink
    - May need to pass nasogastric tube in those who cannot cooperate
  - Only need 6 images for normal exam: You do not need multiple images of stomach and duodenal bulb as in adults
    - 1. Supine position (more likely to drink): Frontal view of esophagus while drinking
    - 2. Turn patient right side down: Lateral view of esophagus while drinking
    - 3. With right side still down, wait for contrast to pass into duodenum: Lateral view documenting that pylorus is normal and that duodenum passes posteriorly
    - 4. Quickly turn infant supine: Frontal view as contrast passes through distal duodenum and proximal jejunum - to document the position of the duodenojejunal junction (Ligament of Treitz)
    - 5. Oblique view obtained with left side down: Air-filled antrum and bulb
    - 6. Fluoroscopic spot or overhead radiograph of entire abdomen to document progression of contrast into the nondilated jejunal loops
  - Most important aspect of UGI in children is documentation of normal duodenojejunal junction and exclusion of malrotation
    - Timing is crucial for steps 3 and 4 and comes with experience
    - If you turn child to supine too early, contrast may not pass into distal duodenum
    - If you turn child to supine too late, contrast may pass into more distal loops and obscure visualization (worst case scenario)
  - Rule out gastrointestinal reflux
    - Many requests for infant UGI will be labeled as "rule out reflux"
    - Although good idea to document reflux when encountered, not a good idea to do maneuvers with fluoroscopy to search for reflux
    - Parents and physicians know infant is refluxing because they bear witness to the infant throwing up
    - Purpose of UGI is really to exclude an important anatomic cause for excessive reflux (such as an obstruction)

GASTROINTESTINAL

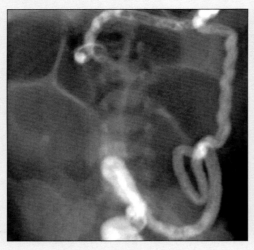

Contrast enema in neonate with distal obstruction shows microcolon and nonopacified, air-filled dilated small bowel loops. Constellation of findings consistent with ileal atresia.

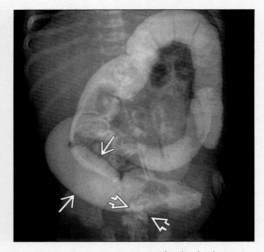

Contrast enema in neonate with distal obstruction shows lack of microcolon with sigmoid (arrows) > rectum (open arrows) = Hirschsprung disease. Note sigmoid in right lower quadrant.

Imaging Guided Reduction Of Intussusception
- Various techniques can be used for imaging guided reduction of intussusception
  - Contrast with fluoroscopic guidance, air with fluoroscopic guidance, water with sonographic guidance
  - At our institution, we use air reduction
    - Inflation device secured in place, adequate rectal seal created, air insufflated
    - Maximum pressure 120 mmHg (will be higher during Valsalva and crying)
    - Success rates of 80-90%
    - Recurrent in 5-10%
- Contraindications
  - Peritonitis on physical examination
  - Free air seen on radiographs (very rare)

Abdominal CT
- Radiosensitivity
  - Infants and young children up to 10x more radiosensitive than adults
  - CT only when indicated
  - Weight based methods should be utilized to use appropriate mAs for patient size
    - Less radiation needed to penetrate body of small child and create adequate image in contrast to adult sized patients
- Slice thickness
  - Slice thickness should be adjusted to patient size
  - 5 mm adequate for most pediatric abdominal work
  - May wish to drop to 1.25-2.5 mm for abdominal CT arteriography or when imaging very small babies

Age Related Anatomic Appearances

Position Of Sigmoid Colon
- Sigmoid colon is often long & redundant in young children
- Lies within RLQ in 43% of young children
- Often overlies region of cecum
- Bowel gas in redundant sigmoid can be mistaken for air in cecum when evaluating for intussusception

Degree Of Mesenteric Fat
- Children often have very little mesenteric and retroperitoneal fat
- Can make CT studies more difficult to interpret and more reliant on optimal intravenous contrast-enhancement

Bowel Gas After Birth
- In neonates, it can take several hours before gas is seen through out gastrointestinal tract
- During first several hours after birth, gas may normally only be seen in proximal bowel
- "Stool" like bubbly appearance is not normally seen in neonates
  - Should raise suspicion of pneumatosis or obstruction

Appearance Of Bowel
- Often is difficult to differentiate small from large bowel when multiple dilated loops of bowel on radiography in young children
- Typical haustral patterns not present

MR Splenic Signal
- At birth, white pulp < red pulp as compared to later in life
- On T2 weighted images in older children and adults, spleen is very high in signal
- During first week of life, spleen normally low in signal related to lack of white pulp
  - Do not confuse normal appearance as suspicious for hemachromatosis or iron overload
- Becomes moderately hyperintense as compared to liver by 8 months of age

Related References
1. Donnelly LF: Fundamentals of Pediatric Radiology. Philadelphia: W.B. Saunders, 2001

GASTROINTESTINAL

IMAGE GALLERY

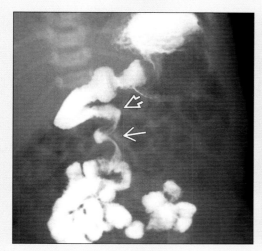
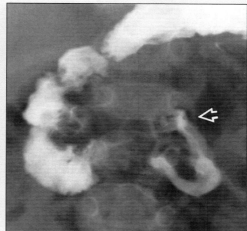

(Left) Upper GI in vomiting infant shows "corkscrew" appearance of proximal jejunum (arrow) consistent with volvulus and duodenojejunal junction not meeting normal criteria (open arrow). *(Right)* Upper GI shows borderline position of duodenojejunal junction (just to left of spine, not as superior as duodenal bulb). Best to follow contrast and prove cecum in right lower quadrant.

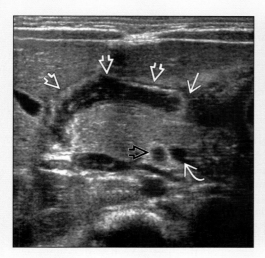
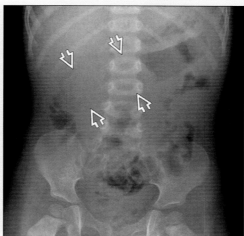

(Left) Axial ultrasound obtained in infant to exclude pyloric stenosis shows normal pylorus (arrow) but dilated duodenum (open white arrows) and reversed superior mesenteric artery (open black arrow)/superior mesenteric vein (curved arrow) relationship = suspicious for malrotation. *(Right)* Radiograph in 8 month old shows soft tissue mass (arrows) in region of transverse colon, highly suspicious for intussusception.

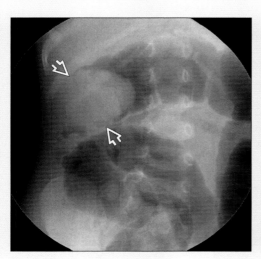
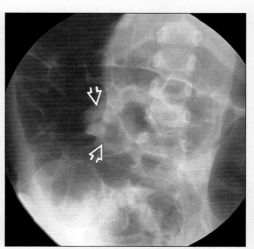

(Left) Air enema in same patient as above right shows intussusception as soft tissue mass (arrows) being reduced to level of hepatic flexure. *(Right)* Air enema later in same patient shows resolution of soft tissue mass, reflux of gas into small bowel, and residual edematous ileocecal valve (arrows). Intussusception reduced.

MIDGUT VOLVULUS

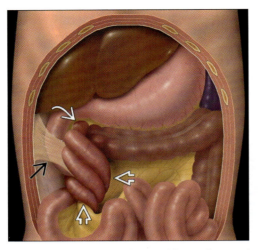

Graphic shows volvulus with twisted loops of proximal small bowel (open arrows) and Ladd band (black arrow). The cecum (curved arrow) is malpositioned within the right upper quadrant.

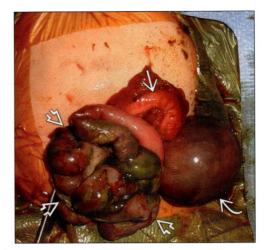

Surgical photograph shows volvulus with twisted and infarcted small bowel (open arrows) to right of colon (arrow). Note incidental ovarian cyst (curved arrow).

TERMINOLOGY

Definitions
- Malrotation: Abnormal fixation of small bowel mesentery resulting in short mesenteric base that is prone to twisting
- Volvulus: Abnormal twisting of small bowel about the superior mesenteric artery that can result in bowel obstruction and bowel ischemia/necrosis
- Ligament of Treitz: Duodenojejunal junction (DJJ), where duodenum passes through transverse mesocolon and becomes jejunum
- Ladd Bands: Abnormal fibrous peritoneal bands that can cause duodenal obstruction
- Bilious vomiting: Green/yellow vomit typically from obstruction of duodenum distal to ampulla of Vater

IMAGING FINDINGS

General Features
- Best diagnostic clue
  ○ Malrotation: Abnormal position of duodenojejunal junction
    ▪ Abnormal position of cecum by small bowel follow through or barium enema
  ○ Volvulus: Cork screw or "Z"shaped appearance of the duodenum which does not cross to the left of midline
- Morphology
  ○ Twisting of the mesentery occurs about the superior mesenteric artery which can cause venous obstruction, bowel wall ischemia and necrosis
  ○ Ladd band may cause duodenal obstruction

Radiographic Findings
- Radiography
  ○ May be normal
  ○ May show distended stomach and proximal duodenum
    ▪ Duodenal bulb should not be markedly enlarged with acute volvulus
    ▪ Markedly enlarged bulb indicative of long-standing obstruction as seen in duodenal atresia or in-utero volvulus
  ○ May show diffuse bowel distention from ischemia/necrosis
    ▪ Such children will be extremely ill
  ○ Pneumatosis, portal venous gas, free peritoneal air

Fluoroscopic Findings
- Upper GI
  ○ Diagnosis of malrotation made on upper GI when criteria for normal position of DJJ (ligament of Treitz) are not met

DDx: Vomiting Infant

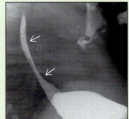

Esophageal Reflux

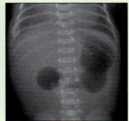

Duodenal Atresia

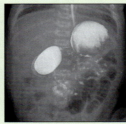

Duodenal Stenosis

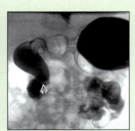

Duodenal Web

MIDGUT VOLVULUS

Key Facts

Terminology
- Malrotation: Abnormal fixation of small bowel mesentery resulting in short mesenteric base that is prone to twisting
- Volvulus: Abnormal twisting of small bowel about the superior mesenteric artery that can result in bowel obstruction and bowel ischemia/necrosis

Imaging Findings
- Abnormal position of cecum by small bowel follow through or barium enema
- Volvulus: Cork screw or "Z"shaped appearance of the duodenum which does not cross to the left of midline
- Diagnosis of malrotation made on upper GI when criteria for normal position of DJJ (ligament of Treitz) are not met
- DJJ is at the same level or more superior than duodenal bulb
- On lateral view, duodenum typically courses posterior then inferiorly

Pathology
- With normal embryonic rotation, both the duodenojejunal and ileocolic portions of the bowel rotate counterclockwise 270 degrees around the axis of the omphalomesenteric vessels
- Etiology: Development anomaly resulting in narrow mesenteric pedicle secondary to abnormal fixation and rotation of bowel

Clinical Issues
- Most common signs/symptoms: Classic presentation: Bilious vomiting

---

- Criteria for normal DJJ
  - AP supine positioning
  - DJJ: Where 4th portion of duodenum turns left and becomes jejunum
  - DJJ is to the left of the spine
  - DJJ is at the same level or more superior than duodenal bulb
- Obvious cases - duodenum coursing into RUQ - never crossing spine
- In borderline cases, small bowel follow through is often helpful to document position of cecum
- With near normal DJJ and RLQ cecum, probably not at risk for volvulus (long small bowel mesentery)
- DJJ is mobile in children and can be "factitiously" moved into normal or abnormal position by distended bowel, masses, or indwelling NJ tube
- On lateral view, duodenum typically courses posterior then inferiorly
  - With malrotation, may not initially course posteriorly
- Goal of upper GI in neonate with bilious vomiting is to exclude or demonstrate findings of malrotation (not necessarily with volvulus)
- In an infant with bilious vomiting, findings of malrotation considered a surgical emergency, even if radiographic findings of volvulus not identified
- Volvulus: Duodenum and jejunum appear as corkscrew or as complete duodenal obstruction
- Malrotation may be an incidental finding
- Contrast enema
  - Cecum not in right lower quadrant
  - Cecum may be in the right upper quadrant (RUQ), left upper quadrant (LUQ) or even the left lower quadrant
  - Cecal location in RUQ or LUQ has greatest prognostic implication for volvulus or obstructing Ladd bands

CT Findings
- CECT
  - Relationship of superior mesenteric vein (SMV) and artery (SMA)
    - Normally SMV to right of SMA
    - SMA: Smaller, rounder, surrounded by fat
    - SMV: Larger, thinner walled
  - With malrotation, often SMV to left of SMA
    - Finding is not specific or sensitive
    - Abnormal relationship can be seen with normal rotation and vice versa
  - With volvulus, swirling pattern of bowel about SMA
  - May have small bowel distention
  - Pneumatosis, portal venous gas and free peritoneal air may be present

Ultrasonographic Findings
- If US done to exclude hypertrophic pyloric stenosis (HPS) and HPS not identified, look for findings of malrotation/volvulus
  - US not done in cases of suspected malrotation, UGI performed
- SMV may be identified to the left of the SMA
- May demonstrate swirling of bowel about the mesenteric vessels
- Proximal duodenum may be persistently fluid filled

Imaging Recommendations
- Best imaging tool
  - Infant with bilious vomiting indication for emergency upper GI
  - Small bowel follow through (SBFT) or barium enema (BE) for borderline DJJ to document position of cecum
- Protocol advice
  - AP supine positioning
  - Image in the lateral view
  - Document location of DJJ
    - DJJ is at the same level or more superior than duodenal bulb
  - Imaging of first pass of barium helpful to avoid DJJ being obscured by contrast in antrum or jejunum

DIFFERENTIAL DIAGNOSIS

Prominent gastroesophageal reflux (GER)
- Non-bilious vomiting

MIDGUT VOLVULUS

- Very common and clinical finding leading to most UGI performed in infants

Spectrum of congenital duodenum obstruction
- Spectrum of related abnormalities: Duodenal atresia, duodenal stenosis, annular pancreas, duodenal web (often coexisting)
- Tend to have distention of proximal duodenum 2nd to chronic obstruction

PATHOLOGY

General Features
- General path comments
  - With normal embryonic rotation, both the duodenojejunal and ileocolic portions of the bowel rotate counterclockwise 270 degrees around the axis of the omphalomesenteric vessels
  - An understanding of the embryogenesis is emphasized, but understanding result more important
  - With normal rotation, duodenojejunal junction positioned in left upper quadrant and cecum positioned in right lower quadrant
    - Result in long, fixed base between ligament of Treitz and cecum that keeps mesentery from twisting
  - If duodenojejunal and ileocecal junctions not in normal positions (malrotation), base of small bowel mesentery may be short and predisposed to twisting (volvulus)
  - Malrotation may also be associated with duodenal obstruction from
    - Ladd bands (abnormal fibrous peritoneal bands)
    - Paraduodenal hernias
- Etiology: Development anomaly resulting in narrow mesenteric pedicle secondary to abnormal fixation and rotation of bowel
- Epidemiology
  - 2.86/10,000 new births
  - Incidence inversely proportional to maternal age
- Associated abnormalities
  - Entities associated with malrotation
    - Congenital diaphragmatic hernia
    - Abdominal wall defects: Gastroschisis, omphalocele
    - Abdominal heterotaxies

Gross Pathologic & Surgical Features
- Abnormal location of DJJ and cecum with short mesenteric base
- Abnormal fibrous peritoneal bands, Ladd bands
- Twisting of small bowel about the superior mesenteric vessels

Microscopic Features
- Ischemic or necrotic bowel

CLINICAL ISSUES

Presentation
- Most common signs/symptoms: Classic presentation: Bilious vomiting
- Other signs/symptoms
  - Acute abdominal pain
  - Vomiting, crampy abdominal pain
  - Failure to thrive
  - Patients may be asymptomatic, have atypical or chronic symptoms

Demographics
- Age
  - 39% present within first 10 days of life
  - > 90% present within first 3 months of life
  - Can occur at any age
- Gender: Slightly higher incidence in boys
- Ethnicity: > In Asian populations

Natural History & Prognosis
- Potential volvulus leading to bowel necrosis
- Possible midgut volvulus is one of few true emergencies in pediatric GI

Treatment
- Surgical emergency
- Ladd procedure: Reduction of volvulus, resect nonviable bowel, transect Ladd bands (if present), place small bowel in right and colon in left abdomen

DIAGNOSTIC CHECKLIST

Consider
- Delay in diagnosis can result in diffuse bowel necrosis or death
- Infant with bilious vomiting indication for emergency upper GI
- Borderline cases of DJJ location, SBFT or BE should be performed to document the location of the cecum

Image Interpretation Pearls
- DJJ should be at the same level or more superior than duodenal bulb
- On lateral view, duodenum typically courses posterior then inferiorly

SELECTED REFERENCES
1. Patino MO et al: Utility of the sonographic whirlpool sign in diagnosing midgut volvulus in patients with atypical clinical presentations. J Ultrasound Med. 23(3):397-401, 2004
2. Strouse PJ: Disorders of intestinal rotation and fixation ("malrotation"). Pediatr Radiol. 34(11):837-51, 2004
3. Millar AJ et al: Malrotation and volvulus in infancy and childhood. Semin Pediatr Surg. 12(4):229-36, 2003
4. Buonomo C: Neonatal gastrointestinal emergencies. Radiol Clin North Am. 35:845-64, 1997
5. Long FR et al: Radiographic patterns of intestinal malrotation in children. Radiographics. 16(3):547-56; discussion 556-60, 1996
6. Berdon WE et al: Midgut malrotation and volvulus. Which films are most helpful? Radiology. 96:375-84, 1970

MIDGUT VOLVULUS

IMAGE GALLERY

Typical

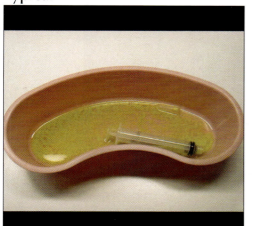 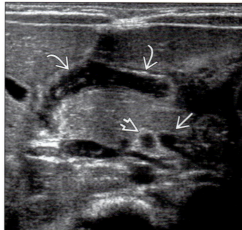

(Left) Clinical photograph shows appearance of bilious emesis. *(Right)* Transverse ultrasound of volvulus shows SMA (open arrow) to right of SMV (arrow). Note fluid filled proximal duodenum (curved arrows). Patient sent to UGI.

Typical

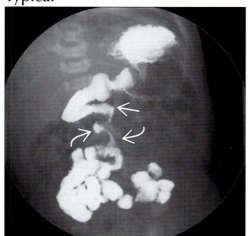 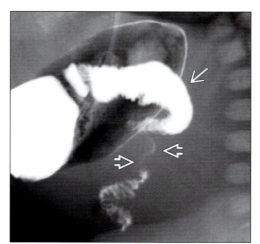

(Left) Anteroposterior upper GI in same patient as above right shows abnormal positioned DJJ (arrow), corkscrew appearance of proximal bowel (curved arrows), and jejunum on right. *(Right)* Lateral upper GI image in same patient shows mild dilatation of proximal duodenum (arrow) and corkscrew appearance of more distal bowel (open arrows).

Typical

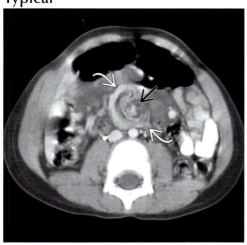 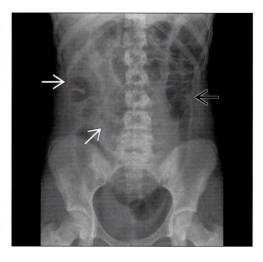

(Left) Axial CECT shows swirling or whirlpool appearance of the bowel and mesenteric pedicle (curved arrows) about the superior mesenteric vessels (arrow). *(Right)* Radiograph in malrotation shows diffuse distention of bowel throughout the abdomen. Loops of small bowel (white arrows) are seen on the right with colon only seen on the left (black arrow).

DUODENAL ATRESIA OR STENOSIS

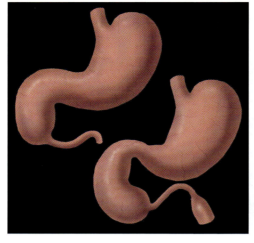

Graphic shows artists rendition of the dilation of the stomach and duodenum to the level of duodenal atresia (upper left) and to the level of duodenal stenosis (lower right).

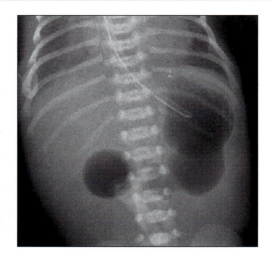

Anteroposterior radiograph Shows dilation of the stomach and duodenum with no distal gas, the so-called "double bubble" sign of duodenal atresia.

TERMINOLOGY

Abbreviations and Synonyms
- Duodenal atresia (DA), duodenal stenosis (DS)

Definitions
- Congenital atresia/stenosis of the duodenum
- Duodenal maldevelopment not an ischemic insult
- Most common upper bowel obstruction in neonate

IMAGING FINDINGS

General Features
- Best diagnostic clue: "Double bubble"
- Location
  - 2nd or 3rd portion of the duodenum
  - In the region of the Ampulla of Vater
- Size: Large stomach and proximal duodenum
- Morphology: Dilated stomach and duodenum proximal to atresia

Radiographic Findings
- Radiography
  - Gaseous distention of stomach and duodenum
    - Dilated duodenum of DA implies long-standing obstruction, midgut volvulus very unlikely
  - Atresia: No distal gas
  - Stenosis: Some distal gas; must exclude midgut volvulus

Fluoroscopic Findings
- Not usually performed for DA, plain films diagnostic
- If upper gastrointestinal (UGI) performed, either
  - Duodenal obstruction
  - Partial duodenal obstruction
- If DA with pancreas divisum, distal contrast possible
  - Bile duct drains on either side of atretic segment

MR Findings
- T1WI: Fetal: Low signal in dilated stomach and duodenum
- T2WI: Fetal: High signal in dilated stomach and duodenum

Ultrasonographic Findings
- Grayscale Ultrasound
  - Anechoic, dilated, fluid-filled stomach and duodenum
  - Associated abdominal findings that can be seen
    - Annular pancreas, preduodenal portal vein, biliary anomalies
  - Prenatal sonography
    - Dilated stomach and duodenum
    - Polyhydramnios in 40%
    - Gastric duplication may mimic duodenal atresia in utero

DDx: Duodenal Obstruction

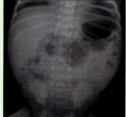
Midgut Volvulus

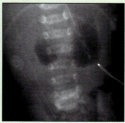
Duodenal Web

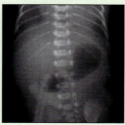
Malrotation And DA

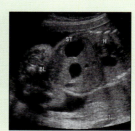
Duodenal Atresia

DUODENAL ATRESIA OR STENOSIS

Key Facts

Terminology
- Most common upper bowel obstruction in neonate

Imaging Findings
- Best diagnostic clue: "Double bubble"
- In the region of the Ampulla of Vater
- Duodenal obstruction
- If "double bubble" on plain film, no further studies required
- If distal gas, upper GI

Top Differential Diagnoses
- Malrotation and midgut volvulus: Extrinsic
- Duodenal web (DW) or diaphragm: Intrinsic
- Other anomalies associated with Intrinsic duodenum obstruction
- Annular pancreas in 33%
- Preduodenal portal vein

Pathology
- Failure of vacuolization (recanalization)
- 30% with DA have Down syndrome (trisomy 21)
- Malrotation: 28%
- Annular pancreas: 33%
- Other intestinal atresias, congenital heart disease, anorectal anomalies, biliary anomalies, renal anomalies, absence of the gallbladder and situs abnormalities, preduodenal portal vein
- Type I: Most common in DA

Clinical Issues
- Onset of vomiting within hours of birth
- Duodenoduodenostomy most common operation

Echocardiographic Findings
- Echocardiogram
  - Associated congenital heart disease
  - If Down syndrome
    - Atrial septal defect (ASD)
    - Ventriculoseptal defect (VSD)
    - Patent ductus arteriosis (PDA)
    - Atrioventricular (AV) canal

Imaging Recommendations
- Best imaging tool
  - Plain film radiography for atresia
  - UGI if distal gas
- Protocol advice
  - If "double bubble" on plain film, no further studies required
  - If distal gas, upper GI
  - Use barium by nasogastric tube for pre-op upper GI
    - Aspirate stomach first, then inject barium
    - Puff small amount of air if suspect stenosis
  - Sometimes enema to exclude other atresias pre-operatively
  - Initial post-op upper GI use isotonic water-soluble contrast
    - To exclude post-op leak

DIFFERENTIAL DIAGNOSIS

Extrinsic vs. intrinsic considerations
- May often be differentiated only at surgery

Malrotation and midgut volvulus: Extrinsic
- Proximal duodenum is typically not dilated in acute volvulus
- In-utero volvulus may cause duodenal dilation
- Upper GI: Malpositioned duodenal jejunal junction (DJJ), corkscrew appearance of duodenum/jejunum
- May involve Ladd bands

Duplication cyst: Extrinsic
- Sonography may show diagnostic double ring sign
- "Gut signature" (hyperechoic inner, hypoechoic outer wall)

Duodenal web (DW) or diaphragm: Intrinsic
- Later presentation
- Windsock appearance

Other anomalies associated with Intrinsic duodenum obstruction
- Annular pancreas in 33%
- Preduodenal portal vein

PATHOLOGY

General Features
- General path comments
  - 2 theories of duodenal maldevelopment
    - Failure of vacuolization (recanalization)
    - Inadequate endodermal proliferation
  - Most DA is the membranous type
  - Spectrum of disease
    - No canalization, blind ending: DA
    - Partial canalization: DS or duodenal web
  - Duodenum most common site of intestinal atresia
- Genetics
  - Several reports of familial occurrence
  - Strong association with Down syndrome
  - Feingold syndrome
    - Combination of hand and foot anomalies, microcephaly, tracheo-esophageal fistula, esophageal/duodenal atresia, short palpebral fissures and developmental delay
  - Partial monosomy 10q with partial trisomy 11q
  - 2q24.3: Quarter deletion
  - Of 265 fetal karyotypes, 43% with DA abnormal
- Etiology
  - Unknown
  - 50% associated with other malformations
  - Developmental error in early period of gestation
  - Different from other atresias which are due to vascular accidents late in development

DUODENAL ATRESIA OR STENOSIS

- Epidemiology: Incidence 1:7,500 to 1:40,000 live births
- Associated abnormalities
  - 50% of patients with DA
  - 30% with DA have Down syndrome (trisomy 21)
    - 11 pairs of ribs, macroglossia, flat acetabular angles, cardiomegaly with shunt vascularity (ASD, VSD, PDA, AV canal)
  - Malrotation: 28%
  - Annular pancreas: 33%
  - Other intestinal atresias, congenital heart disease, anorectal anomalies, biliary anomalies, renal anomalies, absence of the gallbladder and situs abnormalities, preduodenal portal vein

Gross Pathologic & Surgical Features
- Dilated duodenum with an otherwise intact wall
- Usually well perfused, not ischemic at operation

Staging, Grading or Classification Criteria
- Type I: Most common in DA
  - Intact intestinal wall and mesentery
  - Septal or membranous luminal obstruction
  - Diameter proximal > > distal segment
- Type II
  - Intestinal segments separated by fibrous cord
- Type III
  - Two blind ends without intervening cord
  - With wedge-shaped mesenteric defect

CLINICAL ISSUES

Presentation
- Most common signs/symptoms
  - DA/DS present in the newborn
  - Onset of vomiting within hours of birth
    - 85% bilious
    - 15% nonbilious: Proximal to Ampulla of Vater
  - Scaphoid abdomen
  - Feeding intolerance
- Other signs/symptoms: Dehydration, weight loss, electrolyte imbalance, bile-stained aspirates from orogastric tube

Demographics
- Age
  - Newborn in DA/DS
  - 46% were premature in large series

Natural History & Prognosis
- Untreated, dehydration, severe electrolyte abnormalities, death
- With surgical treatment, survival rate > 90%

Treatment
- Surgical repair
  - If radiographically diagnostic of DA surgical repair urgent but not emergent unless clinically warranted
  - Partial duodenal obstructions in which malrotation is not excluded are treated emergently
- Duodenoduodenostomy most common operation
  - Side-to-side vs. diamond-shaped technique
- Contraindications to immediate surgical repair
  - Electrolyte or fluid balance disturbances
  - Severe cardiac defects repaired first
  - Severe respiratory insufficiency

DIAGNOSTIC CHECKLIST

Consider
- Presence or absence of distal bowel gas
- Associated anomalies
- Rare causes of distal gas

Image Interpretation Pearls
- "Double bubble" on radiography/sonography
- If distal gas, think
  - Midgut volvulus, DS/DW, or pancreas divisum

SELECTED REFERENCES

1. Forrester MB et al: Population-based study of small intestinal atresia and stenosis, Hawaii, 1986-2000. Public Health. 118(6):434-8, 2004
2. Sugimoto T et al: Choledochal cyst and duodenal atresia: a rare combination of malformations. Pediatr Surg Int. 20(9):724-6, 2004
3. Doray B et al: Esophageal and duodenal atresia in a girl with a 12q24.3-qter deletion. Clin Genet. 61(6):468-71, 2002
4. Haeusler MC et al: Prenatal ultrasonographic detection of gastrointestinal obstruction: results from 18 European congenital anomaly registries. Prenat Diagn. 22(7):616-23, 2002
5. Pumberger W et al: Duodeno-jejunal atresia with volvulus, absent dorsal mesentery, and absent superior mesenteric artery: a hereditary compound structure in duodenal atresia? Am J Med Genet. 109(1):52-5, 2002
6. Rothenberg SS: Laparoscopic duodenoduodenostomy for duodenal obstruction in infants and children. J Pediatr Surg. 37(7):1088-9, 2002
7. Sencan A et al: Symptomatic annular pancreas in newborns. Med Sci Monit. 8(6):CR434-7, 2002
8. Mordehai J et al: Preduodenal portal vein causing duodenal obstruction associated with situs inversus, intestinal malrotation, and polysplenia: A case report. J Pediatr Surg. 37(4):E5, 2002
9. Maruyama K et al: Partial monosomy 10q with partial trisomy 11q due to paternal balanced translocation. J Paediatr Child Health. 37(2):198-200, 2001
10. Dalla Vecchia LK et al: Intestinal atresia and stenosis: a 25-year experience with 277 cases. Arch Surg. 133(5):490-6; discussion 496-7, 1998
11. Grosfeld JL: Jejunoileal atresia and stenosis. In: O'neal JA, Rowe MI, Grosfeld JL, eds. Pediatric Surgery, 3rd ed. St Louis: Mosby. 1145-1158, 1998
12. Buonomo C: Neonatal gastrointestinal emergencies. Radiol Clin North Am. 35:845-64, 1997
13. Courtens W et al: Feingold syndrome: report of a new family and review. Am J Med Genet. 73(1):55-60, 1997
14. Lemire EG et al: A familial disorder with duodenal atresia and tetralogy of Fallot. Am J Med Genet. 66(1):39-44, 1996
15. Long FR et al: Intestinal malrotation in children: tutorial on radiographic diagnosis in difficult cases. Radiology. 198:775-80, 1996
16. Nicolaides KH et al: Fetal gastro-intestinal and abdominal wall defects: associated malformations and chromosomal abnormalities. Fetal Diagn Ther. 7(2):102-15, 1992

DUODENAL WEB

IMAGE GALLERY

Typical

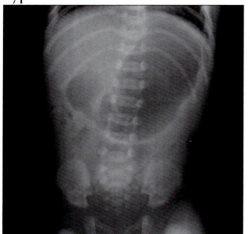
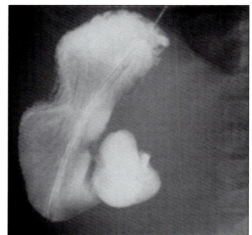

(Left) Anteroposterior radiograph of a newborn with bilious emesis shows a "double bubble" with distal gas which was a tight DW at surgery; it could have been DS or even midgut volvulus. *(Right)* Lateral upper GI shows the contrast halting at the region of the ampulla, the bolus ending with a central "teat" configuration, the region of the tiny orifice in this case of duodenal web.

Typical

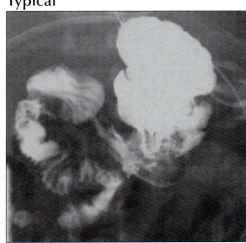
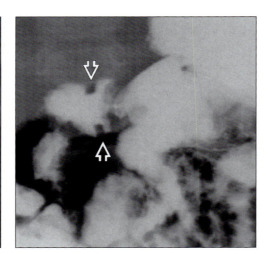

(Left) Anteroposterior upper GI in the patient of image above shows the typical post-op appearance after duodenoduodenostomy with mild residual proximal duodenal dilation; there was malrotation as well. *(Right)* Anteroposterior upper GI shows a circumferential duodenal web (arrows) in the duodenal bulb, an atypical location for a duodenal web, in this patient who presented with recurrent non-bilious emesis.

Variant

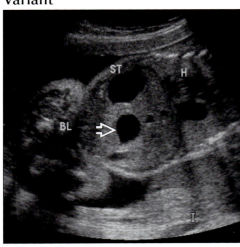
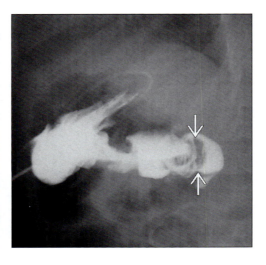

(Left) Coronal ultrasound In utero shows sonographic "double bubble," a dilated stomach (ST) and duodenum (arrow), in this patient who had a tight duodenal web at birth. *(Right)* Lateral upper GI through the G-port of a gastrojejunostomy (GJ) tube in a 3 year old with Down syndrome shows a filling defect (arrows) across the duodenum beyond the bulb; a duodenal web was found at endoscopy.

JEJUNOILEAL ATRESIA

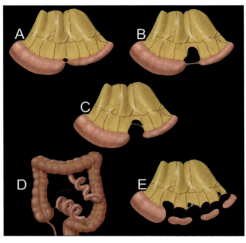

Graphic shows representative examples of the types of jejunoileal atresia; type 1 (A), type 2 (B), type 3a (C), type 3b (D), and type 4 (E).

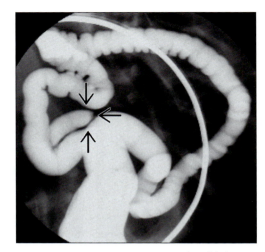

Anteroposterior contrast enema in 1 day old shows a microcolon, contrast refluxing into the terminal ileum, and an abrupt termination of the contrast (arrows) in ileal atresia.

TERMINOLOGY

Abbreviations and Synonyms
- Ilea atresia (IA), ileal stenosis (IS), jejuno-ileal atresia (J-IA), jejunal atresia (JA)

Definitions
- Congenital absence or complete occlusion of the intestinal lumen of a segment of jejunum or ileum
- Stenosis is a forme fruste of atresia
- Distal ileal atresia: Distal obstruction
- Jejunal or proximal ileal atresia: Proximal obstruction

IMAGING FINDINGS

General Features
- Best diagnostic clue
  - Multiple dilated bowel loops on radiography associated with
    - Microcolon in distal ileal atresia
    - Normal to slightly small colon in jejunal and proximal ileal atresia
- Location: Jejunum or ileum
- Size: Dilated small bowel proximal to atresia, out of proportion to colonic distention
- Morphology
  - Diffuse, similarly dilated, multiple loops of bowel proximal to distal ileal obstruction
  - Several massively dilated loops in jejunal or proximal ileal atresia

Radiographic Findings
- Radiography
  - Multiple dilated loops of bowel: Distal obstruction
  - Cannot reliably distinguish small from large bowel on radiographs in neonates
  - Number of dilated loops reflects level of obstruction
    - Many loops: Distal obstruction (ileal or colonic)
    - Few loops: Upper obstruction (jejunal or proximal ileal)
  - Contrast enema to
    - Limit differential diagnosis of distal bowel obstruction
    - Assess for additional atresias in cases of jejunal atresia
  - Soft tissue mass or curvilinear calcification suggests complicated obstruction
    - Perforation, pseudocyst formation, segmental volvulus, ischemia
  - Stenosis more difficult to diagnose

Fluoroscopic Findings
- Water-soluble contrast enema
  - Microcolon (small unused colon)
    - Spectrum of small colon

DDx: Distal Bowel Obstruction

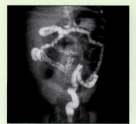
Meconium Ileus

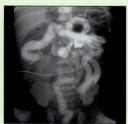
Total Colonic HD

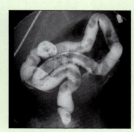
Immature Colon

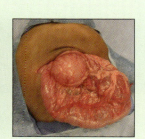
Ileal Duplication

JEJUNOILEAL ATRESIA

Key Facts

Terminology
- Congenital absence or complete occlusion of the intestinal lumen of a segment of jejunum or ileum
- Distal ileal atresia: Distal obstruction
- Jejunal or proximal ileal atresia: Proximal obstruction

Imaging Findings
- Multiple dilated bowel loops on radiography associated with
- Microcolon in distal ileal atresia
- Normal to slightly small colon in jejunal and proximal ileal atresia
- Initial imaging with supine and left lateral decubitus plain radiographs
- If distal obstruction without signs of perforation, then a contrast enema performed
- Water-soluble ionic contrast (nearly isosmotic to body fluids)
- Avoids fluid shifts into or out of bowel, especially premature infants
- If proximal obstruction (only few loops dilated) no imaging necessary
- If enema normal (rare), barium upper evaluation to exclude midgut volvulus
- Small amount of barium through nasogastric (NG) tube near pylorus

Clinical Issues
- Distal IA: Failure to pass meconium, abdominal distention, bilious emesis
- JA, proximal IA: Bilious emesis

- The earlier in gestation the obstruction occurs: The smaller the caliber of colon
- In distal obstruction, either IA, meconium ileus (MI), or total colonic Hirschsprung disease (HD)
- In proximal obstruction, predicts additional distal atresias
- Normal or near normal size colon
  - Seen in jejunal and proximal ileal atresias
  - Colon receives succus entericus from remaining small bowel
  - Rarely late in utero midgut volvulus with small bowel ileus mimics distal obstruction: Colon normal
  - Rarely ileal duplication causes distal obstruction ileal stenosis
- Reflux into normal caliber distal ileum which ends blindly: IA
- Dilated loops of unopacified small bowel proximal to obstruction

MR Findings
- T1WI and T2WI: In utero; progressive dilation of bowel during gestation

Ultrasonographic Findings
- Prenatal ultrasound
  - Dilated bowel loops may be echogenic
  - Calcifications if perforated (meconium peritonitis)

Imaging Recommendations
- Best imaging tool
  - For distal obstruction: Water-soluble contrast enema
  - For proximal obstruction: No imaging necessary except
    - +/- Enema to exclude distal atresias pre-operatively
- Initial imaging with supine and left lateral decubitus plain radiographs
- If distal obstruction without signs of perforation, then a contrast enema performed
  - Water-soluble ionic contrast (nearly isosmotic to body fluids)
    - Avoids fluid shifts into or out of bowel, especially premature infants
- If proximal obstruction (only few loops dilated) no imaging necessary
- Much debate concerning optimal contrast used for enema
- Barium not used, can impede evacuation of meconium
- If enema normal (rare), barium upper evaluation to exclude midgut volvulus
  - Small amount of barium through nasogastric (NG) tube near pylorus
  - Mimics distal obstruction due to ischemia induced ileus
  - These infants will usually be very ill

DIFFERENTIAL DIAGNOSIS

Meconium ileus
- Microcolon
- Meconium pellets obstructing terminal ileum
- Can opacify proximal loops with contrast

Meconium plug syndrome (small left colon syndrome)
- Proximal colon dilated rather than microcolon
- +/- Meconium plugs in colon
- Small caliber left colon to splenic flexure

Hirschsprung disease (total colonic HD)
- Recto/sigmoid ratio < 1
- +/- Meconium plugs
- Transition zone colonic or small bowel

Ileal duplication cyst
- Enema and upper gastrointestinal (GI) usually essentially normal
- Sonography usually makes diagnosis: Cyst with "gut signature" of wall

PATHOLOGY

General Features
- General path comments

JEJUNOILEAL ATRESIA

- More common in distal ileum and proximal jejunum than middle small bowel (SB)
- Etiology different than duodenal atresia (DA)
  - J-IA: In utero ischemia
  - Ischemia by primary vascular causes or in utero volvulus
- J-IA more common than stenosis
- Rare hereditary forms
  - Apple-peel or Christmas tree
  - Multiple intestinal atresias: French Canadian
- IA: Fewer associated anomalies compared to DA
- Can occur with meconium ileus complicated by in utero segmental volvulus
- Genetics
  - Reports of isolated IA in siblings
  - French Canadian ancestry in multiple intestinal atresias
  - Christmas tree atresia
- Etiology
  - Many theories
  - In utero vascular accident: Most accepted theory
    - Volvulus, occlusion of superior mesenteric artery, intussusception
- Associated abnormalities
  - In 10% of J-IA cases
    - Malrotation, volvulus, omphalocele, meconium ileus, gastroschisis
  - Higher incidence in JA than IA
  - Rare: Total colonic HD, biliary atresia, ano-rectal malformation

Staging, Grading or Classification Criteria
- Atresia: Surgical grading system
  - Type 1: Membranous atresia: Web or diaphragm
    - No mesenteric defect, no short bowel
  - Type 2: Blind ends separated by fibrous cord
    - No mesenteric defect, no short bowel
  - Type 3a: Blind ends but complete disconnection
    - V-shaped mesenteric gap, bowel short
  - Type 3b: Apple-peel or Christmas tree deformity (rare hereditary)
    - Large mesenteric defect, bowel short
    - Associated with prematurity, malrotation, short bowel
  - Type 4: Multiple small bowel atresias
- Stenosis: Narrow lumen, irregular muscularis, thick submucosa

CLINICAL ISSUES

Presentation
- Most common signs/symptoms
  - Distal IA: Failure to pass meconium, abdominal distention, bilious emesis
  - JA, proximal IA: Bilious emesis
  - Stenosis: Delayed presentation; intermittent emesis, failure to thrive
- Other signs/symptoms
  - Dilated bowel on prenatal sonography
  - Proximal obstruction: Normal or scaphoid abdomen

Demographics
- Age: In utero to first days of life

Natural History & Prognosis
- Prognosis dependent on amount of residual functional bowel
  - 40 cm is considered adequate
- JIA: Prognosis not as good due to other associated abnormalities
- Potential complications
  - Short gut syndrome, dysmotility, functional obstruction

Treatment
- Full resuscitation prior to surgical correction unless perforated or volvulus
- Surgical resection of affected bowel including very dilated segments
- +/- Tapering enteroplasty if bowel length limited

DIAGNOSTIC CHECKLIST

Consider
- Level of obstruction on radiography
- Differential diagnosis based on enema
- Associated abnormalities

Image Interpretation Pearls
- JA: Few, very dilated, loops with air/fluid levels: Normal size colon
- IA: Many dilated bowel loops with air fluid levels: Microcolon

SELECTED REFERENCES

1. Cho FN et al: Prenatal sonographic findings in a fetus with congenital isolated ileal atresia. J Chin Med Assoc. 67(7):366-8, 2004
2. Sangkhathat S et al: Ileal atresia and total colonic aganglionosis. J Med Assoc Thai. 85(10):1130-4, 2002
3. Rattan KN et al: Intrauterine intussusception--a cause for ileal atresia. Indian J Pediatr. 67(11):851-2, 2000
4. Hasegawa T et al: Ileal atresia associated with an omphalomesenteric duct remnant. Pediatr Surg Int. 13(2-3):182-3, 1998
5. Asabe K et al: Anorectal malformation with ileal atresia. Pediatr Surg Int. 12(4):302-4, 1997
6. Buonomo C: Neonatal gastrointestinal emergencies. Radiol Clin North Am. 35(4):845-64, 1997
7. Janik JP et al: Ileal atresia with total colonic aganglionosis. J Pediatr Surg. 32(10):1502-3, 1997
8. Neal MR et al: Neonatal ultrasonography to distinguish between meconium ileus and ileal atresia. J Ultrasound Med. 16(4):263-6; quiz 267-8, 1997
9. Jackman S et al: A lesson in intestinal atresias. J Pediatr Surg. 23(9):852-3, 1988
10. Kullendorff CM: Atresia of the small bowel. Ann Chir Gynaecol. 72(4):192-5, 1983
11. Gaisie G et al: The bulbous bowel segment: a sign of congenital small bowel obstruction. Radiology. 14:380-3, 1980
12. Daneman A et al: A syndrome of multiple intestinal atresias with intraluminal calcification. A report of a case and review of the literature. Pediatr Radiol 8:227-31, 1979
13. Berdon WE et al: Microcolon in newborn infants with intestinal obstruction. Its correlation with the level and time of onset of obstruction. Radiology 90:878-85, 1968

JEJUNOILEAL ATRESIA

IMAGE GALLERY

Typical

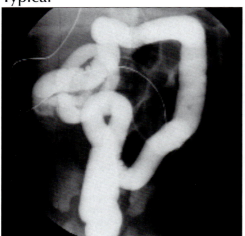 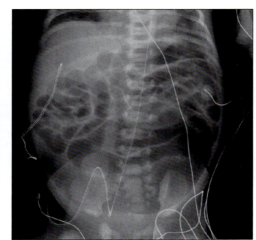

(Left) Anteroposterior contrast enema in a 2 day old shows a small colon with reflux into several loops of ileum; contrast failed to proceed into dilated bowel and ileal atresia found at surgery. *(Right)* Anteroposterior radiograph in a 1 day old with ileal atresia shows the typical appearance of distal bowel obstruction which could be due to various small bowel or colon causes.

Variant

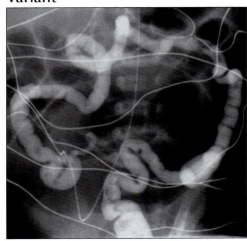 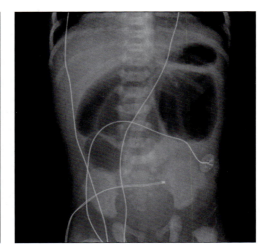

(Left) Anteroposterior contrast enema in a 2 day old shows a microcolon, however, contrast would not reflux into terminal ileum; this enema is indeterminate and at surgery, ileal atresia was found. *(Right)* Anteroposterior radiograph of 1 day old male with bilious emesis shows several moderately dilated loops of bowel suggestive of upper bowel obstruction, likely jejunal atresia.

Typical

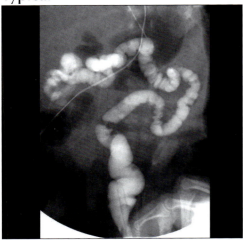 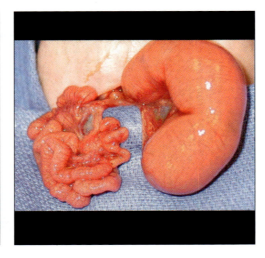

(Left) Anteroposterior contrast enema in same patient as above right shows a microcolon, suggesting a distal atresia in addition to the jejunal atresia, which was confirmed at surgery. *(Right)* Surgical photograph shows the dilated jejunum up to the atretic segment; the distal bowel is decompressed and when the bowel was run, a distal ileal atresia was noted, explaining the microcolon.

HIRSCHSPRUNG DISEASE

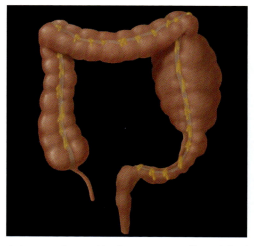

Anteroposterior graphic shows narrow caliber of distal colon through the rectum with transition to dilated proximal colon at the sigmoid, characteristic of low segment Hirschsprung disease.

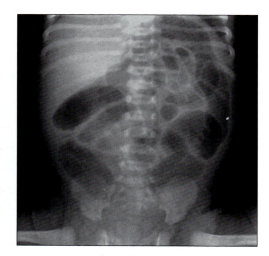

Anteroposterior radiograph in a 2 day old male shows multiple loops of dilated bowel consistent with distal obstruction, requiring a water-soluble contrast enema for further evaluation.

TERMINOLOGY

Abbreviations and Synonyms
- Hirschsprung disease (HD), colonic aganglionosis, total colonic HD, total colonic aganglionosis, total intestinal HD, total intestinal aganglionosis, congenital megacolon (CM)

Definitions
- Functional obstruction of the bowel due to lack of intrinsic enteric ganglion cells
- Described by Ruysch 1691, Hirschsprung 1886

IMAGING FINDINGS

General Features
- Best diagnostic clue: Recto-sigmoid (R/S) ratio < 1 on contrast enema
- Location: Colon
- Morphology
  o Denervated colon is small, narrow, spasmodic
  o Innervated more proximal bowel is dilated
  o Affected portion always includes the anus and variable length of contiguous colon
  o Continuous disease, no proximal without distal involvement

Radiographic Findings
- Radiography
  o Multiple loops of dilated bowel
  o Paucity of gas in the rectum

Fluoroscopic Findings
- Contrast enema findings
  o Rectum smaller than sigmoid (R/S ratio < 1)
  o Transition zone from abnormally small distal to dilated proximal colon
  o Fasciculations or sawtooth appearance of mucosa of involved colon: Spasm
  o Thickened, ulcerated colon in patients with associated colitis
  o Microcolon: Total colonic disease
  o Normal
    ▪ Especially in delayed diagnosis or very low segment disease
    ▪ Dilated distal bowel rarely ischemic: Midgut volvulus

Imaging Recommendations
- Best imaging tool
  o Neonates: Water-soluble contrast enema
  o Infants and children: Barium enema
- If bowel obstruction suspected clinically
  o Plain radiography: 2 view abdomen
- If distal obstruction

DDx: Distal Bowel Obstruction

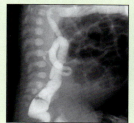
Small Left Colon

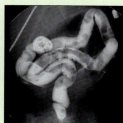
Immature Colon

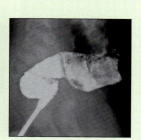
Milk Allergy Colitis

HIRSCHSPRUNG DISEASE

Key Facts

Terminology
- Functional obstruction of the bowel due to lack of intrinsic enteric ganglion cells

Imaging Findings
- Best diagnostic clue: Recto-sigmoid (R/S) ratio < 1 on contrast enema
- Denervated colon is small, narrow, spasmodic
- Innervated more proximal bowel is dilated
- Multiple loops of dilated bowel
- Transition zone from abnormally small distal to dilated proximal colon
- Neonates: Water-soluble contrast enema
- Infants and children: Barium enema
- Critical views: Lateral and AP of Rectosigmoid colon during early filling

Pathology
- Absence of both myenteric and submucosal plexus
- Most cases sporadic
- Familial HD in about 8-10% of HD
- Defective craniocaudal migration of vagal neural crest cells 5-12 weeks gestation

Clinical Issues
- Failure to pass meconium 24-48 hours
- Abdominal distention
- Bilious vomiting
- Constipation since birth
- 90% diagnosed in newborn
- Untreated, HD can lead to toxic megacolon, enterocolitis, sepsis and death
- Surgical resection of affected colon

  - Neonate: Water soluble enema
  - Infants and children: Barium enema
- Contrast enema
  - Critical views: Lateral and AP of Rectosigmoid colon during early filling
  - Compare rectum to sigmoid and more proximal colon
  - If enema normal, consider upper gastrointestinal (UGI) to exclude midgut volvulus

DIFFERENTIAL DIAGNOSIS

No microcolon: Meconium plug (small left colon) syndrome
- Benign reversible functional obstruction
- Resolves: Often after contrast enema
- R/S ratio usually > 1
- Abrupt transition zone at splenic flexure
- Differentiation made on rectal biopsy

No microcolon: Allergic (milk allergy) colitis
- Onset in first weeks of life
- Usually associated with formula feeding
- Enema shows R/S ratio < 1 and sometimes colitis
- Eosinophilia on rectal biopsy with normal ganglion cells

Microcolon (not total colonic HD): Meconium ileus
- Meconium pellets obstructing terminal ileum

Microcolon (not total colonic HD): Ileal atresia
- Abrupt cutoff of contrast in terminal ileum

Microcolon (not total colonic HD): Immature colon
- Premature infant with small colon throughout

Microcolon (not total colonic HD): Colonic atresia
- Small colon which usually ends abruptly in left colon

PATHOLOGY

General Features
- General path comments
  - Aganglionosis always involves anus, continues proximally
  - Absence of both myenteric and submucosal plexus
  - Reduced bowel peristalsis and function
- Genetics
  - Most cases sporadic
  - Several possible genetic mutations: Variable penetrance
    - RET proto-oncogene (RET) on chromosome 10 - MEN 2 and familial & sporadic HD
    - ZFHX1B(SIP1) gene mutation
    - Long segment HD - RET, GDNF glial-cell-line derived neurotrophic growth factor, EDNRB endothelin B receptor gene, EDN3 endothelin3, and Sry-related transcription factor SOX10
  - Familial HD in about 8-10% of HD
    - 20% ultrashort, 20% short, 20% long segment, 40% total colonic
    - Associated abnormalities in 25%
    - Enterocolitis: 35%
- Etiology
  - Precise mechanism unknown
    - Deficiency of nitric oxide and carbon monoxide (inhibitory neurotransmitters) in HD bowel
    - Altered cytoskeleton in smooth muscle of HD bowel
  - Defective craniocaudal migration of vagal neural crest cells 5-12 weeks gestation
  - Increased smooth muscle tone: Loss of tonic neural inhibition
  - Persistent, unopposed contraction of involved bowel: Functional obstruction

HIRSCHSPRUNG DISEASE

- Epidemiology: Frequency in USA 1:5,400-7,200 newborns
- Associated abnormalities
  - Down syndrome: 10-15% of patients with HD
  - Congenital heart disease
  - Genitourinary anomalies
  - Congenital deafness
  - Central hypoventilation (Ondine curse) and neurocristopathy
    - 1.5% of HD
    - 10% with total colonic HD
  - Ileal atresia

Gross Pathologic & Surgical Features
- Small spasmodic bowel from anus proximally
- Dilated bowel is normally innervated

Microscopic Features
- Absence of ganglion cells in myenteric (Auerbach) and submucosal (Meissner) plexus
- Diagnosis made by rectal biopsy: Absent ganglion cells
  - Suction biopsy: At bedside; not reliable as full thickness
  - Full thickness biopsy: Definitive
  - Acetylcholinesterase staining
  - Findings necrotizing colitis often superimposed on HD
- Disease continuous without skip areas
  - Case report: Segmental aganglionosis

Staging, Grading or Classification Criteria
- Short segment: Transition rectosigmoid; 70-80%
- Long segment: Transition above rectosigmoid; 15-25%
- Total colonic: Transition usually distal ileal; 1-4%
- Ultrashort segment: Transition at anorectal verge; very rare
- Total intestinal: Very rare

CLINICAL ISSUES

Presentation
- Most common signs/symptoms
  - Failure to pass meconium 24-48 hours
  - Abdominal distention
  - Bilious vomiting
- Other signs/symptoms
  - Constipation since birth
  - Enterocolitis
    - Enemas avoided in those who are ill
    - Increased risk of causing sepsis, perforation

Demographics
- Age
  - 90% diagnosed in newborn
  - 10% later, rarely adolescent or adult
    - Usually ultrashort segment disease, chronic constipation
- Gender: Males > females 4:1 (except long segment and total colonic 1:1)

Natural History & Prognosis
- Untreated, HD can lead to toxic megacolon, enterocolitis, sepsis and death
- Treated: 90% satisfactory outcome
  - Down syndrome patients have poorer outcome
  - Permanent colostomy in about 1% of surgical cases
- Long term outcome difficult to determine; issues are constipation and incontinence

Treatment
- Surgical resection of affected colon
  - Swenson procedure: Original surgical procedure
  - Duhamel procedure: 1956; modified Swenson
  - Soave (endorectal) procedure: 1960s; pull through procedure

DIAGNOSTIC CHECKLIST

Consider
- UGI to exclude midgut volvulus if enema normal
- Consider omphalomesenteric duct anomaly if enema and UGI normal
- Milk allergy colitis in patients beyond newborn period
- Total colonic HD if intraluminal calcifications

Image Interpretation Pearls
- Rectosigmoid ratio < 1 in HD
- Colitis in newborn, HD until proven otherwise
- Intraluminal calcifications: Total colonic HD, anorectal anomalies, ileal atresia

SELECTED REFERENCES

1. Lewis NA et al: Diagnosing Hirschsprung's disease: increasing the odds of a positive rectal biopsy result. J Pediatr Surg. 38(3):412-6; discussion 412-6, 2003
2. Teitelbaum DH et al: Primary pull-through for Hirschsprung's disease. Semin Neonatol. 8(3):233-41, 2003
3. Markham LA: Total colonic aganglionosis: a case study. Neonatal Netw. 20(2):23-9, 2001
4. Rogers J: Hirschsprung's disease: diagnosis and management in children. Br J Nurs. 10(10):640-9, 2001
5. Shanske A et al: Hirschsprung disease in an infant with a contiguous gene syndrome of chromosome 13. Am J Med Genet. 102(3):231-6, 2001
6. Lall A et al: Neonatal Hirschsprung's disease. Indian J Pediatr. 67(8):583-8, 2000
7. Martucciello G et al: Pathogenesis of Hirschsprung's disease. J Pediatr Surg. 35(7):1017-25, 2000
8. Valioulis I et al: A complex chromosomal rearrangement associated with Hirschsprung's disease. A case report with a review of the literature. Eur J Pediatr Surg. 10(3):207-11, 2000
9. Bloom DA et al: Allergic colitis: a mimic of Hirschsprung disease. Pediatr Radiol. 29(1):37-41, 1999
10. Croaker GD et al: Congenital central hypoventilation syndrome and Hirschsprung's disease. Arch Dis Child. 78(4):316-22, 1998
11. Janik JP et al: Ileal atresia with total colonic aganglionosis. J Pediatr Surg. 32(10):1502-3, 1997
12. Buonomo C: Neonatal gastrointestinal emergencies. Radiol Clin North Am. 35(4):845-64, 1997
13. Martin LW et al: Hirschsprung's disease with skip area (segmental aganglionosis). J Pediatr Surg. 14(6):686-7, 1979
14. Berdon WE et al: The roentgenographic diagnosis of Hirschsprung disease in infancy. AJR. 93:432-46, 1965

HIRSCHSPRUNG DISEASE

IMAGE GALLERY

Typical

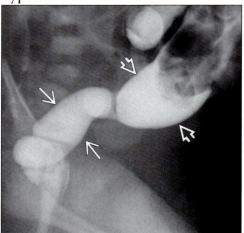
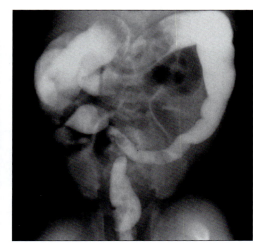

(Left) Lateral contrast enema in 2 day old with water soluble contrast shows small rectum (arrows) with transition to dilated rectosigmoid (open arrows) and a R/S ratio < 1, in biopsy proven HD. *(Right)* Anteroposterior contrast enema in 2 day old shows R/S ratio < 1 with broad transition zone distal to the splenic flexure of the colon, suggestive of Hirschsprung disease; + rectal biopsy.

Variant

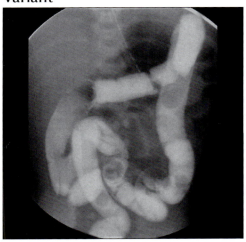
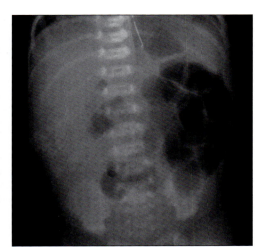

(Left) Anteroposterior contrast enema in 2 day old shows equivocal R/S ratio and smallish colon with no transition in this case which was called possible total colonic HD, confirmed by biopsy. *(Right)* Anteroposterior radiograph in 3 day old male shows round calcific densities in the right abdomen with multiple dilated loops of bowel; considerations included total colonic HD and enema performed (see next image).

Variant

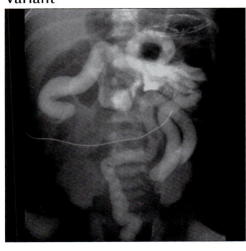
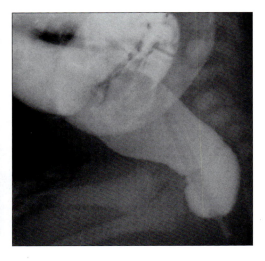

(Left) Anteroposterior contrast enema of previous case shows a small colon and no reflux into terminal ileum; at surgery, there were no ganglion cells in the intestine, the rare total intestinal HD. *(Right)* Lateral contrast enema shows low rectal transition zone, biopsy proven Hirschsprung disease, that could be obscured by a larger catheter if it is placed too deep into the rectum.

MECONIUM PLUG SYNDROME

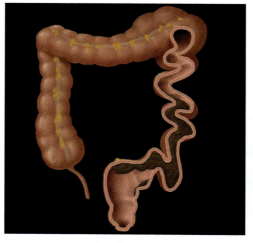

Anteroposterior graphic shows meconium plug (small left colon) syndrome, also known as functional immaturity of the colon. Note small left colon with plugs of meconium, usually to splenic flexure.

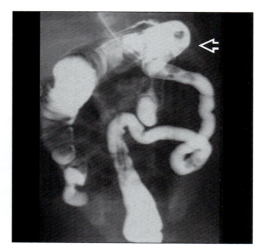

Anteroposterior contrast enema shows a normal R/S ratio, small left colon to about the splenic flexure (arrow), and several meconium plugs within the small left and dilated proximal colon.

TERMINOLOGY

Abbreviations and Synonyms
- Meconium plug syndrome (MPS), small left colon syndrome (SLCS), functional immaturity of the colon (FIC)

Definitions
- Transient functional obstruction of the newborn colon
- Common cause of distal neonatal bowel obstruction

IMAGING FINDINGS

General Features
- Best diagnostic clue
  - Multiple dilated bowel loops in neonate
  - Contrast enema findings include
    - Normal recto-sigmoid (R/S) ratio: Usually
    - Small left colon to the splenic flexure
    - Abrupt zone of transition to dilated proximal colon at the splenic flexure
    - Multiple meconium plugs in the colon
- Location: Left colon
- Size: Small left colon with transition to dilated proximal bowel at splenic flexure
- Morphology: Small but otherwise normal left colon

Radiographic Findings
- Radiography
  - Multiple dilated loops of bowel
  - Cannot differentiate dilated large from small bowel loops in neonates
  - Findings nonspecific, cannot differentiate from other causes of distal bowel

Fluoroscopic Findings
- Contrast enema
  - Recto-sigmoid ratio usually > 1
  - Small caliber left colon to the splenic flexure
  - Abrupt transition to dilated proximal colon
  - Multiple filling defects may fill left colon, but not required
  - Frequent passage of meconium plugs during enema

Other Modality Findings
- Contrast enema
  - R/S ratio usually > 1
  - Descending and sigmoid colon small in caliber
  - Abrupt zone of caliber transition in region of splenic flexure
  - +/- Filling defects (meconium plugs) within colon
  - Ascending and transverse colon increased in caliber
  - Difficult to differentiate from long segment Hirschsprung disease

DDx: Neonatal Distal Bowel Obstruction

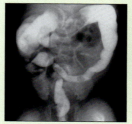
Hirschsprung Disease

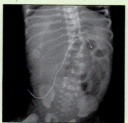
Colonic Atresia

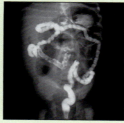
Meconium Ileus

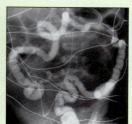
Ileal Atresia

MECONIUM PLUG SYNDROME

Key Facts

Terminology
- Meconium plug syndrome (MPS), small left colon syndrome (SLCS), functional immaturity of the colon (FIC)
- Transient functional obstruction of the newborn colon
- Common cause of distal neonatal bowel obstruction

Imaging Findings
- Multiple dilated bowel loops in neonate
- Small left colon to the splenic flexure
- Abrupt zone of transition to dilated proximal colon at the splenic flexure
- Multiple filling defects may fill left colon, but not required
- Difficult to differentiate from long segment Hirschsprung disease
- Best imaging tool: Water-soluble contrast enema

Pathology
- Distal colon spastic and narrowed, causes functional obstruction usually at the splenic flexure
- Genetics: No association with cystic fibrosis
- Etiology: Probably immaturity of ganglion cells or hormonal receptors
- Associated abnormalities: Most with MPS do not have associated abnormalities

Clinical Issues
- Abdominal distention
- Delayed or failed passage of meconium (> 24-48 hours)
- Bilious emesis
- Condition resolves over time, hastened by enemas

○ Enema often therapeutic; passage of meconium plugs during or just after enema

Imaging Recommendations
- Best imaging tool: Water-soluble contrast enema
- In neonate with abdominal distention, failure to pass meconium, bilious emesis
  ○ Abdominal radiograph: 2 views
    ▪ If multiple dilated loops: Suspect distal bowel obstruction
    ▪ If distal obstruction: Water-soluble contrast enema
  ○ Enema
    ▪ Non-balloon tipped catheter
    ▪ ionic, water-soluble agents, isosmotic to body fluids
    ▪ Barium avoided in neonate; etiology of obstruction unknown
    ▪ Initial lateral film of rectum and sigmoid through the splenic flexure
    ▪ If enema shows normal colon (rare) but dilated small bowel loops then perform upper gastrointestinal (GI) to exclude midgut volvulus (malrotation)

DIFFERENTIAL DIAGNOSIS

Hirschsprung disease
- Rectum smaller than sigmoid diameter, serrated mucosa
- May be difficult to differentiate from meconium plug syndrome
- Broad cone-like zone of transition near splenic flexure

Ileal atresia
- Microcolon
- Portions of ileum opacified are collapsed and blind ends
- Cannot opacify dilated loops (proximal to atresia)

Meconium ileus
- Microcolon
- Distal ileum filled with meconium pellets
- Small bowel proximal to meconium filled segment is dilated
- Nearly all have cystic fibrosis

Colonic atresia
- Microcolon to level of atresia
- Very rare
- Distal obstruction with a single disproportionately dilated loop

Midgut volvulus
- Normal caliber colon on enema: Perform upper GI
- Mimics distal obstruction: Late presentation
- Dilated bowel loops due to ischemia not obstruction
- Upper GI shows
  ○ Abnormal duodenal jejunal junction
  ○ Obstruction at 2nd to 3rd portion duodenum
  ○ Corkscrew, spiral appearance

PATHOLOGY

General Features
- General path comments
  ○ Transient functional disorder of the colon
  ○ No pathologic or laboratory abnormality
  ○ Clinical and radiographic disorder only
  ○ Distal colon spastic and narrowed, causes functional obstruction usually at the splenic flexure
- Genetics: No association with cystic fibrosis
- Etiology: Probably immaturity of ganglion cells or hormonal receptors
- Epidemiology
  ○ Predisposing factors: Infants of
    ▪ Diabetic mothers
    ▪ Mothers treated with magnesium sulfate for preeclampsia
- Associated abnormalities: Most with MPS do not have associated abnormalities

Gross Pathologic & Surgical Features
- Not a pathologic or surgical abnormality

MECONIUM PLUG SYNDROME

CLINICAL ISSUES

Presentation
- Most common signs/symptoms
  - Abdominal distention
  - Delayed or failed passage of meconium (> 24-48 hours)
  - Bilious emesis
- Other signs/symptoms: Otherwise well infant
- Most frequent encountered diagnosis in neonates who fail to pass meconium
- Increased incidence of meconium plug syndrome
  - Infants of diabetic mothers
  - Mothers who receive magnesium sulfate for eclampsia
  - Meconium plug syndrome and meconium ileus (cystic fibrosis) are distinct entities not to be confused
    - Meconium plug syndrome: Zone of transition splenic flexure of colon
    - Meconium ileus: Microcolon with obstructing meconium plugs in terminal ileum

Demographics
- Age: Neonates
- Gender: No gender predilection
- Ethnicity: No known ethnicity predilection

Natural History & Prognosis
- Temporary phenomenon: Usually resolves with benign course
- Prognosis excellent
- Potential complications: Rare
  - Perforation due to unresolved obstruction
  - If hypertonic water-soluble contrast used for enema
    - Rapid fluid shift into the colon causing potentially severe, life-threatening hypotension
    - Electrolyte imbalance

Treatment
- Condition resolves over time, hastened by enemas
- Often resolves after diagnostic water-soluble contrast enema
- Suction rectal biopsy to exclude Hirschsprung disease, especially if persistent symptoms

DIAGNOSTIC CHECKLIST

Consider
- Hirschsprung disease
- Immature colon if premature infant

Image Interpretation Pearls
- Normal R/S ratio (> 1)
- Small left colon +/- meconium plugs
- Transition point to dilated bowel at splenic flexure

SELECTED REFERENCES

1. Burge D et al: Meconium plug obstruction. Pediatr Surg Int. 20(2):108-10, 2004
2. Hajivassiliou CA: Intestinal obstruction in neonatal/pediatric surgery. Semin Pediatr Surg. 12(4):241-53, 2003
3. De Backer AI et al: Radiographic manifestations of intestinal obstruction in the newborn. JBR-BTR. 82(4):159-66, 1999
4. Lassmann G et al: Transient functional obstruction of the colon in neonates: examination of its development by manometry and biopsies. Prog Pediatr Surg. 24:202-16, 1989
5. Hall SL et al: Neonatal intussusception associated with neonatal small left colon syndrome. Clin Pediatr (Phila). 26(4):191-3, 1987
6. Amodio J et al: Microcolon of prematurity: a form of functional obstruction. AJR Am J Roentgenol. 146(2):239-44, 1986
7. Ellerbroek C et al: Neonatal small left colon in an infant with cystic fibrosis. Pediatr Radiol. 16(2):162-3, 1986
8. Johnson JF et al: Localized bowel distension in the newborn: a review of the plain film analysis and differential diagnosis. Pediatrics. 73(2):206-15, 1984
9. Rosenfield NS et al: Hirschsprung disease: accuracy of the barium enema examination. Radiology. 150(2):393-400, 1984
10. Cohen MD et al: Neonatal small left colon syndrome in twins. Gastrointest Radiol. 7(3):283-6, 1982
11. Dunn V et al: Infants of diabetic mothers: radiographic manifestations. AJR Am J Roentgenol. 137(1):123-8, 1981
12. Rangecroft L: Neonatal small left colon syndrome. Arch Dis Child. 54(8):635-7, 1979
13. Berdon WE et al: Neonatal small left colon syndrome: its relationship to aganglionosis and meconium plug syndrome. Radiology. 125(2):457-62, 1977
14. Ferrara TP et al: The radiology corner. Neonatal small left colon syndrome. Am J Gastroenterol. 68(6):608-12, 1977
15. Stewart DR et al: Neonatal small left colon syndrome. Ann Surg. 186(6):741-5, 1977
16. Davis WS et al: Neonatal small left colon syndrome. Occurrence in asymptomatic infants of diabetic mothers. Am J Dis Child. 129(9):1024-7, 1975
17. Davis WS et al: Neonatal small left colon syndrome. AJR. 120:322-9, 1974
18. Berdon WE et al: Microcolon in newborn infants with intestinal obstruction. Its correlation with the level and time of onset of obstruction. Radiology. 90:878-88, 1968

MECONIUM PLUG SYNDROME

IMAGE GALLERY

Typical

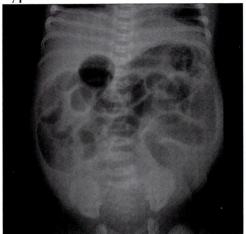
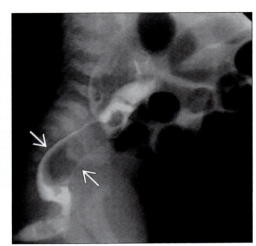

(Left) Anteroposterior radiograph in a 2 day old female with failure to pass meconium and abdominal distention shows multiple dilated bowel loops consistent with distal bowel obstruction. *(Right)* Lateral contrast enema at initial filling of rectum and sigmoid colon shows filling defect (meconium) in rectum (arrows), normal R/S ratio and multiple dilated loops of bowel.

Typical

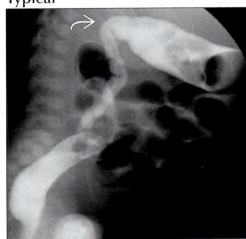
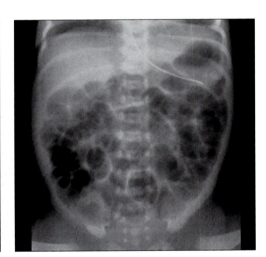

(Left) Lateral contrast enema in same patient as above shows abrupt caliber change of the colon at the splenic flexure (arrow) suggestive of meconium plug (small left colon) syndrome. *(Right)* Anteroposterior radiograph of same patient 2 days after the enema shows resolution of the functional obstruction, typical in the natural history of small left colon syndrome.

Typical

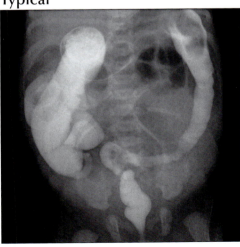
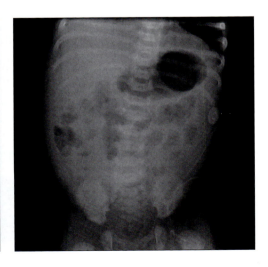

(Left) Anteroposterior contrast enema immediately following the radiograph on previous image shows a small left colon with a somewhat blunted transition near the splenic flexure; biopsy of the rectum was normal. *(Right)* Anteroposterior radiograph on the day following the enema on previous image shows resolution of the functional distal bowel obstruction, typical of functional immaturity of the colon, also known as SLCS and MPS.

MECONIUM ILEUS

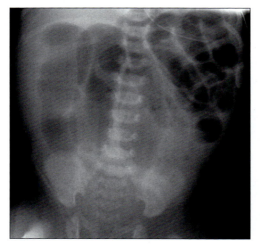

Anteroposterior radiograph in full term neonate who failed to pass meconium shows multiple dilated bowel loops consistent with distal bowel obstruction; no free air or calcifications noted.

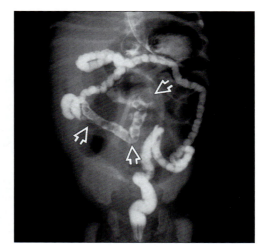

Anteroposterior contrast enema shows smallest microcolon with multiple obstructing meconium pellets in the terminal ileum (arrows), findings pathognomonic for meconium ileus.

TERMINOLOGY

Abbreviations and Synonyms
- Meconium ileus (MI)

Definitions
- Neonatal obstruction of the distal ileum due to abnormally thick, tenacious meconium
  - Essentially all patients with MI have cystic fibrosis (CF)
  - Presenting illness in approximately 15% of CF patients

IMAGING FINDINGS

General Features
- Best diagnostic clue: Distal bowel obstruction with microcolon on enema and meconium-filled terminal ileum (TI)
- Location: Terminal ileum obstruction
- Size: Microcolon (dis-use), small TI, dilated proximal small bowel
- Morphology: Small but morphologically normal TI and colon

Radiographic Findings
- Radiography
  - Difficult to distinguish neonatal large vs. small bowel
  - Uncomplicated MI
    - Multiple dilated bowel loops
    - +/- Bubbly lucencies right lower quadrant (RLQ)
    - Few, if any air-fluid levels (sticky meconium)
    - Contrast enema to diagnose cause of obstruction
  - Complicated MI
    - Soft tissue mass or gasless abdomen
    - +/- Intrauterine perforation and peritonitis
    - Curvilinear calcifications on peritoneal surface or lining pseudocyst
    - Enemas for treatment usually fail, microcolon suggests diagnosis
    - Almost all eventually require surgical treatment

Fluoroscopic Findings
- Water-soluble contrast enema
  - Smallest of microcolons
  - Reflux contrast into TI
  - Meconium pellets in TI; not much in colon
  - Can be therapeutic in uncomplicated MI

Ultrasonographic Findings
- Grayscale Ultrasound
  - Dilated, thick-walled, echogenic bowel loops
  - If perforation: Echogenic ascites or pseudocyst, calcification
- Prenatal Ultrasound

DDx: Microcolon

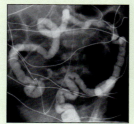
Ileal Atresia

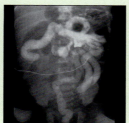
Total Colonic HD

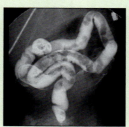
Immature Colon

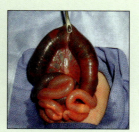
Meconium Ileus

MECONIUM ILEUS

Key Facts

Terminology
- Neonatal obstruction of the distal ileum due to abnormally thick, tenacious meconium
- Essentially all patients with MI have cystic fibrosis (CF)

Imaging Findings
- Best diagnostic clue: Distal bowel obstruction with microcolon on enema and meconium-filled terminal ileum (TI)
- Uncomplicated MI
- Multiple dilated bowel loops
- Complicated MI
- Soft tissue mass or gasless abdomen
- +/- Intrauterine perforation and peritonitis
- Water-soluble contrast enema
- Smallest of microcolons
- Dilated, thick-walled, echogenic bowel loops
- Best imaging tool: Water-soluble enema

Top Differential Diagnoses
- Ileal atresia
- Total colonic Hirschsprung disease (HD)

Pathology
- Mutations in CFTCRG, faulty electrolyte transport across epithelium

Clinical Issues
- Most common signs/symptoms: Failure to pass meconium, abdominal distention, bilious emesis
- Uncomplicated MI: Serial hyperosmotic, water-soluble enemas vs. surgery
- Complicated MI: Surgery

  - Dilated echogenic bowel especially RLQ, peritoneal calcifications, pseudocyst

Imaging Recommendations
- Best imaging tool: Water-soluble enema
- If distal bowel obstruction on radiographs: Contrast enema
- Enemas performed with non-balloon tip catheter
- Dilute, ionic, water-soluble agents
- Much debate concerning optimal contrast used
- Meglumine diatrizoate (Gastrografin): High osmolar agent for treatment of MI
  - Controversial
  - Full-strength dangerous secondary to fluid shifts
- If enema shows no abnormalities (rare), upper gastrointestinal (GI)
  - Exclude midgut volvulus with diffuse ischemia

DIFFERENTIAL DIAGNOSIS

Ileal atresia
- Microcolon
- Portions of ileum opacified collapse
- Cannot opacify bowel proximal to atresia

Total colonic Hirschsprung disease (HD)
- Microcolon
- Meconium plugs in colon +/- TI
- Abnormal rectosigmoid index, smallish colon, serrated mucosa
- Very rare

Meconium plug syndrome (small left colon syndrome)
- Not closely associated with cystic fibrosis
- Colon dilated proximal to splenic flexure; no microcolon
- Meconium plugs predominantly in colon not TI
- Enema often curative

PATHOLOGY

General Features
- General path comments
  - Cystic fibrosis gene (chromosome 7) results in failure of cell membrane chloride pump
  - This failure results in abnormally thick, tenacious meconium
    - Occludes distal ileum and results in bowel obstruction
  - Obstruction can also result in perforation, meconium peritonitis
  - Twisting of meconium-filled loops: In utero bowel volvulus and atresia
- Genetics
  - Autosomal recessive, chromosome 7
  - Mutation of cystic fibrosis transmembrane conductance regulator gene (CFTCRG)
- Etiology
  - Mutations in CFTCRG, faulty electrolyte transport across epithelium
    - Dehydration of luminal contents; obstruction of glands and ducts
    - Pancreas, intestine and lung are organs most affected
- Epidemiology
  - 15% of CF present with MI
  - CF: 1:3,000 live births
  - Caucasian children
- Associated abnormalities
  - Lung disease: Upper lobe predominance
    - Bronchiectasis
    - Mucous plugging
    - Pneumonia atypical pathogens
  - Exocrine pancreas failure: Enzyme deficiency
  - Biliary disease: Obstruction, cholangitis
  - Concurrent GI manifestations: 50% with MI
    - Meconium peritonitis, small intestinal atresia/stenoses, duplication, segmental volvulus, mesenteric bands or adhesions

MECONIUM ILEUS

Gross Pathologic & Surgical Features
- Uncomplicated: Distal small bowel obstruction, obstructing meconium in TI
- Complicated
  - Meconium peritonitis
  - Giant cystic meconium peritonitis
  - Volvulus of dilated bowel segment
  - Atresia in region of segmental volvulus or perforation
  - Obstructing mesenteric bands

Staging, Grading or Classification Criteria
- Uncomplicated MI: 50%
- Complicated MI: 50%
  - Perforation
    - Ascites with diffuse peritonitis
    - Giant cystic meconium peritonitis
    - Calcification: Speckled or curvilinear
  - Segmental volvulus
  - Atresia

CLINICAL ISSUES

Presentation
- Most common signs/symptoms: Failure to pass meconium, abdominal distention, bilious emesis

Demographics
- Age
  - Newborn; sometimes premature newborns
    - Immature colon can mimic MI
- Gender: Male = female
- Ethnicity: Predominantly Caucasian disease

Natural History & Prognosis
- Poor prognosis if obstruction not treated
- MI associated with the worst survival and lung disease outcomes in CF patients
- 1 year survival in patients presenting with MI: 1993 data
  - Uncomplicated: 92%
  - Complicated: 89%
- Estimated probability of long term survival for patients with CF
  - Without MI: 62% +/- 14%
  - With MI: 32% +/- 18%

Treatment
- Uncomplicated MI: Serial hyperosmotic, water-soluble enemas vs. surgery
  - Success rate of enemas 70-80% in experienced centers
  - Perforation rate of enema 1-3%
    - Greatest with injection and use of rectal balloon
  - Surgical if patient decompensates, enemas fail, or if perforation
    - Enterotomy, removal of obstructing meconium, primary closure
- Complicated MI: Surgery
  - Resect abnormal bowel, remove meconium, primary anastamosis
  - If giant meconium cyst: Enterostomy and delayed take down
- Testing for cystic fibrosis

DIAGNOSTIC CHECKLIST

Consider
- Causes of distal obstruction and microcolon
- Hyperosmolar water-soluble contrast if presumed uncomplicated MI
- Enema therapy rarely curative in complicated MI

SELECTED REFERENCES

1. Lai HJ et al: Association between initial disease presentation, lung disease outcomes, and survival in patients with cystic fibrosis. Am J Epidemiol. 159(6):537-46, 2004
2. Eckoldt F et al: Meconium peritonitis and pseudo-cyst formation: prenatal diagnosis and post-natal course. Prenat Diagn. 23(11):904-8, 2003
3. Hajivassiliou CA: Intestinal obstruction in neonatal/pediatric surgery. Semin Pediatr Surg. 12(4):241-53, 2003
4. Burke MS et al: New strategies in nonoperative management of meconium ileus. J Pediatr Surg. 37(5):760-4, 2002
5. Oliveira MC et al: Effect of meconium ileus on the clinical prognosis of patients with cystic fibrosis. Braz J Med Biol Res. 35(1):31-8, 2002
6. De Backer AI et al: Radiographic manifestations of intestinal obstruction in the newborn. JBR-BTR. 82(4):159-66, 1999
7. Feingold J et al: Genetic comparisons of patients with cystic fibrosis with or without meconium ileus. Clinical Centers of the French CF Registry. Ann Genet. 42(3):147-50, 1999
8. Mushtaq I et al: Meconium ileus secondary to cystic fibrosis. The East London experience. Pediatr Surg Int. 13(5-6):365-9, 1998
9. Buonomo C: Neonatal gastrointestinal emergencies. Radiol Clin North Am. 35(4):845-64, 1997
10. Murshed R et al: Meconium ileus: a ten-year review of thirty-six patients. Eur J Pediatr Surg. 7(5):275-7, 1997
11. Neal MR et al: Neonatal ultrasonography to distinguish between meconium ileus and ileal atresia. J Ultrasound Med. 16(4):263-6; quiz 267-8, 1997
12. Kao SC et al: Nonoperative treatment of simple meconium ileus: a survey of the Society for Pediatric Radiology. Pediatr Radiol. 25(2):97-100, 1995
13. Stringer MD et al: Meconium ileus due to extensive intestinal aganglionosis. J Pediatr Surg. 29(4):501-3, 1994
14. Docherty JG et al: Meconium ileus: a review 1972-1990. Br J Surg. 79(6):571-3, 1992
15. Fakhoury K et al: Meconium ileus in the absence of cystic fibrosis. Arch Dis Child. 67(10 Spec No):1204-6, 1992
16. Hussain SM et al: Plain film diagnosis in meconium plug syndrome, meconium ileus and neonatal Hirschsprung's disease. A scoring system. Pediatr Radiol. 21(8):556-9, 1991
17. Leonidas JC et al: Meconium ileus and its complications. A reappraisal of plain film roentgen diagnostic criteria. AJR. 108:598-609, 1970
18. Berdon WE et al: Microcolon in newborn infants with intestinal obstruction. Its correlation with the level and time of onset of obstruction. Radiology. 90:878-85, 1968

MECONIUM ILEUS

IMAGE GALLERY

Typical

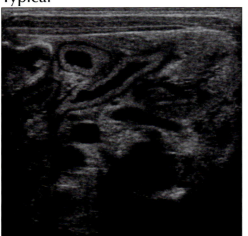
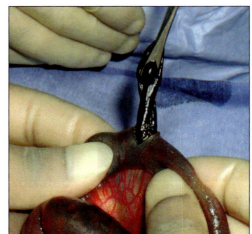

(Left) Transverse ultrasound image in patient with neonatal distal bowel obstruction shows thick-walled, echogenic, fluid-filled small bowel which is commonly seen in patients with meconium ileus. *(Right)* Intra-operative photograph shows manual removal of inspissated meconium through an enterotomy in this patient with MI who had serial water-soluble contrast enemas that were unsuccessful.

Typical

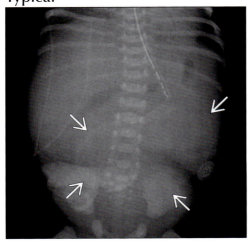
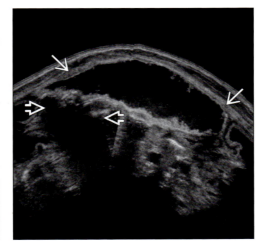

(Left) Anteroposterior radiograph of newborn abdomen shows paucity of gas, rim calcification (arrows) of abdominal mass, likely due to in utero perforation, not uncommon in complicated MI. *(Right)* Transverse ultrasound with extended view of patient at left shows giant meconium cyst (arrows) filled with echogenic contents and shadowing calcification (open arrows).

Typical

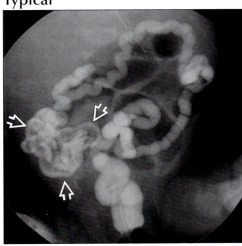
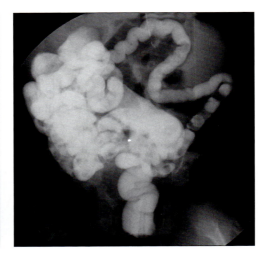

(Left) Anteroposterior contrast enema shows tiny microcolon with reflux of contrast into meconium-filled TI (arrows), most consistent with MI; treatment followed with 1/2 strength Gastrografin. *(Right)* Anteroposterior contrast enema in neonate shows contrast proximal to TI meconium; later images showed decompression of obstruction and passage of meconium, successful non-invasive therapy.

NECROTIZING ENTEROCOLITIS

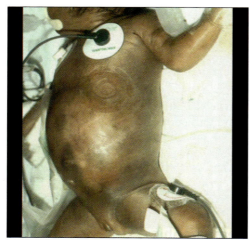

Oblique clinical photograph shows distended abdomen and discoloration of the thin abdominal skin which covers the dilated ischemic and/or necrotic bowel in this patient with advanced NEC.

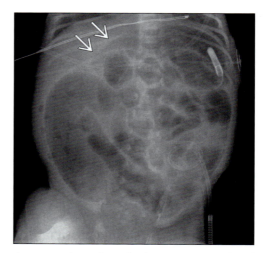

Anteroposterior radiograph shows asymmetric bowel distention, persistently large dilated loop, probable pneumatosis and free air (arrows).

TERMINOLOGY

Abbreviations and Synonyms
- Necrotizing enterocolitis (NEC)

Definitions
- Idiopathic enterocolitis in very low birth weight premature infants most likely related to some combination of infection and ischemia characterized by coagulative and hemorrhagic necrosis and inflammation of portions of the small and large intestine

IMAGING FINDINGS

General Features
- Best diagnostic clue: Pneumatosis
- Location: Most common right colon and terminal ileum; but can occur anywhere in gastrointestinal (GI) tract
- Morphology
  ○ Acutely either normal caliber or dilated bowel
  ○ Chronically may be narrow caliber or stricture, single or multiple; a complication of NEC

Radiographic Findings
- Radiography
  ○ Findings range from normal to suggestive to diagnostic
  ○ Normal
  ○ Suggestive findings
    ■ Asymmetric bowel dilation
    ■ Featureless "unfolded" bowel loops
    ■ Separation of bowel loops
    ■ Fixed configuration of bowel loop(s) over serial films
  ○ Definitive finding: Pneumatosis (50-75% of patients)
    ■ Most common right lower quadrant (RLQ) abdomen, can occur anywhere
    ■ Bubble-like (submucosal) or curvilinear (serosal) lucencies
    ■ Mimics meconium or stool (which is not typically seen in premature infants)
  ○ Definitive finding: Portal venous gas (PVG)
    ■ Branching lucencies over the liver
    ■ More peripheral extension than biliary gas
  ○ Definitive finding: Free intraperitoneal air
    ■ Triangles of anterior lucency, cross-table lateral radiographs
    ■ Lucency adjacent to liver, left lateral decubitus radiographs
    ■ Overall increased lucency, supine radiographs
    ■ Air on both sides of bowel wall (Rigler sign)
    ■ Outline of falciform ligament (football sign)

DDx: Premature Bowel Obstruction

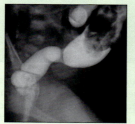
Hirschsprung

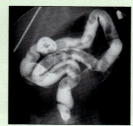
Immature Colon

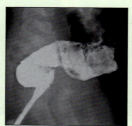
Allergic Colitis

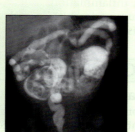
RLQ NEC Stricture

ANORECTAL MALFORMATION

Key Facts

Terminology
- Anorectal malformation (ARM), imperforate anus, cloacal malformation

Imaging Findings
- Multiple dilated bowel loops; clinically no anal opening
- Distal bowel obstruction, intraluminal calcification
- Bladder findings
- Normal; vesicoureteral reflux (VUR); wall-thickening; neurogenic bladder; fistula to rectum
- Urethral findings
- Opens to cloaca, fistula from rectum to posterior > bulbous > penile urethra
- Vaginal findings
- Normal; rectovaginal fistula; congenital anomalies (septate, duplicated, etc.)
- Document connection to urethra, bladder, or vagina
- Pelvic musculature, neorectum, and anal sphincter position/integrity
- Ultrasound (US) hypoechoic rectal pouch-perineal distance

Pathology
- Currarino triad (ARM, sacral deformity, presacral mass)
- Classification: Location of pouch relative to levator ani muscle (PCL on lateral pelvis)

Clinical Issues
- Most common signs/symptoms: Absent/abnormal anal opening, failure to pass meconium, meconium per vagina or urethra

---

- +/- Cloacagram
- Catheter into cloaca (single perineal orifice)
  - Enters bladder, vagina, or colon
- Bladder findings
  - Normal; vesicoureteral reflux (VUR); wall-thickening; neurogenic bladder; fistula to rectum
- Urethral findings
  - Opens to cloaca, fistula from rectum to posterior > bulbous > penile urethra
- Vaginal findings
  - Normal; rectovaginal fistula; congenital anomalies (septate, duplicated, etc.)
- Fistulagram
  - Aka: Distal colostogram
  - Several months after colostomy prior to repair
  - 8-12 Fr Foley catheter in defunctionalized colon stoma
  - Inject water soluble contrast to opacify fistula
  - Key view is lateral
  - Document connection to urethra, bladder, or vagina

MR Findings
- Pelvis
  - Pelvic musculature, neorectum, and anal sphincter position/integrity
    - Normal to absent levator muscle
    - Normal to absent anal sphincter complex
    - Prognosticator of post-op bowel continence
  - Muscle complex malpositioned or atrophic
- Spine
  - Tethered cord, spinal dysraphism, sacral agenesis

Ultrasonographic Findings
- Grayscale Ultrasound
  - Ultrasound (US) hypoechoic rectal pouch-perineal distance
    - < 10 mm: Low lesion; > 10-15 mm - high or intermediate
    - Reliability similar to radiography with similar inaccuracies
    - Evaluate genital structures and urinary structures

Imaging Recommendations
- Best imaging tool
  - Initial diagnosis: Plain radiography or US but unreliable
  - For fistula: Colostogram after diverting colostomy
  - For pre-op anorectoplasty planning: MRI pelvis
    - Development sphincter muscle complex
- Protocol advice
  - Initial abdominal radiographs low vs. high lesion, but unreliable
    - Calcified intraluminal meconium in boy - rectourethral fistula - high lesion
  - Initial US can differentiate low from high but unreliable
  - Renal and bladder US prior to surgery
  - Radiography and US +/- MRI evaluation of spine
  - MRI
    - Rectal pouch relative to puborectalis
    - Pelvic musculature and sphincter muscle complex
    - Fistulae: Low sensitivity for detection (requires T2 imaging)
    - Vertebral and spinal cord anomalies
  - Distal colostogram: High or intermediate lesions prior to definitive operation
    - High sensitivity for fistula detection
  - Voiding cystogram: Vesicoureteral reflux (VUR)?
  - Genitogram/vaginogram/cloacagram
  - If post-op incontinence, MRI pelvis
    - Pelvic/anal musculature, position of neo-anus/rectum

DIFFERENTIAL DIAGNOSIS

Neonatal distal bowel obstruction
- Small left colon
- Hirschsprung disease
- Meconium Ileus
- Ileal atresia

Cloacal exstrophy
- Pubic symphysis diastasis, short colon

ANORECTAL MALFORMATION

- Most severe midline fusion abnormality
- Closed, less severe form looks like ARM

PATHOLOGY

General Features
- Genetics
  - Currarino syndrome
    - Haplotype reconstruction: 7q36 region
  - VATER, VACTERL sequence
- Etiology
  - Unknown
  - Abnormal separation GU system from hindgut
- Epidemiology: 1:5000 births
- Associated abnormalities
  - Some low lesions, 50-66% of high
    - Genitourinary: Horseshoe, agenesis, hypoplasia, hydronephrosis, VUR, bicornuate uterus, uterine didelphys, vaginal septum
    - Skeletal (especially lumbosacral spine)
    - Congenital heart disease: Tetrology of Fallot, ventricular septal defect
    - Esophageal atresia with tracheoesophageal fistula, duodenal atresia, Hirschsprung
    - VATER, VACTERL, caudal regression syndrome
  - Currarino triad (ARM, sacral deformity, presacral mass)

Gross Pathologic & Surgical Features
- Perineal fistula
  - Rectum opens small stenotic orifice
  - Anterior to center sphincter
  - Only lesion treated as newborn, no colostomy
- Imperforate anus
  - Rectourethral fistula: Most males (50%)
    - Prostatic: Poor sacrum and sphincters
    - Bulbar: Good sacrum and sphincters
  - Rectobladder-neck fistula: 10% of males
    - Requires laparotomy
    - Poor sacrum and sphincter
  - No fistula: Male and female; 5% all cases
    - Rectum 2 cm deep to perineum
    - Usually good sacrum and sphincter
    - Frequent in Down syndrome
- Rectal atresia or stenosis: Male and female; 1% all cases
  - Two forms of same malformation
  - Atresia between anus and rectum
  - Normal sacrum and sphincter
- Rectovestibular fistula
  - Most frequent defect in female: 25% female cases
  - Rectum opens between hymen and perineal skin
  - Most good sacrum and sphincter
- Persistent cloaca: Common channel drains rectum/vagina/urethra
  - Single perineal orifice: Wide spectrum
  - 90% have significant urologic defect
  - 40-50% require surgical abdominal approach as well as posterior sagittal anorectoplasty (PSARP)
  - \> 50% septate genitalia and hydrocolpos, leading to urinary obstruction
  - Common channel < 3 cm length: PSARP only, good prognosis for continence, sexual function
  - Common channel > 3 cm length: Laparotomy + PSARP, some fecal and GU sequelae

Staging, Grading or Classification Criteria
- Classification: Location of pouch relative to levator ani muscle (PCL on lateral pelvis)
  - High: Formerly anorectal agenesis (supralevator)
    - Pouch above PCL
  - Intermediate (translevator)
    - End of pouch below PCL and above levator
  - Low (infralevator)
    - Preserved anal sphincter
    - Fistula to perineum, anterior to sphincter (75%)

CLINICAL ISSUES

Presentation
- Most common signs/symptoms: Absent/abnormal anal opening, failure to pass meconium, meconium per vagina or urethra
- Other signs/symptoms: Abdominal distention

Demographics
- Age: Neonatal
- Gender: Slight male predominance

Treatment
- Goals
  - Maximize fecal and urinary continence, sexual function
  - Recognize and preserve all muscle structures, rectum, GU tract
  - Locate rectum surrounded by striated muscle
- Low: Anoplasty +/- PSARP at birth
- High and Intermediate: Colostomy with delayed PSARP +/- laparotomy

SELECTED REFERENCES
1. Levitt MA et al: Outcomes from the correction of anorectal malformations. Curr Opin Pediatr. 17(3):394-401, 2005
2. Georgeson KE et al: Minimally invasive surgery in the neonate: review of current evidence. Semin Perinatol. 28(3):212-20, 2004
3. Sydorak RM et al: Laparoscopic repair of high imperforate anus. Semin Pediatr Surg. 11(4):217-25, 2002
4. Pena A et al: Advances in the management of anorectal malformations. Am J Surg. 180(5):370-6, 2000
5. Kluth D et al: Current concepts in the embryology of anorectal malformations. Semin Pediatr Surg. 6(4):180-6, 1997
6. Lerone M et al: The genetics of anorectal malformations: a complex matter. Semin Pediatr Surg. 6(4):170-9, 1997
7. Pena A: Anorectal malformations. Semin Pediatr Surg. 4(1):35-47, 1995
8. Pena A: Management of anorectal malformations during the newborn period. World J Surg. 17(3):385-92, 1993

ANORECTAL MALFORMATION

IMAGE GALLERY

Typical

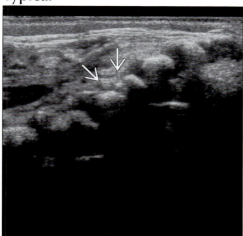
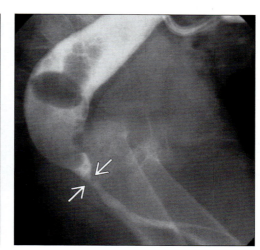

(Left) Sagittal ultrasound of the lower spine in prone position of the same patient as above shows an irregularly shaped S2 vertebral segment *(arrows)* which is not uncommon in patients with VATER. *(Right)* Lateral fistulagram or colostogram via injection of defunctionalized colon shows a rectourethral fistula *(arrows)* in this 3 month old male *(left)* with sigmoid colostomy for imperforate anus.

Variant

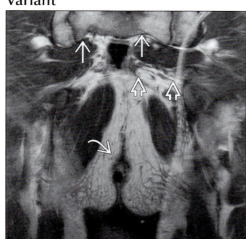
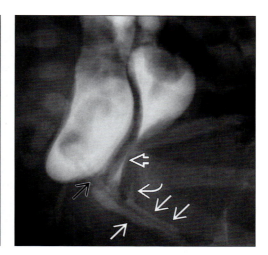

(Left) Coronal T1WI MR in repaired closed cloacal exstrophy variant shows partial sacral agenesis *(arrows)*, absence of left coccygeus *(open arrows)* and a deficient anal sphincter *(curved arrow)*. *(Right)* Lateral cloacagram shows catheter through a large posterior recto-cloaca fistula *(black arrow)*; proceeding anteriorly is the vagina *(open arrow)*, and urethra *(curved arrow)*; cloaca *(white arrows)*.

Typical

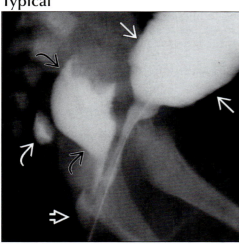
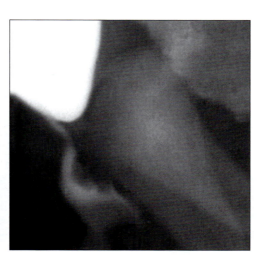

(Left) Lateral voiding cystourethrogram/genitogram through cloaca *(open arrow)* shows catheter inside bladder *(arrows)*, in the vagina *(black curved arrows)*, and minimal rectal contrast *(white curved arrow)*. *(Right)* Sagittal oblique voiding cystourethrogram of patient on left after surgical repair shows urethra that has been brought to the perineum through its own orifice.

ESOPHAGEAL ATRESIA AND TE FISTULA

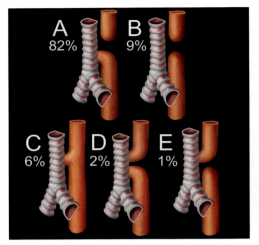

Graphic shows the 5 main types esophageal atresia with tracheoesophageal fistula (EA-TEF), including type C which is an isolated TEF without fistula, the so-called H-type fistula.

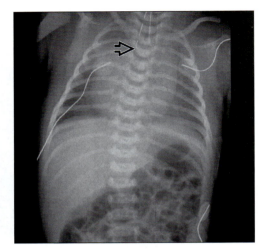

Anteroposterior radiograph day 1 of life shows enteric feeding tube just below the thoracic inlet (arrow) with distal bowel gas consistent with EA with distal TEF which was found at surgery.

TERMINOLOGY

Abbreviations and Synonyms
- Esophageal atresia and tracheoesophageal fistula (EA-TEF), tracheoesophageal fistula (TEF), esophageal atresia (EA)

Definitions
- Faulty division of the foregut into tracheal and esophageal channels during the first month of embryogenesis
- Multiple (5) anatomic variations of EA-TEF

IMAGING FINDINGS

General Features
- Best diagnostic clue: Distended pharyngeal pouch with tip of enteric tube within it
- Location
  ○ Variable levels of esophagus and trachea depending on type of EA-TEF (5)
  ○ EA: Atretic between junction of proximal and middle thirds
- Size: Fistula usually small; atretic segments variable in length
- Morphology: Variable forms (5)

Radiographic Findings
- Radiography
  ○ Air-filled, distended pharyngeal pouch
  ○ Enteric tube tip near thoracic inlet
  ○ If TEF present, bowel gas in distal gastrointestinal (GI) tract; if no TEF, no distal gas
  ○ Signs of other congenital anomalies
    ■ Heart size, vertebral anomalies, distal bowel obstruction
  ○ Side of aortic arch important for surgical repair; thoracotomy opposite side of arch

Fluoroscopic Findings
- Fluoroscopy rarely for diagnosis of EA: Clinical/radiographic diagnosis
- Fistula from esophagus to trachea in H-type TEF
- Contrast study prior to final stage of 2 stage repair
  ○ Air or water-soluble nonionic contrast in upper pouch and lower pouch
  ○ Surgical bougies into upper and lower pouches
  ○ Measure distance between upper and lower pouches
- Upper GI for difficulties following EA-TEF repair (long term)
  ○ Esophageal stricture; short segment at level of EA repair
  ○ Recurrent TEF
  ○ Esophageal leak at site of repair (immediate post-operative)

DDx: Esophageal Atresia With TE Fistula

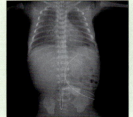

Esophageal Perforation

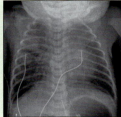

Aspiration

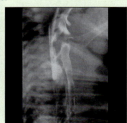

Laryngotracheal Cleft

ESOPHAGEAL ATRESIA AND TE FISTULA

Key Facts

Terminology
- Faulty division of the foregut into tracheal and esophageal channels during the first month of embryogenesis

Imaging Findings
- Best diagnostic clue: Distended pharyngeal pouch with tip of enteric tube within it
- Best imaging tool: Radiography for initial diagnosis +/- air in proximal pouch by fluoroscopy
- Upper GI for isolated (H-type) TEF
- Lateral position for H-type

Pathology
- Faulty division of the foregut into tracheal and esophageal channels, first month gestation
- 50-75% of those have associated abnormalities

- EA with distal TEF: 82%
- EA with no TEF: 9%
- Isolated (H-type) TEF: 6%
- EA with proximal and distal TEF: 2%
- EA with proximal TEF: 1%

Clinical Issues
- Most common signs/symptoms: Excessive oral and pharyngeal secretions or choking, cyanosis, or coughing during first attempt at feeding
- H-type fistula
- Coughing or choking during feeding
- Recurrent pneumonia
- Postsurgical survival: 75-95% (dependent on associated cardiac defects)
- Surgical

- o Esophageal dysmotility in near 100%
- o Gastroesophageal reflux
- Videofluoroscopic swallowing studies due to swallowing dysfunction

MR Findings
- T1WI and T2WI
  - o Non-visualization of fetal stomach; polyhydramnios

Ultrasonographic Findings
- Fetal ultrasound findings
  - o Nonvisualization of fetal stomach; intermittent filling of esophageal pouch, polyhydramnios > 30%

Imaging Recommendations
- Best imaging tool: Radiography for initial diagnosis +/- air in proximal pouch by fluoroscopy
- Protocol advice
  - o Upper GI for isolated (H-type) TEF
    - Optimal positioning and technique required
    - Lateral position for H-type
    - Swallow barium in most cases; rarely requires direct esophageal injection
    - If contrast injected, 5 or 8 French feeding tube: Distend esophagus in expected region of fistula
    - When imaging, fluoroscope continuously in lateral; field of view from pharynx to past carina
    - No images until visually convinced of normal or fistula
    - Do not mistake aspirated contrast for missed fistula
    - Image stomach to duodenojejunal (DJJ) to exclude malrotation, if patient stable
  - o Post-op esophagram: Evaluate for leak or other complication
    - Swallow or tube injection of non-ionic water-soluble contrast lateral view
    - If no obvious leak with water-soluble, use barium to increase detection of subtle leaks

DIFFERENTIAL DIAGNOSIS

Esophageal atresia
- Traumatic pharyngeal perforation with orogastric tube
  - o Inject air via orogastric tube; differentiate air-filled pharyngeal pouch vs. pneumomediastinum
- Laryngotracheal cleft
  - o High fistulous connection

H-type fistula (chronic or recurrent pneumonia)
- Gastroesophageal reflux with aspiration
- Aspirated foreign body
- Underlying immunodeficiency or cystic fibrosis
- Infected congenital lung mass (cystic adenomatoid malformation)

PATHOLOGY

General Features
- General path comments
  - o Faulty division of the foregut into tracheal and esophageal channels, first month gestation
  - o Esophagus is atretic for a variable length, usually at the junction of the proximal and middle thirds
  - o EA can occur in presence or absence of TEF
  - o Rarely, TEF can occur without EA: H-type fistula
- Epidemiology: 1:3,000 live births, sporadically
- Associated abnormalities
  - o 50-75% of those have associated abnormalities
    - Musculoskeletal 14-24%, cardiovascular 11-49%, gastrointestinal 20%, genitourinary,12-50%, craniofacial 10%, neurologic 7%, pulmonary 2%
    - 45%: VACTERL (vertebral, anal, cardiac, tracheoesophageal, renal, limb (radial array) anomalies)
    - Congenital cystic adenomatoid malformation, diaphragmatic hernia, duodenal atresia, biliary atresia, sirenomelia, intracardiac epithelial cyst

ESOPHAGEAL ATRESIA AND TE FISTULA

Gross Pathologic & Surgical Features
- Upper esophagus is blind pouch
- Fistula from anterior esophagus to trachea at or near carina
- Isolated fistula; posteroinferior to anterosuperior
  - Usually just above level of carina
  - Can occur with other types of EA-TEF
  - Rarely esophagobronchial fistula

Microscopic Features
- Squamous metaplasia of trachea and bronchi: 80%
- Tracheobronchial remnants in esophagus
- Pneumonia with foreign body reaction due to aspiration

Staging, Grading or Classification Criteria
- EA with distal TEF: 82%
- EA with no TEF: 9%
- Isolated (H-type) TEF: 6%
- EA with proximal and distal TEF: 2%
- EA with proximal TEF: 1%

CLINICAL ISSUES

Presentation
- Most common signs/symptoms: Excessive oral and pharyngeal secretions or choking, cyanosis, or coughing during first attempt at feeding
- Esophageal atresia
  - Poor feeding since birth
  - Drooling, coughing, choking with most swallows
  - Failure to pass enteric tube into stomach
- H-type fistula
  - Coughing or choking during feeding
  - Recurrent pneumonia

Demographics
- Age
  - Newborn or early childhood
  - 35% Premature

Natural History & Prognosis
- Recurrent infections and dysphagia in patients with undiagnosed isolated TEF
- Long term post-surgical issues
  - Esophageal stricture
    - Short segment at level of EA repair
  - Recurrent TEF: Up to 10% of cases
  - Esophageal dysmotility in near 100%
  - Gastroesophageal reflux; esophagitis in 51%, Barret esophagus 6%
  - Respiratory infections
  - Tracheomalacia; tracheal stenosis in 1/3
- Postsurgical survival: 75-95% (dependent on associated cardiac defects)

Treatment
- Surgical
  - Extrapleural transection of fistula and anastomosis of esophageal segments
  - If EA without fistula, ends often not close enough for primary repair: Staged operation
  - Immediate post-surgical complications
    - Anastamotic leak/obstruction, additional TEFs not seen initially either at imaging or operatively, gastroesophageal reflux

DIAGNOSTIC CHECKLIST

Consider
- Tracheal aspiration, gastroesophageal reflux, additional TEFs (especially on post-op imaging)

Image Interpretation Pearls
- Always fluoroscope esophagus in lateral view first
- Fluoroscope continuously before taking images to differentiate aspiration from TEF

SELECTED REFERENCES

1. Kovesi T et al: Long-term complications of congenital esophageal atresia and/or tracheoesophageal fistula. Chest. 126(3):915-25, 2004
2. Orford J et al: Advances in the treatment of oesophageal atresia over three decades: the 1970s and the 1990s. Pediatr Surg Int. 20(6):402-7, 2004
3. Crabbe DC: Isolated tracheo-oesophageal fistula. Paediatr Respir Rev. 4(1):74-8, 2003
4. Dahms, BB: The Gastrointestinal tract. In Pediatric Pathology 2nd ed. Eds Stocker JT and Dehner LP, Lippincott Williams & Wilkins, Philadelphia. 633-34, 2001
5. Clark DC: Esophageal atresia and tracheoesophageal fistula. Am Fam Physician. 59(4):910-6, 919-20, 1999
6. De Felice C et al: Congenital cystic adenomatoid malformation of the lung associated with esophageal atresia and tracheoesophageal fistula. Pediatr Surg Int. 15(3-4):260-3, 1999
7. Imaizumi K et al: Association of microphthalmia with esophageal atresia: report of two new patients and review of the literature. Am J Med Genet. 87(2):180-2, 1999
8. del Rosario JF et al: Common pediatric esophageal disorders. Gastroenterologist. 6(2):104-21, 1998
9. Thakral CL et al: Concurrent right diaphragmatic hernia and esophageal atresia. Pediatr Surg Int. 14(1-2):96-7, 1998
10. al-Salem AH et al: Concurrent left congenital diaphragmatic hernia and esophageal atresia: case report and review of the literature. J Pediatr Surg. 32(5):772-4, 1997
11. Sapin E et al: Coexisting left congenital diaphragmatic hernia and esophageal atresia with tracheoesophageal fistula: successful management in a premature neonate. J Pediatr Surg. 31(7):989-91, 1996
12. Snyder CL et al: Esophageal duplication cyst with esophageal web and tracheoesophageal fistula. J Pediatr Surg. 31(7):968-9, 1996
13. Benjamin B et al: Diagnosis of H-type tracheoesophageal fistula. J Pediatr Surg. 26:667-71, 1991
14. Berdon WE et al: Radiographic findings in esophageal atresia with proximal pouch fistula. Pediatr Radiol. 3:70-4, 1975
15. Kirkpatrick JA et al: A complex of anomalies associated with tracheoesophageal fistula and esophageal atresia. AJR. 95:208-11, 1965

ESOPHAGEAL ATRESIA AND TE FISTULA

IMAGE GALLERY

Typical

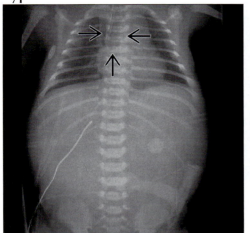
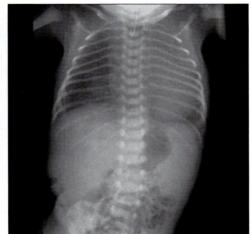

(Left) Anteroposterior radiograph on first day of life shows enteric tube in long upper esophageal pouch (arrows) and no distal bowel gas consistent with esophageal atresia and no distal TEF. *(Right)* Anteroposterior radiograph shows enteric tube tip in proximal pouch, distal bowel gas, cardiomegaly, and thin ribs in EA with distal fistula associated with other congenital anomalies.

Typical

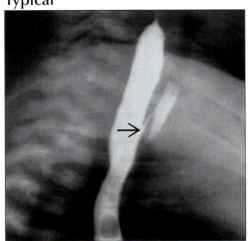
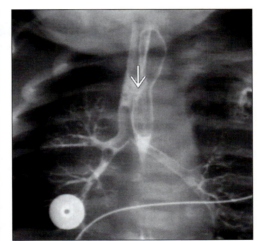

(Left) Lateral upper GI in a newborn turning "blue" with every feed shows an H-type tracheoesophageal fistula which extends from the esophagus (arrow) anterosuperiorly to the trachea. *(Right)* Anteroposterior upper GI after demonstrating the H-type TEF shows contrast in the esophagus, tracheobronchial tree and fistula (arrow), mid way between the thoracic inlet and carina.

Other

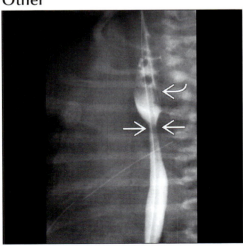
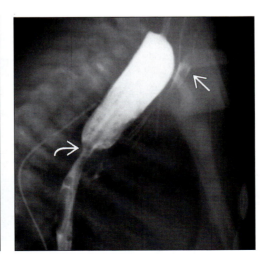

(Left) Lateral upper GI by tube (curved arrow) shows anastomotic narrowing after EA repair, likely due to post-op edema at the surgical site (arrows), not too unexpected soon after repair; no leak. *(Right)* Lateral upper GI post-op EA-TEF repair shows tight anastamosis (curved arrow), no leak but considerable aspiration (arrow), not uncommon since these patients lack swallowing experience.

GASTROESOPHAGEAL REFLUX

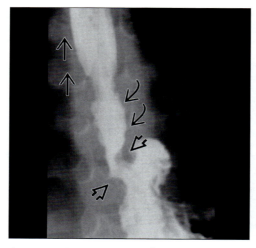

Anteroposterior upper GI shows hiatal hernia, gastroesophageal (GE) junction (open arrows) above the diaphragm, GE reflux (arrows) and esophagitis (curved arrows).

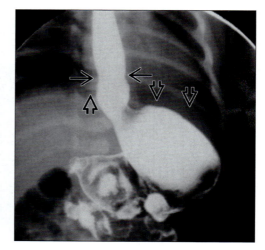

Anteroposterior upper GI shows elevation of the gastroesophageal junction (arrows) above the diaphragm (open arrows) in this patient with a sliding-type hiatal hernia.

TERMINOLOGY

Abbreviations and Synonyms
- Gastroesophageal reflux (GER), gastroesophageal reflux disease (GERD)

Definitions
- GER is a normal physiologic phenomenon occurring intermittently, particularly after meals
- GERD occurs when the amount of GER causes symptoms +/- esophagitis

IMAGING FINDINGS

General Features
- Best diagnostic clue: Retrograde flow of contrast or radiopharmaceutical from the stomach into the esophagus
- Location: Esophagus
- Morphology
  - Normal
  - Hiatal hernia: Gastroesophageal junction (GEJ) above diaphragm

Radiographic Findings
- Radiography
  - Normal
  - Round retrocardiac lucency (hiatal hernia)

Fluoroscopic Findings
- Upper GI
  - Normal
  - Reflux of contrast into esophagus of varying degree
  - GEJ above the diaphragm: Hiatal hernia
  - Disordered peristalsis: Esophageal dysmotility
    - Columning, to-fro movement of contrast
  - Swallowing dysfunction
    - Delayed initiation, vestibular penetration, tracheal aspiration
  - Mid-distal esophageal stricture
  - Schatzki ring
  - Post-op fundoplication
    - Satisfactory post-operative fundoplication
    - Contrast into wrap but no reflux or herniation of the wrap above the diaphragm
    - Recurrent GER
    - Transhiatal, paraesophageal herniation of the wrap
    - Hiatal herniation of the wrap and stomach

Ultrasonographic Findings
- Grayscale Ultrasound: Retrograde flow of stomach contents into esophagus

Nuclear Medicine Findings
- Tc-99m Sulfur Colloid

DDx: Non-Bilious Vomiting

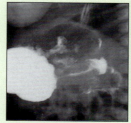

Pyloric Stenosis

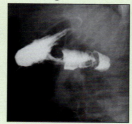

Duodenal Web

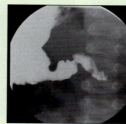

Antral Web

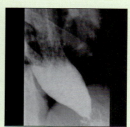

Achalasia

GASTROESOPHAGEAL REFLUX

Key Facts

Terminology
- GER is a normal physiologic phenomenon occurring intermittently, particularly after meals
- GERD occurs when the amount of GER causes symptoms +/- esophagitis

Imaging Findings
- Best diagnostic clue: Retrograde flow of contrast or radiopharmaceutical from the stomach into the esophagus
- Normal
- Reflux of contrast into esophagus of varying degree
- Disordered peristalsis: Esophageal dysmotility
- Swallowing dysfunction
- Mid-distal esophageal stricture
- Technetium99m-labeled sulfur colloid meal

- Upper GI to exclude anatomic upper GI abnormalities such as obstruction, not to identify reflux

Pathology
- Potentially a number of physiologic and anatomic factors
- Epidemiology: Frequency: US; about 7% of population - daily symptoms

Clinical Issues
- Effortless regurgitation, sometimes forceful vomiting
- Vomiting: Nonbilious
- Recurrent pulmonary problems
- Most infantile GER resolves by age 1-2
- About 1% treated surgically

- Radiopharmaceutical activity above the level of GEJ during period of observation
- Potentially delayed gastric emptying

Imaging Recommendations
- Best imaging tool
  - Technetium99m-labeled sulfur colloid meal
    - Directly evaluate gastric emptying and GER
  - Esophagram or upper gastrointestinal (UGI) evaluation
    - Good anatomic evaluation of gastrointestinal (GI) tract
    - Note any incidental GER that occurs
- Protocol advice
  - Upper GI to exclude anatomic upper GI abnormalities such as obstruction, not to identify reflux
    - GER is intermittent, sometimes seen on UGI
    - Provocatory maneuvers not performed in children
    - Extensive fluoroscopic monitoring not performed in children, radiation dose ALARA
    - Evaluate swallowing and esophageal motility
    - Post-op Nissen: Evaluate for reflux, anatomy, and esophageal emptying
  - Radionuclide scintigraphy: Technetium99m-labeled sulfur colloid meal
    - Most sensitive radiologic test for GER (pH probe is gold standard)
    - Evaluation of gastric emptying

DIFFERENTIAL DIAGNOSIS

Pyloric stenosis
- 2 weeks to 3 months

Duodenal stenosis/web
- Preampullary

Antral web
- Vomiting when eating solids

Achalasia
- Childhood to adolescence

Esophagitis
- Any cause

PATHOLOGY

General Features
- Etiology
  - Potentially a number of physiologic and anatomic factors
    - Abnormal length, pressure, increased number transient relaxations of lower esophageal sphincter (LES)
    - Supradiaphragmatic location of GEJ
    - Sub-optimal anatomic relationships of esophagus, diaphragm, stomach
    - Esophageal dysmotility
    - Delayed gastric emptying
  - Certain foods, medications, hormones
  - Obesity
- Epidemiology: Frequency: US; about 7% of population - daily symptoms
- Associated abnormalities
  - Acute life threatening event (ALTE)
  - Esophageal atresia after repair
  - Duodenal atresia after repair
  - Mental retardation
  - Cystic fibrosis
  - Chronic lung disease of prematurity
  - Asthma
  - Obesity

Gross Pathologic & Surgical Features
- Few have hiatal hernia, esophagitis, or stricture

Microscopic Features
- Reflux esophagitis
  - Intraepithelial inflammation: Lymphocytes, polymorphonuclear leukocytes, eosinophils
  - Basal cell hyperplasia
  - Basal cell spongiosis and nuclear enlargement
  - Papillary elongation, balloon cells and telangiectasia

GASTROESOPHAGEAL REFLUX

CLINICAL ISSUES

Presentation
- Most common signs/symptoms
  - Infants
    - Effortless regurgitation, sometimes forceful vomiting
    - Excessive irritability: Possibly due to chest discomfort
    - Failure to thrive: Caloric losses
    - Reactive airways disease
  - Children
    - Poorly localized abdominal or chest pain: Heartburn
    - Vomiting: Nonbilious
    - Reactive airways disease: Reflux into airways
    - Dysphagia: 1/3 have esophageal dysmotility
- Other signs/symptoms
  - Atypical symptoms
    - Cough and/or wheezing
    - Hoarseness: Irritation of vocal cords; usually in the morning
  - Recurrent pulmonary problems
  - Bloating and fullness after meals

Demographics
- Age: All ages but most under age 2 or over age 40
- Gender: No preference
- Ethnicity: Caucasians higher risk of Barrett esophagus and adenocarcinoma

Natural History & Prognosis
- Natural history
  - Most infantile GER resolves by age 1-2
  - About 4% have persistent GER
  - About 1% treated surgically
- Mortality/morbidity
  - Reflux esophagitis (50%)
    - Grade I - erythema
    - Grade II - linear nonconfluent erosions
    - Grade III - circular confluent erosions
    - Grade IV - stricture or Barrett esophagus (8-15%)
  - Barrett esophagus
    - One of most serious complications
    - May progress to cancer by adult years
    - Low LES pressure, severe dysmotility, lots GER
    - Periodic surveillance endoscopy even after fundoplication
  - Pneumonia, asthma, idiopathic pulmonary fibrosis; laryngitis, cancer; otitis media, tooth decay
- Other tests
  - Esophageal manometry - evaluates LES and peristalsis
  - pH monitoring/impedance probe- gold standard
- Prognosis
  - Most improve with medication
  - Predict early those who develop complications - early surgery
  - Alleviation of symptoms in 94% after fundoplication

Treatment
- Non-surgical: About 99% of refluxers
  - Elevate head of bed
  - Hypoallergenic formula, thickening feeds
  - Prokinetic agents, antacids and proton pump inhibitors (PPI)
- Surgical: About 1% of all refluxing patients
  - Indications: Many factors to consider
    - Failed medical therapy, 1 time therapy, Barrett esophagus, extraesophageal symptoms
  - Fundoplication: Mostly laparoscopic today
    - Fundus wrapped around distal esophagus
    - 1) reduce hernia 2) mobilize fundus 3) narrow hiatus 4) 360 degree wrap
    - 94% effective in symptom resolution

DIAGNOSTIC CHECKLIST

Consider
- Anatomic causes for vomiting
- Non-GI causes for recurrent vomiting

SELECTED REFERENCES

1. Dahms BB: Reflux esophagitis: sequelae and differential diagnosis in infants and children including eosinophilic esophagitis. Pediatr Dev Pathol. 7(1):5-16, 2004
2. Gold BD: Review article: epidemiology and management of gastro-oesophageal reflux in children. Aliment Pharmacol Ther. 19 Suppl 1:22-7, 2004
3. Henry SM: Discerning differences: gastroesophageal reflux and gastroesophageal reflux disease in infants. Adv Neonatal Care. 4(4):235-47, 2004
4. Poets CF: Gastroesophageal reflux: a critical review of its role in preterm infants. Pediatrics. 113(2):e128-32, 2004
5. Salvatore S et al: The natural course of gastro-oesophageal reflux. Acta Paediatr. 93(8):1063-9, 2004
6. Sood MR et al: Gastroesophageal reflux in adolescents. Adolesc Med Clin. 15(1):17-36, vii-viii, 2004
7. Davidson G: The role of lower esophageal sphincter function and dysmotility in gastroesophageal reflux in premature infants and in the first year of life. J Pediatr Gastroenterol Nutr. 37 Suppl 1:S17-22, 2003
8. Gold BD: Outcomes of pediatric gastroesophageal reflux disease: in the first year of life, in childhood, and in adults...oh, and should we really leave Helicobacter pylori alone? J Pediatr Gastroenterol Nutr. 37 Suppl 1:S33-9, 2003
9. Orenstein SR: Tests to assess symptoms of gastroesophageal reflux in infants and children. J Pediatr Gastroenterol Nutr. 37 Suppl 1:S29-32, 2003
10. Rudolph CD: Are proton pump inhibitors indicated for the treatment of gastroesophageal reflux in infants and children? J Pediatr Gastroenterol Nutr. 37 Suppl 1:S60-4, 2003
11. Rudolph CD: Supraesophageal complications of gastroesophageal reflux in children: challenges in diagnosis and treatment. Am J Med. 115 Suppl 3A:150S-156S, 2003
12. Strople J et al: Pediatric gastroesophageal reflux disease--current perspectives. Curr Opin Otolaryngol Head Neck Surg. 11(6):447-51, 2003
13. Wenzl TG: Evaluation of gastroesophageal reflux events in children using multichannel intraluminal electrical impedance. Am J Med. 115 Suppl 3A:161S-165S, 2003
14. Rothenberg SS: Laparoscopic Nissen procedure in children. Semin Laparosc Surg. 9(3):146-52, 2002
15. Wasowska-Krolikowska K et al: Asthma and gastroesophageal reflux in children. Med Sci Monit. 8(3):RA64-71, 2002

GASTROESOPHAGEAL REFLUX

IMAGE GALLERY

Typical

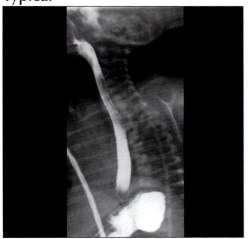 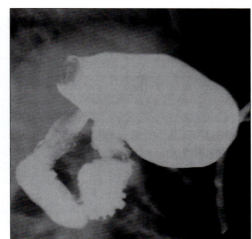

(Left) Lateral upper GI shows column of barium in the esophagus of this 1 week old infant with non-bilious emesis; these findings suggest esophageal dysmotility likely related to GER. *(Right)* Oblique upper GI shows a filling defect in the region of the cardia of the stomach, a satisfactory appearance after Nissen fundoplication; notice there is no GER, and good gastric emptying.

Typical

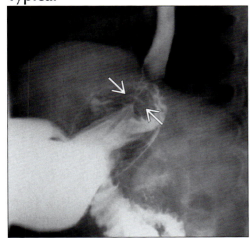 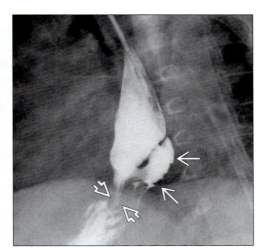

(Left) Lateral upper GI shows normal emptying of the esophagus into the stomach, the GEJ below the diaphragm (arrows), and a satisfactory appearance after Nissen fundoplication. *(Right)* Oblique upper GI shows transhiatal paraesophageal herniation of the Nissen wrap (arrows) with GEJ below the diaphragm (open arrows), compared to typical hiatal hernia in which it is above.

Typical

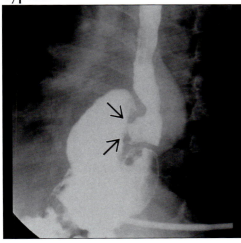 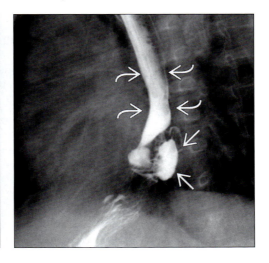

(Left) Oblique upper GI shows gastric fundus and GEJ (arrows) in the chest, in this patient status-post Nissen fundoplication with complication of hiatal hernia. *(Right)* Oblique upper GI image after esophageal tube injection shows small paraesophageal hernia of Nissen wrap (arrows) and distended esophagus to the tight Nissen wrap (curved arrows).

HYPERTROPHIC PYLORIC STENOSIS

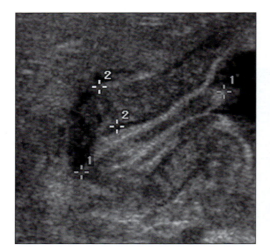 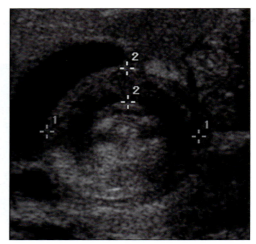

Axial oblique ultrasound shows elongation of the pyloric channel (cursor #1) and thickening of the hypoechoic muscular wall (cursor #2) in an infant with hypertrophic pyloric stenosis.

Transverse ultrasound shows a cross-sectional view of the thickened pyloric channel; diameter is measured between cursors #1 and single wall thickness measured with cursor #2.

TERMINOLOGY

Abbreviations and Synonyms
- Pyloric stenosis, hypertrophic pyloric stenosis (HPS)

Definitions
- Idiopathic thickening of pyloric muscle in infancy which creates progressive gastric outlet obstruction
- Typically seen in 2-12 week old infants with worsening projectile vomiting
- HPS is the cause of vomiting in 1 of every 5 infants referred for imaging
- Incidence of ~2 per 1,000 live births

IMAGING FINDINGS

General Features
- Best diagnostic clue
  - Near complete gastric outlet obstruction due to enlarged and thickened pyloric muscle
  - Ultrasound reveals hypertrophied muscle and decreased gastric emptying on dynamic exam
  - Upper GI shows minimal barium passing through pyloric channel and mass effect of pylorus on antrum and underside of duodenal bulb
- Location: Position of pylorus varies with degree of gastric distention; occasionally located in right lower quadrant

Radiographic Findings
- Radiography
  - Overdistended stomach and minimal bowel gas distally
  - Stomach may be collapsed if infant has recently vomited

Fluoroscopic Findings
- Overdistended stomach
- Caterpillar stomach: Exaggerated gastric motility
- Tram track or string sign of barium within the narrowed channel
- Shoulders of pyloric muscle create an impression on distal antrum
- Teat or beak of barium trying to enter pyloric channel
- Mushroom sign of hypertrophied muscle indenting the base of duodenal bulb

CT Findings
- CECT
  - Occasionally seen on CT scan performed for trauma or other indications
  - Consider pylorospasm as CT does not provide dynamic evaluation of gastric emptying

DDx: Other Causes of Vomiting

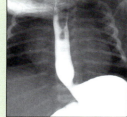 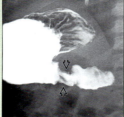 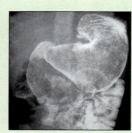 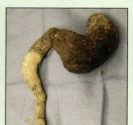

GE Reflux — *Edema Post-Op* — *Gastric Bezoar* — *Trichobezoar*

HYPERTROPHIC PYLORIC STENOSIS

Key Facts

Terminology
- Idiopathic thickening of pyloric muscle in infancy which creates progressive gastric outlet obstruction
- Typically seen in 2-12 week old infants with worsening projectile vomiting
- HPS is the cause of vomiting in 1 of every 5 infants referred for imaging

Imaging Findings
- Caterpillar stomach: Exaggerated gastric motility
- Tram track or string sign of barium within the narrowed channel
- Shoulders of pyloric muscle create an impression on distal antrum
- Teat or beak of barium trying to enter pyloric channel
- Mushroom sign of hypertrophied muscle indenting the base of duodenal bulb
- Abnormal measurements of thickened muscle and elongated pyloric channel vary by author
- Commonly accepted threshold values for HPS
- Single wall thickness of pylorus > 3 mm
- Pyloric channel length > 16 mm
- Pyloric diameter > 15 mm

Top Differential Diagnoses
- Pylorospasm
- Gastroesophageal (GE) reflux
- Malrotation with midgut volvulus
- Gastric bezoar

Clinical Issues
- Surgical: Pyloromyotomy
- Nonsurgical: Atropine and frequent small feedings are an alternative to surgery

Ultrasonographic Findings
- Grayscale Ultrasound
  - Abnormal measurements of thickened muscle and elongated pyloric channel vary by author
  - In general, higher threshold measurements increase specificity but decrease sensitivity
  - Commonly accepted threshold values for HPS
    - Single wall thickness of pylorus > 3 mm
    - Pyloric channel length > 16 mm
    - Pyloric diameter > 15 mm
  - Echogenic mucosal lining also tends to hypertrophy, becomes redundant
  - Gastric hyperperistalsis and obliterated pyloric lumen on dynamic exam
  - Feeding glucose water or formula helpful to assess gastric emptying, define the pyloric channel
  - When duodenal bulb is easily identified distended with fluid, diagnosis of HPS is unlikely
- Color Doppler: Increased flow has been demonstrated in both the muscle and mucosa of infants with HPS

Imaging Recommendations
- Best imaging tool
  - Ultrasound is exam of choice when HPS is strongly clinically suspected
  - Barium studies used when history atypical or if emesis is bilious
- Protocol advice
  - Begin the ultrasound scan with the patient rolled onto their right side in order to pool gastric fluids in the antrum
  - Give glucose water in small aliquots, as overdistending the stomach may push the pylorus into an unfavorable imaging plane (directed posteriorly or displaced into right lower quadrant)
  - Watch for gastric peristaltic waves to propel fluid through the pyloric channel
  - Gastric contractions which are vigorous in the body and antrum, but do not open the pylorus suggest the diagnosis of HPS
  - Formula or glucose water will "swirl" against the thickened pylorus with each wave of gastric peristalsis in HPS

DIFFERENTIAL DIAGNOSIS

Pylorospasm
- Typically seen in irritable infants, resolves with time, wait and re-image

Gastroesophageal (GE) reflux
- Cause of vomiting in 2/3 of all infants referred to radiology
- Presumed diagnosis when ultrasound is normal

Malrotation with midgut volvulus
- A true imaging and surgical emergency
- Emesis is classically greenish from bile
- Best diagnosed fluoroscopically

Gastric bezoar
- Caused by accumulation of undigested matter in stomach
- Trichobezoar: Composed of hair and sometimes nails
- Phytobezoar: Composed of plant or vegetable fiber

Other causes of gastric outlet obstruction
- Duodenal or antral web or stenosis
- Antral polyps
- Annular pancreas
- Choledochocele
- Mass in right upper quadrant

PATHOLOGY

General Features
- General path comments
  - Idiopathic hypertrophy of circular muscle bundles in pylorus
    - Gradually progressive and spontaneously remits after many weeks

HYPERTROPHIC PYLORIC STENOSIS

- Abnormal muscle tone/electrophysiology of the gastroduodenal junction shown in HPS
- Associated with erythromycin exposure prenatally and postnatally via breast milk
- Higher incidence of HPS in patients with cystic fibrosis
- Genetics
  - Tends to run in families, not truly inherited
  - Discordant incidence among monozygotic twins favors environmental factors over genetic predisposition
- Etiology: Unclear: Idiopathic, prostaglandin induced, neural mediated, familial
- Associated abnormalities: Eosinophilic gastritis, prostaglandin induced antral mucosal hyperplasia, hypergastrinemia, nasoenteric tubes, erythromycin

Gross Pathologic & Surgical Features
- Hypertrophy of muscular layers of pylorus
- Thickening of mucosa in antrum and pylorus, to approximately 1/3 diameter of pylorus

CLINICAL ISSUES

Presentation
- Most common signs/symptoms
  - Progressive vomiting in an infant who previously tolerated feedings
  - Palpable "olive" is 97% specific in experienced hands

Demographics
- Age: 2-12 weeks, or later in premature infants
- Gender: M:F = 4-5:1
- Ethnicity: Slightly more common in Caucasians

Natural History & Prognosis
- Weight loss and parental concerns typically prompt imaging
- Excellent prognosis following surgery or conservative medical management
  - No significant GI disturbances seen in German study of infants treated surgically or medically 16-26 years after diagnosis

Treatment
- Surgical: Pyloromyotomy
  - Pyloromyotomy splits the thickened muscle longitudinally and reapproximates edges transversely thereby opening the channel
  - Laparoscopic pyloromyotomy does not appear to offer significant advantages over the open procedure
- Nonsurgical: Atropine and frequent small feedings are an alternative to surgery
  - Treatment takes several weeks before resuming normal feeding without medications

DIAGNOSTIC CHECKLIST

Image Interpretation Pearls
- Pylorospasm mimics HPS, but is typically transient

SELECTED REFERENCES

1. Cohen HL et al: The sonographic double-track sign: not pathognomonic for hypertrophic pyloric stenosis; can be seen in pylorospasm. J Ultrasound Med. 23(5):641-6, 2004
2. Hall NJ et al: Meta-analysis of laparoscopic versus open pyloromyotomy. Ann Surg. 240(5):774-8, 2004
3. Helton KJ et al: The impact of a clinical guideline on imaging children with hypertrophic pyloric stenosis. Pediatr Radiol. 34(9):733-6, 2004
4. Huang YC et al: Medical treatment with atropine sulfate for hypertrophic pyloric stenosis. Acta Paediatr Taiwan. 45(3):136-40, 2004
5. Yagmurlu A et al: Comparison of the incidence of complications in open and laparoscopic pyloromyotomy: a concurrent single institution series. J Pediatr Surg. 39(3):292-6; discussion 292-6, 2004
6. Hernanz-Schulman M et al: Hypertrophic pyloric stenosis in infants: US evaluation of vascularity of the pyloric canal. Radiology. 229(2):389-93, 2003
7. Hernanz-Schulman M: Infantile hypertrophic pyloric stenosis. Radiology. 227(2):319-31, 2003
8. Sorensen HT et al: Risk of infantile hypertrophic pyloric stenosis after maternal postnatal use of macrolides. Scand J Infect Dis. 35(2):104-6, 2003
9. Kakish KS: Cystic fibrosis and infantile hypertrophic pyloric stenosis: is there an association? Pediatr Pulmonol. 33(5):404-5, 2002
10. Hernanz-Schulman M et al: In vivo visualization of pyloric mucosal hypertrophy in infants with hypertrophic pyloric stenosis: is there an etiologic role? AJR Am J Roentgenol. 177(4):843-8, 2001
11. Kawahara H et al: Motor abnormality in the gastroduodenal junction in patients with infantile hypertrophic pyloric stenosis. J Pediatr Surg. 36(11):1641-5, 2001
12. Kobayashi H et al: Pyloric stenosis: new histopathologic perspective using confocal laser scanning. J Pediatr Surg. 36(8):1277-9, 2001
13. Cohen HL et al: Vomiting in infants up to 3 months of age. American College of Radiology Appropriateness Criteria. Radiology. 215 Suppl:779-86, 2000
14. Aktug T et al: Analyzing the diagnostic efficiency of olive palpation for hypertrophic pyloric stenosis. J Pediatr Surg. 34(10):1585-6, 1999
15. Callahan MJ et al: The development of hypertrophic pyloric stenosis in a patient with prostaglandin-induced foveolar hyperplasia. Pediatr Radiol. 29(10):748-51, 1999
16. Bisset GS 3rd et al: Pediatric imaging perspective: the vomiting infant. J Pediatr. 133(2):306-7, 1998
17. Rohrschneider WK et al: Pyloric muscle in asymptomatic infants: sonographic evaluation and discrimination from idiopathic hypertrophic pyloric stenosis. Pediatr Radiol. 28:429-34, 1998
18. Yamamoto A et al: Ultrasonographic follow-up of the healing process of medically treated hypertrophic pyloric stenosis. Pediatr Radiol. 28(3):177-8, 1998
19. Schechter R et al: The epidemiology of infantile hypertrophic pyloric stenosis. Paediatr Perinat Epidemiol. 11(4):407-27, 1997
20. Babyn P et al: Radiologic features of gastric outlet obstruction in infants after long-term prostaglandin administration. Pediatr Radiol. 25(1):41-3; discussion 44, 1995
21. Hernanz-Schulman M et al: Hypertrophic pyloric stenosis in the infant without a palpable olive: accuracy of sonographic diagnosis. Radiology. 193:771-6, 1994
22. Ludtke FE et al: Gastric emptying 16 to 26 years after treatment of infantile hypertrophic pyloric stenosis. J Pediatr Surg. 29(4):523-6, 1994

HYPERTROPHIC PYLORIC STENOSIS

IMAGE GALLERY

Typical

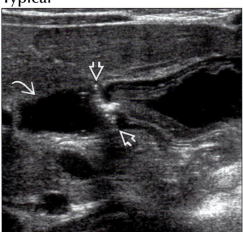
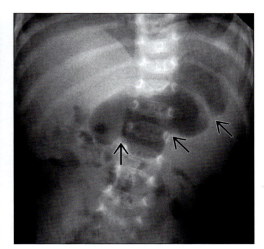

(Left) Ultrasound shows a normal pylorus between open arrows with anechoic fluid in gastric antrum and in distended duodenal bulb (curved arrow). *(Right)* Radiograph in HPS shows hyperperistalsis in gas filled stomach as muscular contractions (arrows) try to push gastric contents through narrowed, hypertrophied pylorus. Note minimal distal bowel gas.

Typical

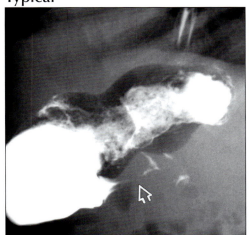
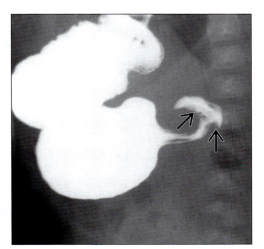

(Left) Lateral upper GI shows thin track of barium (arrow) in elongated pyloric channel. Note the retained formula mixed with barium in the body and fundus despite 4 hour fasting. *(Right)* Lateral upper GI shows parallel tracks of barium in the elongated and narrowed pyloric canal. Note the impression on the underside of the bulb caused by the thickened muscle, the "mushroom" sign (arrows).

Other

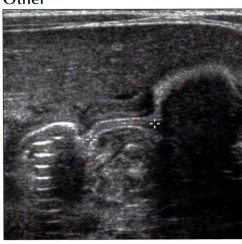
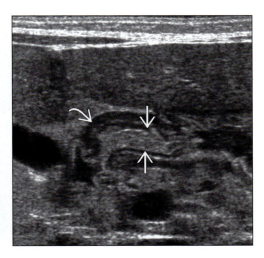

(Left) Ultrasound shows pylorospasm which can mimic HPS, but typically does not meet measurement criteria and usually resolves with time and glucose water feeding. Channel length is marked by cursors. *(Right)* Axial oblique ultrasound in antritis shows mucosal thickening between arrows in the gastric antrum without thickening of the hypoechoic muscular wall (curved arrow). This is not HPS.

GASTRIC VOLVULUS

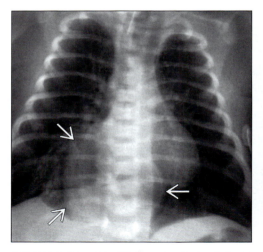

Anteroposterior upper GI fluoroscopic scout image shows air-filled, distended retrocardiac opacity (arrows), the intrathoracic stomach due to hernia with volvulus and acute obstruction.

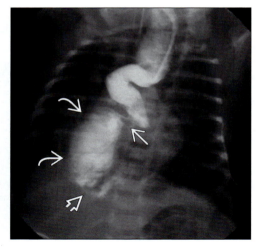

Anteroposterior upper GI shows OAV small amount of contrast entering the stomach at GEJ (arrow) and less exiting the pylorus (open arrow); (curved arrows - greater curvature).

TERMINOLOGY

Abbreviations and Synonyms
- Gastric volvulus (GV), organoaxial volvulus (OAV), mesenteroaxial volvulus (MAV)

Definitions
- Rotation all or part of stomach > 180 degrees, +/- closed-loop obstruction, possible strangulation
  - It is the rotation and not the obstruction which defines the presence of volvulus

IMAGING FINDINGS

General Features
- Best diagnostic clue
  - Mesenteroaxial volvulus
    - Spherical, distended stomach, 2 air-fluid levels (inferior fundus and superior antrum)
    - Beak-like, inferior gastroesophageal junction (GEJ)
  - Organoaxial volvulus
    - Difficult diagnosis on radiography
    - Paucity of gas beyond stomach
    - Low GEJ, marked gastric dilation, slow passage barium
- Location: Predominantly left upper abdomen

- Types of GV: Organoaxial (most common); mesenteroaxial; mixed
  - Organoaxial volvulus (OAV): Rotation around longitudinal axis (most common)
    - Around line extending from cardia to pylorus
    - Stomach twists anteriorly or posteriorly
    - Antrum moves inferior to superior
  - Mesenteroaxial volvulus (MAV): Rotation about mesenteric axis
    - Axis running across stomach right angles to lesser & greater curves
    - Rotation right to left or left to right about gastrohepatic omentum
  - Mixed volvulus: Combination of OAV & MAV

Radiographic Findings
- Radiography
  - Abdominal plain films; patient upright
    - Double air-fluid level
    - Large, distended stomach; spheric viscus displaced upward to left
    - Elevation of diaphragm
    - Small bowel collapsed; paucity distal gas
    - +/- Intramural emphysema gastric wall
  - Chest X-ray: Intrathoracic up-side down stomach
    - Retrocardiac fluid level; 2 air-fluid interfaces different heights

DDx: Intrathoracic Stomach

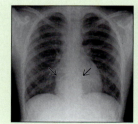
Hiatal Hernia

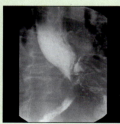
Post-Operative

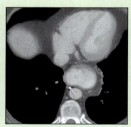
Post-Operative

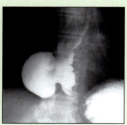
Epi Diverticulum

GASTRIC VOLVULUS

Key Facts

Terminology
- Rotation all or part of stomach > 180 degrees, +/- closed-loop obstruction, possible strangulation

Imaging Findings
- Organoaxial volvulus (OAV): Rotation around longitudinal axis (most common)
- Around line extending from cardia to pylorus
- Mesenteroaxial volvulus (MAV): Rotation about mesenteric axis
- Axis running across stomach right angles to lesser & greater curves
- Double air-fluid level
- Inversion of stomach
- Greater curvature above lesser
- Cardia & pylorus at same level
- Downward pointing pylorus & duodenum
- Incomplete/absent entrance or exit of contrast to/from stomach; acute obstructive GV

Top Differential Diagnoses
- Hiatal hernia
- Post-operative

Pathology
- Large esophageal or paraesophageal hernia
- Diaphragmatic eventration or paralysis

Clinical Issues
- Complications: Intramural emphysema; perforation
- Mortality rate: 30%
- Detorse stomach
- Repair of associated defects
- Prevent recurrence

- Simultaneous fluid levels above & below diaphragm

Fluoroscopic Findings
- Massively distended stomach left upper quadrant +/- extending into chest
- Inversion of stomach
  - Greater curvature above lesser
  - Cardia & pylorus at same level
  - Downward pointing pylorus & duodenum
- May see "beaking" at point of twist
- OAV: 2 points of twist; luminal obstruction
- Incomplete/absent entrance or exit of contrast to/from stomach; acute obstructive GV
- Contrast in stomach may not pass beyond pylorus
- MAV: Antrum & pylorus lie above gastric fundus

CT Findings
- Not generally performed for GV
- Incidental finding on CT done for nonspecific indication
- CT appearance may be variable
  - Depends on extent of gastric herniation, points of torsion, position of stomach
  - May be linear septum within gastric lumen (area of torsion)
- CT chest & abdomen
  - Detect associated malformation or malposition
  - Presence of unattached herniated peritoneal sac
- Large hiatal hernia accompanied by partial GV
  - "Pseudothrombosis" of inferior vena cava on CT
- False positives/negatives
  - Difficult to distinguish paraesophageal hernia without torsion

MR Findings
- Similar to CT findings
  - 2 different signal intensities reflect point of torsion

Angiographic Findings
- Acute upper gastrointestinal hemorrhage
- Gastric vascular supply displaced according to position of stomach

Imaging Recommendations
- Best imaging tool
  - Fluoroscopic upper gastrointestinal (UGI)
    - Demonstrate volvulus, anatomic detail
  - Fluoroscopic guidance to advance feeding tube into obstructed stomach
    - Attempt decompression; stabilize patient
  - CT; complementary role

DIFFERENTIAL DIAGNOSIS

Hiatal hernia
- Stomach enters thorax through esophageal hiatus
- GEJ above diaphragmatic hiatus (type I, sliding)
- GE junction below diaphragm (type II; paraesophageal)
  - Herniation of fundus through hiatus
- Giant paraesophageal hernia: Up to 1/3 of stomach in chest
  - +/- Herniation of small bowel/colon
- Traction or torsion of stomach at or near level of hiatus (volvulus)

Post-operative
- Esophagectomy with gastric pull through
  - Complete mobilization of stomach, resection of lower esophagus, pyloroplasty, transhiatal dissection
  - Intrathoracic stomach

Epiphrenic diverticulum
- Retrocardiac mass +/- air-fluid level

PATHOLOGY

General Features
- General path comments
  - Point of anatomic fixation: Second portion of duodenum, retroperitoneal
  - Ligaments normally anchor stomach

OMPHALOCELE

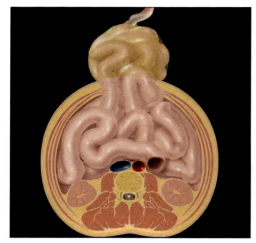

Axial graphic shows a midline abdominal wall defect with herniation of small bowel. It is covered by a membrane with the umbilical cord inserting directly on the mass.

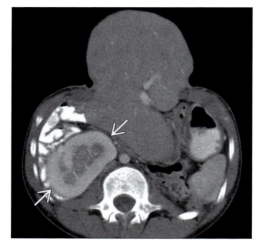

Axial CECT shows liver within persistent omphalocele in a 9 year old. Contrast-filled upper small bowel on right side, indicating malrotation. Single kidney (arrows) with crossed, fused ectopia.

TERMINOLOGY

Definitions
- Herniation of abdominal viscera into the umbilical cord

IMAGING FINDINGS

General Features
- Liver and small bowel most common omphalocele contents
  - Spleen, bladder, stomach, and large bowel less common

Radiographic Findings
- Radiography
  - Anterior mass protruding from midline abdominal wall
    - Gas inside omphalocele: Within small bowel or stomach
  - Cleft sternum
  - Pulmonary hypoplasia
  - Ectopia cordis
  - Left lower lobe collapse due to left mainstem bronchus narrowing
  - Lumbar lordosis
  - Lumbar spine duplication
  - Absent radial ray
- IVP
  - Renal ectopia, solitary kidney
  - Hydronephrosis, ureteropelvic junction obstruction

Fluoroscopic Findings
- Gastroesophageal reflux; bowel malrotation

CT Findings
- NECT
  - Liver or stomach protrusion into omphalocele
  - Malrotation
- CECT: Pelvic ectopia of liver
- CTA: Absent inferior vena cava; ventricular diverticulum; aortic coarctation

MR Findings
- Liver protrusion into the omphalocele
- Gallbladder absent

Ultrasonographic Findings
- Grayscale Ultrasound
  - Can be diagnosed at 15 weeks gestational age when midgut should have returned from base of cord back to abdomen
    - Umbilical cord inserts directly into omphalocele
    - Umbilical cord cysts may also be present

Echocardiographic Findings
- Echocardiogram

DDx: Ventral Herniations

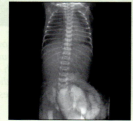
Gastroschisis

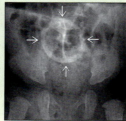
Umbilical Hernia

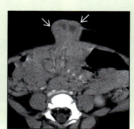
Umbilical Hernia

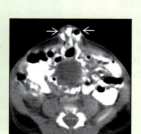
Umbilical Hernia

OMPHALOCELE

Key Facts

Terminology
- Herniation of abdominal viscera into the umbilical cord

Imaging Findings
- Liver and small bowel most common omphalocele contents

Pathology
- Failure of central migration of lateral mesodermal body folds
- Most omphaloceles are sporadic
- Chromosomal abnormalities in 50%
- Incidence: 0.8-9 per 10,000 live births
- 3-fold excess risk after in vitro fertilization
- 3-fold excess risk when mother obese
- 4-fold excess risk in mothers with bicornuate uterus
- Structural anomalies in addition to omphalocele in 62%
- Anomalies more likely if omphalocele contains liver
- Genitourinary anomalies in 40%
- Gastrointestinal and respiratory anomalies in 40%
- Congenital cardiac defects in 30-40%
- Musculoskeletal anomalies in 20%
- Omphalocele covered by both peritoneum and amnion with Wharton jelly in between
- Part of spectrum of midline defects including ectopia cordis, bladder extrophy, epispadias, and cloacal extrophy

Clinical Issues
- Survival as high as 80-90% if normal chromosomes, no other anomalies

---

- Pentalogy of Cantrell
  - Ventricular diverticulum
  - Pericardial effusion
  - Various cardiac defects

DIFFERENTIAL DIAGNOSIS

Gastroschisis
- Abdominal wall defect is off midline, usually on the right
- Fetal ultrasound: Free-floating loops of bowel in amniotic fluid
- Cord insertion or umbilicus position on abdominal wall normal and not into defect
- No membrane covering the hernia
- Liver not involved
- Incidence of omphalocele vs. gastroschisis: 3:2

Umbilical hernia
- Midline defect in linea alba
- 20% African-American infants
- 3% Caucasian infants
- 5% premature infants

PATHOLOGY

General Features
- General path comments
  - Embryology
    - Failure of central migration of lateral mesodermal body folds
    - Additional failure of migration of the cephalic mesodermal folds: Ectopia cordis
- Genetics
  - Most omphaloceles are sporadic
  - Familial omphalocele rare
    - Autosomal dominant or X-linked recessive trait
  - Chromosomal abnormalities in 50%
    - Trisomy 13, 18, and 21, Triploidy, Turner syndrome (45X)
    - Increased incidence if omphalocele contains liver
    - Turner, Kleinfelter syndromes
- Epidemiology
  - Incidence: 0.8-9 per 10,000 live births
    - Incidence increases with advanced maternal age
  - 3-fold excess risk after in vitro fertilization
  - 3-fold excess risk when mother obese
  - 4-fold excess risk in mothers with bicornuate uterus
- Associated abnormalities
  - Structural anomalies in addition to omphalocele in 62%
    - Anomalies more likely if omphalocele contains liver
  - Genitourinary anomalies in 40%
    - OEIS complex
    - Ureteropelvic junction (UPJ) obstruction, renal ectopia, solitary kidney, cryptorchidism, cloacal extrophy
    - Cryptorchidism, solitary kidney
    - Prune-belly syndrome
  - Gastrointestinal and respiratory anomalies in 40%
    - Tracheoesophageal fistula, imperforate anus, malrotation
    - Absent gallbladder
    - Enteric duplication, atresia
    - Torsion of accessory hepatic lobe
    - Meckel diverticulum present 28% when omphalocele small and only 4% when large
    - Thoracoschisis
  - Congenital cardiac defects in 30-40%
    - Septal defects, transposition, ectopia, tetralogy of Fallot, absent inferior vena cava
  - Musculoskeletal anomalies in 20%
    - Camptomelic dysplasia
    - Scoliosis, vertebral abnormalities
    - Lymphatic malformation
    - Clubfoot
  - Central nervous system (CNS) anomalies
    - Encephalocele, holoprosencephaly, cerebellar hypoplasia
  - Acrocephalopolydactylous dysplasia (Elejalde syndrome)
    - Omphalocele

OMPHALOCELE

- Acrocephaly, polydactyly, craniosynostosis
- Large birth weight
- Microtia, hypoplastic nose, genitourinary (GU) anomalies
○ Beckwith-Weideman syndrome in 5-10%
- Omphalocele, umbilical hernia, diastasis recti
- Cranio-facial dysmorphism
- Gigantism, visceromegaly, hemihypertrophy
- Increased incidence of neoplasms
○ Garonchi-Baruch syndrome
- Omphalocele
- Diaphragmatic hernia
- Liver cyst
- Radial ray defects
- Heart defects
○ OEIS complex
- Omphalocele
- Extrophy of bladder
- Imperforate anus
- Spinal defects
○ PAGOD syndrome
- Pulmonary artery and tract anomalies
- Agonadism
- Omphalocele
- Diaphragmatic defects and dextrocardia
○ Pentalogy of Cantrell
- Omphalocele
- Ectopia cordis
- Bifid sternum
- Anterior diaphragmatic hernia
- Pericardial defect
- Also umbilical hernia, diastasis recti, cardiac defects

Gross Pathologic & Surgical Features
- Omphalocele covered by both peritoneum and amnion with Wharton jelly in between

Staging, Grading or Classification Criteria
- Small omphalocele < 5 cm
  ○ 82% survive infancy
  ○ May contain just intestine
  ○ Higher frequency of chromosomal anomalies than when omphalocele large
- Large or giant omphalocele > 5 cm
  ○ 48% survive infancy
  ○ Contains liver (extracorporeal liver)
  ○ Small thorax, pulmonary hypoplasia
- Part of spectrum of midline defects including ectopia cordis, bladder extrophy, epispadias, and cloacal extrophy

CLINICAL ISSUES

Presentation
- Most common signs/symptoms
  ○ Detected by prenatal ultrasound in developed regions
    - Diagnosis obvious at birth elsewhere
- Other signs/symptoms: Elevated maternal serum alpha-fetoprotein (70%)

Demographics
- Age: Increased incidence with advanced maternal age
- Gender: Equal occurrence in males and females
- Ethnicity
  ○ Pacific islanders at low risk
  ○ African-American infants twice as likely to survive as Caucasians and/or Hispanics

Natural History & Prognosis
- Premature birth in 42%
- Survival as high as 80-90% if normal chromosomes, no other anomalies
- Associated structural or chromosomal abnormalities: Mortality 80-100%
- Maternal polyhydramnios or oligohydramnios: Prognosis poor
- Respiratory distress at birth: Prognosis poor

Treatment
- Fetus: Amniocentesis for karyotype
  ○ Delivery at tertiary care facility
- Birth: Benefits of cesarean section controversial
  ○ Not indicated if multiple associated anomalies
- After birth: Surgical and/or gradual (pressure) reduction
  ○ Often not possible to completely reduce large omphaloceles containing mostly liver

SELECTED REFERENCES

1. Blazer S et al: Fetal omphalocele detected early in pregnancy: associated anomalies and outcomes. Radiology. 232(1):191-5, 2004
2. Hwang PJ et al: Omphalocele and gastroschisis: an 18-year review study. Genet Med. 6(4):232-6, 2004
3. Salihu HM et al: Omphalocele and gastroschisis: Black-White disparity in infant survival. Birth Defects Res Part A Clin Mol Teratol. 70(9):586-91, 2004
4. Wilson RD et al: Congenital abdominal wall defects: an update. Fetal Diagn Ther. 19(5):385-98, 2004
5. Halbertsma FJ et al: Cardiac diverticulum and omphalocele: Cantrell's pentalogy or syndrome. Cardiol Young. 12(1):71-4, 2002
6. Macayran JF et al: PAGOD syndrome: eighth case and comparison to animal models of congenital vitamin A deficiency. Am J Med Genet. 108(3):229-34, 2002
7. Salihu HM et al: Omphalocele and gastroschisis. J Obstet Gynaecol. 22(5):489-92, 2002
8. Ericson A et al: Congenital malformations in infants born after IVF: a population-based study. Hum Reprod. 16(3):504-9, 2001
9. Headley BM et al: Left-lung-collapse bronchial deformation in giant omphalocele. J Pediatr Surg. 36(6):846-50, 2001
10. Puthenpurayil K et al: Pelvic ectopia of the liver in an adult associated with omphalocele repair as a neonate. AJR Am J Roentgenol. 177(5):1113-5, 2001
11. Nagaya M et al: Lordosis of lumbar vertebrae in omphalocele: an important factor in regulating abdominal cavity capacity. J Pediatr Surg. 35(12):1782-5, 2000
12. Koivusalo A et al: Cryptorchidism in boys with congenital abdominal wall defects. Pediatr Surg Int. 13(2-3):143-5, 1998
13. Martinez-Frias ML et al: Congenital anomalies in the offspring of mothers with a bicornuate uterus. Pediatrics. 101(4):E10, 1998

OMPHALOCELE

IMAGE GALLERY

Typical

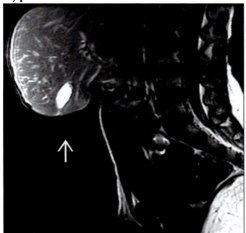 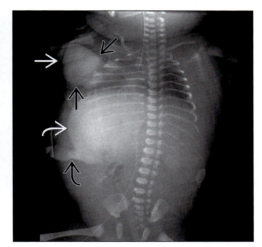

(Left) Sagittal FSE T2 MR shows liver and gallbladder *(arrow)* within the omphalocele. *(Right)* Anteroposterior radiograph shows anterior ectopia cordis *(arrows)* in pentalogy of Cantrell. Omphalocele *(white curved arrow)* is just beneath heart and gives rise to umbilical cord *(black curved arrow)*. Hydrops due to heart failure.

Typical

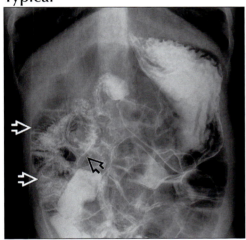 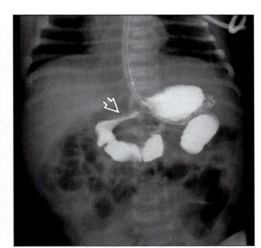

(Left) Anteroposterior radiograph shows malrotation with jejunum *(arrows)* on the right in a 19 year old. Central diaphragm is abnormally elevated. *(Right)* Anteroposterior radiograph in child with previous repair shows superior pressure deformity of duodenal bulb *(arrow)* caused by dysmorphic liver in 2 day old with repaired omphalocele.

Typical

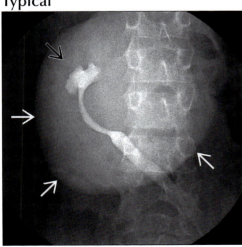 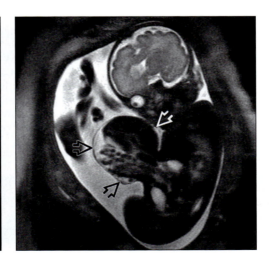

(Left) Anteroposterior IVP shows a solitary ectopic kidney *(black arrow)* in a child with an omphalocele *(white arrows)*. *(Right)* Sagittal T2WI MR shows omphalocele *(arrows)* containing most of the liver in a 30 week fetus.

GASTROSCHISIS

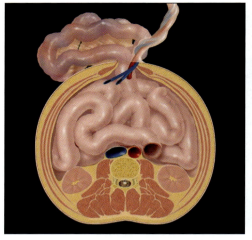

Graphic shows an abdominal wall defect with herniation of small bowel. The defect is adjacent to the normally inserted umbilical cord.

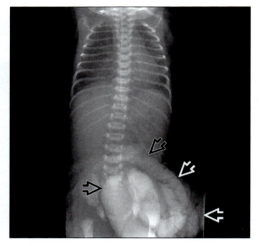

Anteroposterior radiograph shows anterior herniation of dilated, thick-walled intestine (arrows). The abdomen is small.

TERMINOLOGY

Definitions
- Congenital defect in anterior para-umbilical abdominal wall, almost always on the right side
  - Defect involves full thickness of the abdominal wall
  - Midgut herniates into amniotic cavity via defect
  - Midgut floats freely in amniotic fluid; not covered with membrane as in omphalocele
  - "Gastroschisis minor": Defect is small and only omentum protrudes

IMAGING FINDINGS

General Features
- Best diagnostic clue: Prenatal US: Color Doppler shows umbilical cord insertion in normal location beside herniated intestine
- Herniated contents generally small bowel
  - Large bowel and stomach also reported

Radiographic Findings
- Radiography: Pneumatosis intestinalis when necrotizing enterocolitis

Fluoroscopic Findings
- Intestinal hypomotility following repair
  - Marked delay in small bowel transit time
  - May also develop bowel obstruction related to adhesions: Hard to differentiate from hypomotility

Ultrasonographic Findings
- No covering membrane
- Bowel wall may be thickened, echogenic, and nodular due to edema and fibrinous serosal deposits
- Bowel dilatation
  - Both intra- and extra-abdominal loops may be dilated
  - Greater dilatation, poorer prognosis
- Stomach often malpositioned
- Oligohydramnios more common than polyhydramnios
  - Polyhydramnios suggests associated gut atresia
- Intrauterine growth restriction common

Other Modality Findings
- Upper gastrointestinal series: Midgut malrotation
- Fetal MR: Intestine protruded into amnion without covering membrane

Imaging Recommendations
- Document cord insertion with normal abdominal wall on both sides
- Close US follow-up for fetal complications
  - Progressive bowel dilatation, intra-uterine growth retardation

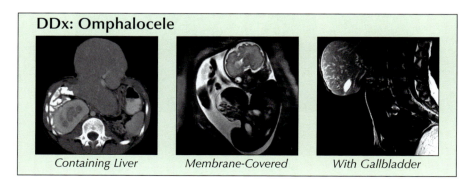

DDx: Omphalocele — Containing Liver — Membrane-Covered — With Gallbladder

GASTROSCHISIS

Key Facts

Terminology
- Congenital defect in anterior para-umbilical abdominal wall, almost always on the right side

Imaging Findings
- Best diagnostic clue: Prenatal US: Color Doppler shows umbilical cord insertion in normal location beside herniated intestine
- Bowel wall may be thickened, echogenic, and nodular due to edema and fibrinous serosal deposits
- Polyhydramnios suggests associated gut atresia
- Intrauterine growth restriction common

Pathology
- No known genetic basis for gastroschisis
- Mothers < 20 years 9 times more likely to have gastroschisis babies

- Closed gastroschisis: Abdominal wall defect closes around prolapsed gut causing midgut infarction and resorption (vanishing midgut) or mummification, abdominal wall may subsequently appear normal
- Defect usually to right of cord; only 7 cases of left-sided gastroschisis reported
- Intestine becomes edematous, inflamed, and matted together with prolonged exposure to amniotic fluid
- Midgut malrotation and malfixation ≈ 100%

Clinical Issues
- Mean age at diagnosis is 17 weeks gestational age
- Elevated α-fetal protein in maternal serum (95%)
- Sepsis commonest cause of death

---

  o Oligohydramnios

DIFFERENTIAL DIAGNOSIS

Omphalocele
- Cord inserts on hernia mass
- Mass covered by peritoneum
- Ruptured omphalocele difficult to differentiate prenatally
- Liver present in the hernia mass

Body stalk anomaly
- Fetus adherent to placenta
- No free floating umbilical cord
- Scoliosis

Bladder/cloacal exstrophy
- Umbilical cord inserts above defect
- Absent bladder is hallmark

Physiologic gut herniation
- Bowel returns to abdomen by 12 weeks
- Gut should not extend more than 1 cm into the cord
- Herniation always midline

PATHOLOGY

General Features
- Genetics
  o No known genetic basis for gastroschisis
  o Familial cases reported rarely
    ▪ 3-5% recurrence risk for siblings
- Etiology
  o Cause unknown: Three theories to explain defect
    ▪ Right umbilical vein: Abnormal involution with subsequent abdominal wall defect
    ▪ Omphalomesenteric (vitelline) artery: Occlusion leads to necrosis of the right side of umbilical ring
    ▪ Omphalocele: Prenatal rupture of omphalocele

  o Possible environmental teratogens: Radiation, aspirin, pseudoephedrine, acetaminophen, cocaine, smoking
- Epidemiology
  o 1:3,000-10,000 births
    ▪ Antenatal diagnosis made by US in 98% in developed countries
    ▪ 2:1 ratio of omphalocele to gastroschisis babies
  o Mean maternal age 23 years
    ▪ Mothers < 20 years 9 times more likely to have gastroschisis babies
  o Significant association with poor maternal education, low maternal socio-economic status, more than 1 abortion, short interval between menarche and first pregnancy
  o Mortality rate of African-American infants twice that of Caucasians
- Associated abnormalities
  o Other anomalies in 15%
    ▪ Hypoplastic gall bladder, hiatal hernia, Meckel diverticulum
    ▪ Hydronephrosis, bladder herniation into the defect
    ▪ Congenital cardiac defect

Gross Pathologic & Surgical Features
- Defect usually < 4 cm
  o Tight, constricted defect: Damage due to venous and lymphatic obstruction
    ▪ Closed gastroschisis: Abdominal wall defect closes around prolapsed gut causing midgut infarction and resorption (vanishing midgut) or mummification, abdominal wall may subsequently appear normal
  o Stomach, colon, bladder, fallopian tube, testis may also herniate
  o Defect usually to right of cord; only 7 cases of left-sided gastroschisis reported
- Intestinal atresia in 8-21%
  o 80% atresias are in jejunum or ileum
    ▪ Colonic atresia is rare
  o Many have subsequent short-gut syndrome

GASTROSCHISIS

- Bowel injury depends upon the duration of the herniation
  - Intestine becomes edematous, inflamed, and matted together with prolonged exposure to amniotic fluid
    - Bowel becomes coated with inflammatory, fibrotic peel
    - Bowel wall thickened
  - Amniotic fluid irritates fetal intestines
    - Amniotic fluid inflammatory cells increased
    - Amniotic fluid proinflammatory cytokine interleukin-8 elevated
    - Meconium in amniotic fluid
- Short-bowel syndrome
  - Bowel resection due to atresia
  - Bowel loss due to necrotizing enterocolitis
  - Volvulus
- Midgut malrotation and malfixation ≈ 100%
- Cryptorchidism in 31%

CLINICAL ISSUES

Presentation
- Most common signs/symptoms
  - Recognized during prenatal US
    - Mean age at diagnosis is 17 weeks gestational age
  - Elevated α-fetal protein in maternal serum (95%)
    - Elevation significant by 2nd trimester
    - Levels greater than in omphalocele
  - Diagnosis obvious at birth
    - Open herniation of intestine
    - Abdominal wall defect on right side of normal umbilical cord
- Intrauterine growth restriction
  - 70% below 50th percentile
- Oligohydramnios

Demographics
- Gender: 1.5x more frequent in males

Natural History & Prognosis
- Perinatal factors
  - Oligohydramnios common; may be polyhydramnios if gut atresia
  - Prematurity in 57%
  - Infants are small for their gestational age
  - Increased chance of intrauterine death
    - Cord compression by dilated bowel
- Bowel complications more frequent than in omphalocele
  - Amniotic fluid irritation factor leading to atresia, bowel edema, poor peristalsis
- 94% survival if no atresia
- 77% survival if atresia
- 10-15% persistent disability
  - Short-gut syndrome
  - Motility disorders
    - 10% incidence of hypoperistalsis syndrome
    - 50% have gastroesophageal reflux
- Inguinal hernias: Develop in most due to increased intra-abdominal pressure
- Sepsis commonest cause of death

Treatment
- Amniotic fluid exchange transfusion with normal saline may improve prognosis (experimental finding)
  - Decreases concentration of irritants in amniotic fluid
- Close fetal monitoring in 3rd trimester because of increased probability of intra-uterine death
- Delivery at tertiary care center
- Early delivery considered if worsening bowel dilatation (controversial)
- Vertex presentation: Caesarian section has no advantage over vaginal delivery
- Immediate surgical repair
  - Primary abdominal wall closure preferred
    - Primary closure feasible if intra-abdominal pressure < 20 mmHg (assessed by measurement of intra-gastric or intra-vesicle pressure) when external contents returned to abdominal cavity
    - If intra-abdominal pressure excessive: Inferior vena cava compression, urethral obstruction, bowel ischemia, respiratory compromise
    - Silo created if primary closure not possible
  - Large defects may require delayed secondary fascial closure
  - Mechanical ventilation after repair for 2-3 days because of increased intra-abdominal pressure
  - Delayed recovery of bowel function expected if intestines edematous and matted together
- Intestinal motility sluggish
  - Intravenous alimentation until intestinal function returns
- Necrotizing enterocolitis
  - Onset may be late; suspect if bloody stools

SELECTED REFERENCES

1. Salihu HM et al: Omphalocele and gastroschisis: Black-White disparity in infant survival. Birth Defects Res A Clin Mol Teratol. 70(9):586-91, 2004
2. Wilson RD et al: Congenital abdominal wall defects: an update. Fetal Diagn Ther. 19(5):385-98, 2004
3. Basaran UN et al: Prenatally closed gastroschisis with midgut atresia. Pediatr Surg Int. 18(5-6):550-2, 2002
4. Salihu HM et al: Omphalocele and gastroschisis. J Obstet Gynaecol. 22(5):489-92, 2002
5. Luton D et al: Effect of amnioinfusion on the outcome of prenatally diagnosed gastroschisis. Fetal Diagn Ther. 14:152-5, 1999
6. Chen CP et al: Prenatal diagnosis and perinatal aspects of abdominal wall defects. Am J Perinatol. 13(6):355-61, 1996
7. Quirk JG Jr et al: Outcomes of newborns with gastroschisis: the effects of mode of delivery, site of delivery, and interval from birth to surgery. Am J Obstet Gynecol. 174(4):1134-8; discussion 1138-40, 1996
8. Beaudoin S et al: Gastroesophageal reflux in neonates with congenital abdominal wall defect. Eur J Pediatr Surg. 5(6):323-6, 1995
9. Nelson TC et al: Familial gastroschisis: a case of mother-and son occurrence. J Pediatr Surg. 30(12):1706-8, 1995
10. Hoyme HE et al: The vascular pathogenesis of gastroschisis: intrauterine interruption of the omphalomesenteric artery. J Pediatr. 98(2):228-31, 1981

GASTROSCHISIS

IMAGE GALLERY

Typical

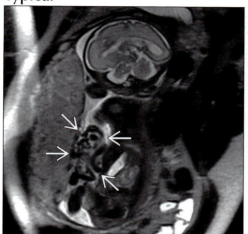
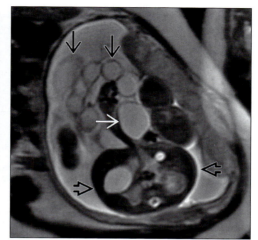

(Left) Sagittal T2WI fetal MR shows non-dilated intestine *(arrows)* free-floating in amnion. Oligohydramnios is present. *(Right)* Axial T2WI fetal MR shows multiple dilated bowel loops *(arrows)* free-floating in amnion. The abdomen *(open arrows)* is small.

Typical

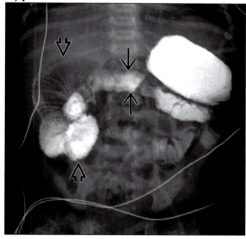
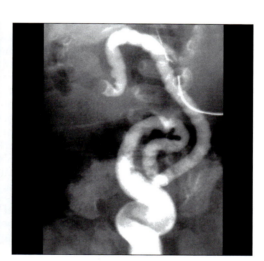

(Left) Anteroposterior radiograph following repair shows dilated duodenal bulb *(arrows)* and proximal jejunum *(open arrows)* in the right upper quadrant indicating malrotation. *(Right)* Anteroposterior radiograph shows microcolon due to ileal atresia.

Typical

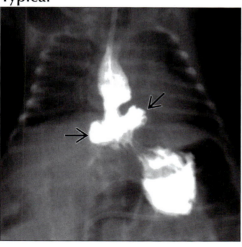
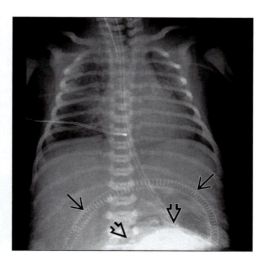

(Left) Anteroposterior radiograph shows a concentric herniation *(arrows)* of the stomach upward through the esophageal hiatus. *(Right)* Anteroposterior radiograph shows intra-abdominal retaining spring *(arrows)* of a silicone elastomer silo bag *(open arrows)* containing the extra-abdominal intestine.

APPENDICITIS

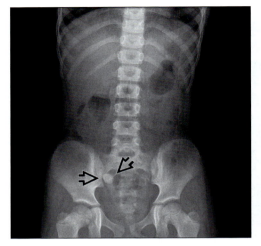

Radiograph shows large calcified appendicolith (arrows) in the right lower quadrant. Note bowel displaced out of right lower quadrant raising possibility of perforation.

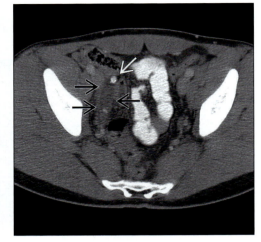

Axial CECT shows appendicolith (white arrow) in the right lower quadrant and dilated appendix distally (black arrows). Periappendiceal soft tissue stranding is present.

TERMINOLOGY

Definitions
- Acute obstruction of the appendiceal lumen results in distention of the appendix, superimposed infection, ischemia, and eventually perforation
- Goals of imaging
  o Decrease negative laparotomy rate
  o Increase rapidity of diagnosis: Decrease perforation rate
  o Identify alternative diagnoses (particularly non-surgical)

IMAGING FINDINGS

General Features
- Best diagnostic clue: Appendicolith
- Location: Normally right lower quadrant (RLQ), but can be in left lower quadrant with malrotation, rarely
- Size: Diameter greater than 6 mm is suggestive
- Morphology: Dilated enhancing tubular structure in RLQ with associated mesoappendix soft tissue stranding

Radiographic Findings
- Radiography
  o Nonperforated appendicitis appendicolith in 5-10% of patients
    ■ Appendicolith in 5-10% of patients
    ■ Air-fluid levels within bowel in right lower quadrant
    ■ Splinting
    ■ Loss of the right psoas margin
    ■ Free peritoneal air very uncommon
    ■ May be normal
  o With perforation
    ■ Small bowel obstruction
    ■ Right lower quadrant extraluminal gas
    ■ Displacement of bowel loops from RLQ

Fluoroscopic Findings
- Barium enema
  o Not commonly used with availability of CT & US
  o Nonfilling of the appendix is suggestive especially if associated with extrinsic mass effect on cecum

CT Findings
- CECT
  o Controversy and debate about appropriate CT protocol: Oral, rectal, IV, no contrast?
  o Appendicolith
  o Periappendiceal soft tissue stranding
  o Wall thickening of the cecum or terminal ileum
  o Diameter of appendix > 6 mm suggestive
  o Appendiceal wall enhances/thickened

DDx: RLQ Pain

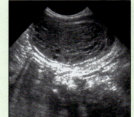
Ovarian Torsion

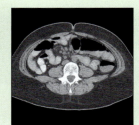
Mesenteric Adenitis

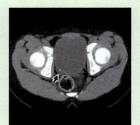
UVJ Stone

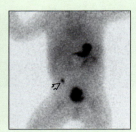
Meckel Diverticulum

APPENDICITIS

Key Facts

Terminology
- Acute obstruction of the appendiceal lumen results in distention of the appendix, superimposed infection, ischemia, and eventually perforation

Imaging Findings
- Best diagnostic clue: Appendicolith
- Location: Normally right lower quadrant (RLQ), but can be in left lower quadrant with malrotation, rarely
- Morphology: Dilated enhancing tubular structure in RLQ with associated mesoappendix soft tissue stranding
- Noncompressible blind-ending tubular structure over 6 mm in diameter
- Much debate concerning imaging algorithms for appendicitis

Top Differential Diagnoses
- Mesenteric adenitis
- Girls: Right ovarian pathology

Pathology
- Most common reason for abdominal surgery in children
- 15-20% of specimens may be negative

Clinical Issues
- Classic symptoms in older children with nonperforated appendicitis
- Pain begins in periumbilical region
- Migration to right lower quadrant
- Tenderness over McBurney's point

- Appendiceal lumen may be dilated
- Right lower quadrant lymphadenopathy
- Common for nonfilling of lumen of appendix, if transit of oral contrast to cecum at time of imaging
- Focal ileus RLQ
- With perforation
  - Small bowel obstruction
  - Inflammatory fluid collections most commonly in RLQ or dependent pelvis (cul-de-sac)

Ultrasonographic Findings
- Grayscale Ultrasound
  - Graded compression/high frequency transducer
  - Shadowing, echogenic appendicolith
  - Noncompressible blind-ending tubular structure over 6 mm in diameter
  - Right lower quadrant fluid, phlegmon, abscess
  - May be limited by rigid abdomen, overlying bowel gas, gas in abscess

Imaging Recommendations
- Best imaging tool
  - Primary imaging test: Ultrasound vs. CT?
  - Much debate concerning imaging algorithms for appendicitis
- Protocol advice
  - Factors that may influence choice of test
    - Ultrasound more accurate in thin patients
    - CT more accurate in heavier patients
    - Ultrasound may also demonstrate ovarian pathology in girls
    - Ultrasound requires a more experienced operator
    - If perforation suspected, CT more accurate in demonstrating fluid collections
  - Technical factors for CT: Oral and IV contrast, rectal and IV contrast, just rectal contrast, just IV contrast, no contrast
  - CT may require sedation in younger children

DIFFERENTIAL DIAGNOSIS

Mesenteric adenitis
- Other common cause of right lower quadrant pain/similar presentation
- Clinical entity related to benign inflammation of mesenteric nodes
- CT: Enlarged and clustered lymphadenopathy in mesentery and RLQ
- May also have ileal wall thickening

Girls: Right ovarian pathology
- Hemorrhagic cyst, ovarian torsion

Meckel diverticulum
- May cause RLQ inflammation and pain
- Usually symptomatic if contains ectopic gastric mucosa: Bleeding, ulceration
- Can also serve as a lead point for intussusception

Inflammatory bowel disease
- Crohn disease may mimic appendicitis with RLQ inflammatory changes

Omental infarction
- Focal infarction of omental fat
- Nonsurgical disease
- Inflammatory changes in anterior RLQ adjacent to colon

PATHOLOGY

General Features
- General path comments: Acute obstruction of the appendiceal lumen results in distention of the appendix, superimposed infection, ischemia, and eventually perforation
- Epidemiology
  - Most common reason for abdominal surgery in children
  - Common etiology for RLQ pain

APPENDICITIS

Gross Pathologic & Surgical Features
- inflamed, dilated appendix
- Mural thickening and suppurative exudate covering the serosa
- 15-20% of specimens may be negative

Microscopic Features
- Inflammatory infiltrate of the muscularis and neutrophil exudate
- Microabscess may form within the wall and focal ulceration and necrosis of the mucosa precedes perforation

CLINICAL ISSUES

Presentation
- Most common signs/symptoms
  - Right lower quadrant abdominal pain
  - Nausea, vomiting, diarrhea
- Other signs/symptoms
  - Classic symptoms in older children with nonperforated appendicitis
    - Pain begins in periumbilical region
    - Migration to right lower quadrant
    - Tenderness over McBurney's point
  - Anorexia
  - Fever
  - Guarding, rebound tenderness
  - Episodic abdominal pain
- Clinical presentation nonspecific in up to 1/3 of patients
  - Diagnosis more often delayed
  - Higher rate of perforation
  - Patients in which imaging plays a role

Demographics
- Age
  - May affect any age group
  - Mean age: Late teens, early twenties
  - Nonspecific presentation >> in young children
- Gender: Males slightly greater than females

Natural History & Prognosis
- Benign course in most cases especially if classic symptoms and prompt surgery
- Goal is for early diagnosis and appendectomy
- Morbidity and mortality increases with perforation
- At presentation up to 40% may have perforation, risk increases with delay in diagnosis
- Post-operative imaging may be preformed to evaluate for intra-abdominal abscess formation
- Hepatic abscess and pyophlebitis have been reported

Treatment
- Goals of imaging in appendicitis
  - Decrease the negative laparotomy rate
  - Increase rapidity of diagnosis: Decrease perforation rate
  - Identify alternative diagnoses
- If classic symptoms, surgery without imaging
- Nonspecific symptoms → documentation with imaging → appendectomy
  - Perforated appendicitis sometimes managed with antibiotics, percutaneous drainage of fluid collections, and interval appendectomy
- Appendectomy by laparoscopy or open
  - May need to convert to open secondary to location of appendix, body habitus, or perforation/degree of inflammatory reaction

DIAGNOSTIC CHECKLIST

Consider
- Controversies
  - Primary imaging modality: US vs. CT
  - Role of abdominal radiographs
  - CT techniques: Oral and IV contrast, rectal and IV contrast, just rectal contrast, just IV contrast, no contrast

Image Interpretation Pearls
- CT
  - Appendicolith
  - Dilated appendiceal lumen unopacified by oral or rectal contrast with diameter greater than 6 mm
  - Periappendiceal soft tissue stranding
- Ultrasound
  - Noncompressible blind-ending tubular structure over 6 mm in diameter
  - Shadowing, echogenic appendicolith

SELECTED REFERENCES

1. Acosta R et al: CT can reduce hospitalization for observation in children with suspected appendicitis. Pediatr Radiol. 2005
2. Garcia Pena BM et al: Selective imaging strategies for the diagnosis of appendicitis in children. Pediatrics. 113(1 Pt 1):24-8, 2004
3. Hagendorf BA et al: The optimal initial management of children with suspected appendicitis: a decision analysis. J Pediatr Surg. 39(6):880-5, 2004
4. Ikeda H et al: Laparoscopic versus open appendectomy in children with uncomplicated and complicated appendicitis. J Pediatr Surg. 39(11):1680-5, 2004
5. Kapfer SA et al: Intestinal malrotation-not just the pediatric surgeon's problem. J Am Coll Surg. 199(4):628-35, 2004
6. Kaiser S et al: Impact of radiologic imaging on the surgical decision-making process in suspected appendicitis in children. Acad Radiol. 11(9):971-9, 2004
7. Kaneko K et al: Ultrasound-based decision making in the treatment of acute appendicitis in children. J Pediatr Surg. 39(9):1316-20, 2004
8. Kosloske AM et al: The diagnosis of appendicitis in children: outcomes of a strategy based on pediatric surgical evaluation. Pediatrics. 113(1 Pt 1):29-34, 2004
9. Moraitis D et al: Laparoscopy in complicated pediatric appendicitis. JSLS. 8(4):310-3, 2004
10. Ponsky TA et al: Hospital- and patient-level characteristics and the risk of appendiceal rupture and negative appendectomy in children. JAMA. 292(16):1977-82, 2004
11. Garcia Pena BM et al: Ultrasonography and limited computed tomography in the diagnosis and management of appendicitis in children. JAMA. 15:282:1041-6, 1999
12. Johnson JF et al: Plain film diagnosis of appendiceal perforation in children. Semin Ultrasound CT MR. 10:306-13, 1989

APPENDICITIS

IMAGE GALLERY

Typical

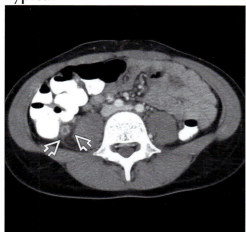
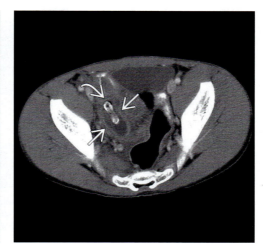

(Left) Axial CECT shows dilated appendix (arrows) with thickened, enhancing wall and periappendiceal soft tissue stranding. *(Right)* Axial CECT shows dilated, tubular appendix (arrows) containing a large elongated appendicolith (curved arrow).

Typical

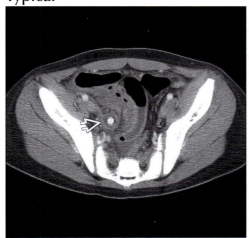
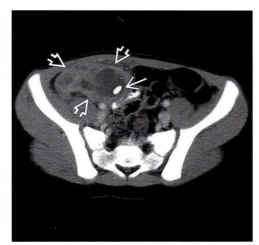

(Left) Axial CECT shows dilated appendix containing appendicolith (arrow). Note adjacent soft tissue stranding. *(Right)* Axial CECT shows perforated appendicitis with RLQ fluid collection (open arrows) containing appendicolith (arrow).

Typical

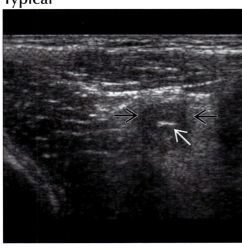
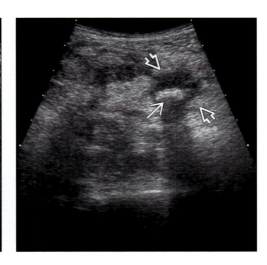

(Left) Transverse ultrasound shows dilated, distended appendix in short axis (black arrows) in the right lower quadrant containing an echogenic appendicolith (white arrow). *(Right)* Transverse ultrasound shows markedly distended appendix (open arrows) containing echogenic material and an area of acoustic shadowing related to an appendicolith (white arrow).

ILEOCOLIC INTUSSUSCEPTION (IDIOPATHIC)

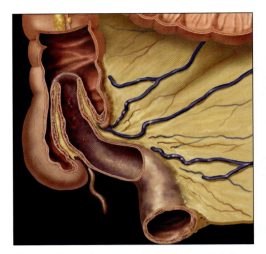

Graphic shows intussusception with terminal ileum invaginating into cecum and ascending colon. Note vascular congestion of intussusceptum.

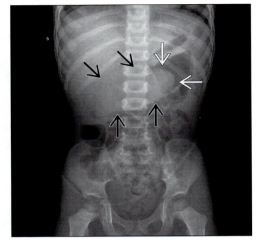

Radiograph shows a soft tissue prominence over ascending and transverse colon (black arrows) with visible large soft tissue mass (white arrows) surrounded by meniscus of gas.

TERMINOLOGY

Definitions
- Intussusception: Forward peristalsis results in invagination of more proximal bowel (the intussusceptum) into lumen of more distal bowel (the intussuscipiens) in a telescope-like manner

IMAGING FINDINGS

General Features
- Best diagnostic clue: Meniscus of soft tissue mass outlined in air-filled colon
- Location
  - Most common site: Terminal ileum/ileocecal valve
  - 90% ileocolic
- Size
  - May involve small segment of terminal ileum and ileocecal valve
  - May progress to involve a large segment of ileum with extension into the transverse or descending colon
  - Invagination may begin with telescoping of ileum into distal ileum and then into cecum or ascending colon, ileo-ileocolic intussusception

Radiographic Findings
- Radiography
  - Rarely completely normal
  - Paucity of right lower quadrant (RLQ) gas
  - Non-visualization of air-filled cecum
  - Left-side-down decubitus/prone views can be helpful in showing lack of air-filled cecum
  - Meniscus of soft tissue mass outlined in air-filled colon
  - Small bowel obstruction

Fluoroscopic Findings
- Air contrast enema
  - Intussusception easily recognized as round mass that moves retrograde with increased pressure
  - Reflux of gas into small bowel and resolution of soft tissue mass denotes successful reduction
- Liquid contrast enema
  - Similar findings as with air enema but with positive contrast

CT Findings
- CECT
  - Not advocated as diagnostic tool for suspected intussusception but intussusception may be encountered on abdominal CT performed for nonspecific abdominal pain

DDx: Abdominal Pain

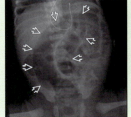
RLQ Sigmoid

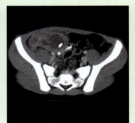
Appendicitis

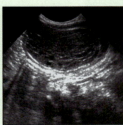
Ovarian Pathology

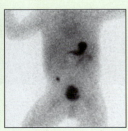
Meckel Diverticulum

ILEOCOLIC INTUSSUSCEPTION (IDIOPATHIC)

Key Facts

Terminology
- Intussusception: Forward peristalsis results in invagination of more proximal bowel (the intussusceptum) into lumen of more distal bowel (the intussuscipiens) in a telescope-like manner

Imaging Findings
- Best diagnostic clue: Meniscus of soft tissue mass outlined in air-filled colon
- Most common site: Terminal ileum/ileocecal valve

Pathology
- Bowel wall congestion from venous obstruction may lead to bowel ischemia and necrosis
- Seasonal occurrence (winter, spring) with viral illnesses

Clinical Issues
- Alternating lethargy and irritability
- Colic
- Most common between 3 months-1 year of age
- Surgery reserved for cases of reduction failure
- Success rates 80-90% with air reduction
- Risk of perforation 0.5%

Diagnostic Checklist
- Left-side-down decubitus/prone views can be helpful in showing lack of air-filled cecum
- CT: Colonic mass with alternating rings of high and low attenuation
- May not be located in RLQ if intussusception has progressed distally

---

- Colonic mass with alternating rings of high and low attenuation
- May be able to appreciate continuity with adjacent mesenteric fat and areas of low attenuation within the bowel lumen
- May not be located in RLQ if intussusception has progressed distal

Ultrasonographic Findings
- Grayscale Ultrasound
  - Can be used in cases in which radiographs or history are inconclusive
  - Mass with alternating rings of hyper- and hypoechogenicity
  - "Pseudo-kidney" appearance on longitudinal images
  - May not be located in RLQ if intussusception has progressed distal
    - Need to scan entire left and right abdomen

Imaging Recommendations
- Best imaging tool: Radiography and ultrasound
- Protocol advice
  - Radiography for initial evaluation of abdominal pain
  - Ultrasound for cases with equivocal history or radiographic findings
  - Reduction enema: Used to both confirm and treat intussusception

DIFFERENTIAL DIAGNOSIS

Normal position of sigmoid colon
- In infants and young children, sigmoid colon may be in right lower quadrant of abdomen 43% of time
- May be misinterpreted as air in cecum and falsely exclude intussusception

Appendicitis
- May present with similar symptoms of abdominal pain, typically older age group
- Identification of appendicolith is helpful
- In cases of perforation, there may be extrinsic mass effect on the cecum mimicking soft tissue mass

Gastroenteritis
- Plain film typically shows multiple air fluid levels within mildly distended bowel loops
- Air fluid levels in colon support gastroenteritis and make intussusception unlikely

Ovarian pathology
- May present as fussiness or pain in young child

Meckel diverticulum
- May serve as lead point for intussusception, cause gastrointestinal (GI) bleeding, or abdominal pain

PATHOLOGY

General Features
- General path comments
  - 90% ileocolic
  - Bowel wall congestion from venous obstruction may lead to bowel ischemia and necrosis
  - Bowel perforation may occur during reduction attempt
- Etiology
  - 90% idiopathic variety (2nd to lymphoid hyperplasia)
  - May be preceded by viral illness
- Epidemiology
  - Relatively common cause of abdominal pain in children 3 months to 1 year of age
  - Seasonal occurrence (winter, spring) with viral illnesses
  - If > 3 years of age, think pathologic lead point, such as lymphoma, Meckel diverticulum, Henoch-Schönlein purpura (wall hematoma)

Gross Pathologic & Surgical Features
- Telescoping to terminal ileum and ileocecal valve into the cecum or ascending colon

ILEOCOLIC INTUSSUSCEPTION (IDIOPATHIC)

CLINICAL ISSUES

Presentation
- Most common signs/symptoms
  - Alternating lethargy and irritability
  - Colic
  - Palpable right-sided abdominal mass
  - May have empty RLQ, Dance's sign
- Other signs/symptoms
  - Bloody diarrhea, ("currant jelly") stools
  - Crampy abdominal pain
  - Vomiting, may be bilious

Demographics
- Age
  - Most common between 3 months-1 year of age
  - If greater than 3 years: Pathologic lead point?
- Gender: Girls > boys

Natural History & Prognosis
- Medical urgency: Can infarct bowel if not reduced
- If bowel necrosis, perforation can occur leading to peritonitis, shock and even death
- In a small number there may be spontaneous reduction, usually more common in small bowel intussusception
- Intussusception recurs after successful reduction in 5-10%
- Most recurrences within first 72 hours

Treatment
- Imaging guided pressure reduction is treatment of choice
- Surgery reserved for cases of reduction failure
- Air insufflation or liquid contrast with fluoroscopic guidance most common methods
- Hydrostatic reduction under ultrasound guidance
- Contraindications: Peritonitis - exam, free peritoneal air - radiography (rare)
- Findings associated with decreased success rate but not contraindications
  - Small bowel obstruction
  - Prolonged history of symptoms (days)
  - Poor clinical condition: Lethargy
- Preparation guidelines: Adequate hydration, IV access, physical examination, pediatric surgery consultation (in case of perforation)
- If child appears not well (lethargic), good idea to have surgery present at time of reduction
- Guidelines: Good rectal seal, 120 mmHg maximal pressure at rest but can be greater during crying/Valsalva, typically three attempts during any one sitting, after rest period additional attempts can be made
- Intussusception encountered as round mass that moves retrograde with increased pressure
- Success: Reflux of gas into small bowel, resolution of soft tissue mass
- Mass most likely to "get stuck" at ileocecal valve
- If initial progression of mass on initial attempts but not able to reduce beyond ileocecal valve, a period of an hour may allow for edema to decrease and increased chance of success
- May be difficult at times to differentiate edematous ileocecal valve from persistent intussusception: Follow clinically
  - Edematous ileocecal valve may predispose to recurrence
- Success rates 80-90% with air reduction
- Risk of perforation 0.5%
- Recurrences can be treated on up to three occurrences prior to considering surgical exploration for potential pathological lead point

DIAGNOSTIC CHECKLIST

Image Interpretation Pearls
- Left-side-down decubitus/prone views can be helpful in showing lack of air-filled cecum
- CT: Colonic mass with alternating rings of high and low attenuation
- US: Mass with alternating rings of hyper- and hypoechogenicity, "pseudo-kidney" appearance on longitudinal image
- May not be located in RLQ if intussusception has progressed distally

SELECTED REFERENCES

1. Daneman A et al: Intussusception. Part 2: An update on the evolution of management. Pediatr Radiol. 34(2):97-108; quiz 187, 2004
2. Navarro O et al: Intussusception. Part 3: Diagnosis and management of those with an identifiable or predisposing cause and those that reduce spontaneously. Pediatr Radiol. 34(4):305-12; quiz 369, 2004
3. Melcher ML et al: Ileoilocolic intussusception in an adult. J Am Coll Surg. 197(3):518, 2003
4. Daneman A et al: Intussusception. Part 1: a review of diagnostic approaches. Pediatr Radiol. 33(2):79-85, 2003
5. Strouse PJ et al: Transient small-bowel intussusception in children on CT. Pediatr Radiol. 33(5):316-20, 2003
6. Khong PL et al: Ultrasound-guided hydrostatic reduction of childhood intussusception: technique and demonstration. Radiographics. 20(5):E1, 2000
7. Kornecki A et al: Spontaneous reduction of intussusception: clinical spectrum, management and outcome. Pediatr Radiol. 30(1):58-63, 2000
8. Nokes S et al: CT scans are helpful in acute abdomen cases. Ileocolic intussusception. J Ark Med Soc. 97(4):125-6, 2000
9. Chan KL et al: Childhood intussusception: ultrasound-guided Hartmann's solution hydrostatic reduction or barium enema reduction? J Pediatr Surg. 32(1):3-6, 1997
10. Peh WC et al: Ileoileocolic intussusception in children: diagnosis and significance. Br J Radiol. 70(837):891-6, 1997
11. Peh WC et al: Sonographically guided hydrostatic reduction of childhood intussusception using Hartmann's solution. AJR Am J Roentgenol. 167(5):1237-41, 1996
12. Strouse PJ et al: Ileocolic intussusception presenting with bilious vomiting due to extrinsic duodenal obstruction. Pediatr Radiol. 25 Suppl 1:S167-8, 1995
13. Shiels WE II et al: Air enema for the diagnosis and reduction of intussusception: clinical experience and pressure correlates. Radiology. 181:169-72, 1991
14. Eklof O et al: Reliability of the abdominal plain film diagnosis in pediatric patients with suspected intussusception. Pediatr Radiol. 9:199-206, 1980

ILEOCOLIC INTUSSUSCEPTION (IDIOPATHIC)

IMAGE GALLERY

Typical

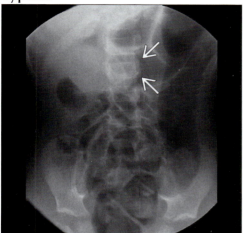
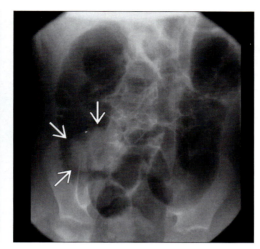

(Left) Air enema (initial image) shows air-filled descending colon with large soft tissue mass *(arrows)* confirming intussusception in transverse colon. *(Right)* Air enema (later image) shows soft tissue mass *(arrows)* moving retrograde distal to ileocecal valve.

Typical

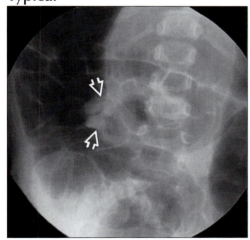
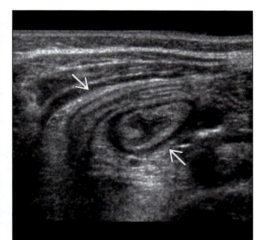

(Left) Air enema shows resolution of soft tissue mass and reflux of gas into small bowel consistent with reduced intussusception. Note persistent edematous ileocecal valve *(arrows)*. *(Right)* Transverse ultrasound image shows mass filling cecum and ascending colon with characteristic appearance of alternating rings of hyper- and hypo-echogenicity *(arrows)*.

Typical

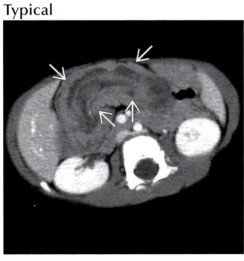
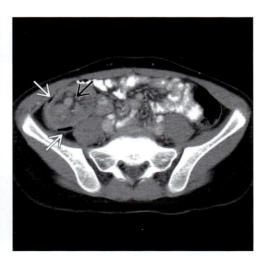

(Left) Axial CECT shows intussusception in transverse colon *(arrows)* with alternating layers of high and low attenuation. *(Right)* Axial CECT shows mass in location of ascending colon with thin rim of gas *(white arrows)* and centrally containing invaginated mesenteric fat *(black arrow)*.

MECKEL DIVERTICULUM

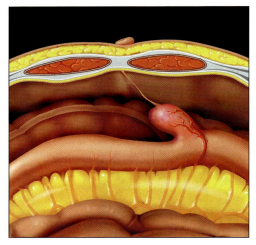

Graphic shows an inflamed Meckel diverticulum growing off the antimesenteric border of the intestine with the obliterated remnant of the omphalomesenteric duct extending from its tip.

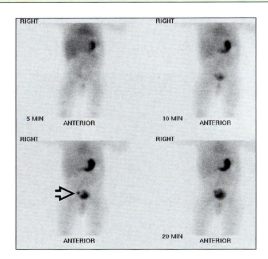

Anterior images from Tc-99m pertechnetate scan show intense, focal radioisotope accumulation in the right lower quadrant (arrow), initially with some mass effect on the adjacent bladder.

TERMINOLOGY

Definitions
- Remnant of the omphalomesenteric duct, can cause bleeding (when contains ectopic gastric mucosa), intussusception, bowel obstruction or perforation
- Rule of 2's: Incidence 2% of general population, found within 2 feet of ileocecal valve, most have clinical symptoms before age 2 years
- Most common end result of the spectrum of omphalomesenteric duct anomalies, which also include umbilicoileal fistula, umbilical sinus, umbilical cyst, and a fibrous cord connecting the ileum to the umbilicus

IMAGING FINDINGS

General Features
- Best diagnostic clue
  - Classic imaging appearance on nuclear pertechnetate scan is focal accumulation in right lower quadrant that is coincident with, and as intense as, gastric uptake, and increases in visibility with time
  - Nuclear scintigraphy is most accurate: Radiographs, sonography, CT scan or barium studies show nonspecific signs of a right lower quadrant inflammatory process
- Location
  - Within 2 feet of ileocecal valve
  - Right lower quadrant or midline/periumbilical in location
- Size: 5-6 cm in length, though inflammatory mass may be much larger

Radiographic Findings
- Radiography
  - Abdominal films may show a right lower quadrant mass or displacement of bowel loops, obstruction, or be normal
  - Enteroliths are occasionally reported in Meckel diverticulum

Fluoroscopic Findings
- Barium studies show indirect evidence of mass and inflammatory changes in adjacent bowel

CT Findings
- CECT
  - Findings very similar to appendicitis; thick walled blind ending structure near cecum with surrounding inflammation
  - If perforated may see abscess and free air

DDx: Clinical Mimickers Of Meckel Diverticulum

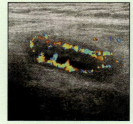
Acute Appendicitis

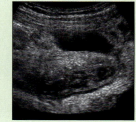
Perforated Appendicitis

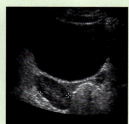
Right Ovarian Torsion

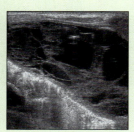
Meconium Pseudocyst

MECKEL DIVERTICULUM

Key Facts

Terminology
- Remnant of the omphalomesenteric duct, can cause bleeding (when contains ectopic gastric mucosa), intussusception, bowel obstruction or perforation
- Rule of 2's: Incidence 2% of general population, found within 2 feet of ileocecal valve, most have clinical symptoms before age 2 years

Imaging Findings
- Classic imaging appearance on nuclear pertechnetate scan is focal accumulation in right lower quadrant that is coincident with, and as intense as, gastric uptake, and increases in visibility with time
- Nuclear scintigraphy is most accurate: Radiographs, sonography, CT scan or barium studies show nonspecific signs of a right lower quadrant inflammatory process
- Findings very similar to appendicitis; thick walled blind ending structure near cecum with surrounding inflammation
- The most specific test for Meckel diverticulum is the Tc-99m pertechnetate scan: Accuracy ~90%
- Pertechnetate accumulates in mucous cells when they are in an acidic environment, in this case in ectopic gastric mucosa
- Pharmacologic enhancement of pertechnetate scans by using subcutaneous pentagastrin, oral or intravenous ranitidine or cimetidine, and IM glucagon is advocated by some

Top Differential Diagnoses
- Appendicitis
- Intestinal duplication containing gastric mucosa
- Hemangioma

- CT is more accurate in diagnosing Meckel diverticulum than arteriography when presenting symptom is gastrointestinal bleeding in pediatric patients
- Non-inflamed Meckel diverticula can move slightly with the bowel in the lower abdomen on sequential imaging

Ultrasonographic Findings
- Grayscale Ultrasound
  - Heterogeneous echotexture mass in right lower quadrant, may mimic appendicitis
  - Thick walled tubular structure or hyperemic bowel loops in right lower quadrant
  - Case reports of cystic masses when gastric mucosa also secretes mucus
  - Inflamed Meckel diverticulum may present as a cyst, but with mucosal layer more irregular than typically found in an intestinal duplication
- Color Doppler: Hyperemia related to inflammatory process

Nuclear Medicine Findings
- Tc-99m pertechnetate scan
  - The most specific test for Meckel diverticulum is the Tc-99m pertechnetate scan: Accuracy ~90%
  - Pertechnetate accumulates in mucous cells when they are in an acidic environment, in this case in ectopic gastric mucosa
  - The diverticulum typically does not communicate with the bowel lumen, so the radiotracer does not appear to move downstream in bowel unless there is active bleeding
  - Pharmacologic enhancement of pertechnetate scans by using subcutaneous pentagastrin, oral or intravenous ranitidine or cimetidine, and IM glucagon is advocated by some
  - However, given the high sensitivity of unenhanced scans, additional medications may be reserved for repeat studies in patients with high clinical suspicion of Meckel diverticular disease and normal initial scans
  - False negative pertechnetate scans
    - Lack of any or sufficient gastric mucosa to localize radiotracer
    - Secondary ischemia due to volvulus or intussusception

Imaging Recommendations
- Best imaging tool: Tc-99m pertechnetate scan

DIFFERENTIAL DIAGNOSIS

Appendicitis
- Hyperemia may cause early increase in pertechnetate activity at the lesion

Intestinal duplication containing gastric mucosa
- Also common in right lower quadrant, also need to be surgically removed

Hemangioma
- Hemangioma can also cause bleeding, obstruction, or intussusception

Inflammatory bowel disease
- Hyperemia causes mildly increased accumulation of pertechnetate

Ovarian pathology
- Negative on pertechnetate scans, but in the same lower quadrant on other imaging studies

Meconium pseudocyst
- Negative on pertechnetate scans, but in the same lower quadrant on other imaging studies

PATHOLOGY

General Features
- General path comments
  - Remnant of the omphalomesenteric duct found in 2-3% of autopsy series

MECKEL DIVERTICULUM

- Small percentage of Meckel become symptomatic, typically due to the presence of ectopic gastric mucosa
- Rarely, the diverticulum contains rests of pancreatic tissue
- Embryology-anatomy
  - Omphalomesenteric duct was the connection between the yolk sac and primitive digestive tract in early fetal life
  - Meckel diverticulum is the most common end result of the spectrum of omphalomesenteric duct anomalies, which also include umbilicoileal fistula, umbilical sinus, umbilical cyst, and a fibrous cord connecting the ileum to the umbilicus

Gross Pathologic & Surgical Features
- Typically 5-6 cm in length, positioned within 2 feet proximal to the ileocecal valve
- Enteroliths are found in the lumen in some cases

Microscopic Features
- Composed of same layers as adjacent small bowel but with the addition of heterotopic gastric or pancreatic rests

CLINICAL ISSUES

Presentation
- Most common signs/symptoms: Gastrointestinal (GI) bleeding, ulceration, abdominal pain, or mass
- Other signs/symptoms
  - May present as intermittent abdominal pain, occult fecal blood, frank blood in stool, small bowel obstruction, intussusception, volvulus, or perforation
  - Perforation of Meckel diverticulum with hemoperitoneum in children is a rare and serious complication
  - Torsion of a Meckel diverticulum may present with nonspecific abdominal pain and mass

Demographics
- Age
  - Most often become symptomatic before two years of age
  - 60% of patients come to medical attention before 10 years of age, with the remainder of cases manifesting in adolescence and adulthood
  - Older patients more likely to present with intussusception or small bowel obstruction than with GI bleeding
- Gender
  - Males = females in true incidence
  - Bleeding and other symptoms/complications are more common in males

Natural History & Prognosis
- Presentation as described above
- Prognosis is excellent

Treatment
- Surgical resection, incidental appendectomy usually also performed
- Meckel diverticula are generally removed when found incidentally on imaging or in the operating room

SELECTED REFERENCES

1. Baldisserotto M: Color Doppler sonographic findings of inflamed and perforated Meckel diverticulum. J Ultrasound Med. 23(6):843-8, 2004
2. Bennett GL et al: CT of Meckel's diverticulitis in 11 patients. AJR Am J Roentgenol. 182(3):625-9, 2004
3. Levy AD et al: From the archives of the AFIP. Meckel diverticulum: radiologic features with pathologic Correlation. Radiographics. 24(2):565-87, 2004
4. Ojha S et al: Meckel's diverticulum with segmental dilatation of the ileum: radiographic diagnosis in a neonate. Pediatr Radiol. 34(8):649-51, 2004
5. Rerksuppaphol S et al: Ranitidine-enhanced 99mtechnetium pertechnetate imaging in children improves the sensitivity of identifying heterotopic gastric mucosa in Meckel's diverticulum. Pediatr Surg Int. 20(5):323-5, 2004
6. Segal SD et al: Rare mesenteric location of Meckel's diverticulum, a forgotten entity: a case study aboard USS Kitty Hawk. Am Surg. 70(11):985-8, 2004
7. Singh MV et al: A fading Meckel's diverticulum: an unusual scintigraphic appearance in a child. Pediatr Radiol. 34(3):274-6, 2004
8. Adams BK et al: A moving Meckel's diverticulum on Tc-99m pertechnetate imaging in a patient with lower gastrointestinal bleeding. Clin Nucl Med. 28(11):908-10, 2003
9. Baldisserotto M et al: Sonographic findings of Meckel's diverticulitis in children. AJR Am J Roentgenol. 180(2):425-8, 2003
10. Danzer D et al: Bleeding Meckel's diverticulum diagnosis: an unusual indication for computed tomography. Abdom Imaging. 28(5):631-3, 2003
11. Onen A et al: When to resect and when not to resect an asymptomatic Meckel's diverticulum: an ongoing challenge. Pediatr Surg Int. 19(1-2):57-61, 2003
12. Jelenc F et al: Meckel's diverticulum perforation with intraabdominal hemorrhage. J Pediatr Surg. 37(6):E18, 2002
13. Mortele KJ et al: Giant Meckel's diverticulum containing enteroliths: typical CT imaging findings. Eur Radiol. 12(1):82-4, 2002
14. Sy ED et al: Meckel's diverticulum associated with ileal volvulus in a neonate. Pediatr Surg Int. 18(5-6):529-31, 2002
15. Farris SL et al: Axial torsion of Meckel's diverticulum presenting as a pelvic mass. Pediatr Radiol. 31(12):886-8, 2001
16. Neidlinger NA et al: Meckel's diverticulum causing cecal volvulus. Am Surg. 67(1):41-3, 2001
17. Oguzkurt P et al: Cystic Meckel's diverticulum: A rare cause of cystic pelvic mass presenting with urinary symptoms. J Pediatr Surg. 36(12):1855-8, 2001
18. O'Hara SM: Pediatric gastrointestinal nuclear imaging. Radiol Clin North Am. 34(4):845-62, 1996
19. Wilton G et al: The "false-negative" Meckel's scan. Clin Nuc Med. 7:441, 1982
20. Sfakianakas GN et al: Detection of ectopic gastric mucosa in Meckel's diverticulum and in other aberrations by scintigraphy.I Pathophysiology and 10-year clinical experience. J Nucl Med. 22:647-52, 1981

MECKEL DIVERTICULUM

IMAGE GALLERY

Typical

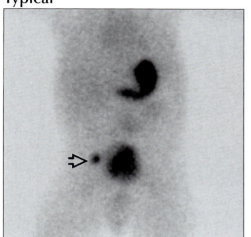
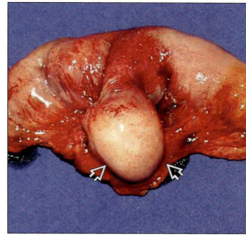

(Left) Close-up of delayed image during Tc-99m pertechnetate scan shows focal uptake in the right lower quadrant (arrow), in a Meckel diverticulum. *(Right)* Gross pathology shows pedunculated Meckel diverticulum (arrows) extending from the antimesenteric border of the ileum, twisted at its inflamed base with tip lying on segment of resected mesentery.

Typical

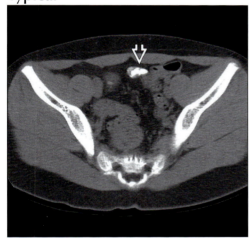
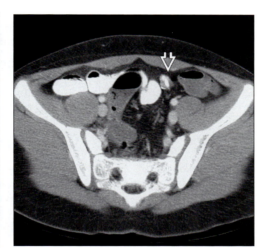

(Left) Axial NECT shows triangular calcification (arrow) in the midline pelvis surrounded by soft tissue. At surgery this was found to be an enterolith in a Meckel diverticulum. *(Right)* Axial CECT shows slight leftward movement of the enterolith and Meckel diverticulum (arrow) following oral and intravenous contrast administration. There was no inflammation at the time of the scan.

Typical

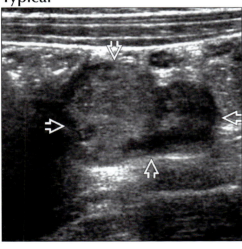
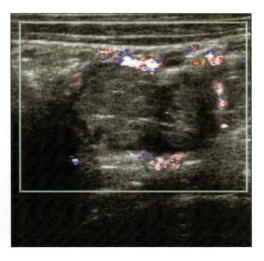

(Left) Transverse ultrasound shows heterogeneous echoes in a noncompressible soft tissue mass (arrows) in the right lower quadrant, later found to represent a Meckel diverticulum. *(Right)* Transverse color Doppler ultrasound shows hyperemia surrounding the Meckel diverticulum in a patient thought to have appendicitis. The ultrasound findings can mimic appendicitis.

HEPATOBLASTOMA

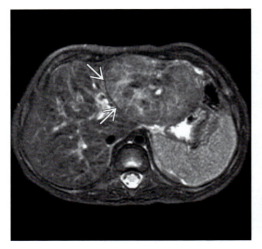

Axial T2WI MR shows hepatoblastoma as well-defined mass in left hepatic lobe displacing the falciform ligament (arrows). Mass is heterogeneous with small foci of high signal intensity.

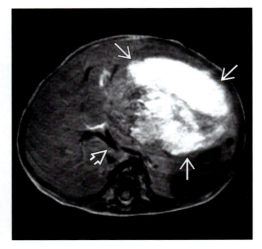

Axial T2WI MR shows hepatoblastoma (arrows) with high signal intensity mass displacing adjacent hepatic vasculature (open arrow).

TERMINOLOGY

Definitions
- Malignant embryonic hepatic tumor composed of epithelial cells and occasionally a mixture of epithelial and mesenchymal cells

IMAGING FINDINGS

General Features
- Best diagnostic clue: Large, well-defined and heterogeneous liver mass in an infant
- Location
  ○ Liver
  ○ More commonly located in the right hepatic lobe: > 60%
- Size: Large, 10-12 cm
- Morphology
  ○ Tend to be well-defined masses
  ○ May be lobulated
  ○ Tend to displace rather than invade adjacent hepatic structures such as falciform ligament
  ○ Usually single contiguous mass
  ○ May be multifocal
  ○ Rarely, diffuse infiltrative masses
  ○ May be heterogeneous in consistency secondary to areas of hemorrhage or necrosis
  ○ In very large masses, organ of origin may be difficult to determine
  ○ Calcifications in up to half of the patients

Radiographic Findings
- Radiography
  ○ Homogeneous soft tissue mass in right upper quadrant displacing bowel gas
  ○ May see dense, chunky calcification

CT Findings
- NECT
  ○ Well-defined, heterogeneous lesion predominantly hypoattenuating compared to normal liver parenchyma
  ○ As many as 50% of lesions have calcification
  ○ Mass typically large at presentation (10-12 cm)
- CECT
  ○ Mass typically well-defined and heterogeneous
  ○ May be lobulated
  ○ Enhancement nonuniform and less than normal liver parenchyma
  ○ Reports of peripheral rim-enhancement
  ○ Coarse calcifications common, osseous matrix if mixed type
  ○ Metastatic disease is common
    ▪ Lung
    ▪ Periaortic lymph nodes
    ▪ Brain, rare

DDx: Hepatic Mass In Young Child

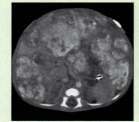
Hemangioendothelioma

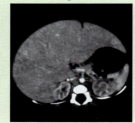
Neuroblastoma Mets

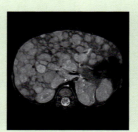
Neuroblastoma Mets

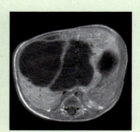
MH

HEPATOBLASTOMA

Key Facts

Terminology
- Malignant embryonic hepatic tumor composed of epithelial cells and occasionally a mixture of epithelial and mesenchymal cells

Imaging Findings
- Best diagnostic clue: Large, well-defined and heterogeneous liver mass in an infant
- More commonly located in the right hepatic lobe: > 60%
- May be heterogeneous in consistency secondary to areas of hemorrhage or necrosis
- Calcifications in up to half of the patients
- Color Doppler: Mass typically hypervascular on Doppler sonography
- Protocol advice: Major goal of imaging is to define anatomic extent of disease and relationship to hepatic lobar anatomy for pre-operative planning/monitor response to chemotherapy

Pathology
- Usually no history of underlying liver disease
- Most common hepatic malignancy in children

Clinical Issues
- Painless abdominal mass
- Serum alpha-fetoprotein levels are elevated in more than 90% of patients
- Gender: 2:1 = M:F predilection
- Poor prognosis

MR Findings
- T1WI
  - Low signal intensity
  - Can have high signal related to hemorrhage
- T2WI
  - Signal on T2WI typically high but variable secondary to amounts of hemorrhage and necrosis
  - May have hypointense fibrous bands
- T1 C+: Heterogeneous enhancement

Ultrasonographic Findings
- Grayscale Ultrasound
  - Well-defined, solid mass
  - May have spoked-wheel appearance
    - Related to fibrous septa
  - Heterogeneous echogenicity from hemorrhage/necrosis
  - Areas of acoustic shadowing due to calcifications
  - Cystic areas may represent necrosis or extramedullary hematopoiesis
- Color Doppler: Mass typically hypervascular on Doppler sonography

Angiographic Findings
- Conventional
  - Mass with dense blush due to neovascularity
  - Typically no arteriovenous shunting
  - Vascular structures draped over, displaced by mass
  - May have inferior vena cava (IVC) invasion
    - Unresectable

Nuclear Medicine Findings
- Bone Scan
  - May have increased uptake secondary to osteoid
  - Sulfur colloids
    - Photopenic defect

Imaging Recommendations
- Best imaging tool
  - Infants who present with abdominal mass often initially evaluated with ultrasound
    - Determine if mass present
    - Whether it is solid mass or other causes such as hydronephrosis
  - Whether definitive imaging study is MRI or CT is controversial
  - Typically no pathognomonic features of hepatic malignancies
- Protocol advice: Major goal of imaging is to define anatomic extent of disease and relationship to hepatic lobar anatomy for pre-operative planning/monitor response to chemotherapy

DIFFERENTIAL DIAGNOSIS

Hemangioendothelioma
- Presentation with congestive heart failure or thrombocytopenia
- Prominent vascular structures
- Negative serum alpha-fetoprotein

Neuroblastoma metastasis
- Usually multiple liver masses or diffuse liver heterogeneity
- Adrenal mass typically present

Mesenchymal hamartoma (MH)
- Well-defined, multilobulated, cystic mass

Hepatocellular carcinoma
- Most common hepatic malignancy in children over 5 years of age
- Rarely occurs under 3 years of age

PATHOLOGY

General Features
- General path comments
  - Well-defined borders with pseudocapsule
  - Usually no history of underlying liver disease
  - Positive serum alpha-fetoprotein
- Genetics
  - May be familial

HEPATOBLASTOMA

- Short arm chromosome 11
  - Similar to rhabdomyosarcoma and Wilms tumor
- Etiology: Congenital hepatic malignancy
- Epidemiology
  - Hepatic masses constitute only 5-6% of all intraabdominal masses in children
  - Primary hepatic neoplasms are 0.5-2% of all pediatric malignancies
  - 3rd most common abdominal malignancy
    - After neuroblastoma and Wilms tumor
  - Most common primary liver tumor of childhood (43% of liver masses)
  - Most common hepatic malignancy in children
- Associated abnormalities
  - Predisposing conditions
    - Beckwith-Wiedemann syndrome
    - Hemihypertrophy
    - Familial polyposis coli
    - Gardner syndrome
    - Fetal alcohol syndrome
    - Wilms tumor
    - Biliary atresia

Gross Pathologic & Surgical Features
- Fleshy, nodular lesion with fibrous bands throughout
  - Reason for spoked-wheel appearance
- May contain areas of necrosis or hemorrhage

Microscopic Features
- Epithelial type
  - Fetal
  - Embryonal
  - Macro trabecular
  - Small cell
- Mixed type with epithelial and foci of mesenchymal cells
  - Cartilage, muscle or fibrous tissue may be present
  - Osteoid

CLINICAL ISSUES

Presentation
- Most common signs/symptoms
  - Painless abdominal mass
  - Hepatomegaly
- Other signs/symptoms
  - Weight loss
  - Nausea
  - Vomiting
  - Anemia
  - Usually no history of underlying liver disease
  - May be present at birth
  - Serum alpha-fetoprotein levels are elevated in more than 90% of patients
  - Precocious puberty
  - More common in boys
  - Usually present in infancy: Most commonly under 3 years of age

Demographics
- Age
  - Most common in infants
  - Range: Newborn to 15 years
  - Peak: 1-2 years of age
- Gender: 2:1 = M:F predilection

Natural History & Prognosis
- Poor prognosis
- Overall survival rate 63-67%
- Better prognosis than hepatoma
- 60% of lesions resectable
- Better prognosis for epithelial type compared to mixed type

Treatment
- Chemotherapy
  - Neoadjuvant therapy has improved resectability rates
- Surgical resection
- Boiled Ethiodol and chemotherapy embolization
- Radiofrequency ablation
- Liver transplantation for nonresectable tumor

DIAGNOSTIC CHECKLIST

Image Interpretation Pearls
- Classic imaging appearance: Large, well-defined and heterogeneous liver mass in an infant
- Include CT of chest for evidence of metastatic disease during initial CT evaluation
- Note if IVC invasion

SELECTED REFERENCES

1. Woodward PJ et al: From the archives of the AFIP: a comprehensive review of fetal tumors with pathologic correlation. Radiographics. 25(1):215-42, 2005
2. Albrecht S et al: Allelic loss but absence of mutations in the polyspecific transporter gene BWR1A on 11p15.5 in hepatoblastoma. Int J Cancer. 111(4):627-32, 2004
3. Alobaidi M et al: Malignant cystic and necrotic liver lesions: a pattern approach to discrimination. Curr Probl Diagn Radiol. 33(6):254-68, 2004
4. Fiegel HC et al: Stem-like cells in human hepatoblastoma. J Histochem Cytochem. 52(11):1495-501, 2004
5. Hemming AW et al: Combined resection of the liver and inferior vena cava for hepatic malignancy. Ann Surg. 239(5):712-9; discussion 719-21, 2004
6. Xianliang H et al: Cure of hepatoblastoma with transcatheter arterial chemoembolization. J Pediatr Hematol Oncol. 26(1):60-3, 2004
7. Wang JN et al: Invasion of the cardiovascular system in childhood malignant hepatic tumors. J Pediatr Hematol Oncol. 24(6):436-9, 2002
8. Shih JC et al: Antenatal diagnosis of congenital hepatoblastoma in utero. Ultrasound Obstet Gynecol. 16(1):94-7, 2000
9. Boechat MI et al: Primary liver tumors in children: comparison of CT and MR imaging. Radiology 169:727-32, 1998
10. Donnelly LF et al: Pediatric liver imaging. Radiol Clin North Am. 36:413-27, 1998
11. Powers C et al: Primary liver neoplasms: MR imaging with pathologic correlation. RadioGraphics 14:459-482, 1994
12. Dachman AH et al: Hepatoblastoma: radiologic-pathologic correlation in 50 cases. Radiology. 164(1):15-9, 1987

HEPATOBLASTOMA

IMAGE GALLERY

Typical

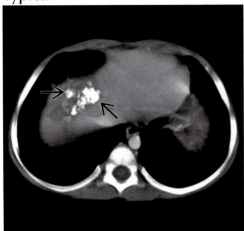
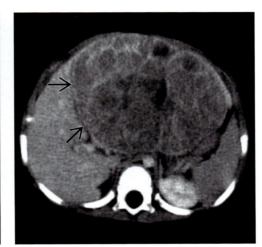

(Left) Axial CECT shows an area of dense calcifications (arrows) within a mass that is relatively lower in attenuation than normal surrounding hepatic parenchyma. (Right) Axial CECT shows a large, heterogeneous mass with well-defined borders (arrows). Mass has diffuse, heterogeneous enhancement that is less than normal hepatic parenchyma.

Typical

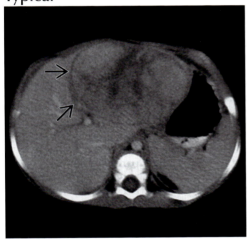
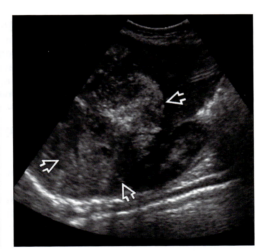

(Left) Axial CECT shows large, more homogeneous mass in left lobe of liver displacing rather than invading falciform ligament (arrows). (Right) Ultrasound shows a large, well-defined mass (arrows) in right hepatic lobe with heterogeneous echogenicity due to areas of hemorrhage/necrosis.

Typical

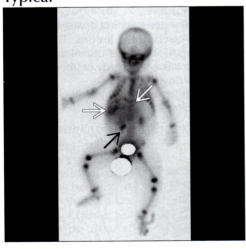
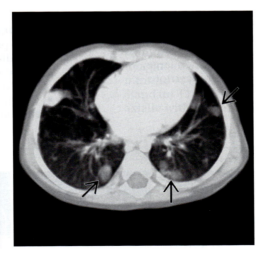

(Left) Bone scan shows a large mass (white arrows) within the liver with increased uptake due to calcification within the tumor. The mass is displacing the right kidney (black arrow). (Right) Axial CECT shows multiple peripheral metastatic soft tissue noncalcified nodules (arrows) throughout the lungs.

BILIARY ATRESIA

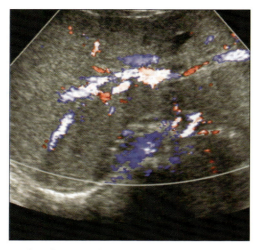

Axial color Doppler ultrasound shows anteriorly positioned portal vein and a transverse liver in a patient with biliary atresia.

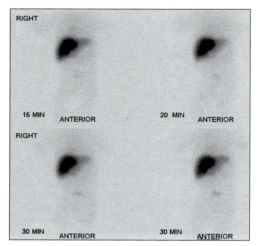

Anterior images from hepatobiliary scan show lack of radioisotope in biliary tree or intestinal tract, relatively high background activity and urinary excretion. Image at 24 hours was unchanged.

TERMINOLOGY

Abbreviations and Synonyms
- Biliary atresia (BA)

Definitions
- Absent or severely deficient extrahepatic biliary tree
- Affects 1 in 10,000-13,000 newborn infants

IMAGING FINDINGS

General Features
- Best diagnostic clue
  ○ Hepatobiliary scans show lack of radiotracer excretion into the intestines
  ○ Initially, hepatocyte function is preserved, but with prolonged symptoms hepatocyte function deteriorates
- Morphology
  ○ Often confused with neonatal hepatitis, a non-surgical disease
  ○ Gallbladder is present in up to 25%

CT Findings
- CECT
  ○ Seldom used when biliary atresia is suspected
  ○ Would show variable liver density depending on degree of hepatocyte dysfunction/child's age
  ○ May show presence of gallbladder, but should not show dilated ducts in biliary atresia
  ○ Is useful in excluding obstructive causes of jaundice: Choledochal malformation, stone disease, masses, dilated biliary tree

MR Findings
- T2WI
  ○ MRCP (magnetic resonance cholangiopancreatography) can be used, but has limitations
  ○ MRCP requires sedation or general anesthesia, and has sensitivity of 90%, specificity of 77% and accuracy of 82%

Ultrasonographic Findings
- Grayscale Ultrasound
  ○ Liver echotexture is typically normal though the organ may be enlarged
  ○ Gallbladder may be present in 25%, though the common bile duct is never seen
  ○ Extrahepatic bile ducts are not visible in cases of biliary atresia; replaced by an echogenic triangular cord sign which is thought to be the fibrotic remnant of the common duct

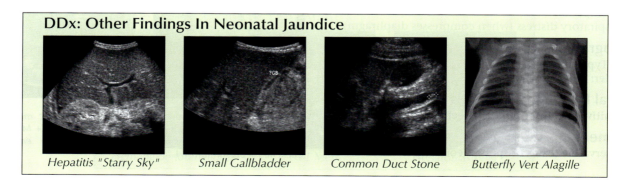

DDx: Other Findings In Neonatal Jaundice

Hepatitis "Starry Sky" | Small Gallbladder | Common Duct Stone | Butterfly Vert Alagille

BILIARY ATRESIA

Key Facts

Terminology
- Absent or severely deficient extrahepatic biliary tree
- Affects 1 in 10,000-13,000 newborn infants

Imaging Findings
- Hepatobiliary scans show lack of radiotracer excretion into the intestines
- Often confused with neonatal hepatitis, a non-surgical disease
- Gallbladder is present in up to 25%
- Extrahepatic bile ducts are not visible in cases of biliary atresia; replaced by an echogenic triangular cord sign which is thought to be the fibrotic remnant of the common duct
- Lack of excretion into the intestines on 24 hour delayed images is highly suggestive of biliary atresia or other extrahepatic occlusion
- Hepatobiliary scans have high sensitivity ~100%, but specificity of 87% and accuracy of 91%
- DDx: Neonatal hepatitis, choledochal malformation, Alagille's, bile plug, stone disease

Clinical Issues
- Most common signs/symptoms: Progressive conjugated (direct) hyperbilirubinemia in the neonatal period
- Prompt diagnosis is crucial to surgical success
- Kasai portoenterostomy is 90% effective if performed before 2 months of age, drops to less than 50% effective if performed after 3 months of age

---

  - Irregular gallbladder shape and wall thickness has also been associated with biliary atresia; this finding improves sonographic diagnostic accuracy
- Color Doppler
  - Doppler is useful to demonstrate the main portal vein and hepatic artery when searching for the triangular cord sign
  - Doppler is also useful to search for associated anomalies: Preduodenal portal vein, transverse liver (showing continuity of portal veins in leftward hepatic tissue), interrupted inferior vena cava (IVC), and cardiac anomalies

Nuclear Medicine Findings
- Hepatobiliary scan
  - Tc-99m disofenin (DISIDA) and mebrofenin (BRIDA) have the highest hepatic extraction rate and shortest transit time of the hepatobiliary radiotracers
  - Pretreat with oral phenobarbital (5mg/kg/day in divided doses x 5 days) which is a choleretic drug shown to improve scintigraphic accuracy
  - Phenobarbital is a potent inducer of hepatic microsomal enzymes and enhances biliary excretion
  - Ursodeoxycholic acid (UDCA) has also been used as a choleretic pre-scintigraphy (20 mg/kg every 12 hours for 48-72 hours) with good results
  - Hepatocyte uptake and extraction of radiotracer from the blood pool is usually preserved in the first 2-3 months of life, later deteriorates
  - Lack of excretion into the intestines on 24 hour delayed images is highly suggestive of biliary atresia or other extrahepatic occlusion
  - Visualization of the gallbladder is not helpful sign; it is seen in 25%
  - Excretion into the intestines effectively excludes biliary atresia
  - Hepatobiliary scans have high sensitivity ~100%, but specificity of 87% and accuracy of 91%

Other Modality Findings
- ERCP is invasive, requires general anesthesia, uses ionizing radiation, and has significant morbidity (1-7%) and failure rates (3-14%)
- Analysis of duodenal drainage is difficult to perform, is not yet standardized, and has sensitivity ~97% and specificity ~93%

Imaging Recommendations
- Best imaging tool
  - Typically, sonography is performed first to search for other causes of jaundice
  - If a gallbladder is seen, some surgeons will proceed directly to intra-operative cholangiogram and definitive surgery if patent ducts are not demonstrated
  - Hepatobiliary scintigraphy requires 5 days pretreatment with phenobarbital for optimal accuracy
  - DDx: Neonatal hepatitis, choledochal malformation, Alagille's, bile plug, stone disease

DIFFERENTIAL DIAGNOSIS

Neonatal hepatitis
- Very common entity, usually self-limited medical disease, though it can also be caused by Hep A, Hep B, cytomegalovirus, rubella, toxoplasmosis, alpha1-antitrypsin deficiency, familial recurrent cholestasis, or other metabolic disorders

Bile-plug syndrome
- Due to cystic fibrosis, dehydration, sepsis, hemolytic disorders, or total parenteral nutrition (TPN)

Biliary hypoplasia or Alagille syndrome
- Paucity of intrahepatic ducts, arteriohepatic dysplasia

Choledochal malformation
- Five subtypes of localized dilation of the extrahepatic biliary tree

PATHOLOGY

General Features
- General path comments

BILIARY ATRESIA

- o Hypoplastic, atretic, or fibrosed extrahepatic ducts which worsen in the perinatal period
- o Approximately 12% have patent proximal ducts and can have simple re-anastomosis surgery, 88% require Kasai procedure to anastomose a loop of small bowel to the dissected porta hepatis
- Genetics: Recessive inheritance when associated with polysplenia syndrome
- Etiology
  - o Congenital biliary atresia is suspected to originate from prenatal biliary duct inflammation of unknown etiology
  - o A proposed mechanism in the pathogenesis of biliary atresia involves an initial virus-induced, progressive T cell-mediated inflammatory obliteration of bile ducts
- Associated abnormalities: Associated with pre-duodenal portal vein, interrupted IVC, congenital heart disease, and polysplenia

Gross Pathologic & Surgical Features
- Absent extrahepatic ducts, cirrhosis if diagnosis is delayed

Microscopic Features
- Absent extrahepatic bile ducts, absence of multinucleated giant cells within the liver, periportal fibrosis, proliferation of small intrahepatic ducts
- Feathery degeneration of hepatocytes, dilated bile canaliculi with retained bile, and Kupffer cell phagocytosis of bile that has leaked into the sinusoidal space, are all nonspecific findings in many types of cholestasis

Staging, Grading or Classification Criteria
- Type I: Common bile duct atresia
- Type II: Common hepatic duct atresia
- Type III: Right & left hepatic duct atresia

CLINICAL ISSUES

Presentation
- Most common signs/symptoms: Progressive conjugated (direct) hyperbilirubinemia in the neonatal period
- Other signs/symptoms
  - o Bilirubin is conjugated in biliary atresia versus unconjugated in sepsis, hepatitis, and metabolic hepatocellular diseases
  - o 10-25% of patients with biliary atresia have co-existing congenital anomalies most commonly involving the heart, abdomen and genitourinary tract

Demographics
- Age: Jaundice becomes evident in the immediate perinatal period
- Gender: No gender or racial predilection

Natural History & Prognosis
- Prompt diagnosis is crucial to surgical success
- Kasai portoenterostomy is 90% effective if performed before 2 months of age, drops to less than 50% effective if performed after 3 months of age
- 4 year survival rate in neonates undergoing Kasai portoenterostomy is ~40%
- Most patients require liver transplantation as teenagers or young adults
- Less than 18% of patients with biliary atresia who have prompt Kasai procedures avoid liver transplantation 20 or more years later

Treatment
- Surgical: Kasai portoenterostomy
- Intestinal loop is anastomosed to dissected surface of porta hepatis

SELECTED REFERENCES

1. Davenport M et al: The outcome of the older (> or =100 days) infant with biliary atresia. J Pediatr Surg. 39(4):575-81, 2004
2. Kahn E: Biliary atresia revisited. Pediatr Dev Pathol. 7(2):109-24, 2004
3. Metreweli C et al: Magnetic resonance cholangiography in children. Br J Radiol. 77(924):1059-64, 2004
4. Poddar U et al: Ursodeoxycholic acid-augmented hepatobiliary scintigraphy in the evaluation of neonatal jaundice. J Nucl Med. 45(9):1488-92, 2004
5. Weerasooriya VS et al: Hepatic fibrosis and survival in biliary atresia. J Pediatr. 144(1):123-5, 2004
6. Aktas S et al: Quantitative analysis of ductus proliferation, proliferative activity, Kupffer cell proliferation and angiogenesis in differential diagnosis of biliary atresia and neonatal hepatitis. Hepatogastroenterology. 50(54):1811-3, 2003
7. Kanegawa K et al: Sonographic diagnosis of biliary atresia in pediatric patients using the "triangular cord" sign versus gallbladder length and contraction. AJR Am J Roentgenol. 181(5):1387-90, 2003
8. Lee HJ et al: Objective criteria of triangular cord sign in biliary atresia on US scans. Radiology. 229(2):395-400, 2003
9. Wildhaber BE et al: The Kasai portoenterostomy for biliary atresia: A review of a 27-year experience with 81 patients. J Pediatr Surg. 38(10):1480-5, 2003
10. Vanderdood K et al: Biliary atresia and cerebellar hypoplasia in polysplenia syndrome. Pediatr Radiol. 33(9):652-4, 2003
11. Benya EC: Pancreas and biliary system: imaging of developmental anomalies and diseases unique to children. Radiol Clin North Am. 40(6):1355-62, 2002
12. Norton KI et al: MR cholangiography in the evaluation of neonatal cholestasis: initial results. Radiology. 222(3):687-91, 2002
13. Bezerra JA et al: Cholestatic syndromes of infancy and childhood. Semin Gastrointest Dis. 12(2):54-65, 2001
14. Larrosa-Haro A et al: Duodenal tube test in the diagnosis of biliary atresia. J Pediatr Gastroenterol Nutr. 32(3):311-5, 2001
15. Iinuma Y et al: The role of endoscopic retrograde cholangiopancreatography in infants with cholestasis. J Pediatr Surg. 35(4):545-9, 2000
16. Tan Kendrick AP et al: Making the diagnosis of biliary atresia using the triangular cord sign and gallbladder length. Pediatr Radiol. 30(2):69-73, 2000
17. O'Hara SM: Pediatric gastrointestinal nuclear imaging. Radiol Clin North Am. 34(4):845-62, 1996
18. Kasai M et al: Technique and results of operative management of biliary atresia. World J Surg. 2:571-9, 1978

BILIARY ATRESIA

IMAGE GALLERY

Typical

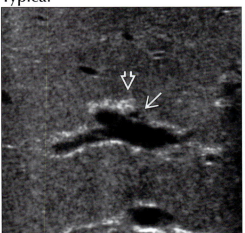
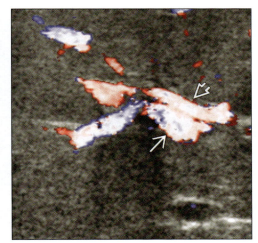

(Left) Axial ultrasound shows echogenic area (open arrow) adjacent to main hepatic artery (arrow) and portal vein which is felt to represent the obliterated common duct: Triangular cord sign. *(Right)* Axial color Doppler ultrasound shows absence of common bile duct adjacent to the main portal vein (arrow) and main hepatic artery (open arrow).

Typical

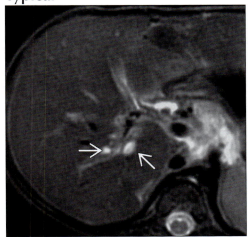
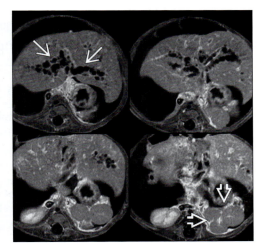

(Left) Axial T2WI MR shows hyperintense masses (arrows) surrounding the right portal vein branch, "biliary cyst" a known entity occurring in biliary atresia patients with cholangitis. *(Right)* Axial T1WI MR post-gadolinium shows beaded appearance of dilated bile ducts (arrows) s/p Kasai for biliary atresia - chronic cholangitis. Note polysplenia (open arrows).

Typical

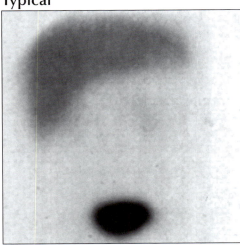
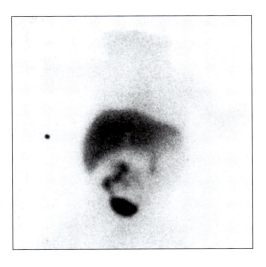

(Left) 24 hour delayed hepatobiliary scan shows retention in liver, but no biliary tree or intestinal activity. Excretion is solely via the urinary tract. *(Right)* Following Kasai procedure radioisotope enters the roux loop promptly. This scan was performed to assess adequacy of biliary drainage.

CHOLEDOCHAL CYST

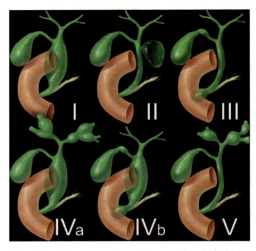

Graphic shows various types of choledochal malformation. Note the anomalous pancreaticobiliary junction; pancreatic duct inserts into the common bile duct proximal to the sphincter of Oddi.

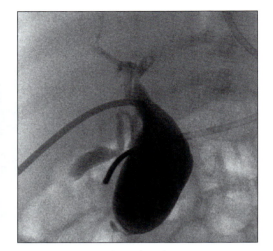

Anteroposterior radiograph during percutaneous cholangiogram shows fusiform dilation of the common bile duct with rapid change in caliber at the sphincter of Oddi, confirming a type I choledochal cyst.

TERMINOLOGY

Abbreviations and Synonyms
- Choledochal malformations, common bile duct cyst or diverticulum, choledochocele

Definitions
- Choledochal cysts are a spectrum of malformations of the extrahepatic and intrahepatic bile ducts
- One in 100,000-150,000 live births in US versus 1 in 1,000 live births in Japan
- Cholangiocarcinoma is a worrisome long-term complication

IMAGING FINDINGS

General Features
- Best diagnostic clue: Dilation of biliary tree
- Location: May involve intrahepatic bile ducts, extrahepatic ducts, or both
- Morphology: Refer to Todani classification of 5 types discussed in pathology section

CT Findings
- Helpful to define relationship of dilated ducts to portal vein, duodenum, and pancreas
- CT cholangiogram has been replaced by MR cholangiogram in pediatric patients

MR Findings
- T2 weighted images very useful in demonstrating fluid filled ducts and the common channel of pancreatic and biliary drainage when this malformation is present
- MR cholangiogram (MRCP) has virtually replaced percutaneous cholangiogram in preoperative planning

Ultrasonographic Findings
- Grayscale Ultrasound
  o Best first test to demonstrate dilated biliary tree and extent of ductal involvement
  o Pitfalls related to cholelithiasis or intestinal gas obscuring anatomic detail
  o Bile duct measuring > 10 mm nearly always related to a choledochal malformation in childhood
- Color Doppler: Useful demonstrating position and displacement of adjacent vessels

Other Modality Findings
- Endoscopic retrograde cholangiopancreatography (ERCP) and percutaneous cholangiogram usually reserved for difficult or complex cases

Imaging Recommendations
- Best imaging tool

DDx: Biliary Ductal Dilation

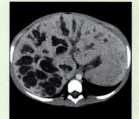
Caroli Disease

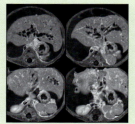
Chronic Cholangitis

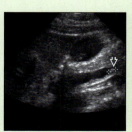
Obstructing Stone

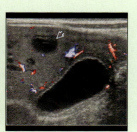
Liver Abscess

CHOLEDOCHAL CYST

Key Facts

Terminology
- Choledochal malformations, common bile duct cyst or diverticulum, choledochocele
- Choledochal cysts are a spectrum of malformations of the extrahepatic and intrahepatic bile ducts

Imaging Findings
- Ultrasound is best initial screening test
- Other cross sectional imaging (CT, MRI) for additional anatomic detail

Top Differential Diagnoses
- Chronic cholangitis
- Obstructing cholelithiasis
- Pancreatic pseudocyst
- Hydatid cyst

Pathology
- Type I cysts are characterized by segmental or diffuse fusiform dilatation of the common bile duct; they are the most common variety, accounting for 75-95% of cases
- Type II cysts represent a diverticulum of the duct, usually protruding from the lateral wall
- Type III cysts represent a choledochocele that most often occurs within the duodenal wall and protrudes as mass into duodenal lumen
- Type IV designates the presence of multiple extrahepatic bile duct cysts; this can be seen alone (type IV B) or in association with Caroli-type intrahepatic biliary cysts (type IV A)
- Type V is cystic dilatation of the intrahepatic bile ducts equivalent to Caroli disease

---

  ○ Ultrasound is best initial screening test
  ○ Other cross sectional imaging (CT, MRI) for additional anatomic detail
  ○ Hepatobiliary scans for functional evaluation

DIFFERENTIAL DIAGNOSIS

Chronic cholangitis
- Bile ducts thicken, dilate, and stenose due to chronic inflammation

Obstructing cholelithiasis
- Stone disease may cause obstruction at several levels

Pancreatic pseudocyst
- Fluid filled pseudocyst mimics dilated distal end of biliary tree

Hydatid cyst
- An important consideration in areas of endemic Echinococcal disease

Caroli disease
- Congenital nonobstructive dilatation of the large intrahepatic bile ducts
- Localized saccular ectasia, producing multiple cyst-like structures of varying size; these ducts are in continuity with the remainder of the biliary tract, and as a result, are predisposed to bile stasis, bacterial cholangitis, intrahepatic pigment stone formation, and cholangiocarcinoma

PATHOLOGY

General Features
- Genetics: Caroli disease/syndrome is often associated with autosomal recessive polycystic kidney disease (ARPKD) and is rarely associated with autosomal dominant polycystic kidney disease (ADPKD)
- Etiology
  ○ Most prevalent of the current theories involves the anomalous junction of the common biliary and pancreatic ducts which provides conduit for mixing of pancreatic juices and bile
  ○ Several studies have documented the activation of pancreatic enzymes within the common bile duct of patients with an anomalous junction
  ○ Animal studies have documented dilatation and structural weakness of the common bile duct and destruction of the elastic fibers of the duct when pancreatic secretions were allowed to reflux
  ○ Proof of anomalous junction causing biliary cysts is not definitive; the two may be only associated findings
  ○ Additional theories in the pathogenesis of bile duct cysts: Decrease in the number of ganglion cells in the narrow portion of the bile duct causing increased intraluminal pressure, reovirus infection, familial pattern of inheritance, failure of recanalization, and duodenal duplication
- Epidemiology
  ○ More common in the far East (orient) than in Western countries
  ○ Approximately 1/3 of all reported cases occur in Japanese patients

Gross Pathologic & Surgical Features
- Range in diameter from a few centimeters to over 15 cm
- Cyst wall is thickened, fibrotic, and occasionally calcified in adults

Microscopic Features
- Histologically: Varying degrees of chronic inflammation and scattered elastic and smooth muscle fibers
- Biliary epithelium lining the cyst is often intact in infants
- Goblet-cell metaplasia and epithelial dysplasia with nuclear hyperchromasia, irregularity, and loss of polarity have been described and may play a role in subsequent development of carcinoma

CHOLEDOCHAL CYST

- Type III cysts (choledochoceles) are usually lined by duodenal mucosa, but occasionally may have biliary epithelium

Staging, Grading or Classification Criteria
- Classification modified by Todani in 1977
- Type I cysts are characterized by segmental or diffuse fusiform dilatation of the common bile duct; they are the most common variety, accounting for 75-95% of cases
- Type II cysts represent a diverticulum of the duct, usually protruding from the lateral wall
- Type III cysts represent a choledochocele that most often occurs within the duodenal wall and protrudes as mass into duodenal lumen
- Type IV designates the presence of multiple extrahepatic bile duct cysts; this can be seen alone (type IV B) or in association with Caroli-type intrahepatic biliary cysts (type IV A)
- Type V is cystic dilatation of the intrahepatic bile ducts equivalent to Caroli disease
- Caroli syndrome (large and small bile duct ectasia with congenital hepatic fibrosis) is much more common than Caroli disease (large bile duct ectasia only)

CLINICAL ISSUES

Presentation
- Most common signs/symptoms
  - Prolonged neonatal cholestasis, so-called infantile obstructive cholangiopathy
  - Jaundice, acholic stools, hepatomegaly, and a palpable abdominal mass are frequent in infants
  - In adults, symptoms include upper abdominal pain, jaundice, cholangitis, and cirrhosis
- Other signs/symptoms: Adult patients tend to present with recurrent cholangitis, pancreatitis, or rarely portal hypertension

Demographics
- Age: 2/3 of all choledochal malformations are diagnosed before 10 years of age
- Gender: More common in females; 3 or 4:1 ratio

Natural History & Prognosis
- Low-grade biliary obstruction may develop and can potentially result in cirrhosis and portal hypertension
- Prevalence of cancer, usually adenocarcinoma, arising in choledochal cysts varies from 2-18%, corresponding to roughly 5-35x increased risk
- Both Caroli disease and Caroli syndrome are associated with risk of cholangiocarcinoma at a rate of 100x that of the general population
- Complications: Bile duct perforation, biliary stone formation, bacterial cholangitis with subsequent hepatic abscess and sepsis, or the development of bile duct carcinomas

Treatment
- Complete surgical excision of type I cysts followed by biliary drainage procedure, typically Roux-en-Y choledochojejunostomy
- Type II choledochal cysts can usually be excised entirely, and the defect in the common bile duct can be closed primarily over a T-tube: This approach can be used because, typically, type II choledochal cysts are lateral diverticula of the bile duct
- Type III cysts, choledochoceles with a diameter < 3 cm may be approached endoscopically with sphincterotomy: Those > 3 cm often associated with some degree of duodenal obstruction, are excised surgically by using a transduodenal approach
- For type IV choledochal cysts, the dilatated extrahepatic duct is completely excised, and a biliary-enteric drainage procedure is performed: No surgery is specifically directed at the intrahepatic ductal disease
- Type V choledochal cyst, or Caroli disease, when limited to a single hepatic lobe, usually the left, may be resected: In diffuse disease when liver failure develops liver transplantation is necessary
- Internal and external drainage, without cyst excision, led to an unacceptably high rate of cholangitis and did not alter the malignant potential of the cyst

SELECTED REFERENCES

1. Chen CP et al: Prenatal diagnosis of choledochal cyst using ultrasound and magnetic resonance imaging. Ultrasound Obstet Gynecol. 23(1):93-4, 2004
2. Hamada Y et al: Magnetic resonance cholangiopancreatography on postoperative work-up in children with choledochal cysts. Pediatr Surg Int. 20(1):43-6, 2004
3. Jordan PH Jr et al: Some considerations for management of choledochal cysts. Am J Surg. 187(3):434-9, 2004
4. Sood A et al: Spontaneous rupture of a choledochal cyst and the role of hepatobiliary scintigraphy. Clin Nucl Med. 29(6):392-3, 2004
5. Varadarajulu S et al: Technical outcomes and complications of ERCP in children. Gastrointest Endosc. 60(3):367-71, 2004
6. Haliloglu M et al: Choledochal cysts in children: evaluation with three-dimensional sonography. J Clin Ultrasound. 31(9):478-80, 2003
7. Sugiyama M et al: Anomalous pancreaticobiliary junction shown on multidetector CT. AJR Am J Roentgenol. 180(1):173-5, 2003
8. Benya EC: Pancreas and biliary system: imaging of developmental anomalies and diseases unique to children. Radiol Clin North Am. 40(6):1355-62, 2002
9. Casaccia G et al: Cystic anomalies of biliary tree in the fetus: is it possible to make a more specific prenatal diagnosis? J Pediatr Surg. 37(8):1191-4, 2002
10. de Vries JS et al: Choledochal cysts: age of presentation, symptoms, and late complications related to Todani's classification. J Pediatr Surg. 37(11):1568-73, 2002
11. Guy F et al: Caroli's disease: magnetic resonance imaging features. Eur Radiol. 12(11):2730-6, 2002
12. Levy AD et al: Caroli's disease: radiologic spectrum with pathologic correlation. AJR Am J Roentgenol. 179(4):1053-7, 2002
13. Krause D et al: MRI for evaluating congenital bile duct abnormalities. J Comput Assist Tomogr. 26(4):541-52, 2002
14. Todani T et al: Congenital bile duct cysts: Classification, operative procedures, and review of thirty-seven cases including cancer arising from choledochal cyst. Am J Surg. 134(2): 263-9, 1977

CHOLEDOCHAL CYST

IMAGE GALLERY

Typical

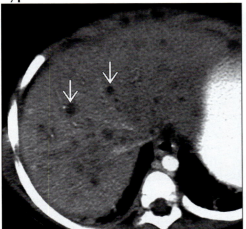
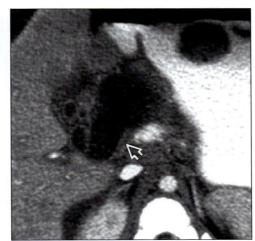

(Left) Axial CECT shows intrahepatic biliary ductal dilation (arrows), low density structures paired with enhancing vessels. *(Right)* Axial CECT shows fusiform dilation of the common bile duct (arrow) at the level of the porta hepatis.

Typical

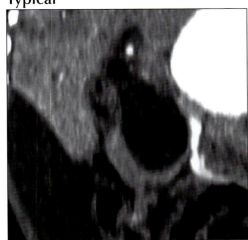
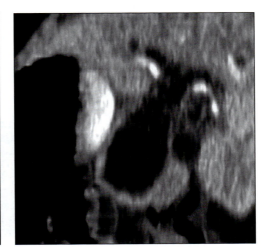

(Left) Coronal CECT reconstructed images show intrahepatic biliary ductal dilation as well as fusiform dilation of the common bile duct. *(Right)* Sagittal CECT reconstructed image shows intrahepatic biliary ductal dilation as well as fusiform dilation of the common bile duct in this type I choledochal cyst.

Variant

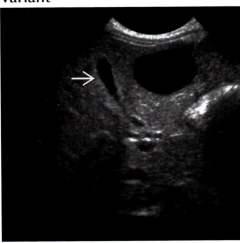
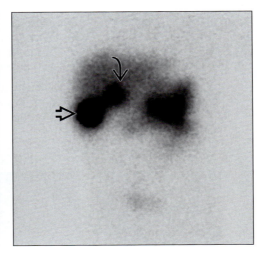

(Left) Transverse ultrasound shows a round cyst medial to the gallbladder (arrow) surrounded by hepatic tissue. There was no color flow in the lesion in this infant being evaluated for antenatally diagnosed liver cyst. *(Right)* Anteroposterior hepatobiliary scan shows radiotracer accumulation medial to the gallbladder (open arrow) in this congenital bile lake (curved arrow), a variant of intrahepatic choledochal cyst.

CAROLI DISEASE

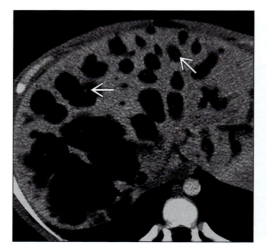

Axial CECT shows "central dot" sign (arrows) of enhancing portal vein radicle surrounded by the massively dilated intrahepatic bile ducts.

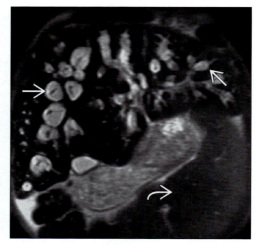

Coronal T2WI MR (SSFSE) shows hyperintense saccular dilation of the intrahepatic biliary tree (arrows) & splenomegaly (curved arrow), in this patient with Caroli syndrome. (Hepatic fibrosis + Caroli disease).

TERMINOLOGY

Abbreviations and Synonyms
- Communicating cavernous ectasia of intrahepatic ducts, type V choledochal cyst (Todani)

Definitions
- Congenital, multifocal, segmental, saccular nonobstructive dilatation of intrahepatic bile ducts (IHBD)
- Caroli syndrome = Caroli disease + congenital hepatic fibrosis

IMAGING FINDINGS

General Features
- Best diagnostic clue
  - "Central dot" sign
    - CECT: Strong enhancing, tiny dots (portal radicles completely surrounded by dilated bile ducts) within dilated IHBDs
  - Classic imaging appearance
    - Cholangiography: Bulbous dilatations of peripheral IHBD
- Location: Segmental, diffuse, or lobar
- Size: Extrahepatic ducts dilated in 1/2, IHBD; mms up to several cms
- One type of fibropolycystic disease (spectrum of variable fibrosis & cysts in liver & kidneys)
  - Autosomal dominant polycystic liver disease
  - Choledochal cyst
  - Congenital hepatic fibrosis
  - Caroli disease
    - Cystic dilation of intrahepatic ducts +/- common bile duct (CBD)
  - Biliary hamartoma (von Meyenburg complex)
- Todani classification of choledochal cysts
  - Type I: Cystic dilation of the CBD
  - Type II: Diverticulum of the CBD
  - Type III: Choledochocele: Intraduodenal diverticulum
  - Type IV: Cystic, fusiform, or saccular dilation of CBD, +/- IHBD
  - Type V: Caroli (others no renal association & not hereditary)
- 2 Types of Caroli disease both autosomal recessive
  - Simple type: Bile duct ectasia
  - Complex (periportal fibrosis) type: Hepatic fibrosis &/or portal hypertension
  - Both types are frequently associated with renal tubular ectasia

CT Findings
- NECT: Multiple, rounded, hypodense areas inseparable from dilated IHBD

DDx: Hepatic Cysts Or Cyst-Like Dilation Of IHBDs

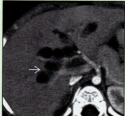
Choledochal Cyst

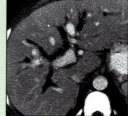
PSC

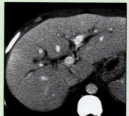
Cholangitis

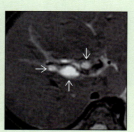
Biliary Cysts

CAROLI DISEASE

Key Facts

Terminology
- Communicating cavernous ectasia of intrahepatic ducts, type V choledochal cyst (Todani)
- Congenital, multifocal, segmental, saccular nonobstructive dilatation of intrahepatic bile ducts (IHBD)

Imaging Findings
- "Central dot" sign
- CECT: Strong enhancing, tiny dots (portal radicles completely surrounded by dilated bile ducts) within dilated IHBDs
- Consider abscess if cyst higher attenuation than other IHBD

Top Differential Diagnoses
- Polycystic liver disease (ADPCKD)
- Choledochal cyst
- Primary sclerosing cholangitis (PSC)
- Ascending cholangitis and/or hepatic abscess
- Recurrent pyogenic cholangitis (RPG)
- Biliary hamartoma
- "Biliary cysts"

Clinical Issues
- Most common signs/symptoms: Intermittent abdominal pain, right upper quadrant (RUQ)
- Cholangiocarcinoma in 7% of patient (100x increased risk)

Diagnostic Checklist
- Other disease with multiple liver cysts +/- IHBD dilation

- CECT
  - Enhancing tiny dot (portal radicle) within dilated IHBD
  - Consider abscess if cyst higher attenuation than other IHBD
  - Splenomegaly in patients with hepatic fibrosis

MR Findings
- T1WI: Multiple, small, hypointense, saccular dilatations of IHBDs
- T2WI: Hyperintense
- T1 C+: Central dot of enhancement (portal radicle) surrounded by dilated biliary tree
- Coronal half-Fourier rapid acquisition with relaxation enhancement (RARE)
  - Kidney: Multiple fluid-containing foci in papillae
  - Medullary sponge kidney or renal tubular ectasia
- MR Cholangiopancreatography (MRCP) findings
  - Multiple hyperintense oval-shaped structures
  - Continuity with IHBDs
  - Luminal contents of bile ducts appear hyperintense in contrast to portal vein, which appears as signal void

Ultrasonographic Findings
- Grayscale Ultrasound
  - Intraductal sludge or calculi
  - "Intraluminal portal vein sign"
    - Portal vein radicles surrounded by IHBDs, best seen on color Doppler imaging
  - Intraductal bridging septa: Echogenic septa completely or incompletely transversing dilated IHBDs
    - Similar finding on cholangiography
  - +/- Dilated gallbladder (GB) or CBD
  - Abscess (less common)

Other Modality Findings
- Percutaneous (PTC) or endoscopic retrograde cholangiopancreatogram (ERCP) findings
  - Segmental saccular, beaded dilatations of IHBDs, stones, strictures
  - Bridge formation across dilated IHBDs
  - Communicating hepatic abscesses

Imaging Recommendations
- Best imaging tool: ERCP or PTC (diagnostic), complication rate: 3% or MRCP
- Protocol advice: NECT + CECT, 3-dimensional MRCP, PTC & ERCP

DIFFERENTIAL DIAGNOSIS

Polycystic liver disease (ADPCKD)
- Hepatic cysts, no communication with biliary tract nor biliary dilation
- Multiple cysts (>10 & many cases innumerable)
- Patients with this disease often harbor renal cysts, not confined to medulla

Choledochal cyst
- Extrahepatic (90%)
- Type IV: Cystic dilation of CBD +/- intrahepatic ducts (Type IVa)
- Not inherited & no renal disease

Primary sclerosing cholangitis (PSC)
- History of ulcerative colitis
- Dilatation of both IHBD & extrahepatic bile ducts
- Ductal dilatation is not as great as Caroli disease & not saccular type
- PSC often shows isolated obstructions of IHBDs; Caroli disease does not

Ascending cholangitis and/or hepatic abscess
- Intrahepatic abscesses communicate with bile ducts
  - Mimics Caroli disease
- However, margins of abscesses are irregular
- Extrahepatic bile duct dilatation noted due to an obstructing stone or tumor

Recurrent pyogenic cholangitis (RPG)
- Dilatation of both intra- & extrahepatic bile ducts & is not of saccular type

CAROLI DISEASE

- Sludge, calculi, pneumobilia & abscesses

Biliary hamartoma
- Variant of fibropolycystic disease
- Cyst-like hepatic nodules (typically < 1.5 cm)
- No communication to biliary tree
- Cystic → solid

"Biliary cysts"
- ↑ Biliary atresia (18%), history of cholangitis

PATHOLOGY

General Features
- General path comments
  - Embryology-Anatomy
    - Incomplete remodeling of ductal plate → persistence of embryonic biliary ductal structures, known as ductal plate malformation
    - If affected larger bile ducts: Caroli disease
    - If affected smaller bile ducts: Congenital hepatic fibrosis
    - Both affected: Caroli syndrome
- Genetics: Inherited as an autosomal recessive pattern
- Etiology
  - Potential etiologies: Perinatal hepatic arterial occlusion or hypo/aplasia of fibromuscular wall components
  - Simple type: Malformation of ductal plate of large central IHBDs
  - Periportal fibrosis type: Malformation of ductal plates of central IHBDs + smaller peripheral bile ducts
    - Latter leading to development of fibrosis
- Epidemiology: Rare
- Associated abnormalities: Hepatic fibrosis, medullary sponge kidney (80%), ADPCKD

Gross Pathologic & Surgical Features
- Dilated, ectatic IHBDs

Microscopic Features
- Simple type
  - Dilation or segmental IHBDs with normal hepatic parenchyma
- Complex (periportal fibrosis) type
  - Segmental dilation of IHBDs with proliferation of bile ductules & fibrosis

CLINICAL ISSUES

Presentation
- Most common signs/symptoms: Intermittent abdominal pain, right upper quadrant (RUQ)
- Other signs/symptoms
  - Simple type
    - RUQ pain, recurrent attacks of cholangitis, fever & jaundice
  - Complex (periportal fibrosis) type:
    - Pain, hepatosplenomegaly, hematemesis (varices)
- Complications
  - Simple type
    - Stone formation (95%), recurrent cholangitis & hepatic abscess
  - Complex (periportal fibrosis) type
    - Cirrhosis → portal hypertension → varices → hemorrhage
  - Cholangiocarcinoma in 7% of patient (100x increased risk)

Demographics
- Age: Children & 2nd-3rd decade, occasionally infancy
- Gender: M = F

Natural History & Prognosis
- Long term prognosis for Caroli disease is poor, especially after cholangitis

Treatment
- Conservative: Ursodeoxycholic acid (↓ cholelithiasis) & broad-spectrum antibiotics for cholangitis
- Localized to lobe/segment: Hepatic lobectomy or segmentectomy
- Decompression of biliary tract: External drainage & biliary-enteric anastomoses are effective
- Extracorporeal shock wave lithotripsy
- Liver transplantation (usually from refractory cholangitis)

DIAGNOSTIC CHECKLIST

Consider
- Other disease with multiple liver cysts +/- IHBD dilation

Image Interpretation Pearls
- ERCP: Saccular or fusiform dilation or ectasia of IHBDs nonobstructive communication with the biliary tree
- "Central dot" sign: Portal radicle surrounded by dilated bile ducts

SELECTED REFERENCES

1. Levy AD et al: Caroli's disease: radiologic spectrum with pathologic correlation. AJR Am J Roentgenol. 179(4):1053-7, 2002
2. Asselah T et al: Caroli's disease: a magnetic resonance cholangiopancreatography diagnosis. Am J Gastroenterol. 93(1):109-10, 1998
3. Betz BW et al: MR imaging of biliary cysts in children with biliary atresia: clinical associations and pathologic correlation. AJR Am J Roentgenol. 162(1):167-71, 1994
4. Ros E et al: Ursodeoxycholic acid treatment of primary hepatolithiasis in Caroli's syndrome. Lancet. 342(8868):404-6, 1993
5. Toma P et al: Sonographic patterns of Caroli's disease: report of 5 new cases. J Clin Ultrasound. 19(3):155-61, 1991
6. Choi BI et al: Caroli disease: Central dot sign in CT. Radiology. 174:161-3, 1990
7. Summerfield JA et al: Hepatobiliary fibropolycystic diseases. A clinical and histological review of 51 patients. J Hepatol. 2(2):141-56, 1986
8. Mittelstaedt CA et al: Caroli's disease: sonographic findings. AJR Am J Roentgenol. 134(3):585-7, 1980

CAROLI DISEASE

IMAGE GALLERY

Typical

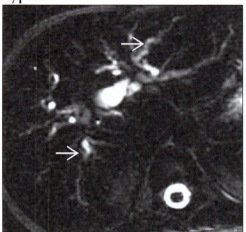
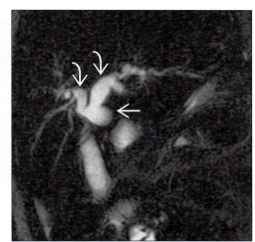

(Left) Axial MRCP shows beaded, dilated intrahepatic biliary tree (arrows) in this patient with Caroli disease. *(Right)* Coronal MRCP in the same patient shows dilated extrahepatic biliary tree, common bile duct (arrow) right & left hepatic ducts (curved arrows).

Typical

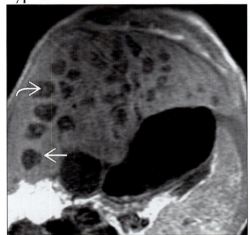
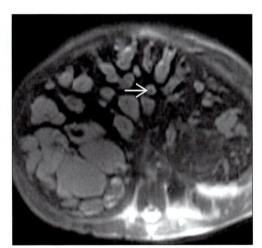

(Left) Coronal T1WI MR shows multiple hypointense cystic dilated intrahepatic biliary tree (arrow) surrounding isointense "central dot", portal vein radicle (curved arrow). *(Right)* Axial T2WI MR (SSFSE) shows hypointense portal vein radicle in a dilated bile duct (arrow). Diffuse intrahepatic biliary dilation is seen throughout the liver in this patient.

Typical

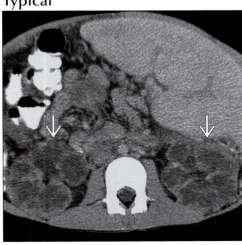
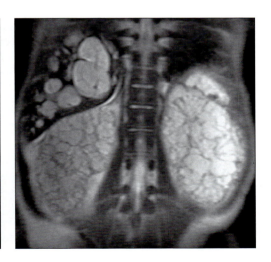

(Left) Axial CECT shows bilateral cystic kidneys (arrows) with splenomegaly in this patient with Caroli syndrome. *(Right)* Coronal CECT (SSFSE) shows Caroli disease in the liver with markedly enlarged cystic kidneys.

LIVER TRANSPLANT COMPLICATIONS

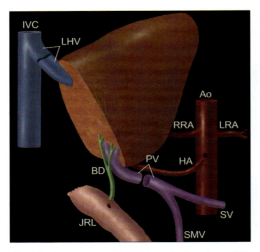

Graphic shows segmental liver transplant anatomy. BD, jejunal Roux loop (JRL), PV, superior mesenteric vein (SMV), splenic vein (SV), HA, Ao, right and left renal arteries (RRA & LRA), IVC, LHV.

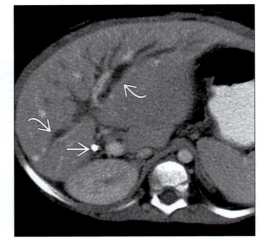

Axial CECT shows diffuse intrahepatic biliary dilatation (curved arrows) in segmental liver transplant in child with symptoms of cholangitis. Note internal biliary stent (arrow).

TERMINOLOGY

Abbreviations and Synonyms
- Segmental liver transplant = partial liver transplant, split liver transplant, reduced-size liver transplant

Definitions
- Segmental liver transplant
  - In children, usually left lobe or lateral segment of the left lobe of the liver is transplanted
  - Developed to increase supply of liver transplants for children
  - Usually adult donor → cadaver or living
- Vascular complications
  - Hepatic arterial thrombosis (HAT) or stenosis
  - Hepatic artery (HA) pseudoaneurysm at infrarenal anastomosis with aorta (Ao)
  - Portal vein stenosis (PVS) and thrombosis
  - Hepatic vein stenosis (HVS)
  - Anastomotic bleeding
- Biliary complications
  - Anastomotic
    - Biliary stenosis (BS) or leak
  - Nonanastomotic
    - Intrahepatic biliary stenosis → dilatation
    - Biloma
    - Intraductal sludge or stone
- Extrahepatic fluid collection
  - Hematoma, seroma, bile leak, abscess
  - Usually found soon after surgery
- Posttransplant lymphoproliferative disease (PTLD)
- Infection
- Organ rejection

IMAGING FINDINGS

CT Findings
- CECT
  - Hepatic artery thrombosis (HAT) or stenosis
    - Peripheral wedge-shaped low attenuation regions
    - Unopacified hepatic artery
    - Sequelae: Biloma, intrahepatic biliary dilation due to biliary strictures
  - Hepatic artery pseudoaneurysm at anastomosis with infrarenal aorta
    - Abnormally dilated hepatic artery near anastomosis with aorta
  - Portal vein stenosis (PVS) and thrombosis
    - Stenosis: Focal narrowing, usually with poststenotic dilation
    - Thrombosis: Unopacified portal vein, portosystemic shunts, splenomegaly, ascites
  - Hepatic vein stenosis (HVS)
    - Distended hepatic veins
    - Congested liver with delayed enhancement

DDx: Treatment Of Complications

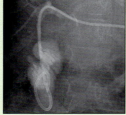
PBD

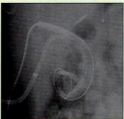
BS Balloon + PBD

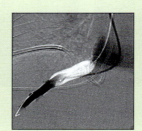
HVS Balloon

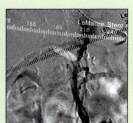
PVS Balloon

LIVER TRANSPLANT COMPLICATIONS

Key Facts

Terminology
- Segmental liver transplant
- In children, usually left lobe or lateral segment of the left lobe of the liver is transplanted
- Developed to increase supply of liver transplants for children

Pathology
- Hepatic artery thrombosis (HAT)
- Leading cause of graft loss and retransplantation (4-26%)
- PV thrombosis
- High risk in segmental liver transplant because of short pulmonary vein segment from donor
- HV stenosis occurs at anastomosis with IVC
- Anastomotic bleeding
- Biliary complications

- Most frequent liver transplantation complication
- Higher incidence in segmental liver transplants +/-
- PTLD: More common in children than adults due to higher rate of EBV(-) before transplantation
- Infection: Leading cause of death (43%)

Clinical Issues
- Vascular complication
- Balloon dilation +/- stent, or surgery
- Biliary complication
- Balloon dilation +/- placement of percutaneous biliary drain (PBD) or surgery
- Biloma
- Drain if infected
- PTLD
- Reduce immunosuppression +/- chemotherapy

- Biliary strictures
  - Dilated ducts caused by obstruction from strictures
- Extrahepatic fluid collection
  - Hematoma, bile, abscess, or seroma
  - Aspiration required for determination of contents
- PTLD
  - Wide range of appearances: Adenopathy or masses almost anywhere in body
- Infection
  - Wide range of appearances, from abnormal fluid collections, solid or visceral organ lesions, dilated bile ducts (BD) (cholangitis)
- Organ rejection
  - Nonspecific, biopsy required for diagnosis
- CTA: Similar findings to CECT, but better detail of vascular structures

MR Findings
- MRA
  - HAT: Signal loss beyond thrombus due to absent flow
  - Hepatic artery pseudoaneurysm: High signal focal enlargement of artery near anastomosis with aorta
- MRCP: Biliary dilatation: High signal dilated bile ducts

Ultrasonographic Findings
- Grayscale Ultrasound
  - HAT: No direct signs → Doppler
  - Hepatic artery pseudoaneurysm: Round anechoic structure near hepatic artery anastomosis with aorta
  - PV stenosis: Narrowing, usually at anastomosis, poststenotic dilation
  - PV thrombosis: Soft tissue filling defect in portal vein lumen
  - HV stenosis: Distended hepatic veins
  - Biliary complications: Biliary dilation
  - PTLD: Adenopathy, mass within or outside abdominal organs
- Color Doppler
  - HAT: No arterial flow or dampened systolic upstroke and high diastolic flow
  - Hepatic artery pseudoaneurysm: Color flow filling dilated hepatic artery lumen
  - PV stenosis: Focal narrowing
  - PV thrombosis: Absent flow in region of thrombus
  - HV stenosis: Dampened waveforms

Angiographic Findings
- DSA
  - Hepatic artery thrombosis: Cut off of hepatic artery
  - Hepatic artery stenosis: Focal narrowing of artery, commonly at anastomosis
  - Hepatic artery pseudoaneurysm: Focal dilation of hepatic artery, usually near aorta
  - HV stenosis: Narrowing at HV anastomosis with inferior vena cava (IVC)

Non-Vascular Interventions
- Transhepatic Cholangiography
  - Biliary strictures: Anastomotic or nonanastomotic → biliary dilation proximal to stricture
  - Biliary sludge/stones: Intraluminal filling defects → proximal biliary dilation

Imaging Recommendations
- Best imaging tool
  - Vasculature and biliary system
    - First line screening: Ultrasound with Doppler
    - HAT: Angiogram
    - PV stenosis/thrombosis: Percutaneous transhepatic portogram (PTP)
    - HV stenosis: Venogram
    - Biliary stenosis: Percutaneous transhepatic cholangiogram (PTC)
  - Biloma or fluid collection: CECT
  - PTLD or Infection: CECT
- Protocol advice
  - Ultrasound liver transplant with Doppler
  - CECT Abdomen: IV and oral contrast

LIVER TRANSPLANT COMPLICATIONS

PATHOLOGY

General Features
- Etiology
  - Biliary complications
    - Depends on surgical reconstruction technique, length of cold ischemia time, immunological reactions, hepatic arterial thrombosis (HAT), CMV infection, ABO blood group incompatibility
  - Anastomotic biliary strictures
    - Anastomotic leak, ABO incompatibility, HAT (results in ischemia to bile ducts)
  - Nonanastomotic biliary strictures
    - ABO incompatibility, HAT
  - PTLD
    - Epstein-Barr virus (EBV) related in 90%, usually EBV(-) transplant recipient who develops EBV infection after transplant
- Epidemiology
  - Hepatic artery thrombosis (HAT)
    - Leading cause of graft loss and retransplantation (4-26%)
    - Interposition grafts or anastomosis with recipient aorta may decrease HAT incidence with small arteries (< 3 mm), although controversial
    - Increased risk in pediatrics because of small size
    - Children do better than adults with HAT because of higher rate of recruitment of collateral arteries
  - PV thrombosis
    - High risk in segmental liver transplant because of short pulmonary vein segment from donor
    - Higher risk in patients with decreased PV flow because of splenectomy, portosystemic collaterals
    - Usually develops slowly after liver transplant → signs of portal venous hypertension (collateral veins, splenomegaly, ascites)
  - HV stenosis/thrombosis or IVC obstruction
    - HV stenosis occurs at anastomosis with IVC
    - Frequently due to twisting when transplant moves/dislocates
  - Anastomotic bleeding
    - Occurs early after transplant and usually requires surgical repair
  - Biliary complications
    - Most frequent liver transplantation complication
    - Higher incidence in segmental liver transplants +/-
    - May lead to chronic graft failure with secondary biliary cirrhosis
  - PTLD: More common in children than adults due to higher rate of EBV(-) before transplantation
    - 1-20% incidence
  - Infection: Leading cause of death (43%)

CLINICAL ISSUES

Presentation
- Most common signs/symptoms
  - Depends on complication
    - HAT: Elevated LFTs
    - PVS: GI bleeding from portosystemic collaterals, splenomegaly, ascites
    - Biliary strictures: Jaundice, cholangitis
    - PTLD: Nonspecific and variable, EBV seroconversion
    - Infection: Fever

Treatment
- Vascular complication
  - Hepatic artery stenosis
    - Balloon dilation +/- stent
    - Surgical repair if balloon resistant
  - Hepatic artery thrombosis
    - Thrombectomy if early
    - May require retransplantation
  - Portal vein stenosis
    - Percutaneous transhepatic portogram (PTP) → balloon dilation +/- stent
    - Surgical revision if necessary
  - Hepatic vein stenosis
    - Balloon dilation +/- stent, or surgery
- Biliary complication
  - Anastomotic biliary stricture
    - Balloon dilation +/- placement of percutaneous biliary drain (PBD) or surgery
    - Metal stent of questionable long term patency rate
  - Nonanastomotic biliary stricture
    - Percutaneous biliary drain placement and balloon dilation
  - Biliary obstruction
    - 20% have no biliary dilation that show obstruction with percutaneous transhepatic cholangiogram (PTC)
    - Thus, if patient jaundiced with ↑ liver function tests (LFTs) → PTC and possible percutaneous biliary drain (PBD)
  - Biloma
    - Drain if infected
  - Biliary leak
    - If large, requires surgical repair
    - If small, may heal with biliary drain
  - Biliary sludge/stones
    - Remove percutaneously
    - May place PBD
- PTLD
  - Reduce immunosuppression +/- chemotherapy
- Infection
  - Antibiotics, antifungals, +/- drainage

SELECTED REFERENCES

1. Unsinn KM et al: Spectrum of imaging findings after pediatric liver transplantation: part 1, posttransplantation anatomy. AJR Am J Roentgenol. 181(4):1133-8, 2003
2. Unsinn KM et al: Spectrum of imaging findings after pediatric liver transplantation: part 2, posttransplantation complications. AJR Am J Roentgenol. 181(4):1139-44, 2003
3. Buell JF et al: Long-term venous complications after full-size and segmental pediatric liver transplantation. Ann Surg. 236(5):658-66, 2002
4. Donnelly LF et al: Unique imaging issues in pediatric liver disease. Clin Liver Dis. 6(1):227-46, viii, 2002
5. Jain A et al: Pediatric Liver Transplantation. A Single Center Experience Spanning 20 Years. Transplantation. 73:941-7, 2002
6. Ametani F et al: Spectrum of CT findings in pediatric patients after partial liver transplantation. Radiographics. 21(1):53-63, 2001

LIVER TRANSPLANT COMPLICATIONS

IMAGE GALLERY

Typical

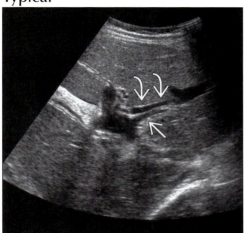
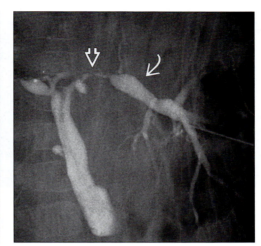

(Left) Axial ultrasound shows intrahepatic biliary dilatation (curved arrows) caused by bile duct sludge in child after liver transplant. The portal vein is deep to the bile duct (arrow). *(Right)* Anteroposterior radiograph during PTC shows long stricture of left central bile duct (open arrow) causing peripheral biliary dilatation (curved arrow). This was later treated with a PBD.

Typical

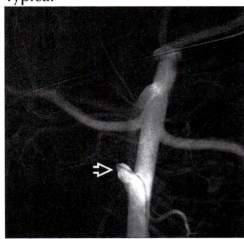
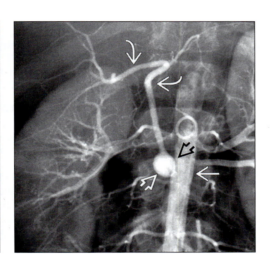

(Left) Oblique angiography shows complete occlusion of hepatic artery near anastomosis with infrarenal aorta (arrow). The patient also had dampened arterial waveforms in the liver by Doppler. *(Right)* Oblique angiography shows a focal pseudoaneurysm (open arrows) of the transplant hepatic artery (curved arrows) near the anastomosis with the infrarenal aorta (arrow).

Typical

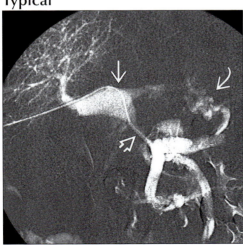
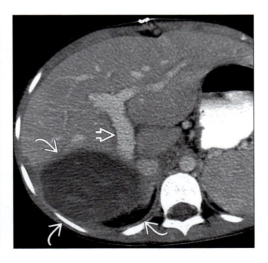

(Left) Oblique DSA shows a portal vein stenosis (open arrow) with post stenotic dilatation (arrow) during a PTP. Note filling of portosystemic collaterals (curved arrow). *(Right)* Axial CECT shows a bile leak from cut edge of liver in child after segmental liver transplant presenting as large ovoid low attenuation mass (curved arrows). Left portal vein (open arrow).

MESENTERIC ADENITIS

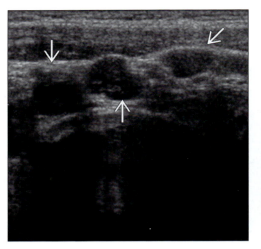

Transverse ultrasound shows numerous enlarged lymph nodes in right lower quadrant (arrows).

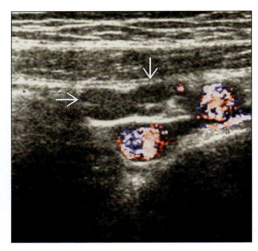

Axial color Doppler ultrasound shows enlarged hypovascular lymph nodes anterior to the right iliac vessel (anterior to the psoas muscle) (arrows).

TERMINOLOGY

Abbreviations and Synonyms
- Mesenteric lymphadenitis

Definitions
- Self-limiting benign inflammation of lymph nodes in the bowel mesentery
- Diagnosis of exclusion

IMAGING FINDINGS

General Features
- Best diagnostic clue
  - 3 or more clustered lymph nodes that measure ≥ 5 mm in short axis diameter
  - Normal appendix
- Location: Mesentery: Diffuse or focal right lower quadrant (RLQ)
- Size
  - ≥ 5 mm in size
  - Cluster of ≥ 3 enlarged lymph nodes
- Mimics appendicitis: Similar presenting signs & symptoms
- Most frequent alternative diagnosis at surgery for appendicitis

Radiographic Findings
- Radiography
  - Typically normal
  - May have focal bowel wall thickening &/or regional ileus RLQ

CT Findings
- Cluster of ≥ 3 lymph nodes in RLQ mesentery
  - ≥ 5 mm in short axis diameter
  - Most commonly anterior to right psoas muscle
  - 1/2 in small bowel mesentery
  - Appendicitis also associated with RLQ lymph nodal enlargement (40-82%)
    - Average: 9 mm
    - Average: 11 mm in mesenteric adenitis
    - More numerous lymph nodes throughout the mesentery in mesenteric adenitis
- Normal appendix
- Ileal wall thickening (up to 33%)
  - More common < 5 year olds
  - ≥ 3 mm over at least 5 cm
- Colonic wall thickening (up to 18%)
  - More common < 5 year olds

Ultrasonographic Findings
- Graded compression procedure of choice of ultrasound (US)
- May have RLQ pain with compression

DDx: Right Lower Quadrant Pain

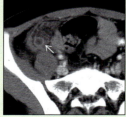
Appendicitis

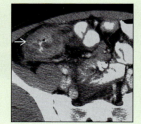
Crohn Disease

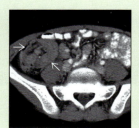
Intussusception

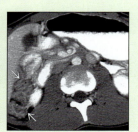
Salmonella

MESENTERIC ADENITIS

Key Facts

Terminology
- Self-limiting benign inflammation of lymph nodes in the bowel mesentery

Imaging Findings
- 3 or more clustered lymph nodes that measure ≥ 5 mm in short axis diameter
- Normal appendix
- ≥ 5 mm in size
- Cluster of ≥ 3 enlarged lymph nodes
- Mimics appendicitis: Similar presenting signs & symptoms
- Appendicitis also associated with RLQ lymph nodal enlargement (40-82%)
- More numerous lymph nodes throughout the mesentery in mesenteric adenitis
- Graded compression US
- Preferred due to radiation exposure of CECT

Top Differential Diagnoses
- Appendicitis
- Infectious enteritis
- Crohn disease
- Intussusception

Clinical Issues
- Most common signs/symptoms: Diffuse or focal RLQ tenderness & pain +/- rebound
- Children & young adults

Diagnostic Checklist
- When appendix is normal & a cluster of 3 or more enlarged RLQ lymph nodes

---

- Numerous RLQ or diffuse mesenteric enlarged lymph nodes (≥ 5 mm)
- Normal appendix (< 7 mm & compressible)
- +/- Ileal or ileocolonic wall thickening
- No abscess or phlegmon

Nuclear Medicine Findings
- Indium 111-labeled white blood cells (wbc) scan
  - Not often useful
  - Questionable utility in patients with a prolonged coarse of symptoms

Imaging Recommendations
- Best imaging tool
  - Graded compression US
    - Preferred due to radiation exposure of CECT
    - Normal appendix can be seen
    - Numerous enlarged lymph nodes in the RLQ or diffusely in the small bowel mesentery

DIFFERENTIAL DIAGNOSIS

Appendicitis
- Dilated appendix
  - ≥ 7 mm in diameter
  - Noncompressible on US
- Abscesses or phlegmon common
- Also causes ileal or colonic wall thickening
- Less numerous lymph nodes

Infectious enteritis
- Yersinia: Typically terminal ileum (TI)
- TB: Narrowed cecum & TI
- Others: Salmonella (colon), amebiasis, shigella (distal colon), CMV, herpes & fungal

Crohn disease
- Entire GI tract
  - From mouth to anus, segmental & skip lesions
- Transmural, eccentric, sinuses, fissures, fistulas
- Aphthoid ulcers (mucosa) to deep ulcers (submucosa)
  - Cobblestoning: Longitudinal & transverse ulcers
- US & CECT
  - Mural thickening of cecum & TI
  - Average: 11 mm

Intussusception
- Invagination of one segment of bowel into another
- Idiopathic (typical)
- 2 months → 3 years
  - Younger & older patient consider pathologic lead point
- Mostly ileocolic
- US: Pseudokidney sign
  - Hypoechoic layers with echogenic internal mesenteric fat
- "Coiled spring" sign: Bowel invaginating into bowel
- Also can follow upper respiratory infection (URI) or gastroenteritis
- May have blood in stool, "currant jelly" stool

Pseudomembranous colitis
- Usually related to antibiotic therapy & overgrowth of clostridium difficile bacteria
- Pancolitis (typical)
- CECT
  - "Accordion sign": Trapped enteric contrast between thickened large bowel folds
  - "Target sign": Intensely enhancing mucosa surrounded by diminished attenuation mural thickening

Ulcerative colitis
- Chronic, idiopathic inflammatory disease that primarily involves the colorectal mucosa & submucosa
- Diffuse, continuous, concentric & symmetric wall thickening of the colon
- "Collar button" ulcers
- "Leadpipe" colon
  - Shortened, rigid & symmetric narrowing of the lumen
- Backwash ileitis
  - Distal 5-25 cm of ileum is inflamed (10-40%)

Pelvic inflammatory disease
- Complex adnexal mass

MESENTERIC ADENITIS

- Sexually active girls
- Common bacteria
  - Neisseria gonorrhea
  - Chlamydia trachomatis
- Laboratory findings
  - Leukocytosis with a left shift
  - ↑ Erythrocyte sedimentation rate
- Cervical motion tenderness
- Lower abdominal &/or pelvic pain

Epiploic appendagitis
- Acute
  - Infarction: Torsion or venous thrombosis
  - Inflammation of the epiploic appendages
- Hyperdense ring surrounding an internal hypodense (fat) nodule
- Left > right
- Older age group
  - Typically 2nd decade or later
- Symptoms usually spontaneously resolve by 1 week

PATHOLOGY

General Features
- Etiology
  - Yersinia enterocolitica (most common)
    - Yersinia infections: Meat, milk & water contamination
  - Yersinia pseudotuberculosis, Helicobacter jejuni, Salmonella, Shigella, Campylobacter, Staphylococcal
  - Viral: Coxsackievirus & adenovirus
  - Following Streptococcal URI
- Epidemiology: Most frequent alternative diagnosis to appendicitis
- Associated abnormalities: Streptococcal URI (25%)

Microscopic Features
- Hyperplastic cortical & paracortical pulp with dilated sinuses
- ↑ Plasma cells & immunoblasts

CLINICAL ISSUES

Presentation
- Most common signs/symptoms: Diffuse or focal RLQ tenderness & pain +/- rebound
- Other signs/symptoms
  - Nausea
  - Vomiting
  - Diarrhea
  - Laboratory: Leukocytosis (50%)
  - During or following URI
    - Cervical adenopathy (20%)

Demographics
- Age
  - Children & young adults
  - Most common < 15 years old
  - Ileocolitis usually < 5 years old
- Gender: Yersinia more common in boys

Natural History & Prognosis
- Symptoms typically resolve by 2 weeks
- Diagnosis sometimes not made until after surgery

Treatment
- Conservative
- Self-limiting

DIAGNOSTIC CHECKLIST

Consider
- When appendix is normal & a cluster of 3 or more enlarged RLQ lymph nodes
- Diagnosis of exclusion

SELECTED REFERENCES

1. Lee CC et al: Mesenteric adenitis caused by Salmonella enterica serovar Enteritidis. J Formos Med Assoc. 103(6):463-6, 2004
2. Burke BB et al: Mesenteric Adenitis. eMedicine. Apr, 2003
3. Likitnukul S et al: Appendicitis-like syndrome owing to mesenteric adenitis caused by Salmonella typhi. Ann Trop Paediatr. 22(1):97-9, 2002
4. Macari M et al: Mesenteric adenitis: CT diagnosis of primary versus secondary causes, incidence, and clinical significance in pediatric and adult patients. AJR Am J Roentgenol. 178(4):853-8, 2002
5. Lamps LW et al: The role of Yersinia enterocolitica and Yersinia pseudotuberculosis in granulomatous appendicitis: a histologic and molecular study. Am J Surg Pathol. 25(4):508-15, 2001
6. Lee JH et al: The etiology and clinical characteristics of mesenteric adenitis in Korean adults. J Korean Med Sci. 12(2):105-10, 1997
7. Rao PM et al: Sensitivity and specificity of the individual CT signs of appendicitis: experience with 200 helical appendiceal CT examinations. J Comput Assist Tomogr. 21(5):686-92, 1997
8. Rao PM et al: CT diagnosis of mesenteric adenitis. Radiology. 202(1):145-9, 1997
9. Van Noyen R et al: Causative role of Yersinia and other enteric pathogens in the appendicular syndrome. Eur J Clin Microbiol Infect Dis. 10(9):735-41, 1991
10. Tertti R et al: Clinical manifestations of Yersinia pseudotuberculosis infection in children. Eur J Clin Microbiol Infect Dis. 8(7):587-91, 1989
11. Black RE et al: Yersinia enterocolitica. Infect Dis Clin North Am. 2(3):625-41, 1988
12. Puylaert JB: Mesenteric adenitis and acute terminal ileitis: US evaluation using graded compression. Radiology. 161(3):691-5, 1986
13. Marriott DJ et al: Yersinia enterocolitica infection in children. Med J Aust. 143(11):489-92, 1985
14. Saebo A: The Yersinia enterocolitica infection in acute abdominal surgery. A clinical study with a 5-year follow-up period. Ann Surg. 198(6):760-5, 1983
15. Constantinides CG et al: Suppurative mesenteric lymphadenitis in children. Case reports. S Afr Med J. 60(16):629-31, 1981
16. Schapers RF et al: Mesenteric lymphadenitis due to Yersinia enterocolitica. Virchows Arch A Pathol Anat Histol. 390(2):127-38, 1981
17. Kohl S: Yersinia enterocolitica infections in children. Pediatr Clin North Am. 26(2):433-43, 1979
18. Gilmore OJ et al: Appendicitis and mimicking conditions. A prospective study. Lancet. 2(7932):421-4, 1975

MESENTERIC ADENITIS

IMAGE GALLERY

Typical

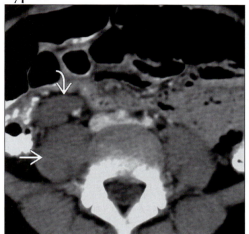
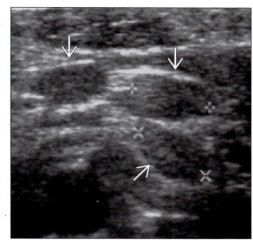

(Left) Axial CECT shows enlarged lymph node *(curved arrow)* anterior to the right psoas muscle *(arrow)*. Numerous other enlarged lymph nodes were seen on other axial images with a normal appearing appendix. *(Right)* Transverse ultrasound shows enlarged lymph nodes in the left lower quadrant mesentery *(arrows)*. Numerous enlarged but smaller lymph nodes were noted diffusely in this patient.

Typical

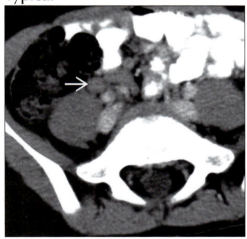
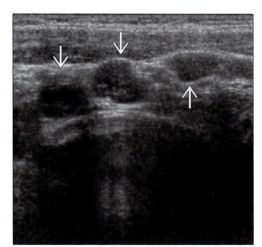

(Left) Axial CECT shows numerous right lower quadrant lymph nodes *(arrow)* anterior to the psoas & iliac vessels. *(Right)* Transverse ultrasound shows enlarged hypoechoic masses *(arrows)* in the right lower quadrant, most consistent with lymphadenopathy in this patient with mesenteric adenitis.

Typical

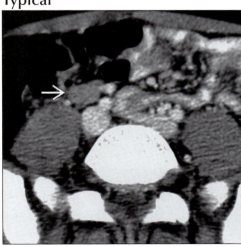
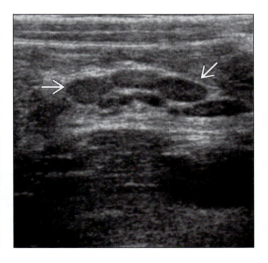

(Left) Axial CECT shows enlarged hypodense mass anterior to the right iliac vessels, lymphadenopathy *(arrow)* in this patient with mesenteric adenitis. *(Right)* Ultrasound image shows cluster of numerous enlarged lymph nodes *(arrows)*. This patient's symptoms resolved over a period of 3 days. The appendix was not identified on this study.

MESENTERIC LYMPHATIC MALFORMATIONS

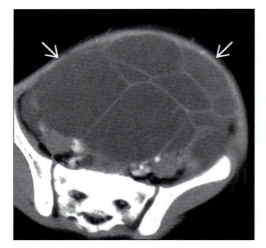

Axial CECT shows thin walled multiseptated cystic mass (arrows), consistent with a small bowel mesenteric cyst. (Courtesy of Alan Brody, MD).

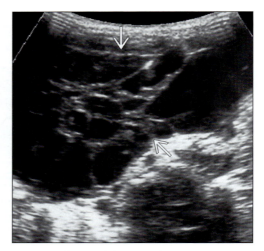

Transverse ultrasound shows anechoic cystic mass with thin septations (arrows) in this patient with a small bowel mesenteric cyst. (Courtesy of Alan Brody, MD).

TERMINOLOGY

Abbreviations and Synonyms
- Mesenteric cyst, omental cyst, mesenteric lymphangioma

Definitions
- Proliferation of lymphatic tissue that fails to communicate with the central lymphatic system, arising from the mesentery

IMAGING FINDINGS

General Features
- Best diagnostic clue: Cystic mass in the small bowel mesentery
- Location
  - Duodenal to rectal mesentery
  - Lymphatic malformations
    - Neck & axillae (95%)
  - 5%: Mediastinum, omentum, mesentery & extremities
  - Mesenteric: Small bowel: 60%, colonic: 24%
  - Retroperitoneal: 14.5%
- Size: Few mm to 40 cm
- Morphology: Unilocular, multilocular, or multiple

Radiographic Findings
- Normal, soft tissue mass, displaced bowel loops, small bowel obstruction

CT Findings
- Well-defined fluid-filled mass +/- septations, attenuation of the fluid will varying on the composition of the cyst [fat (chylous) → serous fluid → hemorrhage]
- Fine calcifications of cyst wall have been described

Ultrasonographic Findings
- Mostly anechoic multiloculated mass with thin septations
- Can be complex with debris, hemorrhage, infection, or fat/fluid levels

Imaging Recommendations
- Best imaging tool: Ultrasound or CECT

DIFFERENTIAL DIAGNOSIS

Pancreatic pseudocyst
- Collection of pancreatic fluid & exudate contained by a fibrous capsule, visible wall
- History of pancreatitis, develops > 4 weeks after episode of pancreatitis

DDx: Cystic Abdominal Masses

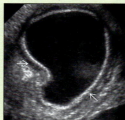

Duplication Cyst

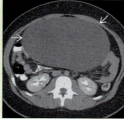

Ovarian Cystadenoma

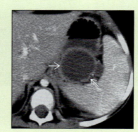

Pancreatic Pseudocyst

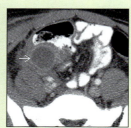

Abscess

MESENTERIC LYMPHATIC MALFORMATIONS

Key Facts

Terminology
- Proliferation of lymphatic tissue that fails to communicate with the central lymphatic system, arising from the mesentery

Imaging Findings
- Neck & axillae (95%)
- Mesenteric: Small bowel: 60%, colonic: 24%
- Retroperitoneal: 14.5%
- Size: Few mm to 40 cm

- Best imaging tool: Ultrasound or CECT

Top Differential Diagnoses
- Pancreatic pseudocyst
- Ovarian cystic mass
- Duplication cyst

Pathology
- Rare: 1/100,000 to 1/250,000 hospital admissions
- 1/20,000 pediatrics hospital admissions

- Most commonly in lesser sac, 1/3 elsewhere

Ovarian cystic mass
- Dermoid cyst
- Serous cystadenoma (unilocular > multilocular)
  - Thin walled cyst up to 20 cm in size

Duplication cyst
- Ultrasound typically possess "double wall" sign (gut signature)
  - Inner echogenic mucosa + outer hypoechoic muscular wall
- Most present during 1st year of life

Other pseudocysts
- Ventriculoperitoneal shunt, loculated ascites, peritoneal inclusion, abscess, hematoma

PATHOLOGY

General Features
- Epidemiology
  - Rare: 1/100,000 to 1/250,000 hospital admissions
  - 1/20,000 pediatrics hospital admissions

Gross Pathologic & Surgical Features
- Thin walled septated unilocular, multilocular or multiple cystic spaces (chylous → serous → hemorrhagic cysts)
- Along the mesenteric side of the bowel wall +/- attachment to adjacent bowel wall
- Jejunal: Chylous fluid; ileal or colonic: Serous fluid

CLINICAL ISSUES

Presentation
- Most common signs/symptoms
  - Abdominal distension (71%), pain (50%), pain & distension (43%), vomiting (50%)
  - Commonly asymptomatic, acute abdomen

Demographics
- Age
  - Pediatric patient (1/3 of all mesenteric cysts)
    - Average age 6 years old, most < 5 years old

Natural History & Prognosis
- Complications
  - Small bowel obstruction, hemorrhage, volvulus, rupture, infection, torsion
  - Rarely obstruct adjacent biliary tree or urinary system
- Recurrence rate: 0-13.6%

Treatment
- Laparoscopic enucleation +/- bowel resection (50%)
- Larger masses: Marsupialization

DIAGNOSTIC CHECKLIST

Consider
- Other cystic masses

SELECTED REFERENCES

1. Mason JE et al: Laparoscopic excision of mesenteric cysts: a report of two cases. Surg Laparosc Endosc Percutan Tech. 11(6):382-4, 2001
2. O'Brien MF et al: Mesenteric cysts--a series of six cases with a review of the literature. Ir J Med Sci. 168(4):233-6, 1999
3. Egozi EI et al: Mesenteric and omental cysts in children. Am Surg. 63(3):287-90, 1997
4. Liew SC et al: Mesenteric cyst. Aust N Z J Surg. 64(11):741-4, 1994
5. Ros PR et al: Mesenteric and omental cysts: histologic classification with imaging correlation. Radiology. 164(2):327-32, 1987
6. Estourgie RJ et al: Mesenteric cysts. Z Kinderchir. 32(3):223-30, 1981

IMAGE GALLERY

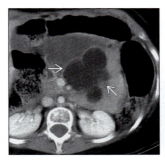 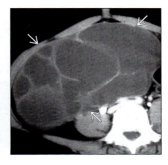

(Left) Axial CECT shows low density mass (arrows) consistent with chylous fluid in this jejunal mesenteric cyst. *(Right)* Axial CECT shows a multiseptated mass containing low density fluid in the right lower quadrant (arrows), consistent with a small bowel mesenteric cyst.

HYPOPERFUSION COMPLEX

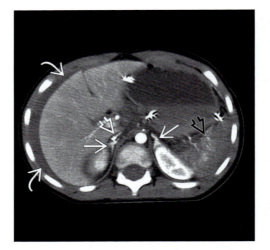 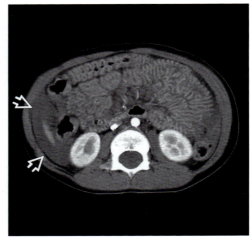

Axial CECT shows abnormal enhancing adrenals (arrows), small and dense IVC (white open arrow), ascites (curved arrows), and splenic laceration (black open arrow).

Axial bone CT in same patient shows diffuse small bowel wall thickening and enhancement, densely enhancing IVC and aorta, dense kidneys, and ascites (arrows).

TERMINOLOGY

Abbreviations and Synonyms
- Shock bowel
- Shock abdomen
- Hypoperfusion complex (HC)

Definitions
- Hypoperfusion complex: A combination of CT findings seen in the abdomen of children with compensated shock
  - Most commonly encountered in young children who have significant hemorrhage after trauma
  - Associated with tenuous hemodynamic state and poor prognosis

IMAGING FINDINGS

General Features
- Best diagnostic clue: Diffuse bowel wall enhancement and thickening associated with abnormal enhancement of solid organs and abnormal enhancement and small caliber of vessels

CT Findings
- Best imaging clue: Diffuse bowel wall enhancement and thickening associated with abnormal enhancement of solid organs and abnormal enhancement and small caliber of vessels
- Abnormal intense enhancement of
  - Bowel wall
    - Diffuse bowel wall enhancement involving large portions of bowel
    - In contrast to focal bowel wall enhancement seen with bowel injury
  - Mesentery
  - Adrenal glands
    - Adrenal glands normally soft tissue attenuation similar to muscle
    - With shock, adrenal glands enhance similar in attenuation to aorta
  - Liver
  - Kidneys
  - Pancreas
- Intense enhancement and decreased caliber
  - Inferior vena cava
    - Inferior vena cava will have a flat, "pancake" appearance
  - Aorta
- Diffuse bowel wall thickening

DDx: Bowel Wall Thickening/Enhancement

| Bowel Injury | GVHD | HSP | SB Intussusception |

HYPOPERFUSION COMPLEX

Key Facts

Imaging Findings
- Best imaging clue: Diffuse bowel wall enhancement and thickening associated with abnormal enhancement of solid organs and abnormal enhancement and small caliber of vessels
- Abnormal intense enhancement of
- Bowel wall
- Mesentery
- Adrenal glands
- Liver
- Kidneys
- Pancreas
- Intense enhancement and decreased caliber
- Inferior vena cava
- Aorta
- Diffuse bowel wall thickening
- Diffuse bowel dilatation
- Unexplained ascites
- CT findings may be apparent before clinical findings of shock

Clinical Issues
- In one series, progressive hypotension developed within 10 minutes of CT in 19% of children
- In same series, mortality rate associated with presence of hypoperfusion complex was 85%, compared with 2% of all children who suffered blunt trauma
- Immediately transfer child from CT to more supportive area or operating room
- Intense monitoring
- Fluid/blood volume replacement

  - Involving large portions of small and occasionally large bowel
  - In contrast to bowel injury, in which thickening will often involve only a focal area of bowel
- Diffuse bowel dilatation
- Unexplained ascites
- CT findings may be apparent before clinical findings of shock

Ultrasonographic Findings
- Ultrasound may be used in "FAST" scanning of the abdomen for potential abdominal trauma screening
- May show peritoneal fluid
- Diffuse fluid-filled and dilated bowel
- Bowel wall thickening

Imaging Recommendations
- Immediate removal of child from CT scanner and transfer to intensive care area or operating room

DIFFERENTIAL DIAGNOSIS

Bowel trauma
- Trauma to bowel associated with focal bowel wall thickening, wall enhancement, and dilatation
- Diffuse bowel involvement favors hypoperfusion complex
- Extra-bowel findings such as adrenal enhancement and small inferior vena cava (IVC) caliber favor shock bowel over direct bowel trauma
- Unexplained peritoneal fluid
- Mesenteric soft tissue stranding adjacent to involved bowel
- Both may coexist

Transient small bowel (SB) intussusception
- With increased use of CT, transient small bowel intussusceptions are being visualized at increased frequency
- Believed to be incidental "normal" findings that resolve spontaneously and have no clinical relevance
- Seen with higher frequency in trauma patients than in patients with CT performed for other indications
- CT shows area of small bowel with alternating rings of high and low attenuation
- Bowel not diffusely abnormal

Henoch-Schönlein purpura (HSP)
- Small vessel vasculitis of unknown origin
- Purpuric rash, abdominal pain, may have arthritis and nephritis
- 3-7 years old, boys more commonly affected
- Typically resolves spontaneously
- Edema and hemorrhage of bowel wall
  - CT shows multiple areas of bowel wall thickening, increased attenuation, and enhancement
- May also be areas of small bowel intussusception

Graft vs. host disease (GVHD)
- GVHD may have similar bowel findings as compared to hypoperfusion complex
  - Diffuse bowel wall enhancement and mild bowel wall thickening
  - Small bowel more often involved than large bowel
  - Increased soft tissue attenuation within mesenteric fat
  - Peritoneal fluid
- Clinical history of bone marrow transplant and absent history of trauma is obviously essential

Other bowel inflammatory processes
- Pre-existing conditions may be present in setting of trauma
- Other inflammatory causes of bowel wall thickening and enhancement
  - Pseudomembranous colitis: Diffuse pancolitis, severe bowel wall thickening with disproportionately small amount of pericolonic inflammatory change, related to antibiotic use
  - Crohn disease: Marked thickening typically of terminal ileum and cecum, "creeping fat"
  - Infectious enterocolitis: Shigella, E. coli, etc. - abnormal bowel wall thickening, dilatation, and wall enhancement

HYPOPERFUSION COMPLEX

PATHOLOGY

General Features
- General path comments
  - Unlike in adults, in children with hypovolemic shock, compensation can occur in which increased sympathetic stimulation maintains adequate blood pressure and cardiac output
    - Differential vasospasm causes perfusion of vital organs
  - Child with hypovolemic shock may have normal blood pressures despite significant reductions in circulating blood volume
    - This may lead to patient appearing stable and having CT imaging
    - However, in children, transition from stable shock to decompensation is abrupt, not gradual
  - Increased sympathetic activity and resultant altered pathways of arterial flow result in findings seen at CT with hypoperfusion complex
    - Small caliber aorta and inferior vena cava are related to vasospasm and hypovolemia
    - Bowel dilatation and enhancement related to mesenteric vasoconstriction
    - Intense enhancement of adrenal glands related to central role of adrenal in generating sympathetic response to hypovolemic shock
- Epidemiology
  - Findings of hypoperfusion complex can be seen in compensated shock at any age
  - However, CT findings more common and more striking in young children
- Associated abnormalities
  - Findings of parenchymal organ hemorrhage - from liver, spleen, or kidney
  - Active extravasation from parenchymal organ
    - High attenuation material (similar in attenuation to aorta) surrounding an injured organ
  - Bowel injury may also be present

CLINICAL ISSUES

Presentation
- Most common signs/symptoms
  - Clinical findings of compensated shock
  - Children may be normotensive but often are tachycardic in an attempt to maintain adequate blood pressure
- Other signs/symptoms
  - CT findings seen most commonly in trauma patient but can occur with shock of any cause
  - CT findings often recognized prior to clinical recognition of severity of shock

Demographics
- Age
  - CT findings more common and more striking with shock seen in young children
  - CT findings, however, can be seen at any age

Natural History & Prognosis
- In one series, progressive hypotension developed within 10 minutes of CT in 19% of children
- In same series, mortality rate associated with presence of hypoperfusion complex was 85%, compared with 2% of all children who suffered blunt trauma
  - In other series, the mortality has been as low as 17%

Treatment
- Immediately transfer child from CT to more supportive area or operating room
- Intense monitoring
- Fluid/blood volume replacement
- Surgical management when necessary for underlying injuries

DIAGNOSTIC CHECKLIST

Consider
- When diffuse bowel wall enhancement, dilatation, and thickening: Think hypoperfusion complex
  - Look for supporting signs of intense enhancement of other organs and small caliber and intense enhancement of IVC and aorta

SELECTED REFERENCES

1. Strouse PJ et al: CT of bowel and mesenteric trauma in children. Radiographics. 19(5):1237-50, 1999
2. O'Hara SM et al: Intense contrast enhancement of the adrenal glands: another abdominal CT finding associated with hypoperfusion complex in children. AJR Am J Roentgenol. 173(4):995-7, 1999
3. Levine CD et al: CT in patients with blunt abdominal trauma: clinical significance of intraperitoneal fluid detected on a scan with otherwise normal findings. AJR Am J Roentgenol. 164(6):1381-5, 1995
4. Mirvis SE et al: Diffuse small-bowel ischemia in hypotensive adults after blunt trauma (shock bowel): CT findings and clinical significance. AJR Am J Roentgenol. 163(6):1375-9, 1994
5. Sivit CJ et al: CT in children with rupture of the bowel caused by blunt trauma: diagnostic efficacy and comparison with hypoperfusion complex. AJR Am J Roentgenol. 163(5):1195-8, 1994
6. Hara H et al: Significance of bowel wall enhancement on CT following blunt abdominal trauma in childhood. J Comput Assist Tomogr. 16(1):94-8, 1992
7. Sivit CJ et al: Posttraumatic shock in children: CT findings associated with hemodynamic instability. Radiology. 182(3):723-6, 1992
8. Jeffrey RB Jr et al: The collapsed inferior vena cava: CT evidence of hypovolemia. AJR Am J Roentgenol. 150(2):431-2, 1988
9. Taylor GA et al: Hypovolemic shock in children: abdominal CT manifestations. Radiology. 164(2):479-81, 1987

HYPOPERFUSION COMPLEX

IMAGE GALLERY

Typical

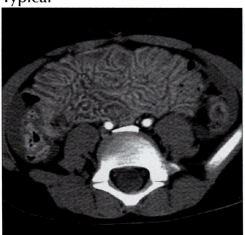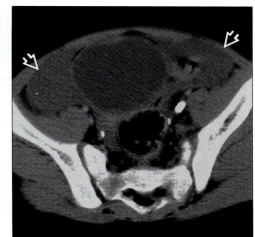

(Left) Axial CECT shows abnormal enhancement and thickening of bowel wall diffusely. There is also a small amount of ascites. *(Right)* Axial CECT in same patient shows unexplained ascites (arrows) in the pelvis.

Typical

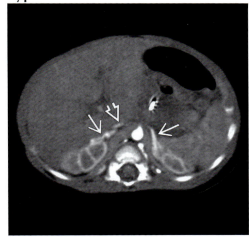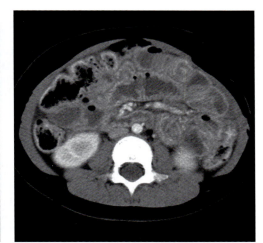

(Left) Axial CECT small and densely enhancing IVC (open arrow), and densely enhancing aorta, kidneys and adrenal glands (arrows). *(Right)* Axial CECT shows diffuse abnormal enhancement and thickening of small and large bowel wall.

Typical

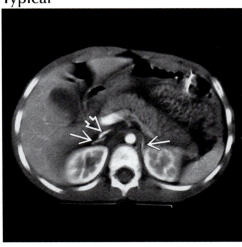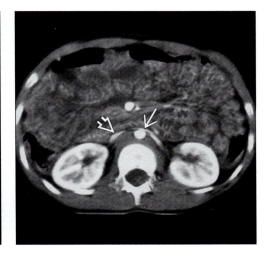

(Left) Axial CECT shows densely enhancing and small caliber IVC (open arrow) and enhancement of the adrenal glands (arrows) and kidneys. *(Right)* Axial CECT in same patient as on left shows diffuse bowel wall thickening and enhancement, densely enhancing kidneys, and small caliber and dense IVC (open arrow) and aorta (arrow).

BOWEL INJURY

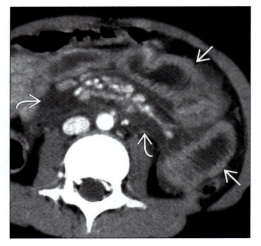

Axial CECT shows abnormal enhancing thickened jejunum (arrows) with free fluid/hematoma (curved arrows) in this patient with a jejunal perforation.

Axial CECT shows moderate jejunal wall enhancement (arrows). Mesenteric & retroperitoneal fluid/hematoma (curved arrows) is evident from a jejunal transection.

TERMINOLOGY

Abbreviations and Synonyms
- Intestinal injury, injury to bowel, bowel wall hematoma

IMAGING FINDINGS

General Features
- Best diagnostic clue: Bowel wall enhancement, thickening +/- enteric contrast extravasation & pneumoperitoneum
- Location
  ○ Most common
    ▪ Duodenum & jejunum (just distal to ligament of Treitz)
- Morphology
  ○ Most common mechanism
    ▪ Small bowel (SB) compression against vertebral column
    ▪ Acceleration-deceleration injury with mesenteric tear
    ▪ Sudden dramatic increase in intraabdominal pressure
  ○ Lap belt injuries
    ▪ Lap belt ecchymosis over skin
    ▪ May not be clinically apparent for hours
    ▪ Lap belt may be abnormally positioned high riding over the abdomen rather than over the anterosuperior iliac spine → higher center of gravity → shearing force or acute flexion
    ▪ Associated with Chance fractures or bladder injury
- Common etiologies
  ○ Bicycle handlebar
    ▪ Bicycle accidents account for 5-14% of blunt trauma in children
    ▪ Usually focal injury
  ○ Motor vehicle accident
    ▪ Blunt trauma or lap belt & deceleration injuries
  ○ Child abuse
    ▪ Direct blow: Bowel compressed between force & spinal column
  ○ Iatrogenic
    ▪ Endoscopic biopsy
  ○ Penetrating injuries
    ▪ Gunshot
    ▪ Stabbing
- Other general features
  ○ Laparotomies for blunt trauma
    ▪ < 10% incidence of SB & mesenteric injuries
  ○ Trauma leading cause of death (1-40 year olds)

Radiographic Findings
- Small or large bowel dilation
  ○ Ileus or obstruction secondary to peritonitis

DDx: Edema Or Hemorrhage In The Small Bowel Wall

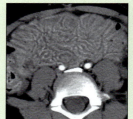 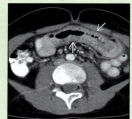 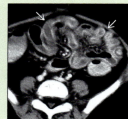 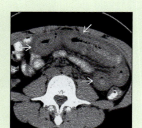

"Shock Bowel" | HSP | GVHD | SLE

BOWEL INJURY

Key Facts

Terminology
- Intestinal injury, injury to bowel, bowel wall hematoma

Imaging Findings
- Best diagnostic clue: Bowel wall enhancement, thickening +/- enteric contrast extravasation & pneumoperitoneum
- Bicycle handlebar
- Motor vehicle accident
- Child abuse
- Trauma leading cause of death (1-40 year olds)
- Focal bowel wall thickening (> 2-3 mm) or hematoma
- Pneumoperitoneum
- Extraluminal contrast extravasation
- Most specific sign, rare

Top Differential Diagnoses
- Hypoperfusion complex (shock bowel)
- Vasculitis
- Graft verses host disease (GVHD)
- Inflammatory bowel disease

Clinical Issues
- Abdominal tenderness, guarding, rigidity +/- absent bowel sounds
- Surgery: Perforation or infarction

Diagnostic Checklist
- Lap belt ecchymosis: Associated bowel, urinary bladder or spinal injuries

---

- Soft tissue mass displacing or narrowing bowel gas column
- Retroperitoneal air
  - Duodenal tear, transection or laceration
    - Outlines psoas, right kidney or crus of right hemidiaphragm
  - Ascending or descending colonic injury
- Pneumoperitoneum
  - Ruptured hollow viscus
  - Upright or left lateral decubitus (less sensitive than CT)
    - Can detect as little as 1-2 ml of air
  - Without history of peritoneal lavage, air introduced from bladder catheter (or a ruptured bladder) or pneumomediastinum (rare cause)
  - "Rigler" sign: Supine image, air on both sides of bowel wall
  - "Falciform ligament" sign: Supine image, linear density in right upper quadrant outlined by air
  - "Football" sign: Peritoneal cavity as an oval gas shadow
  - "Inverted-V" sign: Outlined with air the medial umbilical folds in the pelvis
- "Flank-stripe" sign: Peritoneal fluid separating ascending or descending colon from the peritoneal reflection or properitoneal fat
- "Dog's ear" sign: Pelvic fluid separating bowel from bladder
- Splinting: Scoliosis curvature toward injury

Fluoroscopic Findings
- Bowel wall hematoma
  - Mass effect → narrowing → obstruction
  - Most commonly 2nd or 3rd portion of duodenum
- Contrast extravasation

CT Findings
- Important viewing study with lung windows also
- Focal bowel wall thickening (> 2-3 mm) or hematoma
  - Most common CT finding of bowel injury
  - Focal thickening, abnormal enhancement & peritoneal fluid: Highly suggests bowel injury
  - Diffuse bowel wall thickening may occur late with peritonitis
- Pneumoperitoneum
  - 30-40%
  - Other causes: Peritoneal lavage/laparotomy, bladder rupture (air instilled during bladder catheterization), mechanical ventilation, pneumomediastinum & pneumothorax
  - Most common location: Mid abdomen, anterior peritoneal surface of liver
- Peritoneal fluid
  - Concerning for mesenteric or bowel injury when lacking solid organ injury or pelvic fractures
  - Unusual as only manifestation of bowel injury
- Extraluminal contrast extravasation
  - Most specific sign, rare
- Retroperitoneal free air
  - High suspicion of duodenal transection
  - Also seen in colon and bladder tears/transection
- Hyperdense enhancement of the bowel wall
  - > Psoas muscle in Hounsfield units (HU)
- Mesenteric fluid, hematoma &/or infiltration
  - Sentinel clot sign adjacent to bowel (> 60 HU)
  - Polygonal collections between bowel segments & mesenteric folds
- Bowel wall discontinuity (rare)
- Active hemorrhage
  - = HU to enhancing vessels
- Mesenteric pseudoaneurysm

Ultrasonographic Findings
- Free fluid FAST scanning of Morison pouch, splenorenal recess, pouch of Douglas & pericolonic gutters
- Nonspecific finding

Angiographic Findings
- Control active bleeding & therapy for pseudoaneurysms & arteriovenous fistulas

Imaging Recommendations
- Best imaging tool: Helical multislice CECT +/- oral contrast

BOWEL INJURY

DIFFERENTIAL DIAGNOSIS

Hypoperfusion complex (shock bowel)
- Overlaps imaging findings with bowel injury
- Diffuse bowel wall thickening (rather than focal seen in bowel injury)
- Dilated bowel with intense enhancement of the bowel mucosa
- Intense enhancement of the adrenal gland, pancreas & mesenteric vessels
- ↓ Enhancement of spleen (can simulate splenic injury)
- ↓ Size of aorta & inferior cava
- Diffuse bowel wall thickening with secondary findings favors hypoperfusion complex over bowel trauma
- Poor clinical outcome

Vasculitis
- Henoch-Schönlein purpura (HSP)
  - No trauma history, usually begins as upper respiratory infection
  - Focal or multifocal bowel wall thickening
  - Purpuric rash on legs or extensor surface of the upper extremities
  - Rash may occur after abdominal symptoms
  - Colicky abdominal pain, gastrointestinal (GI) bleeding, intussusceptions & arthralgias
- Systemic lupus erythematosus (SLE)
  - Connective tissue disease, systemic
  - GI bleeding
  - Mesenteric ischemia: Thumbprinting, nodular folds, colitis, necrosis & perforation

Graft verses host disease (GVHD)
- Bone marrow transplantation patients
- Small bowel fold thickening or effacement ("ribbon bowel")
- Diffuse enhancing mucosa of both large & small bowel

Inflammatory bowel disease
- No history of trauma
- Colicky abdominal pain, recurrent diarrhea, weight loss, perianal disease, malabsorption
- Most commonly terminal ileal involvement
  - Thickened nodular folds, aphthous ulcers, cobblestone mucosa

Coagulopathy
- Bleeding into the bowel wall
- Idiopathic thrombocytopenia purpura & Hemophilia

PATHOLOGY

General Features
- Etiology
  - Blunt trauma
    - Lap belt
    - Bicycle handlebar
    - Child abuse
  - Penetrating trauma
- Epidemiology: < 10% of blunt trauma at laparotomy
- Associated abnormalities
  - Liver, spleen, adrenal, kidney & pancreas injuries
  - Lap belt: Associated with spine & bladder injuries

Gross Pathologic & Surgical Features
- Contusion, hematoma, laceration or transection

CLINICAL ISSUES

Presentation
- Most common signs/symptoms
  - Abdominal tenderness, guarding, rigidity +/- absent bowel sounds
  - Hypotension & tachycardia
  - Delayed presentation of symptoms > 24 hours
- Positive diagnostic peritoneal lavage (DPL)
  - Aspiration of free flowing blood
  - Aspiration of feces
  - Bloody lavage fluid from catheter, urinary catheter, or chest tube containing
    - Rbc: > 100,00/mm3
    - Wbc: > 500/mm3 or gram stain with bacteria present
    - Amylase: > 175 w/dl

Natural History & Prognosis
- Complications
  - Peritonitis, abscess, death
- Prognosis good with early recognition
- Prognosis poor with delayed recognition
  - Morbidity & mortality ↑ up to 65%

Treatment
- Surgery: Perforation or infarction
- CT findings influence decisions concerning triage of patient (discharge, admission, length and intensity of observation)
- Decisions to go to surgery usually based more on clinical condition of patient than CT findings

DIAGNOSTIC CHECKLIST

Consider
- Lap belt ecchymosis: Associated bowel, urinary bladder or spinal injuries

SELECTED REFERENCES

1. Emery KH: Lap belt iliac wing fracture: a predictor of bowel injury in children. Pediatr Radiol. 32(12):892-5, 2002
2. Strouse PJ et al: CT of bowel and mesenteric trauma in children. Radiographics. 19(5):1237-50, 1999
3. Sivit CJ et al: CT in children with rupture of the bowel caused by blunt trauma: diagnostic efficacy and comparison with hypoperfusion complex. AJR Am J Roentgenol. 163(5):1195-8, 1994
4. Hara H et al: Significance of bowel wall enhancement on CT following blunt abdominal trauma in childhood. J Comput Assist Tomogr. 16(1):94-8, 1992
5. Mirvis SE et al: Rupture of the bowel after blunt abdominal trauma: diagnosis with CT. AJR Am J Roentgenol. 159(6):1217-21, 1992
6. Sivit CJ et al: Blunt trauma in children: significance of peritoneal fluid. Radiology. 178(1):185-8, 1991

BOWEL INJURY

IMAGE GALLERY

Typical

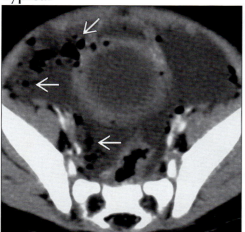
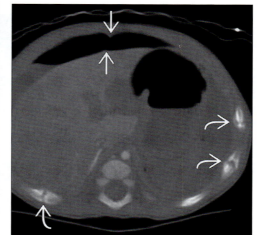

(Left) Axial CECT shows multiple extraluminal air bubbles (arrows), free air & complex fluid in this child with a sigmoid perforation from child abuse. *(Right)* Axial CECT in the same patient shows "falciform ligament" sign; falciform ligament (arrows) surrounded by free air. Notice the multiple healing rib fractures (curved arrows) from abuse.

Typical

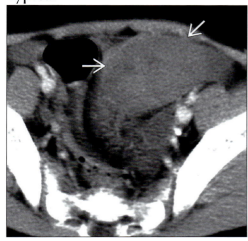
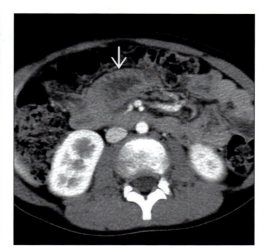

(Left) Axial CECT shows a large hyperdense mass, sigmoid mesocolon hematoma (arrows). *(Right)* Axial CECT shows focal thickened small bowel segment (arrow) from blunt trauma.

Typical

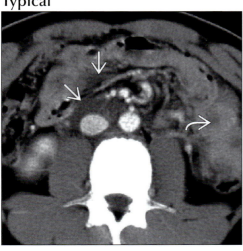
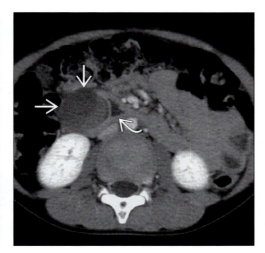

(Left) Axial CECT shows hypodense mass in the mesentery & retroperitoneum (arrows) with mild proximal small bowel wall thickening (curved arrow) in this patient with a jejunal transection. *(Right)* Axial CECT shows a hypodense intramural mass (arrows) in the duodenum with mild eccentric luminal narrowing (curved arrow), consistent with a hematoma from recent biopsy.

LIVER TRAUMA

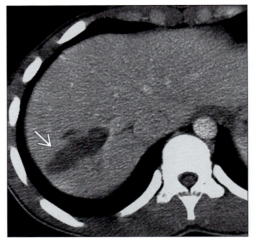

Axial CECT shows hypodense band along the posterior liver (arrow), consistent with a laceration. This patient had a grade III liver injury.

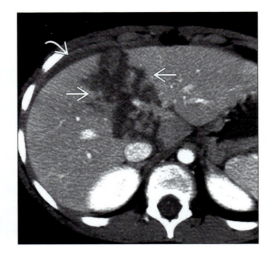

Axial CECT shows hypodense stellate region in the liver consistent with a laceration (arrows). There is also perihepatic hematoma (curved arrow) in this patient with a handlebar trauma.

TERMINOLOGY

Abbreviations and Synonyms
- Synonym(s): Liver or hepatic laceration, fracture, injury

IMAGING FINDINGS

General Features
- Best diagnostic clue
  - CECT
    - Linear or branching intraparenchymal regions of ↓ attenuation
    - Perihepatic blood
- Location
  - Right lobe > left lobe; 3:1
    - Most commonly posterior segment of right lobe
    - Fixed by coronary ligament
    - Limits motion, while remainder of liver can move
- Key concepts
  - Liver is the most common solid organ injured
    - Hemoperitoneum in 2/3
    - 10-30% of blunt trauma
    - 50% of deaths from blunt abdominal trauma in children
  - Blunt > penetrating trauma
  - Iatrogenic (liver biopsy)
  - Trauma leading cause of death 1-40 year olds

CT Findings
- CECT
  - Subcapsular hematoma
    - Collection that compresses convex shaped lateral margin of parenchyma
    - Lenticular shaped
    - Anterolateral to right lobe most common
  - Parenchymal laceration
    - Jagged linear area of hypodensity due to hematoma
    - Usually peripheral
  - Intraparenchymal hematoma
    - Irregular ↑ attenuation clotted blood surrounded by ↓ attenuation hematoma
  - Unclotted blood (35-45 Hounsfield units (HU))
    - ↓ Attenuation compared to liver parenchyma
  - Clotted blood
    - 60-90 HU
  - Active extravasation/bleeding or pseudoaneurysm
    - 85-300 HU
    - ↑ Attenuation focus isodense to aortic enhancement; surrounded by ↓ attenuation clot or hematoma
  - Infarction
    - Wedge shaped without perihepatic hematoma
  - Periportal edema

DDx: Hypodense Liver Lesions

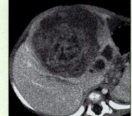
Hepatoblastoma

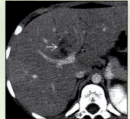
Hepatic Abscesses

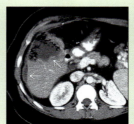
Infarct & Abscess

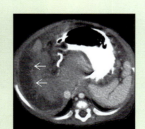
Hepatic Infarct

LIVER TRAUMA

Key Facts

Terminology
- Synonym(s): Liver or hepatic laceration, fracture, injury

Imaging Findings
- Right lobe > left lobe; 3:1
- Most commonly posterior segment of right lobe
- Fixed by coronary ligament
- 50% of deaths from blunt abdominal trauma in children
- Blunt > penetrating trauma
- Active extravasation/bleeding or pseudoaneurysm
- 85-300 HU
- ↑ Attenuation focus isodense to aortic enhancement; surrounded by ↓ attenuation clot or hematoma
- Conventional: Therapy: Embolization of active extravasation or pseudoaneurysms

Top Differential Diagnoses
- Hepatic abscesses
- Artifacts: Beam hardening artifact or motion
- Primary or metastatic disease
- Liver infarction

Pathology
- Blunt > penetrating trauma
- 45% associated splenic injury

Clinical Issues
- Age: Vehicular injuries: Most common cause of death in 15-25 year olds
- Excellent prognosis with early diagnosis and intervention
- Liver grades do not predict prognosis or outcome in children

---

- 25% of children
- Fluid hydration & distended lymphatics (most likely etiology)
- Bile or blood tracking up biliary tree
○ Biliary injury
  - Hematobilia
  - Biloma
  - Biliary ascites
  - Bile duct disruption

MR Findings
- Adds very little additional information
- MRCP can be useful in evaluation of pancreatic duct or biliary tree

Ultrasonographic Findings
- Grayscale Ultrasound
  ○ Subcapsular hematoma: Compresses lateral margin of liver
  ○ Variable echogenicity of lacerations depending on time of imaging
    - Anechoic (initially) → echogenic (1 day) → hypoechoic (4-5 days)
  ○ Intraparenchymal hematoma
  ○ Bilomas
    - Cystic mass near gallbladder in echogenicity
  ○ Sensitive for grade III injury or greater

Angiographic Findings
- Conventional: Therapy: Embolization of active extravasation or pseudoaneurysms

Nuclear Medicine Findings
- Hepatobiliary Scan: For biliary leaks

Imaging Recommendations
- Best imaging tool: CECT technique of choice

DIFFERENTIAL DIAGNOSIS

Hepatic abscesses
- Rounded, septated or irregular
- ↓ Attenuation lesion

Artifacts: Beam hardening artifact or motion
- Streaks of low density extending from ribs
- Excessive patient motion

Primary or metastatic disease
- Can simulate intraparenchymal hematoma
- Primary tumor may rupture or bleed
  ○ Hepatic adenoma or hepatocellular carcinoma most common

Liver infarction
- Thrombus or embolus most common cause
- Peripheral wedge-shaped
- Sometimes appears rounded or central
- Sometimes the result of trauma

PATHOLOGY

General Features
- Etiology
  ○ Blunt > penetrating trauma
    - Deceleration or shearing injury
    - Compression against ribs/spine/abdominal wall (anterior & posterior)
  ○ Iatrogenic, usually liver biopsy
    - Usually subcapsular hematoma
- Epidemiology: 50% of intraabdominal injuries in children are isolated liver injury
- Associated abnormalities
  ○ 45% associated splenic injury
  ○ 33% rib fractures
  ○ Duodenal hematoma or pancreatic injury

Gross Pathologic & Surgical Features
- Lacerations, intraparenchymal hematoma, subcapsular hematoma, vascular avulsion

Staging, Grading or Classification Criteria
- American Association of Surgery of Trauma (AAST)
- Grade I
  ○ Hematoma
    - Subcapsular, < 10% surface area

LIVER TRAUMA

- Laceration
  - Capsular tear, < 1 cm parenchymal depth
- Grade II
  - Hematoma
    - Subcapsular, 10-50% surface area
    - Intraparenchymal, < 10 cm in diameter
  - Laceration
    - 1-3 cm parenchymal depth, < 10 cm in length
- Grade III
  - Hematoma
    - Subcapsular, > 50% surface area or expanding; ruptured subcapsular or parenchymal hematoma
    - Intraparenchymal hematoma > 10 cm or expanding
  - Laceration
    - > 3 cm parenchymal depth
- Grade IV
  - Laceration
    - Parenchymal disruption involving 25-75% of hepatic lobe or 1-3 Couinaud segments within a single lobe
- Grade V
  - Laceration
    - Parenchymal disruption involving > 75% of hepatic lobe or > 3 Couinaud segments within a single lobe
  - Vascular
    - Juxtahepatic venous injuries; i.e., retrohepatic vena cava (ivc)/central major hepatic veins
- Grade VI
  - Vascular
    - Hepatic avulsion

CLINICAL ISSUES

Presentation
- Most common signs/symptoms
  - Blunt abdominal trauma
  - Right upper quadrant pain, guarding, tenderness
  - Asymptomatic → death
  - Hypotension
    - Decreased hematocrit
  - Hematemesis or melena
  - ↑ Liver enzymes

Demographics
- Age: Vehicular injuries: Most common cause of death in 15-25 year olds
- Gender: M > F

Natural History & Prognosis
- Complications
  - Biloma
  - Delayed hemorrhage
  - Hemobilia
  - Hepatic infarcts
  - Pseudoaneurysm
  - Arteriovenous fistula
- Excellent prognosis with early diagnosis and intervention
- Liver grades do not predict prognosis or outcome in children

- Grades used for description & helps guide clinician/surgeon in decision making
- Associated injuries affect prognosis
- Mortality up to 25%
  - 1/2 from liver injury
  - Rest from the associated injuries

Treatment
- CT findings often affect decisions concerning disposition of patient
  - Discharge versus admission
  - Level of intensity for observation: Intensive care vs. standard floor
- Non-operative management for minor injuries
- Active extravasation/active bleeding or blush ideally observed in intensive care unit
  - Increased risk of rebleed
  - Angiographic embolization if active arterial extravasation & hemobilia
- Surgical intervention for shock and biliary peritonitis
  - Interventional radiology or gastroenterology (ERCP) with stent placement

SELECTED REFERENCES

1. Yoon W et al: CT in blunt liver trauma. Radiographics. 25(1):87-104, 2005
2. Paddock HN et al: Management of blunt pediatric hepatic and splenic injury: similar process, different outcome. Am Surg. 70(12):1068-72, 2004
3. Schmidt B et al: Blunt liver trauma in children. Pediatr Surg Int. 20(11-12):846-50, 2004
4. Tas F et al: The efficacy of ultrasonography in hemodynamically stable children with blunt abdominal trauma: a prospective comparison with computed tomography. Eur J Radiol. 51(1):91-6, 2004
5. Al-Mulhim AS et al: Non-operative management of blunt hepatic injury in multiply injured adult patients. Surgeon. 1(2):81-5, 2003
6. Eubanks JW 3rd et al: Significance of 'blush' on computed tomography scan in children with liver injury. J Pediatr Surg. 38(3):363-6; discussion 363-6, 2003
7. Munshi IA et al: Bicycle handlebar injury. J Emerg Med. 24(2):215-6, 2003
8. Gaines BA et al: Abdominal and pelvic trauma in children. Crit Care Med. 30(11 Suppl):S416-23, 2002
9. Lau BH et al: Management of hemobilia with transarterial angiographic embolization: report of one case. Acta Paediatr Taiwan. 43(2):96-9, 2002
10. Sharif K et al: Benefits of early diagnosis and preemptive treatment of biliary tract complications after major blunt liver trauma in children. J Pediatr Surg. 37(9):1287-92, 2002
11. Resende V et al: Helical computed tomography characteristics of splenic and hepatic trauma in children subjected to nonoperative treatment. Emerg Radiol. 9(6):309-13, 2002
12. Delgado Millan MA et al: Computed tomography, angiography, and endoscopic retrograde cholangiopancreatography in the nonoperative management of hepatic and splenic trauma. World J Surg. 25(11): 1397-1402, 2001
13. Pryor JP et al: Severe blunt hepatic trauma in children. J Pediatr Surg. 36(7):974-9, 2001
14. Richards JR et al: Sonographic detection of blunt hepatic trauma: hemoperitoneum and parenchymal patterns of injury. J Trauma. 47(6):1092-7, 1999

LIVER TRAUMA

IMAGE GALLERY

Typical

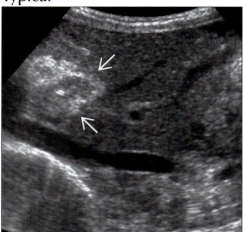
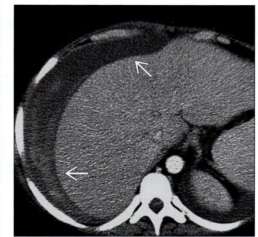

(Left) Ultrasound longitudinal image shows an ill-defined hyperechoic lesion *(arrows)* in the liver, in this case an intraparenchymal hematoma. *(Right)* Axial CECT shows a mixed attenuation subcapsular hematoma *(arrows)* in this coagulopathic child.

Typical

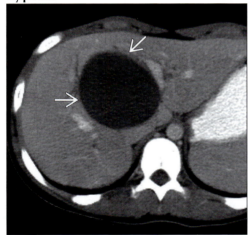
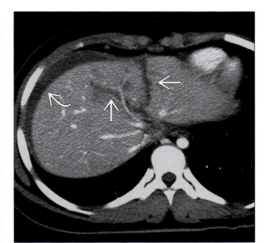

(Left) Axial CECT shows a low density rounded intraparenchymal mass *(arrows)* with HU measurements near water in attenuation, most consistent with a biloma. *(Right)* Axial CECT shows jagged hypodense laceration extending to the hepatic/IVC confluence consistent with a hematoma *(arrows)* with a perihepatic hematoma *(curved arrow)*.

Variant

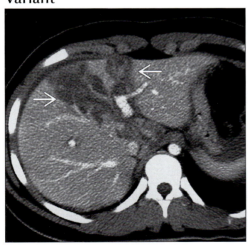
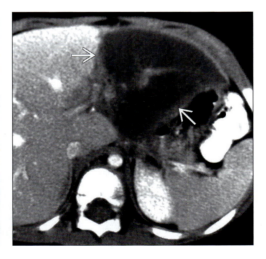

(Left) Axial CECT shows hypodense liver laceration *(arrows)* in this patient with a grade IV injury. *(Right)* Axial CECT shows wedge shaped, geographic low density region in the left lobe of the liver *(arrows)*, hepatic infarction in this patient with trauma.

SPLEEN TRAUMA

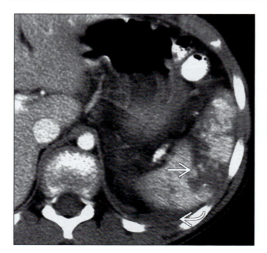

Axial CECT shows hypodense jagged branching lacerations (arrow) throughout the spleen in this patient with a grade III injury & perisplenic hematoma (curved arrow).

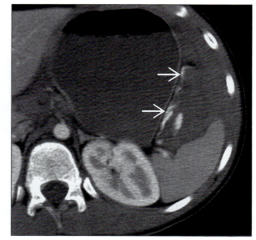

Axial CECT shows a blush (arrows) from active contrast extravasation/active bleeding into a perisplenic hematoma in this patient with hemophilia & trauma.

TERMINOLOGY

Abbreviations and Synonyms
- Splenic laceration, splenic fracture, splenic injury, blunt injury to spleen, subcapsular hematoma

Definitions
- Parenchymal injury to spleen with or without capsular disruption

IMAGING FINDINGS

General Features
- Best diagnostic clue
  - Low attenuation laceration or subcapsular hematoma
  - Surrounding perisplenic hematoma [> 30 Hounsfield units (HU)]
  - Classic imaging appearance
    - Low density intraparenchymal hematoma
    - Subcapsular hematoma flattens or compresses outer splenic margin
    - Active arterial extravasation diagnosed when high attenuation focus isodense to aorta is seen within an area of low density hematoma
- Morphology
  - Laceration: Jagged linear area due to hematoma
  - Intraparenchymal hematoma: Clotted blood surrounded by unclotted blood
  - Fracture: Deep laceration extending from outer capsule through splenic hilum
  - Subcapsular hematoma: Lenticular hematoma that compresses lateral margin of parenchyma

Radiographic Findings
- Radiography
  - Triad
    - Elevated left hemidiaphragm
    - Pleural effusion
    - Left lower lobe atelectasis or collapse
    - Not reliable or a common finding in splenic injuries
  - Left lower rib fractures
    - Most common association, 44% of patients
  - Medial displacement of stomach bubble
  - Inferiorly displaced splenic flexure
  - Findings of retroperitoneal hematoma
    - Obscured left kidney & psoas shadows
    - Ill-defined inferior splenic shadow
    - Displacement of descending colon medially

CT Findings
- NECT
  - Hemoperitoneum > 25-30 HU
  - Clot > 45 HU
- CECT

DDx: Splenic Lesions Mimicking Trauma

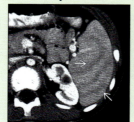
Bolus Artifact

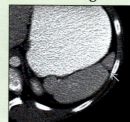
Splenic Cleft

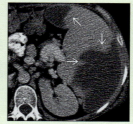
Splenic Infarcts

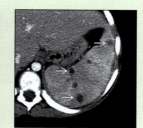
Splenic Abscesses

SPLEEN TRAUMA

Key Facts

Terminology
- Parenchymal injury to spleen with or without capsular disruption

Imaging Findings
- Low attenuation laceration or subcapsular hematoma
- Surrounding perisplenic hematoma [> 30 Hounsfield units (HU)]
- Classic imaging appearance
- Low density intraparenchymal hematoma
- Subcapsular hematoma flattens or compresses outer splenic margin
- Active arterial extravasation diagnosed when high attenuation focus isodense to aorta is seen within an area of low density hematoma
- CT accuracy: 98%; sensitivity: 95%

Top Differential Diagnoses
- Bolus artifact
- Splenic cleft
- Splenic infarct
- Splenic abscess

Pathology
- Etiology: Blunt trauma; (MVA #1 & handle-bar injuries)

Diagnostic Checklist
- Bolus artifact or congenital cleft in patients lacking perisplenic hematoma

---

- When perisplenic attenuation > 60 HU think laceration even when not seen
- CT accuracy: 98%; sensitivity: 95%
- Laceration
  - Nonenhancing variable configuration; linear branching, irregular or jagged low attenuation bands
- Intraparenchymal hematoma
  - Clotted blood (↑ attenuation) surrounded by not clotted blood (↓ attenuation)
- Fracture
  - Laceration from outer capsule extending through hilum
- Subcapsular hematoma
  - Lenticular shaped with compression of convex shaped outer margin of parenchyma
- Active extravasation
  - High attenuation focus isodense to aorta is seen within an area of ↓ density hematoma
- Differential for hyperdense region
  - Active extravasation or active bleeding
  - Arteriovenous (AV) fistula
  - Pseudoaneurysm
    - Sign of non-operative failure
    - Almost 3/4 not seen on initial CECT

Ultrasonographic Findings
- Laceration, hematoma
- Subcapsular hematoma of variable echogenicity
- No ascites or hemoperitoneum (25%)

Angiographic Findings
- Hemodynamically stable patient
  - Active extravasation or pseudoaneurysm

Imaging Recommendations
- Best imaging tool: CECT technique of choice

DIFFERENTIAL DIAGNOSIS

Bolus artifact
- Heterogeneous enhancement of the spleen
- Corrugated appearance on CECT or MR C+ T1WI
  - Differences in enhancement of the red & white pulp
- Most commonly during 1st minute of the CECT study
  - Most commonly during arterial phase
- 95% resolve by 70 seconds

Splenic cleft
- Congenital variant in contour of spleen
- Linear ↓ attenuation area without evidence of hemorrhage
- Smooth verses irregular contour with lacerations

Splenic infarct
- Triangular or wedge-shaped ↓ attenuation region with apex toward hilum
- Associated with splenomegaly
- Systemic embolization

Splenic abscess
- Rounded, irregular, ↓ attenuation lesion
- Chemical signs of infection

PATHOLOGY

General Features
- Etiology: Blunt trauma; (MVA #1 & handle-bar injuries)
- Associated abnormalities: Frequently associated with other abdominal injuries

Gross Pathologic & Surgical Features
- Intraparenchymal or subcapsular hematoma
- Laceration or fracture
- Intraperitoneal hemorrhage
- Retroperitoneal hemorrhage
  - Usually laceration or fracture that extend to hilum
  - Extends into anterior pararenal space & along pancreas

Staging, Grading or Classification Criteria
- American association for surgery of trauma (AAST)

SPLEEN TRAUMA

- Grade I
  - Hematoma
    - Subcapsular, < 10% surface area
  - Laceration
    - Capsular tear, < 1 cm parenchymal depth
- Grade II
  - Hematoma
    - Subcapsular, 10-50% surface area: Intraparenchymal, < 5 cm in diameter
  - Laceration
    - 1-3 cm parenchymal depth; which does not involve trabecular vessels
- Grade III
  - Hematoma
    - Subcapsular, < 50% surface area or expanding; ruptured subcapsular or parenchymal hematoma
    - Intraparenchymal hematoma > 5 cm or expanding
  - Laceration
    - > 3 cm parenchymal depth or involving trabecular vessels
- Grade IV
  - Laceration
    - Laceration involving segmental or hilar vessels producing major devascularization
    - > 25% of spleen
- Grade V
  - Laceration
    - Completely shattered
  - Vacular
    - Hilar vascular injury which devascularizes spleen

CLINICAL ISSUES

Presentation
- Most common signs/symptoms
  - Blunt abdominal trauma
  - Abdominal distension & tenderness
  - Left upper quadrant pain
  - Hypotension (25-30%)
- Other signs/symptoms
  - Rib pain: Left lower posterior rib fractures
  - Ecchymosis
    - Signs of retroperitoneal bleed
    - Appearance can be delayed for days
    - Grey Turner sign: Flank
    - Cullen sign: Umbilicus
  - Not clinically apparent (10-20%)

Demographics
- Age: Trauma leading cause of death in 1-40 year olds
- Gender: M > F

Natural History & Prognosis
- Excellent prognosis with early diagnosis & intervention
- Grading system (AAST) is predictive of outcome in adults
- Best for description in children
  - Not a predictor of outcome
- Nor is amount of hemoperitoneum
- Predictor of outcome: Other associated injuries
- Non-operative management in children is the standard of care in hemodynamically stable patient
  - Post splenectomy sepsis, complication of laparotomies, ↓ blood transfusions, shorter hospital stay
- CT findings of active extravasation originally stated as indication for surgery: Can often be managed conservatively
- Complications
  - Pseudocyst (20-30 HU), pseudoaneurysm, delayed rupture (bleed > 48 hours after trauma)

Treatment
- Non-operative management for minor injuries
- Splenectomy or splenorrhaphy when surgery required
- Follow-up CECT (unless clinical indications) do not change outcome or management of patients

DIAGNOSTIC CHECKLIST

Consider
- Bolus artifact or congenital cleft in patients lacking perisplenic hematoma

SELECTED REFERENCES

1. Cloutier DR et al: Pediatric splenic injuries with a contrast blush: successful nonoperative management without angiography and embolization. J Pediatr Surg. 39(6):969-71, 2004
2. Lutz N et al: The significance of contrast blush on computed tomography in children with splenic injuries. J Pediatr Surg. 39(3):491-4, 2004
3. Paddock HN et al: Management of blunt pediatric hepatic and splenic injury: similar process, different outcome. Am Surg. 70(12):1068-72, 2004
4. Yardeni D et al: Splenic artery embolization for post-traumatic splenic artery pseudoaneurysm in children. J Trauma. 57(2):404-7, 2004
5. Upadhyaya P: Conservative management of splenic trauma: history and current trends. Pediatr Surg Int. 19(9-10):617-27, 2003
6. Koren JP et al: Management of splenic trauma in the pediatric hemophiliac patient: Case series and review of the literature. J Pediatr Surg. 37(4):568-71, 2002
7. Minarik L et al: Diagnostic imaging in the follow-up of nonoperative management of splenic trauma in children. Pediatr Surg Int. 18(5-6):429-31, 2002
8. Erez I et al: Abdominal injuries caused by bicycle handlebars. Eur J Surg. 167(5):331-3, 2001
9. Leone RJ Jr et al: Nonoperative management of pediatric blunt hepatic trauma. Am Surg. 67(2):138-42, 2001
10. Shanmuganathan K et al: Nonsurgical management of blunt splenic injury: use of CT criteria to select patients for splenic arteriography and potential endovascular therapy. Radiology. 217(1):75-82, 2000
11. Donnelly LF et al: Heterogeneous splenic enhancement patterns on spiral CT images in children: minimizing misinterpretation. Radiology. 210(2):493-7, 1999
12. Davis KA et al: Improved success in nonoperative management of blunt splenic injuries: embolization of splenic artery pseudoaneurysms. J Trauma. 44(6):1008-13; discussion 1013-5, 1998
13. Emery KH: Splenic emergencies. Radiol Clin North Am. 35(4):831-43, 1997
14. Sarioglu A et al: Aneurysmatic arteriovenous fistula complicating splenic injury. Eur J Pediatr Surg. 6(3):183-5, 1996

SPLEEN TRAUMA

IMAGE GALLERY

Typical

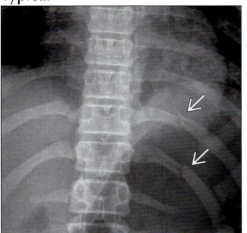
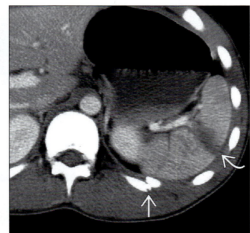

(Left) Anteroposterior radiograph shows multiple lower posterior rib fractures *(arrows)* in this patient with a splenic laceration. *(Right)* Axial CECT in the same patient shows a hypodense splenic laceration *(curved arrow)* with an associated rib fracture *(arrow)*.

Variant

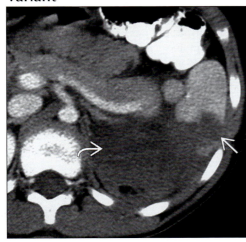
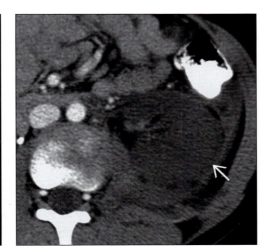

(Left) Axial CECT shows hypodense laceration along inferior spleen *(arrow)* with a large pararenal space hematoma *(curved arrow)* in this patient with a grade III splenic laceration. *(Right)* Axial CECT in the same patient shows lack of contrast-enhancement, an associated devascularization injury to the left kidney *(arrow)* & pararenal space hematoma.

Variant

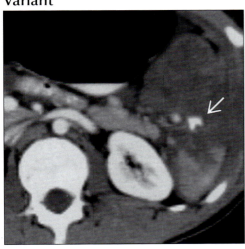
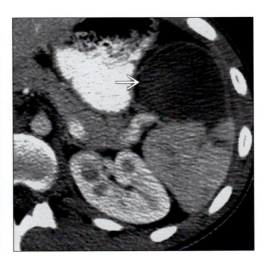

(Left) Axial CECT shows blush of active extravasation or bleeding *(arrow)* with HU values equal to aorta. This patient was treated non-operatively. *(Right)* Axial CECT follow-up image in the same patient shows development of an early splenic pseudocyst *(arrow)*, near water in attenuation.

DUODENAL HEMATOMA

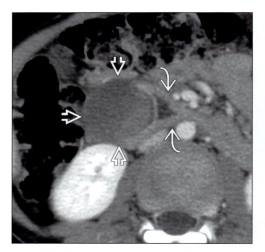

Axial CECT shows a well-circumscribed low attenuation mass (open arrows) located at 2nd and 3rd portion of duodenum (curved arrows) in 6 year old with blunt trauma from a bicycle handlebar.

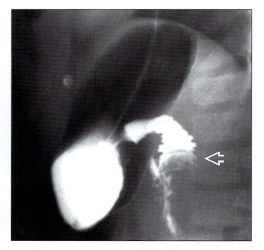

Lateral upper GI (same child) shows a partially obstructing rounded intraluminal mass (open arrow) in 2nd portion of duodenum caused by a large duodenal hematoma.

TERMINOLOGY

Definitions
- Intramural duodenal hematoma due to
  - Blunt trauma (most common)
  - Child abuse
  - Iatrogenic
  - Bleeding disorder
  - Henoch-Schönlein purpura (HSP)

IMAGING FINDINGS

General Features
- Best diagnostic clue
  - CECT: Mass 2nd or 3rd portion of duodenum in child with trauma, esophagogastroduodenoscopy (EGD), or bleeding disorder
  - Upper gastrointestinal (UGI): Intraluminal filling defect or obstruction of duodenum
- Location: Most commonly 2nd or 3rd portion of duodenum
- Size: Variable
- Morphology
  - Variable
    - Eccentric: Tends to be round or ovoid
    - Circumferential: Thickened duodenal wall
- Most common site of bowel injury in blunt abdominal trauma (25%)
- Important to assess for duodenal perforation (requires emergency surgical repair)
  - Extraluminal enteric contrast: 100% specific for perforation
  - Extraluminal gas
  - Retroperitoneal fluid
- Frequently associated with pancreatic injury in cases of blunt trauma

Fluoroscopic Findings
- Upper GI
  - Intraluminal filling defect or obstruction in duodenum
  - Variable appearances
    - Eccentric hematoma: Rounded intraluminal filling defect
    - Circumferential hematoma: Short or long segment luminal narrowing with thickened duodenal folds
    - Coil spring appearance

CT Findings
- CECT
  - Eccentric or circumferential bowel wall thickening
  - 2nd or 3rd portion of duodenum most common
  - Luminal narrowing
  - Hematoma initially high attenuation → gradually decreases in attenuation as hematoma evolves

DDx: Duodenal Obstruction

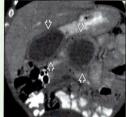
Duplication Cysts

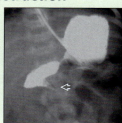
Midgut Volvulus

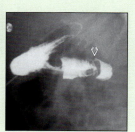
Duodenal Web

DUODENAL HEMATOMA

Key Facts

Imaging Findings
- CECT: Mass 2nd or 3rd portion of duodenum in child with trauma, esophagogastroduodenoscopy (EGD), or bleeding disorder
- Upper gastrointestinal (UGI): Intraluminal filling defect or obstruction of duodenum
- Most common site of bowel injury in blunt abdominal trauma (25%)
- Important to assess for duodenal perforation (requires emergency surgical repair)
- Frequently associated with pancreatic injury in cases of blunt trauma

Top Differential Diagnoses
- Enteric duplication cyst
- Small bowel malrotation/midgut volvulus

Clinical Issues
- Vomiting
- Abdominal pain
- Excellent prognosis
- Supportive care
- Resolves spontaneously
- Surgical repair
- If conservative management fails

Diagnostic Checklist
- Duodenal hematoma in vomiting child with
- Blunt abdominal trauma (most common)
- EGD with biopsy
- Bleeding disorder
- HSP

- High association with pancreatic trauma
- Proximal distention of small bowel and stomach due to obstruction

MR Findings
- T1 C+
  - Mass does not enhance
  - Thin rim-enhancement
- T1WI, T2WI
  - Duodenal mass with variable signal intensity
    - Signal depends on age of hematoma and state of degradation of blood

Ultrasonographic Findings
- Grayscale Ultrasound
  - Hypoechoic heterogeneous mass in duodenum
    - Becomes more hypoechoic with increased through transmission with time
  - Well-circumscribed
  - Most commonly found in 2nd or 3rd portion of duodenum
- Color Doppler: No color flow within hematoma

Imaging Recommendations
- Best imaging tool
  - CECT abdomen
    - Oral contrast → ↑ sensitivity and specificity for duodenal perforation
- Protocol advice: Routine CECT abdomen + oral contrast

DIFFERENTIAL DIAGNOSIS

Enteric duplication cyst
- Well-circumscribed cystic mass along medial wall of 2nd or 3rd portion of duodenum
- 12% occur in gastroduodenal location
- Similar appearance to eccentric duodenal hematoma
- US: Cyst wall frequently has "gut-signature"
- Abnormality of recanalization of duodenal lumen

Small bowel malrotation/midgut volvulus
- Bilious vomiting
- May have duodenal obstruction due to midgut volvulus or congenital peritoneal bands
- CT
  - Duodenum does not cross midline
  - Superior mesenteric vein (SMV) left of superior mesenteric artery (SMA)
  - Colon may be on left side
- UGI
  - Midgut volvulus: May see abrupt occlusion of duodenum or
    - "Corkscrew" appearance of small bowel
    - Abnormal location of duodenal jejunal junction
    - Surgical emergency because bowel may become ischemic

Crohn disease
- Involves duodenum in 5-20% of patients
- Duodenal ulcer or stricture
- Duodenal inflammation/wall thickening
- May form fistula with adjacent large or small bowel

Duodenal web
- Similar symptoms: Vomiting, feeding intolerance
- No history of trauma
- Presents early or later in childhood
- Higher incidence in Down syndrome and children with other congenital abnormalities

Duodenal ulcer/duodenitis
- Rare in children
- Duodenal wall edema
- May perforate →
  - Extraluminal gas
  - Extraluminal fluid
- May cause duodenal stricture and gastric outlet obstruction
- If distal to duodenal bulb, consider
  - Zollinger-Ellison syndrome
  - Crohn disease

Small bowel malignancy
- Very rare in children

DUODENAL HEMATOMA

- Gastrointestinal stromal tumor (GIST), lipoma, adenoma, adenocarcinoma, lymphoma, metastases
- Typically enhance with intravenous contrast, unlike hematoma
- May cause duodenal obstruction and vomiting

Pancreatitis
- Inflamed pancreas/pancreatic pseudocysts → mass effect or inflammation of duodenum → narrowing of duodenal lumen → obstruction → vomiting
- Abdominal pain

Annular pancreas
- May present in first decade of life with duodenal stenosis and vomiting
- 50% not diagnosed until adulthood
- May be difficult to appreciate by CT

Pancreatic tumor
- Rare
- Mass effect may compress duodenum

PATHOLOGY

General Features
- Etiology
  - Blunt trauma
    - Compression of duodenum against vertebral body
    - Sudden blow to epigastrium
    - Lap belts, bicycle handlebar, child abuse (punching child in stomach)
    - In children < 4 years old, duodenal injury most often due to child abuse
    - Visceral trauma is the second leading cause of death in child abuse behind central nervous system (CNS) trauma
  - Iatrogenic
    - Upper endoscopic biopsy
    - Ph probe placement
  - Bleeding disorder
    - Iatrogenic (Warfarin or Heparin)
    - Chemotherapy → thrombocytopenia
    - Liver disease → abnormal coagulation factors and abnormal platelet function
    - Hemophilia
    - Other causes of abnormal coagulation or thrombocytopenia
  - Henoch-Schönlein purpura (HSP)
    - Systemic hypersensitivity disease of unknown etiology
    - Abnormal permeability of small blood vessels caused by deposition of immune complexes within small vessels throughout body
    - Purpuric rash, glomerulonephritis, and gastrointestinal (GI) tract hemorrhage
    - May see multifocal areas of bowel wall thickening and mesenteric edema

Gross Pathologic & Surgical Features
- Intramural hematoma

CLINICAL ISSUES

Presentation
- Most common signs/symptoms
  - Vomiting
  - Abdominal pain

Demographics
- Gender
  - M > F
    - Likely due to association with trauma

Natural History & Prognosis
- Spontaneously resolves over several weeks
- Excellent prognosis

Treatment
- Supportive care
  - Feeding tube to bypass obstruction caused by hematoma
  - Resolves spontaneously
  - May have delayed perforation or stricture
- Surgical repair
  - If conservative management fails
    - Persistent pain
    - Signs of infection
    - Perforation of duodenal wall
  - Percutaneous drainage may be a less invasive alternative

DIAGNOSTIC CHECKLIST

Consider
- Duodenal hematoma in vomiting child with
  - Blunt abdominal trauma (most common)
  - EGD with biopsy
  - Bleeding disorder
  - HSP

SELECTED REFERENCES

1. Gullotto C et al: CT-guided percutaneous drainage of a duodenal hematoma. AJR Am J Roentgenol. 184(1):231-3, 2005
2. Gaines BA et al: Duodenal injuries in children: beware of child abuse. J Pediatr Surg. 39(4):600-2, 2004
3. Desai KM et al: Blunt duodenal injuries in children. J Trauma. 54(4):640-5; discussion 645-6, 2003
4. Jayaraman MV et al: CT of the duodenum: an overlooked segment gets its due. Radiographics. 21 Spec No:S147-60, 2001
5. Brody JM et al: CT of blunt trauma bowel and mesenteric injury: typical findings and pitfalls in diagnosis. Radiographics. 20(6):1525-36; discussion 1536-7, 2000
6. Strouse PJ et al: CT of bowel and mesenteric trauma in children. Radiographics. 19(5):1237-50, 1999
7. Kurkchubasche AG et al: Blunt intestinal injury in children. Diagnostic and therapeutic considerations. Arch Surg. 132(6):652-7; discussion 657-8, 1997
8. Kunin JR et al: Duodenal injuries caused by blunt abdominal trauma: value of CT in differentiating perforation from hematoma. AJR Am J Roentgenol. 160(6):1221-3, 1993

DUODENAL HEMATOMA

IMAGE GALLERY

Typical

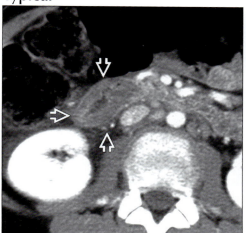
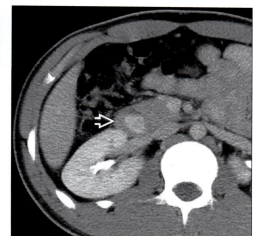

(Left) Axial CECT shows a circumferential hematoma at junction between 2nd and 3rd portions of the duodenum (open arrows), a common location. *(Right)* Axial CECT shows a small round high attenuation mass in duodenal wall, representing a duodenal hematoma (open arrow).

Typical

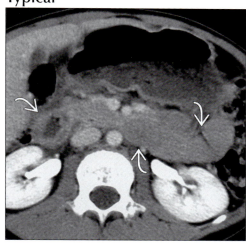
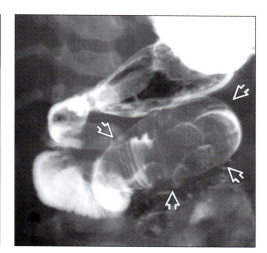

(Left) Axial CECT shows long duodenal hematoma in 3rd portion of duodenum with homogeneous intermediate attenuation (curved arrows), a less common location of a duodenal hematoma. *(Right)* Anteroposterior upper GI shows a long filling defect (open arrows) distending the distal duodenum and proximal jejunum caused by a large intramural hematoma.

Typical

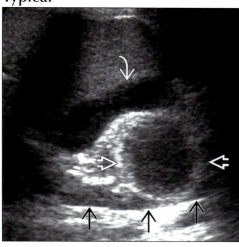
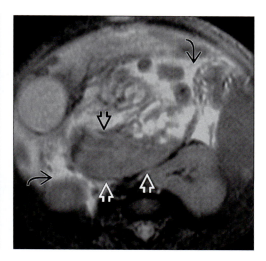

(Left) Sagittal ultrasound shows duodenal hematoma as round hypoechoic mass (open arrows) with increased through-transmission, located between gall bladder (curved arrow) and IVC (arrows). *(Right)* Axial T2WI MR shows an intermediate signal intensity hematoma filling the 3rd portion of duodenum (open arrows) in patient with liver disease and EGD biopsy. Note ascites (curved arrows).

LYMPHOPROLIFERATIVE DISORDER

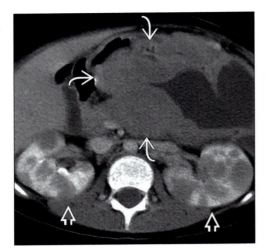

Axial CECT shows extensive PTLD as multiple low attenuation lesions in both kidneys (open arrows) and stomach wall (curved arrows) in 8 year old with liver transplant for hepatoblastoma.

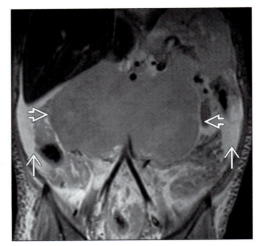

Coronal STIR MR shows large mass at mesenteric root (open arrows) in 3 year old with heart transplant for hypoplastic left heart. Biopsy: EBV+ Burkitt lymphoma. Ascites (arrows).

TERMINOLOGY

Abbreviations and Synonyms
- Posttransplantation lymphoproliferative disorder (PTLD)
- Posttransplant lymphoproliferative disorder (PTLD)

Definitions
- Spectrum of abnormal lymphoid proliferation in transplant patient that straddles the border between malignancy and infection

IMAGING FINDINGS

General Features
- Best diagnostic clue: Lymphadenopathy or solid mass anywhere in organ transplant patient
- Location
  - Virtually anywhere, any organ system
  - More often near transplant organ
  - Not infrequently located in transplant organ
- Size: Variable
- Morphology
  - Variable, "protean"
    - Adenopathy
    - Discrete masses
    - Infiltrative masses

CT Findings
- CECT
  - CT Abdomen
    - Adenopathy
    - Discrete mass or masses of variable sizes
    - Splenomegaly
    - Hepatomegaly
    - Extranodal (parenchymal organ) masses more common than adenopathy or splenic involvement (different from lymphoma in nontransplant patient)
  - CT Chest
    - Parenchymal opacity
    - Mediastinal mass
    - Cardiac mass (heart transplant)
  - CT Neck
    - Nonspecific adenopathy
    - Enlarged tonsils
  - CT Head
    - Low attenuation parenchymal lesions surrounded by vasogenic edema
    - +/- Enhancement

MR Findings
- T1WI: Usually intermediate signal intensity
- T2WI: Usually high signal intensity
- T1 C+ FS: Usually enhance

DDx: Abdominal Pain In Children With Transplants

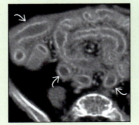

GVHD

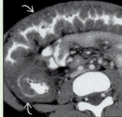

Pseudom Colitis

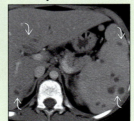

Fungal Abscesses

LYMPHOPROLIFERATIVE DISORDER

Key Facts

Terminology
- Posttransplant lymphoproliferative disorder (PTLD)
- Spectrum of abnormal lymphoid proliferation in transplant patient that straddles the border between malignancy and infection

Imaging Findings
- Best diagnostic clue: Lymphadenopathy or solid mass anywhere in organ transplant patient
- Variable, "protean"
- Adenopathy
- Discrete masses
- Infiltrative masses

Pathology
- Ebstein-Barr virus (EBV) infects lymphoid cells in immunosuppressed transplant patient →
- Unregulated expansion of lymphoid cells = PTLD
- Most cases of PTLD occur in children who are seronegative for EBV (EBV-) at time of transplantation and subsequently develop primary EBV infection and become seropositive (EBV+)
- Higher incidence also associated with cytomegalovirus (CMV) infection
- Incidence higher in transplants that require more immunosuppression
- Heart, lung, liver, small bowel > kidney transplants
- Range from lymphoid hyperplasia to malignant lymphoid proliferation

Clinical Issues
- Nonspecific, requires high level of clinical suspicion
- Reduced immunosuppression
- Chemotherapy

Ultrasonographic Findings
- Grayscale Ultrasound: Solid masses with variable echogenicity

Nuclear Medicine Findings
- PET
  - Variable uptake with fluoro-deoxy-glucose (FDG)
  - Little data to date

Imaging Recommendations
- Best imaging tool
  - Body (neck, chest, abdomen, and pelvis): CECT
  - Brain and spine: MRI without and with contrast
- Protocol advice: Routine protocols with contrast typically sufficient

DIFFERENTIAL DIAGNOSIS

Graft versus host diseases (GVHD)
- Allogenic bone marrow transplant patients
- Lymphocytes from donor attack the recipient's tissues
- May involve small bowel and large bowel
- May have similar symptoms, including diarrhea which is sometimes bloody, abdominal pain and cramping
- CT: Diffuse bowel wall enhancement with mild bowel wall thickening (small and large bowel)
- CT or small bowel follow through (SBFT): Featureless "ribbon-like" appearance of small bowel due to diffuse luminal narrowing
- Treatment → ↑ immunosuppression

Colitis
- Fever
- Diarrhea
  - Watery, bloody
- Abdominal pain
- CT: Circumferential colonic wall thickening
- Abdominal radiograph: "Thumbprinting" of colon wall
- Types: Pseudomembranous, neutropenic, other infectious
- If severe infection, may be associated with pneumatosis, perforation, and pericolonic fluid

Fungal infection
- Candida most common type to infect gastrointestinal (GI) tract, liver, and spleen
  - May cause esophagitis
    - Esophagram: Dysmotility, "shaggy mucosa", "cobblestone" appearance
    - Nonspecific appearance that cannot be radiographically distinguished from other infectious etiologies
  - May cause microabscess in liver, spleen, and kidneys
    - US: Multiple hypoechoic lesions, some with hyperechoic centers → "target" or "bull's eye"
    - CT: Multiple low attenuation lesions
    - Image guided aspiration may be performed for diagnosis
- Aspergillus may involve lungs, sinuses or brain
  - Lungs: Invasive aspergillosis: Best to surgically resect if possible
- Present with fever

PATHOLOGY

General Features
- Etiology
  - Normal immune surveillance, lost in immunosuppressed patients, is essential for
    - Control of viral infection
    - Prevention of neoplasm
  - Ebstein-Barr virus (EBV) infects lymphoid cells in immunosuppressed transplant patient →
    - Unregulated expansion of lymphoid cells = PTLD
- Epidemiology
  - Most cases of PTLD occur in children who are seronegative for EBV (EBV-) at time of transplantation and subsequently develop primary EBV infection and become seropositive (EBV+)
    - EBV plays pivotal role (85-90%) in most pediatric PTLD
    - EBV acquired from donor organ or community
    - Most are EBV+ B-cell

LYMPHOPROLIFERATIVE DISORDER

- Remainder are T-cell, myeloma, or EBV- B-cell lymphoma
- Higher incidence also associated with cytomegalovirus (CMV) infection
- Incidence increases with increased immunosuppression
  - Range: 1-20% of children with organ transplants
- Incidence higher in transplants that require more immunosuppression
  - Heart, lung, liver, small bowel > kidney transplants
- Adults are more likely to be EBV+ at time of transplantation → immune system better able to control EBV infection → lower rate of PTLD

Microscopic Features
- Range from lymphoid hyperplasia to malignant lymphoid proliferation

Staging, Grading or Classification Criteria
- American Society of Hematopathology: 3 general categories
  - Hyperplastic
    - Preservation of normal tissue architecture
    - Benign end of spectrum
  - Polymorphic
    - Effacement and destruction of normal tissue architecture
    - Lymphoid infiltrates of varying shapes and sizes
  - Monomorphic
    - Destructive lymphoid infiltrate
    - Cells closely resemble lymphoma

CLINICAL ISSUES

Presentation
- Most common signs/symptoms
  - Nonspecific, requires high level of clinical suspicion
  - Depends on location of mass
    - Neuro: Seizure or focal neurological deficit
    - Head and neck: Mononucleosis-like symptoms including fever, malaise, adenopathy, pharyngitis
    - Chest: May be asymptomatic with incidental parenchymal opacity on chest radiograph, fever, decreased pulmonary function tests
    - Abdomen: Abdominal pain, distention, bloody stool, intussusception, multisystem organ failure

Demographics
- Age: Children > adults

Natural History & Prognosis
- Better prognosis with early detection
  - Median onset 4 months to 7 years following transplant
  - Earlier onset if EBV+ transplant organ → EBV- transplant recipient
- Universally fatal if not treated
- Prognosis depends on degree of immunosuppression
  - More immunosuppressed → poorer prognosis
- Histology
  - Best Prognosis
    - Polymorphic
    - Polyclonal
    - Confined to lymph node or single organ
    - Responds to decreased immunosuppression
  - Worst prognosis
    - Monomorphic → similar to lymphoma, usually requires chemotherapy

Treatment
- 2 primary methods
  - Reduced immunosuppression
    - When detect EBV seroconversion or primary EBV infection
    - Works best in polymorphic PTLD (recover natural immune surveillance)
    - Must balance with risk of transplant rejection
  - Chemotherapy
    - For overt malignancy (Burkitt lymphoma)
    - If inadequate response to reduced immunosuppression
- Second line treatment
  - IVIG (anti-EBV antibodies)
  - Anti-B-cell monoclonal antibodies
  - Cellular immunotherapy
  - Interferon alpha
  - Chemotherapy
  - Surgery

DIAGNOSTIC CHECKLIST

Consider
- PTLD in transplant patient with fever, nonspecific symptoms, EBV seroconversion
- PTLD in transplant patient with adenopathy or mass

Image Interpretation Pearls
- Adenopathy or mass in transplant patient = PTLD until proven otherwise
- Imaging plays key role in detecting disease and guiding biopsy for definitive diagnosis

SELECTED REFERENCES

1. Green M et al: Posttransplantation lymphoproliferative disorders. Pediatr Clin North Am. 50(6):1471-91, 2003
2. Lim GY et al: Posttransplantation lymphoproliferative disorder: manifestations in pediatric thoracic organ recipients. Radiology. 222(3):699-708, 2002
3. Pickhardt PJ et al: Posttransplantation lymphoproliferative disorder in children: clinical, histopathologic, and imaging features. Radiology. 217(1):16-25, 2000
4. Pickhardt PJ et al: Posttransplantation lymphoproliferative disorder of the abdomen: CT evaluation in 51 patients. Radiology. 213(1):73-8, 1999
5. Praghakaran K et al: Rational management of posttransplant lymphoproliferative disorder in pediatric recipients. J Pediatr Surg. 34(1):112-5; discussion 115-6, 1999
6. Donnelly LF et al: Lymphoproliferative disorders: CT findings in immunocompromised children. AJR Am J Roentgenol. 171(3):725-31, 1998
7. Rowe DT et al: Use of quantitative competitive PCR to measure Epstein-Barr virus genome load in the peripheral blood of pediatric transplant patients with lymphoproliferative disorders. J Clin Microbiol. 35(6):1612-5, 1997

LYMPHOPROLIFERATIVE DISORDER

IMAGE GALLERY

Typical

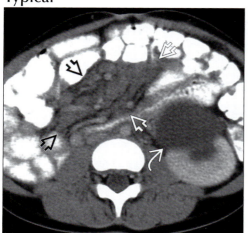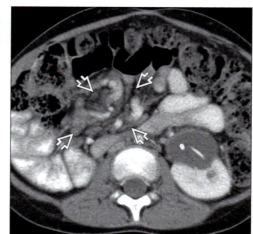

(Left) Axial CECT in 6 year old with liver transplant shows PTLD presenting as mesenteric adenopathy (open arrows) and GI bleed. Incidental ureteropelvic junction (UPJ) obstruction (curved arrow). *(Right)* Axial CECT (same patient) shows dramatic decrease in size of mesenteric nodes (open arrows) after reduced immunosuppression. Biopsy (before treatment): EBV+ atypical lymphoid hyperplasia.

Typical

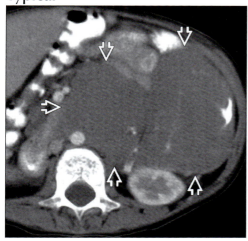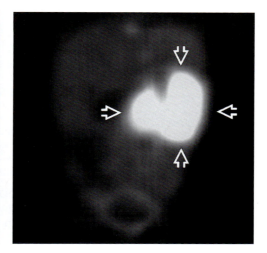

(Left) Axial CECT shows PTLD as large retroperitoneal and colon wall mass (open arrows) in 4 year old with liver transplant 3 years prior. Presented with abdominal pain and bloody stool. *(Right)* Coronal PET shows (same patient as left) with increased FDG uptake in large PTLD mass (open arrows). Biopsy: EBV+ monomorphic Burkitt-like B-cell lymphoma.

Variant

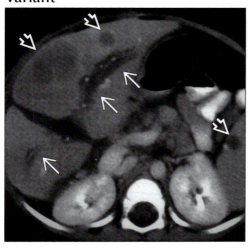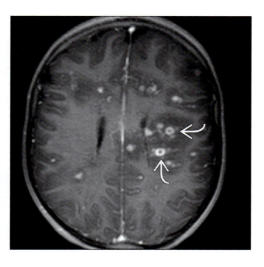

(Left) Axial CECT shows liver and splenic lesions (open arrows) in liver transplant patient. Note low attenuation masses along portal vein branches (arrows), a pattern typical for PTLD. *(Right)* Axial T1 C+ MR shows multiple ring enhancing lesions (curved arrows) throughout brain in child with renal transplant. Biopsy revealed EBV+ PTLD. Uncommon, especially with renal transplants.

PSEUDOMEMBRANOUS COLITIS

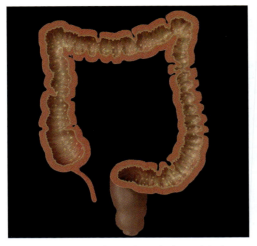

Graphic shows pancolitis with marked mural thickening with multiple elevated yellow-white plaques (pseudomembranes).

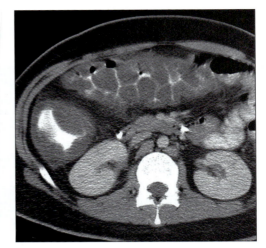

Axial CECT shows marked pancolitis with enteric contrast trapped between thickened haustral folds ("accordian sign").

TERMINOLOGY

Abbreviations and Synonyms
- Common acronym: Pseudomembranous colitis (PMC)
- Antibiotic associated colitis, clostridium difficile (C. difficile) colitis & necrotizing colitis

Definitions
- Inflammation of colon caused by clostridium difficile & toxins A & B produced by this organism
- PMC is usually associated with antibiotic use; especially ampicillin in children, clindamycin in adults
  - Antibiotics alter the normal bowel flora & allow overgrowth of certain bacteria

IMAGING FINDINGS

General Features
- Best diagnostic clue: Classic imaging appearance: Colonic submucosal edema causing wall thickening & nodularity
- Location
  - Usually pancolitis
  - Rectum & sigmoid colon: Up to 95% of cases
  - Proximal colon only: 10-20%
- Morphology: Plaque-like necrotic tissue with mucus on damaged colonic mucosa

Radiographic Findings
- Radiography
  - Thickened nodular haustral folds
  - Thumbprinting
    - Most commonly transverse colon
  - Small bowel ileus: 20-25%
  - Fulminant cases
    - Toxic megacolon: Mortality when presents as high as 35%
    - Perforation

Fluoroscopic Findings
- Barium enema (BE) studies
  - Small nodular filling defects
  - Contraindicated in severe or fulminant cases of PMC due to risk of perforation

CT Findings
- CECT
  - CT 88% positive predictive value with the highest sensitivity & specificity
    - Treatment may be merited based on CT findings alone
  - Pancolitis is most common
  - Right colon may be involved exclusively in select cases of PMC

DDx: Other Causes of Colitis

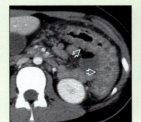
Crohn

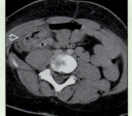
Typhlitis

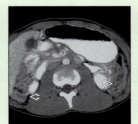
Salmonella

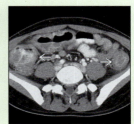
UC

PSEUDOMEMBRANOUS COLITIS

Key Facts

Terminology
- Common acronym: Pseudomembranous colitis (PMC)
- Antibiotic associated colitis, clostridium difficile (C. difficile) colitis & necrotizing colitis

Imaging Findings
- Best diagnostic clue: Classic imaging appearance: Colonic submucosal edema causing wall thickening & nodularity
- Usually pancolitis
- "Accordion sign"
- "Target sign"

Top Differential Diagnoses
- Infectious colitis
- Crohn disease: Granulomatous colitis
- Ulcerative colitis (UC)
- Typhlitis

Pathology
- Antibiotic or chemotherapy alters gut flora permitting C. difficile overgrowth with release of toxins produced by organism causing symptoms
- C. difficile in bowel flora in 2-5% of healthy adults & 50-70% of healthy infants

Clinical Issues
- Most common signs/symptoms: Profuse foul smelling watery diarrhea

Diagnostic Checklist
- Marked colonic bowel wall thickening
- Wall thickening disproportionately greater compared to degree of pericolonic edema

---

- Colonic wall thickening, nodularity & mural plaques
  - Mural thickening > 3-4 mm
  - Thickening more ill-defined in PMC than in Crohn's disease
- "Accordion sign"
  - Alternating bands of higher attenuation enteric contrast & lower attenuation thickened haustral folds
  - Think PMC
  - 50-70%
- "Target sign"
  - Hyperemic enhancing mucosa surrounded by thickened low attenuation submucosa edema
- Pericolonic stranding is often present but disproportionately less severe compared to degree of bowel wall thickening because PMC is mucosal disease
- Ascites: Unusual in other forms of inflammatory bowel disease
- Pneumoperitoneum

Other Modality Findings
- Indium-labeled leukocytes: Nonspecific inflammation of the colon

Imaging Recommendations
- Best imaging approach is CECT with 2 hour oral contrast prep

DIFFERENTIAL DIAGNOSIS

Infectious colitis
- Has less wall thickening than PMC
- May be indistinguishable form PMC
- Right colon predominant: Shigella & Salmonella
- Diffuse colonic involvement: E. Coli
- Others: Campylobacter, Yersinia (TI and cecum), Amebiasis, TB (TI & cecum +/- ascending & transverse colon), CMV

Crohn disease: Granulomatous colitis
- Concurrent small bowel disease is norm
- Segmental distribution, skip lesions
- Cobblestoning, transmural (asymmetric bowel wall involvement), fissures & fistulas
- "Creeping fat": Fibrofatty proliferation of the mesentery on CT, fibrosis & strictures

Ulcerative colitis (UC)
- Pancolitis with "collar button" ulcerations of BE
- Wall thickening < 10 mm
- Symmetric wall thickening, inflammatory polyps & pseudopolyps

Typhlitis
- History of neutropenia

Ischemic colitis
- May also be focal or diffuse
- More commonly seen in watershed area
- Has less wall thickening than PMC

Colonic Non-Hodgkin lymphoma (NHL)
- Any condition that has "thumbprinting" can mimic PMC including NHL, carcinoma, amyloid infiltration & typhlitis

PATHOLOGY

General Features
- Etiology
  - Antibiotic or chemotherapy alters gut flora permitting C. difficile overgrowth with release of toxins produced by organism causing symptoms
    - PMC usually presents 4-9 days after starting antibiotic therapy
    - Up to 1/3 present after antibiotics therapy has ended
    - Antibiotic therapy can be up to 6 months prior in selected cases
- Epidemiology
  - 1-10 cases per 1,000 patient discharges from hospital

PSEUDOMEMBRANOUS COLITIS

- 1 case per 10,000 antibiotic prescriptions written outside hospital
- C. difficile in bowel flora in 2-5% of healthy adults & 50-70% of healthy infants

Gross Pathologic & Surgical Features
- Inflamed colon with discrete or confluent, raised, tan-black nodules that are 2-20 mm in size = pseudomembranes
- When removed during endoscopy, reveals erythematous, inflamed mucosa

Microscopic Features
- Colonization of colon by c. difficile present
- Mild-early: Focal necrosis of surface epithelial cells in glandular crypts with neutrophilic infiltration
  - Fibrin plugging of the capillaries in the lamina propria & mucus hypersecretion in adjacent crypts
- Moderate: Crypt abscesses
- Severe-late: Necrosis & denudation of mucosa with thrombosis of submucosal venules

CLINICAL ISSUES

Presentation
- Most common signs/symptoms: Profuse foul smelling watery diarrhea
- Most common sign/symptom
  - Asymptomatic state: Carrier
    - Up to 25% of inpatients on antibiotic therapy
  - Antibiotic associated diarrhea: 20% of all antibiotic associated diarrhea
  - PMC
    - Watery diarrhea, abdominal pain & cramping, bloody stools, ileus, leukocytosis (50%), fever (up to 50%)
  - Fulminant Colitis: 3%
    - Toxic Megacolon
    - Perforation
- Diagnosis made from stool assay: C. difficile cytotoxin
  - Typically takes 48 hours (2-5 days)
- Endoscopy can detect pseudomembranes but there is risk of perforation
  - May also be only isolated right colon involvement
- High risk groups: ICU patients, uremia, burn, c-section, cancer, recent abdominal surgery

Demographics
- Age
  - Rare in infants < 12 months due to passive protection by maternal antibodies
  - Elderly are higher risk for developing PMC & recurrent PMC than young
- Gender
  - M = F
  - Women have a higher recurrence rate

Natural History & Prognosis
- If treated early, full recovery expected
- Severe cases may need colectomy
- Untreated cases can lead to perforation, acute abdomen & death

Treatment
- Carrier state: No treatment
- Mild cases: Discontinuing or changing antibiotics is usually sufficient (most patients recover by 10 days)
  - Supportive therapy, avoid narcotics, avoid antidiarrheal drugs, enteric isolation
- More severe cases: Metronidazole (Flagyl) or oral vancomycin recommended therapy
  - Metronidazole = drug of choice (higher side effects)
  - Bacitracin
- In severe cases with megacolon, colectomy may become necessary (< 1%)

DIAGNOSTIC CHECKLIST

Consider
- Patients with a history of antibiotic therapy or high risk groups

Image Interpretation Pearls
- Pancolitis typical
- Marked colonic bowel wall thickening
- Wall thickening disproportionately greater compared to degree of pericolonic edema
- "Accordion sign": Enteric contrast trapped between thickened haustral folds
- "Target sign": Hyperemic mucosa surrounded by ↓ density submucosa

SELECTED REFERENCES

1. Oldfield EC 3rd: Clostridium difficile-associated diarrhea: risk factors, diagnostic methods, and treatment. Rev Gastroenterol Disord. 4(4):186-95, 2004
2. Hussain SZ et al: Clostridium difficile colitis in children with cystic fibrosis. Dig Dis Sci. 49(1):116-21, 2004
3. Jabbar A et al: Gastroenteritis and antibiotic-associated diarrhea. Prim Care. 30(1):63-80, vi, 2003
4. Spivack JG et al: Clostridium difficile-associated diarrhea in a pediatric hospital. Clin Pediatr (Phila). 42(4):347-52, 2003
5. Lembcke B et al: Antibiotic-associated diarrhea: therapeutic aspects and practical guidelines--an interdisciplinary approach to a common problem. Schweiz Rundsch Med Prax. 92(17):809-16, 2003
6. Beaugerie L et al: Antibiotic-associated diarrhoea and Clostridium difficile in the community. Aliment Pharmacol Ther. 17(7):905-12, 2003
7. Gronczenski CA. Katz JP: Clostridium Difficile Colitis. eMedicine Nov. 11, 2003
8. Iseman DT et al: Pseudomembranous (Clostridium difficile) colitis. Gastrointest Endosc. 56(6):907, 2002
9. Hurley BW et al: The spectrum of pseudomembranous enterocolitis and antibiotic-associated diarrhea. Arch Intern Med. 162(19):2177-84, 2002
10. Yassin SF: Pseudomembranous Colitis. eMedicine Nov.11, 2002
11. Kirkpatrick IDC et al: Evaluating the CT diagnosis of Clostridium difficile colitis: Should CT guide therapy? AJR 176:635-9, 2001
12. Fishman EK et al: Pseudomembranous colitis: CT evaluation in 26 cases. Radiology 180:57-60, 1991
13. Stanley RJ et al: The spectrum of radiographic findings in antibiotic related pseudomembranous colitis. Radiology 111:519-24, 1974

PSEUDOMEMBRANOUS COLITIS

IMAGE GALLERY

Typical

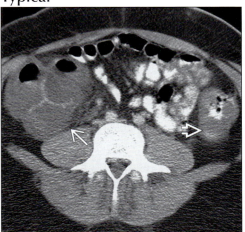
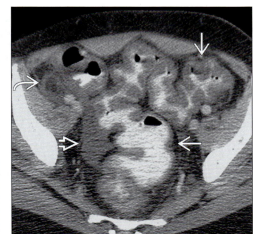

(Left) Axial CECT shows the typical massive mural plaques, submucosal edema of the cecum *(arrow)* & descending colon *(open arrow)*. *(Right)* Axial CECT shows typical pancolitis, marked thickening of the entire colon *(arrows)*, ascites *(open arrow)*, & pericolonic stranding *(curved arrow)* along the cecum.

Typical

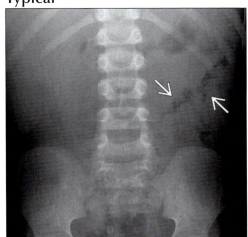
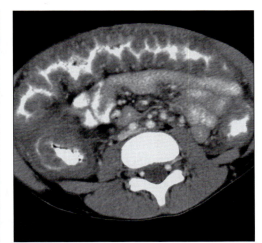

(Left) Anteroposterior radiograph shows marked thickening of the transverse colon *(arrows)* and very little bowel gas elsewhere. *(Right)* Axial CECT shows severe pancolitis with contrast trapped between haustra & marked mural thickening ("accordian sign") with pericolonic stranding.

Typical

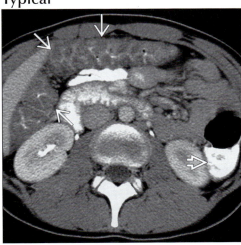
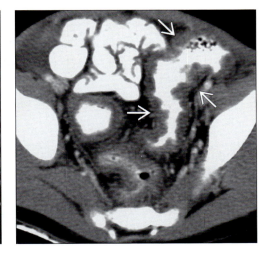

(Left) Axial CECT shows a variant example of mild mural thickening of the right colon *(arrows)* with sparing of the descending colon *(open arrow)*. *(Right)* Axial CECT shows marked mural thickening of the rectum and sigmoid colon *(arrow)*. The right colon in this case was spared.

NEUTROPENIC COLITIS

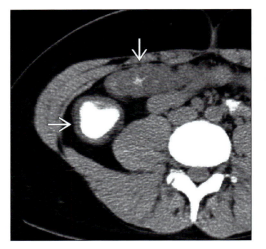

Axial CECT in this leukemic patient shows typical circumferential thickening of the wall of the cecum & ascending colon (arrows).

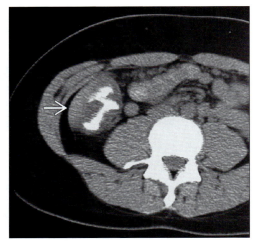

Axial CECT in this ALL patient shows irregular thickening of the cecum (arrow) & moderate luminal narrowing.

TERMINOLOGY

Abbreviations and Synonyms
- Synonym(s): Typhlitis, ileocecal syndrome, cecitis & necrotizing enteropathy

Definitions
- Inflammatory or necrotizing process that involves cecum, ascending colon & occasionally terminal ileum or appendix
- Classic imaging appearance
  - Massive mural thickening of wall of cecum/ascending colon
- Other general features
  - Children: Acute myelocytic leukemia (AML) or acute lymphocytic leukemia (ALL)
  - Usually seen in neutropenic patients after chemotherapy
  - Adults: Malignancy (mainly leukemia & lymphoma), aplastic anemia, organ & bone marrow transplantation, ischemia & infection
  - Clinical syndrome
    - Fever + right lower quadrant tenderness in immunosuppressed host
    - Typhlitis first reported in leukemic children undergoing chemotherapy

IMAGING FINDINGS

General Features
- Best diagnostic clue
  - Mural thickening of the cecum, +/- ascending colon, +/- terminal ileum (TI)
  - Diagnosis is made on basis of clinical & imaging findings after excluding other pathologic entities
- Location
  - Patterns
    - Cecum only
    - Cecum & ascending colon (most common)
    - Cecum, ascending colon & ileum
    - Cecum & sporadic ulcers through gastrointestinal (GI) tract
- Morphology: Cecal dilation or mural thickening & narrowing

Radiographic Findings
- Radiography
  - Ileocecal dilatation with air-fluid levels
  - Soft-tissue mass in right lower quadrant (RLQ)
  - Localized thumbprinting of ascending colon due to bowel edema
  - Distended small bowel (SB)
  - ± Pneumatosis: Seen as speckled or linear pattern (uncommon)

DDx: Causes Of Cecal Bowel Wall Thickening

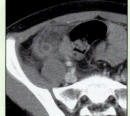
Appendicitis

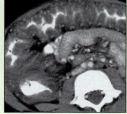
PMC

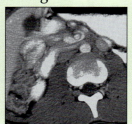
Salmonella

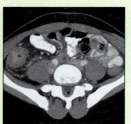
Crohn

NEUTROPENIC COLITIS

Key Facts

Terminology
- Synonym(s): Typhlitis, ileocecal syndrome, cecitis & necrotizing enteropathy
- Inflammatory or necrotizing process that involves cecum, ascending colon & occasionally terminal ileum or appendix
- Classic imaging appearance
- Massive mural thickening of wall of cecum/ascending colon

Imaging Findings
- Circumferential symmetric wall thickening of cecum +/- ascending colon & distal ileum
- Heterogeneous enhancement of bowel wall
- High attenuation regions reflect hemorrhage
- Helical NE + CECT
- Study of choice for diagnosis of typhlitis
- Contrast enema & colonoscopy
- Contraindicated due to ↑ risk of perforation

Top Differential Diagnoses
- Crohn disease
- Appendicitis
- Infectious colitis
- Pseudomembranous colitis (PMC)
- Ischemic
- Acute graft versus host (GVH)

Diagnostic Checklist
- In any child with neutropenia & RLQ symptoms, especially in a child with AML & ALL, bone marrow transplantation & chemotherapy history
- Cecal thickening or dilation in a severely neutropenic child

Fluoroscopic Findings
- Fluoroscopic guided contrast enema: Barium or water-soluble contrast findings
  - Mural thickening & mucosal thumbprinting
  - Luminal narrowing or dilatation of cecum
  - ± Dilatation of adjacent bowel loops (due to paralytic ileus)
  - Shallow or deep ulcerations
- Not recommended: ↑ Incidence of bowel perforation

CT Findings
- NECT
  - Cecal luminal distention or narrowing
    - Fluid-filled cecum or wall thickening
  - Circumferential symmetric wall thickening of cecum +/- ascending colon & distal ileum
    - > 3-4 mm
  - ↓ Bowel-wall attenuation (due to edema)
  - ↑ Attenuation of pericecal fat & thickening of fascial planes (inflammatory stranding or pericolonic inflammation)
  - +/- Intramural pneumatosis, pneumoperitoneum & pericolic fluid collection
  - +/- Dilatation of adjacent bowel loops (due to paralytic ileus)
- CECT
  - Heterogeneous enhancement of bowel wall
    - High attenuation regions reflect hemorrhage

Ultrasonographic Findings
- Grayscale Ultrasound
  - Hypoechoic or hyperechoic mural thickening
  - Anechoic free fluid; +/- mixed echoic abscess
  - Increased color flow, hypervascularity
  - "Target sign"

Imaging Recommendations
- Best imaging tool
  - Helical NE + CECT
    - Study of choice for diagnosis of typhlitis
  - Contrast enema & colonoscopy
    - Contraindicated due to ↑ risk of perforation

DIFFERENTIAL DIAGNOSIS

Crohn disease
- Transmural noncaseating granulomas & skip lesions (up to 90%), discontinuous GI involvement
- Anywhere from mouth to anus
  - Most common involvement of TI
- Bowel wall thickening: Average thickness of 11 mm, 1-2 cm
- Aphthous ulcers (up to 5 mm), cobblestone mucosa (longitudinal & transverse ulcers)
- Fissures, sinuses & fistulas (anywhere, most common entero-enteric)
- "String sign", strictures (20%), perirectal/anal disease (up to 80%)

Appendicitis
- Clinical mimicker
- Appendix can be inflamed in both
- Lack of mural thickening or thumbprinting differentiates from typhlitis

Infectious colitis
- TB: Narrowed cecum & TI
- Salmonella, amebiasis, cytomegalovirus (CMV), herpes & fungal
- Yersinia: Typically TI

Pseudomembranous colitis (PMC)
- Due to Clostridium difficile bacteria, also seen in the neutropenic patient population
- Clinical history of antibiotic therapy with laboratory correlation
- Typically pancolitis, right colon only 10-20%
- Mesenteric infiltration & ascites similar to neutropenic colitis
- Mean bowel wall thickness of 11-12 mm, greater fold thickening & wall nodularity
  - "Accordion sign": Trapped enteric contrast between thickened haustral folds

Ischemic
- Also must be considered in patients with pneumatosis

NEUTROPENIC COLITIS

Acute graft versus host (GVH)
- Also a complication of neutropenia
- Mean bowel wall thickness of 5 mm, < 7 mm
- More common hyperintense mucosal enhancement & bowel dilation

PATHOLOGY

General Features
- General path comments: Hemorrhage (intramural & intraluminal), edema, ulceration, +/- transmural necrosis from ischemic injury to the cecum
- Etiology
  - Neutropenia predisposing factors
    - Aplastic anemia
    - Immunosuppression, bone marrow or solid organ transplantation
    - Chemotherapy or cytotoxic drugs
    - Myelodysplastic syndrome
    - Infection: Acquired immunodeficiency syndrome (AIDS) & CMV; pseudomonas, clostridia, E. coli, Enterobacter or candida
  - Other causes of typhlitis
    - Leukemic or lymphomatous infiltrate
    - Ischemia
  - Mechanism
    - Multifactorial
    - Cytotoxic drugs & antibiotics → immunosuppression → neutropenia → infection → typhlitis
    - Ischemia → infection → typhlitis
    - Infiltration of bowel wall by neoplastic cells
    - Cecal dilation compromising blood flow leading to ischemia
    - All lead to the endpoint of mucosal injury & compromised bowel integrity, allowing for bacterial invasion & penetration into the bowel wall leading to submucosal necrosis and intraluminal hemorrhage

Gross Pathologic & Surgical Features
- Dilated cecum with thickened irregular wall +/- pericecal inflammation

Microscopic Features
- Inflammatory, hemorrhagic, ischemic, necrotic (transmural) & ulcerative changes

CLINICAL ISSUES

Presentation
- Most common signs/symptoms
  - Fever, RLQ pain, watery diarrhea, +/- hematochezia
  - Fullness; palpable mass; RLQ pain (+/- rebound)
  - Mimics acute appendicitis
- Lab: Severe neutropenia (< 1,000 cells/microliter), leukopenia; +/- fecal occult blood
- Complications
  - Abscess, sepsis, perforation or death

Demographics
- Age: Incidence: Children > adults
- Gender: M = F

Natural History & Prognosis
- Early stage: Good
- Late stage: Poor
  - In 10% of leukemic children undergoing chemotherapy who die
- Usually reflects a relapse in a patient with leukemia
- Mortality rate: 40-50% medical only, 20% surgical intervention
  - Usually related to cecal necrosis, perforation & sepsis
- Prognosis related to the degree of neutropenia

Treatment
- Early recognition & treatment may affect outcome
- Early aggressive medical support
  - High dose of broad spectrum antibiotics; covering gram negative, anaerobic (clostridium) & fungal
  - Bowel rest, supplemental nutrition & IV fluids
  - Granulocyte transfusions
  - Avoid antidiarrheal or narcotics (can ↑ symptoms)
- Complicated case
  - Surgical resection of affected bowel
    - Uncontrollable GI bleeding (after correction of clotting abnormalities & improved neutropenia)
    - Perforation, abscess, obstruction & sepsis
    - Clinical deterioration
  - Granulocyte transfusions

DIAGNOSTIC CHECKLIST

Consider
- In any child with neutropenia & RLQ symptoms, especially in a child with AML & ALL, bone marrow transplantation & chemotherapy history

Image Interpretation Pearls
- Cecal thickening or dilation in a severely neutropenic child

SELECTED REFERENCES

1. Kirkpatrick ID et al: Gastrointestinal complications in the neutropenic patient: characterization and differentiation with abdominal CT. Radiology. 226(3):668-74, 2003
2. Horton KM et al: CT evaluation of the colon: Inflammatory disease. RadioGraphics. 20: 399-418, 2000
3. Sloas MM et al: Typhlitis in children with cancer: a 30-year experience. Clin Infect Dis. 17(3):484-90, 1993
4. Moir CR et al: Typhlitis: selective surgical management. Am J Surg. 151(5):563-6, 1986
5. Shamberger RC et al: The medical and surgical management of typhlitis in children with acute nonlymphocytic (myelogenous) leukemia. Cancer. 57(3):603-9, 1986
6. Adams GW et al: CT detection of typhlitis. Journal of Computed Assisted Tomography. 9: 363-5, 1985
7. Frick MP et al: Computed tomography of neutropenic colitis. AJR. 143: 763-5, 1984

ESOPHAGEAL STRICTURES

Key Facts

Imaging Findings
- Contrast esophagram demonstrates stricture
- Contrast-enhanced CT useful for complications

Top Differential Diagnoses
- Achalasia
- Foreign body in esophagus
- Vascular anomalies may cause extrinsic compression
- Cricopharyngeal achalasia
- Retropharyngeal abscess
- Gastroesophageal reflux and esophagitis

Pathology
- Post-operative esophageal atresia anastomotic stricture
- Caustic esophagitis and strictures
- Epidermolysis bullosa
- Infective esophagitis
- Dermatomyositis primarily affects the striated muscle of pharynx and upper esophagus
- Eosinophilic esophagitis
- Scleroderma is a mixed collagen disorder which has esophageal dysmotility
- Post-operative Nissen fundoplication
- Specific diagnosis may be made by biopsy or culture

Clinical Issues
- Infants present with eating and feeding problems
- Balloon dilatation is used for many conditions

- Chronic strictures appear tapered with smooth mucosa although they may have shouldered appearance
  - Infective esophagitis
    - Double-contrast esophagogram done in older children with possible esophagitis
    - Mucosal irregularities can be seen as raised mounds within esophagus
    - Lower two thirds may have mucosal irregularities and decreased motility and spasm
    - Severe infections esophagitis may progress to strictures
    - Tuberculosis esophagitis is very rare but may develop fistulous tracts or compression from adenopathy

DIFFERENTIAL DIAGNOSIS

Achalasia
- Failure of relaxation of lower esophageal sphincter
- Neuromuscular abnormality with thickening of circular and longitudinal muscles
- Children present with dysphagia and may have pulmonary disease
- Esophagus is dilated and air-fluid levels in upright position

Foreign body in esophagus
- Coins may be ingested and lodge in esophagus at thoracic inlet and at level of aortic arch
- Non-verbal child is not able to communicate or articulate
- Clinically they present with transient airway problems, drooling, or refusal to eat

Vascular anomalies may cause extrinsic compression
- May causes dysphagia and symptoms
- Classic patterns on esophagram demonstrate the differential diagnosis

Cricopharyngeal achalasia
- Failure of relaxation of the cricopharyngeal dysfunction may lead to feeding problems or aspiration
- Entity not well understood

Retropharyngeal abscess
- Young children present with fever, drooling and refusal to swallow
- Lateral radiograph demonstrates increase in retropharyngeal soft tissues with displacement of airway
- Computed tomography may demonstrate an abscess or phlegmon

Gastroesophageal reflux and esophagitis
- Commonly occurs in newborns to six months of age
- Persistent gastroesophageal reflux may cause esophagitis
- Esophagus becomes enlarged with decreased tone
- Children may or may not vomit and usually not associated with failure to thrive

PATHOLOGY

General Features
- Etiology
  - Post-operative esophageal atresia anastomotic stricture
    - Probably the most frequent cause of esophageal stricture
    - Children may have retained foreign bodies in proximal pouch
  - Caustic esophagitis and strictures
    - Accidental ingestion of household cleaners, lye ingestion, acid cleaning substance
    - Burns in the mouth and throat which cause swallowing difficulty and possible aspiration
    - Complications include acute perforation and mediastinitis

ESOPHAGEAL STRICTURES

- Strictures occur in 30% and incidence of reflux is high
- Epidermolysis bullosa
  - Hereditary disorder which has both an autosomal dominant and recessive form
  - Congenital hereditary disorder affecting squamous epithelium affecting skin and mucous membranes
  - Numerous bullous lesions, sloughing and then healing
  - Loss of motility, mucosal irregularity, ulceration, and stenosis
  - Scarring occurs after the vesicles have ruptured which lead to contractures, and esophageal strictures
- Foreign bodies in esophagus
  - Certain batteries can cause caustic burn injuries in esophagus within hours of ingestion
  - Chronic foreign bodies in the esophagus can erode, perforate and cause strictures
  - Large pills may lodge in esophagus and cause pain, erosions but rarely strictures
- Infective esophagitis
  - Children that are immunocompromised are at risk
  - AIDS patients may have moniliasis, cytomegalovirus, Herpes virus
  - Candida albicans is most common
  - Tuberculosis esophagitis has irregular mucosa often eccentric in position, extrinsic compressions from adjacent nodes and occasional fistulous tract
- Dermatomyositis primarily affects the striated muscle of pharynx and upper esophagus
  - Swallowing disorder and proximal esophagitis, strictures
  - Spontaneous perforation secondary to vasculitis
- Eosinophilic esophagitis
  - Peripheral eosinophilia and infiltration of the gastrointestinal tract
  - Dysphagia with abnormal manometry
  - Biopsy shows irregular mucosa and stricture formation
- Scleroderma is a mixed collagen disorder which has esophageal dysmotility
  - Affects the smooth muscle of the lower two thirds of the esophagus
  - Abnormal peristalsis of distal esophagus with reflux and esophagitis
- Post-operative Nissen fundoplication
  - Complication of the procedure occurs when the wrap is too tight
  - Proximal esophagus dilates secondary to stricture or tight wrap
- Crohn disease
  - Rarely affects the esophagus in children
  - Older children or adults may have mucosal ulcerations which lead to stricture formation
- Graft vs. host disease
  - Esophageal involvement may cause esophagitis and stricture

Microscopic Features
- Depends on the etiology
- Specific diagnosis may be made by biopsy or culture

CLINICAL ISSUES

Presentation
- Most common signs/symptoms
  - Infants present with eating and feeding problems
    - Foreign bodies in the esophagus can present with drooling
  - Airway symptoms such as wheezing, recurrent coughing episodes
    - Post-operative esophageal atresia patients have tracheomalacia
    - As esophagus dilates, it imprints the posterior wall of the trachea
  - Systemic diseases such as scleroderma, dermatomyositis, epidermolysis bullosa have multi-organ involvement
    - Many systemic diseases have skin findings, diffuse multi-organ involvement

Demographics
- Age
  - Depends on the disease process
  - Systemic disease may occur in older children
- Gender: Depends on the disease

Natural History & Prognosis
- Acute phase the injury or involvement occurs to the esophagus
- Healing at the injury sites occurs
- Scar and strictures may occur at that site
- Strictures are dilatated
- Recurrent strictures may occur in similar site

Treatment
- Balloon dilatation is used for many conditions
  - Post-operative anastomotic stricture in esophageal atresia
  - Caustic injuries
  - Systemic diseases with strictures such as dermatomyositis, epidermolysis bullosa
  - Usually children have multiple dilatations depending on symptoms
- Complications of balloon dilation
  - Perforation, mediastinitis

SELECTED REFERENCES

1. Liacouras CA et al: Eosinophilic esophagitis. Curr Opin Pediatr. 16(5):560-6, 2004
2. Sant'Anna AM et al: Eosinophilic Esophagitis in Children: Symptoms, Histology and pH Probe Results. J Pediatr Gastroenterol Nutr. 39(4):373-377, 2004
3. Schlesinger AE et al: Acquired Esophageal Lesions. In: Kuhn JP, Slovis TL and Haller JO (eds). Caffey's Pediatric Diagnostic Imaging (10th edition). Mosby, Philadelphia. pp. 1561-8, 2004
4. Fasulakis S et al: Balloon dilatation in children for oesophageal strictures other than those due to primary repair of oesophageal atresia, interposition or restrictive fundoplication. Pediatr Radiol. 33(10):682-7, 2003
5. Kottamasu SR et al: Pharynx and Esophagus In: Stringer DA and Babyn PS (eds). Pediatric Gastrointestinal Imaging and Intervention. B.C. Decker Inc. Canada, (2nd edition). pp 161-236, 2000

ESOPHAGEAL STRICTURES

IMAGE GALLERY

Typical

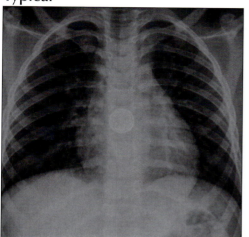
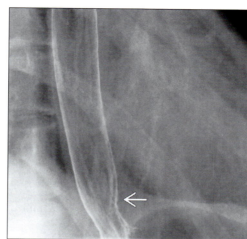

(Left) Anteroposterior radiograph shows rounded radiopaque foreign body which was a large battery disc. Batteries lodged in esophagus may cause corrosive injury within hours of ingestion and subsequent stricture development. *(Right)* Double-contrast esophagram in an adolescent with dysphagia demonstrating mild irregularity of the distal esophagus (arrow). Biopsy was positive for eosinophilic esophagitis.

Typical

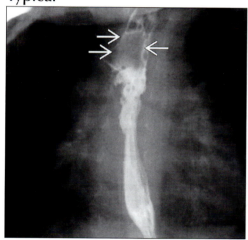
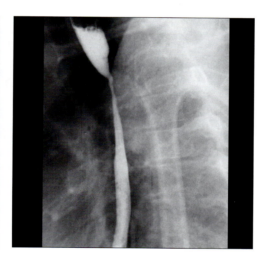

(Left) Anteroposterior esophagram in a young child who had esophageal atresia repair and gastroesophageal reflux. Child has piece of meat (arrows) proximal to mild area of narrowing of esophagus. *(Right)* Lateral upper GI shows dilatation of the esophagus proximal to moderate long segment narrowing secondary to epidermolysis bullosa in an adolescent child.

Typical

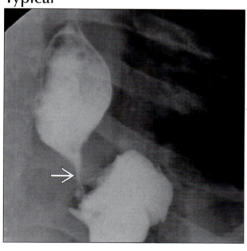
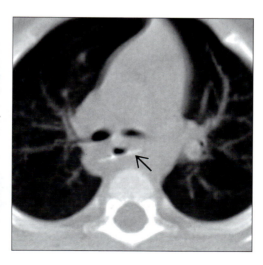

(Left) Oblique esophagram shows dilatation of the distal esophagus, narrowing of esophagus (arrow) at surgical site of Nissen fundoplication. Nissen was too tight and required balloon dilatation. *(Right)* Axial NECT shows leak of contrast (arrow) from the posterior portion of the esophagus into mediastinum following removal of a chronic foreign body from the inflamed and narrowed esophagus.

SMALL BOWEL INTUSSUSCEPTION

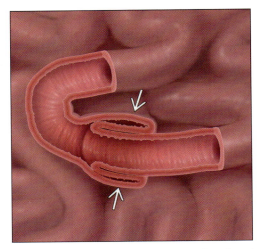

Graphic shows small bowel-small bowel intussusception. Note small bowel invaginating (arrows) into more distal bowel in direction of peristalsis.

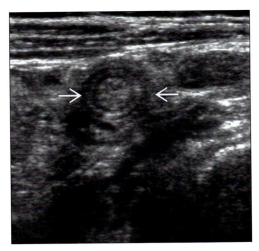

Axial ultrasound shows "bull's eye", "target" or doughnut sign of an intussusception (arrows), in this case SB-SB.

TERMINOLOGY

Abbreviations and Synonyms
- Enteroenteric intussusceptions [small bowel-small bowel (SB)]

Definitions
- Telescoping or invagination of proximal bowel (intussusceptum) into a contiguous bowel segment (intussuscipiens)

IMAGING FINDINGS

General Features
- Best diagnostic clue
  - "Target" sign
    - Internal mesenteric fat with vessels surrounded by higher attenuation bowel wall
  - "Layered" appearance
    - Alternating high attenuation (enhancing bowel wall) & lower attenuation (mesenteric fat)
- Location
  - Enteroenteric (SB-SB) uncommon
    - Ileoileal most common in adults
    - SB-SB: Up to 40% of intussusceptions in adults
  - Ileocolic (90%), ileoileocolic 2nd most common
- Size
  - SB-SB: Size smaller than ileocolic intussusceptions
  - Average: 2 cm
    - Length important in determining self-limiting verses surgical (< 3.5 cm)
- Morphology
  - SB-SB intussusceptions
    - Transient in children
    - Adults more likely pathologic lead point (benign > malignant)
    - Usually detected as an incidental finding when CECT performed for other reasons
  - Intussusceptions (ileocolic)
    - Children account for the majority of intussusceptions (90-95%)
    - Common, 2nd to acute appendicitis for causing acute abdomen
    - Idiopathic (90-95%)
    - Possibly related to lymphoid hyperplasia

Fluoroscopic Findings
- Air Enema: Mostly normal

CT Findings
- Intussusceptions: (General)
  - "Target" sign: Early
    - Mass with internal mesenteric fat & blood vessels
  - Crescent of gas or fluid may insinuate between intussusceptum and intussuscipiens

DDx: Other Causes Of Intussusception

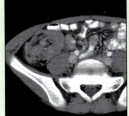
Ileocolic

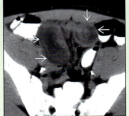
Meckel Diverticulum

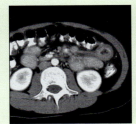
HSP

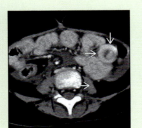
Pancreatitis

SMALL BOWEL INTUSSUSCEPTION

Key Facts

Terminology
- Telescoping or invagination of proximal bowel (intussusceptum) into a contiguous bowel segment (intussuscipiens)

Imaging Findings
- Enteroenteric (SB-SB) uncommon
- Length important in determining self-limiting verses surgical (< 3.5 cm)
- SB-SB intussusceptions
- Transient in children
- SB-SB: Smaller than ileocolic intussusceptions
- Small size, (-) wall edema, short segment, preserved wall motion

Top Differential Diagnoses
- Ileocolic intussusception
- Meckel diverticulum
- Henoch-Schönlein purpura (HSP)
- Duplication cyst
- Intra-abdominal inflammation
- Cystic fibrosis
- Malabsorption syndromes
- Non-Hodgkin lymphoma most common

Pathology
- SB-SB: Uncommon

Clinical Issues
- 2 → 20 years in children
- Average age 11 years
- Gender: M > F

- Rim of enteric contrast between the intussusceptum & intussuscipiens
- Long axis image, sausage shaped mass (later stage)
  - "Layered" appearance
  - Alternating bands of high (enhancing bowel wall) & low (mesenteric fat & blood vessels) attenuation
- Reniform mass
  - Bowel wall thickening or edema
- Small bowel obstruction: Uncommon

MR Findings
- Coiled spring or bowel-within-bowel
- Usually incidental finding

Ultrasonographic Findings
- Intussusceptions: (General)
  - "Target" or "bull's eye" sign
    - Alternating hypoechoic & hyperechoic concentric rings
    - Hypoechoic outer edematous wall of intussuscipiens
    - Hyperechoic middle ring of mesenteric fat
    - Hypoechoic inner ring of the intussusceptum
  - "Pseudokidney" sign
    - Hypoechoic bowel segment on each side of echogenic central mesenteric fat
  - SB-SB: Smaller than ileocolic intussusceptions
    - Small size, (-) wall edema, short segment, preserved wall motion

Imaging Recommendations
- Best imaging tool: Ultrasound (US) or CECT performed for abdominal pain or for some other indication

DIFFERENTIAL DIAGNOSIS

Ileocolic intussusception
- 2 months → 3 year olds
- Larger than enteroenteric intussusceptions
- Idiopathic, ileocolic (90%)
- Intermittent abdominal pain, vomiting or diarrhea
- Currant jelly stool
- US for diagnosis (no radiation)
- Air contrast enema for diagnosis & therapy (barium contrast enema studies also)

Meckel diverticulum
- Remnant of omphalomesenteric duct
- Rule of 2's
  - 2% of population, 2 feet from ileocecal valve, presents < 2 years old, length 2 inches
- 15% contain gastric mucosa
- Complications (20%): Obstruction, bleeding, perforation & intussusception
- Mass fluid attenuation surrounded by collar of soft tissue
- Technetium 99m pertechnetate: For diagnosis in those containing gastric mucosa
- Mostly asymptomatic

Henoch-Schönlein purpura (HSP)
- Systemic hypersensitivity reaction with a small vessel vasculitis
- Purpuric rash on legs or extensor surface of arms
- Abdominal pain &/or bloody diarrhea may precede rash
- Mural bleed predisposes to intussusceptions
- Complications: Bowel infarction, perforation or intussusceptions (3%)

Duplication cyst
- Most common terminal ileum & ileocecal area
- Contain both mucosa & muscular layers ("double wall" sign on US)
- Complication: Bleeding, intussusception & volvulus

Intra-abdominal inflammation
- Any diffuse abdominal process that causes inflammation of the bowel wall
- Diverticulitis, pancreatitis, etc.

Cystic fibrosis
- Autosomal recessive, ↑ Caucasian
- 1% incidence of intussusception
- Meconium ileus

SMALL BOWEL INTUSSUSCEPTION

- Distal intestinal obstruction syndrome = meconium ileus equivalent

Malabsorption syndromes
- Celiac disease ↑ incidence
  - Nontropical sprue, gluten enteropathy
  - Diarrhea (hallmark of disease): 90%
  - Reversal of jejunum & ileal fold pattern

Lymphoma
- Non-Hodgkin lymphoma most common
- Must consider in children > typical age for ileocolic intussusceptions
- Aneurysmal dilation of bowel
- Nodular, polypoid mucosa, infiltrating mass with adenopathy

PATHOLOGY

General Features
- Etiology
  - Abnormal peristalsis leading to invagination of bowel segment with mesenteric fat into a contiguous bowel segment
  - Most adult intussusceptions are transient, non-obstructing & no lead point
    - Adults higher incidence of lead point than children
  - Most children intussusceptions are ileocolic & idiopathic
    - SB-SB: Uncommon, self-limiting, idiopathic & no lead point
  - Meckel diverticulum, Henoch-Schönlein purpura, duplication cyst, inflammatory process, malabsorption syndromes, cystic fibrosis, adhesions, polyps, intramural hematoma, foreign body, lipoma, neurofibroma
  - Post-operative abdominal surgery
    - Small bowel more common
  - Appendiceal stump granuloma
    - Small bowel more common
  - Gastrojejunal enteric tubes
- Epidemiology
  - SB-SB: Uncommon
  - Intussusception (general)
    - Children >> adults
    - Idiopathic: 85-90% (most commonly lymphoid hyperplasia)
    - Children: Ileocolic & ileoileocolic comprise 90% of intussusceptions

Gross Pathologic & Surgical Features
- 3 layers
  - Intussuscipiens: Receiving the intussusception (outer loop)
  - Intussusceptum: 2 layers, entering & exiting bowel segment
- If lead point specific pathology for that diagnosis

CLINICAL ISSUES

Presentation
- Most common signs/symptoms: Most commonly asymptomatic
- Other signs/symptoms: Intermittent abdominal pain

Demographics
- Age
  - 2 → 20 years in children
    - Average age 11 years
- Gender: M > F

Natural History & Prognosis
- SB-SB
  - Transient
  - Majority resolve
  - Recurrent, multiple or persistent
    - Further evaluation
    - Repeat US to assure resolution
    - Small bowel follow through or enteroclysis to evaluate for lead point
    - Surgical referral

Treatment
- SB-SB
  - Conservative
  - Usually resolve without treatment

SELECTED REFERENCES

1. Kim JH: US features of transient small bowel intussusception in pediatric patients. Korean J Radiol. 5(3):178-84, 2004
2. Sandrasegaran K et al: Proximal small bowel intussusceptions in adults: CT appearance and clinical significance. Abdom Imaging. 29(6):653-7, 2004
3. Lvoff N et al: Distinguishing features of self-limiting adult small-bowel intussusception identified at CT. Radiology. 227(1):68-72, 2003
4. Strouse PJ et al: Transient small-bowel intussusception in children on CT. Pediatr Radiol. 33(5):316-20, 2003
5. Gayer G et al: Pictorial review: adult intussusception--a CT diagnosis. Br J Radiol. 75(890):185-90, 2002
6. Harris JP et al: Sonographic diagnosis of multiple small-bowel intussusceptions in Peutz-Jeghers syndrome: a case report. Pediatr Radiol. 32(9):681-3, 2002
7. Ko SF et al: Small bowel intussusception in symptomatic pediatric patients: experiences with 19 surgically proven cases. World J Surg. 26(4):438-43, 2002
8. Hughes UM et al: Further report of small-bowel intussusceptions related to gastrojejunostomy tubes. Pediatr Radiol. 30(9):614-7, 2000
9. Kornecki A et al: Spontaneous reduction of intussusception: clinical spectrum, management and outcome. Pediatr Radiol. 30(1):58-63, 2000
10. Mushtaq N et al: Small bowel intussusception in celiac disease. J Pediatr Surg. 34(12):1833-5, 1999
11. Catalano O: Transient small bowel intussusception: CT findings in adults. Br J Radiol. 70(836):805-8, 1997
12. Merine D et al: Enteroenteric intussusception: CT findings in nine patients. AJR Am J Roentgenol. 148(6):1129-32, 1987

SMALL BOWEL INTUSSUSCEPTION

IMAGE GALLERY

Typical

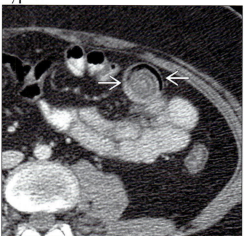 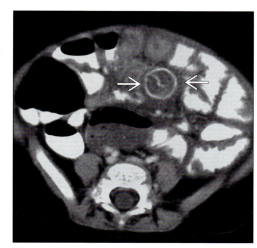

(Left) Axial CECT shows a typical small sized, nonobstructing short segment small bowel intussusception *(arrows)* with a small amount of air encircling the intussusceptum. *(Right)* Axial CECT shows a crescent of enteric contrast encircling the intussusceptum *(arrows)*.

Typical

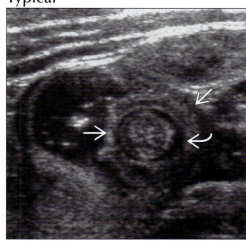 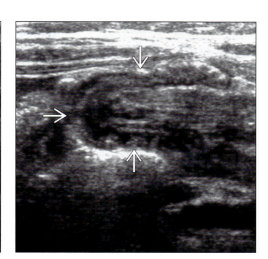

(Left) Transverse ultrasound shows "bull's eye" sign of an intussusception *(arrows)*, small bowel. There is a small amount of fluid trapped between the intussusceptum & the intussuscipiens *(curved arrow)*. *(Right)* Ultrasound longitudinal image in the same patient shows "pseudokidney" or hay fork sign of a small bowel intussusception *(arrows)*.

Variant

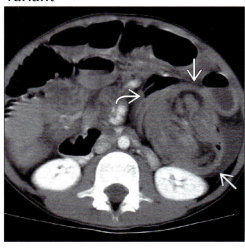 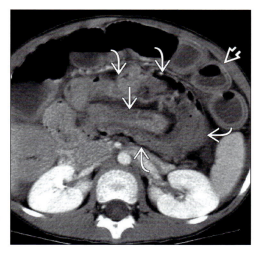

(Left) Axial CECT shows a pathologic lead point (lymphoma) in this SB-SB intussusception *(arrows)* with layered coiled-spring appearance *(curved arrow)* & small bowel obstruction. *(Right)* Axial CECT in the same patient shows a large (> 3.5 cm) reniform mass, the intussusceptum *(arrow)* telescoping into the intussuscipiens *(curved arrows)* with edematous SB *(open arrow)*.

GENITOURINARY

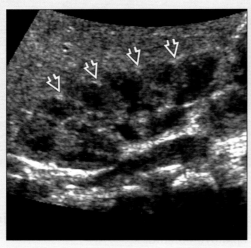

Ultrasound shows normal neonatal kidney with fetal lobulation. Note cortical indentations (arrows) are between medullary pyramids. Also note prominence of medullary pyramids.

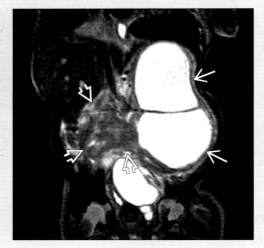

Coronal T2WI MR shows multiple congenital genitourinary problems including horseshoe kidney (open arrows) with dilated obstructed left collecting system (arrows).

Imaging Techniques

Urinary Tract Infections (UTI)
- UTI is the most common problem of genitourinary system in children
  - 2nd most common site of infection, after respiratory tract
- Goals of imaging in UTI
  - Identifying underlying congenital anomalies
  - Identifying vesicoureteral reflux (VUR)
  - Identifying renal cortical damage
  - Providing a baseline of renal size for documentation of subsequent growth
  - Establishing prognosticating factors
  - Overall goal: Reduce chance of renal damage and chronic renal insufficiency
- Modalities commonly used in evaluation of UTI: Ultrasound, voiding cystourethrography
  - Controversy about when to image
    - Boys: After first infection, girls: After second infection

Renal Ultrasound
- Transverse and longitudinal images obtained of both kidneys and bladder
- Kidney images obtained in both supine and prone positions
  - Renal lengths measured in both positions
  - Prone measurements often more accurate
- Important to compare renal length with tables of age-related normal length
  - Length: Within 2 standard deviations of mean
  - Length: Within 1 cm of contralateral kidney
    - Discrepant length indicates either one kidney too small (scarring) or one kidney too big (pyelonephritis, duplication)

Voiding Cystourethrography (VCUG)
- Most commonly performed for UTI but also for voiding dysfunction, enuresis, hydronephrosis
- Demonstrates presence or absence of VUR, documents anatomic abnormalities of bladder and urethra
- Related to bladder catheterization, exams can be stressful for child and parents
  - Education of parents & child, effective communication, and child friendly environment essential to optimizing patient's experience
- Technical factors
  - Performed under fluoroscopy with patient awake
  - Catheterized under sterile conditions typically with 8 French catheter
  - Views obtained (can use last image hold)
    - Pre-contrast scout - calcifications, bowel gas pattern baseline - not to be mistaken for VUR later
    - Early filling view - to exclude a ureterocele which can be compressed/obscured later
    - Bilateral oblique views with bladder full - to demonstrate regions of of ureterovesicular junction, obtained with collimation open top to bottom with bladder inferiorly to show potential contrast filled ureter, if VUR present
    - Voiding image of uretra - male urethra imaged in oblique projection - exclude posterior ureteral valves
    - Post void - image over pelvis and kidneys to document presence or absence of reflux and show any post void residual contrast in bladder
  - May be difficult to get young child to void while laying on table - almost all children eventually do but it takes a great deal of patience
    - Maneuvers to help patient void: Warm water on perineum or toes, warm wet washcloth on lower abdomen, tipping table head up, running water in a sink so patient can hear it, dimming the lights
  - Bladder capacity of small children can be calculated by adding 2 to the patient's age in years and multiplying that number by 30 ml

Age Related Normal Appearance

Infant Kidney Ultrasound Appearance
- Normal infant kidneys appear different than older children and adults

GENITOURINARY

Common Pediatric Genitourinary Problems

Common Congenital Anomalies
- Vesiculoureteral reflux
- Ureteropelvic junction obstruction
- Ureteropelvic duplications
- Renal ectopia and fusion

Renal Cystic Disease In Children
- Autosomal recessive polycystic renal disease (infantile)
- Autosomal dominant polycystic renal disease (adult)
- Solitary simple cyst
- Multicystic dysplastic kidney
- Syndrome related cysts
- Cystic neoplasms
- Calyceal diverticulum

Renal Tumors
- Wilm tumor
- Multilocular cystic nephroma
- Mesoblastic nephroma
- Angiomyolipoma
- Renal cell carcinoma

Neuroblastoma (As Compared To Wilm Tumor)
- Patients younger (typically < 2 years)
- Calcifications more common (85% vs. 20%)
- Grows invasively engulfing rather than displacing vessels
- Suprarenal: Displaces rather than arises from kidney
- Lung metastasis uncommon

- Prominent undulating contour = fetal lobulation
  - Not to be confused with scarring in which indentations in cortex are over medullary pyramids
  - With fetal lobulation, "thinned" areas of cortex between medullary pyramids
- Prominence of hypoechoic renal pyramids
  - In contrast to echogenic renal cortex, should not be confused with hydronephrosis

Prenatally Detected Hydronephrosis
- Prenatally diagnosed hydronephrosis becoming more common scenario with increasing use of prenatal US, MRI
- Postnatal evaluation usually includes US and VCUG
- Controversy around timing of US examination
  - Relative state of dehydration occurs after 1st 24 hours of life
  - During the period of relative dehydration, US can underestimate or fail to detect hydronephrosis
  - Recommendation: Postnatal US either during 1st 24 hours of life or after 1 week of age

Common Congenital Anomalies

Ureteropelvic Junction Obstruction (UPJ)
- Most common congenital obstruction: Urinary tract
- Increased incidence of other congenital GU anomalies
- Imaging: Dilated renal collecting system but not ureter

Ureteropelvic Duplications
- Range of anatomic malformations: Incomplete more common than complete
- Incomplete: Bifid renal pelvis with/without duplicated proximal ureter but one distal ureter
  - US: Column of tissue similar to cortex separating echogenic central renal fat
  - Often no significance
- Complete: Two completely separate ureters
  - Predisposed to UTI, obstruction from associated ureterocele, VUR, and scarring

Renal Ectopia And Fusion
- Failure of separation or migration of kidneys during development
- Renal ectopia: Abnormal position of kidney
- Renal fusion: Abnormal connection between two kidneys

Renal Cystic Disease in Children

Autosomal Recessive Polycystic Renal Disease (Infantile)
- Rare
- Microcystic disease of kidneys
- Associated with hepatic fibrosis
- Often presents prenatally or during infancy with markedly enlarged, echogenic kidneys
  - Discrete cysts often not seen due to small size

Autosomal Dominant Polycystic Renal Disease (Adult)
- Typically presents during early adulthood with hypertension, hematuria, or renal failure
- Cysts can present in childhood and increase with age
- Multiple cysts with normal intervening renal tissue

Solitary Simple Cyst
- Can occur in children, but << common than in adults
- When single solitary simple cyst encountered in child, often of no clinical significance

Multicystic Dysplastic Kidney (MCDK)
- Congenital lesion: Related to fetal obstruction
- "Grape-like" collection of varying sized cysts that do not appear to communicate
- Lacks a dominant central cyst
- No renal function
- Associated with other congenital GU anomalies
- Slowly decrease in size over time

Syndromes Associated With Cysts
- Tuberous sclerosis

GENITOURINARY

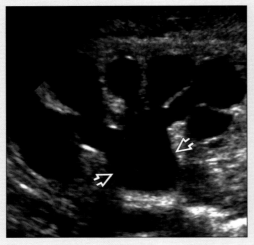

Ultrasound shows ureteropelvic junction obstruction. Note multiple dilated calyces are seen to connect to central renal pelvis (arrows). No dilated ureter was identified.

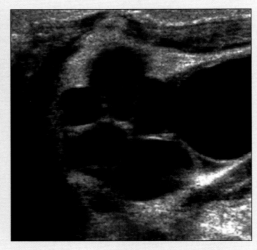

Ultrasound shows multicystic dysplastic kidney. Note multiple, disorganized collection of variable sized cysts without central dominant cyst. Cysts do not appear to connect.

- von Hippel-Lindau disease
- Meckel-Gruber syndrome

Cystic Neoplasms
- Wilm tumor
- Multilocular cystic nephroma

Calyceal Diverticulum
- May fill with contrast on excretory phase of IVP or CT

Renal Tumors

Wilm Tumor
- Most common pediatric renal malignancy
- Approximately 8% of all childhood malignant tumors

Nephroblastomatosis
- Rare entity
- Persistence of nephrogenic rests within the renal parenchyma
- Plaque-like peripheral renal lesions/medullary rests
- Can degenerate into Wilm tumor

Renal Cell Carcinoma
- 2nd most common renal malignancy in children
- Most common cause of renal malignancy in older children
- Calcifications in 25%

Multilocular Cystic Nephroma
- Cystic mass with multiple septae
- Mainly affects young boys and adult women

Mesoblastic Nephroma
- Most common renal mass encountered in neonates
- Mean age of diagnosis 3 months
- Nonspecific solid renal mass

Angiomyolipoma
- Tumor that contains mixed elements including fat: Key diagnostic imaging finding
- Occurs most commonly in patients with tuberous sclerosis

- Can spontaneously hemorrhage when > than 4 cm in size

Focal Pyelonephritis
- Can appear very mass-like and be confused with tumor
- Often multiple, wedge-shaped, peripheral

Uncommon Pediatric Renal Masses
- Renal lymphoma: Often multifocal
- Clear cell carcinoma
- Rhabdoid tumor
- Renal medullary carcinoma (sickle cell anemia)

Wilm vs. Neuroblastoma

Neuroblastoma
- Most common in children < 2 years of age
- Calcifications common (85% on CT)
- Invasive growth: Surrounds and engulfs vessels
- Suprarenal: Displaces and rotates kidney
- Lung metastasis uncommon
- No venous vascular invasion

Wilm Tumor
- Mean age at diagnosis 3 years
- Calcifications uncommon (15% on CT)
- Grows like ball: Displaces vessels
- Arises from kidney: Claw sign
- Lung metastasis common (20%)
- Invasion of renal vein, inferior vena cava

Related References
1. Donnelly LF: Fundamentals of Pediatric Radiology. W.B. Saunders company, Philadelphia, 2001

GENITOURINARY

IMAGE GALLERY

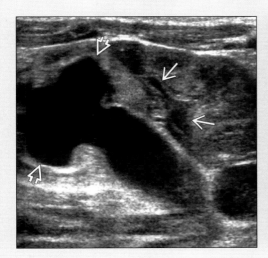
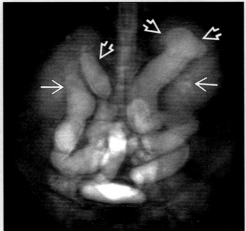

(Left) Ultrasound shows duplicated left kidney with dilated/obstructed upper pole (open arrows) and slight dilation and urothelial thickening of lower pole collecting system (arrows) related to VUR. *(Right)* MR urography shows bilateral renal duplication with dilated, obstructed upper pole collecting systems (open arrows) and dilated, refluxing lower pole collecting systems (arrows).

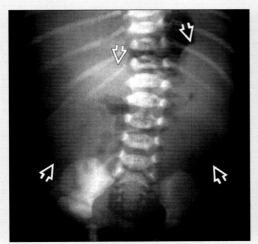
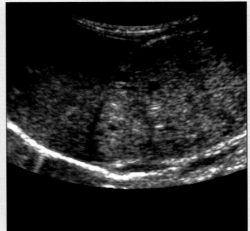

(Left) Radiograph shows markedly enlarged kidneys (arrows) in neonate with autosomal recessive polycystic renal disease (ARPRD). *(Right)* Ultrasound in same patient with ARPRD shows enlarged, echogenic kidney with several small visible cysts. Note kidney is hyperechoic as compared to adjacent liver.

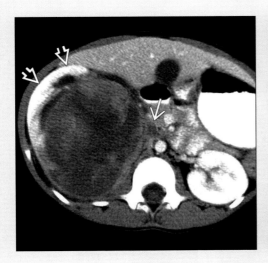
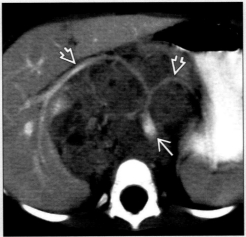

(Left) CECT shows Wilm tumor: Note large mass arising from kidney with claw of renal tissue (open arrows), tumor grows like ball with displacement of vessels. Also note IVC invasion (arrow). *(Right)* CECT shows neuroblastoma: Note mass engulfs and surrounds branches of celiac artery (open arrows) and completely surrounds and elevates aorta (arrow). Mass is heterogeneous in density.

VESICOURETERAL REFLUX

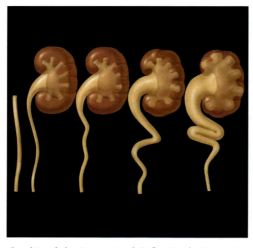

Graphic of the International Reflux Study Committee grading system. Note the progressive level of reflux, dilatation, caliceal blunting and intrarenal reflux from grade I on the left to grade V on the right.

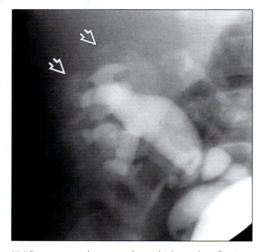

Voiding cystourethrogram shows high grade reflux into the right kidney, with dilated tortuous ureter, blunted calyces, and intra-renal reflux into the tubules (arrows), constituting grade V vesicoureteral reflux.

TERMINOLOGY

Abbreviations and Synonyms
- Vesicoureteric reflux (VUR), reflux

Definitions
- Retrograde flow of urine from the bladder toward the kidney

IMAGING FINDINGS

General Features
- Best diagnostic clue: Contrast instilled into the bladder opacifies the ureter and may reach the intrarenal collecting system, often only seen transiently

Fluoroscopic Findings
- Voiding cystourethrography (VCUG) performed fluoroscopically
- Requires bladder catheterization
- Preliminary scout film is useful, especially when there has been prior surgery or urolithiasis
- Early filling image of the bladder is best to show intraluminal abnormalities: Ureterocele, polyp, mass
- Iodinated contrast seen in ureter and renal collecting system confirms vesicoureteral reflux
- Oblique views of the distended bladder helpful to show periureteral diverticula and ureteric insertion into bladder in cases of reflux
- Ectopic ureters that insert below the bladder neck will only reflux during voiding
- Voiding images of the urethra performed to exclude distal pathology, which may contribute to back pressure or bladder outlet obstruction
- In cases of high grade reflux, a delayed upright image can be used to assess drainage from the upper tract and exclude concomitant ureteropelvic junction obstruction

Ultrasonographic Findings
- Normal ultrasound without dilatation in no way excludes significant reflux
- Ultrasound contrast agents are being instilled into the bladder for sonographic cystograms outside the United States
  - These contrast agents are not FDA approved
  - Bladder catheterization is still required; no ionizing radiation is a benefit
  - Color Doppler is sometimes used to show movement of contrast agents in the ureter
  - Urethral evaluation is possible with ultrasound probe on perineum

Nuclear Medicine Findings
- Scintigraphy

DDx: Other Findings Associated With Vesicoureteral Reflux

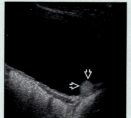
Deflux Injection

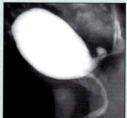
Periureteral Divertic

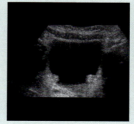
Ureteral Re-Implants

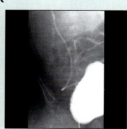
Neurogenic Bladder

VESICOURETERAL REFLUX

Key Facts

Terminology
- Retrograde flow of urine from the bladder toward the kidney

Imaging Findings
- Best diagnostic clue: Contrast instilled into the bladder opacifies the ureter and may reach the intrarenal collecting system, often only seen transiently
- VCUG preferred whenever anatomic detail of the upper tracts is needed and in all cases when urethral anatomy is being evaluated
- Nuclear cystogram preferred when anatomy is known and for follow-up studies
- Cystosonography performed in countries where ultrasound contrast agents are available

Pathology
- Shortened or abnormally angulated insertion of ureter into bladder is theorized to result in VUR
- The vast majority (80%) of pediatric patients outgrow VUR, presumably due to changes at the level of the ureterovesicle junction, often associated with a growth spurt
- Clear association with acute pyelonephritis
- INTERNATIONAL REFLUX STUDY COMMITTEE grading system of vesicoureteral reflux
- I: Reflux into ureter not reaching the renal pelvis
- II: Reflux reaching pelvis but no blunting of calyces
- III: Mild caliceal blunting
- IV: Progressive caliceal and ureteral dilation
- V: Very dilated and tortuous collecting system, intrarenal reflux

---

- ○ Study performed with gamma camera, radioisotope instilled into bladder via catheter
- ○ Radiotracer activity extends cephalad from bladder in varying amounts
- ○ Imaging is performed throughout bladder filling and voiding
- ○ Though anatomic detail is less than with VCUG, continuous imaging increases detection of transient VUR, so that nuclear cystogram is a more sensitive exam
- ○ Nuclear cystogram historically had up to 1/100th radiation exposure compared with fluoroscopic VCUG
  - ▪ With state-of-the-art, pulsed, low dose fluoroscopy units, radiation exposure is now almost equivalent
- ○ Nuclear cystogram gives no information about urethral abnormalities

Imaging Recommendations
- Best imaging tool
  - ○ VCUG preferred whenever anatomic detail of the upper tracts is needed and in all cases when urethral anatomy is being evaluated
  - ○ Nuclear cystogram preferred when anatomy is known and for follow-up studies
  - ○ Cystosonography performed in countries where ultrasound contrast agents are available

DIFFERENTIAL DIAGNOSIS

Fluoroscopic mimics of VUR
- Normal bowel wall surrounded by air, contrast in bowel, or the bony iliopectineal line can mimic contrast in ureter, clarify with oblique views
- Ventriculoperitoneal tubing and other intra-abdominal catheters can resemble contrast filled ureter

Radiopaque stones or staghorn calculus
- Density may simulate contrast in the renal pelvis
- Check scout image or watch for drainage on post-void

Sonographic mimics of VUR
- Normally peristalsing ureter or renal pelvis
- Distended distal ureter in patients with very full bladders

PATHOLOGY

General Features
- General path comments
  - ○ Shortened or abnormally angulated insertion of ureter into bladder is theorized to result in VUR
  - ○ May also result from periureteral (Hutch) diverticulum, ureterocele, bladder outlet obstruction, voiding dysfunction, or neurogenic bladder
  - ○ Embryology-anatomy
    - ▪ The vast majority (80%) of pediatric patients outgrow VUR, presumably due to changes at the level of the ureterovesicle junction, often associated with a growth spurt
- Etiology
  - ○ Clear association with acute pyelonephritis
  - ○ Probable association of sterile reflux with renal scarring
- Epidemiology
  - ○ Incidence varies, reported as low as < 1% and as high as 1-2% of general population
  - ○ VUR seen in 25-40% of children evaluated for acute pyelonephritis
  - ○ VUR seen in 5-50% of asymptomatic siblings of children with documented reflux
  - ○ Females > > males
- Associated abnormalities
  - ○ Multicystic dysplastic kidney
  - ○ Ectopic kidneys
    - ▪ Note that reflux most commonly involves the contralateral orthotopic kidney
  - ○ Repaired bladder exstrophy
  - ○ Neurogenic bladder
  - ○ Voiding dysfunction: Many varieties

VESICOURETERAL REFLUX

Gross Pathologic & Surgical Features
- Deficiency or immaturity of longitudinal muscle in submucosal ureter
- Distortion of ureteral insertion by adjacent bladder anomaly
- Abnormal angle of ureteral insertion through bladder wall which tends to correct as ureter grows and elongates

Staging, Grading or Classification Criteria
- International Reflux Study Committee grading system of vesicoureteral reflux
  - I: Reflux into ureter not reaching the renal pelvis
  - II: Reflux reaching pelvis but no blunting of calyces
  - III: Mild caliceal blunting
  - IV: Progressive caliceal and ureteral dilation
  - V: Very dilated and tortuous collecting system, intrarenal reflux

CLINICAL ISSUES

Presentation
- Most common signs/symptoms
  - Most often discovered during work-up of urinary tract infection
  - Higher grades of reflux may be suspected on prenatal ultrasound

Demographics
- Age
  - VUR most common in children less than 2 years old
  - 0.5 times as likely in those 3-6 years old
  - 0.3 times as likely in those 7-11 years old
  - 0.15 times as likely in those 12-21 years old
- Gender: Female to male ratio 2:1
- Ethnicity: Caucasian children much more often affected than African-American children, varies with study between 3:1 and 20:1 ratio

Natural History & Prognosis
- 80% outgrow VUR before puberty
- Prognosis dependent on the severity of reflux, duration, urinary tract infections (UTIs), and scarring
- With higher grade VUR, longer standing VUR, more numerous UTIs, and subsequent renal scarring, the incidence of renal insufficiency, hypertension, and end-stage renal disease increases

Treatment
- Prophylactic antibiotic therapy (medical management)
- Ureteral reimplantation surgery (surgical management)
- Endoscopic periureteral injections (minimally invasive endoscopic management) utilizing
  - Polydimethylsiloxane (PDS), Macroplastique, Uroplasty BV, Geleen, the Netherlands
  - Deflux, dextranomer/hyaluronic acid copolymer, Q-Med Scandinavia, Inc., Princeton, New Jersey
  - Autologous chondrocytes
  - Previously used autologous blood, silicone, Teflon, polytetrafluoroethylene (PTFE), and bovine cross-linked collagen have fallen out of favor
- Note that reduced grade of reflux is considered "success" in many of these endoscopic procedure studies
- The presence of voiding dysfunction was identified as a limiting factor in the success of endoscopic treatment
- Treatment-induced hydroureteronephrosis following endoscopic procedures is uncommon and usually self-limited

SELECTED REFERENCES

1. Berrocal T et al: Vesicoureteral reflux: can the urethra be adequately assessed by using contrast-enhanced voiding US of the bladder? Radiology. 234(1):235-41, 2005
2. Casale P et al: Symptomatic refluxing distal ureteral stumps after nephroureterectomy and heminephroureterectomy. What should we do? J Urol. 173(1):204-6; discussion 206, 2005
3. Gonzalez E et al: Impact of vesicoureteral reflux on the size of renal lesions after an episode of acute pyelonephritis. J Urol. 173(2):571-4; discussion 574-5, 2005
4. Taskinen S et al: Post-pyelonephritic renal scars are not associated with vesicoureteral reflux in children. J Urol. 173(4):1345-8, 2005
5. Ardissino G et al: Long-term outcome of vesicoureteral reflux associated chronic renal failure in children. Data from the ItalKid Project. J Urol. 172(1):305-10, 2004
6. Capozza N et al: The role of endoscopic treatment of vesicoureteral reflux: a 17-year experience. J Urol. 172(4 Pt 2):1626-8; discussion 1629, 2004
7. DeFoor W et al: Results of tapered ureteral reimplantation for primary megaureter: extravesical versus intravesical approach. J Urol. 172(4 Pt 2):1640-3; discussion 1643, 2004
8. Fanos V et al: Antibiotics or surgery for vesicoureteric reflux in children. Lancet. 364(9446):1720-2, 2004
9. Guarino N et al: The incidence of associated urological abnormalities in children with renal ectopia. J Urol. 172(4 Pt 2):1757-9; discussion 1759, 2004
10. Mingin GC et al: Abnormal dimercapto-succinic acid scans predict an increased risk of breakthrough infection in children with vesicoureteral reflux. J Urol. 172(3):1075-7; discussion 1077, 2004
11. Paltiel HJ et al: Endoscopic treatment of vesicoureteral reflux with autologous chondrocytes: postoperative sonographic features. Radiology. 232(2):390-7, 2004
12. Papachristou F et al: Urinary bladder volume and pressure at reflux as prognostic factors of vesicoureteral reflux outcome. Pediatr Radiol. 34(7):556-9, 2004
13. Sjostrom S et al: Spontaneous resolution of high grade infantile vesicoureteral reflux. J Urol. 172(2):694-8; discussion 699, 2004
14. van Capelle JW et al: The long-term outcome of the endoscopic subureteric implantation of polydimethylsiloxane for treating vesico-ureteric reflux in children: a retrospective analysis of the first 195 consecutive patients in two European centres. BJU Int. 94(9):1348-51, 2004
15. Kraus SJ: Genitourinary imaging in children. Pediatr Clin North Am. 48:1381-424, 2001
16. Fernbach SK et al: Pediatric voiding cystourethrography: A pictorial guide. Radiographics. 20:155-68, 2000
17. Smellie JM et al: Childhood reflux and urinary infection: a follow-up of 10-41 years in 226 adults. Pediatr Nephrol. 12:727-36, 1998

VESICOURETERAL REFLUX

IMAGE GALLERY

Typical

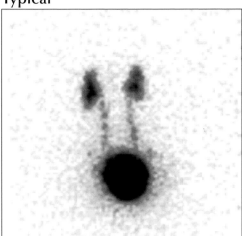
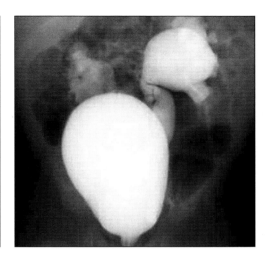

(Left) Nuclear cystogram shows radiotracer extending cephalad in both ureters reaching the renal pelves, comparable to radiographic grade II-III vesicoureteral reflux. *(Right)* Voiding cystourethrogram shows bilateral grade IV vesicoureteral reflux with dilated tortuous ureters and blunted calyces.

Typical

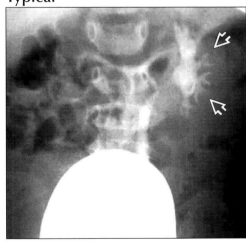
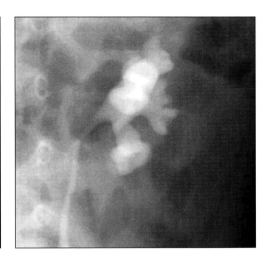

(Left) Voiding cystourethrogram shows grade II vesicoureteral reflux on the left without blunting of the calyces; there is no reflux on the right side. *(Right)* Voiding cystourethrogram shows grade III reflux on the left with blunted calyces. Compare the shape and thickness of calyces in this case to the prior case, an example of grade II VUR.

Typical

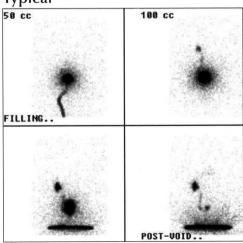
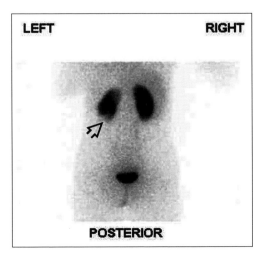

(Left) Nuclear cystogram shows radiotracer extending cephalad in the left ureter (posterior image) reaching the renal pelvis, corresponding to grade II vesicoureteral reflux. *(Right)* Tc 99m glucoheptonate scan shows left lower pole scar (arrow) from chronic reflux and/or infection in the same patient as adjacent nuclear cystogram. Progressive scarring prompted surgery in this case.

URETEROPELVIC JUNCTION OBSTRUCTION

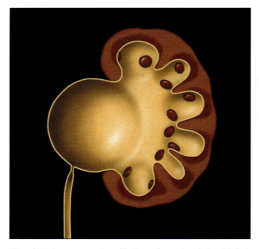

Graphic shows massive dilation of renal pelvis which is disproportionately large compared to dilated calyces. Note focal narrowing at UPJ and the proximal ureter which is not dilated.

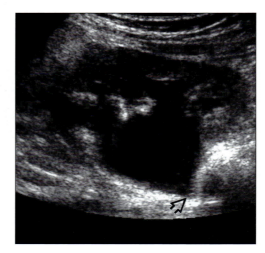

Sagittal ultrasound shows dilated calyces and renal pelvis with rapid tapering of the renal pelvis at the junction with the proximal ureter (arrow) in this case of UPJ obstruction.

TERMINOLOGY

Abbreviations and Synonyms
- UPJ obstruction, UPJO, pelviureteric obstruction (PUJO)

Definitions
- UPJ obstruction is the most common form of urinary tract obstruction in pediatrics
- Variable degree of obstruction to urine flow at the level of the ureteropelvic junction
- Patients may be diagnosed antenatally with sonography or present with UTI, intermittent abdominal pain, vomiting, hematuria
  - A few are found incidentally during evaluation for trauma

IMAGING FINDINGS

General Features
- Best diagnostic clue
  - Classic imaging appearance: Marked hydronephrosis that ends abruptly at the ureteropelvic junction with normal caliber ureter downstream
  - Disproportionate enlargement of the renal pelvis and variable drainage of the collecting system
- Morphology: UPJO has been likened to Hirschsprung's disease of the ureter, with focal transition zone and aperistaltic segment

Radiographic Findings
- Radiography: May see mass effect from enlarged hydronephrotic kidney and splinting
- IVP
  - Delayed nephrogram which depends on degree of obstruction
  - Contrast excretion into dilated collecting system
  - Contrast gradually opacifying a distended renal pelvis that tapers abruptly

Fluoroscopic Findings
- Intraoperative retrograde ureterogram used to confirm the focal narrowing or crossing vessel

CT Findings
- CECT
  - Delayed nephrogram in an enlarged kidney
  - Delayed contrast excretion into the collecting system
  - Marked renal pelvic dilation with normal or non-visualized ureter

MR Findings
- Hydronephrosis without hydroureter

DDx: Mimickers of UPJ Obstruction

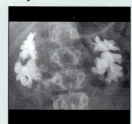
MCDK

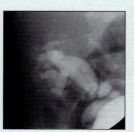
Megacalycosis

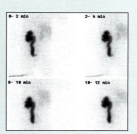
High Grade Reflux

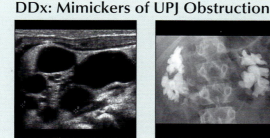
Megaureter

URETEROPELVIC JUNCTION OBSTRUCTION

Key Facts

Terminology
- UPJ obstruction is the most common form of urinary tract obstruction in pediatrics
- Variable degree of obstruction to urine flow at the level of the ureteropelvic junction
- Patients may be diagnosed antenatally with sonography or present with UTI, intermittent abdominal pain, vomiting, hematuria

Imaging Findings
- Classic imaging appearance: Marked hydronephrosis that ends abruptly at the ureteropelvic junction with normal caliber ureter downstream
- Renal pelvis is typically disproportionately enlarged compared to calyces
- Abrupt tapering of pelvis at ureteropelvic junction
- Nuclear renal scans are typically performed with a diuretic challenge and show hydronephrosis with poor drainage despite hydration and diuretic washout
- The time to half of peak activity (T½) is one measure of the severity of obstruction:
- T ½ < 10 min is normal
- T ½ > 20 min is obstructed
- T ½ between 10 and 20 minutes is indeterminate

Top Differential Diagnoses
- Multicystic Dysplastic Kidney
- Megacalycosis or Congenital Megacalyces
- Hydronephrosis of other etiologies
- Megaureter

Clinical Issues
- May improve or deteriorate spontaneously

Ultrasonographic Findings
- Grayscale Ultrasound
  - Moderate to severe hydronephrosis without hydroureter
  - Renal pelvis is typically disproportionately enlarged compared to calyces
  - Abrupt tapering of pelvis at ureteropelvic junction
- Color Doppler
  - Careful search for crossing aberrant vessels at the site of obstruction is mandatory, as this has important implications for surgical approach
  - Ureteral jets are useful in excluding complete obstruction
  - Qualitative assessment for dampened, infrequent or abnormally angulated jets is difficult
- Pulsed Doppler
  - Attempts to correlate resistive indices (RI's) with degree of obstruction can be helpful when the contralateral kidney is normal and can serve as an internal standard
  - Because renal resistive indices change with age, strict cutoff value for an obstructive RI is not applicable in pediatrics

Nuclear Medicine Findings
- Scintigraphy
  - Nuclear renal scans are typically performed with a diuretic challenge and show hydronephrosis with poor drainage despite hydration and diuretic washout
  - Nuclear studies are used to follow differential renal function and quantify changing renal function and degree of obstruction
  - The time to half of peak activity (T½) is one measure of the severity of obstruction:
    - T ½ < 10 min is normal
    - T ½ > 20 min is obstructed
    - T ½ between 10 and 20 minutes is indeterminate
  - Study should be performed in standardized fashion with adequate hydration and bladder drainage

Other Modality Findings
- Whitaker tests (pressure monitoring during direct fluid infusion into collecting system) were once the gold standard, but now are less commonly performed

Imaging Recommendations
- Best imaging tool: Sonography is usually performed first, then nuclear renal scan is used to grade the degree of obstruction and determine when surgical intervention or percutaneous drainage is needed
- Protocol advice
  - Obstruction is most often partial and can improve or worsen over time
  - These children typically have serial exams every 6-12 months (if they remain asymptomatic) to determine when to intervene
  - Occasionally UPJO is diagnosed when cystograms are performed to assess vesicoureteral reflux
    - UPJ obstruction is suggested during cystogram by:
    - Blockage of refluxed contrast material at the UPJ,
    - Contrast dilution in the renal pelvis,
    - Slow renal pelvic drainage

DIFFERENTIAL DIAGNOSIS

Multicystic Dysplastic Kidney
- These cysts do not interconnect as dilated calyces would
- The largest cyst in MCDK is not typically centrally located as the renal pelvis would be in UPJO

Megacalycosis or Congenital Megacalyces
- Idiopathic dilation of calyces without enlarged renal pelvis
- Drainage in megacalycosis is normal or minimally delayed
- Hematuria after minor trauma is often presenting complaint

Hydronephrosis of other etiologies
- Can be related to vesicoureteral reflux, UVJ obstruction, ureterocele, etc.

URETEROPELVIC JUNCTION OBSTRUCTION

Megaureter
- Can mimic UPJO proximally, but need to search for dilated ureter
- Megaureters can be obstructed, or non-obstructed and refluxing or non-refluxing

PATHOLOGY

General Features
- General path comments
  - Theoretical etiology of obstruction at the UPJ
    - Abnormal smooth muscle arrangement impairs distensibility
    - Abnormal innervation of proximal ureter - Hirschsprung's equivalent
    - Crossing vessel or fibrous scar at the UPJ
- Etiology: At surgical resection massively dilated pelvis is too distorted to confirm any single theory
- Epidemiology
  - Higher incidence of UPJO associated with multicystic dysplastic kidneys
  - These patients require prompt surgical intervention, since the MCDK is nonfunctional and the UPJ may compromise remaining renal function

Gross Pathologic & Surgical Features
- Disproportionate enlargement of the renal pelvis giving rise to normal caliber ureter

Microscopic Features
- Obstructive nephropathy leads to tubulointerstitial fibrosis and loss of renal function
- Nerve fibers are depleted in the muscular layers in the ureteric walls
- Denervation results in dysfunction / atrophy of muscle fibers & increased collagen fibers within the muscle layers
- Abnormal accumulations of intercellular and interstitial collagen are also seen pathologically

Staging, Grading or Classification Criteria
- Anteroposterior pelvic diameter (APPD) > 10 mm in 3rd trimester fetus or newborn suggests obstruction

CLINICAL ISSUES

Presentation
- Most common signs/symptoms: Antenatally detected on fetal sonogram or MRI
- Other signs/symptoms
  - Infants and children can present with urinary tract infection, intermittent abdominal pain, flank pain or hematuria
  - In older children who present with symptomatic UPJO, a crossing vessel is the cause in ~50%

Natural History & Prognosis
- May improve or deteriorate spontaneously
- Prognosis is excellent if renal function has not been compromised by longstanding, high-grade obstruction
- Pelvicaliectasis persists for years on sonography following successful surgery
- Appropriate renal growth and good drainage on nuclear scans are measures of surgical success

Treatment
- Pyeloplasty (open or laparoscopic surgery)
  - Tapered dismembered pyeloplasty has been the classic surgery used to correct the abnormality
  - Narrowed segment at UPJ is resected or crossing vessel is re-routed
  - Ureteral stents are often left in place, crossing the surgical anastomosis, for several weeks post-op
  - Open or laparoscopic procedures are preferable when crossing vessels or aberrant vessels are recognized; endoscopic hemorrhagic complications are increases in these cases
- Endoscopic incision, also known as endopyelotomy
- Endopyeloplasty which is horizontal percutaneous suturing of a conventional longitudinal endopyelotomy incision
- Ureterocalicostomy is a reconstructive option in the rare patient with surgically failed UPJ repair or difficult anatomy due to fibrosis or other concurrent problems
- Percutaneous drainage as a temporizing measure, especially if infected

SELECTED REFERENCES

1. Desai MM et al: Endopyeloplasty versus endopyelotomy versus laparoscopic pyeloplasty for primary ureteropelvic junction obstruction. Urology. 64(1):16-21; discussion 21, 2004
2. Gill IS et al: Laparoscopic ureterocalicostomy: initial experience. J Urol. 171(3):1227-30, 2004
3. Stauss J et al: Dynamic renal scintigraphy in children with vesicoureteral reflux and suspected coexisting ureteropelvic junction obstruction. J Urol. 170(5):1966-70, 2003
4. Khaira HS et al: Helical computed tomography for identification of crossing vessels in ureteropelvic junction obstruction-comparison with operative findings. Urology. 62(1):35-9, 2003
5. Brkljacic B et al: Doppler sonographic renal resistance index and resistance index ratio in children and adolescents with unilateral hydronephrosis. Eur Radiol. 12(11):2747-51, 2002
6. Cvitkovic Kuzmic A et al: Doppler visualization of ureteric jets in unilateral hydronephrosis in children and adolescents. Eur J Radiol. 39(3):209-14, 2001
7. Rooks VJ et al: Extrinsic ureteropelvic junction obstruction from a crossing renal vessel: demography and imaging. Pediatr Radiol. 31(2):120-4, 2001
8. Frauscher F et al: Crossing vessels at the ureteropelvic junction: detection with contrast-enhanced color Doppler imaging. Radiology. 210(3):727-31, 1999
9. Park JM et al: The pathophysiology of UPJ obstruction. Current concepts. Urol Clin North Am. 25(2):161-9, 1998
10. Amling CL et al: Ultrasound changes after pyeloplasty in children with ureteropelvic junction obstruction: long-term outcome in 47 renal units. J Urol 156:2020-4, 1996
11. Flashner SC et al: Nonobstructive dilatation of upper urinary tract may later convert to obstruction. Urology. 42(5):569-73, 1993
12. Gordon et al: Antenatal diagnosis of pelvic hydronephrosis: assessment of renal function and drainage as a guide to management. J Nuc Med 32:1649-54, 1991

URETEROPELVIC JUNCTION OBSTRUCTION

IMAGE GALLERY

Typical

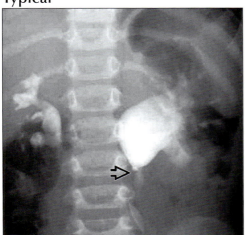
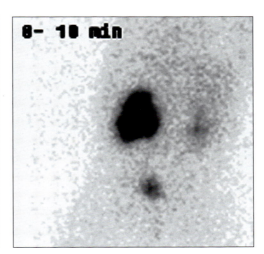

(Left) IVP shows dilated left collecting system and abrupt narrowing at the junction of the left renal pelvis and ureter (arrow). *(Right)* Tc-99m MAG3 scan shows no significant washout from the left renal pelvis despite a diuretic challenge.

Typical

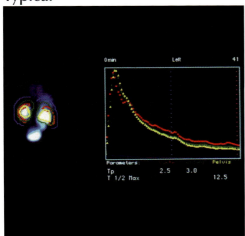
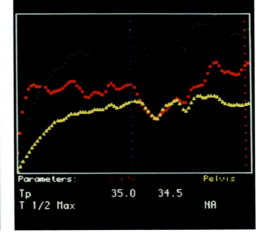

(Left) Standard regions of interest are drawn around the renal cortex (red), whole kidney (green), and renal pelvis (yellow). The time-activity curve shown is normal with short time to peak activity and rapid washout. *(Right)* Time-activity curves in a patient with UPJO show continual rise in counts 20 minutes after Lasix challenge (blue vertical dotted line). Time to half max activity can not be calculated.

Typical

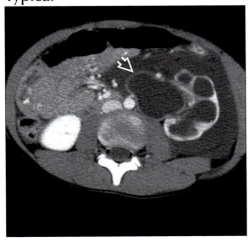
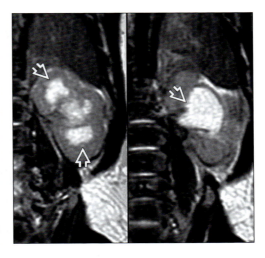

(Left) Axial CECT shows marked hydronephrosis of the left kidney with enlarged renal pelvis (arrow), cortical thinning and perinephric fluid in a 12 year-old involved in car accident. This left UPJO ruptured in the collision. *(Right)* Coronal T2WI MR shows dilated calyces and renal pelvis (arrows) in this patient with proven ureteropelvic junction obstruction.

URETEROPELVIC DUPLICATIONS

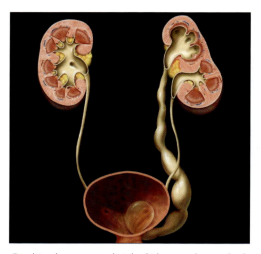

Graphic shows normal right kidney and completely duplicated left kidney, with poorly draining ectopic ureterocele seen in the bladder, medial and inferior to the lower pole ureteral orifice.

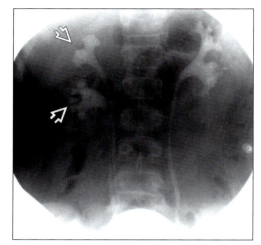

Voiding cystourethrogram shows complete duplication of ureter and intra-renal collecting system on the right (arrows). The left kidney is normal, not duplicated.

TERMINOLOGY

Abbreviations and Synonyms
- Duplicated kidney, duplex collecting system, partial/incomplete/complete duplication, bifid pelvis

Definitions
- The presence of two separate pelvicaliceal collecting systems in one kidney
- Two draining ureters may join above the bladder (partial duplication) or insert into the bladder separately (complete duplication)
- The ureter draining the cephalad portion of the kidney tends to insert in the bladder inferior and medial to the ureter draining the lower segment of the kidney (Weigert-Meyer rule)
- Corollary to Weigert-Meyer rule
  - The upper pole tends to obstruct
  - The lower pole tends to have vesicoureteral reflux
- Upper pole ureteral orifice is, by definition, ectopic in location & often associated with ureterocele

IMAGING FINDINGS

General Features
- Best diagnostic clue: Identification of two renal pelves or proximal ureters on any imaging modality
- Location: The duplication process can involve the entire urinary tract: From renal parenchyma to urethra
- Size: Duplicated kidneys tend to be larger than non-duplex, even when there is no hydronephrosis
- Morphology
  - Normal renal parenchyma, more than 10 calyces, two renal pelves, 1 or 2 ureters
  - More than one renal artery and vein are very common

Fluoroscopic Findings
- Voiding Cystourethrogram
  - Look for reflux, which occurs into the lower pole more often than the upper pole
  - Saddle reflux or yo-yo reflux is unique to partial duplications which have a single distal ureter
    - The term refers to refluxed contrast first entering one component of the upper tract collecting system, draining, and then refluxing into the second component

CT Findings
- Contrast-enhanced CT useful to demonstrate course of ureters and locate renal arteries
- Presence of supranumerary calyces and bifid pelvis can be more challenging to detect on axial imaging

DDx: Duplications: High & Low

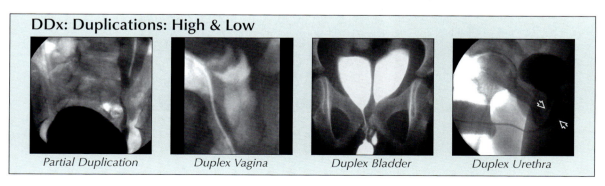

Partial Duplication | Duplex Vagina | Duplex Bladder | Duplex Urethra

URETEROPELVIC DUPLICATIONS

Key Facts

Terminology
- The presence of two separate pelvicaliceal collecting systems in one kidney
- Two draining ureters may join above the bladder (partial duplication) or insert into the bladder separately (complete duplication)
- The ureter draining the cephalad portion of the kidney tends to insert in the bladder inferior and medial to the ureter draining the lower segment of the kidney (Weigert-Meyer rule)

Top Differential Diagnoses
- Column of Bertin
- Partial or incomplete duplication
- Segmental multicystic dysplastic kidney (MCDK)
- Upper pole renal mass or adrenal mass

Pathology
- Incidence is 12-15% in general population
- Left-sided > > right
- Genital anomalies found in 1/2 of affected females

Clinical Issues
- Most common signs/symptoms: Most often discovered antenatally or incidentally on imaging studies performed for other reasons
- Complete duplications much more common in women
- Prognosis varies with type and severity of complications
- Chronic obstruction, infection, scarring may lead to secondary hypertension and renal insufficiency

MR Findings
- T2 weighted urography series are useful to show fluid within the collecting system
- This is often the best test when an ectopic ureter cannot be demonstrated with other imaging
- Coronal thick slab series are often the most useful

Ultrasonographic Findings
- Grayscale Ultrasound
  - Look for a band of renal cortex crossing the medullary portion of the kidney
  - Separate renal pelves are often visible along with separate proximal ureters
  - Distal ureters can be more difficult to identify due to bowel gas near the bladder
  - Look for ureterocele, assess for presence and location of ureteral jets
  - Remember to survey for concomitant genital anomalies, especially uterine anomalies
  - While a dilated distal ureter may be suggestive of vesicular ureteral reflux
    - Lack of dilatation of the ureter and collecting system in no way excludes the presence of reflux
    - Many cases of even severe reflux do not show dilatation at ultrasound
- Color Doppler
  - Doppler useful to define arterial anatomy
  - Doppler also used to confirm lack of blood-flow in renal pelves

Nuclear Medicine Findings
- Occasionally nuclear study is the first to suggest a renal duplication
- Renal scans used to show differential function, drainage, and scarring
- Results guide surgical intervention when there is obstruction, reflux, or ongoing scarring

Other Modality Findings
- Intravenous pyelogram (IVP) useful test to delineate ectopic ureter and show relative function
- Other modalities without ionizing radiation are preferred in pediatric patients: Ultrasound, MR
- When the upper pole is hydronephrotic, it exerts mass effect on the lower pole displacing it inferiorly
  - "Drooping lily" refers to the classic appearance of the opacified lower pole collecting system on IVP or VCUG, displaced by "mass-like" upper pole hydronephrosis
  - Now this finding may also be seen on coronal reformat CT, coronal MR, and ultrasound
  - Beware that true suprarenal masses can also create this appearance

Imaging Recommendations
- Best imaging tool
  - Ultrasound, IVP, CT, and MR all demonstrate this normal variant well
  - VCUG is useful when reflux is present
  - Nuclear renal scans useful for assessing differential renal function, drainage, and scarring
- Protocol advice: When searching for ureter from poorly functioning, chronically obstructed upper pole, consider IVP or MR urography

DIFFERENTIAL DIAGNOSIS

Column of Bertin
- Normal variant of junctional parenchyma, typically in the mid pole region, looks like focally thickened cortex; not truly hypertrophied tissue nor is it a hamartoma

Partial or incomplete duplication
- Determine if there is one or more renal pelvis & ureter

Segmental multicystic dysplastic kidney (MCDK)
- Upper pole MCDK can mimic an obstructed, hydronephrotic upper pole moiety

URETEROPELVIC DUPLICATIONS

Upper pole renal mass or adrenal mass
- Can mimic the "drooping lily" sign by displacing the collecting system inferiorly

PATHOLOGY

General Features
- Genetics
  - Not inherited
  - Some familial tendency has been reported
- Etiology
  - Early branching of the ureteric bud or two ureteral buds arising from the Wolffian duct
  - Each bud induces formation of its own nephrons when it meets the metanephric blastema
  - Abnormal branching of ureteric bud can also give rise to a supranumerary kidney or triplicate collecting system (both very rare)
- Epidemiology
  - Incidence is 12-15% in general population
  - Left-sided > > right
- Associated abnormalities
  - Genital anomalies found in 1/2 of affected females
  - Duplications of bladder, urethra, and genital structures are associated with renal duplication
  - Ureteropelvic junction obstruction is more common in duplicated kidneys

Gross Pathologic & Surgical Features
- Almost always has two renal arteries and veins; often with separate renal artery orifice from aorta
- Renal parenchyma and collecting system tissue are normal, in the absence of complications

Microscopic Features
- Depend on complications: Scarring, hydronephrosis, fibrosis

CLINICAL ISSUES

Presentation
- Most common signs/symptoms: Most often discovered antenatally or incidentally on imaging studies performed for other reasons
- Other signs/symptoms: Symptomatic duplications may show: Infection, obstruction, calculi, scarring, hematuria, abdominal or flank pain, voiding dysfunction, urinary retention

Demographics
- Age
  - Congenital, usually discovered early in life
  - Incidence of 12-15% in general population, but only 1% found de novo in cadaveric renal donors
- Gender
  - Complete duplications much more common in women
  - Partial duplications have no gender predilection

Natural History & Prognosis
- Prognosis varies with type and severity of complications
- Chronic obstruction, infection, scarring may lead to secondary hypertension and renal insufficiency

Treatment
- Depends on the complications that arise
  - Associated ureteroceles are incised, unroofed, resected, or reimplanted
  - Hydronephrosis is treated surgically to improve drainage
    - Higher degrees of upper pole cortical thinning and diminished relative function on nuclear scans, correlate with histopathologic changes of fibrosis, scarring, and dysplasia
    - Cortical thinning and relative function are used to determine surgical course: Salvage versus resection
  - Infections are treated with antibiotics and evaluated for urine stasis and reflux
  - Reflux can be managed conservatively (medically), or treated surgically
  - Calculi are removed, fragmented, or monitored
  - Voiding dysfunction is assessed to exclude ectopic ureterocele, prolapsing cecoureterocele, and bladder dyskinesia

SELECTED REFERENCES

1. Castagnetti M et al: Transurethral incision of duplex system ureteroceles in neonates: does it increase the need for secondary surgery in intravesical and ectopic cases? BJU Int. 93(9):1313-7, 2004
2. Davidovits M et al: Unilateral duplicated system: comparative length and function of the kidneys. Clin Nucl Med. 29(2):99-102, 2004
3. Perez-Brayfield M et al: Endoscopic treatment with dextranomer/hyaluronic acid for complex cases of vesicoureteral reflux. J Urol. 172(4 Pt 2):1614-6, 2004
4. Wah TM et al: Lower moiety pelvic-ureteric junction obstruction (PUJO) of the duplex kidney presenting with pyonephrosis in adults. Br J Radiol. 76(912):909-12, 2003
5. Whitten SM et al: Accuracy of antenatal fetal ultrasound in the diagnosis of duplex kidneys. Ultrasound Obstet Gynecol. 21(4):342-6, 2003
6. De Caluwe D et al: Fate of the retained ureteral stump after upper pole heminephrectomy in duplex kidneys. J Urol. 168(2):679-80, 2002
7. Husmann DA et al: Is endoscopic decompression of the neonatal extravesical upper pole ureterocele necessary for prevention of urinary tract infections or bladder neck obstruction? J Urol. 167(3):1440-2, 2002
8. Kupeli B et al: Extracorporeal shockwave lithotripsy in anomalous kidneys. J Endourol. 13(5):349-52, 1999
9. Decter RM: Renal duplication and fusion anomalies. Pediatr Clin North Am. 44(5):1323-41, 1997
10. Stylianos S et al: Complex colon duplication mimicking an obstructed, non-functioning kidney in a newborn with imperforate anus and spinal dysraphism. Pediatr Radiol. 25(4):269-71, 1995
11. Avni EF et al: Renal duplications: the impact of perinatal ultrasound on diagnosis and management. Eur Urol. 20(1):43-8, 1991
12. Pollak R et al: Anatomic abnormalities of cadaver kidneys procured for purposes of transplantation. Am Surg. 52(5):233-5, 1986

URETEROPELVIC DUPLICATIONS

IMAGE GALLERY

Typical

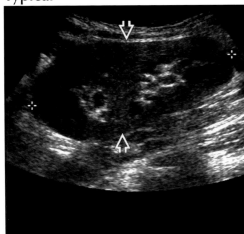
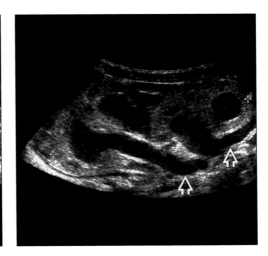

(Left) Coronal ultrasound shows duplicated left kidney with a band of parenchyma (arrows) splitting the central sinus fat. There is no dilation of either the upper or lower collecting system in this case. *(Right)* Coronal ultrasound shows another case of duplication, but with dilation of the intra-renal collecting system and proximal ureters (arrows) in this patient.

Typical

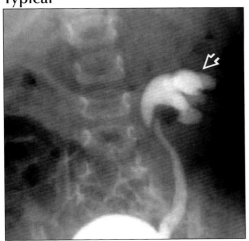
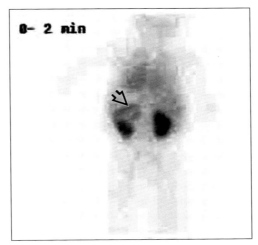

(Left) Voiding cystourethrogram shows vesicoureteral reflux (grade 3) into a lower pole collecting system in the left kidney (arrow). The upper pole is obstructed, mass-like and pushes downward on the lower pole, so called "drooping lily" sign. *(Right)* Posterior image from Tc 99m MAG3 scan shows normal right kidney and poorly functioning, hydronephrotic upper pole (arrow) of the left kidney in the same patient with "drooping lily" sign on VCUG.

Typical

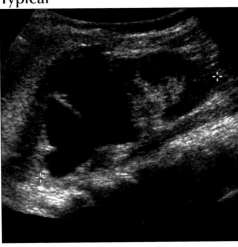
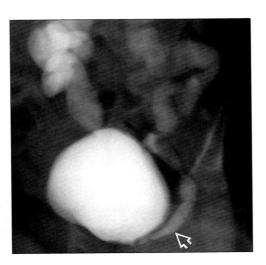

(Left) Coronal ultrasound shows dilation of the upper pole moiety and cortical thinning in another case of duplication. The lower pole is normal; neither ureter is dilated. *(Right)* Oblique voiding cystourethrogram shows high grade vesicoureteral reflux bilaterally and ectopic insertion of a left-sided ureter into the bladder neck (arrow). This ureter is draining the left upper pole.

URETEROCELE

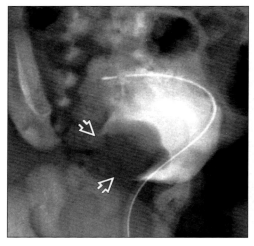

Oblique voiding cystourethrogram shows a radiolucent filling defect (arrows) in the bladder base, consistent with a ureterocele. Note that ureteroceles are best seen on early filling images.

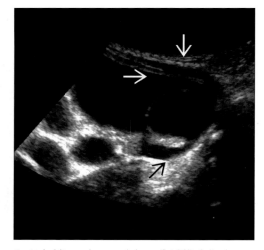

Sagittal oblique ultrasound shows fluid filled distal ureter (black arrow) and ureterocele (white arrows) within the bladder in this patient with a duplicated left kidney.

TERMINOLOGY

Abbreviations and Synonyms
- Bladder cyst, cobra head ureter, cecoureterocele

Definitions
- Congenital cystic dilatation of the distal submucosal portion of one or both ureters
- Categorized according to their position
  - Intravesical, when the ureterocele is completely contained inside the bladder
  - Extravesical, when part of the cyst extends to the urethra, bladder neck, or perineum
- Categorized according to their insertion
  - Orthotopic (simple) ureterocele has orifice located in a normal anatomic position in bladder trigone
  - Ectopic ureterocele refers to those ureteroceles whose orifices are located anywhere else
- Categorized according to the type of kidney that they drain
  - Single system ureteroceles are associated with a single kidney, a single collecting system, and a solitary ureter
    - These are typically simple, intravesicle ureteroceles
  - Duplex system ureteroceles are associated with kidneys that have completely duplicated collecting system and 2 ureters
    - These are more likely to be ectopic, extravesicle ureteroceles
- Cecoureteroceles are a unique subtype of ureterocele that is elongated beyond the ureterocele orifice by tunneling under the trigone and the urethra
- Any type may become obstructed and cause hydronephrosis
- Weigert-Meyer rule states that the ureter from the upper moiety of a duplicated kidney inserts inferior and medial to the normal insertion site of the lower pole moiety in the trigone
- Ureteroceles may prolapse in and out of the bladder

IMAGING FINDINGS

General Features
- Best diagnostic clue: A filling defect in the bladder on any imaging modality

Radiographic Findings
- IVP: Filling defect in contrast filled bladder and possible delayed function of upper pole moiety

MR Findings
- T2WI
  - MR urogram sequences are useful when trying to detect a poorly functioning upper pole moiety and its draining ureter

DDx: Other Bladder Abnormalities

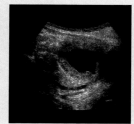

Rhabdomyosarcoma

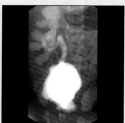

Cystitis

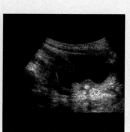

Urethral Valves (PUV)

Distal UVJ Stone

URETEROCELE

Key Facts

Terminology
- Congenital cystic dilatation of the distal submucosal portion of one or both ureters
- Categorized according to their position
- Intravesical, when the ureterocele is completely contained inside the bladder
- Extravesical, when part of the cyst extends to the urethra, bladder neck, or perineum
- Categorized according to their insertion
- Orthotopic (simple) ureterocele has orifice located in a normal anatomic position in bladder trigone
- Ectopic ureterocele refers to those ureteroceles whose orifices are located anywhere else

Imaging Findings
- Best diagnostic clue: A filling defect in the bladder on any imaging modality

Top Differential Diagnoses
- Bladder mass: Rhabdomyosarcoma, hematoma, fungus ball, etc.
- Mass effect from sigmoid colon
- Bladder "Hutch" diverticulum

Clinical Issues
- Antenatal detection is usual method of discovery
- Females >> males, 4-7:1 ratio
- Left side > right
- Bilateral in 10%
- Ectopic, extravesical variety >> orthotopic, simple variety by 3:1 ratio
- Prognosis is excellent if nonobstructed and nonrefluxing
- Prognosis is variable if prolonged obstruction or high grade reflux has compromised renal function

---

  - Some advocate vigorous hydration and diuretic use during the MR scan
  - MR also useful to delineate associated gynecologic abnormalities seen in 50% of women with duplication

Ultrasonographic Findings
- Grayscale Ultrasound
  - Anechoic, thin-walled cyst inside the bladder
  - May be able to demonstrate connection to distal ureter and ureteral jet
  - Look for signs of duplicated kidney, hydronephrosis, and dilated proximal ureter
- Color Doppler
  - Ureteral jets useful to exclude complete obstruction of a ureterocele
  - Velocity of the ureteral jet has been compared to contralateral normal side to estimate degree of obstruction

Nuclear Medicine Findings
- Nuclear Cystogram: Difficult to see on nuclear cystogram unless very large or prolapsing
- Renal Scans
  - Used to assess function of obstructed or poorly functioning upper pole moiety
  - Poor function on nuclear scan is predictive of severe histologic changes in renal parenchyma and helps justify heminephrectomy

Other Modality Findings
- Recognized on almost any imaging modality as a bladder filling defect
- Voiding cystourethrography (VCUG) findings
  - Best seen on early filling image before contrast in bladder is too dense and before intravesical pressure compresses the ureterocele

Imaging Recommendations
- Best imaging tool
  - VCUG and ultrasound are best, first line of imaging
  - Nuclear scans useful to assess differential function in duplicated kidneys
  - MR and IVP reserved for difficult or complex cases
- Protocol advice: VCUG is best test to assess dynamic nature of the ureterocele: Refluxing, prolapsing, everting, causing bladder outlet obstruction

DIFFERENTIAL DIAGNOSIS

Bladder mass: Rhabdomyosarcoma, hematoma, fungus ball, etc.
- These lack communication with distal ureter and are more likely to be solid lesions than simple cystic lesion

Mass effect from sigmoid colon
- Can be confusing on VCUG, check oblique views

Bladder "Hutch" diverticulum
- A periureteral diverticulum of the bladder that does not usually prolapse into the bladder lumen and is separate from the distal ureter

Urethral prolapse or urethral caruncle
- These are more often seen in adult women, especially postmenopausal women

PATHOLOGY

General Features
- General path comments: Normal urothelium which is dilated in it's intramucosal or submucosal segment
- Genetics: Not inherited
- Etiology
  - Embryology-anatomy
    - Thought to result from delayed canalization of Chwalla membrane during embryogenesis which causes obstruction of the ureteral orifice
    - Chwalla membrane is a primitive membrane that separates the ureteral bud from the developing urogenital sinus
- Epidemiology
  - Incidence: Approximately 1 in every 4,000 children, less frequently diagnosed in adults

URETEROCELE

- Incidence of ectopic ureteroceles parallels incidence of renal duplication
- Duplications occur in 1 of 150 in general population
  - Note: Partial duplications have a single ureter and are less likely to have ureterocele
- Associated abnormalities
  - Vesicoureteral reflux (VUR) seen in the lower pole in 50% of cases of ureteroceles
  - VUR seen in the contralateral kidney in 25%

Microscopic Features
- In heminephroureterectomy specimens the following histologic changes are found
  - chronic interstitial inflammation, fibrosis, tubular atrophy, glomerulosclerosis and dysplasia

CLINICAL ISSUES

Presentation
- Most common signs/symptoms
  - Antenatal detection is usual method of discovery
  - Febrile urinary tract infection is the most common postnatal presentation
- Other signs/symptoms
  - Simple ureteroceles may not be diagnosed until adulthood
  - Ectopic ureteroceles are usually diagnosed in infancy or shortly after toilet training and present with hematuria, UTI, chronic "enuresis", or hydronephrosis
  - Rarely, prolapse and acute obstruction of the bladder outlet is the presenting sign
  - Other rare presentations: Failure to thrive, cyclic abdominal pain, ureteral calculus (calculi are seldom seen in children)

Demographics
- Age: Most often detected antenatally
- Gender
  - Females >> males, 4-7:1 ratio
  - Left side > right
  - Bilateral in 10%
  - Ectopic, extravesical variety >> orthotopic, simple variety by 3:1 ratio
- Ethnicity: Most frequent in Caucasians

Natural History & Prognosis
- Classic history of ectopic ureteral insertion below the sphincter in girls is: Never successfully toilet trained or underwear is always damp
- In boys the ectopic ureter may insert into the epididymis, vas deferens, or spermatic cord and cause epididymitis or other scrotal symptomatology
- Prognosis is excellent if nonobstructed and nonrefluxing
- Prognosis is variable if prolonged obstruction or high grade reflux has compromised renal function
- Antenatal diagnosis reported to improve overall course: Fewer infections, fewer surgical procedures
- Ureteroceles diagnosed antenatally should be treated surgically within the first weeks of life, as the rate of urinary tract infection exceeds 50% despite prophylactic antibiotics

Treatment
- Endoscopic incision (puncture or unroofing) especially if infected or obstructed in neonates
  - Note that following endoscopic incision the ureterocele wall typically appears thickened, irregular, even "mass-like"
  - Endoscopic incision may convert an obstructed ureterocele into a refluxing ureterocele
  - Iatrogenic, de novo, VUR occurs in 40-50% of pediatric patients
- Ureteral reimplantation surgery: Extravesical reimplantation, ureteroureterostomy, ureteropyelostomy
  - Patients undergoing bilateral ectopic ureterocele repair are at increased risk for post-operative voiding dysfunction; unclear if risk is present pre-operatively or is a result of trigonal surgery
- Heminephroureterectomy if upper moiety is very poorly functioning
- Antenatally, laser ablation of ureteroceles has been reported in fetuses who have severe bilateral hydronephrosis, bladder outlet obstruction, and oligohydramnios
- Surgical success after a single procedure is greater in non-duplicated ureters; many patients require more than one surgical procedure

SELECTED REFERENCES
1. Gran CD et al: Primary lower urinary tract reconstruction for nonfunctioning renal moieties associated with obstructing ureteroceles. J Urol. 173(1):198-201, 2005
2. Castagnetti M et al: Transurethral incision of duplex system ureteroceles in neonates: does it increase the need for secondary surgery in intravesical and ectopic cases? BJU Int. 93(9):1313-7, 2004
3. Bolduc S et al: The predictive value of diagnostic imaging for histological lesions of the upper poles in duplex systems with ureteroceles. BJU Int. 91(7):678-82, 2003
4. Lebowitz RL: Paediatric urology and uroradiology: changes in the last 25 years. BJU Int. 92 Suppl 1:7-9, 2003
5. Soothill PW et al: Ultrasound-guided laser treatment for fetal bladder outlet obstruction resulting from ureterocele. Am J Obstet Gynecol. 188(4):1107-8, 2003
6. Chavhan GB: The cobra head sign. Radiology. 225(3):781-2, 2002
7. Holmes NM et al: Is bladder dysfunction and incontinence associated with ureteroceles congenital or acquired? J Urol. 168(2):718-9, 2002
8. Upadhyay J et al: Impact of prenatal diagnosis on the morbidity associated with ureterocele management. J Urol. 167(6):2560-5, 2002
9. Pike SC et al: Ureterocele prolapse-rare presentation in an adolescent girl. Urology. 57(3):554, 2001
10. Staatz G et al: Magnetic resonance urography in children: evaluation of suspected ureteral ectopia in duplex systems. J Urol. 166(6):2346-50, 2001
11. Besson R et al: Incidence of urinary tract infection in neonates with antenatally diagnosed ureteroceles. Eur J Pediatr Surg. 10(2):111-3, 2000
12. Keesling CA et al: Sonographic appearance of the bladder after endoscopic incision of ureteroceles AJR. 170:759-63, 1998

URETEROCELE

IMAGE GALLERY

Typical

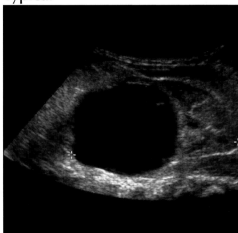
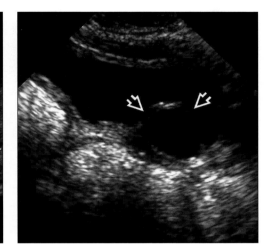

(Left) Sagittal ultrasound shows marked hydronephrosis of the upper pole moiety in this duplicated kidney which had a distal ureterocele that was poorly draining. Ectopic ureteral insertions are often obstructed. *(Right)* Sagittal ultrasound shows a rather thick-walled ureterocele (arrows) in the bladder base. Wall thickness may vary with distention and frequently looks thicker following endoscopic incision.

Typical

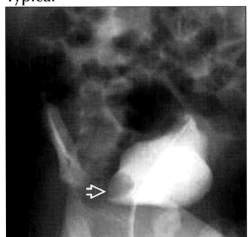
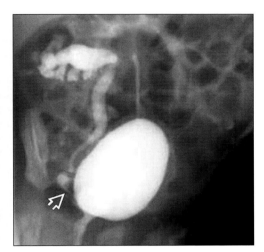

(Left) Oblique voiding cystourethrogram shows a small ureterocele (arrow) at the bladder base during the early filling phase. *(Right)* Oblique voiding cystourethrogram shows the same ureterocele (arrow) everting during voiding when reflux is also noted. Everting ureteroceles and periureteral diverticula can be difficult to discriminate.

Variant

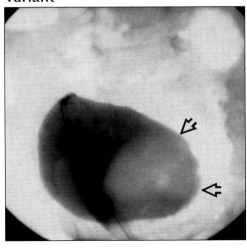
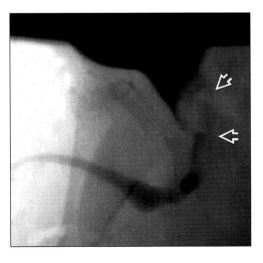

(Left) Oblique voiding cystourethrogram shows a large ureterocele (arrows) in the bladder base in a toddler being evaluated for urinary retention. Note the position of the catheter in urethra in relationship to the ureterocele. *(Right)* Oblique voiding cystourethrogram shows prolapse of the ureterocele into the posterior urethra (arrows) as voiding starts and the catheter is expelled. Voiding stopped seconds later due to urethral obstruction.

RENAL ECTOPIA AND FUSION

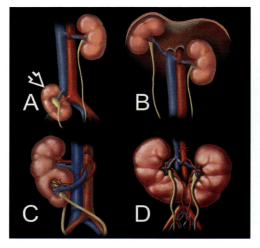

Graphic shows variations of renal ectopia and fusion: A) pelvic kidney (arrow), B) subdiaphragmatic/thoracic kidney C) crossed fused ectopic kidney and D) horseshoe kidney.

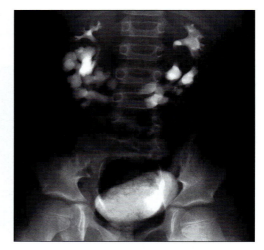

IVP shows classic "U" shape of a horseshoe kidney. Note variable calyceal blunting, abnormal rotation, abnormal renal axis, and at least four renal pelves.

TERMINOLOGY

Abbreviations and Synonyms
- Includes: Horseshoe or pancake kidney, crossed fused ectopia, pelvic, iliac (ptotic) and thoracic kidneys

Definitions
- Normal renal tissue in an abnormal location
- Results from abnormal ascent and rotation of the fetal kidney
- Kidneys form at sacral level and ascend to L1 by term, renal pelvis initially directed anteriorly but rotates 90 degrees medially as it ascends
- Malpositioned kidneys are more susceptible to trauma, iatrogenic injury, obstruction, infection, and stones
- High incidence of aberrant and multiple renal arteries and veins

IMAGING FINDINGS

General Features
- Best diagnostic clue: Normal renal parenchyma with: Abnormal location, axis of orientation, or position of renal pelvis
- Location: Anywhere from presacral to intrathoracic, bilateral or unilateral, may cross the midline
- Size: Overall volume of renal parenchyma is similar to orthotopic kidneys, though longitudinal measurements vary based on shape of ectopic kidney
- Morphology
  o Normal cortex, pyramids, and collecting system, though hydronephrosis is a common association
  o Isthmus or midline junctional zone of a horseshoe kidney may contain functioning renal tissue or fibrotic nonfunctional tissue

Radiographic Findings
- Radiography
  o May simulate a midline or pelvic mass
  o Bowel gas
    ▪ Can be displaced by ectopic kidney
    ▪ Or can occupy the renal fossa; typically splenic and hepatic flexures of colon are repositioned
- IVP
  o Functional renal parenchyma in atypical location, hydronephrosis common
  o Ectopic kidneys, especially thoracic and horseshoe varieties may appear "mass-like" on initial scout view
  o Expect bowel to occupy empty renal fossa
  o Early nephrogram may be missed on tightly coned films, not included in field of view
  o Abnormalities of vasculature and ureter are also common

DDx: Mimickers Of Renal Ectopia

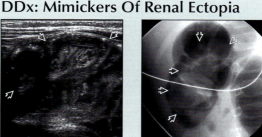
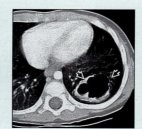
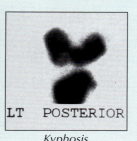

Intussusception | Intuss On Enema | Sequestration | Kyphosis

RENAL ECTOPIA AND FUSION

Key Facts

Terminology
- Normal renal tissue in an abnormal location
- Results from abnormal ascent and rotation of the fetal kidney
- Kidneys form at sacral level and ascend to L1 by term, renal pelvis initially directed anteriorly but rotates 90 degrees medially as it ascends
- Malpositioned kidneys are more susceptible to trauma, iatrogenic injury, obstruction, infection, and stones
- High incidence of aberrant and multiple renal arteries and veins

Imaging Findings
- Ultrasound is typically sufficient to document location and gross morphology of ectopic and fused kidneys
- Contrast enhanced studies (nuclear, IVP, CT, or MRI) used to assess drainage in cases of hydronephrosis, document nephrolithiasis, and locate position of aberrant renal arteries and veins

Top Differential Diagnoses
- Any "mass" typical for ectopic location
- Intussusception or pseudokidney of bowel

Pathology
- Horseshoe kidneys are associated with genital anomalies, VACTERL, Turner, and other syndromes
- Horseshoe incidence 1 in 400 births, most common fusion anomaly
- Crossed fused ectopic kidney less common
- Simple ectopia seen in 1 in 900 autopsy series

- Ureteral insertion site in bladder is a clue to where the kidney initially formed, (i.e. lower pole ureter of crossed fused ectopic kidney inserts into trigone on contralateral side)
- Oblique views are often helpful to profile an abnormally rotated collecting system
- May require fluoroscopic spot views to capture ureteral course
- Pelvic compression devices should be avoided

Fluoroscopic Findings
- Renal ectopia may be noted incidentally during other fluoro procedures: Barium studies, VCUG, or genitograms

CT Findings
- NECT
  - Occasionally initially seen on noncontrast enhanced renal stone CT
  - Soft tissue "mass" identified along with "absent" renal tissue in renal fossa
  - Associated hydronephrosis or stone disease are frequent clues to the correct diagnosis
- CECT
  - Look for abnormal location, rotation, axis, and ureteral course
  - Expect normal renal enhancement and excretion of contrast, except in cases of obstruction
  - Delayed imaging often useful
    - In hydronephrotic kidneys
    - To aid in localizing distal ureters
- CTA: Used occasionally for mapping of aberrant arterial supply pre-operatively

MR Findings
- Similar to other modalities: Abnormal location, axis, rotation
- Coronal and oblique planes useful in malrotated and malpositioned kidneys

Ultrasonographic Findings
- Grayscale Ultrasound
  - Classically described as normal echotexture renal parenchyma in abnormal location, though hydronephrosis and scarring may alter renal echotexture and architecture
  - May be difficult to see pelvic kidneys due to adjacent bowel gas
  - Colon typically occupies the empty renal fossa
- Color Doppler: Useful in detecting aberrant vessels and localizing ureteral jets
- Power Doppler: Useful in cases of pyelonephritis where parenchymal perfusion is decreased in infected segments

Angiographic Findings
- Conventional: Reserved for renal donors or patients undergoing surgery who have abnormalities of renal ascent and rotation, that are not clearly defined by other imaging modalities

Nuclear Medicine Findings
- May be found incidentally on bone scan, PET scan, gallium, labeled white blood cells (WBC), or renal imaging studies
- Nuclear renal studies sometimes specifically requested to document presence of a pelvic kidney which could not be appreciated on ultrasound due to intervening bowel gas
- Expect to see normal uptake of radiopharmaceutical with variable degrees of hydronephrosis

Imaging Recommendations
- Best imaging tool
  - Ultrasound is typically sufficient to document location and gross morphology of ectopic and fused kidneys
  - Contrast enhanced studies (nuclear, IVP, CT, or MRI) used to assess drainage in cases of hydronephrosis, document nephrolithiasis, and locate position of aberrant renal arteries and veins

RENAL ECTOPIA AND FUSION

DIFFERENTIAL DIAGNOSIS

Any "mass" typical for ectopic location
- Characteristic functioning renal tissue and lack of kidney in renal fossa help to confirm correct diagnosis
- Thoracic considerations: Pulmonary sequestration, neuroblastoma, neurenteric duplications, etc.
- Abdominal: Lymphoma, omental cake, desmoid, etc.
- Pelvis: Ovarian tumors, sacrococcygeal teratoma, pelvic rhabdomyosarcoma, etc.

Intussusception or pseudokidney of bowel
- Loops of bowel, especially when intussuscepted can mimic a kidney's echo pattern on ultrasound

Simulated ectopia related to severe kyphoscoliosis
- Mimics horseshoe kidney or crossed fused ectopia, but lacks connection between right and left kidneys
- Cross-sectional imaging or orthogonal views will clarify the difference

PATHOLOGY

General Features
- General path comments
  - Parenchyma is normal pathologically, though secondary changes of obstruction, scarring, nephrolithiasis are not uncommon
  - Embryology-anatomy
    - Results from abnormal ascent and rotation of metanephric blastema after induction by the ureteric bud
    - Multiple supplying vessels and draining ureters are very common
    - The isthmus of a horseshoe kidney may have functioning renal parenchyma or fibrous connective tissue
- Genetics
  - Horseshoe kidneys are associated with genital anomalies, VACTERL, Turner, and other syndromes
  - Other abnormalities of ascent and rotation less frequently associated with syndromes
  - Geographic "hot spots" suggest either a common exposure to teratogenetic factors, or a hereditary condition with variable penetrance
- Epidemiology
  - Horseshoe incidence 1 in 400 births, most common fusion anomaly
  - Crossed fused ectopic kidney less common
  - Simple ectopia seen in 1 in 900 autopsy series
- Associated abnormalities
  - Urologic abnormalities associated with simple ectopia
    - Vesicoureteral reflux 20-30%
    - Contralateral renal dysplasia 4%
    - Cryptorchidism 5%
    - Hypospadias 5%
  - Many syndromes have associated renal ectopia and abnormal fusion
    - VACTERL (vertebral, anorectal, cardiac, tracheoesophageal, renal, limb abnormalities)
  - Adrenal ectopia has been reported in association with renal ectopia
  - Cardiac and skeletal anomalies are common

CLINICAL ISSUES

Presentation
- Most common signs/symptoms
  - May be suspected on antenatal ultrasound
  - Can present later in infancy as palpable mass or with UTI or obstruction

Demographics
- Gender: All types of ectopia are more common in boys than girls

Natural History & Prognosis
- Aside from complications of obstruction, stone formation, UTI, and injury most kidneys function normally
- Primary concern is avoidance of iatrogenic injury to renal parenchyma and supplying vessels during routine surgery - especially laparoscopic surgery
- Slightly increased risk of Wilm and carcinoid tumors in horseshoe kidneys
- Prognosis generally excellent
  - One third of patients with horseshoe kidney are asymptomatic throughout life

Treatment
- Treat complications of obstruction, reflux, and stones

SELECTED REFERENCES

1. Guarino N et al: The incidence of associated urological abnormalities in children with renal ectopia. J Urol. 172(4 Pt 2):1757-9; discussion 1759, 2004
2. Yuksel A et al: Sonographic findings of fetuses with an empty renal fossa and normal amniotic fluid volume. Fetal Diagn Ther. 19(6):525-32, 2004
3. Watanabe T: Reflux nephropathy in a patient with crossed renal ectopia with fusion. Pediatr Nephrol. 17(8):617-9, 2002
4. Buyukdereli G et al: Tc-99m DMSA and Tc-99m DTPA imaging in the diagnosis of crossed renal ectopia. Clin Nucl Med. 26(3):257-8, 2001
5. Jefferson KP et al: Thoracic kidney: a rare form of renal ectopia. J Urol. 165(2):504, 2001
6. Kumar A et al: Live donation of ectopic kidneys: a feasible option under compelling circumstances. J Urol. 165(2):505-6, 2001
7. Rinat C et al: Familial inheritance of crossed fused renal ectopia. Pediatr Nephrol. 16(3):269-70, 2001
8. Colberg JW et al: Unilateral adrenal heterotopia with renal-adrenal fusion. J Urol. 160(1):116, 1998
9. Decter RM et al: Renal duplications and fusion anomalies. Pediatr Clin North Am. 44:1323-41, 1997
10. Saxey R: Sonographic findings in crossed renal ectopia without fusion. AJR Am J Roentgenol. 154(3):657, 1990
11. Slovis TL et al: Imaging of the Pediatric Urinary Tract. Philadelphia, WB Saunders. 69-162, 1989
12. Das S et al: Ureteropelvic junction obstruction with associated renal anomalies. J Urol. 131(5):872-4, 1984
13. Kyrayiannis B et al: Ectopic kidneys with and without fusion. Br J Urol. 51(3):173-4, 1979

RENAL ECTOPIA AND FUSION

IMAGE GALLERY

Typical

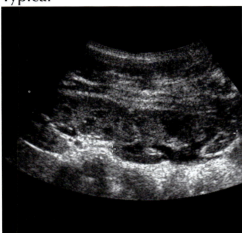
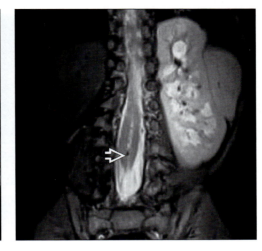

(Left) Ultrasound shows crossed fused ectopic kidney, positioned on the patient's right side. Cursors mark what would have been the patient's left kidney, fused to the lower pole of the orthotopic right kidney. *(Right)* T2WI MR shows crossed fused ectopic kidney on the left, extending in the lower thoracic cavity in this patient with split spinal cord, diastematomyelia. The bony spur of the the diastem is indicated by the arrow.

Typical

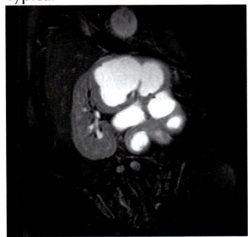
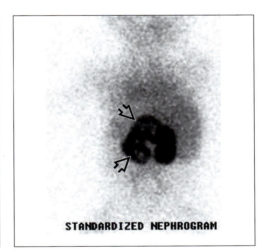

(Left) T2WI MR shows relatively normal appearing right renal moiety fused at the upper pole with a hydronephrotic left kidney in this unusual configuration of a horseshoe or pancake kidney. *(Right)* Tc 99m MAG3 scan shows good function of the right-sided moiety and delayed function in the hydronephrotic left sided portion (arrows) of the same patient shown on adjacent MR image.

Typical

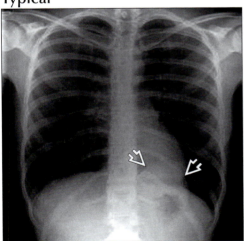
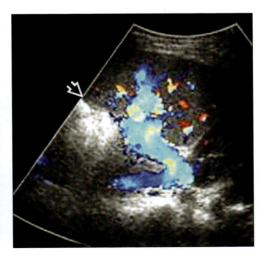

(Left) Radiograph shows soft tissue mass at the left lung base (arrows), which was located posteriorly on the lateral view. Patient had no pulmonary symptoms; routine screening chest X-ray. *(Right)* Axial ultrasound shows vascular pedicle feeding the "mass" at the left lung base, which has normal renal architecture. Note the echogenic interface of renal tissue with the lung (arrow).

PRIMARY MEGAURETER

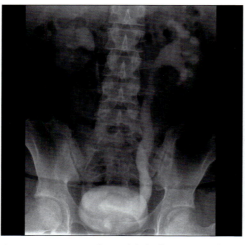

Anteroposterior IVP shows left hydroureteronephrosis with standing column of urine to the adynamic distal ureteral segment, in primary megaureter.

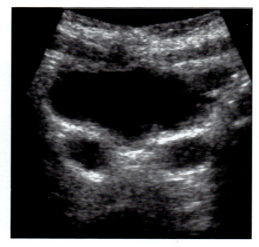

Axial ultrasound of urinary bladder shows bilateral ureteral dilation in this patient with primary megaureter.

TERMINOLOGY

Abbreviations and Synonyms
- Primary obstructive megaureter, functional megaureter, ureteral achalasia

Definitions
- Obstructive ureteral dilation above adynamic, normal caliber, short ureteral segment above ureterovesical junction (UVJ)
- Megaureter - dilated, tortuous ureter without implying cause

IMAGING FINDINGS

General Features
- Best diagnostic clue: Persistent ureteral dilation to just above UVJ on IVP, or diuretic MAG3 renal scan
- Location: Distal ureter just above UVJ
- Size
  ○ Narrow distal ureteral segment
  ○ Variable degree ureteral dilation and hydronephrosis (HN)
- Morphology
  ○ Concentric distal ureteral narrowing
  ○ Dilated curved distal ureter tapers to short segment

Radiographic Findings
- Radiography
  ○ Mostly normal
  ○ Mass effect if severe HN of kidney
- IVP
  ○ Ureteral dilation above distal ureteral segment
  ○ Frequently more ureteral than calyceal dilation
  ○ Ureter not usually as tortuous as reflux
  ○ Dilation persists on post-void, upright image
  ○ Adynamic segment may or may not opacify

Fluoroscopic Findings
- Voiding Cystourethrogram
  ○ Normal
  ○ Reflux into dilated ureter and calyces
    ▪ Delayed drainage of refluxed contrast
    ▪ Short normal-caliber distal ureteral segment
    ▪ Active ureteral peristalsis of dilated ureter

Ultrasonographic Findings
- Grayscale Ultrasound
  ○ Hydroureter +/- hydronephrosis
  ○ Increased real-time to-fro peristalsis

Nuclear Medicine Findings
- Diuretic Tc-99m-MAG3 or -DTPA renal scan
  ○ Intrarenal and ureteral accumulation of radiopharmaceutical

DDx: Hydroureteronephrosis

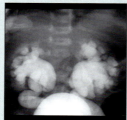
Refluxing Megaureter

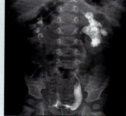
Nonreflux Megaureter

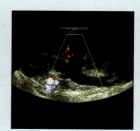
Nonreflux Megaureter

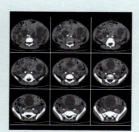
PUV

PRIMARY MEGAURETER

Key Facts

Imaging Findings
- Best diagnostic clue: Persistent ureteral dilation to just above UVJ on IVP, or diuretic MAG3 renal scan
- Ureteral dilation above distal ureteral segment
- Reflux into dilated ureter and calyces
- Delayed drainage of refluxed contrast
- If severe reflux, check ureteral drainage

Pathology
- Associated abnormalities: UPJ obstruction same moiety or opposite kidney

Clinical Issues
- Most common signs/symptoms: Prenatal HUN, urinary tract infection (UTI)
- Severity of obstruction usually stable
- Mild disease improves with time in many cases

- Delayed clearance after Lasix
  - T 1/2 > 20 minutes
  - Intrarenal and ureteral T 1/2

Imaging Recommendations
- Best imaging tool
  - Diuretic MAG3 renal scan - function
  - IVP: Anatomy
- Protocol advice
  - Renal ultrasound (US): Kidneys, ureters, bladder
  - Voiding cystourethrogram (VCUG): Exclude reflux
    - If severe reflux, check ureteral drainage
    - Poor drainage with normal caliber distal segment
  - MAG3 renal scan: Renal function and ? obstruction
  - Sequential sonography for follow-up q6-12 months

DIFFERENTIAL DIAGNOSIS

Refluxing megaureter
- Entire ureter dilated

Nonrefluxing nonobstructive megaureter
- Sequelae of antenatal dilation?

Secondary hydroureter
- Ureteral valves or diverticula, retrocaval ureter, tumors, distended bladder, urolithiasis

Posterior urethral valves
- bilateral or unilateral HUN

PATHOLOGY

General Features
- Etiology
  - Unknown
    - Paucity of ganglion cells
    - Hypoplasia/atrophy muscle fibers
- Associated abnormalities: UPJ obstruction same moiety or opposite kidney

Gross Pathologic & Surgical Features
- HUN of ipsilateral urinary system

Microscopic Features
- Additional smooth muscle collar surrounding terminal ureter

CLINICAL ISSUES

Presentation
- Most common signs/symptoms: Prenatal HUN, urinary tract infection (UTI)

Demographics
- Age: Prenatal to adolescence
- Gender: Both; males > females

Natural History & Prognosis
- Severity of obstruction usually stable
- Mild disease improves with time in many cases
- Some renal dysfunction and need surgical repair

Treatment
- Conservative approach
  - Follow-up: Chemoprophylaxis, imaging studies
- Surgical approach
  - Ureteral reimplant +/- ureteral tapering

SELECTED REFERENCES

1. Shukla AR et al: Prenatally detected primary megaureter: a role for extended followup. J Urol. 173(4):1353-6, 2005
2. Manzoni C: Megaureter. Rays. 27(2):83-5, 2002
3. McLellan DL et al: Rate and predictors of spontaneous resolution of prenatally diagnosed primary nonrefluxing megaureter. J Urol. 168(5):2177-80; discussion 2180, 2002

IMAGE GALLERY

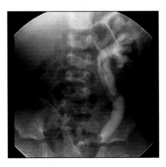 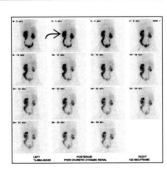

(Left) Anteroposterior voiding cystourethrogram shows high grade VUR into a bifid ureter, with delayed drainage of the ureter and a short, non-dilated distal ureteral segment. *(Right)* Diuresis renal scan shows delayed T1/2 of drainage of left urinary system (arrow) compared to the normal right system in this case of left refluxing primary megaureter.

POSTERIOR URETHRAL VALVES

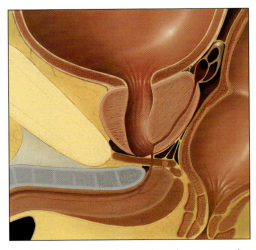

Sagittal graphic of PUV shows enlarged posterior urethra extending through the prostate gland and abrupt change in urethral caliber just distal to the verumontanum at the level of the valve tissue.

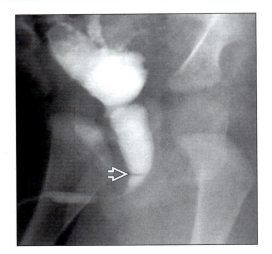

Oblique voiding cystourethrogram shows dilated posterior urethra and thin valve tissue extending from the ventral surface of the urethra (arrow). The urethral caliber narrows just distal to the valve tissue.

TERMINOLOGY

Abbreviations and Synonyms
- Posterior urethral valves (PUV), valves

Definitions
- Varying degree of chronic urethral obstruction due to fusion and prominence of plicae colliculi, normal concentric folds of urethra
- Classic imaging appearance: Abrupt transition on VCUG from dilated posterior urethra to small bulbous urethra at the level of the valves, actual valve tissue may not be visible
- Occurs exclusively in males
- 3 types of valves described
  o Type I: Most common, anterior fusion of plicae colliculi
  o Type II: Rarest, longitudinal folds from verumontanum to bladder neck
  o Type III: Rare, disc or windsock-type tissue distal to verumontanum
- Diagnosis made on voiding cystourethrogram (VCUG), cystoscopy, or cystosonography (outside the United States)

IMAGING FINDINGS

General Features
- Best diagnostic clue
  o Distinct caliber change in urethra at level of valves
  o Actual valve tissue is very thin and may not be directly visible
- Location: Posterior urethra for type I valves

Radiographic Findings
- Radiography: Indirect evidence of bladder obstruction or urinary retention: Bladder pseudomass in pelvis
- IVP
  o IVP is not the first line of imaging for PUV
    ▪ Could see indirect evidence of bladder wall thickening, upper tract obstruction, reflux

Fluoroscopic Findings
- Voiding Cystourethrogram
  o VCUG is the gold standard for imaging posterior urethral valves
  o Hallmark is abrupt, caliber change in posterior urethra
    ▪ Dilated posterior urethra gives rise to small caliber bulbous and penile urethra
    ▪ Actual valve tissue need not be seen on imaging to make diagnosis

DDx: Mimickers Of Posterior Urethral Valves

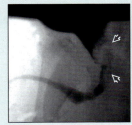
Cecoureterocele

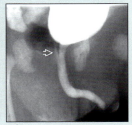
Prostatic Utricle

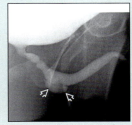
Cowper Syringocele

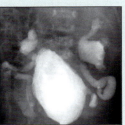
Prune Belly Syndrome

POSTERIOR URETHRAL VALVES

Key Facts

Terminology
- Varying degree of chronic urethral obstruction due to fusion and prominence of plicae colliculi, normal concentric folds of urethra
- Classic imaging appearance: Abrupt transition on VCUG from dilated posterior urethra to small bulbous urethra at the level of the valves, actual valve tissue may not be visible
- Occurs exclusively in males

Imaging Findings
- VCUG is the gold standard for imaging posterior urethral valves
- Associated findings
- Bladder wall trabeculation/muscular hypertrophy
- Vesicoureteral reflux
- Urinary ascites
- Urinoma/perinephric urine collection
- Reflux into utricle or other ducts
- MR is superior to ultrasound in older fetuses whose ossifying pelvic bones obscure visualization of the bladder outlet

Top Differential Diagnoses
- Anterior urethral valves
- Voiding dysfunction
- Cecoureterocele
- Post-surgical or post-traumatic urethral stricture

Pathology
- Incidence between 1 in 8,000 to 25,000 births
- Associated abnormalities: 80% have associated vesicoureteral reflux

---

- Note: Urethral catheter left in place during voiding may "stent" the valve tissue, obscuring caliber change and pushing valve tissue against urethral wall
  - Associated findings
    - Bladder wall trabeculation/muscular hypertrophy
    - Vesicoureteral reflux
    - Urinary ascites
    - Urinoma/perinephric urine collection
    - Reflux into utricle or other ducts

CT Findings
- Urethral abnormality not optimally demonstrated on axial CT images
- Associated findings are well-demonstrated on contrast-enhanced CT

MR Findings
- Best imaging test for antenatal diagnosis
  - MR is superior to ultrasound in older fetuses whose ossifying pelvic bones obscure visualization of the bladder outlet
  - Keyhole appearance of bladder is classic finding in PUV
  - In the fetus also look for
    - Oligohydramnios
    - Urine ascites or urinoma
    - Variable degrees of hydronephrosis and hydroureter
    - Variable degrees of renal dysplasia
    - Bladder wall thickening
    - Megacystis

Ultrasonographic Findings
- Grayscale Ultrasound
  - Angling the transducer toward the bladder neck may reveal a dilated posterior urethra
  - Cystosonography is gaining popularity in countries where ultrasound contrast agents are available
    - Exam is performed from a transperineal approach
    - Bladder catheterization and voiding while being imaged are still required
  - Sonography can also look for associated signs of reflux, urinary ascites, and renal dysplasia

Nuclear Medicine Findings
- Nuclear renogram studies may be performed to assess degree of renal dysplasia related to chronic obstruction and vesicoureteral reflux
- Nuclear cortical imaging useful in detecting scarring and differential renal function

Other Modality Findings
- At direct cystoscopy the valve tissue is translucent and may be pushed back against the outer walls of the urethra by inflowing irrigation fluid
- Similar drawbacks exist for fluoroscopic retrograde urethrogram which may not show the dynamic change in urethral caliber

Imaging Recommendations
- Best imaging tool
  - VCUG is exam of choice
  - Cystosonography being used outside the US, where ultrasound contrast agents are available

DIFFERENTIAL DIAGNOSIS

Anterior urethral valves
- Prominent semilunar fold in urethra more distal to the verumontanum, uncommon

Voiding dysfunction
- Detrusor external sphincter dyssynergia can resemble PUV transiently, but does not show persistent discrepancy in urethral caliber

Cecoureterocele
- Ureterocele prolapsing into the posterior urethra causing obstruction

Megalourethra
- Rare, entire length of urethra is enlarged, due to absence of corpus spongiosum

POSTERIOR URETHRAL VALVES

Post-surgical or post-traumatic urethral stricture
- History is key to making this diagnosis

PATHOLOGY

General Features
- General path comments: Related to abnormal thickening and/or fusion of normal circular mucosal folds in the urethra
- Epidemiology
  - Seen only in males
  - Incidence between 1 in 8,000 to 25,000 births
- Associated abnormalities: 80% have associated vesicoureteral reflux

Gross Pathologic & Surgical Features
- Valve tissue is typically very thin but functions like a sail, causing near-complete obstruction to antegrade flow of urine

Microscopic Features
- Valve tissue is thin, normal urothelium
- Bladder wall will show muscular hypertrophy and fibrosis
- Kidneys may show tubulointerstitial fibrosis and dysplasia

Staging, Grading or Classification Criteria
- Type I: Most common, anterior fusion of plicae colliculi
- Type II: Rarest, longitudinal folds from verumontanum to bladder neck
- Type III: Rare, disc or windsock-type tissue distal to verumontanum

CLINICAL ISSUES

Presentation
- Most common signs/symptoms
  - Severity of obstruction determines age at presentation and clinical symptoms
  - Oligohydramnios, hydronephrosis, urine ascites, urinoma, pulmonary hypoplasia antenatally
  - Urinary tract infection, sepsis, urinary retention, poor urinary stream, failure to thrive in infancy
  - Abnormal voiding patterns, hesitancy, straining, poor stream, large post-void residual, renal insufficiency/failure in childhood
  - Approximately 1/3 present at each stage

Demographics
- Age: Congenital, but age of presentation varies with degree of bladder outlet obstruction
- Gender: Males only

Natural History & Prognosis
- Varies with degree of renal dysplasia related to chronic obstruction and vesicoureteral reflux
- Unilateral reflux and urinary ascites are protective for contralateral kidney (relieve pressure)
- 10-15% of pediatric renal transplants are a result of PUV
- 30% of patients with PUV will eventually develop end stage renal disease
- Long-term problems with poor bladder compliance, small capacity bladder, and voiding dysfunction are also issues
- Plasma renin activity has been reported to be an early indicator of renal damage

Treatment
- Endoscopic valve ablation
- Fetal surgery sometimes performed in cases of severe oligohydramnios
  - Fetal therapies
  - Amnioinfusion to restore normal amniotic fluid volume
  - Serial bladder aspirates
  - A vesico-amniotic shunt can placed fetoscopically
  - Sequelae of pulmonary hypoplasia still are life threatening
  - Complications of shunting include limb entrapment, intestinal injury, hernia, and shunt migration
- Secondary bladder surgeries often needed: Bladder augmentation or continent diversion (Mitrofanoff)
- Long term follow-up is necessary in patients with PUV to monitor renal function and bladder compliance

SELECTED REFERENCES

1. Bajpai M et al: Posterior urethral valves: preliminary observations on the significance of plasma Renin activity as a prognostic marker. J Urol. 173(2):592-4, 2005
2. Berrocal T et al: Vesicoureteral reflux: can the urethra be adequately assessed by using contrast-enhanced voiding US of the bladder? Radiology. 234(1):235-41, 2005
3. Adams J et al: Pediatric renal transplantation and the dysfunctional bladder. Transpl Int. 17(10):596-602, 2004
4. Eckoldt F et al: Posterior urethral valves: prenatal diagnostic signs and outcome. Urol Int. 73(4):296-301, 2004
5. Ghanem MA et al: Long-term bladder dysfunction and renal function in boys with posterior urethral valves based on urodynamic findings. J Urol. 171(6 Pt 1):2409-12, 2004
6. Strand WR: Initial management of complex pediatric disorders: prunebelly syndrome, posterior urethral valves. Urol Clin North Am. 31(3):399-415, vii, 2004
7. Ylinen E et al: Prognostic factors of posterior urethral valves and the role of antenatal detection. Pediatr Nephrol. 19(8):874-9, 2004
8. DeFoor W et al: Successful renal transplantation in children with posterior urethral valves. J Urol. 170(6 Pt 1):2402-4, 2003
9. Mercado-Deane MG et al: US of renal insufficiency in neonates. Radiographics. 22(6):1429-38, 2002
10. Perks AE et al: Posterior urethral valves. J Pediatr Surg. 37(7):1105-7, 2002
11. Yohannes P et al: Current trends in the management of posterior urethral valves in the pediatric population. Urology. 60(6):947-53, 2002
12. Kraus SJ et al: Genitourinary Imaging in Children. Pediatr Clin North Am 48:1381-424, 2001
13. Fernbach SK et al: Pediatric voiding cystourethrography: A pictorial guide. Radiographics 20:155-68, 2000
14. Slovis TL et al: Imaging of the Pediatric Urinary Tract. Philadelphia, WB Saunders. 69-162, 1989

POSTERIOR URETHRAL VALVES

IMAGE GALLERY

Typical

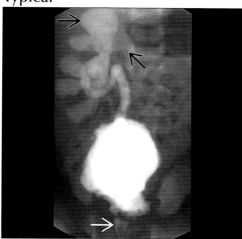
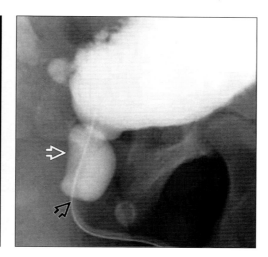

(Left) Voiding cystourethrogram shows high grade reflux into the right kidney (black arrows), irregular bladder wall thickening, bladder overdistention, and dilated posterior urethra (white arrow). *(Right)* Voiding cystourethrogram shows marked dilation of the posterior urethra, with a filling defect at white arrow representing the verumontanum. The valve tissue is located at the level of the black arrow, but is not visible.

Typical

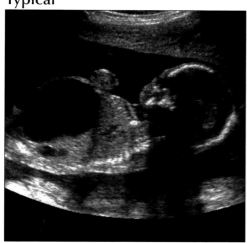
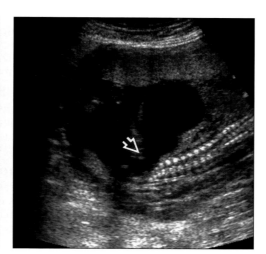

(Left) Fetal ultrasound shows massive cystic structure in the abdomen which appears distended. Bilateral hydronephrosis was also noted on images in different planes. *(Right)* Ultrasound shows additional scanning of the fetus revealed the cystic structure was a dramatically enlarged urinary bladder with a "keyhole" appearance caudally (arrow); later found to represent posterior urethral valves.

Typical

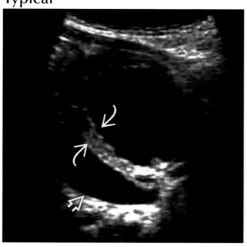
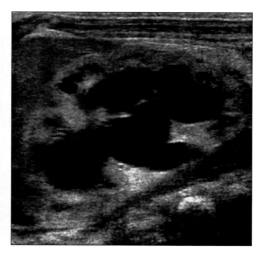

(Left) Coronal ultrasound shows dilated distal ureter (open arrow) and bladder wall thickening (between curved arrows) in a patient with posterior urethral valves. Distal hydroureter may be due to reflux or UVJ obstruction. *(Right)* Sagittal ultrasound from a prone, posterior approach shows marked hydronephrosis and cortical thinning in an infant with posterior urethral valves. The contralateral kidney was normal.

URACHAL ABNORMALITIES

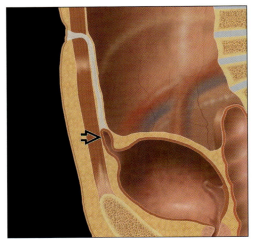 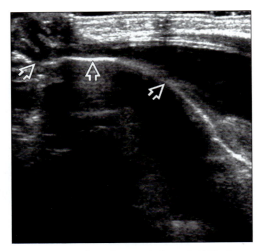

Graphic shows urachal diverticulum (arrow) and fibrotic tract to the umbilicus, which is called a patent urachus when it remains open. Urachal sinus and urachal cyst are additional variations discussed below.

Longitudinal midline ultrasound shows fluid-filled tract marked with arrows between dome of bladder and umbilicus in this newborn with a draining patent urachus.

TERMINOLOGY

Abbreviations and Synonyms
- Patent urachus, urachal fistula, urachal remnant, urachal cyst, urachal sinus, urachal diverticulum

Definitions
- Persistence of all or a portion of the connection between the bladder dome and the umbilicus, a remnant of the fetal allantoic stalk

IMAGING FINDINGS

General Features
- Best diagnostic clue: Fluid or cyst along the tract between bladder dome and umbilicus
- Location: Midline between dome of bladder and umbilicus
- Size: Variable
- Morphology
  - Patent urachus or urachal fistula
    - Open channel from bladder to navel through which urine can leak
  - Urachal sinus
    - Persistence of superficial segment of the channel opening onto the skin surface
  - Urachal diverticulum
    - Persistence of deep segment creating a point or diverticulum off the anterior-superior bladder wall
  - Urachal cyst
    - Persistence of the intermediary segment, fibrous attachments to bladder and navel

Radiographic Findings
- Radiography
  - Cross-table lateral film in neonate may be first test ordered to exclude hernia
  - In general, radiography not very useful

Fluoroscopic Findings
- Voiding Cystourethrogram
  - Best test to document patency of urachus
  - Inflammation along the tract can intermittently block the lumen
  - Voiding cystourethrogram (VCUG) tends to underestimate the length or extent of the remnant
  - True lateral views are necessary
  - Radiopaque marker on umbilicus can be helpful

CT Findings
- Occasionally recognized incidentally on CT scans performed for other reasons
- Infected urachal cyst may present with "rule out abscess"
- Look for solid or tubular structure extending through anterior aspect of peritoneal cavity to umbilicus

DDx: Other Umbilical Abnormalities

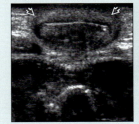 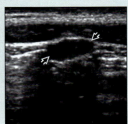 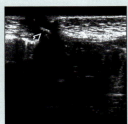 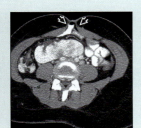

Granulation Tissue   *Palpable Node*   *Umbilical Hernia*   *Umbilical Hernia*

URACHAL ABNORMALITIES

Key Facts

Terminology
- Persistence of all or a portion of the connection between the bladder dome and the umbilicus, a remnant of the fetal allantoic stalk

Imaging Findings
- Best diagnostic clue: Fluid or cyst along the tract between bladder dome and umbilicus
- Patent urachus or urachal fistula
  - Open channel from bladder to navel through which urine can leak
- Urachal sinus
  - Persistence of superficial segment of the channel opening onto the skin surface
- Urachal diverticulum
  - Persistence of deep segment creating a point or diverticulum off the anterior-superior bladder wall
- Urachal cyst
  - Persistence of the intermediary segment, fibrous attachments to bladder and navel
- Helpful hints when scanning for urachal remnants with ultrasound
  - Bladder should be fairly full
  - Begin scanning at bladder level and sweep the transducer upward toward umbilicus
  - Gentle pressure on bladder dome can push fluid into a patent tract to aid in visualization

Top Differential Diagnoses
- Granulation tissue of umbilical stump
- Omphalitis
- Umbilical hernia
- Hemangioma of umbilical cord

- Surrounding inflammatory changes are common
- Localized cystic structure may also be seen when proximal and distal segments are fibrotic
- Fluid-debris levels may be present in urachal cysts

MR Findings
- Similar findings as CT
- Incidental finding on MR scan performed for other indications

Ultrasonographic Findings
- Grayscale Ultrasound
  - Typically has thick, well-defined wall
  - May or may not contain fluid
  - Size & shape depend on type of remnant present and presence of inflammation
  - Diverticulum is contiguous with anterior superior aspect of the bladder
  - Fluid-debris levels may be present in urachal cysts
- Color Doppler
  - Doppler useful in
    - Assessing degree of hyperemia when infected
    - And in excluding hemangioma
- Helpful hints when scanning for urachal remnants with ultrasound
  - Bladder should be fairly full
  - Patient should be calm; Valsalva can squeeze fluid out of a patent tract
  - Begin scanning at bladder level and sweep the transducer upward toward umbilicus
  - Gentle pressure on bladder dome can push fluid into a patent tract to aid in visualization

Imaging Recommendations
- Best imaging tool
  - Ultrasound defines the static anatomy well
  - Voiding cystourethrography (VCUG) useful to show flow dynamics, confirm patency

DIFFERENTIAL DIAGNOSIS

Granulation tissue of umbilical stump
- Most often confused with urachal remnants, especially urachal sinus
- Imaging can differentiate between the two by showing deeper extent of urachal remnant

Omphalitis
- Can be present in conjunction with urachal remnant
- In severe cases, may need to treat with antibiotics and re-evaluate

Umbilical hernia
- Usually readily discerned by physical exam and by imaging
- Hernia may contain peristalsing bowel or omentum
- When fluid appears in the hernia, it is surrounded by bowel wall signature on ultrasound

Hemangioma of umbilical cord
- Doppler ultrasound will show blood-flow rather than stagnant fluid

PATHOLOGY

General Features
- Genetics: Not inherited
- Etiology
  - Embryologically the allantois
    - Forms from the caudal end of the yolk sac
    - Functions as the primitive bladder as well as a blood forming organ
    - Normally involutes by 2nd month of gestation
    - Fibrotic cord remnant forms median umbilical ligament
    - Persistent segments of the allantoic channel are called urachal remnants
  - The urachus lies in the space of Retzius
    - Between the transversalis fascia anteriorly and the peritoneum posteriorly
- Epidemiology

URACHAL ABNORMALITIES

- Incidence of patent urachus is 1 in 40,000
- Other urachal anomalies are more common, though reliable statistics are not available
- Associated abnormalities
  - Peri-umbilical associations
    - Omphalocele
    - Omphalomesenteric remnant
  - Bladder outlet associations
    - Posterior urethral valves
    - Urethral atresia
    - Cloacal anomalies
    - Urogenital sinus malformation
  - Miscellaneous associations
    - Meningomyelocele (perhaps because of neurogenic bladder)
    - Unilateral kidney & other renal anomalies
    - Vaginal atresia

Gross Pathologic & Surgical Features
- Well-defined stalk with mucosal lining and varying degrees of fibrosis/lumen obliteration

Microscopic Features
- Cellular histology varies, not simple urothelium
  - Transitional cell epithelium
  - Columnar epithelium
  - Glandular epithelium
  - Squamous epithelium
- Varied cell types explain the variety of malignant cell lines found in adults urachal tumors

CLINICAL ISSUES

Presentation
- Most common signs/symptoms
  - Clinical presentation varies with type of urachal remnant
    - Patent urachus presents with drainage from umbilicus, urinary tract infection, and relapsing periumbilical inflammation
    - Occasionally, the urachus remains patent in response to bladder outlet obstruction (posterior urethral valves, pelvic mass, etc.) and will close when outlet is repaired
    - Urachal sinus presents with periumbilical tenderness, a wet umbilicus, or non-healing granulation tissue at the base of the umbilicus
    - Urachal cyst presents in childhood or adolescence with suprapubic mass, fever, pain, and irritative voiding symptoms
    - Urachal diverticula generally are asymptomatic and discovered incidentally; rarely they enlarge, fail to drain during urination, and become predisposed to infection or stone formation

Demographics
- Age
  - Patent urachus seen in newborns primarily
  - Urachal sinus also typically diagnosed within first few months of life
  - Urachal cysts may go undetected until childhood or adulthood
  - Urachal diverticulum often undetected, autopsy finding
- Gender
  - Males > females
  - 2:1 ratio

Natural History & Prognosis
- Generally prognosis is excellent
  - Urachal tract is resected; no further follow-up needed
- Risk of malignancy if not resected
  - Adenocarcinoma
  - Mucinous cystadenocarcinoma
  - Villous adenoma in urachal remnants
- Urachal malignancies account for < 1% of all bladder cancers
- Typically occur in patients 40-70 years of age
- Majority of cancers occur in men (~75%)
- Present with hematuria or mucinous micturition
- Many also present with vague abdominal pain related to local invasion
- Local tumor invasion is common at time of urachal cancer diagnosis
- Imaging generally performed: CT

Treatment
- Resection of the entire tract
  - Open surgery was previously the rule
  - Laparoscopic resection gaining popularity
- Often performed in staged fashion
  - Inflammation and infection are treated and allowed to heal
  - Delayed definitive surgery is performed
- When accompanied by bladder outlet obstruction
  - Surgery to relieve the outlet obstruction must be performed first
  - Patent urachus is serving as a pop-off valve in these cases
  - Following correction of bladder outlet problems, allow up to one year for patent urachus to close independently
  - If drainage persists, reassess bladder outlet function, and if functioning well, resect the tract

SELECTED REFERENCES

1. Nobuhara KK et al: The giant umbilical cord: an unusual presentation of a patent urachus. J Pediatr Surg. 39(1):128-9, 2004
2. Ozel SK et al: An unusual presentation of patent urachus: report of a case. Eur J Pediatr Surg. 14(3):206-8, 2004
3. Amano Y et al: MR imaging of umbilical cord urachal (allantoic) cyst in utero. AJR Am J Roentgenol. 180(4):1181-2, 2003
4. McCollum MO et al: Surgical implications of urachal remnants: Presentation and management. J Pediatr Surg. 38(5):798-803, 2003
5. Ueno T et al: Urachal anomalies: ultrasonography and management. J Pediatr Surg. 38(8):1203-7, 2003
6. Cothren C et al: Urachal carcinoma: key points for the general surgeon. Am Surg. 68(2):201-3, 2002
7. Yu JS et al: Urachal remnant diseases: spectrum of CT and US findings. Radiographics. 21(2):451-61, 2001
8. Clapuyt P et al: Urachal neuroblastoma: first case report. Pediatr Radiol. 29(5):320-1, 1999

URACHAL ABNORMALITIES

IMAGE GALLERY

Typical

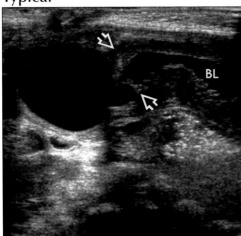
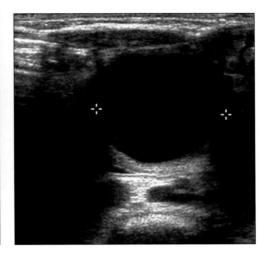

(Left) Longitudinal midline ultrasound shows cephalad tenting of the bladder dome (between arrows) just inferior to a well-defined urachal cyst. This cyst did not communicate with the bladder or umbilicus at surgical resection. *(Right)* Transverse ultrasound of the midline abdomen between the bladder and umbilicus shows the same urachal cyst between cursors in orthogonal plane.

Typical

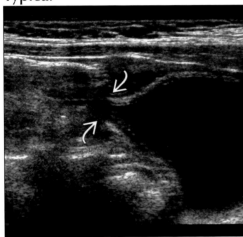
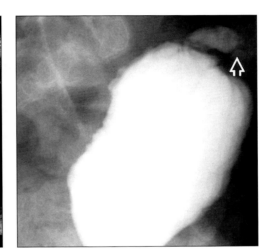

(Left) Longitudinal midline ultrasound shows cephalad pointing of the bladder dome (arrows), but no fluid-filled tract to the umbilicus, in this patient with urachal diverticulum. *(Right)* Lateral view during VCUG shows contrast filling a tubular outpouching (arrow) from the dome of the bladder, a urachal diverticulum, in this patient with neurogenic bladder.

Typical

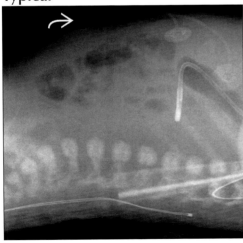
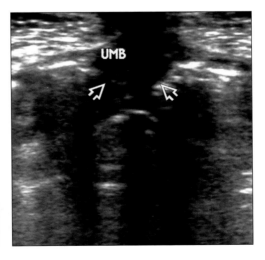

(Left) Lateral abdominal radiograph shows a dressing (arrow) overlying the umbilicus in this patient who had intermittent drainage from the umbilicus. There is no evidence of hernia on this cross-table view. *(Right)* Transverse ultrasound in the same patient shows a shallow, blind ending sinus at the base of the umbilical stump, a urachal sinus marked by arrows.

MULTICYSTIC DYSPLASTIC KIDNEY

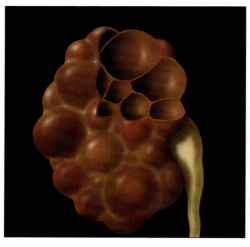

Graphic shows multiple cysts of varying size with minimal intervening dysplastic tissue. A ureter may or may not be recognizable at the renal hilum on imaging studies.

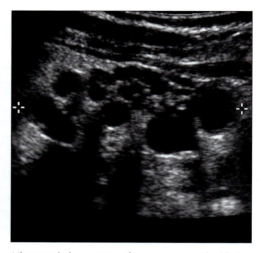

Ultrasound shows cysts of varying size embedded in echogenic tissue which roughly has the contour of a kidney, but lacks other renal architectural features. Upper and lower margins marked by cursors.

TERMINOLOGY

Abbreviations and Synonyms
- Multicystic dysplastic kidney (MCDK)

Definitions
- A non-functional kidney, replaced by multiple cysts and dysplastic tissue, can vary in size from 10-15 cm to only 1-2 cm
- MCDK is the second most common abdominal mass in a neonate
  - Hydronephrosis is the most common neonatal mass
- Classic imaging appearance: 2 forms generally recognized
  - Pelvoinfundibular MCDK, more common type, theoretically results from atresia of ureter or renal pelvis; cysts are remnants of dilated calyces
  - Hydronephrotic type of MCDK, occurs less frequently, results from atretic segment of ureter; cysts are the entire pelvocaliceal system
- Up to 40% of patients with MCDK have contralateral abnormality
  - Ureteropelvic junction obstruction (UPJO) and vesicoureteral reflux are most common
- Tend to involute with time, cysts shrink and residual tissue does not have a reniform shape
- Can be segmental in duplicated kidneys
- Incidence
  - 0.03% in autopsy series
  - 1 in 4,300 live births

IMAGING FINDINGS

General Features
- Best diagnostic clue
  - Typically discovered with ultrasound prenatally or perinatally when palpated
  - Ultrasound may not be conclusive for diagnosis when cysts mimic hydronephrosis
  - Nuclear scintigraphy documents lack of renal function, confirms the diagnosis of MCDK
    - If some excretion is present, consider poorly functioning hydronephrosis
- Location: Renal fossa most common, but can occur ectopically from pelvis to chest
- Size: Wide range: 10-15 cm in length to only 1-2 cm after years of involution
- Morphology
  - Numerous cysts of varying size with echogenic intervening parenchyma
  - No recognizable corticomedullary architecture
  - Renal contour may or may not be preserved

Radiographic Findings
- Radiography: Indirect evidence of MCDK is space occupying lesion in the flank

DDx: Mimickers Of MCDK

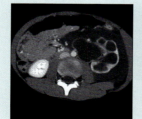
UPJO With Rupture

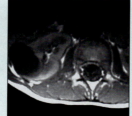
Cystic Wilm Tumor

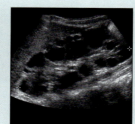
Tuberous Sclerosis

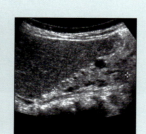
ESRD

MULTICYSTIC DYSPLASTIC KIDNEY

Key Facts

Terminology
- A non-functional kidney, replaced by multiple cysts and dysplastic tissue, can vary in size from 10-15 cm to only 1-2 cm
- MCDK is the second most common abdominal mass in a neonate
- Up to 40% of patients with MCDK have contralateral abnormality
- Tend to involute with time, cysts shrink and residual tissue does not have a reniform shape
- Can be segmental in duplicated kidneys

Imaging Findings
- Ultrasound may not be conclusive for diagnosis when cysts mimic hydronephrosis
- Nuclear scintigraphy documents lack of renal function, confirms the diagnosis of MCDK
- Cysts of varying size that do not interconnect as massive hydronephrosis would
- Intervening parenchyma tends to be echogenic fibrous tissue

Top Differential Diagnoses
- Hydronephrosis
- Wilm tumor
- Tuberous sclerosis
- End-stage renal disease (ESRD)
- Congenital mesoblastic nephroma (CMN)

Clinical Issues
- Typically discovered antenatally or in infancy as a palpable mass
- Vast majority involute with time and remain asymptomatic

- IVP
  - Tissue is not functioning, therefore will not see excretion of iodinated contrast
  - May see transient blush during contrast bolus infusion because tissue is perfused
  - IVP's are seldom performed in pediatric patients

CT Findings
- NECT: Low density cysts (though some cysts may contain debris) replacing normal renal parenchyma
- CECT: Minimal or no contrast enhancement and lack of excretion on delayed images

MR Findings
- T1WI
  - Cysts replacing normal renal parenchyma
  - Usually noted incidentally on MR performed for other indications
- T2WI: High signal intensity fluid in cysts, irregular lobulated contour

Ultrasonographic Findings
- Grayscale Ultrasound
  - Cysts of varying size that do not interconnect as massive hydronephrosis would
  - Largest cyst is not generally central in position
  - Intervening parenchyma tends to be echogenic fibrous tissue
  - Outer contour often lobulated with outer cyst walls forming the margins of the mass
  - Often followed with annual ultrasound scans to
    - Assess growth of contralateral kidney
    - Confirm involution of MCDK (very large MCDK's may be surgically removed due to mass effect)
    - Watch for unusual growth of MCDK that has been reported with Wilm tumor arising in these lesions
- Color Doppler: Minimal flow in parenchyma, central hilar vessels tend to be small

Nuclear Medicine Findings
- Scintigraphy
  - MAG3, DTPA, glucoheptonate are typically agents of choice
  - Initial blood flow images show perfusion of the MCDK, but sequential images document lack of any excretory function
  - Note that Tc 99m DMSA may localize to the renal cortex in MCDK due to the presence of tubular cells, but this is different than true excretion of radiopharmaceutical

Other Modality Findings
- Retrograde ureterogram will show blind ending ureter, different from rapid change in caliber of ureter and communication with calyces seen in UPJO or other causes of hydronephrosis

Imaging Recommendations
- Best imaging tool
  - Ultrasound for initial identification
  - Nuclear scan to document non function of MCDK and assess drainage of contralateral kidney

---

DIFFERENTIAL DIAGNOSIS

Hydronephrosis
- Calyces should communicate with each other in hydronephrosis, look for connections on ultrasound
- UPJO is a common finding in the contralateral kidney

Wilm tumor
- Can be difficult to separate by US, absent excretory function is key

Tuberous sclerosis
- Kidneys may have cysts and/or angiomyolipomas

End-stage renal disease (ESRD)
- Kidneys tend to be small, echogenic and can resemble old, involuted MCDK
- ESRD is bilateral whereas MCDK is unilateral

Congenital mesoblastic nephroma (CMN)
- Included in this differential because it is a neonatal renal mass, but CMN is seldom cystic

MULTICYSTIC DYSPLASTIC KIDNEY

- CMN is the most common solid renal tumor of infancy
- Solid renal tumors in infancy are, in general, very rare

PATHOLOGY

General Features
- Genetics: Generally considered sporadic, though there are reports of familial cases where inheritance is autosomal dominant with variable expression and penetrance
- Etiology: Probably due to atresia of ureter or ureteropelvic junction during the metanephric stage of intrauterine development
- Associated abnormalities
  o Genitourinary abnormalities in 25-40%
    - Contralateral ureteropelvic or ureterovesical obstruction
    - Megaureter
    - Cystic dysplasia of testis
    - Vesicoureteral reflux in 12-26%
  o Non-urologic abnormalities
    - Cardiac and musculoskeletal most common
  o Associated syndromes
    - Turner syndrome
    - Trisomy 21
    - Chromosome 22 deletions
    - Waardenburg syndrome
    - Others

Gross Pathologic & Surgical Features
- Walls of cysts vary in thickness, fibrotic dysplastic tissue replaces normal renal stroma, may be quite large and non-reniform in shape

CLINICAL ISSUES

Presentation
- Most common signs/symptoms
  o Typically discovered antenatally or in infancy as a palpable mass
  o Can have delayed presentation as incidental finding when
    - Symptoms of contralateral UPJ obstruction are evaluated
    - Patient evaluated for urinary tract infection
    - Patient imaged for a traumatic injury

Demographics
- Age: Congenital abnormality, usually presents in infancy
- Gender: Equal incidence in males and females

Natural History & Prognosis
- Vast majority involute with time and remain asymptomatic
  o Approximately half show complete involution by 7 years of age
- Can have complications of infection or mass effect
- Though case reports of hypertension exist in patients with unilateral MCDK, the overall risk is extremely low
  o In patients treated with nephrectomy for hypertension, blood pressure normalized in only half, suggesting the source was not the MCDK
- Prognosis is excellent when uncomplicated
  o Still excellent even when surgery required
- If contralateral kidney has delayed diagnosis of UPJO or UVJO, renal insufficiency can be a problem
- VUR into the kidney contralateral to a MCDK is associated with smaller size of that kidney during the first year of life
- Reports of small incidence of Wilm tumor developing in MCDK

Treatment
- Surgical excision when complicated by focal enlargement (potential Wilm tumor), recurrent infections, mass effect, or hypertension
- Otherwise, serial sonograms for 3-5 years are used to monitor

SELECTED REFERENCES

1. Farnham SB et al: Pediatric urological causes of hypertension. J Urol. 173(3):697-704, 2005
2. Narchi H: Risk of Wilms' tumour with multicystic kidney disease: a systematic review. Arch Dis Child. 90(2):147-9, 2005
3. Kaneyama K et al: Associated urologic anomalies in children with solitary kidney. J Pediatr Surg. 39(1):85-7, 2004
4. Abidari JM et al: Serial followup of the contralateral renal size in children with multicystic dysplastic kidney. J Urol. 168(4 Pt 2):1821-5; discussion 1825, 2002
5. Aubertin G et al: Prenatal diagnosis of apparently isolated unilateral multicystic kidney: implications for counselling and management. Prenat Diagn. 22(5):388-94, 2002
6. Belk RA et al: A family study and the natural history of prenatally detected unilateral multicystic dysplastic kidney. J Urol. 167(2 Pt 1):666-9, 2002
7. Mercado-Deane MG et al: US of renal insufficiency in neonates. Radiographics. 22(6):1429-38, 2002
8. Suzuki K et al: Segmental multicystic dysplastic kidney in an adult woman. Urol Int. 66(1):51-4, 2001
9. Snodgrass WT: Hypertension associated with multicystic dysplastic kidney in children. J Urol. 164(2):472-3;discussion 473-4, 2000
10. Srivastava T et al: Autosomal dominant inheritance of multicystic dysplastic kidney. Pediatr Nephrol. 13(6):481-3, 1999
11. John U et al: Kidney growth and renal function in unilateral multicystic dysplastic kidney disease. Pediatr Nephrol. 12(7):567-71, 1998
12. Kessler OJ et al: Involution rate of multicystic renal dysplasia. Pediatrics. 102(6):E73, 1998
13. Zerin JM et al: The impact of vesicoureteral reflux on contralateral renal length in infants with multicystic dysplastic kidney. Pediatr Radiol. 28(9):683-6, 1998
14. Homsy YL et al: Wilms tumor and multicystic dysplastic kidney disease. J Urol. 158(6):2256-9; discussion 2259-60, 1997
15. Beckwith JB: Wilms tumor in MCDK. Dialogues in Pediatric Urology. 19:3-5, 1996
16. Strife JL et al: Multicystic dysplastic kidney in children: US follow up. Radiology. 186:785-8, 1993
17. Slovis TL et al: Imaging of the Pediatric Urinary Tract. Philadelphia, WB Saunders. 69-162, 1989

MULTICYSTIC DYSPLASTIC KIDNEY

IMAGE GALLERY

Typical

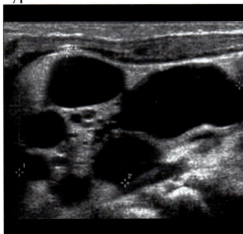
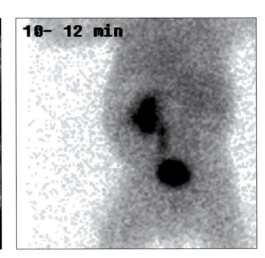

(Left) Sagittal ultrasound shows cursors roughly marking the borders of this multicystic dysplastic kidney. Note that the largest cyst is in the lower pole, not in the expected location of the renal pelvis. *(Right)* Posterior planar image from Tc 99m MAG3 study shows normally functioning left kidney in this patient with a right-sided MCDK. High radiotracer concentration in the normal kidney can mimic hydronephrosis.

Typical

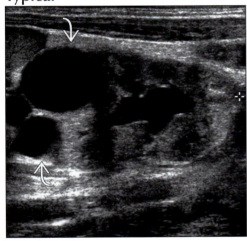
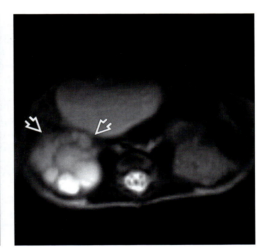

(Left) Ultrasound shows upper pole segmental MCDK (arrows) in this duplicated left kidney. The cursor marks the inferior margin of the normal lower pole cortex. *(Right)* Axial T2WI MR shows a right MCDK (arrows) with variable size cysts and normal left kidney in a newborn being evaluated for tethered spinal cord.

Typical

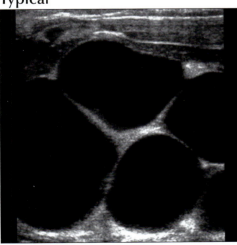
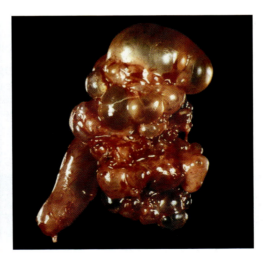

(Left) Ultrasound shows near complete replacement of renal parenchyma with cysts in MCDK. Cortex is barely visible in some areas and the outer contour is lobular. *(Right)* Gross pathology shows numerous cysts replacing the renal parenchyma and distorting the renal contour. Note that the largest cyst in this specimen is in the upper pole, not in the renal hilum.

POLYCYSTIC RENAL DISEASE, RECESSIVE

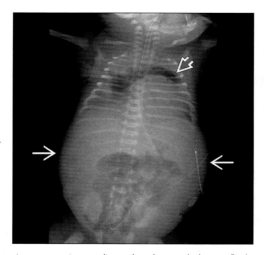

Anteroposterior radiograph shows bulging flanks (arrows) in a patient with Potter's facies, severe respiratory distress, and air-block complication (open arrow), due to ARPKD.

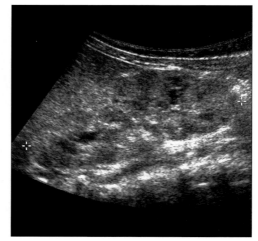

Sagittal ultrasound shows a newborn kidney measuring 9 cm (between cursors) with poor corticomedullary differentiation and globally increased echotexture in a patient with ARPKD.

TERMINOLOGY

Abbreviations and Synonyms
- Autosomal recessive polycystic kidney disease (ARPKD), infantile polycystic kidney disease

Definitions
- Single gene disorder characterized by bilateral, symmetric cystic renal disease involving distal convoluted tubules and collecting ducts

IMAGING FINDINGS

General Features
- Best diagnostic clue
  - Bilaterally enlarged hyperechoic kidneys in a newborn
  - History of fetal oligohydramnios is supportive evidence
- Location: Massive kidneys fill the flanks and displace adjacent organs
- Size: 2-4 standard deviations above the mean size in majority of patients
- Morphology
  - Reniform shape generally maintained
  - Loss of normal intra-renal architecture

Radiographic Findings
- Radiography
  - Bilateral flank "masses"
  - Pulmonary hypoplasia or respiratory compromise common
- IVP
  - Seldom performed today
  - Classic appearance was persistence of iodinated contrast in dilated tubules for hours after injection, with minimal or absent contrast excretion

CT Findings
- NECT
  - Enlarged, symmetric kidneys
  - Punctate calcifications may be seen and correlate with worsening renal function
- CECT
  - Iodinated contrast is trapped in dilated tubules in the medullary portion of the kidney
  - Minimal excretion of contrast into collecting system
  - Bladder typically empty or small
  - Small cysts may be present, generally < 3 cm in size

MR Findings
- General Features
  - Large kidneys of uniform high signal intensity on T2 weighted series
    - Small, discrete cysts may be discerned

DDx: Other Cystic Diseases

MCDK | ADPKD | Tuberous Sclerosis | Cystic Dysplasia

POLYCYSTIC RENAL DISEASE, RECESSIVE

Key Facts

Terminology
- Single gene disorder characterized by bilateral, symmetric cystic renal disease involving distal convoluted tubules and collecting ducts

Imaging Findings
- Bilaterally enlarged hyperechoic kidneys in a newborn
- History of fetal oligohydramnios is supportive evidence
- Poor or absent corticomedullary differentiation
- Small cysts may be present, generally < 1 cm in diameter, seen in roughly half of patients
- Diffuse microcystic appearance also described
- Tiny, punctate hyperechoic foci develop with time and correlate with renal failure

Top Differential Diagnoses
- Bilateral multicystic dysplastic kidney
- Autosomal dominant polycystic kidney disease (ADPKD)
- Cystic renal dysplasia
- Meckel-Gruber
- Tuberous sclerosis

Pathology
- Ectatic distal convoluted tubules & collecting ducts
- Gene is called polycystic kidney and hepatic disease 1 (PKHD1)

Clinical Issues
- More severe disease typically presents in infancy
- Milder forms of ARPKD can present in childhood and survive to adulthood

---

  - Uniform or grainy hypointense signal on T1 weighted series
  - On MR urography series radially arranged dilated tubules visible in medullary portion of kidney
  - No urine in bladder

Ultrasonographic Findings
- Grayscale Ultrasound
  - Enlarged, hyperechoic kidneys
  - Poor or absent corticomedullary differentiation
  - Dilated tubules, radially arranged in kidney are seen in 2/3 with high resolution linear transducers
  - Focal rosettes consisting of a cluster of the radially oriented, dilated collecting tubules also reported
  - Small cysts may be present, generally < 1 cm in diameter, seen in roughly half of patients
  - Cysts > 1 cm seen only in a minority of cases
  - Diffuse microcystic appearance also described
  - Tiny, punctate hyperechoic foci develop with time and correlate with renal failure
    - Etiology is likely calcium deposits, which can be confirmed on CT scans
    - Calcium citrate and calcium oxalate crystals have been found histologically
    - Echogenic foci do not cause posterior acoustic shadowing, but may cause ring-down artifact
  - Prenatal ultrasound findings
    - Kidneys > 2 standard deviation (SD) above mean for gestational age
    - Renal enlargement may not occur until mid 2nd trimester
    - Cysts may be visible but do not predominate
    - Normal hypoechoic cortex is present
    - Look for thin rim around echogenic medulla
    - Oligohydramnios
    - Fetal bladder not visible
    - Associated musculoskeletal abnormalities due to mechanics; oligohydramnios limits movement

Nuclear Medicine Findings
- Hepatobiliary Scan: Enlarged left liver lobe, a delay in maximal hepatocyte uptake, delayed tracer excretion into the biliary tree and gut

- Tc 99m DMSA renal cortical scans
  - Loss of kidney outline and internal structure, patchy tracer uptake with focal defects throughout the kidneys

Imaging Recommendations
- Best imaging tool: Ultrasound
- Protocol advice
  - High frequency linear transducer in infants
  - Serial renal measurements in fetuses at risk
  - Ratio renal circumference to abdominal circumference
    - > 2 SD above mean
  - Amniotic fluid assessment
    - 1st or 2nd trimester oligohydramnios carries a poor prognosis

DIFFERENTIAL DIAGNOSIS

Bilateral multicystic dysplastic kidney
- Visible macroscopic cysts dominant feature

Autosomal dominant polycystic kidney disease (ADPKD)
- Check family history and scan kidneys of parents
- May have asymmetric renal enlargement
- Rare in utero
  - Cysts may be visible late 3rd trimester
- Amniotic fluid normal
- Renal echogenicity normal

Cystic renal dysplasia
- Usually related to chronic obstruction, infection, or vascular compromise
- These kidneys are small, have numerous cysts and echogenic intervening parenchyma

Meckel-Gruber
- Encephalocele, large polycystic kidneys and polydactyly
  - Microcephaly is a clue if oligohydramnios limits views

POLYCYSTIC RENAL DISEASE, RECESSIVE

Tuberous sclerosis
- Rhabdomyoma: Echogenic cardiac mass
- Tubers: Subependymal nodules in brain may be difficult to detect in newborn
- Renal cysts: Not usually seen in utero
- Angiomyolipomas: Not usually seen in newborn

PATHOLOGY

General Features
- General path comments
  - Ectatic distal convoluted tubules & collecting ducts
    - Increased volume of medulla leads to renal enlargement
    - Increase in reflective interfaces from the dilated tubules creates high echogenicity
- Genetics
  - Autosomal recessive
  - Maps to proximal chromosome 6p
  - Gene is called polycystic kidney and hepatic disease 1 (PKHD1)
  - Risk of recurrence in subsequent pregnancies is 25%
- Epidemiology
  - 1:20,000 births
  - Heterozygous carrier state of 1 in 70
- Associated abnormalities: Musculoskeletal abnormalities related to fetal packing

Gross Pathologic & Surgical Features
- Enlarged kidneys with preserved reniform shape

Microscopic Features
- Ectatic distal convoluted tubules and collecting ducts
- Tubules originally described as "saccular or cylindrically enlarged"

CLINICAL ISSUES

Presentation
- Most common signs/symptoms: Bilateral renal enlargement and renal insufficiency
- Other signs/symptoms: Respiratory distress common and may be severe, life-limiting
- Fetal Presentation: Enlarged kidneys at imaging
  - Majority detected > 24 weeks
  - Diagnosis reported at 16 weeks in at-risk fetus
    - Most kidneys look normal up to 20 weeks
  - May look normal up to late in 2nd trimester
    - Reports of delayed onset oligo after 28 weeks
- Marked nephromegaly may cause dystocia at birth

Demographics
- Age
  - More severe disease typically presents in infancy
  - Milder forms of ARPKD can present in childhood and survive to adulthood
- Gender: M = F

Natural History & Prognosis
- Perinatal form
  - Severe renal disease
  - Pulmonary hypoplasia
  - Minimal hepatic fibrosis
  - Worst prognosis, high mortality in 1st month of life
- Juvenile form
  - More mild renal disease, more severe hepatic fibrosis
  - Liver disease more relevant in survivors
    - Portal hypertension and fibrosis develop in approximately half of patients
  - Survival rate has increased for milder form to 82% at age 3 years, and 79% at 15 years
- Fetal diagnosis: Majority stillborn or neonatal death
- Perinatal survivors will require renal replacement therapy (dialysis or transplant)
  - If prolonged survival, liver disease becomes relevant
  - Liver transplant currently only available treatment for hepatic component of this disease
  - Long term survivors have had combined renal and hepatic transplants
- Severity and outcomes vary within affected families
- Systemic hypertension seen in 75%
- Chronic ventilatory support in 30-50%

Treatment
- Karyotype
- Deliver at tertiary center
- Monitor fetal abdominal circumference: Risk of dystocia
- Encourage autopsy confirmation if demise or termination
- Renal replacement therapy: Dialysis or transplant
- Liver transplant when associated with progressive hepatic fibrosis

SELECTED REFERENCES
1. Bergmann C et al: Clinical consequences of PKHD1 mutations in 164 patients with autosomal-recessive polycystic kidney disease (ARPKD). Kidney Int. 67(3):829-48, 2005
2. Traubici J et al: High-resolution renal sonography in children with autosomal recessive polycystic kidney disease. AJR Am J Roentgenol. 184(5):1630-3, 2005
3. Zerres K et al: New options for prenatal diagnosis in autosomal recessive polycystic kidney disease by mutation analysis of the PKHD1 gene. Clin Genet. 66(1):53-7, 2004
4. Guay-Woodford LM et al: Autosomal recessive polycystic kidney disease: the clinical experience in North America. Pediatrics. 111(5 Pt 1):1072-80, 2003
5. Stein-Wexler R et al: Sonography of macrocysts in infantile polycystic kidney disease. J Ultrasound Med. 22(1):105-7, 2003
6. Zerres K et al: Autosomal recessive polycystic kidney disease (ARPKD). J Nephrol. 16(3):453-8, 2003
7. Avni FE et al: Hereditary polycystic kidney diseases in children: changing sonographic patterns through childhood. Pediatr Radiol. 32(3):169-74, 2002
8. Khan K et al: Morbidity from congenital hepatic fibrosis after renal transplantation for autosomal recessive polycystic kidney disease. Am J Transplant. 2(4):360-5, 2002
9. Zagar I et al: The value of radionuclide studies in children with autosomal recessive polycystic kidney disease. Clin Nucl Med. 27(5):339-44, 2002
10. Kern S et al: Appearance of autosomal recessive polycystic kidney disease in magnetic resonance imaging and RARE-MR-urography. Pediatr Radiol. 30(3):156-60, 2000

POLYCYSTIC RENAL DISEASE, RECESSIVE

IMAGE GALLERY

Typical

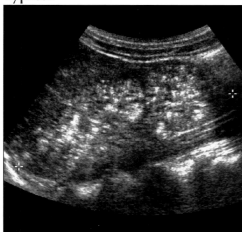
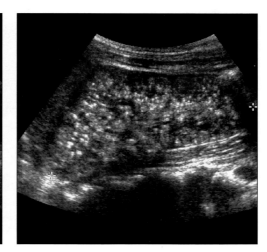

(Left) Sagittal ultrasound shows an enlarged echogenic kidney (between cursors) with no discernible corticomedullary differentiation and innumerous punctate hyperechoic foci in a 3 year old patient with ARPKD. *(Right)* Sagittal ultrasound shows similar findings in the opposite kidney of the same patient. This child had progressive renal failure and worsening appearance of the kidneys on serial ultrasound exams.

Typical

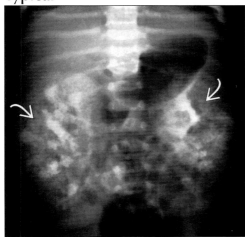
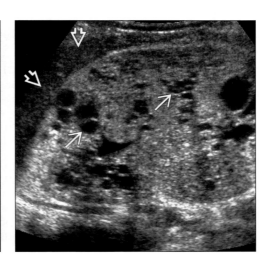

(Left) Anteroposterior IVP shows persistent contrast in dilated tubules (arrows) in the medullary portions of each kidney 3 hours post injection. Note minimal contrast excretion into the collecting system. *(Right)* Sagittal ultrasound shows newborn with massive kidneys due to ARPKD. Note the numerous small cysts (arrows) and overall increased renal echotexture compared to the liver (open arrows).

Typical

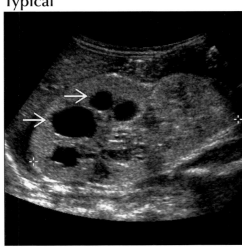
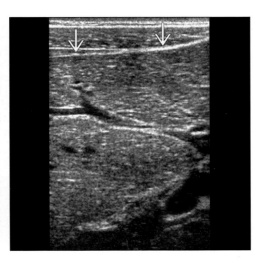

(Left) Sagittal ultrasound shows an unusual case of ARPKD with macrocysts (arrows) in the upper pole of a kidney which is enlarged and has globally increased echotexture. *(Right)* Transverse ultrasound shows increased echotexture in a patient with ARPKD and hepatic fibrosis. Arrows mark the anterior margin of the liver.

POLYCYSTIC RENAL DISEASE, DOMINANT

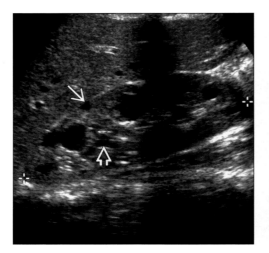

Sagittal ultrasound shows numerous, variably sized cysts occupying all areas of the kidney, from subcapsular (arrow), to central or medullary (open arrow) in this teenager with ADPKD.

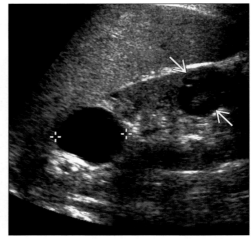

Sagittal ultrasound shows an uncomplicated anechoic cyst between cursors and a complicated cyst (arrows) containing debris in the same kidney. Several very tiny cysts are visible in the subcapsular region.

TERMINOLOGY

Abbreviations and Synonyms
- Autosomal dominant polycystic kidney disease (ADPKD), adult polycystic kidney disease

Definitions
- Hereditary disorder characterized by multiple renal cysts & various other systemic manifestations
- Cystic organ involvement
  - Kidneys (100%), liver (50%), pancreas (9%), brain/ovaries/testis (1%)
- Non-cystic manifestations
  - Cardiac valvular disorders (26%), hernias (25%), colonic diverticula
  - Aneurysms: Cerebral "berry" aneurysms (5-10%), aortic or coronary aneurysms less common

IMAGING FINDINGS

General Features
- Best diagnostic clue: Enlarged kidneys with innumerable macrocysts
- Location: Always involves the kidneys, other organs variably involved
- Size: Cysts tend to be larger than 1 cm diameter
- Morphology: Renal size is within 2 standard deviations of normal at time of diagnosis in half of pediatric patients

Radiographic Findings
- Radiography
  - In young children kidneys often normal in size and contour, with few cysts
  - May see curvilinear, dystrophic cyst wall calcification, renal calculi, or enlarged kidneys
- IVP
  - Mildly to markedly enlarged kidneys
  - Cyst wall calcification and calculi typically only seen in adults
  - Smooth or bosselated (lumpy) renal contour
  - "Swiss cheese" enhancement pattern
    - Smoothly marginated radiolucencies in cortex & medulla seen on nephrographic phase
  - Normal or effaced collecting system

CT Findings
- NECT
  - Early stage: Kidneys are normal in size & contour
  - Later stage: Increasing size & number of cysts increases renal volume; ± asymmetrical kidneys
    - Bosselated kidneys refers to multiple cysts projecting beyond renal contours
  - Cysts: Multiple well-defined round/oval; variable in size, generally bilateral

DDx: Bilateral Renal Enlargement

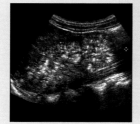
ARPKD

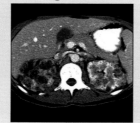
Tuberous Sclerosis

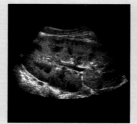
Renal Lymphoma

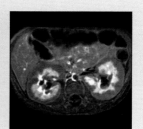
Nephroblastomatosis

POLYCYSTIC RENAL DISEASE, DOMINANT

Key Facts

Terminology
- Hereditary disorder characterized by multiple renal cysts & various other systemic manifestations

Imaging Findings
- Morphology: Renal size is within 2 standard deviations of normal at time of diagnosis in half of pediatric patients
- In young children kidneys often normal in size and contour, with few cysts

Top Differential Diagnoses
- Autosomal recessive polycystic kidney disease
- Multiple simple cysts
- Acquired cystic disease of dialysis
- Tuberous sclerosis
- Other causes of bilateral renal enlargement

Pathology
- 90% autosomal dominant; 10% spontaneous mutations
- 50% chance of child inheriting mutant gene from ADPKD parent

Clinical Issues
- Cyst visibility increases with age
- 54% appear in first decade of life
- 72% occur within second decade
- Prognosis is excellent in childhood
- Prognosis in adulthood variable: Renal insufficiency and hypertension primary issues
- Fourth leading cause of chronic renal failure in the world

- Hypodense cysts have fluid attenuation with thin walls
- Location may be cortex, medulla, or subcapsular
- CECT
  - Normal renal tissue enhancement
  - No enhancement of uncomplicated cysts, hypodense relative to enhanced normal renal tissue
  - Complicated (hemorrhagic) cysts
    - Hyperdense cysts (60-90 HU)
    - Location more often subcapsular
    - May have associated perinephric hematomas due to rupture
    - May see curvilinear mural calcification or calculi within cysts
  - Complicated (infected) cysts
    - Hypodense, may see gas within infected cyst
    - Thick irregular wall and thickened adjacent renal fascia
    - Variable wall enhancement

MR Findings
- T1WI
  - Uncomplicated & infected cysts: Hypointense
  - Complicated (hemorrhagic cysts)
    - Varied signal intensity (depending on age of hemorrhage)
    - Hyperintense (met Hb- paramagnetic + short T1 relaxation time)
    - ± Fluid-iron levels, hyperintense material layers posteriorly
- T2WI
  - Uncomplicated cysts: Hyperintense contents with thin wall
  - Complicated (infected cysts): Hyperintense with marked mural thickening
  - Complicated (hemorrhagic cysts): Varied signal intensity

Ultrasonographic Findings
- Grayscale Ultrasound
  - Multiple well-defined round anechoic areas in both kidneys
  - Renal contour typically normal early in life, may become lumpy as more cysts form
  - Renal size and echotexture typically normal in young patients, aside from the few cysts
- Color Doppler
  - Vessels typically displaced by large cysts
  - Cysts distort normal vascular architecture and have minimal vascular supply to their walls

Imaging Recommendations
- Best imaging tool
  - Ultrasound (sensitivity 97%; specificity 100%; accuracy 98%)
  - CT and MR scans also useful, but involve ionizing radiation, iodinated contrast exposure, +/or sedation
- Protocol advice: Use high frequency linear transducer

DIFFERENTIAL DIAGNOSIS

Autosomal recessive polycystic kidney disease
- Look for dilated tubules and hyperechoic intervening parenchyma

Multiple simple cysts
- Normal renal function

Acquired cystic disease of dialysis
- Early stage: Small kidneys with multiple cysts
- Advanced stage: Indistinguishable from ADPKD

Tuberous sclerosis
- Look for renal angiomyolipomas as well

Other causes of bilateral renal enlargement
- Lymphoma
- Nephroblastomatosis
- Glomerulonephritis
- Renal vein thrombosis
- Radiation nephritis

POLYCYSTIC RENAL DISEASE, DOMINANT

PATHOLOGY

General Features
- General path comments: Abnormal rate of tubule divisions and hypoplasia of tubule segments leads to cystic dilation of Bowman capsule, loop of Henle, and proximal convoluted tubules, intermixed with normal renal parenchyma
- Genetics
  - 90% autosomal dominant; 10% spontaneous mutations
  - 50% chance of child inheriting mutant gene from ADPKD parent
  - Three types of ADPKD based on gene location
    - PKD1: Short arm of chromosome 16 (90%)
    - PKD2: Long arm of chromosome 4 (10%)
    - PKD3: Gene poorly defined
  - Family history lacking in almost half of patients due to variable expressivity and spontaneous mutations
- Etiology
  - Hereditary: Autosomal dominant
  - Abnormal gene → tubular proliferation → diverticula of nephrons
- Epidemiology
  - One of the most common monogenetic disorders
  - Incidence: 1 in 400 to 1000 persons in US
  - Prevalence in US: Higher than cystic fibrosis, hemophilia, sickle cell disease, or muscular dystrophy
- Associated abnormalities
  - Cystic changes in other organs including liver, pancreas, spleen, thyroid, lung, brain, gonads, and bladder
  - Cardiac and aortic abnormalities include valvular disease, coarctation, and aneurysms
  - Slightly increased risk of renal cell carcinoma
  - 10% of patients with ADPKD die from rupture of intracranial berry aneurysm

Gross Pathologic & Surgical Features
- Variably enlarged kidneys
- Cysts may only be seen on cut specimens
- Cysts filled with clear, serous, turbid, or hemorrhagic fluid

Microscopic Features
- Cysts lined by simple flattened/cuboidal epithelium; ± wall calcification
- Cysts communicate with nephrons and collecting tubules on microdissection
- Cyst fluid more closely resembles urine than plasma-like fluid of simple renal cysts

CLINICAL ISSUES

Presentation
- Most common signs/symptoms
  - Typically asymptomatic in childhood
    - Discovered incidentally or found when screening children of affected adults
- Other signs/symptoms
  - Flank pain, hematuria, hypertension, and renal failure also reported in children
  - Hypertension precedes renal failure

Demographics
- Age
  - Variable age at diagnosis: Childhood to 8th decade
  - Cyst visibility increases with age
    - 54% appear in first decade of life
    - 72% occur within second decade
    - 86% visible by third decade
- Gender: M = F

Natural History & Prognosis
- Complications: Hemorrhage, infection, rupture, malignancy, renal failure
- Prognosis is excellent in childhood
- Prognosis in adulthood variable: Renal insufficiency and hypertension primary issues
- Fourth leading cause of chronic renal failure in the world

Treatment
- Treat symptoms & complications: Hypertension, pain, renal infection
- Renal transplantation

SELECTED REFERENCES

1. de Mattos AM et al: Autosomal-dominant polycystic kidney disease as a risk factor for diabetes mellitus following renal transplantation. Kidney Int. 67(2):714-20, 2005
2. Lang EK et al: Autosomal dominant polycystic disease with renal cell carcinoma. J Urol. 173(3):987, 2005
3. Nagaba Y et al: Spontaneous rupture of a left gastroepiploic artery aneurysm in a patient with autosomal-dominant polycystic kidney disease. Clin Nephrol. 63(2):163-6, 2005
4. Paterson AD et al: Progressive loss of renal function is an age-dependent heritable trait in type 1 autosomal dominant polycystic kidney disease. J Am Soc Nephrol. 16(3):755-62, 2005
5. Rohatgi R et al: Cyst fluid composition in human autosomal recessive polycystic kidney disease. Pediatr Nephrol. 20(4):552-3, 2005
6. Grubb RL 3rd et al: Transitional cell carcinoma of the renal pelvis associated with hypercalcemia in a patient with autosomal dominant polycystic kidney disease. Urology. 63(4):778-80, 2004
7. Kanne JP et al: Autosomal dominant polycystic kidney disease presenting as subarachnoid hemorrhage. Emerg Radiol. 11(2):110-2, 2004
8. Persu A et al: Comparison between siblings and twins supports a role for modifier genes in ADPKD. Kidney Int. 66(6):2132-6, 2004
9. Ramunni A et al: Renal vascular resistance and renin-angiotensin system in the pathogenesis of early hypertension in autosomal dominant polycystic kidney disease. Hypertens Res. 27(4):221-5, 2004
10. Wong H et al: Patients with autosomal dominant polycystic kidney disease hyperfiltrate early in their disease. Am J Kidney Dis. 43(4):624-8, 2004
11. Yanaka K et al: Management of unruptured cerebral aneurysms in patients with polycystic kidney disease. Surg Neurol. 62(6):538-45; discussion 545, 2004
12. Avni FE et al: Hereditary polycystic kidney diseases in children: changing sonographic patterns through childhood. Pediatr Radiol. 32(3):169-74, 2002

POLYCYSTIC RENAL DISEASE, DOMINANT

IMAGE GALLERY

Typical

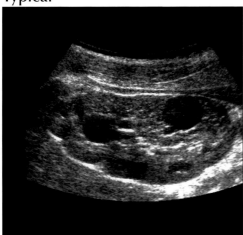
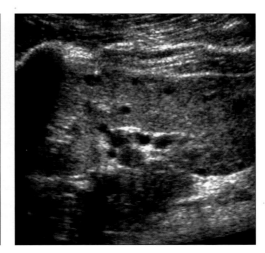

(Left) Sagittal ultrasound shows predominantly large cysts in this child who was being screened for ADPKD. *(Right)* Sagittal ultrasound contrasts with this child who has only tiny cysts scattered throughout the renal parenchyma. This appearance can be difficult to distinguish from ARPKD and may need biopsy or genetic testing.

Typical

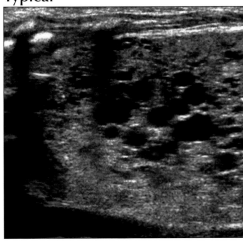
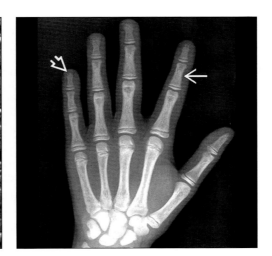

(Left) Sagittal ultrasound shows numerous cysts virtually replacing the renal parenchyma, but not distorting the renal contour in another case of autosomal dominant polycystic kidney disease. *(Right)* Anteroposterior radiograph performed for short stature shows changes of renal osteodystrophy in a patient not previously known to have polycystic kidneys. Note acro-osteolysis (open arrow) and subchondral bone resorption (arrow).

Variant

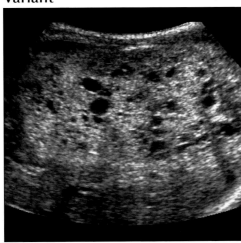
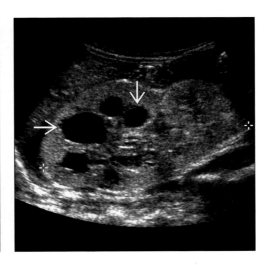

(Left) Sagittal ultrasound shows atypical, but biopsy proven, ADPKD with microcysts and echogenic surrounding parenchyma. Renal function was within normal range at the time of this scan. *(Right)* Sagittal ultrasound shows atypical, but also biopsy proven, ARPKD with macrocysts (arrows) involving only the upper pole of the kidney in this newborn.

CALYCEAL DIVERTICULUM

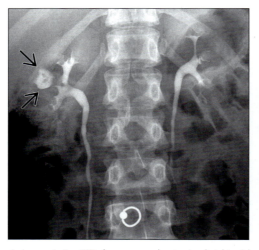

Anteroposterior IVP shows a moderate sized right-mid to upper pole calyceal diverticulum (arrows) with several small filling defects within which were calculi, seen on sonography.

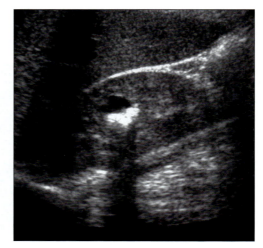

Sagittal ultrasound of the right kidney of patient at left shows small shadowing calculi in an anechoic cystic structure which corresponds to the calyceal diverticulum seen on the IVP.

TERMINOLOGY

Abbreviations and Synonyms
- Calyceal diverticulum (CD)

Definitions
- Urine-filled eventration of calyx into renal parenchyma connected by narrow channel

IMAGING FINDINGS

General Features
- Best diagnostic clue: Contrast filling the diverticulum on contrast-enhanced CT (CECT) or intravenous pyelography (IVP)
- Location
  - Corticomedullary junction of the kidney
    - Minor calyx
    - Major calyx or renal pelvis
- Size: Variable
- Morphology: Smooth, round, thin-walled outpouching of renal calyx

Radiographic Findings
- Radiography
  - Normal
  - Renal calcification(s)
  - Meniscus-like, half-moon-shaped density that changes position (milk of calcium)
- IVP
  - +/- Renal calcification on scout image
  - Contrast-filled outpouching from calyx +/- filling defect/debris
  - Best seen on delayed images - fills retrograde from connecting calyx

Fluoroscopic Findings
- Voiding Cystourethrogram
  - Usually CD incidental finding
  - Outpouching of refluxed contrast from renal calyx

CT Findings
- NECT
  - +/- Calcification or milk of calcium
  - Low attenuation corticomedullary cystic lesion
- CECT: Layering contrast medium in cystic lesion on delayed images

Ultrasonographic Findings
- Grayscale Ultrasound
  - Round, thin walled, anechoic lesion with through transmission
  - +/- Echogenic material layering or shadowing stone within

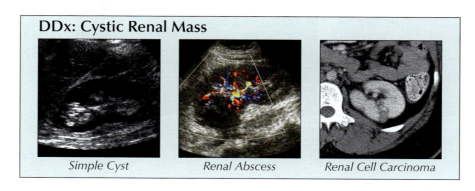

DDx: Cystic Renal Mass — Simple Cyst | Renal Abscess | Renal Cell Carcinoma

CALYCEAL DIVERTICULUM

Key Facts

Terminology
- Urine-filled eventration of calyx into renal parenchyma connected by narrow channel

Imaging Findings
- Best diagnostic clue: Contrast filling the diverticulum on contrast-enhanced CT (CECT) or intravenous pyelography (IVP)
- Morphology: Smooth, round, thin-walled outpouching of renal calyx
- +/- Calcification or milk of calcium
- Renal and bladder sonography
- CECT or IVP with delayed images (15-30 min)

Clinical Issues
- Most common signs/symptoms: Asymptomatic
- Other signs/symptoms: Flank pain, mobile calculi or milk of calcium, pyuria, fever, hematuria, hypertension
- Percutaneous or laparoscopic drainage

Imaging Recommendations
- Best imaging tool: Renal sonography and IVP or CECT
- Protocol advice
  - Renal and bladder sonography
  - CECT or IVP with delayed images (15-30 min)

DIFFERENTIAL DIAGNOSIS

Renal cyst
- No delayed contrast opacification on CT or IVP

Abscess
- Rim-enhancing lesion without delayed opacification on CT

Renal tumor
- Only slight opacification after contrast injection

PATHOLOGY

General Features
- Etiology
  - Probably congenital
    - Failure regression 3rd or 4th division of ureteric buds Wolffian duct
  - May be acquired
    - Abscess, obstruction, infundibular stenosis

Gross Pathologic & Surgical Features
- Type 1
  - Most common
  - Related to minor calyx
- Type 2
  - Related to renal pelvis or major calyx
  - Usually larger, more likely symptomatic

Microscopic Features
- Lined by transitional epithelium
- Surrounded by layer muscularis mucosae

CLINICAL ISSUES

Presentation
- Most common signs/symptoms: Asymptomatic
- Other signs/symptoms: Flank pain, mobile calculi or milk of calcium, pyuria, fever, hematuria, hypertension

Demographics
- Age: Any
- Gender: M = F

Natural History & Prognosis
- Small CD usually asymptomatic
- Stasis of urine - infection, milk of calcium, stone formation - become symptomatic

Treatment
- Percutaneous or laparoscopic drainage
- Possible calyceal resection or partial nephrectomy

SELECTED REFERENCES

1. Canales B et al: Surgical management of the calyceal diverticulum. Curr Opin Urol. 13(3):255-60, 2003
2. Wogan JM: Pyelocalyceal diverticulum: an unusual cause of acute renal colic. J Emerg Med. 23(1):19-21, 2002
3. Chen RN et al: Milk of calcium within a calyceal diverticulum. Urology. 49(4):620-1, 1997
4. Frank RG: Rupture of a large calyceal diverticulum. Urology. 49(2):265-6, 1997
5. Choudhury SR et al: Calyceal diverticula. J Indian Med Assoc. 90(6):159-61, 1992
6. Latiff A: Case profile: calyceal diverticulum causing recurrent urinary tract infection. Urology. 17(6):621, 1981
7. Siegel MJ et al: Calyceal diverticula in children: unusual features and complications. Radiology. 131(1):79-82, 1979

IMAGE GALLERY

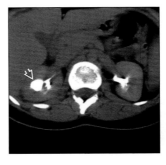 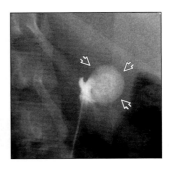

(Left) Axial CECT performed at level of kidneys 15 minutes after contrast injection shows filling of moderate-size calyceal diverticulum *(arrow)*, similar to sonogram/IVP shown on previous page. *(Right)* Oblique percutaneous nephrostogram shows contrast in calyceal diverticulum *(arrows)* with stones within it prior to percutaneous removal of calculi by a combined radiology/urology procedure.

WILM TUMOR

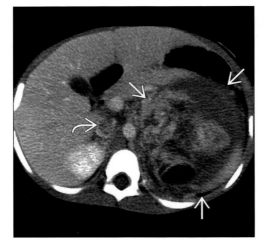

Axial CECT shows a mixed attenuation mass replacing the left kidney (arrows). Note the low density centrally in the vena cava (curved arrow) which represents thrombus in this patient with Wilm tumor.

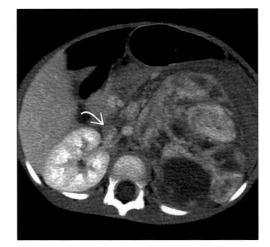

Axial CECT in the same patient shows inferior extension of the tumor, displacement of aorta and mesenteric vessels, and additional low density thrombus in the vena cava (arrow).

TERMINOLOGY

Abbreviations and Synonyms
- Malignant nephroblastoma, embryoma of kidney

Definitions
- A malignant tumor of primitive metanephric blastema
- Most common abdominal neoplasm in children 1-8 years old
- 3rd most common childhood malignancy after leukemia and CNS tumors

IMAGING FINDINGS

General Features
- Best diagnostic clue: Large heterogeneous mass replacing kidney and extending into renal vein and inferior vena cava (IVC)
- Location: Flank mass
- Size: Typically quite large
- Morphology: May show local invasion or have smooth contour

Radiographic Findings
- Radiography
  - Mass displacing adjacent bowel
  - Calcifications less often seen in Wilm than in neuroblastoma
    - Calcium visible on radiographs in 9%, on CT scan in 15%

CT Findings
- NECT: Lung metastases in 20% at time of diagnosis
- CECT
  - Typically large, heterogeneous mass replacing the kidney
  - Displaces adjacent organs
  - Frequently grows into renal vein and IVC
  - Poorly enhancing, heterogeneous
  - Well-defined margins or pseudocapsule
  - Local extension into perirenal fat and local lymph nodes

MR Findings
- T1WI: Typically low signal intensity on T1
- T2WI: High signal on T2, but heterogeneous and frequently containing blood products
- MRA: MR angiography useful in determining vascular spread pre-operatively

Ultrasonographic Findings
- Grayscale Ultrasound
  - Findings similar to CT and MRI: Heterogeneous echotexture, large mass, may see local invasion & adenopathy

DDx: Other Pediatric Renal Tumors

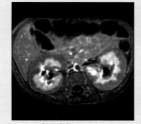
Nephroblastomatosis

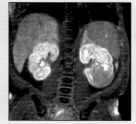
Mesoblastic Nephroma

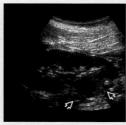
Renal Cell Carcinoma

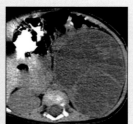
MLCN

WILM TUMOR

Key Facts

Terminology
- A malignant tumor of primitive metanephric blastema
- Most common abdominal neoplasm in children 1-8 years old
- 3rd most common childhood malignancy after leukemia and CNS tumors

Imaging Findings
- Best diagnostic clue: Large heterogeneous mass replacing kidney and extending into renal vein and inferior vena cava (IVC)

Top Differential Diagnoses
- Neuroblastoma
- Multilocular cystic nephroma
- Clear cell sarcoma and rhabdoid tumor of the kidney
- Renal cell carcinoma
- Nephroblastomatosis
- Congenital mesoblastic nephroma

Pathology
- I: Confined to kidney, completely excised
- II: Local extension, completely resected
- III: Incomplete resection, no distant metastases
- IV: Distant metastases to lung, liver, brain, or bone
- V: Bilateral synchronous tumors

Clinical Issues
- 80% of cases in children less than 5 years old
- Cure rate for Wilm tumor
- Is better than 90% with current therapy

  - Tumor mass often difficult to image whole without extended field of view
- Color Doppler: Useful to determine tumor thrombus extension versus compression of veins by bulky mass

Echocardiographic Findings
- Echocardiogram
  - Used to assess intracardiac tumor thrombus
  - Especially in cases where chemotherapy is performed to "shrink" tumor thrombus prior to surgery

Nuclear Medicine Findings
- Bone Scan: Metastatic disease to bone occurs very late; bone scans are not routine
- PET
  - Increasing use in Wilm and all pediatric tumors
  - Primarily has an adjunctive, problem solving role
    - Differentiating scar tissue from residual active tumor

Other Modality Findings
- IVP was once the mainstay of imaging, now seldom performed

Imaging Recommendations
- Best imaging tool
  - Ultrasound is frequently the first exam performed
  - CT or MRI scan is used to supplement sonography per national protocols
  - Chest X-ray or chest CT scan for staging (chest CT specified by NWTS-5)
- Protocol advice: Contralateral kidney should be closely scrutinized for synchronous tumor

DIFFERENTIAL DIAGNOSIS

Neuroblastoma
- Wilm tumor seldom extends behind the aorta as neuroblastoma does
- Neuroblastoma is more often calcified
- Originates from adrenal gland or paraspinal sympathetic neural tissues

Multilocular cystic nephroma
- Similar age distribution and can resemble cystic Wilm tumor

Clear cell sarcoma and rhabdoid tumor of the kidney
- Once considered aggressive forms of Wilm tumor, identical on imaging
- Rhabdoid tumors typically diagnosed in infancy (younger than 1 year)
- Clear cell sarcomas frequently have skeletal metastases at diagnosis

Renal cell carcinoma
- Typically seen in older children

Nephroblastomatosis
- Multiple bilateral nephrogenic rests
- Can be subcortical, medullary, or both
- Associated with bilateral Wilm tumor, Beckwith-Wiedemann, hemihypertrophy

Congenital mesoblastic nephroma
- Most common solid renal tumor in pediatrics
- Commonly diagnosed in infancy

Angiomyolipoma
- Contain fat and enhance with contrast
- Associated with tuberous sclerosis

Renal medullary carcinoma
- Adolescents with sickle cell trait or disease

PATHOLOGY

General Features
- General path comments
  - A tumor of persistent primitive metanephric blastemal elements
  - Embryology-anatomy
    - Metanephric blastema is typically fully differentiated by 34 weeks or term

WILM TUMOR

- Persistence of metanephric blastema is termed nephroblastomatosis
- Patients with nephroblastomatosis are at high-risk for Wilm tumors
- 30-44% of patients with nephroblastomatosis will develop Wilm tumor
- Nephrogenic rests present in 1% of infant autopsies and in 4% of multicystic dysplastic kidney
  - 5-10% of cases are bilateral and associated with nephroblastomatosis
- Genetics
  - Deletion on chromosome #11 (now named WT1) strongly associated
  - Wilm tumor suppressor gene at 11p13 also believed to be important
  - Additional suspects being investigated: 16q, 1p, p53
  - Still only 2% of Wilm tumors are familial
- Epidemiology
  - 500 new cases each year in United States
  - When associated with syndromes, age at tumor occurrence is younger
  - 1/3 of patients with sporadic aniridia have Wilm while 1% of Wilm tumor patients have aniridia
- Associated abnormalities
  - Genitourinary anomalies
  - Overgrowth syndromes (Beckwith-Wiedemann and isolated hemihypertrophy)
  - Sporadic aniridia
  - Trisomy 18
  - Sotos syndrome
  - Bloom syndrome
  - Denys-Drash syndrome
  - WAGR syndrome: Wilm tumor, aniridia, genitourinary anomalies, and mental retardation
    - Contiguous gene deletion syndrome involving the Wilm tumor 1 gene (WT1), the paired box gene 6 (PAX6), and possibly other genes on chromosome 11p13

Microscopic Features
- 4-10% of tumors have unfavorable histology
  - Anaplasia
  - Sarcomatous appearance

Staging, Grading or Classification Criteria
- I: Confined to kidney, completely excised
- II: Local extension, completely resected
- III: Incomplete resection, no distant metastases
- IV: Distant metastases to lung, liver, brain, or bone
- V: Bilateral synchronous tumors

CLINICAL ISSUES

Presentation
- Most common signs/symptoms: Asymptomatic flank mass, hematuria, vomiting, failure to thrive
- Other signs/symptoms: Hypertension, fever from tumor necrosis, anemia

Demographics
- Age
  - 80% of cases in children less than 5 years old
  - Peak age 3.6 years
- Gender: M = F

Natural History & Prognosis
- Prognosis based on stage and histology
- Cure rate for Wilm tumor
  - Was less than 10% in 1920 and
  - Is better than 90% with current therapy
- Collaborative international treatment protocols
  - National Wilm Tumor Study Group (NWTSG)
  - Societe Internationale d'Oncologie Pediatric (SIOP)

Treatment
- Pre-operative chemotherapy for large, otherwise unresectable tumors, bilateral tumors, and tumor thrombus extending above hepatic veins
- Surgical resection
- Radiation and chemotherapy post-operatively
- Bone marrow transplant usually reserved for relapses

SELECTED REFERENCES

1. Akyuz C et al: Cavoatrial tumor extension in children with wilms tumor: a retrospective review of 17 children in a single center. J Pediatr Hematol Oncol. 27(5):267-9, 2005
2. Khoury JD: Nephroblastic neoplasms. Clin Lab Med. 25(2):341-61, vi-vii, 2005
3. Merks JH et al: High incidence of malformation syndromes in a series of 1,073 children with cancer. Am J Med Genet A. 134(2):132-43, 2005
4. Narchi H: Risk of Wilms' tumour with multicystic kidney disease: a systematic review. Arch Dis Child. 90(2):147-9, 2005
5. Perotti D et al: WT1 gene analysis in sporadic early-onset and bilateral wilms tumor patients without associated abnormalities. J Pediatr Hematol Oncol. 27(4):197-201, 2005
6. Scott DA et al: Congenital diaphragmatic hernia in WAGR syndrome. Am J Med Genet A. 134(4):430-3, 2005
7. Varan A et al: Prognostic significance of metastatic site at diagnosis in Wilms' tumor: results from a single center. J Pediatr Hematol Oncol. 27(4):188-91, 2005
8. Zani A et al: Long-term outcome of nephron sparing surgery and simple nephrectomy for unilateral localized Wilms tumor. J Urol. 173(3):946-8; discussion 948, 2005
9. Firoozi F et al: Follow-up and management of recurrent Wilms' tumor. Urol Clin North Am. 30(4):869-79, 2003
10. O'Hara SM: Tumors of the Pediatric Genitourinary System. In Oncologic Imaging 2nd edition. Bragg, Rubin, Hricak editors:chapter 36, 779-811, W B Saunders, Philadelphia, 2002
11. Lonergan GL et al: Nephrogenic rests, nephroblastomatosis, and associated lesions of the kidney. Radiographics. 18:947-68, 1998
12. Wiener JS et al: Current concepts in the biology and management of Wilms tumor. J Urol. 159:1316-25, 1988

WILM TUMOR

IMAGE GALLERY

Typical

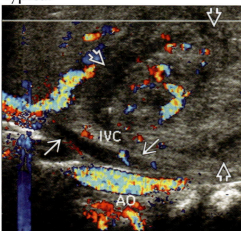
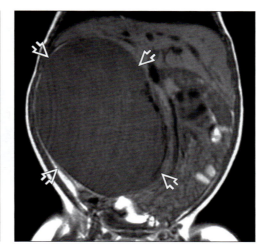

(Left) Sagittal color Doppler ultrasound Shows lack of color flow in the IVC (arrows) in a patient with Wilm tumor (open arrows). Doppler ultrasound and MRI are often used to assess venous invasion of Wilm tumor. *(Right)* Coronal T1WI MR shows huge, homogeneous mass occupying the right flank (arrows), displacing bowel and liver. This Wilm tumor compresses the vena cava along the left margin of the mass, but does not have venous invasion.

Typical

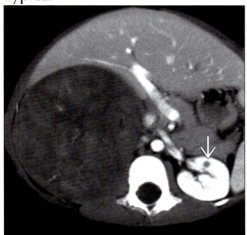
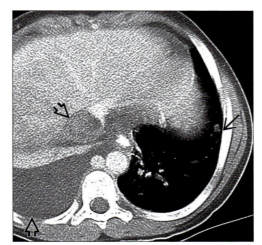

(Left) Axial CECT shows large, poorly enhancing Wilm tumor in the right flank and a small low density area in the contralateral kidney (arrow) which was a synchronous Wilm tumor. *(Right)* Axial CECT Filmed at lung windows shows two round pulmonary metastases (arrow) in the left lung base from Wilm tumor. Note the right pleural effusion and caval thrombus (open arrows) in this patient with stage IV disease.

Typical

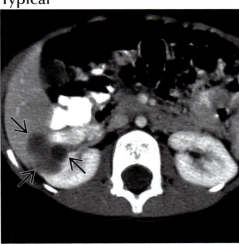
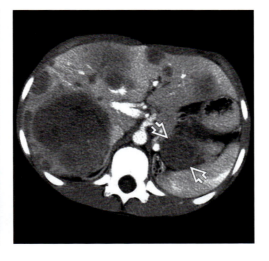

(Left) Axial CECT shows low density, lobulated mass (arrows) in the right kidney which was found to represent a cystic Wilm tumor. *(Right)* Axial CECT shows low density mass in the left flank (arrows) several months after nephrectomy for Wilm tumor. Note metastatic deposits in the liver in this case of relapsed Wilm tumor.

MULTILOCULAR CYSTIC NEPHROMA

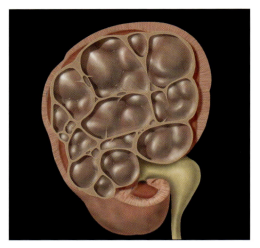

Graphic shows multilocular cystic mass that herniates into the renal hilum.

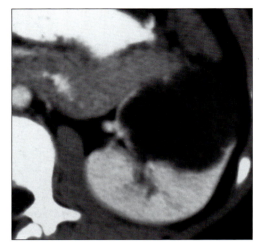

Axial CECT shows a large cyst in the anterior cortex of the left kidney with thin enhancing septa.

TERMINOLOGY

Abbreviations and Synonyms
- Multilocular cystic nephroma (MLCN), cystic nephroma, cyst adenoma

Definitions
- Best classified as one of the 2 types of multilocular cystic renal tumor
  - 1. Cystic nephroma (= MLCN)
  - 2. Cystic partially differentiated nephroblastoma (CPDN)
- Rare nonhereditary benign cystic renal neoplasm
- Indistinguishable from CPDN by imaging, but histologically distinct
  - Both have same excellent prognosis with excision

IMAGING FINDINGS

General Features
- Best diagnostic clue: Large multilocular cystic renal mass
- Location: Typically solitary intraparenchymal cyst
- Size: Few cm to > 30 cm (mean = 10 cm)
- Morphology: Well-circumscribed cystic mass with a thick fibrous capsule ± herniation into renal pelvis

CT Findings
- NECT
  - Large, well-defined multiloculated cystic mass
  - Attenuation equal to/higher than water
  - Small locules (< 1 cm) ± proteinaceous material within cysts → may appear as solid mass
  - ± Calcification
- CECT
  - Capsule: ± Enhancement
  - Separate from collecting system
  - May herniate into renal hilum, distort collecting system, ± obstruction

MR Findings
- T1WI
  - Multiloculated hypointense mass (clear fluid)
  - Variable signal intensity (blood or protein)
- T2WI
  - Hyperintense (clear fluid) or variable (blood or protein)
  - Capsule & septa: Hypointense (fibrous tissue)
- T1 C+: Enhancement of thin septa

Ultrasonographic Findings
- Grayscale Ultrasound
  - Large, well-defined multiloculated cystic mass
  - Innumerable anechoic cysts + hyperechoic septa and fibrous capsule

DDx: Cystic Pediatric Renal Masses

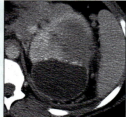

Cystic RCC

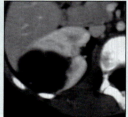

Complex Cyst

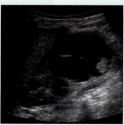

Complex Cyst

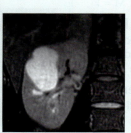

Calyceal Diverticulum

MULTILOCULAR CYSTIC NEPHROMA

Key Facts

Terminology
- Rare nonhereditary benign cystic renal neoplasm
- Indistinguishable from CPDN by imaging, but histologically distinct

Imaging Findings
- Best diagnostic clue: Large multilocular cystic renal mass
- Location: Typically solitary intraparenchymal cyst

Top Differential Diagnoses
- Cortical (simple) cysts
- Malignant cystic renal tumors
- Multicystic dysplastic kidney (MCDK)
- Calyceal diverticulum

Clinical Issues
- Biphasic age and sex distribution
- M > F: 3 months to 2 years (mostly CPDN)
- F >> M: 5th & 6th decades (mostly MLCN)

- Portions of lesion may appear solid due to numerous tiny cysts causing acoustic interfaces

Imaging Recommendations
- CECT, US, or MR + T1 C+

DIFFERENTIAL DIAGNOSIS

Cortical (simple) cysts
- Smooth, sharply marginated water density masses
- Large multiloculated cyst may simulate MLCN

Malignant cystic renal tumors
- Multilocular cystic renal cell carcinoma (RCC); cystic Wilm tumor; clear cell sarcoma with cystic change
- Rare malignant tumors that may be indistinguishable

Multicystic dysplastic kidney (MCDK)
- Usually involves entire kidney, unless duplicated
- Present in newborn and neonate, unlike MLCN

Calyceal diverticulum
- Communicates with collecting system

PATHOLOGY

General Features
- Etiology: Arises from metanephric blastema
- Epidemiology: Rare tumor

Gross Pathologic & Surgical Features
- Thick fibrous capsule
- "Honeycombed" cystic areas of varied sizes

Microscopic Features
- MLCN: Septa have no undifferentiated elements
- CPDN: Septa contain blastemal ± other embryonal elements, more common than MLCN in children

CLINICAL ISSUES

Presentation
- Most common signs/symptoms
  - Children: No pain; palpable abdominal/flank mass
  - Adults: Abdominal/flank pain; ± palpable mass
- ± Hematuria & urinary tract infection (UTI)

Demographics
- Age
  - Biphasic age and sex distribution
    - M > F: 3 months to 2 years (mostly CPDN)
    - F >> M: 5th & 6th decades (mostly MLCN)

Natural History & Prognosis
- Prognosis
  - Cured with complete excision
  - Local recurrence usually due to incomplete excision
  - Malignant transformation extremely rare

Treatment
- Complete or partial nephrectomy

DIAGNOSTIC CHECKLIST

Image Interpretation Pearls
- Unilateral, solitary, multiloculated, cystic mass ± herniation into renal pelvis

SELECTED REFERENCES

1. Hopkins JK et al: Best cases from the AFIP: cystic nephroma. Radiographics. 24(2):589-93, 2004
2. Eble JN et al: Extensively cystic renal neoplasms: cystic nephroma, cystic partially differentiated nephroblastoma, multilocular cystic renal cell carcinoma, and cystic hamartoma of renal pelvis. Semin Diagn Pathol. 15(1):2-20, 1998
3. Agrons GA et al: Multilocular cystic renal tumor in children: radiologic-pathologic correlation. Radiographics. 15(3):653-69, 1995

IMAGE GALLERY

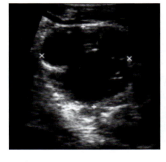 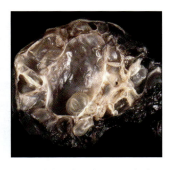

(Left) Axial ultrasound shows MLCN as multiloculated cyst with thin septations. *(Right)* Gross pathology shows MLCN as multiloculated cyst containing cysts of varying sizes.

MESOBLASTIC NEPHROMA

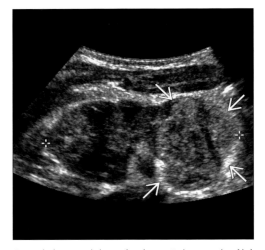

Sagittal ultrasound shows focal mass in lower pole of left kidney (arrows) which distorts renal contour and has heterogeneous increased echotexture. Note the normal echotexture in upper pole of this newborn.

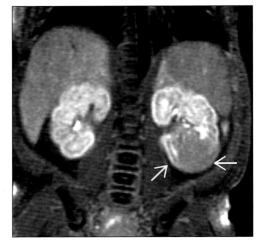

Coronal T1 C+ MR shows focal mass (arrows) in lower pole of left kidney in same patient. Note the poor contrast enhancement and well-defined margins of this solid mass, a congenital mesoblastic nephroma.

TERMINOLOGY

Abbreviations and Synonyms
- Congenital mesoblastic nephroma (CMN), leiomyomatous hamartoma, mesenchymal hamartoma of the kidney, renal fibroma, and Bolande tumor
  - Bolande initially described congenital mesoblastic nephroma as histologically distinct from Wilm tumor

Definitions
- Hamartomatous renal tumor composed predominately of spindle cells, fibroblasts
  - Generally benign
  - Cellular variant potentially more aggressive

IMAGING FINDINGS

General Features
- Best diagnostic clue: Solid, unilateral renal mass in a fetus or newborn
- Location: Intra-renal, though it may replace the entire kidney and cross the midline when large
- Size: Variable, from < 1 cm diameter to > 15 cm
- Morphology
  - Bland, solid tumor
  - Tends to grow in oval or spherical shape
- Pertinent negatives
  - Hemorrhage or necrosis uncommon
  - Hydronephrosis usually not present
  - Cystic areas are very uncommon

Radiographic Findings
- Radiography: Radiographs may show mass effect from large tumor, rarely cardiac enlargement from shunting

CT Findings
- NECT
  - Solid tumor in flank
  - Calcifications are not typically seen
- CECT
  - Variably enhancing mass with smooth contours
  - Cystic areas or foci of necrosis and hemorrhage are uncommon

MR Findings
- T1WI
  - Intermediate to low signal intensity
  - Enhancement is variable after gadolinium
  - Multiplanar imaging useful to confirm renal origin
- T2WI: Bright on T2 weighted sequences, despite the fibrous nature of the lesion

Ultrasonographic Findings
- Grayscale Ultrasound

DDx: Other Pediatric Renal Tumors

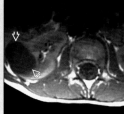

Wilm

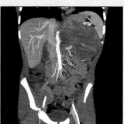

Cystic Wilm

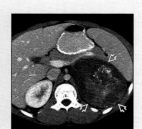

Neuroblastoma

Ganglioneuroma

MESOBLASTIC NEPHROMA

Key Facts

Terminology
- Hamartomatous renal tumor composed predominately of spindle cells, fibroblasts
- Generally benign
- Cellular variant potentially more aggressive

Imaging Findings
- Best diagnostic clue: Solid, unilateral renal mass in a fetus or newborn
- Identify normal adrenal gland to confirm mass has renal origin

Top Differential Diagnoses
- Wilm tumor
- Neuroblastoma or ganglioneuroma
- Adrenal hemorrhage
- Autosomal recessive polycystic kidney disease
- Multicystic dysplastic kidney
- Extrapulmonary sequestration
- Ossifying renal tumor of infancy

Pathology
- Whorled appearance
- Similar to uterine fibroid
- Cut surface usually yellow-tan, solid, rubbery stromal tissue
- 3 types based on histologic features

Clinical Issues
- Flank mass which is palpable
- Prognosis is excellent
- Surgery is typically curative
- Chemotherapy or radiation not usually indicated

- Smaller masses retain reniform shape
  - Infiltrative growth pattern histologically
  - Smooth contours are typical seen on imaging
- Larger masses may fill abdomen displacing bowel
  - Bowel obstruction may occur
  - Venous obstruction may occur
  - Vascular invasion is not typically seen
- Variable echogenicity, relatively homogeneous solid tissue, similar to muscle
- Color Doppler: Vascularity may be normal or increased
- Pulsed Doppler: High diastolic flow has been reported which is atypical for normal newborn renal parenchyma

Imaging Recommendations
- Best imaging tool: Ultrasound is best, both in fetus and newborn
- Protocol advice
  - Identify normal adrenal gland to confirm mass has renal origin
  - In pregnancy, frequent ultrasound scans are performed to assess for
    - Worsening polyhydramnios
    - Enlarging abdominal circumference
    - Fetal hydrops, a very rare complication

DIFFERENTIAL DIAGNOSIS

Wilm tumor
- Imaging appearance may be identical
- Histologic examination needed to differentiate from Wilm
- Wilm is extraordinarily rare in utero
  - Average age at presentation 3.6 years

Neuroblastoma or ganglioneuroma
- Suprarenal location
- Kidney displaced inferiorly
- Normal adrenal gland not identified

Adrenal hemorrhage
- Will evolve over time
- No color flow expected within the hemorrhagic area
- MR can confirm blood products

Autosomal recessive polycystic kidney disease
- Bilateral enlargement

Multicystic dysplastic kidney
- Cystic not solid

Extrapulmonary sequestration
- Look for separate kidneys displaced by the mass

Ossifying renal tumor of infancy
- Extremely rare tumor characterized by ossification/calcification

PATHOLOGY

General Features
- General path comments: Suggested to arise from the metanephric blastema or from secondary mesenchyme
- Genetics
  - Sporadic
  - No recurrence risk in siblings
  - Recent description of a t(12;15)(p13;q25) chromosomal translocation in cellular type CMN
- Epidemiology: Rare
- Associated abnormalities: Low incidence of associated gastrointestinal and genitourinary anomalies

Gross Pathologic & Surgical Features
- Whorled appearance
  - Similar to uterine fibroid
- No capsule
  - Still appears well defined by imaging
- Cut surface usually yellow-tan, solid, rubbery stromal tissue
- Occasionally see cystic areas and foci of necrosis or hemorrhage

MESOBLASTIC NEPHROMA

Microscopic Features
- Proliferation of spindle cells and smooth muscle
- Entrapped normal or immature tubules and glomeruli
- Sporadic calcifications
- Islands of hematopoietic components
- Mitotic cells are typically few
- Lacks a well-defined capsule and may invade adjacent tissues

Staging, Grading or Classification Criteria
- 3 types based on histologic features
  - "Classical" which is most common
  - "Cellular" or "atypical"
  - "Mixed"
  - Cellular type resembles congenital fibrosarcoma in terms of cytogenetic and molecular markers
    - Cellular or atypical tumors have: Worse prognosis, tend to metastasize, treated with chemotherapy, according to Wilm tumor or sarcoma protocols

CLINICAL ISSUES

Presentation
- Most common signs/symptoms
  - Flank mass which is palpable
  - Polyhydramnios common feature and may be severe (etiology uncertain)
    - Some infants with mesoblastic nephroma have hypercalcemia which has been associated with polyuria
  - Potential explanations for increased amniotic fluid
    - Hyperfiltration
    - Hypercalcemia causing polyuria
    - Mechanical obstruction of the intestine or IVC by large mass which impairs amniotic fluid absorption
- Other signs/symptoms
  - In pregnancy
    - Large for dates due to polyhydramnios
    - Preterm labor
  - In newborn
    - Reports of congestive heart failure due to high diastolic flow and arterio-venous shunting within some tumors
    - Case reports of hypertension and hyper-reninemia

Demographics
- Age
  - Newborn
  - Most diagnosed within 3 months of birth
- Gender: M > F
- Ethnicity: No ethnic predisposition

Natural History & Prognosis
- Can show rapid growth despite benign histology
- Large abdominal circumference may result in dystocia at delivery
- Prognosis is excellent
  - Surgery is typically curative
  - Chemotherapy or radiation not usually indicated
- Rare local recurrence or metastases
  - Lung most common site of metastatic disease
  - Liver, heart, brain, and bone metastases also reported

Treatment
- Amnioreduction for polyhydramnios
- Tocolytics for preterm labor
- Referral to pediatric urologist
- Resection in neonatal period
  - Nephrectomy with wide margins usually curative
  - Follow-up imaging performed to exclude unusual cases with local recurrence

SELECTED REFERENCES

1. Leclair MD et al: The outcome of prenatally diagnosed renal tumors. J Urol. 173(1):186-9, 2005
2. Glick RD et al: Renal tumors in infants less than 6 months of age. J Pediatr Surg. 39(4):522-5, 2004
3. Siemer S et al: Prenatal diagnosis of congenital mesoblastic nephroma associated with renal hypertension in a premature child. Int J Urol. 11(1):50-2, 2004
4. Sugimura J et al: Gene expression profiling of mesoblastic nephroma and Wilms tumors--comparison and clinical implications. Urology. 64(2):362-8; discussion 368, 2004
5. Wang J et al: Usefulness of immunohistochemistry in delineating renal spindle cell tumours. A retrospective study of 31 cases. Histopathology. 44(5):462-71, 2004
6. Chen WY et al: Prenatal diagnosis of congenital mesoblastic nephroma in mid-second trimester by sonography and magnetic resonance imaging. Prenat Diagn. 23(11):927-31, 2003
7. Henno S et al: Cellular mesoblastic nephroma: morphologic, cytogenetic and molecular links with congenital fibrosarcoma. Pathol Res Pract. 199(1):35-40, 2003
8. Moore SW et al: The epidemiology of neonatal tumours. Report of an international working group. Pediatr Surg Int. 19(7):509-19, 2003
9. Patel Y et al: Use of sarcoma-based chemotherapy in a case of congenital mesoblastic nephroma with liver metastases. Urology. 61(6):1260, 2003
10. Bell MG et al: Perinephric cystic mesoblastic nephroma complicated by hepatic metastases: a case report. Pediatr Radiol. 32(11):829-31, 2002
11. Daskas N et al: Congenital mesoblastic nephroma associated with polyhydramnios and hypercalcemia. Pediatr Nephrol. 17(3):187-9, 2002
12. Guschmann M et al: Myoid differentiation in mesoblastic nephroma: clinicopathologic and cytogenetic findings of a rare case. J Pediatr Surg. 37(8):E22, 2002
13. Irsutti M et al: Mesoblastic nephroma: prenatal ultrasonographic and MRI features. Pediatr Radiol. 30(3):147-50, 2000
14. Fung TY et al: Polyhydramnios and hypercalcemia associated with congenital mesoblastic nephroma: Case report and a new appraisal. Obstet Gynecol. 85:815-7, 1995

MESOBLASTIC NEPHROMA

IMAGE GALLERY

Typical

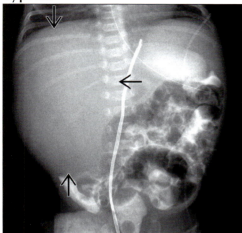
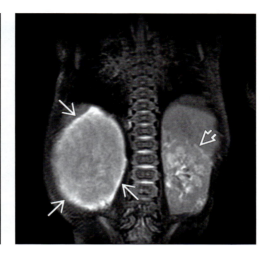

(Left) Anteroposterior radiograph shows a large soft tissue mass (arrows) in the right flank displacing bowel leftward in a newborn infant. *(Right)* Coronal T2WI MR shows large mass (arrows) in the same patient, replacing the right kidney, distending the flank, but still demonstrating sharp margins and signal intensity similar to the normal left kidney (open arrow).

Typical

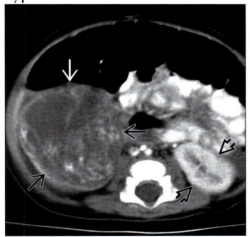
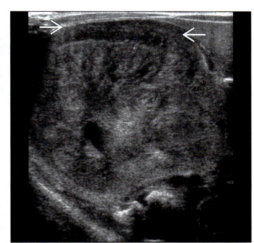

(Left) Axial CECT shows large mesoblastic nephroma replacing the entire right kidney (arrows). Contrast enhancement in this solid tumor is variably decreased compared to normal left kidney (open arrows). *(Right)* Transverse ultrasound shows same tumor in a similar scan plane with ultrasound. Note the heterogeneous echotexture of this solid tumor, with a crescent of subcapsular hematoma in the near field (arrows).

Typical

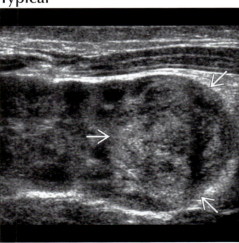
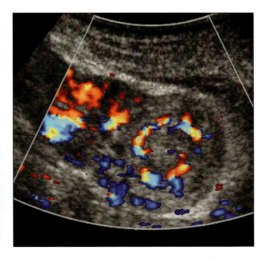

(Left) Sagittal ultrasound shows CMN (arrows) involving only the lower pole of this newborn kidney. Note the hypoechoic pyramids and persistent fetal lobation in the normal upper pole region. *(Right)* Sagittal color Doppler ultrasound shows swirled color flow within the tumor involving lower pole. Vascularity in these tumors is highly variable, but is reliably different from the normal arborization seen in the unaffected kidney.

ANGIOMYOLIPOMA

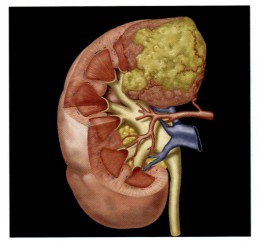

Graphic shows a renal mass which contains fat, abnormal vessels, and soft tissue.

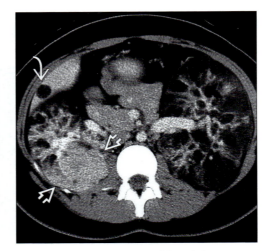

Axial CECT shows extensive bilateral fatty masses (AMLs) replacing both kidneys in patient with TS. AML in right kidney contains less fat (open arrows). AML also in liver (curved arrow).

TERMINOLOGY

Abbreviations and Synonyms
- Angiomyolipoma (AML)

Definitions
- Benign renal tumor consisting of abnormal blood vessels (angio-), smooth muscle (-myo-), and fat (-lipoma)
- Most commonly located in kidney, but also found in liver and many other sites
  - Some series find hepatic AMLs in 13% of tuberous sclerosis (TS) patients with renal AMLs (usually patients with bilateral diffuse renal AMLs)
- Rare in children unless have tuberous sclerosis

IMAGING FINDINGS

General Features
- Best diagnostic clue: Intrarenal fatty mass
- Location
  - Most common: Renal
  - But may be found in liver, lymph nodes, spleen, etc.
- Size: Variable
- Morphology
  - Mass center or periphery may contain fat
  - Mass shape is variable
  - Mass number: Single or multiple; unilateral or bilateral

CT Findings
- NECT
  - Renal mass with intramural fat is diagnostic of AML
    - Variable amounts of fat present
    - May require thin-section CT to see more subtle collections
  - When multiple AMLs seen, suspect tuberous sclerosis
  - ~ 5% have no detectable fat on CT; such AML cannot be diagnosed by CT or other imaging modalities
  - Spontaneous hemorrhage is common complication, but is rarely seen if AML is ≤ 4 cm
  - Calcification extremely rare
    - If calcifications present, must consider renal cell carcinoma (RCC)
    - RCC may rarely "de-differentiate" to form bone and fat
- CECT
  - Lesions may enhance significantly following contrast infusion, depending on extent of vascular component
  - AML does not undergo malignant change, but benign satellite deposits may be present in lymph nodes, liver, and spleen

DDx: Other Pediatric Renal Masses

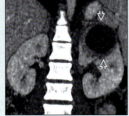

Renal Abscess

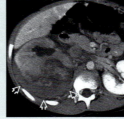

Wilm Hemorrhage

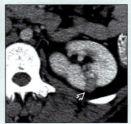

RCC

ANGIOMYOLIPOMA

Key Facts

Terminology
- Benign renal tumor consisting of abnormal blood vessels (angio-), smooth muscle (-myo-), and fat (-lipoma)
- Most commonly located in kidney, but also found in liver and many other sites

Imaging Findings
- Best diagnostic clue: Intrarenal fatty mass
- Renal mass with intramural fat is diagnostic of AML
- When multiple AMLs seen, suspect tuberous sclerosis

Pathology
- Mean age 41 years
- Children: Rare unless have TS
- 80% with TS develop AMLs by age 10
- If have TS, more often bilateral, multifocal, and larger

Clinical Issues
- Most commonly asymptomatic
- If > 4 cm diameter more likely to spontaneously hemorrhage
- Possible life-threatening hemorrhage (Wunderlich syndrome)
- 80% AML are incidental findings on abdominal imaging exams
- 20% of patients with renal AML have tuberous sclerosis
- 80% of patients with tuberous sclerosis develop renal AML
- No malignant potential

Diagnostic Checklist
- Classic imaging appearance: Well-circumscribed intrarenal fatty mass

---

- CTA: Aneurysmal renal vessels may be seen on CT angiography

MR Findings
- T1WI
  - Mass contains high signal (fat)
  - Fat suppression: Low signal (fat)
- T1 C+
  - Variable enhancement
  - If high fat content, may show minimal enhancement
  - If high vascular content, many show marked enhancement
- Varied signal intensity due to variable amounts of vessels, muscle, and fat

Ultrasonographic Findings
- Grayscale Ultrasound
  - Markedly hyperechoic mass relative to normal renal tissue
  - If muscle, vascular elements, or hemorrhage predominate, lesion may be hypoechoic
  - May look similar to small renal cell carcinoma, which may also be hyperechoic

Angiographic Findings
- DSA
  - Characteristic dilated tortuous vessels with aneurysms
    - Vascular mass
    - Multisacculated pseudoaneurysms
    - Absent arteriovenous shunts
    - "Sunburst" appearance of capillary nephrogram
    - "Onion peel" appearance of peripheral vessels in venous phase
  - Some AMLs are hypovascular

Imaging Recommendations
- Best imaging tool: CT
- Protocol advice: Best imaging approach is thin-section (≤ 3 mm) NECT & CECT

DIFFERENTIAL DIAGNOSIS

Wilm tumor
- Most common childhood renal malignant tumor
- Solid renal mass which may contain areas of necrosis and/or hemorrhage
- May invade renal vein, IVC, and right atrium
- Metastases to lymph nodes, liver, lung
- May rarely contain fat
- Increased frequency in certain syndromes
  - Beckwith-Wiedemann
  - Hemihypertrophy
  - Congenital aniridia
  - WAGR syndrome
    - Wilm tumor
    - Aniridia
    - Genitourinary malformations
    - Mental retardation
  - Denys-Drash syndrome
  - Trisomy 18

Renal abscess
- Nonspecific rim-enhancing low attenuation mass
- May have history of pyelonephritis, fevers, costovertebral angle tenderness
- Typically does not contain fat

Renal lymphoma
- Multiple renal masses easily differentiated from multiple fatty AML
- Tuberous sclerosis patients with bilateral AML can simulate renal lymphoma if AML lesions are fat deficient
- Renal lymphoma usually in the setting of widespread disease, with extensive adenopathy

Renal cell carcinoma
- Rare in children
- Rarely reported to contain fat
  - Usually engulfed renal sinus fat
- Calcification in mass highly suggestive of RCC, as calcifications are extremely rare in AML
- If AML is fat deficient, may mimic renal cell carcinoma

ANGIOMYOLIPOMA

Liposarcoma
- Large exophytic AML may simulate well-differentiated retroperitoneal liposarcoma
- Defect in renal parenchyma seen with AML differentiates these lesions
- Reported in teenagers and young adults
- Rare in children: Mean age 50 years
- Most common soft tissue sarcoma in adults

Oncocytoma
- Rare in children: Mean age is 62-68 years
- Rare solid benign renal tumor; rarely contains fat
- Classic spoke-wheel pattern of vessels on angiogram
- Usually resected, because they are indistinguishable from RCC

PATHOLOGY

General Features
- General path comments
  - Epidemiology of lesion
    - 0.3-3% in autopsy series
    - 80% isolated, sporadic AML
    - 20% AML associated with tuberous sclerosis
- Genetics
  - 2 abnormal genes associated with TS
    - TSC1: Band 9q34
    - TSC2: Band 16q13.3
- Etiology: Benign renal tumor with mixed vascular, muscle & fatty elements
- Epidemiology
  - Occur in 80% of TS patients
  - Also associated with neurofibromatosis and von Hippel-Lindau syndrome
  - Mean age 41 years
  - F:M = 4:1
  - Children: Rare unless have TS
  - 80% with TS develop AMLs by age 10
  - If have TS, more often bilateral, multifocal, and larger

Gross Pathologic & Surgical Features
- Round, lobulated, yellow-to-gray color secondary to fat content

Microscopic Features
- Variable amounts of 3 components
  - Angioid (vascular)
  - Myoid (smooth muscle)
  - Lipoid (fatty)

CLINICAL ISSUES

Presentation
- Most common signs/symptoms
  - Most commonly asymptomatic
  - If > 4 cm diameter more likely to spontaneously hemorrhage
    - Flank pain
    - Abdominal pain
    - Hematuria
    - Possible life-threatening hemorrhage (Wunderlich syndrome)
- Other signs/symptoms
  - 80% AML are incidental findings on abdominal imaging exams
  - 20% of patients with renal AML have tuberous sclerosis
    - 80% of patients with tuberous sclerosis develop renal AML

Demographics
- Age: Mean age at presentation is 41 years
- Gender
  - Isolated, sporadic AML M:F = 1:4
  - AML associated with tuberous sclerosis M:F = 1:1

Natural History & Prognosis
- No malignant potential
- Rarely becomes locally aggressive and invades adjacent structures (e.g., IVC and regional lymph nodes)
- AML usually grows slowly
- Massive replacement of renal parenchyma with AML may result in end stage renal disease

Treatment
- Debate exists as to how to manage asymptomatic patients with AML
- If under 4 cm, conservative management with follow-up recommended
- If larger than 4 cm, partial nephrectomy or arterial coil embolization often recommended
- Patients presenting with spontaneous bleeding may be treated with arterial coil embolization

DIAGNOSTIC CHECKLIST

Consider
- Consider tuberous sclerosis in any child with angiomyolipoma

Image Interpretation Pearls
- Classic imaging appearance: Well-circumscribed intrarenal fatty mass
- If see calcifications, more likely RCC and unlikely AML

SELECTED REFERENCES
1. Fricke BL et al: Frequency and imaging appearance of hepatic angiomyolipomas in pediatric and adult patients with tuberous sclerosis. AJR Am J Roentgenol. 182(4):1027-30, 2004
2. Kim JK et al: Angiomyolipoma with minimal fat: differentiation from renal cell carcinoma at biphasic helical CT. Radiology. 230(3):677-84, 2004
3. Logue LG et al: Best cases from the AFIP: angiomyolipomas in tuberous sclerosis. Radiographics. 23(1):241-6, 2003
4. Casper KA et al: Tuberous sclerosis complex: renal imaging findings. Radiology. 225(2):451-6, 2002
5. Yamakado K et al: Renal angiomyolipoma: relationships between tumor size, aneurysm formation, and rupture. Radiology. 225(1):78-82, 2002
6. Lowe LH et al: Pediatric renal masses: Wilms tumor and beyond. Radiographics. 20(6):1585-603, 2000

ANGIOMYOLIPOMA

IMAGE GALLERY

Typical

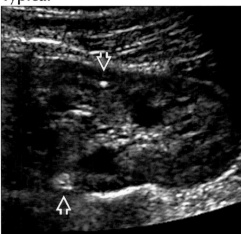
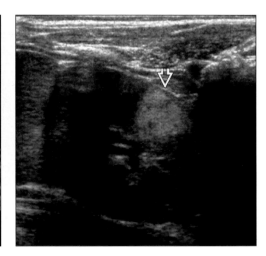

(Left) Sagittal ultrasound shows nonshadowing echogenic renal masses (open arrows) in 3 year old with TS, consistent with angiomyolipomas. *(Right)* Axial ultrasound shows moderate-sized nonshadowing echogenic mass (open arrow) in renal cortex in 2 year old with tuberous sclerosis, consistent with an angiomyolipoma.

Typical

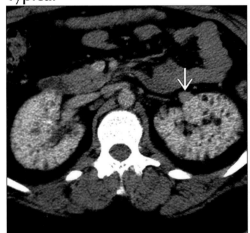
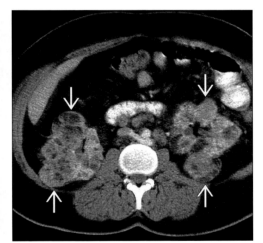

(Left) Axial CECT shows multiple small fatty renal parenchymal masses in 18 year old with TS. While most contain visible fat, the exophytic mass does not (arrow). *(Right)* Axial CECT shows another patient with tuberous sclerosis and multiple bilateral renal masses containing variable amounts of fat, consistent with angiomyolipomas (arrows).

Typical

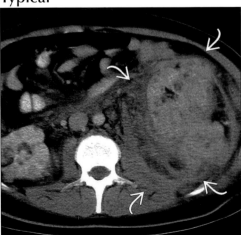
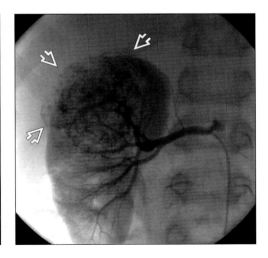

(Left) Axial CECT shows a large spontaneous perinephric hemorrhage (arrows) surrounding the left kidney which contains innumerable fatty masses (AMLs) in a TS patient. *(Right)* Anteroposterior angiography in child with TS shows multiple abnormal tortuous vessels within large right upper pole (arrows) AML. This large AML was embolized to reduce hemorrhage risk.

HYDROMETROCOLPOS

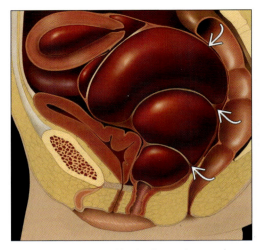

Graphic shows potential levels of vaginal septa (arrows) causing obstruction and hydrometrocolpos. Note that the vagina distends with trapped secretions and blood to a much greater degree than the uterus.

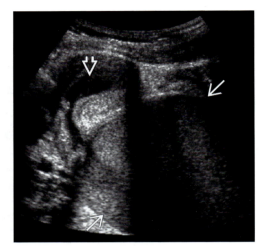

Sagittal ultrasound shows homogeneous echoes distending the vagina (between arrows) and anechoic fluid within the endometrial cavity (open arrow) in this newborn with hydrometrocolpos.

TERMINOLOGY

Abbreviations and Synonyms
- Synonym(s): Hematometrocolpos, hydrometra, hematometra

Definitions
- Dilation of vagina or vagina and uterus secondary to distal stenosis, atresia, transverse vaginal septa, or imperforate membrane
  - Prefix: Hydro meaning fluid, hemato meaning blood
  - Suffix: Metra meaning uterine cavity
  - Suffix: Metrocolpos meaning uterus and vagina

IMAGING FINDINGS

General Features
- Best diagnostic clue: Cystic or debris filled mass in pelvis, separate from bladder and rectum, can cause secondary hydronephrosis
- Location: Between bladder and rectum
- Size: Variable, can be very large and simulate early pregnancy in teenage girls
- Classic imaging appearance: Echogenic debris filling dilated vagina and to a lesser extent uterus creates mass effect in pelvis
  - Vagina has elastic walls and can dilate more than uterus
- Can be associated with Mullerian duct fusion anomalies, particularly uterus didelphys

Radiographic Findings
- Radiography
  - Soft tissue mass in pelvis displacing bowel loops
  - Case reports of peritoneal calcification, presumably from debris spilling out the fallopian tubes

CT Findings
- CECT
  - Fluid-filled cavity with enhancing walls originating deep in pelvis
  - Displaces bladder, rectum, and small bowel
  - Enhancing uterus extends from cephalad aspect of collection
    - Scrutinize the uterus for associated malformations: Didelphys, bicornuate, septate, etc.

MR Findings
- MR findings are similar to CT
- Aging blood components have characteristic signal intensity
- Multiplanar imaging of MR useful to optimally profile uterine and cervical anomalies

DDx: Pelvic "Masses"

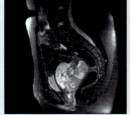
Rhabdomyosarcoma

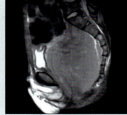
Burkitt

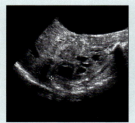
Pelvic Kidney

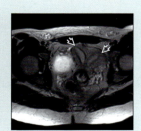
Septate Uterus

HYDROMETROCOLPOS

Key Facts

Terminology
- Synonym(s): Hematometrocolpos, hydrometra, hematometra
- Dilation of vagina or vagina and uterus secondary to distal stenosis, atresia, transverse vaginal septa, or imperforate membrane
- Prefix: Hydro meaning fluid, hemato meaning blood
- Suffix: Metra meaning uterine cavity
- Suffix: Metrocolpos meaning uterus and vagina

Imaging Findings
- Sonographically see echogenic, layering debris in well-defined cavity between bladder and rectum
- Ultrasound is best first imaging study
- MR used when uterine and complex GU anomalies can not be clearly defined with ultrasound

Top Differential Diagnoses
- Pelvic abscess
- Ovarian tumor, torsion, or massive ovarian edema
- Fallopian tube torsion, cyst, or obstruction
- Pelvic rhabdomyosarcoma
- Other pelvic masses

Pathology
- Embryology-anatomy
- Failure of canalization, stenosis, or atresia along the lumen
- Most often associated with anal, renal, vertebral, and cardiac anomalies

Ultrasonographic Findings
- Grayscale Ultrasound
  - Sonographically see echogenic, layering debris in well-defined cavity between bladder and rectum
  - Uterus is frequently visible arising from dome of collection
    - Look for variable uterine distention
    - Uterine anomalies, Mullerian duct fusion anomalies are commonly associated
  - Also check for presence of both kidneys and secondary hydronephrosis
- Color Doppler
  - Useful to confirm lack of blood-flow within debris filled cavities
  - Acute blood may appear "solid" on ultrasound

Other Modality Findings
- Rarely, hysterosalpingography or sonohysterography are performed in the convalescent phase to re-evaluate uterine morphology

Imaging Recommendations
- Best imaging tool
  - Ultrasound is best first imaging study
  - MR used when uterine and complex GU anomalies can not be clearly defined with ultrasound
    - Consider delaying the MR exam to convalescent phase, after fluid and debris have been drained

DIFFERENTIAL DIAGNOSIS

Pelvic abscess
- In newborn hydrometrocolpos much more likely
- In adolescents consider pelvic inflammatory disease and sexually transmitted infection
- Clinical presentation can mimic perforated appendicitis with pelvic abscess

Ovarian tumor, torsion, or massive ovarian edema
- Look for separate ovaries and identify uterus contiguous with mass

Fallopian tube torsion, cyst, or obstruction
- Should be able to separate tube from uterus and vagina on imaging

Pelvic rhabdomyosarcoma
- Hydrocolpos can mimic vagina or pelvic floor rhabdomyosarcoma, history is helpful

Other pelvic masses
- Consider sacrococcygeal teratoma, Burkitt lymphoma, pelvic neuroblastoma & others based on patient age and location/origin of mass

PATHOLOGY

General Features
- General path comments
  - Site of obstruction can be
    - Imperforate hymen
    - Vaginal stenosis or atresia
    - Cervical stenosis or atresia
    - Mass effect from duplications of uterus & vagina (didelphys)
    - Transverse vaginal septum
  - Most common location of transverse vaginal septum is between middle and upper thirds of vagina
    - These patients have a functional uterus though their fertility is often compromised
  - Secondary urinary obstruction can occur at level of
    - Urethra
    - Ureterovesical junction
    - Distal ureter
- Genetics
  - Generally sporadic, not inherited
  - McKusick-Kaufman syndrome

HYDROMETROCOLPOS

- Rare multiple congenital anomaly syndrome comprised of hydrometrocolpos, postaxial polydactyly, and congenital heart malformation, inherited in an autosomal recessive pattern
  - Bardet-Biedl syndrome
    - Also has hydrometrocolpos and postaxial polydactyly with retinitis pigmentosa, obesity, and learning disability becoming apparent by early school age
- Etiology
  - Embryology-anatomy
    - Failure of canalization, stenosis, or atresia along the lumen
- Epidemiology
  - Incidence
    - Transverse vaginal septum 1 in 80,000
    - Imperforate hymen more common
    - Note: Female hymen is the homolog of plica collicularis (valve tissue) in males
- Associated abnormalities
  - Most often associated with anal, renal, vertebral, and cardiac anomalies
  - Also associated with
    - Intestinal aganglionosis
    - Imperforate anus
    - Urogenital sinus
    - Cloacal anomalies
  - Can be associated with Mullerian duct fusion anomalies, particularly uterus didelphys
  - Iatrogenic cases reported due to malposition of artificial urinary sphincter in prepubertal girls

Gross Pathologic & Surgical Features

- Debris contents
  - In fetal life and infancy contents are primarily cervical mucus, mucocolpos or hydrocolpos
    - Maternal estrogen stimulates cervical mucus production and causes swelling of labia minora
  - Peripubertal contents are blood, sloughed endometrial lining, cervical and vagina mucus

CLINICAL ISSUES

Presentation

- Most common signs/symptoms
  - In infancy presents as pelvic mass, sepsis, or utinary tract infection and is related to maternal hormone effects on neonatal uterus and vagina
  - In adolescent girls presents as delayed menarche, cyclic pelvic pain, mass
- Occasionally presents as a prolapsing interlabial mass
- When hydrometrocolpos is massive in fetal life, secondary urinary tract obstruction is problematic
  - Can cause secondary fetal anuria
  - Oligohydramnios with poor fetal lung development
  - Secondary renal dysplasia, renal failure in newborn
  - Occasionally intrauterine drainage/aspiration procedures are attempted

Demographics

- Age
  - Bimodal age presentation
    - Infancy
    - Menarche
- Gender: Females only

Natural History & Prognosis

- Immediate prognosis is excellent
- Compromised fertility and endometriosis are long-term complications in some patients

Treatment

- Typically drained & septum or stenotic segment excised from inferior approach with minimal tissue resected
- Stenoses and focal atresias may require primary anastomosis and perioperative stenting
- Secondary hydronephrosis typically resolves spontaneously without additional intervention

SELECTED REFERENCES

1. Slavotinek AM et al: A female with complete lack of Mullerian fusion, postaxial polydactyly, and tetralogy of fallot: genetic heterogeneity of McKusick-Kaufman syndrome or a unique syndrome? Am J Med Genet A. 129(1):69-72, 2004
2. Seigel MJ et al: in 3rd edition Pediatric Sonography. Lippincott, Williams & Wilkins, Philadelphia:558-64, 2002
3. Geipel A et al: Diagnostic and therapeutic problems in a case of prenatally detected fetal hydrocolpos. Ultrasound Obstet Gynecol. 18(2):169-72, 2001
4. Hu MX et al: An unusual case of neonatal peritoneal calcifications associated with hydrometrocolpos. Pediatr Radiol. 31(10):742-4, 2001
5. Nalaboff KM et al: Imaging the endometrium: disease and normal variants. Radiographics. 21(6):1409-24, 2001
6. Slavotinek AM et al: Phenotypic overlap of McKusick-Kaufman syndrome with bardet-biedl syndrome: a literature review. Am J Med Genet. 95(3):208-15, 2000
7. Amagai T et al: Endoscopic septotomy: a new surgical approach to infantile hydrometrocolpos with imperforate hemivagina and ipsilateral renal agenesis. J Pediatr Surg. 34(4):628-31, 1999
8. Arena F et al: The neonatal management and surgical correction of urinary hydrometrocolpos caused by a persistent urogenital sinus. BJU Int. 84(9):1063-8, 1999
9. Cain MP et al: Vaginal stenosis and hydrometrocolpos: late complication of inadvertent perivaginal placement of an artificial urinary sphincter in prepubertal girls(1). Urology. 54(5):923, 1999
10. David A et al: Hydrometrocolpos and polydactyly: a common neonatal presentation of Bardet-Biedl and McKusick-Kaufman syndromes. J Med Genet. 36(8):599-603, 1999
11. Li YW et al: Unilateral occlusion of duplicated uterus with ipsilateral renal anomaly in young girls: a study with MRI. Pediatr Radiol. 25 Suppl 1:S54-9, 1995
12. Scanlan KA et al: Value of transperineal sonography in the assessment of vaginal atresia. AJR Am J Roentgenol. 154(3):545-8, 1990
13. Blask ARN et al: Obstructed urovaginal anomalies: demonstration with sonography. Part I: neonates and infants. Radiology 179:79-83, 1991
14. Wu A et al: Sonography of pelvic masses in children: diagnostic predictability. AJR Am J Roentgenol. 148(6):1199-202, 1987

HYDROMETROCOLPOS

IMAGE GALLERY

Typical

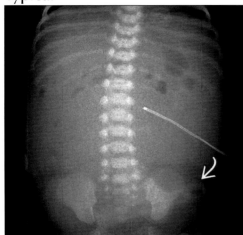
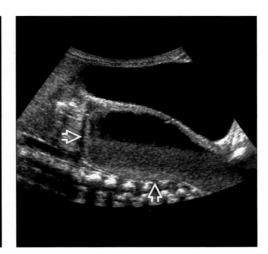

(Left) Abdominal radiograph in an newborn girl shows distended flanks and displacement of bowel loops out of the pelvis. An umbilical cord clamp *(arrow)* and monitor wire overlie the abdomen. *(Right)* Longitudinal extended field of view ultrasound shows urine filled bladder in the nearfield and a fluid-debris level in a well-defined collection *(arrows)* deep to the bladder and anterior to the lumbosacral spine.

Typical

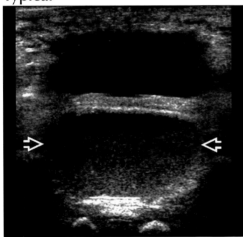
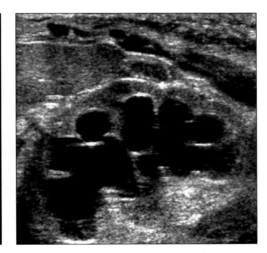

(Left) Transverse ultrasound in the same patient shows bladder in nearfield, collection with relatively thick wall *(arrows)*, and echogenic portions of sacral spine posteriorly in this infant with hydrometrocolpos. *(Right)* Longitudinal ultrasound shows secondary hydronephrosis due to bladder and distal ureteral compression in the same baby girl with imperforate hymen.

Typical

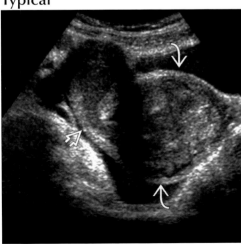
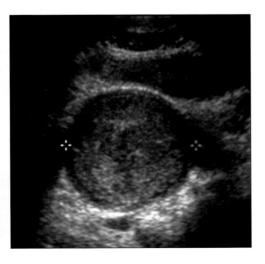

(Left) Longitudinal ultrasound in a teenager with pelvic pain shows acute blood distending the vagina *(between curved arrows)*, extending through the open cervical os *(open arrow)* and filling the endometrial cavity. Note free fluid in the cul-de-sac. *(Right)* Transverse ultrasound in the same teenager shows acute blood between cursors distending the vagina in a case of transverse vaginal septum. Patient was just starting her menses.

NEONATAL ADRENAL GLAND, NORMAL

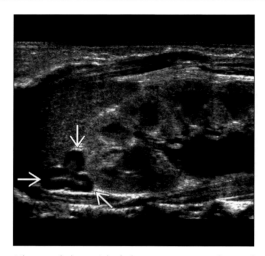

Ultrasound shows 3-leaf clover appearance of normal newborn adrenal gland (arrows). Note the echogenic central medullary stripe and thick, hypoechoic fetal cortex. The renal pelvis is mildly dilated.

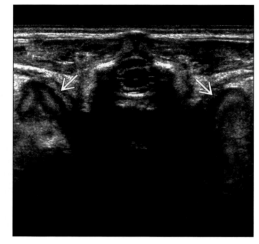

Ultrasound performed transversely over the spine with the baby lying prone shows normal bilateral adrenal glands (arrows) with a chevron or inverted "v" configuration. Shapes resembling "y" and "z" are also common.

TERMINOLOGY

Abbreviations and Synonyms
- Suprarenal gland

Definitions
- Part of the hypothalamic pituitary axis which regulates many body functions and responds to stress
- The adrenal cortex, the largest part of the adrenal gland, produces three major hormones, in three layers which are described from superficial to deep as follows
  o The zona glomerulosa is responsible for making aldosterone, a mineralocorticoid which retains sodium and wastes potassium
    ▪ Regulates fluid and electrolyte balance and helps maintain blood pressure under the influence of ACTH (corticotropin), angiotensin II, and others
  o The zona fasciculata is where glucocorticoids (cortisol mostly) are made
    ▪ Glucocorticoids regulate metabolism of glucose, protein, and fat and allow the body to respond to stress by increasing blood glucose levels and cardiac output
  o The zona reticularis is credited with producing dehydroepiandrosterone, a sex hormone that works much like testosterone: Androgens are responsible for sexual differentiation in the fetus
- The medulla makes and stores epinephrine and norepinephrine in neurosecretory granules: These are the "stress hormones" also known as adrenaline
- The newborn adrenal gland is quite large (5 gm), almost twice the weight of an adult adrenal gland
  o Most of the newborn adrenal is made up of fetal cortex, which functions in utero and continues to grow until term
  o The fetal cortex starts to involute shortly after delivery and gradually decreases in size until it is almost inapparent by 6 months of age

IMAGING FINDINGS

General Features
- Best diagnostic clue
  o Hypoechoic fetal cortex and echogenic central medullary portion in a layered configuration
  o The shape of the newborn adrenal varies, sometimes described as letters "y", "v", or "z"
- Location: Cephalad to the kidney
- Size: 0.9-3.6 cm in length and 0.2-0.3 cm thick
- Morphology
  o Adrenal cortex initially much thicker than medulla, overall contour is convex outward
  o After 2-3 months, cortex and medulla are equivalent thickness, contour starts to flatten

DDx: Abnormal Adrenal Findings In Neonates

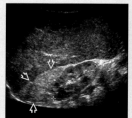
Neuroblastoma + Mets

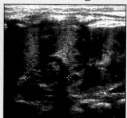
Adrenal Hemorrhage

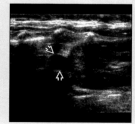
Adrenal Cyst

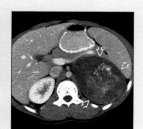
Ganglioneuroma

NEONATAL ADRENAL GLAND, NORMAL

Key Facts

Terminology
- Part of the hypothalamic pituitary axis which regulates many body functions and responds to stress
- The newborn adrenal gland is quite large (5 gm), almost twice the weight of an adult adrenal gland
- Most of the newborn adrenal is made up of fetal cortex, which functions in utero and continues to grow until term
- The fetal cortex starts to involute shortly after delivery and gradually decreases in size until it is almost inapparent by 6 months of age

Imaging Findings
- Hypoechoic fetal cortex and echogenic central medullary portion in a layered configuration
- The shape of the newborn adrenal varies, sometimes described as letters "y", "v", or "z"
- Size: 0.9-3.6 cm in length and 0.2-0.3 cm thick
- Adrenal cortex initially much thicker than medulla, overall contour is convex outward

Top Differential Diagnoses
- Congenital adrenal hyperplasia
- Imaging findings in CAH are an enlarged gland with redundant folds of cortex and medulla creating a pattern that resembles sulci and gyri in the brain, the so called "cerebriform" appearance
- Gland weight may reach 15 grams in CAH; length > 2 cm and width > 4 mm suggests the diagnosis
- Adrenal insufficiency
- Neuroblastoma
- Neonatal adrenal hemorrhage
- Wolman disease

---

   o Around 6 months, corticomedullary differentiation is lost on imaging, contours flatten
   o After 1 year, resembles adult gland with thin limbs and flat or concave margins

Imaging Recommendations
- Best imaging tool: Ultrasound shows the newborn adrenal gland very well
- Protocol advice: When masses or cysts are noted, use Doppler to assess vascularity and exclude neonatal hemorrhage

DIFFERENTIAL DIAGNOSIS

Congenital adrenal hyperplasia
- Synonyms: Congenital adrenal hyperplasia (CAH), adrenogenital syndrome, 21-hydroxylase deficiency
- Definition: A disorder present at birth characterized by a deficiency in the hormones cortisol and aldosterone and an over production of androgen
- CAH is inherited as autosomal recessive gene defects
- CAH is well suited for newborn screening, because it is a common and potentially fatal disease
   o CAH can be easily diagnosed by a simple hormonal measurement in blood
   o 17 alpha-hydroxyprogesterone (17OHP) is measured in filter paper blood spots obtained by a heel puncture preferably between 2 and 4 days after birth
- A severe form of the disease can cause life-threatening "adrenal crisis" in the newborn due to salt wasting
   o In the salt-losing form of adrenogenital syndrome, newborn infants develop symptoms shortly after birth including vomiting, dehydration, electrolyte changes, and cardiac arrhythmias
   o Unrecognized and untreated, this condition can lead to death within 1-2 weeks
- Incidence: 1 in 10,000 to 18,000 children are born with congenital adrenal hyperplasia
- CAH affects both females and males
- In a female newborns with this disorder
   o The clitoris is enlarged with the urethral opening at the base (ambiguous genitalia, often appearing more male-like than female)
   o The ovaries, uterus and Fallopian tubes are normal
   o As she grows older, masculinization of some features occurs, such as deepening of the voice, the appearance of facial hair, and failure to menstruate at puberty
- In a male newborns with CAH
   o No obvious abnormality is present at birth
   o Long before puberty should occur, as early as 2-3 years of age, the child becomes increasingly muscular, the penis enlarges, pubic hair appears, and the voice deepens
   o At puberty, the testes are small
- Imaging findings in CAH are an enlarged gland with redundant folds of cortex and medulla creating a pattern that resembles sulci and gyri in the brain, the so called "cerebriform" appearance
- Gland weight may reach 15 grams in CAH; length > 2 cm and width > 4 mm suggests the diagnosis
- Treatment: Daily administration of forms of cortisol (dexamethasone, fludrocortisone, or hydrocortisone): Additional doses of medicine are required during times of stress such as severe illness or surgery

Adrenal insufficiency
- Primary adrenal insufficiency occurring in the newborn period is very rare and most often due to adrenal hypoplasia congenita and syndromes including triple A and IMAGE
- Congenital aplasia is very rare; found in 10% with unilateral renal agenesis
   o Bilateral hypoplasia is associated with anencephaly and due to lack of ACTH cells; causes adrenal insufficiency
- Unilateral adrenal absence occurs in 1 per 10,000 live births and may be associated with sudden infant death syndrome
- Clinical symptoms of adrenal insufficiency: Weight loss, vomiting, dehydration, severe electrolyte disturbances due to mineralocorticoid deficiency, hypotension, hypoglycemia

NEONATAL ADRENAL GLAND, NORMAL

- Imaging and pathology: Small for age adrenal glands, decreased fetal zone in newborns, scattered cytomegalic cells, cells have decreased lipid
- DDx: Chronic exogenous glucocorticoids causes acquired hypoplasia, look for maternal steroid use

Neuroblastoma
- Suspect neuroblastoma when a hypervascular mass is found in the adrenal
- Neonatal or congenital neuroblastoma tends to have an excellent prognosis, even with disseminated disease (stage 4S)
- Neonatal neuroblastomas are more often cystic than tumors in older children
- Calcification is present in > 85%

Neonatal adrenal hemorrhage
- Perinatal bleeding into normal gland
- Associated with perinatal stress: Asphyxia, sepsis, labile blood pressure, birth trauma, coagulopathy
- Occurs more often in full-term infants and large-for-gestational-age babies
- Hemorrhage is bilateral in 10%; this group is at risk for adrenal insufficiency

Adrenal cysts
- Can be seen as sequelae of prior hemorrhage or in association with Beckwith-Wiedemann

Wolman disease
- Synonym: Primary familial xanthomatosis
- Rare, autosomal recessive lipid storage disorder
- Deficiency of lysosomal acid lipase, causing accumulation of triglycerides and cholesterol esters in liver, spleen and adrenal glands
- Usually causes death by age 6 months to 1 year
- Imaging: Markedly enlarged adrenal glands with dystrophic calcifications, normal histologic architecture

Ganglioneuroma
- Part of the benign spectrum of neural crest tumors

PATHOLOGY

Gross Pathologic & Surgical Features
- The newborn adrenal gland is quite large (5 gm), almost twice the weight of an adult adrenal gland
  - Most of the newborn adrenal is made up of fetal cortex, which functions in utero and continues to grow until term
  - The fetal cortex starts to involute shortly after delivery and gradually decreases in size until it is almost inapparent by 6 months of age

CLINICAL ISSUES

Presentation
- Most common signs/symptoms
  - Prominence of the newborn adrenal gland usually noted during renal ultrasound
  - Awareness of normal newborn adrenal appearance avoids inappropriate work-up

SELECTED REFERENCES

1. Duman N et al: Scrotal hematoma due to neonatal adrenal hemorrhage. Pediatr Int. 46(3):360-2, 2004
2. Kushner BH: Neuroblastoma: a disease requiring a multitude of imaging studies. J Nucl Med. 45(7):1172-88, 2004
3. Merrot T et al: Prenatally detected cystic adrenal mass associated with Beckwith-Wiedemann syndrome. Fetal Diagn Ther. 19(6):465-9, 2004
4. Nebesio TD et al: Infant with classic congenital adrenal hyperplasia (CAH) born to a mother with classic CAH. J Pediatr. 145(2):250-2, 2004
5. Ng PC et al: Transient adrenocortical insufficiency of prematurity and systemic hypotension in very low birthweight infants. Arch Dis Child Fetal Neonatal Ed. 89(2):F119-26, 2004
6. Rahmah R et al: Bilateral adrenal cysts and ectopic pancreatic tissue in Beckwith-Wiedemann syndrome: is a conservative approach acceptable? J Pediatr Endocrinol Metab. 17(6):909-12, 2004
7. Watterberg KL: Adrenocortical function and dysfunction in the fetus and neonate. Semin Neonatol. 9(1):13-21, 2004
8. Olgemoller B et al: Screening for congenital adrenal hyperplasia: adjustment of 17-hydroxyprogesterone cut-off values to both age and birth weight markedly improves the predictive value. J Clin Endocrinol Metab. 88(12):5790-4, 2003
9. Pfluger T et al: Integrated imaging using MRI and 123I metaiodobenzylguanidine scintigraphy to improve sensitivity and specificity in the diagnosis of pediatric neuroblastoma. AJR Am J Roentgenol. 181(4):1115-24, 2003
10. Subhedar NV: Treatment of hypotension in newborns. Semin Neonatol. 8(6):413-23, 2003
11. Sul HJ et al: Congenital neuroblastoma with multiple metastases: a case report. J Korean Med Sci. 18(4):618-20, 2003
12. Tanaka S et al: Prenatally diagnosed cystic neuroblastoma: a report of two cases. Asian J Surg. 26(4):225-7, 2003
13. Walther FJ et al: Adrenal suppression and extubation rate after moderately early low-dose dexamethasone therapy in very preterm infants. Early Hum Dev. 74(1):37-45, 2003
14. Sauvat F et al: Outcome of suprarenal localized masses diagnosed during the perinatal period: a retrospective multicenter study. Cancer. 94(9):2474-80, 2002
15. Manson DE et al: Pitfalls in the sonographic diagnosis of juxtadiaphragmatic pulmonary sequestrations. Pediatr Radiol. 31(4):260-4, 2001
16. Hibbert J et al: The ultrasound appearances of neonatal renal vein thrombosis. Br J Radiol. 70(839):1191-4, 1997
17. Steffens J et al: Neonatal adrenal abscesses. Eur Urol. 31(3):347-9, 1997
18. Westra SJ et al: Imaging of the adrenal gland in children. Radiographics. 14(6):1323-40, 1994
19. Avni EF et al: Sonographic demonstration of congenital adrenal hyperplasia in the neonate: the cerebriform pattern. Pediatr Radiol. 23(2):88-90, 1993
20. Sivit CM et al: Adrenal hemorrhage in infants undergoing ECMO: prevalence and clinical significance. Pediatr Radiol. 23(7):519-21, 1993
21. Demirci A et al: Bilateral adrenal hemorrhage associated with bilateral renal vein and vena cava thrombosis. Pediatr Radiol. 21(2):130, 1991
22. Sivit CJ et al: Sonography in neonatal congenital adrenal hyperplasia. AJR Am J Roentgenol. 156(1):141-3, 1991
23. Willemse AP et al: Magnetic resonance appearance of adrenal hemorrhage in a neonate. Pediatr Radiol. 19(3):210-1, 1989
24. Oppenheimer DA et al: Sonography of the normal neonatal adrenal gland. Radiology. 146(1):157-60, 1983

NEONATAL ADRENAL GLAND, NORMAL

IMAGE GALLERY

Typical

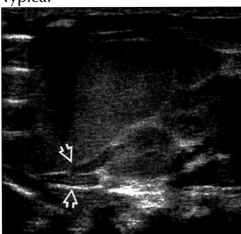
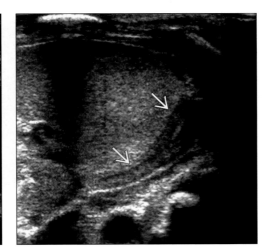

(Left) Ultrasound shows slightly less conspicuous adrenal gland (arrows) in 1 month old infant. Note that hypoechoic fetal cortex has started to involute and appears thinner than in the newborn. *(Right)* Transverse ultrasound of the same left adrenal gland shows similar findings. The adrenal (arrows) is located between the spleen (nearfield) and splenic flexure of colon (shadowing gas).

Typical

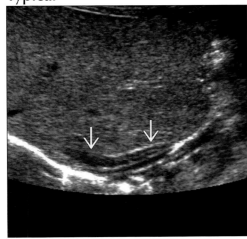
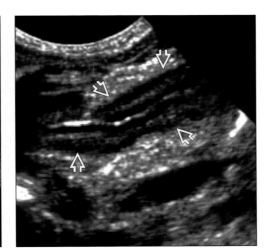

(Left) Ultrasound shows elongated, flat adrenal gland (arrows) in a patient with congenital absence of the ipsilateral kidney. This flat or "lying down" appearance suggests the kidney was never in this renal fossa. *(Right)* Transverse ultrasound in another case of ipsilateral renal agenesis shows the two limbs of the adrenal gland sandwiched together (arrows) with layers of hypoechoic cortex and echogenic medulla.

Other

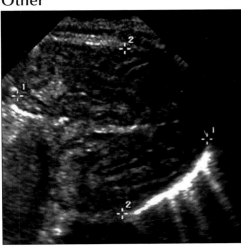
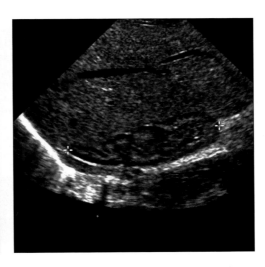

(Left) Transverse ultrasound shows an enlarged newborn adrenal gland with redundant folding of echogenic medulla and hypoechoic cortex in this infant with congenital adrenal hyperplasia. Cursors mark the margins of the gland. *(Right)* Coronal ultrasound shows another case of CAH where the cursors measure the gland length > 4.5 cm. The alternating layers and enfolded pattern are sometimes called "cerebriform".

NEONATAL ADRENAL HEMORRHAGE

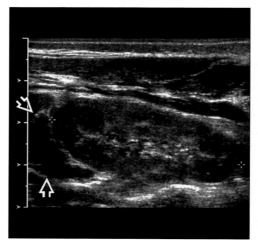

Sagittal ultrasound performed with the infant lying prone shows crescentic mixed echotexture mass (arrows) cephalad to the kidney (marked by cursors) in this infant with a subacute adrenal hemorrhage.

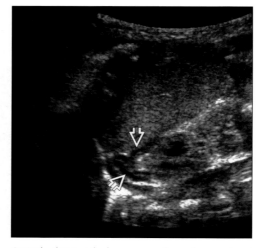

Sagittal ultrasound shows normal newborn adrenal gland (arrows) for comparison. Note the echogenic central medullary portion of the gland surrounded by hypoechoic fetal cortex.

TERMINOLOGY

Abbreviations and Synonyms
- Adrenal hemorrhage, adrenal cortical hematoma

Definitions
- Perinatal bleeding into normal adrenal gland
- Associated with many perinatal stressors: Asphyxia, sepsis, birth trauma, coagulopathies
- Occurs more often in full-term infants and large-for-gestational-age babies
- Bilateral in 10%
- Occurs more often on the right side than the left
- Newborns may present with anemia, dropping hematocrit, jaundice or adrenal insufficiency
- Complications include: Cyst formation, calcification, rarely adrenal insufficiency which can be fatal

IMAGING FINDINGS

General Features
- Best diagnostic clue
  - Echogenic mass replacing or expanding the newborn adrenal gland
  - Bleeding seldom extends outside of gland: Case reports of associated scrotal hematoma
- Location: Suprarenal

Radiographic Findings
- Radiography: May see calcification months to years after hemorrhage

CT Findings
- CECT: Dense (if acute) or hypodense (if chronic) enlargement of the adrenal gland without enhancement

MR Findings
- Used when there is clinical suspicion of neonatal neuroblastoma
- MR shows classic signal intensity pattern of aging blood products
- Gradient echo series shows "bloom" of hemosiderin

Ultrasonographic Findings
- Grayscale Ultrasound
  - Classic imaging appearance varies with timing of ultrasound exam
    - Acutely the hemorrhage appears echogenic and mass-like
    - Subacutely blood products begin to liquefy and contract creating a mixed echotexture mass
    - Chronically the gland resumes normal size and may calcify
- Color Doppler

DDx: Other Neonatal Adrenal Abnormalities

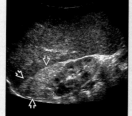
Neuroblastoma + Mets

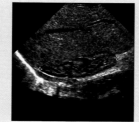
CAH

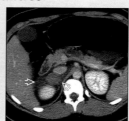
Traumatic Hemorrhage

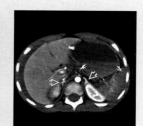
Adrenals in Shock

NEONATAL ADRENAL HEMORRHAGE

Key Facts

Terminology
- Perinatal bleeding into normal adrenal gland
- Associated with many perinatal stressors: Asphyxia, sepsis, birth trauma, coagulopathies
- Occurs more often in full-term infants and large-for-gestational-age babies
- Bilateral in 10%

Imaging Findings
- Radiography: May see calcification months to years after hemorrhage
- MR shows classic signal intensity pattern of aging blood products
- Classic imaging appearance varies with timing of ultrasound exam
- Acutely the hemorrhage appears echogenic and mass-like
- Subacutely blood products begin to liquefy and contract creating a mixed echotexture mass
- Chronically the gland resumes normal size and may calcify
- Doppler is helpful to show avascular nature of the hematoma

Top Differential Diagnoses
- Neuroblastoma
- Congenital adrenal hyperplasia (CAH)
- Wolman disease
- Subdiaphragmatic pulmonary sequestration

Pathology
- Normal involution of fetal adrenal cortical tissue may contribute to the frequency with which neonatal hemorrhage occurs

---

  ○ Doppler is helpful to show avascular nature of the hematoma
  ○ Versus Doppler in neuroblastoma which is typically very vascular
  ○ Doppler is also useful to assess the adjacent renal veins; renal vein thrombosis is associated with adrenal hemorrhage, though a causal relationship has not been established

Other Modality Findings
- Nuclear renal scans occasionally suggest indirect evidence of neonatal adrenal hemorrhage, flattening of the upper pole of the kidney, though this is not the exam of choice

Imaging Recommendations
- Best imaging tool
  ○ Sonography is the imaging modality of choice for initial diagnosis and follow-up
  ○ If lesion appears to increase in size with time, MR is usually performed to document the characteristic signal intensity of aging blood
- Protocol advice: Turn on Doppler to show lack of flow in these mass-like hematomas

DIFFERENTIAL DIAGNOSIS

Neuroblastoma
- Doppler sonography useful to show avascularity of adrenal hemorrhage and sequential exams show decreasing size and cystic evolution
- Look for other signs of neuroblastoma, such as liver metastasis
- Adrenal mass associated with neuroblastoma will distort adrenal architecture

Congenital adrenal hyperplasia (CAH)
- Classically there is bilateral adrenal enlargement and cerebriform contour of the gland

Wolman disease
- A rare autosomal-recessive disorder of lipid metabolism caused by reduced levels of lysosomal acid lipase that causes bilateral adrenal calcification
- It occurs in infancy and is fatal in most cases before the age of 1 year
- Affected infants show signs of lipid storage in most tissues, including hepatosplenomegaly, abdominal distension, vomiting, steatorrhea, failure to thrive, and adrenal calcifications
- Case reports exist of isolated fetal ascites in Wolman disease

Subdiaphragmatic pulmonary sequestration
- Look for systemic vessel feeding homogeneous echotexture mass

Adrenal cysts
- Associated with Beckwith-Wiedemann

PATHOLOGY

General Features
- General path comments
  ○ Normal involution of fetal adrenal cortical tissue may contribute to the frequency with which neonatal hemorrhage occurs
  ○ Embryology-anatomy
    ▪ Fetal adrenal cortex functions in utero to produce corticosteroids and is quite thick at the time of birth creating convex borders
    ▪ The central medullary portion of the gland is brightly echogenic in comparison to the cortex
    ▪ The fetal cortex and overall size of the gland decrease after birth and become almost inapparent by 6 months of age
    ▪ Neonatal adrenal glands are relatively large weighing 8-10 grams, against the adult weight of 5 grams
- Genetics: Not inherited
- Etiology

NEONATAL ADRENAL HEMORRHAGE

- Several proposed mechanisms
  - Fetal compression during birth causes increased venous pressure and rupture of small venules
  - Transient hypoxia or hypotension causes hemorrhage
  - Normal involution of fetal cortex, vacuolization, increases tendency for bleeding
- Epidemiology: Full-term infants, and large-for-gestational-age babies are more prone to neonatal adrenal hemorrhage

Gross Pathologic & Surgical Features
- Hemorrhage into otherwise normal tissues for age
- More common on the right side, up to 85% in one study
- One theoretic risk for greater right-sided incidence is relatively short right adrenal vein

Microscopic Features
- Ischemic necrosis, supporting the theory of involuting fetal cortex as a predisposing factor

CLINICAL ISSUES

Presentation
- Most common signs/symptoms: Anemia, dropping hematocrit, jaundice, or adrenal insufficiency in the perinatal period
- Other signs/symptoms: Occasionally discovered incidentally during work-up of antenatal hydronephrosis

Demographics
- Age
  - Newborn infants
  - Incidence of neonatal adrenal hemorrhage is 1-2 per 1,000 births
- Gender: No gender predilection
- Ethnicity: No racial predilection

Natural History & Prognosis
- Blood products retract and liquefy, dystrophic calcifications may develop, adrenal function is typically preserved especially in unilateral cases
- Prognosis is excellent

Treatment
- Observation
- Occasionally medical therapy for adrenal insufficiency needed transiently
  - Exogenous steroid support of hypotension in the neonate is discussed in detail in several of references listed
  - Adrenal insufficiency is extremely rare, requiring damage to > 90% of adrenal tissue

SELECTED REFERENCES

1. Duman N et al: Scrotal hematoma due to neonatal adrenal hemorrhage. Pediatr Int. 46(3):360-2, 2004
2. Merrot T et al: Prenatally detected cystic adrenal mass associated with Beckwith-Wiedemann syndrome. Fetal Diagn Ther. 19(6):465-9, 2004
3. Rahmah R et al: Bilateral adrenal cysts and ectopic pancreatic tissue in Beckwith-Wiedemann syndrome: is a conservative approach acceptable? J Pediatr Endocrinol Metab. 17(6):909-12, 2004
4. Simm PJ et al: Primary adrenal insufficiency in childhood and adolescence: advances in diagnosis and management. J Paediatr Child Health. 40(11):596-9, 2004
5. Watterberg KL: Adrenocortical function and dysfunction in the fetus and neonate. Semin Neonatol. 9(1):13-21, 2004
6. Arena F et al: Bilateral neonatal adrenal abscess. Report of two cases and review of the literature. Pediatr Med Chir. 25(3):185-9, 2003
7. Drut R et al: Pathology of the umbilical cord in adrenal fusion syndrome. Pediatr Pathol Mol Med. 22(3):243-6, 2003
8. Pfluger T et al: Integrated imaging using MRI and 123I metaiodobenzylguanidine scintigraphy to improve sensitivity and specificity in the diagnosis of pediatric neuroblastoma. AJR Am J Roentgenol. 181(4):1115-24, 2003
9. Subhedar NV: Treatment of hypotension in newborns. Semin Neonatol. 8(6):413-23, 2003
10. Sul HJ et al: Congenital neuroblastoma with multiple metastases: a case report. J Korean Med Sci. 18(5):618-20, 2003
11. Tanaka S et al: Prenatally diagnosed cystic neuroblastoma: a report of two cases. Asian J Surg. 26(4):225-7, 2003
12. Bolt RJ et al: Maturity of the adrenal cortex in very preterm infants is related to gestational age. Pediatr Res. 52(3):405-10, 2002
13. Oguzkurt P et al: Ectopic adrenal tissue: an incidental finding during inguinoscrotal operations in children. Hernia. 6(2):62-3, 2002
14. Patankar JZ et al: Neonatal adrenal haemorrhagic pseudocyst. J Postgrad Med. 48(3):239-40, 2002
15. Sauvat F et al: Outcome of suprarenal localized masses diagnosed during the perinatal period: a retrospective multicenter study. Cancer. 94(9):2474-80, 2002
16. Seigel MJ et al: in 3rd edition Pediatric Sonography. Lippincott Williams & Wilkins. Vol:486-90, 2002
17. Strouse PJ et al: Horseshoe adrenal gland in association with asplenia: presentation of six new cases and review of the literature. Pediatr Radiol. 32(11):778-82, 2002
18. Virdi VS et al: Ventricular tachycardia in congenital adrenal hyperplasia. Anaesth Intensive Care. 30(3):380-1, 2002
19. Manson DE et al: Pitfalls in the sonographic diagnosis of juxtadiaphragmatic pulmonary sequestrations. Pediatr Radiol. 31(4):260-4, 2001
20. Suga K et al: Coexisting renal vein thrombosis and bilateral adrenal hemorrhage: renoscintigraphic demonstration. Clin Nucl Med. 25(4):263-7, 2000
21. Hibbert J et al: The ultrasound appearances of neonatal renal vein thrombosis. Br J Radiol. 70(839):1191-4, 1997
22. Steffens J et al: Neonatal adrenal abscesses. Eur Urol. 31(3):347-9, 1997
23. Westra SJ et al: Imaging of the adrenal gland in children. Radiographics. 14(6):1323-40, 1994
24. Sivit CM et al: Adrenal hemorrhage in infants undergoing ECMO: prevalence and clinical significance. Pediatr Radiol. 23(7):519-21, 1993
25. Sivit CJ et al: Sonography in neonatal congenital adrenal hyperplasia. AJR Am J Roentgenol. 156(1):141-3, 1991
26. Gotoh T et al: Adrenal hemorrhage in the newborn with evidence of bleeding in utero. J Urol. 141:1145-7, 1989
27. Willemse AP et al: Magnetic resonance appearance of adrenal hemorrhage in a neonate. Pediatr Radiol. 19(3):210-1, 1989
28. Oppenheimer DA et al: Sonography of the normal neonatal adrenal gland. Radiology. 146(1):157-60, 1983

NEONATAL ADRENAL HEMORRHAGE

IMAGE GALLERY

Typical

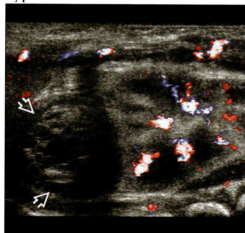
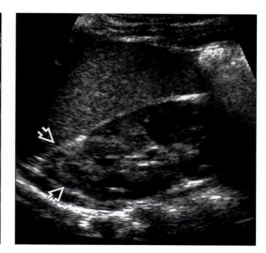

(Left) Coronal color Doppler ultrasound shows subacute adrenal hemorrhage (arrows) with mixed echogenicity which exerts some mass effect on kidney. Note lack of Doppler signal in hematoma. *(Right)* Coronal ultrasound shows nearly normal appearance of the same adrenal gland (arrows) imaged 10 months later. Calcification and cysts may develop in resolving adrenal hematomas.

Typical

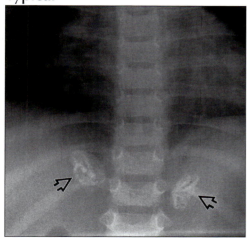
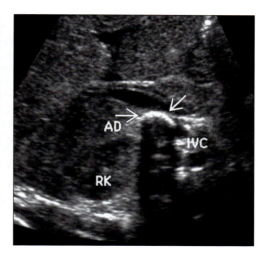

(Left) Radiograph shows bilateral calcifications (arrows) in the upper abdomen in the expected location of the adrenal glands. Chest radiograph was performed for wheezing. *(Right)* Transverse ultrasound shows crescentic calcification (arrows) in the anterior margin of the adrenal gland in the same patient. Shadowing from the calcium necessitates imaging from several directions to exclude a mass.

Other

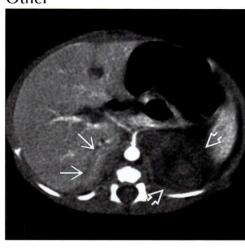
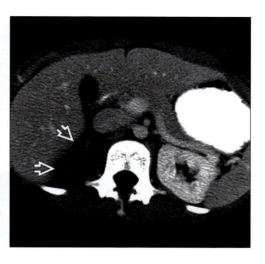

(Left) Axial CECT shows left adrenal hemorrhage (open arrows) in a newborn with rib fractures and hemoperitoneum, due to child abuse. Note the relatively thick, normal right adrenal gland (arrows). *(Right)* Axial CECT shows traumatic right adrenal hemorrhage (arrows) in a 2 year old who fell approximately 12 feet while trying to climb up a rope swing.

NEUROBLASTOMA

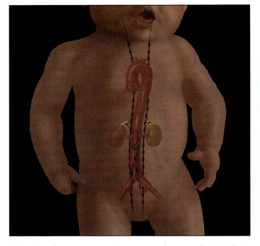

Graphic shows anatomic extent of sympathetic chain (including adrenal glands) from cervical region to inferior pelvis. Neuroblastoma can arise anywhere along sympathetic chain.

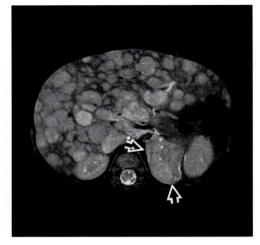

Axial T2WI MR shows left adrenal mass (arrows) with multiple high signal lesions in the liver consistent with diffuse liver mets.

TERMINOLOGY

Definitions
- Malignant tumor of primitive neural crest cells
- Most common extracranial solid malignancy in children
- 3rd most common pediatric malignancy

IMAGING FINDINGS

General Features
- Best diagnostic clue: Invasive suprarenal mass with calcifications
- Location
  - Adrenal medulla (35%)
  - Extraadrenal retroperitoneum (30-35%)
  - Posterior mediastinum (20%)
  - Pelvis (2-3%)
  - Neck (1-5%)
  - Metastatic disease with no primary identified (1%)
- General Imaging Features
  - Most commonly arises from adrenal gland but can arise anywhere along sympathetic chain from neck to pelvis
  - Aggressive tumor with tendency to invade adjacent tissues
  - Surrounds and engulfs, rather than vascular structures such as celiac artery, superior mesenteric artery (SMA), and aorta
  - Tendency to invade into spinal canal via neuroforamina
    - Important to recognize for presurgical planning
  - Metastasizes most commonly to liver and bone
    - Low attenuation liver lesions or diffuse, heterogeneous liver enlargement
    - Destructive bony lesions
  - Prognosis and patterns of disease dependent on age
    - < 1 year of age: Better prognosis, mets to liver and skin
    - > 1 year of age: Worse prognosis, mets to bone
  - Often demonstrate calcifications (74% by CT)

Radiographic Findings
- Radiography
  - Nonspecific soft tissue mass
  - Calcifications: 30% by radiography
  - Widening of inferior thoracic paraspinal soft tissues may be only radiographic finding of upper abdominal mass that extends in retrocrural location
  - Bone metastasis
    - Lucent, sclerotic or mixed lesions
    - Bone metastasis may be presenting clinical or imaging finding

DDx: Suprarenal Mass

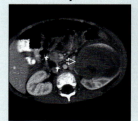
Wilm Tumor

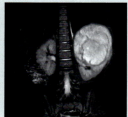
Wilm Tumor

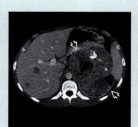
Adrenocortical CA

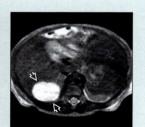
Adrenal Hemorrhage

NEUROBLASTOMA

Key Facts

Terminology
- Malignant tumor of primitive neural crest cells
- Most common extracranial solid malignancy in children
- 3rd most common pediatric malignancy

Imaging Findings
- Most commonly arises from adrenal gland but can arise anywhere along sympathetic chain from neck to pelvis
- Aggressive tumor with tendency to invade adjacent tissues
- Surrounds and engulfs, rather than vascular structures such as celiac artery, superior mesenteric artery (SMA), and aorta
- Tendency to invade into spinal canal via neuroforamina
- Important to recognize for presurgical planning
- Metastasizes most commonly to liver and bone
- Low attenuation liver lesions or diffuse, heterogeneous liver enlargement
- Destructive bony lesions
- Prognosis and patterns of disease dependent on age
- < 1 year of age: Better prognosis, mets to liver and skin
- > 1 year of age: Worse prognosis, mets to bone
- Often demonstrate calcifications (74% by CT)

Pathology
- Continuous spectrum with more benign counterparts: Ganglioneuroma and ganglioneuroblastoma (determined by degree of cellular maturation)

CT Findings
- Mass often heterogeneous from necrosis, hemorrhage
- Calcification seen on CT in up to 85%
- Invasive pattern of growth with engulfing rather than displacing vessels

MR Findings
- Tends to be high in signal on T2 weighted images and low in signal on T1 weighted images
- Heterogeneous signal related to calcification, hemorrhage, and necrosis
- Excellent for detecting extension of tumor into spinal canal: Often obtained in addition to other imaging for this purpose alone

Ultrasonographic Findings
- Typically increased echogenicity, heterogeneous
- Calcification may cause shadowing echogenicities
- Can have varying echogenicity with necrosis/hemorrhage
- Increased vascularity on color Doppler
- Suprarenal rather than arising from kidney
  - In some cases, neuroblastoma may invade the kidney and therefore mimic renal origin

Nuclear Medicine Findings
- Bone Scan
  - Technetium-99m MDP
  - Uptake seen in bony metastasis (both cortical and marrow)
  - Calcified primary mass often also demonstrated uptake in up to 74% of cases
- PET: Role of PET not defined in neuroblastoma, many tumors are PET positive
- MIBG
  - Metaiodobenzylguanidine
  - Avid uptake related to catecholamine production
  - Excellent for following extent of disease in MIBG avid tumors
  - Approximately 30% of neuroblastoma are not MIBG avid

Imaging Recommendations
- Best imaging tool
  - May often be identified with US or CT
  - CT or MRI (controversial which) for defining local extent of disease and organ of origin
  - MIBG and bone scan for determining distal extent of disease
    - PET may play an increasing role in future
- Protocol advice
  - Do not need to do both NECT and CECT through entire abdomen and pelvis
    - Do CECT first
    - If suspect calcification, do repeat, selective, significantly delayed images through are of mass only

DIFFERENTIAL DIAGNOSIS

Wilm tumor
- Mean age = 3 years [neuroblastoma (NBT) < 2 years]
- Calcification uncommon (NBT common)
- Grows like ball: Displaces vessels (NBT surrounds and engulfs vessels)
- Arises from kidney: Claw sign (NBT usually displaces kidney)
- Lung mets in 20% (NBT uncommon)
- Invasion of renal vein and inferior vena cava (IVC) (NBT - does not occur)

Neonatal adrenal hemorrhage
- US: Decreased echogenicity (NBT increased), can follow on serial US
- US: Avascular (NBT vascular)
- MRI: For problematic cases, low T2 weighted signal (NBT increased)

Less common adrenal tumors
- Pheochromocytoma, adrenocortical carcinoma (CA)

RHABDOMYOSARCOMA, GENITOURINARY

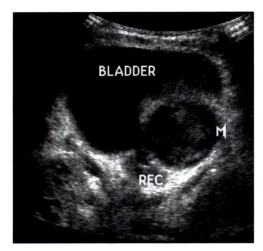

Axial ultrasound shows anechoic bladder, collapsed rectum surrounded by fat, and heterogeneous, solid mass "M" projecting into the bladder lumen in this embryonal bladder rhabdomyosarcoma.

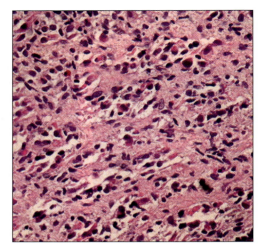

Micropathology shows a mixture of poorly oriented, spindle shaped cells and larger cells with fibrillar eosinophilic cytoplasm which contains cross striation consistent with rhabdomyoblasts.

TERMINOLOGY

Abbreviations and Synonyms
- Genitourinary (GU) rhabdomyosarcoma, botryoid tumor, sarcoma botryoides, embryonal rhabdomyosarcoma

Definitions
- Rhabdomyosarcoma originating from any of the pelvic organs

IMAGING FINDINGS

General Features
- Best diagnostic clue
  - Tumors may be cystic or solid, are typically large and cause significant mass effect
  - Secondary urinary obstruction is common
  - Tumors spread by local extension, via lymphatics, and hematogenous metastases to lungs, liver, and bone
- Location: May originate from bladder, vagina, cervix, uterus, pelvic side walls, prostate and paratesticular tissues
- Size: Tend to be large
- Morphology
  - Heterogeneous, solid tumor typical of embryonal cell type
  - Botryoid variety resembles a bunch of grapes, multiple cysts

Radiographic Findings
- Radiography
  - X-ray of pelvis may show calcifications &/or bone involvement
  - Chest X-ray useful to look for pulmonary metastases
- IVP: Useful to determine level and degree of urinary obstruction

CT Findings
- NECT: Performed of lungs to exclude pulmonary metastases
- CECT
  - CT or MRI of pelvis useful to determine organ of origin and margins of tumor
  - Variable size, heterogeneous enhancing masses
  - Frequently locally invasive
  - Search for adjacent adenopathy
  - Include the liver as this is a frequent site of metastatic disease

MR Findings
- MR findings similar to CT scans
- Signal intensity between muscle and fat
- Enhances with gadolinium

DDx: Other Pediatric Pelvic Masses

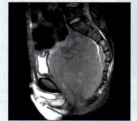

Burkitt

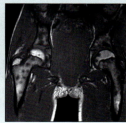

Burkitt & Mets

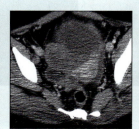

Tubo-Ovarian Torsion

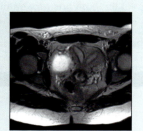

Septate Uterus

RHABDOMYOSARCOMA, GENITOURINARY

Key Facts

Terminology
- Rhabdomyosarcoma originating from any of the pelvic organs

Imaging Findings
- Tumors may be cystic or solid, are typically large and cause significant mass effect
- Secondary urinary obstruction is common
- Tumors spread by local extension, via lymphatics, and hematogenous metastases to lungs, liver, and bone

Top Differential Diagnoses
- Complex ureterocele
- Bladder hematoma
- Ovarian tumor
- Pelvic neuroblastoma
- Pelvic lymphoma/Burkitt
- Hematometrocolpos
- Sacrococcygeal teratoma
- Pelvic inflammatory disease/abscess

Pathology
- Four major histologic types
- Embryonal cell type, accounts for 55%
- Botryoid variant of embryonal type, 5%
- Alveolar rhabdomyosarcoma, 20%
- Undifferentiated type, 20%

Clinical Issues
- Peak incidence 2-6 years old
- Surgery, chemotherapy, and radiation therapy combined

- Useful in cases with intraspinal extension

Ultrasonographic Findings
- Grayscale Ultrasound
  - Often the first imaging study performed to evaluate urinary symptoms
  - Tumor typically large, heterogeneous if solid, multilobulated if cystic
  - Look for secondary evidence of urinary tract obstruction, adenopathy
- Color Doppler
  - Useful to trace displaced and compressed vessels
  - Vascular invasion is unusual

Nuclear Medicine Findings
- Bone Scan: Evaluate for bony metastatic disease
- PET: Increasing use in pediatrics, as an adjunctive test

Other Modality Findings
- VCUG Findings
  - Bladder tumors may mimic large, complex ureterocele or bladder polyp
  - Focal bladder wall thickening is also possible

Imaging Recommendations
- Protocol advice
  - Urinary symptoms typically prompt ultrasound evaluation
  - Followed by CT or MR cross-sectional imaging
  - Finally, staging bone scan

DIFFERENTIAL DIAGNOSIS

Complex ureterocele
- Look for communication with distal ureter or ureteral jet

Bladder hematoma
- Clinical history of instrumentation, cystitis, or chemotherapy

Ovarian tumor
- Differentiation can be difficult, attempt to identify organ of origin

Pelvic neuroblastoma
- Calcifications more often seen in neuroblastoma than sarcoma

Pelvic lymphoma/Burkitt
- Differentiation can be difficult

Hematometrocolpos
- Look for layering debris on cross-sectional imaging

Sacrococcygeal teratoma
- Mass always intimately associated with coccyx

Pelvic inflammatory disease/abscess
- Search for pertinent clinical history

PATHOLOGY

General Features
- General path comments
  - Rhabdomyosarcoma can arise virtually anywhere in the body
  - Four major histologic types
    - Embryonal cell type, accounts for 55%
    - Botryoid variant of embryonal type, 5%
    - Alveolar rhabdomyosarcoma, 20%
    - Undifferentiated type, 20%
  - Botryoid cell type most often located in bladder, vagina, and nasopharynx
  - Prostatic origin is most frequent in boys
  - Rhabdomyosarcoma of paratesticular tissues and vas deferens has one of the best prognoses
- Genetics: Alveolar cell type associated with chromosome translocations
- Etiology: Thought to arise from primitive muscle cells
- Epidemiology: 250 new cases per year in United States
- Associated abnormalities
  - Neurofibromatosis

RHABDOMYOSARCOMA, GENITOURINARY

- Li-Fraumeni syndrome
- Rubinstein-Taybi syndrome
- Beckwith-Wiedemann syndrome
- Environmental factors linked to rhabdomyosarcoma
  - Parental use of marijuana and cocaine
  - In utero radiation exposure
  - Exposure to alkylating agents

Gross Pathologic & Surgical Features
- Botryoid subtype has cysts filled with mucosanguineous fluid
- Can have a transparent gelatinous appearance on gross pathology

Microscopic Features
- One of the small round blue cell tumors
- Rhabdomyoblasts are hallmark
- Not always present, especially in poorly differentiated types
- Histochemical markers for muscle cells are helpful: Desmin, myoglobin, actin
- Disseminated rhabdomyoblasts in bone marrow mimic leukemia

Staging, Grading or Classification Criteria
- Based on tumor invasiveness, tumor size, nodal disease, and metastases
  - Stage 1* = T1 or T2, T size a or b, nodes N0, N1 or Nx, and M0
  - Stage 2 = T1 or T2, T size a, nodes N0 or Nx, and M0
  - Stage 3 = T1 or T2, T size a, nodes N1, and M0
  - Stage 4 = T1 or T2, T size a or b, nodes No or N1, and M1
    - * Genitourinary site excluding the bladder and prostate
    - T (tumor): T1 - confined to organ of origin, T2 - local extension
    - T size: a < or = 5 cm diameter, b > 5 cm diameter
    - N (regional nodes): N0 - not clinically involved, N1 - involved, Nx - unknown
    - M (metastases): M0 - no distant metastases, M1 - distant metastases

CLINICAL ISSUES

Presentation
- Most common signs/symptoms
  - Large pelvic mass
  - Urinary symptoms such as dysuria, hematuria, frequency, urinary retention
  - Pain variably present
- Other signs/symptoms: Vaginal discharge or constipation

Demographics
- Age
  - Peak incidence 2-6 years old
  - 75% are < 5 years old at diagnosis
  - Paratesticular tumors are more common in adolescents
- Gender
  - M:F = 2 or 3:1 for genitourinary tumors
  - Head, neck, and extremity tumors have equal male & female incidence
- Ethnicity: No predilection

Natural History & Prognosis
- Based on stage of disease
- 5 year survival rates
  - Stage 1 is 93%
  - Stage 2 is 81%
  - Stage 3 only about 50%
  - Stage 4 is approximately 30%

Treatment
- Surgery, chemotherapy, and radiation therapy combined
  - Initial surgery includes wide margins (when possible) and lymph node sampling
  - Pelvic exoneration type surgeries have fallen out of favor
    - Organ sparing surgery is now performed
    - Gonads often moved out of radiation field, temporarily
- Protocols through Children's Oncology Group Soft Tissue Sarcoma Committee
  - Formerly the Intergroup Rhabdomyosarcoma Study Group (IRSG)

SELECTED REFERENCES

1. Gruessner SE et al: Management of stage I cervical sarcoma botryoides in childhood and adolescence. Eur J Pediatr. 163(8):452-6, 2004
2. Raney RB et al: Intergroup Rhabdomyosarcoma Study-IV, 1991-1997. Results of treatment of fifty-six patients with localized retroperitoneal and pelvic rhabdomyosarcoma: a report from The Intergroup Rhabdomyosarcoma Study-IV, 1991-1997. Pediatr Blood Cancer. 42(7):618-25, 2004
3. Sanghvi DA et al: Primary rhabdomyosarcoma of the seminal vesicle. Br J Radiol. 77(914):159-60, 2004
4. Nakada K et al: Successful resection of prostatic rhabdomyosarcoma by the posterior sagittal approach combined with preoperative chemotherapy. J Pediatr Surg. 38(7):E6-8, 2003
5. Ng TY et al: Alveolar rhabdomyosarcoma of the cervix. Gynecol Oncol. 91(3):623-6, 2003
6. Ortega JA et al: Presence of well-differentiated rhabdomyoblasts at the end of therapy for pelvic rhabdomyosarcoma: implications for the outcome. J Pediatr Hematol Oncol. 22(2):106-11, 2000
7. Donaldson SS et al: Factors that influence treatment decisions in childhood rhabdomyosarcoma. Radiology. 203:17-22, 1997
8. Silvan AM et al: Organ-preserving management of rhabdomyosarcoma of the prostate and bladder in children. Med Pediatr Oncol. 29(6):573-5, 1997
9. Seigel MJ: Pelvic tumors in childhood. Radiol Clin North Am. 35:1455-75, 1997
10. Duel BP et al: Reconstructive options in genitourinary rhabdomyosarcoma. J Urol. 156(5):1798-804, 1996
11. Breen JL et al: Genital tract tumors in children. Pediatr Clin North Am. 28:355-67, 1981

RHABDOMYOSARCOMA, GENITOURINARY

IMAGE GALLERY

Typical

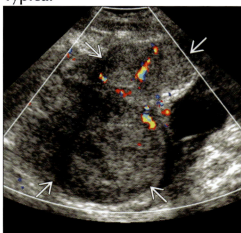
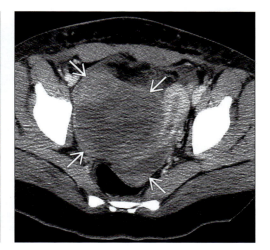

(Left) Transverse color Doppler ultrasound shows bilobed, intermediate echotexture, solid mass in the pelvis (arrows) displacing the urinary bladder to the left. *(Right)* Axial CECT in the same patient shows a large, poorly enhancing mass in the pelvis (arrows), displacing the uterus to the left and compressing the rectum. No adenopathy or bone destruction is seen.

Typical

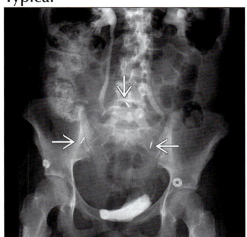
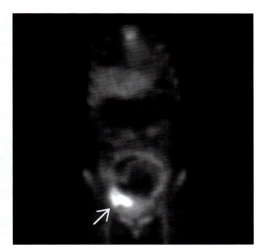

(Left) Anteroposterior IVP image shows surgical clips at the margins of the mass (arrows) to aid in radiation planning and compression of the urinary bladder inferiorly and to the left. *(Right)* Coronal PET shows a minimal rim of F-18-FDG accumulation in the periphery of the tumor following chemotherapy. The largest area of FDG avid tumor in along the lower right margin (arrow).

Typical

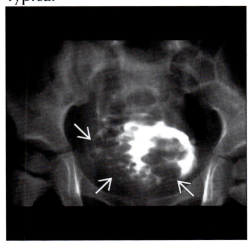
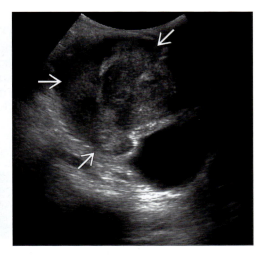

(Left) Anteroposterior IVP film shows numerous small, rounded filling defects (arrows) in the contrast-filled bladder in this patient with sarcoma botryoides. *(Right)* Transverse ultrasound shows a heterogeneous, solid mass (arrows) filling the bladder in a different patient with bladder rhabdomyosarcoma, undifferentiated type.

SACROCOCCYGEAL TERATOMA

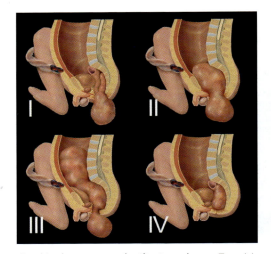

Graphic shows tumor classification scheme: Type I is primarily exophytic, type II has equivalent size masses intra- and extra-abdominally, type III has a larger intra-abdominal component, and type IV is entirely intra-abdominal.

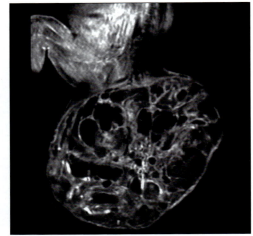

Sagittal T1 C+ MR shows a type I, primarily exophytic, complex, solid and cystic sacrococcygeal teratoma in a newborn. Note the enhancing cyst walls and solid components of the tumor.

TERMINOLOGY

Abbreviations and Synonyms
- Teratoma, germ cell tumor of coccyx, sacrococcygeal teratoma (SCT)

Definitions
- Tumors may contain hair, teeth, cartilage, and fat extending from the coccyx and potentially growing both internally and externally
- Both benign and malignant varieties

IMAGING FINDINGS

General Features
- Best diagnostic clue
  - Classic imaging appearance: Calcifications, mixed solid and cystic components, fat-fluid-debris levels, bone, hair, and cartilage
  - Presence of multiple tissue types: Hair, calcium, bone, fat, fluid levels and involvement of tissues around coccyx
- Location: Origin is always from coccyx, but growth can occur in any direction
- Size: Variable from only a few mL volume to massive, bulky tumor exceeding fetal weight
- Morphology
  - Classically are heterogeneous, containing multiple tissue types
  - Calcification common

Radiographic Findings
- Radiography
  - Typically show large mass extending outside the infant
  - Calcifications may be present

Fluoroscopic Findings
- Type IV SCT may be found incidentally during fluoro studies for constipation or voiding problems

CT Findings
- NECT
  - Demonstrates the fatty components, calcium, and fluid levels well
  - Heterogeneous mass wrapped around the coccyx, but typically without bony destruction
- CECT: Variable enhancement pattern in solid and cystic components

MR Findings
- Similar to CT, mixed signal intensity components, chemical shift artifact at fat/fluid interfaces
- Variable enhancement with gadolinium which does not predict malignancy

DDx: Pediatric Pelvic Masses

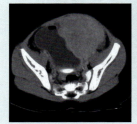
Rhabdomyosarcoma

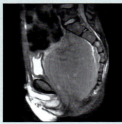
Burkitt

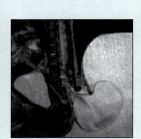
Myelocystocele

SACROCOCCYGEAL TERATOMA

Key Facts

Terminology
- Teratoma, germ cell tumor of coccyx, sacrococcygeal teratoma (SCT)
- Tumors may contain hair, teeth, cartilage, and fat extending from the coccyx and potentially growing both internally and externally
- Both benign and malignant varieties

Imaging Findings
- Classic imaging appearance: Calcifications, mixed solid and cystic components, fat-fluid-debris levels, bone, hair, and cartilage

Top Differential Diagnoses
- Exophytic rhabdomyosarcoma
- Neuroblastoma
- Myelomeningocele or myelocystocele

Pathology
- American Association of Pediatric Surgery Section Classification
- Type I: 47%
- Primarily external in location
- Type II: 34%
- Dumbbell shape, equal int/external components
- Type III: 9%
- Primarily located within the abdomen/pelvis
- Type IV: 10%
- Entirely internal, no external component visible

Clinical Issues
- Prognosis is excellent in benign tumors
- 5% risk of recurrence
- Prognosis is variable in malignant tumors

Ultrasonographic Findings
- Grayscale Ultrasound
  - Ultrasound may be limited due to large size and presence of shadowing calcium and bone elements
  - Heterogeneous echotexture mass
  - Calcification and fat cause highly echogenic areas while cystic areas are hypo to anechoic
- Color Doppler: Areas of normal vascularity, high blood-flow, and necrotic segments may all be present

Nuclear Medicine Findings
- PET
  - Used more often in evaluation of malignant recurrence than in initial diagnosis
  - Expect PET use to increase in the future

Imaging Recommendations
- Best imaging tool
  - Prenatal sonography is most common initial diagnostic modality
  - Post-natally CT or MR to determine full extension of mass and aid surgical planning

DIFFERENTIAL DIAGNOSIS

Exophytic rhabdomyosarcoma
- Presence of calcium, bone and hair suggest teratoma

Neuroblastoma
- May arise in pelvis

Myelomeningocele or myelocystocele
- More than just neural elements and cerebrospinal fluid present on imaging suggest teratoma

Other intra-pelvic masses
- Consider Burkitt lymphoma, ovarian tumors, hematometrocolpos, and abscess

PATHOLOGY

General Features
- General path comments
  - Probably results from rests of pluripotential cells at the caudal end of notochord/spine
  - Malignant characteristics increase with
    - Age at diagnosis
    - Surgical subtype (type IV is worst)
    - Male gender
    - And presence of necrosis or hemorrhage
  - Surgical resection must include the coccyx or risk of recurrence increases
- Genetics: Not inherited
- Epidemiology: Prevalence: 1 in 35,000 to 40,000 births
- Associated abnormalities
  - 10% of sacrococcygeal teratomas are associated with other congenital anomalies, primarily defects of the hindgut and cloacal region, which exceeds the baseline rate of 2.5% expected in the general population
  - SCT are second most common after anterior meningocele in the familial disorder of Currarino (autosomal dominant triad of presacral mass, partial sacral agenesis, and anorectal defects)
  - Familial tendency for these tumors is reported, prompting some to recommend screening asymptomatic siblings

Gross Pathologic & Surgical Features
- Typical of all teratomas: Multiple tissue types in varying stages of maturation and differentiation
- Solid and cystic components are common

Microscopic Features
- Tumors can be mature or immature
- Only 17% of sacrococcygeal tumors have malignant features
- Immature elements frequently include yolk sac tumor, endodermal glands with subnuclear vacuoles, foci of hepatic tissue, and immature intestinal glands

SACROCOCCYGEAL TERATOMA

Staging, Grading or Classification Criteria
- American Association of Pediatric Surgery Section Classification
  - Type I: 47%
    - Primarily external in location
  - Type II: 34%
    - Dumbbell shape, equal int/external components
  - Type III: 9%
    - Primarily located within the abdomen/pelvis
  - Type IV: 10%
    - Entirely internal, no external component visible

CLINICAL ISSUES

Presentation
- Most common signs/symptoms
  - Frequently diagnosed in utero
    - Large fetal tumors require c-section delivery or
    - In utero surgical intervention: Open fetal surgery, fetal radiofrequency or thermal ablation
  - Most other tumors diagnosed within first few days of life
  - Exophytic masses are easily diagnosed
  - Mass that are entirely internal may have delayed diagnosis, presenting with urinary symptoms, urinary retention, or constipation
  - Masses diagnosed after the 1st birthday and located only internally have a worse prognosis, higher malignant potential
  - Serum alpha-fetoprotein is useful tumor marker post-operatively
- Other signs/symptoms
  - In utero complications include polyhydramnios and tumor hemorrhage, which can cause anemia and nonimmune hydrops fetalis
  - Significant atrioventricular shunting can lead to hydrops, as a result of high-output cardiac failure
  - Hydrops which develops before 30 weeks gestation has a dire prognosis, > 90% mortality rate
  - Prognostic indicators of impending fetal distress or demise include
    - Cardiomegaly
    - Fetal hydrops and
    - Increased preload indexes of the fetal venous system are signs of fetal heart failure (pulsatile umbilical vein and abnormal ductus venosus waveform)

Demographics
- Age
  - Typically diagnosed in fetus or newborn
  - Delayed diagnoses possible in first year of life, rarely even later
- Gender
  - Variably reported
    - Older references report SCT as more common in females
    - Newer references report no gender predilection

Natural History & Prognosis
- Prognosis is excellent in benign tumors
  - Gait abnormalities and early arthrosis reported with extensive pelvic muscle resection
- 5% risk of recurrence
- Prognosis is variable in malignant tumors
- Malignant components may be found at presentation or at time of recurrence
  - Yolk sac tumor is most common
  - Embryonal carcinoma is second most common
  - With intensive chemotherapy, 5 year relapse-free survival rate is reported between 76-90%

Treatment
- Complete surgical resection to include the coccyx
- Benign tumors do not require additional therapy
- Malignant tumors are treated with chemotherapy (platinum-based agents) and radiation

SELECTED REFERENCES

1. Heerema-McKenney A et al: Congenital teratoma: a clinicopathologic study of 22 fetal and neonatal tumors. Am J Surg Pathol. 29(1):29-38, 2005
2. Gatcombe HG et al: Primary retroperitoneal teratomas: a review of the literature. J Surg Oncol. 86(2):107-13, 2004
3. Isaacs H Jr: Perinatal (fetal and neonatal) germ cell tumors. J Pediatr Surg. 39(7):1003-13, 2004
4. Neubert S et al: Sonographic prognostic factors in prenatal diagnosis of SCT. Fetal Diagn Ther. 19(4):319-26, 2004
5. Urioste M et al: Malignant degeneration of presacral teratoma in the Currarino anomaly. Am J Med Genet A. 128(3):299-304, 2004
6. Zaccara A et al: Gait analysis in patients operated on for sacrococcygeal teratoma. J Pediatr Surg. 39(6):947-52; discussion 947-52, 2004
7. Graf JL et al: Fetal sacrococcygeal teratoma. World J Surg. 27(1):84-6, 2003
8. Hirose S et al: Fetal surgery for sacrococcygeal teratoma. Clin Perinatol. 30(3):493-506, 2003
9. Huddart SN, et al; Children's Cancer Study Group. Sacrococcygeal teratomas: the UK Children's Cancer Study Group's experience. I. Neonatal. Pediatr Surg Int. 19(1-2):47-51, 2003
10. Avni FE et al: MR imaging of fetal sacrococcygeal teratoma: diagnosis and assessment. AJR Am J Roentgenol. 178(1):179-83, 2002
11. Lam YH et al: Thermocoagulation of fetal sacrococcygeal teratoma. Prenat Diagn. 22(2):99-101, 2002
12. O'Hara SM: Tumors of the Pediatric Genitourinary System. In Oncologic Imaging 2nd edition. Bragg, Rubin, Hricak editors:chapter 36, W B Saunders, Philadelphia, 779-811, 2002
13. Wakhlu A et al: Sacrococcygeal teratoma. Pediatr Surg Int. 18(5-6):384-7, 2002
14. Kamata S et al: Operative management for sacrococcygeal teratoma diagnosed in utero. J Pediatr Surg. 36(4):545-8, 2001
15. Singh SJ et al: Familial presacral masses: Screening pitfalls. J Pediatr Surg. 36(12):1841-4, 2001
16. Wells RG et al: Imaging of sacrococcygeal germ cell tumors. Radiographics. 10:701-13, 1990
17. Altman RP et al: Sacrococcygeal teratoma: American Academy of Pediatrics surgical section survey-1973. J Pediatr Surg. 9:389-98, 1973

SACROCOCCYGEAL TERATOMA

IMAGE GALLERY

Typical

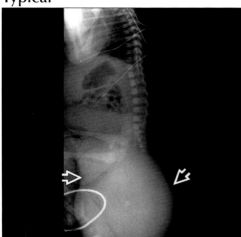
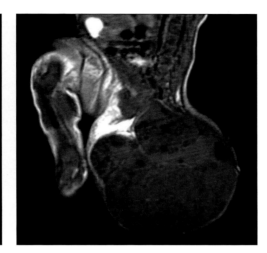

(Left) Lateral radiograph shows large soft tissue mass, a sacrococcygeal teratoma *(arrows)*, extending from the sacrum in this newborn who also has anorectal malformation. *(Right)* Sagittal T1WI MR shows intermediate to low signal intensity exophytic tumor in the same patient. Bulky masses like this one are most often diagnosed in utero.

Typical

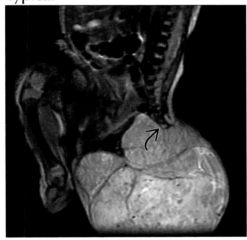
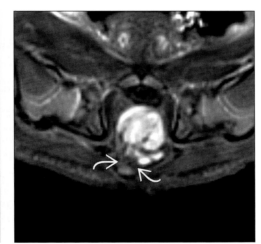

(Left) Sagittal T2WI MR shows primarily solid, intermediate to high signal intensity mass in the same patient. Note how the coccyx is encircled by the tumor *(arrow)*. *(Right)* Axial T2WI MR shows pelvic origin of the tumor with high signal intensity encircling the coccyx *(arrows)*. The coccyx is resected with teratomas to decrease the rate of local recurrence.

Typical

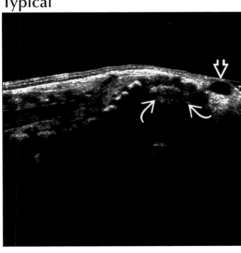
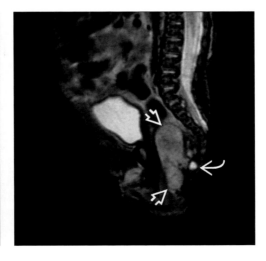

(Left) Sagittal ultrasound performed for "sacral bump" shows cystic mass inferior to the coccyx *(open arrow)* and more subtle soft tissue mass anterior to the sacrum *(curved arrows)* which raised the suspicion of SCT. *(Right)* Sagittal T2WI MR performed to follow-up ultrasound findings confirmed the presacral mass *(open arrows)* with small cystic component inferior to the coccyx *(curved arrow)* in this patient with type IV SCT.

OVARIAN TERATOMA

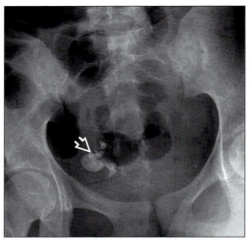

Radiograph shows unusual calcification in the right side of the pelvis (arrow) in a patient with right lower quadrant abdominal pain, suspected to be appendicitis.

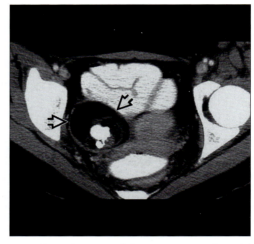

CECT shows the same calcifications in a complex, solid and cystic right adnexal mass (arrows), which was subsequently removed and found to be an ovarian teratoma. Her appendix (not shown) was normal.

TERMINOLOGY

Abbreviations and Synonyms
- Dermoid tumor, dermoid cyst, cystic teratoma

Definitions
- Teratomas are made up of a variety of parenchymal cell types from more than a single germ layer, usually all 3
- These tumors typically are midline or paraxial and arise from totipotential cells
- The term dermoid comes from the skin-like lining found in many of these tumors

IMAGING FINDINGS

General Features
- Best diagnostic clue
  - Heterogeneous pelvic mass, containing calcium, bone, hair, and/or fat
  - Typically well-defined margins without surrounding inflammatory changes
- Location: Pelvis and lower abdomen
- Size
  - Variable, from 1-45 cm diameter
  - Mean diameter 6 cm
- Morphology: Mixed tissue types surrounded by a capsule

Radiographic Findings
- X-ray may show calcifications, bone, and mass effect

CT Findings
- Useful in confirming presence of fat and calcium
- Variable density of tissue components, septations, and fluid-debris levels are hallmarks of teratomas
- CT is useful to exclude inflammatory diseases and regional spread of malignant tumors

MR Findings
- Teratomas demonstrate mixed signal intensity
- Fluid-fat-debris levels may be present
- Low signal intensity from hair, calcium, tooth or bone
- Chemical shift artifact from fat

Ultrasonographic Findings
- Grayscale Ultrasound
  - Heterogeneous echotexture mass
  - Cystic and solid components
  - Calcifications may show posterior shadowing or ring down artifact when very small
  - Fat and hair appear echogenic
  - Fluid-fat-debris levels within cysts
  - Teeth and cartilage may also be discerned

DDx: Other Gynecologic "Masses"

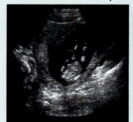
Intrauterine Gestation

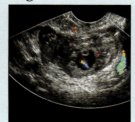
Live Ectopic

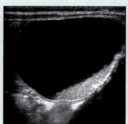
Hemorrhagic Cyst

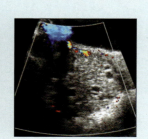
Ovarian Torsion

OVARIAN TERATOMA

Key Facts

Terminology
- Dermoid tumor, dermoid cyst, cystic teratoma
- Teratomas are made up of a variety of parenchymal cell types from more than a single germ layer, usually all 3

Top Differential Diagnoses
- Other ovarian neoplasms
- Endometrioma
- Perforated appendicitis with appendicolith
- Tubo-ovarian abscess
- Pedunculated uterine fibroid
- Ovarian torsion
- Pregnancy
- Pelvic kidney
- Peritoneal cysts

Pathology
- Tissues include hair, teeth, fat, skin, muscle, and endocrine tissue
- Bilateral in up to 15%
- Complications of ovarian teratoma include
- Ovarian torsion
- Rupture, causing chemical peritonitis
- Malignant degeneration seen in ~ 2%

Clinical Issues
- Incidental finding on physical exam or during imaging for unrelated symptoms
- Treatment is surgical resection, ovary sparing surgery
- Laparoscopic surgery preferred

- "Dermoid mesh" appearance refers to linear and punctate hyperechoic interfaces floating within a cystic mass
- "Dermoid plug" refers to crescentic echogenic material, usually positioned dependently within a cyst or attached to the cyst wall
- "Tip of the iceberg sign" refers to a strong echogenic interface at the leading edge of teratoma that blocks the deeper components from view
  - May be caused by calcification, hair, fat, etc.
- Color Doppler: Flow useful in differentiating solid perfused tissue from solid avascular hair, teeth, etc.

Imaging Recommendations
- Best imaging tool
  - Ultrasound generally is best
  - CT and MRI reserved for complex cases or patients who are ill-suited to sonography
- Protocol advice
  - Scan the mass in orthogonal planes, looking for variable tissue and cyst contents
  - Endovaginal scanning is optimal when tolerated
  - Larger masses may require transabdominal scanning and extended field of view

DIFFERENTIAL DIAGNOSIS

Other ovarian neoplasms
- Benign
  - Simple/follicular cysts
  - Cystadenomas
  - Gonadoblastoma
- Malignant
  - Germ cell tumors
  - Stromal tumors
  - Epithelial carcinomas
  - Malignant teratomas

Endometrioma
- Cyclic pain history is useful

Perforated appendicitis with appendicolith
- Can be a close mimicker of ovarian teratoma

Tubo-ovarian abscess
- Fever, cervical tenderness, vaginal discharge are typical

Pedunculated uterine fibroid
- Imaging can distinguish between these diagnoses

Ovarian torsion
- May require surgical exploration to distinguish
- May co-exist with ovarian teratoma

Pregnancy
- Ectopic or intrauterine
- Correlate with beta HCG

Pelvic kidney
- Reniform shape and corticomedullary differentiation are key

Peritoneal cysts
- Lack complex contents seen in teratomas

PATHOLOGY

General Features
- General path comments
  - 3 types of ovarian teratomas
    - Mature cystic teratoma (dermoid cyst)
    - Monodermal teratomas (struma ovarii, carcinoid tumors, neural tumors)
    - Immature teratomas (malignant teratoma)
  - Teratoma distribution
    - Sacrococcygeal (57%)
    - Gonadal (29%), ovarian > testicular
    - Mediastinal (7%)
    - Retroperitoneal (4%)
    - Cervical (3%)
    - Intracranial (3%)
  - Cells differentiate along various germ lines, essentially recapitulating any tissue of the body

TESTICULAR TORSION

- 80-100% if found in patients who present within 6 hours of pain
- Virtually 0% after 12 hours

CLINICAL ISSUES

Presentation
- Most common signs/symptoms
  - Acute scrotal and/or inguinal pain
  - Swollen, erythematous hemiscrotum without recognized trauma
  - Physical examination findings highly predictive of testicular torsion include
    - Elevation of affected testicle
    - Transverse position of testicle
    - Anterior rotation of epididymis
    - Absence of cremasteric reflex
    - Pain relief with successful manual de-torsion
  - In neonates, purple discoloration of swollen scrotum may indicate extravaginal testicular torsion
    - More common in high birth weight babies
    - Can be confused with scrotal hematoma due to birth trauma
- Other signs/symptoms
  - Nausea and vomiting are common
  - Low grade torsion may be tolerated for long periods
  - Almost half of patients have history of similar symptoms that resolved spontaneously
    - Indicating spontaneous torsion and detorsion
- Clinical Profile: Male child with acute scrotal pain

Demographics
- Age
  - Bimodal peak
    - 14 years
    - Neonates
- Gender: Males only
- Incidence of testicular torsion is increased in cold weather months: December and January

Natural History & Prognosis
- Surgical emergency: Testicular infarction if not treated promptly
- Testicular viability depends on
  - Degree of torsion, > 540° worse
  - Duration of symptoms
  - Time to surgical intervention
- Unilateral testicular loss typically does not lead to infertility problems

Treatment
- Surgical exploration; de-torsion; bilateral orchidopexy if viable testicle
  - Non-viable testicle usually removed; anti-sperm antibody theory
  - Higher risk of subsequent torsion on contralateral side justifies contralateral pexy
- Bilateral pexy is advocated in children with intermittent scrotal pain
  - Risk of testicular loss approaches 80% in patients with intermittent torsion
- Note that orchiopexy is not a guarantee against future torsion

DIAGNOSTIC CHECKLIST

Consider
- Pitfall of normal color Doppler flow in early or partial torsion; normal US does not exclude early torsion

Image Interpretation Pearls
- Decreased or absent flow on power and pulsed Doppler

SELECTED REFERENCES

1. Akin EA et al: Ultrasound of the scrotum. Ultrasound Q. 20(4):181-200, 2004
2. Ciftci AO et al: Clinical predictors for differential diagnosis of acute scrotum. Eur J Pediatr Surg. 14(5):333-8, 2004
3. Dogra VS et al: Torsion and beyond: new twists in spectral Doppler evaluation of the scrotum. J Ultrasound Med. 23(8):1077-85, 2004
4. Dogra V et al: Acute painful scrotum. Radiol Clin North Am. 42(2):349-63, 2004
5. Hormann M et al: Imaging of the scrotum in children. Eur Radiol. 14(6):974-83, 2004
6. Kalfa N et al: Ultrasonography of the spermatic cord in children with testicular torsion: impact on the surgical strategy. J Urol. 172(4 Pt 2):1692-5; discussion 1695, 2004
7. Kwong Y et al: A case of traumatic testicular torsion associated with a ruptured epididymis. Int J Urol. 11(5):349-51, 2004
8. Matsumoto A et al: Torsion of the hernia sac within a hydrocele of the scrotum in a child. Int J Urol. 11(9):789-91, 2004
9. Mernagh JR et al: Testicular torsion revisited. Curr Probl Diagn Radiol. 33(2):60-73, 2004
10. Sorensen MD et al: Prenatal bilateral extravaginal testicular torsion--a case presentation. Pediatr Surg Int. 20(11-12):892-3, 2004
11. Candocia FJ et al: An infant with testicular torsion in the inguinal canal. Pediatr Radiol. 33(10):722-4, 2003
12. Diamond DA et al: Neonatal scrotal haematoma: mimicker of neonatal testicular torsion. BJU Int. 91(7):675-7, 2003
13. Dogra VS et al: Sonography of the scrotum. Radiology. 227(1):18-36, 2003
14. Dogra V: Bell-clapper deformity. AJR Am J Roentgenol. 180(4):1176; author reply 1176-7, 2003
15. Kamaledeen S et al: Intermittent testicular pain: fix the testes. BJU Int. 91(4):406-8, 2003
16. Nelson CP et al: The cremasteric reflex: a useful but imperfect sign in testicular torsion. J Pediatr Surg. 38(8):1248-9, 2003
17. Sessions AE et al: Testicular torsion: direction, degree, duration and disinformation. J Urol. 169(2):663-5, 2003
18. Stehr M et al: Critical validation of colour Doppler ultrasound in diagnostics of acute scrotum in children. Eur J Pediatr Surg. 13(6):386-92, 2003
19. Traubici J et al: Original report. Testicular torsion in neonates and infants: sonographic features in 30 patients. AJR Am J Roentgenol. 180(4):1143-5, 2003
20. Williams CR et al: Testicular torsion: is there a seasonal predilection for occurrence? Urology. 61(3):638-41; discussion 641, 2003
21. Lrhorfi H et al: Trauma induced testicular torsion. J Urol. 168(6):2548, 2002
22. Kravchick S et al: Color Doppler sonography: its real role in the evaluation of children with highly suspected testicular torsion. Eur Radiol. 11(6):1000-5, 2001

TESTICULAR TORSION

IMAGE GALLERY

Typical

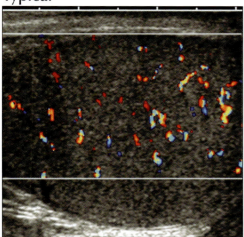
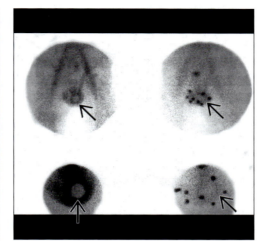

(Left) Color Doppler sonogram of false-negative study for torsion. Note preserved flow to the testis on longitudinal scan. At surgery, testicle was twisted 180° and was only minimally ischemic. *(Right)* Tc-99m pertechnetate scan shows pinhole images of scrotum without (left images) and with markers (right images) in a patient with left-sided "cold" testicle, indicating torsion (arrows).

Typical

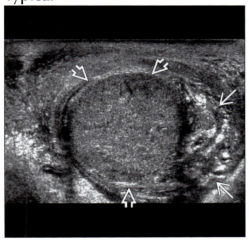
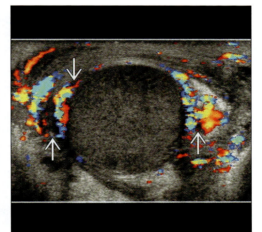

(Left) Transverse grayscale US image in testicular torsion. Note mildly hypoechoic and mildly heterogeneous echotexture of testis (open arrows) and thickened echogenic epididymis (arrows) due to torsion. *(Right)* Transverse color Doppler ultrasound shows peripheral, capsular blood-flow (arrows), but no intratesticular blood-flow. The peripheral blood-flow is supplied by inguinal and scrotal vessels which attempt to, but cannot restore, testicular perfusion.

Typical

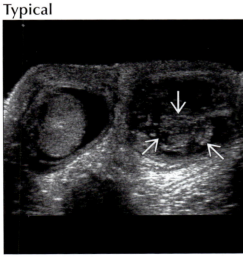
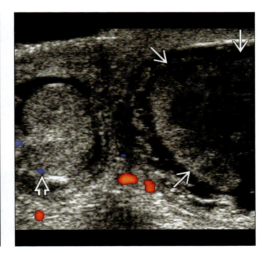

(Left) Transverse ultrasound shows side by side view of neonate with left side extra-vaginal torsion (arrows) which likely occurred in utero. Note that the left testicle is heterogeneous in echotexture due to necrosis. *(Right)* Transverse color Doppler ultrasound in the same patient shows marked size discrepancy and scant but normal blood-flow in the right testis (open arrow) and lack of blood-flow in the left testicle (arrows).

TORSION OF THE TESTICULAR APPENDAGE

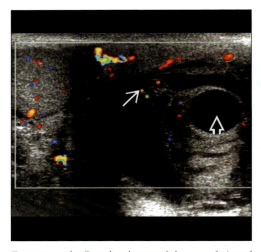

Transverse color Doppler ultrasound shows perfusion of an enlarged epididymal appendage (arrow) surrounded by hydrocele fluid and adjacent to an incidental epididymal cyst (open arrow).

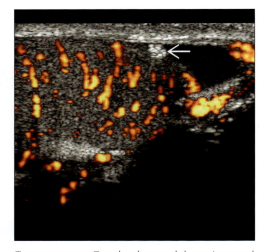

Transverse power Doppler ultrasound shows tiny round echogenic nodule (arrow) which is not perfused in this case of twisted testicular appendage. Note normal blood-flow within the adjacent testicle.

TERMINOLOGY

Abbreviations and Synonyms
- Twisted appendage, appendix testis torsion, torsion of the appendix epididymis, appendiceal torsion

Definitions
- Spontaneous twisting of one of the pedunculated vestigial remnants of tissue extending from the testicle or epididymis, which causes ischemia and pain
- The most common etiology of acute scrotal pain in pediatric patients
- Incidence exceeds epididymoorchitis and testicular torsion

IMAGING FINDINGS

General Features
- Best diagnostic clue
  - Ultrasound showing enlarged appendage, spherical shape and periappendiceal hyperemia
    - Reactive hydrocele is very common
    - Doppler findings can be variable
  - Imaging has higher sensitivity and specificity for diagnosing torsion of testicular or epididymal appendage than
    - Clinical signs alone
    - Imaging for testicular torsion or epididymoorchitis
- Location
  - Most common appendage to twist is testicular remnant of paramesonephric (Müllerian) duct
    - Located between the superior pole of the testis and the epididymis
  - The appendix epididymis is a remnant of the mesonephric (wolffian) duct
    - Most often seen projecting from head of epididymis
  - Other minor appendages of the testicle and epididymis exist, have variable location and may also twist
- Size
  - Appendage larger than 5.6 mm is diagnostic of torsion
    - Sensitivity of 68.2%, and specificity of 100% according to study by Baldisseratto et al
  - Normal appendix is usually tubular, pedunculated and 4 mm or smaller
- Morphology
  - Spherical shape and enlargement are most reliable indicators of appendiceal torsion
  - Echotexture is not predictive of torsion

Ultrasonographic Findings
- Grayscale Ultrasound

DDx: Other Inflammatory Processes

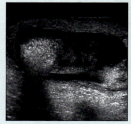
Epididymoorchitis

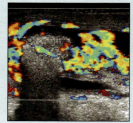
Epididymoorchitis

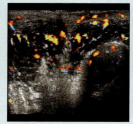
Scrotal Cellulitis

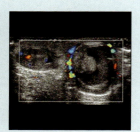
Testicular Torsion

TORSION OF THE TESTICULAR APPENDAGE

Key Facts

Terminology
- Spontaneous twisting of one of the pedunculated vestigial remnants of tissue extending from the testicle or epididymis, which causes ischemia and pain
- The most common etiology of acute scrotal pain in pediatric patients

Imaging Findings
- Ultrasound showing enlarged appendage, spherical shape and periappendiceal hyperemia
- Reactive hydrocele is very common
- Most common appendage to twist is testicular remnant of paramesonephric (Müllerian) duct
- Spherical shape suggests swelling; normally vermiform
- Best imaging tool: Ultrasound with Doppler

Top Differential Diagnoses
- Testicular torsion
- Epididymoorchitis or orchitis
- Scrotal cellulitis
- Complications of hernia
- Testicular tumor
- Testicular trauma

Clinical Issues
- "Blue dot" sign of ischemic appendage seen through the scrotal wall in minority of patients
- Self limited illness, excellent prognosis
- Pain usually resolves within a week
- Analgesics and anti-inflammatory agents for symptomatic relief

---

- ○ Size of appendix is best indicator of torsion, size > 5.6 mm
- ○ Spherical shape suggests swelling; normally vermiform
- ○ Reactive hydrocele common
  - ▪ Consider trauma or infection if debris is present in hydrocele fluid
- Color Doppler
  - ○ Actual appendage often too small to detect blood-flow within parenchyma
    - ▪ Worse in children who are uncooperative and in pain
  - ○ Periappendiceal hyperemia and normal testicular blood-flow are strong indicators of appendiceal torsion
- Power Doppler
  - ○ Useful in younger and uncooperative patients
    - ▪ By definition more sensitive in detecting low flow; directional information is lost

Nuclear Medicine Findings
- Tc-99m pertechnetate scan
  - ○ Scan shows normal testicular uptake, excluding the diagnosis of testicular torsion
  - ○ May show focal increased or decreased uptake in the region of the testicular head indicative of twisted appendix
    - ▪ Focal "hot" spot is equivalent to "blue dot" seen on physical exam
  - ○ Technique is same as for work-up of testicular torsion
    - ▪ Pinhole or low-energy high-resolution collimator
    - ▪ Scrotum supported on towels, penis secured up out of field-of-view
    - ▪ Dynamic acquisition during blood flow or perfusion phase
    - ▪ Static delayed imaging with and without markers
  - ○ Ultrasound is currently preferred over nuclear scanning

Other Modality Findings
- Occasionally incidentally recognized on (CT or MR) imaging performed to evaluate pelvic pain

- ○ May mimic intestinal appendicitis in young or non-verbal boys

Imaging Recommendations
- Best imaging tool: Ultrasound with Doppler
- Protocol advice
  - ○ High frequency linear transducer is best
  - ○ Thick layer of ultrasound gel decreases discomfort during scan
  - ○ Supporting the scrotum on towels and comparing to asymptomatic side are both helpful

DIFFERENTIAL DIAGNOSIS

Testicular torsion
- Doppler useful to show normal flow in adjacent testicle and confirm enlarged spherical appendage

Epididymoorchitis or orchitis
- Look for hyperemia in involved tissue on Doppler exam; global tenderness on physical exam

Scrotal cellulitis
- Imaging and physical findings more global than focal

Complications of hernia
- Incarcerated bowel or hernia sac torsion usually easily differentiated

Testicular tumor
- Look for focal intra-testicular mass

Testicular trauma
- Hematocele, irregular testicular contour, altered testicular echotexture or testicular disruption

PATHOLOGY

General Features
- Genetics: No predilection
- Etiology

TORSION OF THE TESTICULAR APPENDAGE

- Spontaneous twisting most common, occasionally associated with trauma or tumor
- Rising levels of estrogen and androgens early in puberty may account for appendiceal enlargement and predisposition to torsion in this age group
  - Testicular appendage contains variable numbers of both androgen and estrogen receptors
- Epidemiology
  - Incidence much higher than testicular torsion
  - Epididymoorchitis > > torsion of testicular appendage > testicular torsion
  - 1 in 2000 males
  - 80% of cases occur in children aged 7-14 years
- Associated abnormalities
  - The appendix testis contains Müllerian epithelium that theoretically may produce epithelial tumors similar to those that occur in the female genital tract
  - Rare case reports exist of tumors arising in scrotal appendages
    - Though some tumors (rhabdomyosarcoma) likely actually arise from stromal tissues rather than from testicular or epididymal appendages

Gross Pathologic & Surgical Features
- Inflamed, enlarged, ischemic, but otherwise histologically normal testicular or epididymal tissue

Microscopic Features
- Variable degrees of interstitial edema, hemorrhage, and necrosis

CLINICAL ISSUES

Presentation
- Most common signs/symptoms
  - Acute scrotal pain, swelling
  - Small, tender, mobile lump may be felt at the upper pole of the testis
  - "Blue dot" sign of ischemic appendage seen through the scrotal wall in minority of patients
- Other signs/symptoms
  - Torsion of testicular appendage is 2.5 times more commonly the cause of acute scrotum than testicular torsion
  - Metachronous and bilaterally synchronous appendiceal torsion have been reported

Demographics
- Age
  - Mean age 9 years
    - Compared to 14 years for testicular torsion and epididymoorchitis
- Gender: Males only

Natural History & Prognosis
- Self limited illness, excellent prognosis
- Pain usually resolves within a week
- Consider repeat imaging if symptoms persists
  - Rare case reports of secondary infection in infarcted, necrotic tissue

Treatment
- Analgesics and anti-inflammatory agents for symptomatic relief
- Antibiotics are not indicated in routine cases
- During exploratory surgery of acute scrotum, appendices are often removed

SELECTED REFERENCES

1. Baldisserotto M et al: Color Doppler sonography of normal and torsed testicular appendages in children. AJR Am J Roentgenol. 184(4):1287-92, 2005
2. Yang DM et al: Torsed appendix testis: gray scale and color Doppler sonographic findings compared with normal appendix testis. J Ultrasound Med. 24(1):87-91, 2005
3. Ciftci AO et al: Clinical predictors for differential diagnosis of acute scrotum. Eur J Pediatr Surg. 14(5):333-8, 2004
4. Adams BK et al: Tc-99m blood-pool imaging in torsion of an epididymal appendix. Clin Nucl Med. 28(6):526, 2003
5. Boardman J et al: Radiologic-pathologic conference of Keller Army Community Hospital at West Point, the United States Military Academy: torsion of the epiploic appendage. AJR Am J Roentgenol. 180(3):748, 2003
6. Sellars ME et al: Ultrasound appearances of the testicular appendages: pictorial review. Eur Radiol. 13(1):127-35, 2003
7. Samnakay N et al: Androgen and oestrogen receptor status of the human appendix testis. Pediatr Surg Int. 19(7):520-4, 2003
8. McAndrew HF et al: The incidence and investigation of acute scrotal problems in children. Pediatr Surg Int. 18(5-6):435-7, 2002
9. Baker LA et al: An analysis of clinical outcomes using color doppler testicular ultrasound for testicular torsion. Pediatrics. 105(3 Pt 1):604-7, 2000
10. Munden MM et al: Scrotal pathology in pediatrics with sonographic imaging. Curr Probl Diagn Radiol. 29(6):185-205, 2000
11. Johnson DB et al: Mullerian-type epithelial tumor arising within a torsed appendix testis. Urology. 54(3):561, 1999
12. Monga M et al: Metachronous bilateral torsion of the testicular appendices. Int J Urol. 6(11):589-91, 1999
13. Van Glabeke E et al: Acute scrotal pain in children: results of 543 surgical explorations. Pediatr Surg Int. 15(5-6):353-7, 1999
14. Kadish HA et al: A retrospective review of pediatric patients with epididymitis, testicular torsion, and torsion of testicular appendages. Pediatrics. 102(1 Pt 1):73-6, 1998
15. Noske HD et al: Historical milestones regarding torsion of the scrotal organs. J Urol. 159(1):13-6, 1998
16. Jefferson RH et al: Critical analysis of the clinical presentation of acute scrotum: a 9-year experience at a single institution. J Urol. 158(3 Pt 2):1198-200, 1997
17. Strauss S et al: Torsion of the testicular appendages: sonographic appearance. J Ultrasound Med. 16(3):189-92; quiz 193-4, 1997
18. Kwan DJ et al: Testicular microlithiasis in a child with torsion of the appendix testis. J Urol. 153(1):183-4, 1995
19. Yazbeck S et al: Accuracy of Doppler sonography in the evaluation of acute conditions of the scrotum in children. J Pediatr Surg. 29(9):1270-2, 1994
20. Atkinson GO Jr et al: The normal and abnormal scrotum in children: evaluation with color Doppler sonography. AJR Am J Roentgenol. 158(3):613-7, 1992
21. Middleton WD et al: Acute scrotal disorders: prospective comparison of color Doppler US and testicular scintigraphy. Radiology. 177(1):177-81, 1990

TORSION OF THE TESTICULAR APPENDAGE

IMAGE GALLERY

Typical

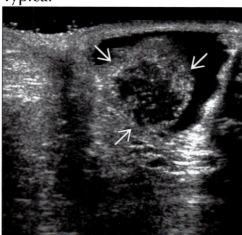
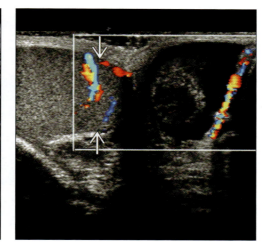

(Left) Transverse ultrasound shows heterogeneous echotexture area (arrows) in superior aspect of scrotum on the left side with surrounding anechoic hydrocele. Patient was exquisitely tender in this area. (Right) Transverse color Doppler ultrasound shows absence of perfusion in the same area, consistent with twisted epididymal appendage. Note that normal blood-flow is seen in contralateral testis (arrows).

Typical

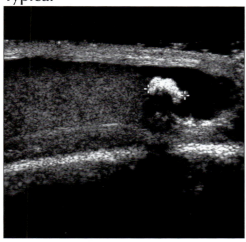
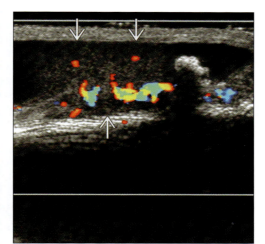

(Left) Sagittal ultrasound shows very echogenic, calcified testicular appendage between cursors, reflecting remote torsion. A small hydrocele is also present making the calcified appendix more visible. (Right) Sagittal color Doppler ultrasound Shows absent blood-flow in the echogenic, shadowing nodule and normal blood-flow in the adjacent testicle (arrows). Sometimes these twisted appendages auto-amputate and become free floating in the scrotum.

Typical

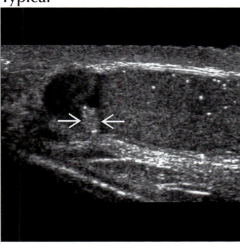
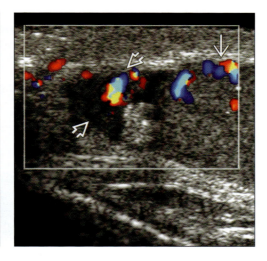

(Left) Sagittal ultrasound shows echogenic nodule (arrows) between the upper pole of the testicle and the epididymis in a patient with incidental testicular microlithiasis (punctate echogenic calcifications). (Right) Sagittal color Doppler ultrasound Shows absent blood-flow in the same area, consistent with a twisted testicular appendage. Note normal blood-flow in the adjacent epididymis (open arrows) and testicle (arrow).

PYELONEPHRITIS

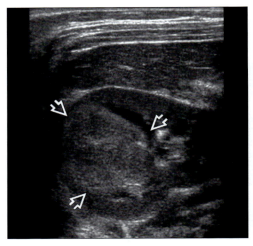

Axial ultrasound shows rounded area of altered echotexture in the lateral aspect of the right kidney.

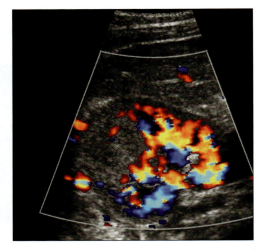

Axial color Doppler ultrasound shows decreased perfusion in the same area.

TERMINOLOGY

Abbreviations and Synonyms
- Acute lobar nephronia, focal bacterial nephritis

Definitions
- Acute infection of the renal parenchyma, often difficult to distinguish from lower urinary tract infection or cystitis
- Overview
  o Classic imaging appearance: Focal swelling and decreased perfusion of the affected parenchyma visible on nuclear scintigraphy, sonography, CT, MR, and IVP
  o Associated with vesicoureteral reflux in approximately 1/3 of cases
  o Permanent scarring more likely complication in children < 2 years old
  o Patients can have variable presentation: Fever, lethargy, irritability, vomiting, abdominal or flank pain, hematuria, or dysuria

IMAGING FINDINGS

General Features
- Best diagnostic clue
  o Marked inflammatory response to the infection causes swelling that effectively decreases radiographic contrast delivery to the site which results in
    - Photopenic area on nuclear cortical scans
    - Decreased perfusion on Doppler imaging and altered echotexture on grayscale ultrasound
    - Striated or wedge-shaped areas of decreased enhancement on CT or IVP
    - Decreased contrast-enhancement following gadolinium on MR
- Morphology: Areas of infection tend to be wedge-shaped, but when very inflamed can assume a more rounded, mass-like appearance

Radiographic Findings
- IVP: Striated nephrogram is classic, though IVPs are currently seldom performed in pediatric patients

CT Findings
- CECT
  o Wedge-shaped or round areas of poor enhancement
  o May have streaky enhancement
  o Inflammatory changes in perirenal fat is an secondary finding
  o Occasionally mass-like, may distort normal renal contour

DDx: Mimickers Of Pyelonephritis

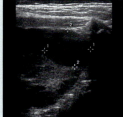
Nephroblastomatosis

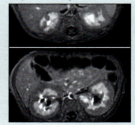
Nephroblastomatosis

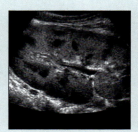
Lymphoma

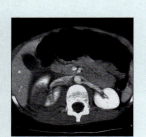
Fractured Kidney

PYELONEPHRITIS

Key Facts

Terminology
- Acute infection of the renal parenchyma, often difficult to distinguish from lower urinary tract infection or cystitis
- Classic imaging appearance: Focal swelling and decreased perfusion of the affected parenchyma visible on nuclear scintigraphy, sonography, CT, MR, and IVP
- Associated with vesicoureteral reflux in approximately 1/3 of cases
- Permanent scarring more likely complication in children < 2 years old
- Patients can have variable presentation: Fever, lethargy, irritability, vomiting, abdominal or flank pain, hematuria, or dysuria

Imaging Findings
- Wedge-shaped or round areas of poor enhancement
- Poor corticomedullary differentiation and focal areas of increased or decreased echogenicity
- Decreased perfusion is noted areas of pyelonephritis on color or power Doppler imaging
- Decreased accumulation of renal cortical agents, typically in a wedge-shaped distribution that points toward the renal hilum
- Ultrasound with Doppler is least invasive and readily available, though nuclear renal cortical scans, CT and MR are slightly more sensitive

Top Differential Diagnoses
- Renal infarction
- Renal scarring
- Renal mass

MR Findings
- T1WI: Often difficult to see on T1WI
- T2WI
  - Due to increased water content show high signal intensity in affected areas of renal parenchyma
  - May also see inflammatory changes in perirenal fat
- STIR
  - Inversion recovery series post gadolinium are reported to be best at detecting pyelonephritis and should be used when the MR exam is being tailored to this diagnosis
  - Areas of pyelonephritis typically show decreased signal on inversion recovery sequences post-gad
  - Inversion recovery sequence is often not included in abdominal MR scans performed for other indications; then T2 weighted series is most informative

Ultrasonographic Findings
- Grayscale Ultrasound
  - Localized or generalized swelling; unilateral renal enlargement may be the only clue to pyelonephritis
  - Poor corticomedullary differentiation and focal areas of increased or decreased echogenicity
  - Occasionally, rounded or mass-like areas of altered echotexture are noted
- Color Doppler
  - Decreased perfusion is noted areas of pyelonephritis on color or power Doppler imaging
  - Adding Doppler to the ultrasound exam significantly improves diagnostic accuracy and sensitivity

Nuclear Medicine Findings
- Nuclear Scintigraphic Findings
  - Decreased accumulation of renal cortical agents, typically in a wedge-shaped distribution that points toward the renal hilum
  - Findings persist for up to 6 weeks after the acute infection
  - Tc 99m DMSA or glucoheptonate are both used
  - Pinhole collimation and SPECT imaging improve diagnostic sensitivity and accuracy

Imaging Recommendations
- Best imaging tool
  - Ultrasound with Doppler is least invasive and readily available, though nuclear renal cortical scans, CT and MR are slightly more sensitive
  - Ultrasound is frequently performed to search for associated complications (abscess, stones, scarring), congenital anomalies, and hydronephrosis

DIFFERENTIAL DIAGNOSIS

Renal infarction
- The wedge-shaped pattern of decreased perfusion mimics ischemic injury, though the clinical symptoms of fever, leukocytosis, flank pain, and positive urine culture help to distinguish pyelonephritis

Renal scarring
- On nuclear scans, scarring tends to be more superficial while pyelonephritis extends deeply into parenchyma toward the hilum

Renal mass
- Acute pyelonephritis may present as a focal, mass-like swelling of the renal cortex
- Consider Wilm tumor, nephroblastomatosis, and lymphoma in these cases

PATHOLOGY

General Features
- General path comments
  - Patchy interstitial suppurative inflammation and tubular necrosis
  - Infection may occur via ascending route, vesicoureteral reflux, hematogenous spread, or related to instrumentation

RENAL INJURY

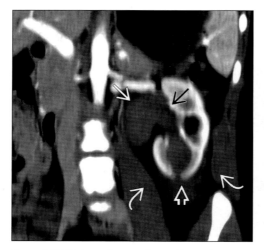

Coronal CECT shows lower pole renal laceration (open arrow) with perinephric blood or urine (curved arrows), and hematoma in collecting system (arrows) in 15 year old after car accident.

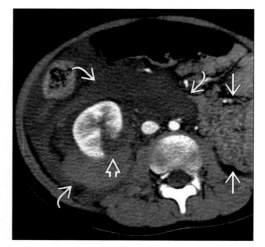

Axial CECT in 5 year old hemodynamically unstable child after bike accident with renal laceration (open arrow) and large perinephric hematoma (curved arrows). Note shock bowel (arrows).

TERMINOLOGY

Definitions
- Types
  - Hematoma
    - Intraparenchymal, subcapsular, perinephric, collecting system
  - Laceration
  - Vascular pedicle injury
  - Collecting system injury

IMAGING FINDINGS

General Features
- Best diagnostic clue: Renal parenchymal defect with perirenal hemorrhage +/- extravasation of urine or blood

CT Findings
- American Association for the Surgery of Trauma (AAST) Classification
- Grade 1
  - Normal imaging with hematuria
  - Intrarenal hematoma/contusion
    - Ill-defined/round/ovoid lesion
    - Parenchymal phase: ↓ Enhancement relative to normal kidney
    - Delayed phase: Hyperdense due to urine stasis + clot filled tubules
  - Nonexpanding subcapsular hematoma
    - Crescentic or elliptical collection (40-70 HU clotted blood) adjacent to renal parenchyma
    - Some deformity of underlying kidney when large
  - Subsegmental cortical infarct
    - Small/sharply demarcated/wedge-shaped ↓ attenuation area
- Grade 2
  - Nonexpanding perinephric hematomas confined to retroperitoneum
    - Ill-defined, often high density fluid between renal parenchyma and Gerota fascia
  - Superficial cortical lacerations < 1 cm in depth without collecting system injury
    - Small linear hypodense areas in periphery of renal cortex
    - May contain blood or clot: Higher attenuation than water, but no enhancement
    - No urinary contrast extravasation
- Grade 3
  - Renal lacerations > 1 cm in depth that do not involve collecting system
    - Linear hypodense area in renal cortex > 1 cm long
- Grade 4
  - Renal lacerations extending through kidney into collecting system

DDx: Pediatric Renal Mass

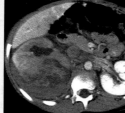
Wilm Hemorrhage

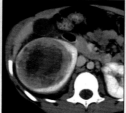
RCC

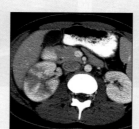
Pyelonephritis

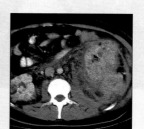
AML Hemorrhage

RENAL INJURY

Key Facts

Imaging Findings
- Best diagnostic clue: Renal parenchymal defect with perirenal hemorrhage +/- extravasation of urine or blood
- Best imaging tool: CECT sensitive and specific in detection and characterization of renal injury
- CECT: Image during late cortical phase or early homogeneous nephrographic phase (approximately 70 seconds) and excretory phase (> 3 minutes after contrast injection)
- Detects vascular injury and collecting system injury

Top Differential Diagnoses
- Pyelonephritis
- Wilm tumor
- Renal cell carcinoma (RCC)
- Angiomyolipoma (AML)

Pathology
- Children: Kidneys relatively large and mobile, thus vulnerable to trauma
- 8-10% of blunt/penetrating abdominal injuries have renal trauma
- 80-90% due to blunt injury rather than penetrating injury
- Severe renal injury usually associated with other abdominal injuries
- Increased risk for injury if have pre-existing renal abnormality

Clinical Issues
- Most common signs/symptoms: Flank pain, hematuria
- Nonoperative management in most renal injuries

- Parenchymal phase: Large/distracted renal fracture (hypodense)
- Excretory phase: Contrast extravasation into perinephric space
- ± Antegrade filling of ureter
- Injuries involving the main renal artery (RA) or renal vein (RV) with contained hemorrhage
  - RA: Nonenhancing wedge-shaped area or entire kidney
  - RV: Mass in renal vein/renal enlargement/delayed renal function
- Segmental renal infarctions without associated lacerations
  - Sharply demarcated, dorsal/ventral segmental wedge-shaped multifocal ↓ enhancement area
  - Due to thrombosis, dissection, or laceration of segmental arteries
- Grade 5
  - Shattered or devascularized kidney = extreme of multiple renal lacerations
    - Segmental infarction (devitalized upper/lower renal pole branch)
    - "Cortical rim" sign: Subacute finding in renal artery thrombosis: Preserved capsular/subcapsular enhancement
    - Global infarction + perinephric hematoma (avulsion of renal artery)
    - Hemoperitoneum (Morrison pouch)/displacement of major vessels
  - UPJ avulsions: Shearing injury at the renal pelvis as kidney pulls on relatively fixed ureter, renal artery and vein
    - Excretion of contrast + medial perinephric extravasation
    - A medial or circumferential urinoma may be seen around affected kidney
    - Partial tear: May see contrast in distal ureter on delayed imaging
  - Complete laceration or thrombus of main renal artery or vein
    - RA: Absent enhancement of kidney
    - RV: Mass in renal vein/renal enlargement/delayed renal function
- Vascular contrast extravasation
  - Early parenchymal phase: Bright enhancement close to the density of nearby arteries within a laceration or around an injured kidney
  - Pseudoaneurysm or contained hemorrhage: Fairly well-circumscribed

MR Findings
- May be used if contraindication for iodinated contrast or CT not available
- Use gadolinium to evaluate for renal injury and collecting system injury

Ultrasonographic Findings
- Grayscale Ultrasound: Insensitive in evaluation for renal trauma

Angiographic Findings
- DSA
  - Rarely used, because vascular injury can usually be assessed less invasively with CECT
  - May perform in conjunction with embolization in hemodynamically stable patients with renal injuries associated with ongoing hemorrhage or arteriovenous fistula or pseudoaneurysm
  - Venography: Rare, to assess renal vein or IVC injury

Non-Vascular Interventions
- Ureteral stent
- Pyelography: Assess ureter and collecting system

Nuclear Medicine Findings
- Renal scintigraphy
  - Occasionally used to evaluate for function of kidney in patients with contraindication to iodinated contrast or following repair of renovascular trauma

Other Modality Findings
- Intravenous urography (IVP) findings
  - Grade 1: Normal
  - Grade 2-5: Variable, delayed/absent excretion/extravasation

RENAL INJURY

Imaging Recommendations
- Best imaging tool: CECT sensitive and specific in detection and characterization of renal injury
- Protocol advice
  - CECT: Image during late cortical phase or early homogeneous nephrographic phase (approximately 70 seconds) and excretory phase (> 3 minutes after contrast injection)
    - Detects vascular injury and collecting system injury
- IVP: Limited urography (to evaluate hemodynamically unstable patient)
  - Obtain abdomen plain film; next administer 100-150 ml of 60% contrast IV; next, obtain "cone down" nephrogram film + full abdomen film after 8 min
  - "One-shot IVP": Used to assess normal kidney/not to evaluate injured kidney

DIFFERENTIAL DIAGNOSIS

Pediatric renal mass
- Pyelonephritis
  - Ill-defined low attenuation foci in kidneys
  - Costophrenic angle pain, fever, urinalysis usually abnormal
- Wilm tumor
  - Solid renal mass/most common renal tumor in children
  - May spontaneously hemorrhage/invade renal vein +/- IVC
- Renal cell carcinoma (RCC)
  - Less common solid renal mass
  - Imaging features similar to WIlm
- Angiomyolipoma (AML)
  - Usually contains fat, commonly associated with tuberous sclerosis
  - Prone to spontaneous hemorrhage when larger than 4 cm

PATHOLOGY

General Features
- Etiology
  - Blunt/penetrating/deceleration injuries
  - Children: Kidneys relatively large and mobile, thus vulnerable to trauma
- Epidemiology
  - 8-10% of blunt/penetrating abdominal injuries have renal trauma
    - 80-90% due to blunt injury rather than penetrating injury
    - 80% are grade 1
  - Severe renal injury usually associated with other abdominal injuries
  - Isolated renal injuries are usually minor
  - Increased risk for injury if have pre-existing renal abnormality
    - E.g. ectopic or horseshoe kidneys, hydronephrosis, extrarenal pelvis, ureteropelvic junction (UPJ) obstruction, renal tumor, renal cyst

Gross Pathologic & Surgical Features
- Contusion/laceration/hematoma/infarct/vascular or ureteropelvic injury

Microscopic Features
- Contusion/laceration/ischemia of corticomedullary or collecting system

CLINICAL ISSUES

Presentation
- Most common signs/symptoms: Flank pain, hematuria
- Other signs/symptoms: Shock, other abdominal trauma
- Complications
  - Early
    - Urinoma, perinephric abscess, sepsis, arteriovenous fistula, pseudoaneurysm
  - Late
    - Hydronephrosis
    - Hypertension ("Page kidney" = chronic compression of kidney by subcapsular hematoma → reactive hypertension)
    - Calculus formation
    - Chronic pyelonephritis

Treatment
- Nonoperative management in most renal injuries
  - As long as hemodynamically stable
- Active bleeding: Angioembolization
- Active urinary extravasation: Consider ureteral stent/catheter drainage
- Surgery frequently indicated in polytrauma patient in shock, shattered kidney, vascular pedicle injury
- If severe injury: Surgical nephrectomy

DIAGNOSTIC CHECKLIST

Consider
- Underlying renal tumor if hemorrhage out of proportion to injury

Image Interpretation Pearls
- Arterial extravasation usually requires catheter embolization to control bleeding
- Urinary extravasation may require ureteral stent +/- catheter drainage of urinoma

SELECTED REFERENCES
1. Smith JK et al: Imaging of renal trauma. Radiol Clin North Am. 41(5):1019-35, 2003
2. Titton RL et al: Urine leaks and urinomas: diagnosis and imaging-guided intervention. Radiographics. 23(5):1133-47, 2003
3. Harris AC et al: CT findings in blunt renal trauma. RadioGraphics. 21: S201-S214, 2001
4. Kawashima A et al: Imaging of renal trauma: A comprehensive review. RadioGraphics. 21: 557-574, 2001

RENAL INJURY

IMAGE GALLERY

Typical

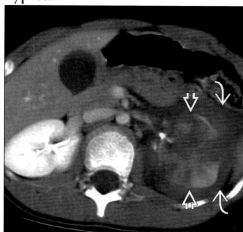
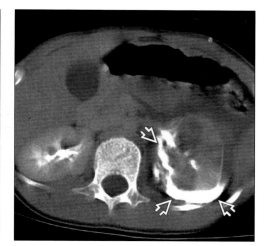

(Left) Axial CECT shows decreased enhancement and several wedge shaped areas of absent parenchymal enhancement (open arrows) with perinephric blood or urine (curved arrows). (Right) Axial CECT delayed imaging in same patient as left shows extravasation of urine into perinephric space (open arrows), suggesting laceration of renal pelvis.

Typical

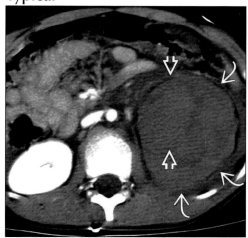
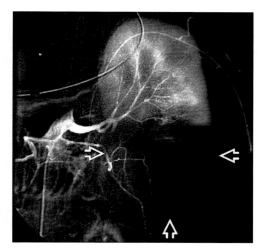

(Left) Axial CECT shows no enhancement of lower pole of left kidney (open arrows) and large perinephric hematoma (curved arrows), suggesting a laceration of segmental renal artery. (Right) Anteroposterior DSA in same unstable patient shows absent perfusion of lower pole of left kidney (open arrows), consistent with devascularization injury. No active extravasation.

Variant

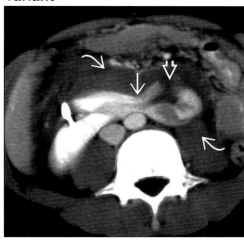
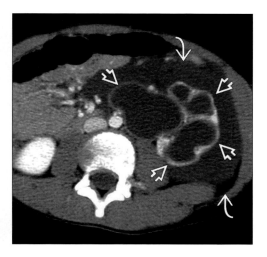

(Left) Axial CECT in 13 year old with horseshoe kidney and trauma shows laceration of the left kidney (open arrow) and perinephric blood or urine (curved arrows). Note renal isthmus (arrow). (Right) Axial CECT in child after 8 ft fall and left flank pain shows large perinephric urine or blood (curved arrows) around congenital UPJ obstruction (open arrows) with marked cortical thinning.

NEUROGENIC BLADDER

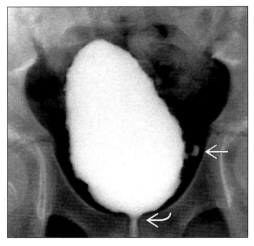

Anteroposterior voiding cystourethrogram in patient with NGB shows trabeculated, towering urinary bladder with a left diverticulum (arrow) and shows leakage into urethra (curved arrow).

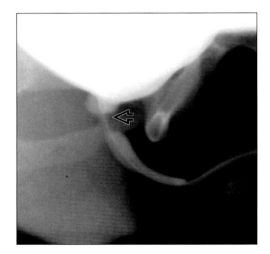

Oblique voiding cystourethrogram shows an incompetent bladder neck and contracted urethral sphincter (arrow) which intermittently relaxes, consistent with detrusor-sphincter dyssynergia.

TERMINOLOGY

Abbreviations and Synonyms
- Neurogenic bladder (NGB)

Definitions
- Malfunctioning bladder due to any type of neurologic disorder

IMAGING FINDINGS

General Features
- Best diagnostic clue: Towering, contracted, thickened or trabeculated bladder, that fills or empties poorly
- Location: Pelvis
- Size: Variable
- Morphology: Towering, trabeculated, thick urinary bladder

Radiographic Findings
- Radiography
  - Normal
  - Sacral anomalies
  - Spina bifida
  - Scoliosis
  - Obstipation

Fluoroscopic Findings
- Modified VCUG
  - Noncompliant bladder - high filling pressure, cessation of infusion flow at low filling volumes
    - Associated VUR
    - Deterioration of upper urinary tract
    - Impaired renal function
  - Leakage around the catheter
    - In relation to current filling volume (estimated bladder pressure)
  - Abrupt and intermittent cessation or reversal of flow - rise in filling pressure
  - Uninhibited detrusor contractions
    - Contrast flowing into posterior urethra stopped by reflex contraction external sphincter or static distal sphincter obstruction
- Three types bladder dysfunction
  - Contractile bladders (hyperreflexive detrusor)
    - Trabeculated, thick-walled bladder
    - Serrated mucosa
    - Prominent interureteric ridge
    - Uninhibited detrusor contraction, sudden bladder neck opening
    - Bulging posterior urethra up to contracted urethral sphincter - detrusor-sphincter dyssynergia (DSD)

DDx: Neurogenic Bladder

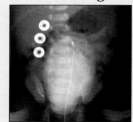
Myelomeningocele

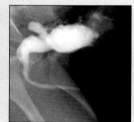
Post Urethral Valve

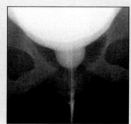
DSD

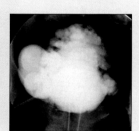
William Syndrome

NEUROGENIC BLADDER

Key Facts

Terminology
- Malfunctioning bladder due to any type of neurologic disorder

Imaging Findings
- Best diagnostic clue: Towering, contracted, thickened or trabeculated bladder, that fills or empties poorly
- Noncompliant bladder - high filling pressure, cessation of infusion flow at low filling volumes
- Leakage around the catheter
- Abrupt and intermittent cessation or reversal of flow - rise in filling pressure
- Uninhibited detrusor contractions
- Autonomic dysreflexia
- Best imaging tool: Modified voiding cystourethrogram

Clinical Issues
- Upper tract deterioration, UTI, and chronic renal failure related to increased bladder pressure
- Without intervention 50% upper urinary tract deterioration in first 5 years of life
- Preservation of renal function
- Avoidance of UTI
- Achieve appliance-free, social continence

Diagnostic Checklist
- Extraurinary findings in patients with clinical suspicion of NGB
- During VCUG
- Monitor contrast flow
- Evaluate bladder contour, sphincter function, bladder filling volume, and degree of emptying

---

- Functional obstruction; deterioration of upper tracts
  - Intermediate bladders
    - Bladder necks closed at early filling
    - Bladder neck opens with increasing volume and bladder pressure
    - No bulging posterior urethra; funnel-like
    - Any descent of bladder neck in boys or mild descent girls - denervation of striated sphincter
  - Acontractile bladders (detrusor areflexia)
    - No signs of radiologically detectable detrusor contractions
    - Bladder neck incontinence, open during entire filling phase
    - Sphincter weakness incontinence - leakage of contrast around catheter, especially during coughing
- Secondary bladder & upper tract abnormalities
  - Trabeculation, pseudodiverticula, dilated upper tracts
  - DSD vs. functional infravesical obstruction
  - VUR in 20-25% cases
- Autonomic dysreflexia
  - During bladder distention in cystography, or during urethral catheterization
  - Spinal lesions above T5
  - Life threatening condition
  - Hypertension, anxiety, sweating, piloerection, headaches, bradycardia
  - Treatment: Evacuate bladder and catheter, elevate head of table, monitor blood pressure, pharmacologic intervention if necessary

Ultrasonographic Findings
- Grayscale Ultrasound
  - Small contracted/large atonic bladder; +/- wall thickening; increased post-void residual
  - Diverticula, pseudodiverticula
  - Urinary tract dilation, unilateral or bilateral

Imaging Recommendations
- Best imaging tool: Modified voiding cystourethrogram
- Protocol advice

- Renal and bladder sonography: Follow-up every 6 months
- Modified voiding cystourethrography: Follow-up yearly
- +/- Videourodynamics (if available)

DIFFERENTIAL DIAGNOSIS

Myelodysplasia
- Detrusor hyperreflexia (early) → areflexia (chronic)
- Relieve obstruction → ↑ function, but never normal

Posterior urethral valves
- Severity of bladder findings dependent on the presence of VUR
  - The higher grade of reflux, the more severe the bladder findings

Detrusor-sphincter dyssynergia
- Usually associated with neurologic spinal lesion
- Dilated posterior urethra to level of contracted urethral sphincter
- No posterior urethral valve on VCUG

Pelvic mass
- Ovarian, vaginal or prostatic rhabdomyosarcoma, sacral teratoma
- No trabeculation; features do not change with voiding

Multiple diverticula
- William syndrome
- Menkes kinky hair syndrome
- Cutis laxa or Ehlers-Danlos

PATHOLOGY

General Features
- Etiology
  - Myelodysplasia
  - Sacral agenesis
  - Cerebral palsy
  - Traumatic spinal cord lesions

NEUROGENIC BLADDER

- Associated abnormalities
  - Myelodysplasia (80-90%)
  - Lipomeningocele
  - Sacral agenesis
  - Occult congenital spinal dysraphisms
  - Cerebral palsy
  - Traumatic causes (rare)

Staging, Grading or Classification Criteria
- Level of neurologic disorder
  - Upper motor neuron lesion (UMNL)
  - Lower motor neuron lesion (LMNL)
- Bladder function
  - Inability to store urine properly
  - Inability to evacuate urine properly
  - Reflexive activity of the detrusor
    - Contractile detrusor (detrusor hyperreflexia) - UMNL
    - Acontractile detrusor (detrusor areflexia) - LMNL
    - Intermediate detrusor (mixed type)

CLINICAL ISSUES

Presentation
- Most common signs/symptoms
  - Failure to empty bladder
  - Frequency, nocturia, urgency, retention, incontinence
  - Urinary tract infection (UTI)
  - Bladder stones
- Other signs/symptoms
  - Detrusor underactivity to overactivity, depending on the site of neurologic insult
  - Sphincter underactivity or overactivity and loss of coordination with bladder function
  - Hyper- or hyporeflexia; impaired or no sensation

Demographics
- Age: Neonatal to adolescence
- Gender: Both

Natural History & Prognosis
- Complications
  - Pyelonephritis
  - Hydronephrosis
  - Urolithiasis
  - Sexual dysfunction
  - Autonomic dysreflexia
- Upper tract deterioration, UTI, and chronic renal failure related to increased bladder pressure
- Without intervention 50% upper urinary tract deterioration in first 5 years of life
- Predictive indicators for deterioration
  - Detrusor-sphincter dyssynergia
  - High bladder-filling pressure
  - Poor bladder compliance
  - High leak-point pressure
  - VUR

Treatment
- Treatment goals
  - Preservation of renal function
  - Avoidance of UTI
  - Achieve appliance-free, social continence
- Therapeutic maneuvers to achieve goals
  - Clean intermittent catheterization
  - Medications
  - Surgical procedures
    - Operation for continence
    - Bladder augmentation
    - Artificial sphincters
- Hyperreflexia
  - ↑ Volume: Cystoplasty, muscular or fascial slings, parasympatholytic drugs, botulinum-a toxin
  - ↑ Voiding: Catheter, transurethral sphincterotomy
- Hyporeflexia
  - Bladder training, catheter, bladder neck resection/denervation, parasympathomimetic drugs

DIAGNOSTIC CHECKLIST

Consider
- Extraurinary findings in patients with clinical suspicion of NGB

Image Interpretation Pearls
- During VCUG
  - Monitor contrast flow
  - Evaluate bladder contour, sphincter function, bladder filling volume, and degree of emptying

SELECTED REFERENCES

1. Lebowitz RL: Paediatric urology and uroradiology: changes in the last 25 years. BJU Int. 92 Suppl 1:7-9, 2003
2. Campioni P et al: The neurogenic bladder: anatomy and neurophysiology. Rays. 27(2):107-14, 2002
3. Campioni P et al: Diagnostic imaging of neurogenic bladder. Rays. 27(2):121-5, 2002
4. Madersbacher H: Neurogenic bladder dysfunction in patients with myelomeningocele. Curr Opin Urol. 12(6):469-72, 2002
5. Salvaggio E et al: Clinical patterns of neurogenic bladder. Rays. 27(2):115-20, 2002
6. Nijman RJ: Neurogenic and non-neurogenic bladder dysfunction. Curr Opin Urol. 11(6):577-83, 2001
7. van Gool JD et al: Bladder-sphincter dysfunction in myelomeningocele. Eur J Pediatr. 160(7):414-20, 2001
8. Bankhead RW et al: Evaluation and treatment of children with neurogenic bladders. J Child Neurol. 15(3):141-9, 2000
9. Agarwal SK et al: Neurogenic bladder. Indian J Pediatr. 64(3):313-26, 1997
10. Jayanthi VR et al: The nonneurogenic neurogenic bladder of early infancy. J Urol. 158(3 Pt 2):1281-5, 1997
11. Fotter R: Neurogenic bladder in infants and children--a new challenge for the radiologist. Abdom Imaging. 21(6):534-40, 1996
12. Fernbach SK et al: Abnormalities of the bladder in children: imaging findings. AJR Am J Roentgenol. 162(5):1143-50, 1994
13. Zawin JK et al: Neurogenic dysfunction of the bladder in infants and children: Recent advances and the role of radiology. Radiology. 182: 297, 1992
14. Ruutu M et al: The value of urethrocystography in the investigation of patients with spinal cord injury. Clinical Radiology. 35: 485-9, 1984

NEUROGENIC BLADDER

IMAGE GALLERY

Variant

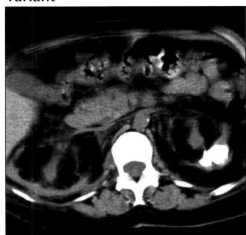
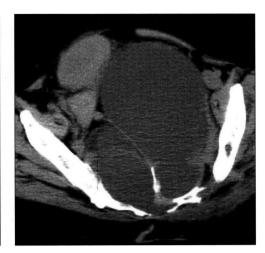

(Left) Axial NECT in an older patient with neurogenic bladder shows bilateral renal cortical atrophy and parenchymal calcification due to chronic reflux. *(Right)* Axial CECT shows distended neurogenic bladder and anterior meningocele in a patient with spina bifida and abnormal sacrum, findings seen in patients with Currarino triad.

Typical

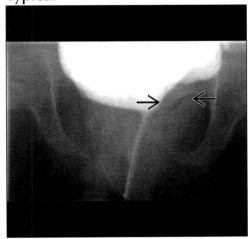
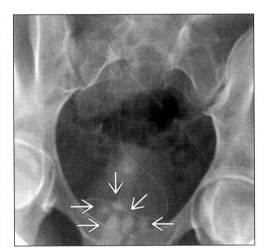

(Left) Anteroposterior voiding cystourethrogram in a patient with spina bifida shows a distended neurogenic bladder with an open bladder neck (arrows). *(Right)* Anteroposterior voiding cystourethrogram scout image shows several radiopaque bladder stones (arrows) not present on the prior VCUG one year previously; catheter was placed via Mitrofanoff.

Variant

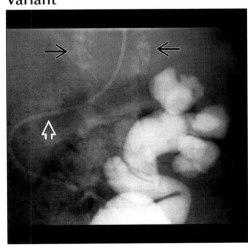
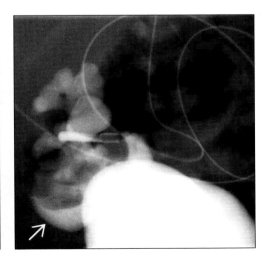

(Left) Anteroposterior voiding cystourethrogram in myelomeningocele patient shows left grade 5 VUR, spinal dysraphism (arrows), ventriculoperitoneal shunt (open arrow), and stool-filled colon. *(Right)* Anteroposterior voiding cystourethrogram shows forniceal rupture (arrow) in 2 week old male with recent myelomeningocele repair who had study performed to evaluate for signs of NGB.

BLADDER DIVERTICULA

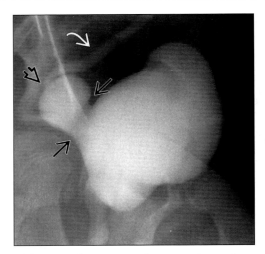

Oblique voiding cystourethrogram shows large, wide-mouthed bladder diverticulum (arrows) which has incorporated the right UVJ (open arrow), resulting in right VUR (curved arrow).

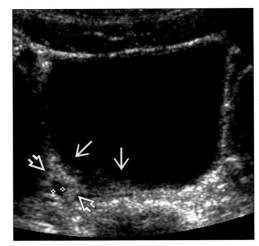

Transverse ultrasound of case at left shows probable diverticulum inverted into the bladder (arrows) with mild ureteral dilation (cursors) and focal bladder wall thickening (open arrows).

TERMINOLOGY

Abbreviations and Synonyms
- Bladder diverticulum (one), bladder diverticula (many), Hutch diverticulum, tic

Definitions
- Protrusion of mucosa through defect in muscular wall of urinary bladder
- Hutch diverticulum: In periureteral location

IMAGING FINDINGS

General Features
- Best diagnostic clue: Contained outpouching of contrast from urinary bladder on voiding cystourethrography (VCUG)
- Location: Most commonly near ureteral orifice of urinary bladder
- Size: Variable, most small
- Morphology: Round outpouching with variable size neck

Radiographic Findings
- Radiography
  - +/- Radiopaque urinary stone within diverticulum
  - +/- Air in diverticulum if catheterized

Fluoroscopic Findings
- Voiding Cystourethrogram
  - Round outpouching of contrast through bladder wall
  - Neck of diverticulum (image tangential to bladder)
  - Variable degrees of size and filling during contrast filling and voiding
    - Sometimes only fills during voiding
    - Volume sometimes bigger than bladder
  - Vesicoureteral reflux
    - Usually caused by larger diverticula
    - As diverticulum enlarges, can incorporate and distort ureteral tunnel, resultant reflux
    - Oblique patient to capture image of ureteral insertion into diverticulum
  - Multiple diverticula
    - William syndrome (WS): Supravalvular aortic stenosis
    - Menkes kinky hair syndrome (MKHS): Osteoporosis
    - Cutis laxa (CL), Ehlers-Danlos (ED): Ligamentous laxity

CT Findings
- Protrusion of mucosa outside bladder
- Rectovesical space cystic mass that connects to bladder

DDx: Diverticula Look-A-Likes

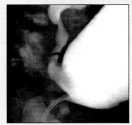

Everting Ureterocele

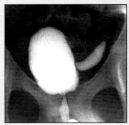

Ureteral Stump

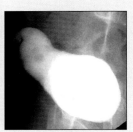

Urachal Diverticulum

BLADDER DIVERTICULA

Key Facts

Terminology
- Protrusion of mucosa through defect in muscular wall of urinary bladder

Imaging Findings
- Best diagnostic clue: Contained outpouching of contrast from urinary bladder on voiding cystourethrography (VCUG)
- Variable degrees of size and filling during contrast filling and voiding
- Vesicoureteral reflux
- Rectovesical space cystic mass that connects to bladder
- Best imaging tool: Fluoroscopic VCUG

Pathology
- Congenital (most) - weakness in bladder wall
- Acquired - bladder outlet obstruction
- Iatrogenic

Clinical Issues
- Asymptomatic
- Urinary tract infection
- Most found incidentally and are asymptomatic
- Complications of diverticula reflect location and size
- Stagnant urine
- Deform ureterovesical junction (UVJ)
- Urethral obstruction - large diverticula

Diagnostic Checklist
- Mimickers of diverticula
- Everting ureterocele
- Ureteral stump more likely if
- Post-operative defect

Ultrasonographic Findings
- Normal
  - Diverticula may be invisible
    - Decompressed just outside bladder wall
    - Within the bladder wall
    - Just inside bladder wall
- Anechoic, roundish fluid collection that may or may not connect to bladder
  - +/- Shadowing calculus
- Focal bladder wall thickening adjacent to ureteral orifice
- Intravesical hypoechoic echogenicity mimicking debris in periureteral location
- Ureteral dilation if ipsilateral VUR

Imaging Recommendations
- Best imaging tool: Fluoroscopic VCUG
- Protocol advice
  - Bladder sonography including kidneys
    - Scan with full bladder
    - Are kidneys duplex?
  - Fluoroscopic VCUG
    - Diverticulum may only fill during voiding
    - Diverticulum may only be seen on post-void image
    - Image the neck of diverticulum
    - If VUR, document site of ureteral insertion in relation to diverticulum
    - Document drainage pattern of diverticulum
  - If nonspecific cystic mass seen incidentally on CT and diverticulum suspected
    - Consider bladder sonography
    - VCUG

DIFFERENTIAL DIAGNOSIS

Everting ureterocele
- Everting ureterocele almost always associated with lower pole VUR
- Hutch diverticulum almost always associated with single system VUR

Ureteral stump
- Often associated with ipsilateral multicystic dysplastic kidney
- Not uncommonly seen in ipsilateral ureter after nephrectomy

Urachal diverticulum
- Located at bladder dome pointing toward umbilicus

PATHOLOGY

General Features
- Genetics
  - Chromosomal links for diverticula associated with syndromes
    - WS: WS critical region: ELN, LIMK1, and GTF2I
    - MKHS : Long arm of the X chromosome at Xq13.3
    - CL: Four genetic forms: Sex-linked, autosomal dominant, and two types of autosomal recessive inheritance
    - ED: Multiple forms of inheritance
- Etiology
  - Congenital (most) - weakness in bladder wall
    - Hutch diverticulum - 50% with VUR
    - Urachal diverticulum
    - Other locations in bladder
  - Acquired - bladder outlet obstruction
    - Posterior urethral valves (PUV)
    - Neurogenic bladder - urethral sphincter (commonly myelomeningocele)
  - Iatrogenic
    - Post-ureteral reimplantation
    - Suprapubic catheter placement
    - Repair of rectovesical fistulae (anorectal malformation)
    - Ureterocele remnant
- Associated abnormalities
  - William syndrome
    - Supravalvular aortic stenosis
    - Hypercalcemia
    - Elfin facies

BLADDER DIVERTICULA

- MKHS
  - X-linked recessive disorder; dysfunction in numerous copper-dependent enzyme systems
  - Structural changes in hair, brain, bones, liver, bladder, arteries, etc.
  - Poor prognosis despite treatment
- Cutis laxa (CL, elastolysis), Ehlers-Danlos (ED)
  - Connective tissue disorders
  - CL: Alterations in the quantity or the morphology of elastin
  - ED: Group of inherited connective-tissue disorders of abnormal collagen structure and function; joint hypermobility, cutaneous fragility, and hyperextensibility
  - Overlapping manifestations - copper metabolism involved in forms of both and MKHS
- Prune belly syndrome (Eagle-Barrett)
  - Mesodermal arrest?
  - Lack abdominal wall musculature
  - Functional bladder outlet obstruction - upper tract dilation

Gross Pathologic & Surgical Features
- Larger diverticula may require extravesical or intravesical approach
- Laparoscopic approach becoming popular

Microscopic Features
- Transitional epithelium

CLINICAL ISSUES

Presentation
- Most common signs/symptoms
  - Asymptomatic
  - Urinary tract infection

Demographics
- Age: Infant to adolescent
- Gender: Both

Natural History & Prognosis
- Most found incidentally and are asymptomatic
- Complications of diverticula reflect location and size
  - Stagnant urine
    - Infection
    - Bleeding
    - Stone formation
  - Deform ureterovesical junction (UVJ)
    - VUR
    - Ureteral obstruction
  - Urethral obstruction - large diverticula

Treatment
- Indications for operative treatment
  - Persistent infection
  - Stone formation
  - Ureteral or urethral obstruction
- 3 surgical approaches
  - Intravesical, extravesical, transurethral
  - Laparoscopic (intra- or extra- vesical)

DIAGNOSTIC CHECKLIST

Consider
- Mimickers of diverticula
  - Everting ureterocele
    - Duplex appearance of the ipsilateral kidney on US
    - Ipsilateral lower pole reflux (axis of kidney toward ipsilateral shoulder)
  - Ureteral stump more likely if
    - History of ipsilateral nephrectomy
    - Ipsilateral multicystic dysplastic kidney
    - Ipsilateral kidney absent on renal sonogram
  - Post-operative defect
    - Check for surgical history
  - Urachal diverticulum
    - Location at dome of bladder

SELECTED REFERENCES

1. Shukla AR et al: Giant bladder diverticula causing bladder outlet obstruction in children. J Urol. 172(5 Pt 1):1977-9, 2004
2. Campioni P et al: The neurogenic bladder: anatomy and neurophysiology. Rays. 27(2):107-14, 2002
3. Kok KY et al: Laparoscopic excision of congenital bladder diverticulum in a child. Surg Endosc. 14(5):501, 2000
4. Pieretti RV et al: Congenital bladder diverticula in children. J Pediatr Surg. 34(3):468-73, 1999
5. Oshio T et al: Urologic abnormalities in Menkes' kinky hair disease: report of three cases. J Pediatr Surg. 32(5):782-4, 1997
6. Maynor CH et al: Urinary bladder diverticula: sonographic diagnosis and interpretive pitfalls. J Ultrasound Med. 15(3):189-94, 1996
7. Schulman SL et al: Increased prevalence of urinary symptoms and voiding dysfunction in Williams syndrome. J Pediatr. 129(3):466-9, 1996
8. Bellah RD et al: Ureterocele eversion with vesicoureteral reflux in duplex kidneys: findings at voiding cystourethrography. AJR Am J Roentgenol. 165(2):409-13, 1995
9. Blane CE et al: Bladder diverticula in children. Radiology. 190(3):695-7, 1994
10. Vates TS et al: Acute urinary retention in an infant: an unusual presentation of a paraureteral diverticulum. Pediatr Radiol. 23(5):371-2, 1993
11. Ozguven M et al: Visualization of bladder diverticulum during Tc-99m DTPA renal scintigraphy. Ann Nucl Med. 6(3):195-8, 1992
12. Levard G et al: Urinary bladder diverticula and the Ehlers-Danlos syndrome in children. J Pediatr Surg. 24(11):1184-6, 1989
13. Bellinger MF et al: Bladder diverticulum associated with ureteral obstruction. Pediatr Radiol. 15(3):207-8, 1985
14. Hernanz-Schulman M et al: The elusiveness and importance of bladder diverticula in children. Pediatr Radiol. 15(6):399-402, 1985
15. Verghese M et al: Urinary retention secondary to congenital bladder diverticula in infants. J Urol. 132(6):1186-8, 1984
16. Blacklock AR et al: The treatment of large bladder diverticula. Br J Urol. 55(1):17-20, 1983
17. Lebowitz RL et al: Neonatal hydronephrosis caused by vesical diverticula. Urology. 13(3):335-41, 1979
18. Stephens FD: The vesicoureteral hiatus and paraureteral diverticula. J Urol. 121(6):786-91, 1979
19. Boechat MI et al: Diverticula of the bladder in children. Pediatr Radiol. 7(1):22-8, 1978

BLADDER DIVERTICULA

IMAGE GALLERY

Typical

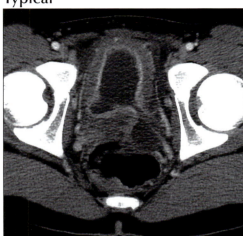
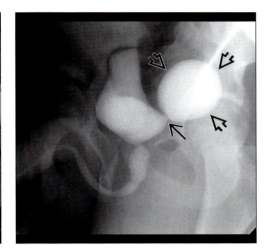

(Left) Axial CECT performed for pain/fever in a teen boy shows cystic mass in the rectovesical space with connection to the bladder; considerations included bladder diverticulum and VCUG performed. (Right) Oblique voiding cystourethrogram shows large left bladder diverticulum (open arrows) with well defined neck (arrow) that filled with bladder filling and enlarged readily with voiding.

Typical

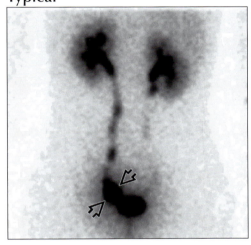
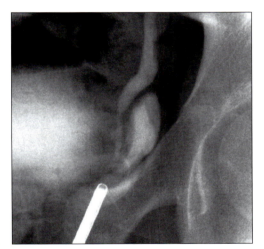

(Left) Posterior anterior view from MAG3 renal scan of the same patient as above shows collection of radiopharmaceutical (arrows) near the left UVJ corresponding to the periureteral diverticulum. (Right) Oblique cystoscopic contrast injection of diverticulum and ureter shows close proximity of diverticulum to the left ureteral orifice; tic enlargement increases risk of ureteral obstruction.

Variant

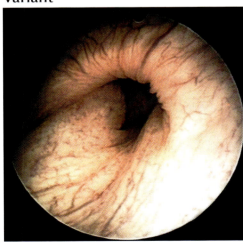
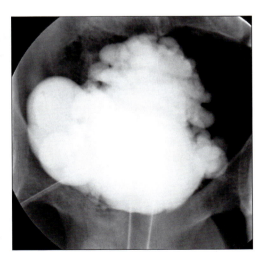

(Left) Intra-operative photograph at cystoscopy showing the diverticulum from inside the bladder; the neck is gaping, not unexpected after seeing immediate filling of diverticulum at VCUG (above). (Right) Anteroposterior voiding cystourethrogram shows multiple diverticula, too numerous to count, throughout the urinary bladder in this patient with William syndrome.

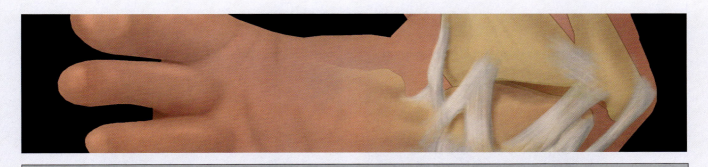

SECTION 6: Musculoskeletal

Introduction and Overview
Musculoskeletal   6-2

Trauma
Physeal Fractures   6-6
Child Abuse, Metaphyseal Fracture   6-10
Incomplete Fractures   6-14
Stress Fracture   6-18
Supracondylar Fracture   6-22
Toddler's Fractures   6-26
Medial Epicondyle Avulsion   6-30
Osgood-Schlatter Lesion   6-34
Chronic Foreign Body   6-38

Infection
Osteomyelitis   6-42
Syphilis, Musculoskeletal   6-46

Soft Tissue Masses
Infantile Hemangioma, Musculoskeletal   6-50
Venous Malformations   6-54
Lymphatic Malformation   6-58
Arteriovenous Malformation   6-62
Aggressive Fibromatosis   6-66
Rhabdomyosarcoma, Musculoskeletal   6-70

Focal Bone Lesions
Ewing Sarcoma   6-74
Osteosarcoma   6-78
Leukemia, Musculoskeletal   6-82
Langerhans Cell Histiocytosis   6-86
Fibroxanthoma   6-90
Osteoid Osteoma   6-94

Abnormalities of the Hip
Developmental Dysplasia of the Hip   6-98
Proximal Focal Femoral Deficiency   6-102
Legg-Calve-Perthes Disease   6-106
Slipped Capital Femoral Epiphysis   6-110

Constitutional Disorders of Bone
Achondroplasia   6-114
Mucopolysaccharidoses (MPS)   6-118
Osteogenesis Imperfecta (OI)   6-122
Osteopetrosis   6-126

Autoimmune Diseases
Juvenile Rheumatoid Arthritis   6-130
Dermatomyositis   6-134

Other Congenital Lesions
Club Foot (Talipes Equinovarus)   6-138
VACRERL Association   6-142
Tarsal Coalition   6-146
Discoid Meniscus   6-150

Miscellaneous
Distal Femoral Metaphyseal Irregularity   6-154
Rickets   6-158
Fibromatosis Colli   6-162
Osteochondritis Dissecans   6-166
Sickle Cell Anemia, Bone   6-170
Scoliosis   6-174
Spondylolysis   6-178

MUSCULOSKELETAL

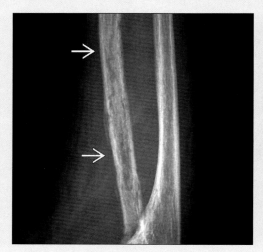

Anteroposterior radiograph shows an aggressive permeative destructive lesion of the radius (arrows), osteomyelitis.

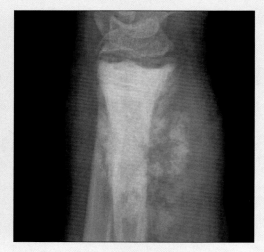

Lateral radiograph shows a large sclerotic distal radial mass with cloud-like matrix in this patient with osteosarcoma.

Normal Variants

Physiologic Periosteal Reaction
- 1-6 months old during periods of rapid growth
- Femur, tibia, humerus, tends to be symmetric
- When asymmetric may need to differentiate from infection or tumor

Dense Metaphyseal Bands
- Dense thickened white line on radiographs along zone of provisional calcification, 2-6 years old
- When proximal fibula involved also consider heavy metal poisoning, especially lead

Ischiopubic Synchondrosis
- Irregular, expanded or ballooned ischiopubic synchondrosis, asymmetric
- May mimic an osseous neoplasm or infection
  - May need MR if high clinical concern

Pseudoepiphysis
- False ossification center, no physis separation from diaphysis
- Typically proximal aspect of 2nd → 5th metacarpals, distal 1st metacarpal
- Associated with hypothyroidism & cleidocranial dysostosis

Fibroxanthoma
- Nonossifying fibroma, benign cortical defect
- Eccentric lucent lesion with sclerotic margin, most commonly distal femur
- MR: Mixed hypointense on T2WI due to hemosiderin or fibrous components
- Multiple: Neurofibromatosis (NF), Jaffe-Campanacci syndrome

Distal Femoral Irregularity
- Lateral > medial femoral condyle, typical: Posterior location
- MR sometimes needed to differentiate from infection or osteochondritis dissecans (OCD)
  - Abnormal cartilage or hyperintense T2WI adjacent marrow signal

Avulsive Cortical Irregularity
- Posterior medial femoral condyle in 10-15 year olds
- Medial head of gastrocnemius origin

Bone Marrow

Occurs In Ordered Pattern
- Hematopoietic → fatty marrow
- Distal → proximal
  - Toes & fingers → hips & shoulders
  - Axial skeleton may occur in adulthood
- Epiphysis → diaphysis → metaphysis
  - Once epiphyseal ossification center appears radiographically, typically fatty replaced by 6 months
  - Proximal humeral or femoral metaphye contain hematopoietic marrow into adulthood
- Predicts disease location
  - Hematopoietic marrow is richly vascularized
    - Metastatic disease, leukemia, infection
  - Fatty marrow less vascularized
    - Bone infarcts or avascular necrosis

Elbow Ossification

Mnemonic For Ossification Center Radiographic Appearance: CRITOE
- Capitellum → Radial head → Internal epicondyle (medial epicondyle) → Trochlea → Olecranon → External epicondyle (lateral epicondyle)

Should Not See Trochlea Without Medial Epicondyle
- Think displaced or entrapped medial epicondyle

Irregular Trochlea Ossification
- Normal variant

MUSCULOSKELETAL

Key Information

CRITOE For Elbow Ossification Appearance
- Trochlear ossification on radiographs without finding medial epicondyle think displaced or entrapped fragment
- Trochlear ossification can be irregular or fragmented

Soft Tissue Masses
- Some masses can be diagnosed with ultrasound
  - Popliteal cyst, ganglion cyst, some vascular malformations, lymph nodes, fibromatosis colli
- Other masses should be evaluated initially with radiographs followed by MR to direct diagnosis & therapy
  - Try placing the mass into either determinate or indeterminate categories by radiographic & MR appearance

Common Malignant Soft Tissue Masses
- By far RMS is the most common
- Extremity RMS is most commonly alveolar subtype, lymph node (+), older age, more often distant metastasis at presentation, thus the poorest prognosis
- Remember some soft tissues sarcomas appear nonaggressive by MR but are highly malignant

Don't Skip The Metastasis
- Large FOV in searching for skip marrow lesions in primary osseous malignancies
- Joint to joint imaging
- Followed by small FOV of the osseous lesion to assess resectability for limb sparing surgery

---

Capitellar Ossification Should Be Smooth
- Irregular: Think Panner disease, OCD or infection

How To Work-Up A Soft Tissue Mass

A Few Soft Tissue Masses Can Be Diagnosed By Clinical Exam
- Lipoma: Superficial dough-like mass
- Ganglion cyst: Near joint or tendon with transillumination
- Vascular malformations

Begin With Conventional Radiograph
- Bone mass extending into soft tissues, bone destruction (more aggressive lesion), foreign body, calcification (synovial cell sarcoma, phleboliths from a venous malformation), fat (lipoma)

MR
- Categorize into indeterminate (can't diagnose with certainty) or determinate (can diagnosis by MR appearance) for management
- Determinate lesions
  - Lipoma
    - Equals fat on all sequences
    - Nodular regions on post-contrast or T2WI cannot differentiate from liposarcoma
    - May demonstrate septal enhancement < 2 mm in thickness
  - Plexiform neurofibroma
    - Target appearance: Hyperintense T2WI surrounding a lower signal neural & fibrous center, also seen on post-contrast with enhancing outer surrounding lower center
  - Ganglion cyst
    - Communicates with tendon sheath or joint space
    - Hypointense T1WI, hyperintense T2WI, may have a thin rim of enhancement
  - Vascular birthmarks
    - Hemangioma: True neoplasm, hyperintense T2WI, high flow with diffuse enhancement (soft tissue)
    - Arteriovenous malformation or fistula: High flow lesion, tangle or vessels, lacks soft tissue
    - Lymphatic malformation: Low flow lesion, cystic, can mimic solid lesion (microcystic), septal enhancement
    - Venous malformation: Low flow lesion, diffuse enhancement, phleboliths or thrombi
    - Combination
  - Hematoma, abscess, myositis ossificans, etc.
  - Therapy: Observe or excise
- Indeterminate lesion
  - Many lesions may appear benign by MR (small size, well-marginated, one tissue compartment, uniform signal intensity, lacks invasion) but highly malignant (synovial sarcoma, liposarcoma, rhabdomyosarcoma)
  - Biopsy for diagnosis then plan therapy

Common Malignant Soft Tissue Neoplasms

Rhabdomyosarcoma (RMS)
- Large heterogeneous soft tissue mass, head & neck (28-40%), extremities (15-20%)
- 70% < 10 years old, embryonal RMS (60-70%); genitourinary or head & neck, alveolar RMS (20%); extremity, trunk & perirectal/perianal, botryoid RMS (10%); vagina, bladder, biliary tree, nasopharynx

Synovial Cell Sarcoma
- Calcifications in 1/3, not articular, but near joint

Fibrosarcoma
- Congenital-infantile fibrosarcoma: Present at birth
- Mostly a tumor of adults

Primitive Neuroectodermal Tumor (PNET) & Extraosseous Ewing Sarcoma
- No calcification, heterogeneous soft tissue mass, looks like RMS

Myxoid Liposarcoma, Malignant Fibrous

MUSCULOSKELETAL

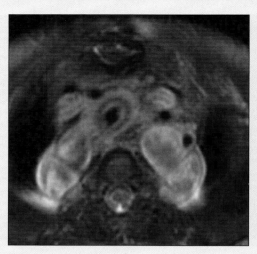

Axial T2WI MR shows target appearance of plexiform neurofibromas, determinate lesions.

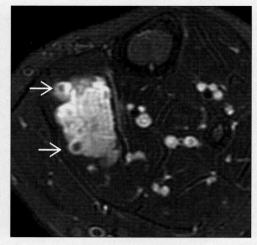

Axial T2WI MR of another determinant shows hypointense foci (arrows) throughout this hyperintense mass, consistent with phleboliths or thrombi in this venous malformation.

Histiocytoma
- Variable appearance: Can look like RMS

Malignant Peripheral Nerve Sheath Tumor (MPNST)
- Malignant schwannoma, neurofibrosarcoma
- >50% are seen in NF patients
  - If rapid enlargement, pain, loss of target, large size (> 5 cm), must consider atypical neurofibroma or malignant degeneration

How To Work-Up A Malignant Bone Lesion

Conventional Radiographs First
- Helpful in determining tumor matrix & cortical bone involvement

MR For Diagnosis & Treatment Planning
- Large field of view (FOV) T1WI from joint to joint (both proximal & distal joints) for skip marrow metastasis
- Then smaller FOV in evaluation of the mass with small parts or surface coil; FSE T2WI FS, STIR, T1WI, post contrast TWI FS
  - Evaluation of neurovascular, joint, epiphyseal, ligament or tendon involvement
- Follow-up MR to assess response to therapy & resectability (+/- limb sparing surgery)
- MRI > CT: Lacks ionizing radiation, better soft tissue contrast resolution, better evaluation of the articular cartilage
- CT > MR: Matrix evaluation, cortical bone involvement
- Chest NECT for staging
- Positron emission tomography (PET) with FDG for metastatic disease &/or response to therapy
- Technetium 99m-MDP bone scan for metastatic disease

Common Primary Malignant Bone Neoplasms

Osteogenic Sarcoma
- Osteoid matrix in 90%, metaphysis, ill-defined lytic lesion with patchy sclerosis, adolescents, most common primary bone malignancy in childhood
- Less commonly purely lytic or sclerotic

Ewing Sarcoma
- Central, diaphyseal or metaphyseal, lytic, lamellated "onion skin" or permeative periosteal reaction, large soft tissue mass
- Child during 2nd decade of life
- Can occur in any bone or soft tissue; upper/lower extremity > pelvis > ribs
- Osteomyelitis can mimic, but tends to have a more rapid progression after onset of symptoms (by 2 weeks on radiographs compared to 6-12 weeks in Ewing sarcoma)

Leukemia
- Variable appearance; osteopenia → permeative → moth eaten bone destruction, sclerosis, periosteal reaction (smooth, lamellated, or sunburst)
- Long bones in children, leukemic lines: 40-53% ALL

Lymphoma
- Mostly solitary, occasional multifocal, soft tissue mass > amount of bone destruction, older age group

Related References
1. Donnelly LF: Fundamentals of Pediatric Radiology. Philadelphia: W.B. Saunders, 2001

MUSCULOSKELETAL

IMAGE GALLERY

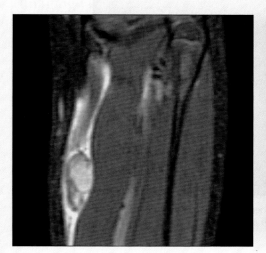
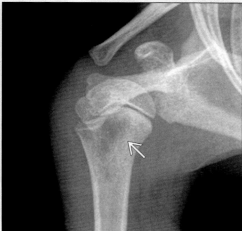

(Left) Coronal STIR MR shows a large soft tissue mass with a tail of tumor extending along a fascial plane. There were flocculent calcifications in this mass prior to the MR on radiographs which gave clues to the diagnosis of synovial cell sarcoma. (Right) Anteroposterior radiograph shows a nonspecific subtle ill-defined lucent lesion proximal metaphysis of the humerus without soft tissue mass or periosteal reaction, biopsy proven lymphoma.

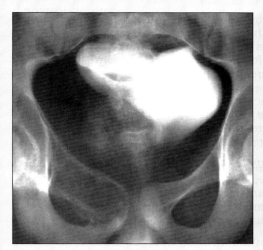
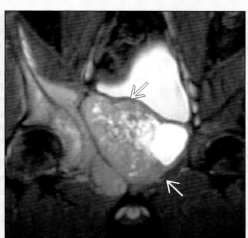

(Left) Anteroposterior radiograph shows expansile lytic lesion of the right superior pubic ramus. (Right) Coronal STIR MR in the same patient shows abnormal hyperintense marrow signal in the right pubic bone, acetabulum, & iliac wing. Notice the very large soft tissue mass (arrows) displacing the urinary bladder, compared to the amount of bone destruction, characteristic of Ewing sarcoma.

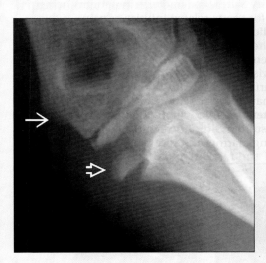
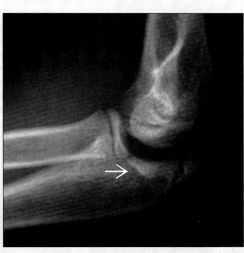

(Left) Anteroposterior radiograph shows lack of medial epicondyle ossification center (arrow) with visualized trochlea & entrapped medial epicondyle (open arrow). (Right) Lateral radiograph shows an entrapped medial epicondyle (arrow).

PHYSEAL FRACTURES

- Surface of metaphyses' and epiphyses' physeal face is irregular or corrugated: Consists of small bony projections, undulations, knobs, and ridges called "mammillary processes"
- Mostly metaphysis and epiphysis receive arterial supply from separate sources: Fracture through the physis does not interfere with blood supply of either epiphysis or metaphysis
  - Exceptions: Femoral capital and radial head epiphyses (because intra-articular)
- Structure of physeal fracture
  - Damage due to shear, grinding, and compression force
  - Fracture plane undulates within proliferative, hypertrophic, and provisional calcification zones
  - Fibrin appears within cleavage, cartilaginous cells continue to grow, epiphyseal plate thickens as cellular columns lengthen
  - By ~21 days fibrin gone and normal growth pattern restored

Staging, Grading or Classification Criteria
- Type 1: Fracture involves only the physis
- Type 2: Fracture involves physis and metaphysis
- Type 3: Fracture involves physis and epiphysis
- Type 4: Fracture involves physis, metaphysis, and epiphysis
- Type 5: Crush fracture involving all or part of physis
  - Rare, usually first recognized when cone epiphyses or partial epiphyseal arrest becomes apparent later
- Type 6-9, as described by Ogden 1981 (all rare)
  - Perichondral ring injury (type 6), intra-epiphyseal fracture not involving physis (type 7), metaphysis fracture not involving physis directly but → ischemic growth disturbance (type 8), periosteal injury → disturbed diaphyseal growth (type 9)

CLINICAL ISSUES

Presentation
- Most common signs/symptoms: Pain, swelling, point tenderness, limited range of motion, inability to bear weight

Demographics
- Age
  - Peak age: 11-12 years
  - Ages 16 and 17: Physeal fractures more common in males just because physes have closed in females
- Gender
  - Average age: Girls = 11 years; boys = 12 years
  - Physeal fractures the same fraction all of all fractures in both boys and girls: 18%

Natural History & Prognosis
- Overall complication rate: ~14%
- Complications: Premature early or complete epiphyseal closure, limb shortening or angulation, persistently trapped periosteum, joint incongruity
- Most substantial complications occur at the knee and ankle
- Prognosis is worse in lower extremities irrespective of the Salter-Harris classification

- Premature epiphyseal closure in lower tibial fractures
  - 27% overall rate
  - 21% in triplane fractures, rare in Tillaux fractures

Treatment
- Casting for low Salter-Harris categories
- Open reduction and internal fixation often required with higher categories
- Prolonged immobilization (3-18 months) may be needed in children with myelodysplasia

DIAGNOSTIC CHECKLIST

Consider
- Follow knee and ankle fractures for at least a year or until skeletal maturity for early detection of premature closure of epiphyses

SELECTED REFERENCES

1. Craig JG et al: The distal femoral and proximal tibial growth plates: MR imaging, three-dimensional modeling and estimation of area and volume. Skeletal Radiol. 33(6):337-44, 2004
2. Swischuk LE et al: Frequently missed fractures in children (value of comparative views). Emerg Radiol. 11(1):22-8, 2004
3. Barmada A et al: Premature physeal closure following distal tibia physeal fractures: a new radiographic predictor. J Pediatr Orthop. 23(6):733-9, 2003
4. Koury SI et al: Recognition and management of Tillaux fractures in adolescents. Pediatr Emerg Care. 15(1):37-9, 1999
5. Carey J et al: MRI of pediatric growth plate injury: correlation with plain film radiographs and clinical outcome. Skeletal Radiol. 27(5):250-5, 1998
6. Rodgers WB et al: Chronic physeal fractures in myelodysplasia: magnetic resonance analysis, histologic description, treatment, and outcome. J Pediatr Orthop. 17(5):615-21, 1997
7. Shih C et al: Chronically stressed wrists in adolescent gymnasts: MR imaging appearance. Radiology. 195(3):855-9, 1995
8. Rogers LF et al: Imaging of epiphyseal injuries. Radiology. 191(2):297-308, 1994
9. Mizuta T et al: Statistical analysis of the incidence of physeal injuries. J Pediatr Orthop. 7(5):518-23, 1987
10. Ogden JA: Injury to the growth mechanisms of the immature skeleton. Skeletal Radiol. 6:237-53, 1981
11. Salter RB et al: Injuries involving the epiphyseal plate. J Bone Joint Surg Am. 45:587-622, 1963

PHYSEAL FRACTURES

IMAGE GALLERY

Typical

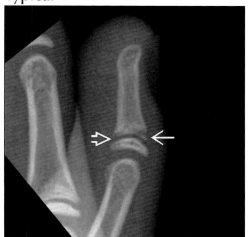
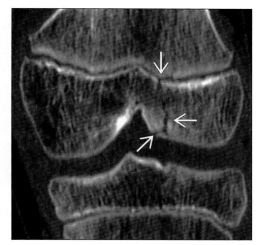

(Left) Lateral radiograph shows Salter-Harris type 2 fracture of 4th finger's distal phalanx. The physis is widened (open arrow) and metaphyseal fracture fragment is seen (arrow) in 15 year old boy. (Right) Coronal reconstruction CT shows Salter-Harris type 3 epiphyseal fracture (arrows) in an 11 year old girl.

Typical

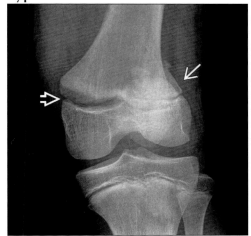
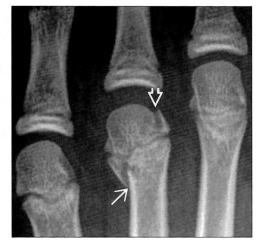

(Left) Anteroposterior radiograph shows Salter-Harris type 2 femoral fracture. The fracture involves physis (open arrow); lateral metaphyseal fragment (arrow) still attached to the epiphysis in an 11 year old boy. (Right) Anteroposterior radiograph shows Salter-Harris type 4 fracture of 4th metatarsal. Fractures of the head (open arrow) and metaphysis (arrow) are seen. The head is offset laterally in an 11 year old girl.

Typical

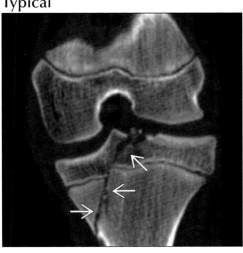
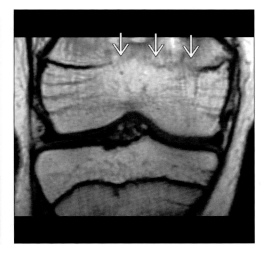

(Left) Coronal-reconstruction CT shows a Salter-Harris type 4 fracture (arrows) of the tibia in an 15 year old boy. (Right) Coronal T1WI MR 11 months later in same lad shows central closure of epiphysis (arrows).

CHILD ABUSE, METAPHYSEAL FRACTURE

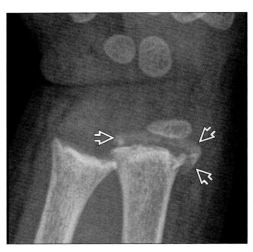

Anteroposterior radiograph shows a bucket-handle fracture (arrows) of the distal radius. The radial epiphysis is offset laterally.

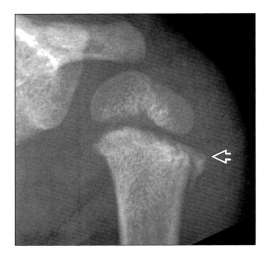

Anteroposterior radiograph shows a corner fracture (arrow) of the upper humoral metaphysis.

TERMINOLOGY

Abbreviations and Synonyms
- Child abuse: Nonaccidental trauma, battered child syndrome
- Metaphyseal corner fracture: Classic metaphyseal lesion, metaphyseal infraction, avulsion fracture, and metaphyseal flag

Definitions
- Child abuse: Injury of a child by a violent act of another human being
  - Children are shaken, squeezed, jerked, twisted, punched, burned, bitten, punctured, and thrown
  - Abuse that is emotional, sexual, or a result of neglect may be devastating but is not an indication for imaging
  - Perpetrators usually have a parental or parent-like relationship to the child
  - A confession by perpetrator is rare, so mechanism of injury usually is not known

IMAGING FINDINGS

General Features
- Best diagnostic clue: Bucket-handle fracture
- Location
  - Metaphyses of long bones
  - Most common in lower femur, upper and lower tibia, upper humerus
- Size: Often subtle

Radiographic Findings
- Radiography
  - Metaphyseal corner fractures are highly specific for child abuse
    - Triangular bit of bone is seen at the corner of a metaphysis close to the physis
    - May be subtle prior to callus formation
  - Radiographic appearance depends upon angle at which fractured metaphyseal rim visualized
    - If viewed tangential to plane of physis, fracture will appear as a corner fracture
    - If viewed obliquely, a corner fracture may turn into a bucket-handle fracture
  - Bucket-handle fractures are similar to corner fractures, but involve more of metaphyseal circumference
    - Bucket-handle fracture may be seen when metaphysis viewed obliquely to the plane of epiphysis
    - Will appear as 1 or 2 corner fractures if X-ray beam parallel to physis

DDx: Diseases With Multiple Fractures Or Fracture-Like Appearance

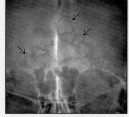

Osteogenesis Imperf

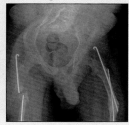

Osteogenesis Imperf

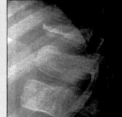

Leukemia

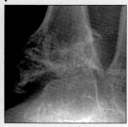

SM Dysplasia

CHILD ABUSE, METAPHYSEAL FRACTURE

Key Facts

Imaging Findings
- Best diagnostic clue: Bucket-handle fracture
- Metaphyseal corner fractures are highly specific for child abuse
- If viewed obliquely, a corner fracture may turn into a bucket-handle fracture
- Bucket-handle fractures are similar to corner fractures, but involve more of metaphyseal circumference
- Bucket-handle fracture may be seen when metaphysis viewed obliquely to the plane of epiphysis
- Fractures highly specific for child abuse in infants are rib, scapula, spinous process, sternum, and metaphysis
- Fractures moderately specific for child abuse in infants and children are multiple fractures (especially bilateral), fractures of different ages, epiphyseal separations, vertebral-body fractures, finger fractures, and complex skull fractures
- Common but of low-specificity are subperiosteal new bone formation; and fractures that are clavicular, long-bone diaphysis, and linear skull
- Bone scan extremely helpful in first week after injury by showing areas of subperiosteal hemorrhage before subperiosteal new bone may become visible
- Bone scan excellent for detecting rib fractures
- Best imaging tool: Skeletal survey using radiographs

Clinical Issues
- Most children < 1 year old at presentation

- Crescentic or annular rim of bone from metaphysis just underneath "periosteal collar" where cortical bone is resorbed as part of bone remodeling during growth
  - May be seen as only a corner fracture when X-ray beam is in plane of epiphysis
- Other bone findings
  - Fractures highly specific for child abuse in infants are rib, scapula, spinous process, sternum, and metaphysis
  - Fractures moderately specific for child abuse in infants and children are multiple fractures (especially bilateral), fractures of different ages, epiphyseal separations, vertebral-body fractures, finger fractures, and complex skull fractures
  - Common but of low-specificity are subperiosteal new bone formation; and fractures that are clavicular, long-bone diaphysis, and linear skull
  - Spiral femoral fractures before walking

CT Findings
- Rib and lung injuries
- Liver, spleen, pancreas injury
- Duodenal hematoma
- Bowel rupture
- Subdural hematoma

MR Findings
- Brain injury
  - Shaken baby syndrome

Ultrasonographic Findings
- Grayscale Ultrasound
  - Subdural hematoma
  - Intracerebral hemorrhage
  - Liver, spleen, kidney, and pancreas injury
  - Duodenal hematoma

Nuclear Medicine Findings
- Bone Scintigraphy
  - Bone scan extremely helpful in first week after injury by showing areas of subperiosteal hemorrhage before subperiosteal new bone may become visible
  - Bone scan excellent for detecting rib fractures
  - Difficult in regions of physes as these are normally high in activity
  - Radiographs are better for skull fractures and metaphyseal fractures

Imaging Recommendations
- Best imaging tool: Skeletal survey using radiographs
- When abuse suspected, skeletal survey obtained to document findings of abuse for legal reasons so that child can be removed from the abuser
- Identification and reporting of radiographic findings of abuse is important task
  - False-positive findings may result in removal of a nonabused child from its family
  - False-negative findings may result in returning a child to a dangerous environment
- Other tests that may be used to document findings of abuse
  - Repeat skeletal survey in 2 weeks will identify healing, previously-occult fractures and subperiosteal new bone formation
  - Skeletal scintigraphy
  - Abdominal and chest CT
  - Brain MR
- Radiographs are better than scintigraphy for finding metaphyseal and skull fractures

DIFFERENTIAL DIAGNOSIS

Entities associated with multiple fractures or fracture-like appearance of metaphyses
- Osteogenesis imperfecta: Multiple fractures, Wormian bones
- Rickets: Metaphyseal irregularity and fractures, subperiosteal new bone formation
- Congenital indifference to pain: Metaphyseal injuries common
- Myelomeningocele: Metaphyseal injuries in leg bones due to decreased pain sensation

INCOMPLETE FRACTURES

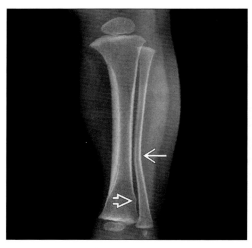

Anteroposterior radiograph shows a tibial buckle fracture (open arrow) and a fibular plastic bowing fracture (arrow) in a 16 month old.

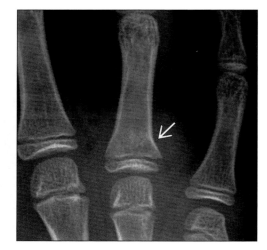

Anteroposterior radiograph shows a buckle fracture (arrow) in the metadiaphysis of the 4th finger's proximal phalanx in a 15 year old.

TERMINOLOGY

Abbreviations and Synonyms
- Buckle, torus, greenstick, plastic bowing, plastic bending, toddlers, impaction, stress, and hairline fractures

Definitions
- Children's bone tends to be more elastic than adult bone and has greater propensity to bow or bend before breaking than does adult bone
- Incomplete fracture: Does not involve entire circumference of a bone
  - Buckle fractures
    - Buckle fracture: Bone cortex bulges out or in on compression side and cortex is usually intact on tension side
    - Bone cortex folds either in or out when it buckles
    - Buckled in (concave): Fracture is just called a "buckle fracture" or "angle buckle fracture"
    - Buckled out (convex): Fracture usually called a "buckle fracture" but it may be termed 'torus fracture" from Latin "bulge, protuberance, lowest convex moulding at base of a column"
  - Plastic bending fractures
    - Plastic bending: Bone bent without cortical deformity (vs. cortical deformity in buckle fractures) or a visible fracture line
  - Greenstick fractures
    - Plastic bowing fracture variant in which one or several hairline (or larger) incomplete fractures occur on tension side
    - Like bending a "green stick"
  - Impaction fractures
    - Due to longitudinal compression
  - Hairline fractures
    - Tiny fractures close to the limit of systems resolution
  - Stress fractures
    - Incomplete fracture at first due to repetitive stress that is either invisible or hairline at symptom-onset
    - May become complete
  - Toddler's fractures
    - An incomplete lower extremity fracture without known trauma in young child who recently began walking
  - Salter-Harris physeal fractures types 2-4 meet the definition of incomplete fractures (do not involve entire bone circumference), but are not thought of as belonging to incomplete-fracture group because joint and physeal involvement demands different orthopedic management

DDx: Bent Bones

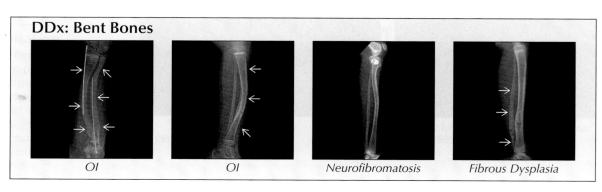

OI   OI   Neurofibromatosis   Fibrous Dysplasia

INCOMPLETE FRACTURES

Key Facts

Terminology
- Incomplete fracture: Does not involve entire circumference of a bone
- Buckle fracture: Bone cortex bulges out or in on compression side and cortex is usually intact on tension side
- Plastic bending: Bone bent without cortical deformity (vs. cortical deformity in buckle fractures) or a visible fracture line
- Plastic bowing fracture variant in which one or several hairline (or larger) incomplete fractures occur on tension side

Imaging Findings
- Monteggia-equivalent fracture: Bending fracture of ulna with anterior dislocation of radial head
- Plastic bending fractures may be subtle: In such cases comparison views of contralateral bones may be helpful in making diagnosis
- Bone scans show increased uptake in all incomplete fractures including plastic bending
- Comparison radiographs of opposite normal side may assist in evaluation of subtle fractures

Pathology
- Absorption of fracture energy may occur along much of length of immature bone → plastic bowing and greenstick fractures

Clinical Issues
- Decreased range of pronation-supination in plastic bending forearm fractures

IMAGING FINDINGS

General Features
- Best diagnostic clue: Cortical bump or angulation at site of pain or injury
- Location
  - Buckle fractures
    - Found most often in humerus, radius, ulna, carpal scaphoid, metacarpals, fingers, tibia, fibula, metatarsals, toes
  - Plastic bending fractures
    - Commonest in radius, ulna, clavicle, fibula
    - Reported to occur in neonatal femur
    - Monteggia-equivalent fracture: Bending fracture of ulna with anterior dislocation of radial head
    - Slow to remodel if untreated, especially in older children
  - Greenstick fractures
    - Most common in forearm
  - Impaction fractures
    - Type 2 toddler's fracture in tibia, cuboid, carpal scaphoid
  - Hairline fractures
    - Small bones of hands and feet, tibial diaphysis, tibial proximal metaphysis, proximal ulna
  - Stress fractures
    - Most common in legs and feet
  - Toddler's fractures
    - Found in legs and feet

Radiographic Findings
- Radiography
  - Buckle fracture
    - Angular deformity or buckle of cortex
    - On cortical side subjected to compression
    - Subtle angulation may be seen at buckle site
  - Plastic bending fracture
    - Typically in midshaft of bones
    - Most commonly radius and ulna
    - Plastic bending fractures may be subtle: In such cases comparison views of contralateral bones may be helpful in making diagnosis
    - Often accompanied by complete or plastic bending fracture of companion bone in forearm and lower-leg fractures
    - Periosteal reaction absent during recovery (neonates may be an exception)
    - Occurs rarely in adults
  - Greenstick fracture
    - Subset of plastic bending fracture in which visible hairline (or even larger) fractures occur in convex cortical side subjected to tension (distraction); bone and periosteum intact on concave (compression) side

CT Findings
- NECT: May be performed when physeal fracture suspected or when evaluating an area of sclerosis in the setting of an unclear subacute fracture

Nuclear Medicine Findings
- Bone Scan
  - Bone scans show increased uptake in all incomplete fractures including plastic bending
    - Due to increased osteoblastic activity

Other Modality Findings
- MR: May be performed when physeal fracture suspected

Imaging Recommendations
- Best imaging tool: Radiographs
- Protocol advice
  - Comparison radiographs of opposite normal side may assist in evaluation of subtle fractures
    - Can be very helpful in plastic bending fractures
    - Contralateral views are not recommended as part of routine imaging

DIFFERENTIAL DIAGNOSIS

Bone bending due to skeletal disease
- Bone dysplasia
  - Osteogenesis imperfecta (OI)
  - Fibrous dysplasia

INCOMPLETE FRACTURES

- Neurofibromatosis, type 1
- Many other dysplasias
• Metabolic bone disease
- Hyperparathyroidism
- Hyperphosphatemia
- Hypophosphatasia
- Rickets

Normal variation
• Comparison views may be helpful

PATHOLOGY

General Features
• General path comments
  - Developing skeleton is more elastic and less brittle than adult bone
    ▪ Absorption of fracture energy may occur along much of length of immature bone → plastic bowing and greenstick fractures
• Etiology
  - Plastic bending fractures
    ▪ Axial load on long bone
  - Fall on hyperextended wrist → scaphoid impaction fracture
  - Buckle fractures: Angular loading, often with rotational component

Microscopic Features
• Torus fracture
  - Periosteum intact but variably elevated due to subperiosteal hemorrhage
  - Cortical fracture propagates through vascular foramina
  - Longitudinal splits along osteoid seams
• Greenstick and plastic bending fractures
  - Splitting and widening of developing Haversian system
  - Compressive distortion along osteoid seams

CLINICAL ISSUES

Presentation
• Most common signs/symptoms
  - Pain, swelling, tenderness
  - Refusal to walk
• Decreased range of pronation-supination in plastic bending forearm fractures

Natural History & Prognosis
• Complete healing is rule
• Development of small subperiosteal post-traumatic cortical defects in radius is rare phenomenon
  - Appear 1-10 months after injury
  - Location: Usually in cortex which has been compressed during injury
  - MR signal consistent with blood or fat in defect
• Remodeling corrects angular bone deformities, may not correct rotational deformities
• Greenstick fracture: Median nerve entrapment and transection may occur

Treatment
• Immobilization (casting)
• Most incomplete fractures heal without internal fixation
• Manipulation of plastic bending forearm fractures to restore full range of pronation-supination
  - Normal range: Supination is 80-120° from neutral; pronation is 50-80° from neutral

SELECTED REFERENCES

1. Sai S et al: Radial head dislocation with acute plastic bowing of the ulna. J Orthop Sci. 10(1):103-7, 2005
2. Swischuk LE et al: Frequently missed fractures in children (value of comparative views). Emerg Radiol. 11(1):22-8, 2004
3. Hernandez JA et al: The angled buckle fracture in pediatrics: a frequently missed fracture. Emerg Radiol. 10(2):71-5, 2003
4. Hernandez JA et al: Scaphoid (navicular) fractures of the wrist in children: attention to the impacted buckle fracture. Emerg Radiol. 9(6):305-8, 2002
5. Roach RT et al: Paediatric post-traumatic cortical defects of the distal radius. Pediatr Radiol. 32(5):333-9, 2002
6. Proubasta IR et al: Entrapment of the median nerve in a greenstick forearm fracture. A case report and review of the literature. Bull Hosp Jt Dis. 58(4):220-3, 1999
7. Noonan KJ et al: Forearm and distal radius fractures in children. J Am Acad Orthop Surg. 6(3):146-56, 1998
8. Sclamberg J et al: Acute plastic bowing deformation of the forearm in an adult. AJR Am J Roentgenol. 170(5):1259-60, 1998
9. Wass AR et al: Cortical bone cyst following a greenstick radial fracture. J Accid Emerg Med. 13(1):63-4, 1996
10. Ogden JA et al: The pathology of acute chondro-osseous injury in the child. Yale J Biol Med. 66(3):219-33, 1993
11. Gordon L et al: Acute plastic deformation of the ulna in a skeletally mature individual. J Hand Surg [Am]. 16(3):451-3, 1991
12. Aponte JE Jr et al: Acute plastic bowing deformity: a review of the literature. J Emerg Med. 7(2):181-4, 1989
13. Zionts LE et al: Plastic bowing of the femur in a neonate. J Pediatr Orthop. 4(6):749-51, 1984
14. Miller JH et al: Scintigraphy in acute plastic bowing of the forearm. Radiology. 142(3):742, 1982
15. Martin W 3rd et al: Acute plastic bowing fractures of the fibula. Radiology. 131(3):639-40, 1979
16. Borden S 4th: Roentgen recognition of acute plastic bowing of the forearm in children. Am J Roentgenol Radium Ther Nucl Med. 125(3):524-30, 1975

INCOMPLETE FRACTURES

IMAGE GALLERY

Typical

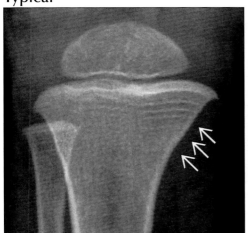
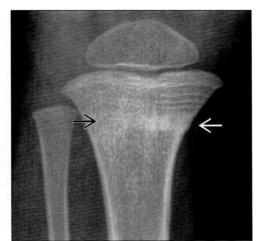

(Left) Anteroposterior radiograph shows cortical bulge of a subtle buckle fracture of tibial metaphysis (arrows) in a 2 year old. *(Right)* Anteroposterior radiograph 23 days later in same child shows a sclerotic band (arrows) formed by callus within healing fracture.

Typical

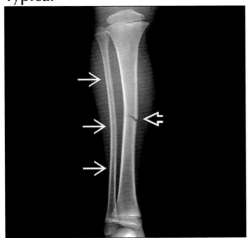
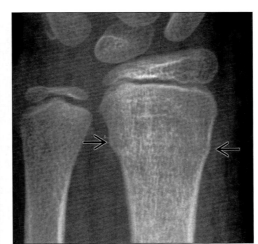

(Left) Anteroposterior radiograph shows tibial greenstick fracture with incomplete transverse fracture (open arrow) on tension side and plastic bowing fracture (arrows) of fibula in a 10 year old. *(Right)* Anteroposterior radiograph shows buckle fracture (arrows) of the radial metaphysis in a 9 year old.

Typical

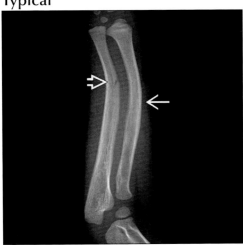
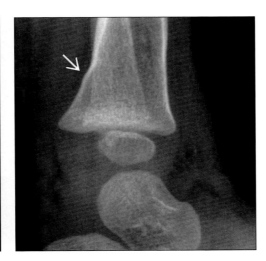

(Left) Lateral-oblique radiograph shows a radial plastic bowing fracture (arrow) and a greenstick fracture of ulna with a single incomplete hairline fracture (open arrow) on the distraction side. 6 year old child. *(Right)* Lateral radiograph shows cortical buckle fracture (arrow) of tibia in a 16 month old.

STRESS FRACTURE

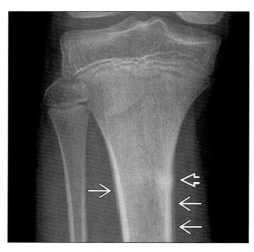

Anteroposterior radiograph shows circumferential periosteal reaction (arrows) and an area of cortical sclerosis (open arrow) in 12 year old's tibia.

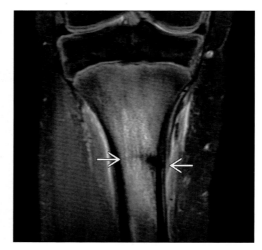

Coronal PD TSE FS MR shows stress fracture as hypointense transverse band (arrows) in same patient. Signal of surrounding marrow and circumferential parosteal tissues is increased.

TERMINOLOGY

Abbreviations and Synonyms
- March, exhaustion, spontaneous, crack, and pseudo-fracture

Definitions
- Fatigue fracture
  - Normal bone subject to repetitive stresses, none of which is by itself capable of producing a fracture, leading to mechanical failure over time
- Insufficiency fracture
  - Results from normal stress applied to abnormal bone
    - Osteopenia/osteoporosis, osteogenesis imperfecta, rickets/osteomalacia, hyperparathyroidism

IMAGING FINDINGS

General Features
- Best diagnostic clue: Persistent pain in an athlete, or refusal to walk in a toddler
- Location
  - Upper extremity: Coracoid process of scapula (trapshooting), scapula (running with hand-held weights), humerus (throwing, racquet sports), olecranon (pitching, javelin throwers, gymnasts, weight lifters), ulna (tennis, gymnastics, volleyball, swimming, softball, wheelchair sports)
  - Axial skeleton: First rib (pitching), ribs 2-10 (rowing, kayaking), pars interarticularis (gymnastics, ballet, soccer, cricket, volleyball, springboard diving), pubic ramus (distance running, ballet)
  - Lower extremity: Femoral neck (distance running, jumping, ballet), femoral shaft (distance running), patella (running, hurdling), tibial plateau (running), tibial shaft (running, ballet), fibula (running, aerobics, race-walking, ballet), medial malleolus (basketball, running)
  - Foot: Calcaneus (baseball, soccer, basketball, gymnastics, military marching), talus (pole vaulting), navicular (sprinting, middle-distance running, hurdling, long- or triple-jumping, football), metatarsals (running, ballet, marching), 2nd metatarsal base (ballet), 5th metatarsal (tennis, ballet), foot sesamoids (running, ballet, basketball, skating)
  - Stress fractures in athletes

DDx: Causes Of Bone Sclerosis

Brodie Abscess | Osteosarcoma | Osteoid Osteoma

STRESS FRACTURE

Key Facts

Terminology
- Normal bone subject to repetitive stresses, none of which is by itself capable of producing a fracture, leading to mechanical failure over time

Imaging Findings
- Subperiosteal new bone at any stage (except earliest) may be the only radiographic sign
- Sclerotic bands: Due to cancellous bone trabecular microcallus
- Pars interarticularis fracture → spondylolysis → spondylolisthesis
- IR, FSE, FS: Areas of marrow hyperintensity against dark background of suppressed fat
- Radiography → bone scan → MR
- CT: Use for high-risk locations such as femoral neck, or when fracture not shown by MR

Pathology
- Stress fractures result when microdamage rate exceeds repair rate
- Track & field: Accounts for 64% of stress fractures in females, 50% in males
- Microfracture → osteoclasts form resorption cavities adjacent to osteons → cavities coalescence → stress fracture
- Microfractures and stress fractures → periosteal stimulation → subperiosteal new bone formation
- Trabecular microfractures → microcallus → sclerotic cancellous bone

Clinical Issues
- Prognosis poorer: Anterior tibial and tarsal navicular fractures

---

- Total number of stress fractures: Tibia: 19-63%, cuboid-calcaneus-talus: 8-63%, fibula: 0-30%, tarsal navicular: 0-29%, femur: 0-23%, pelvis: 0-11%

Radiographic Findings
- Initial subtle poor cortical definition, intracortical lucent striations
  - Due to osteoclastic activity
  - Hairline fracture progresses to complete fracture
- Subperiosteal new bone at any stage (except earliest) may be the only radiographic sign
- Sclerotic bands: Due to cancellous bone trabecular microcallus
- Spine
  - Pars interarticularis fracture → spondylolysis → spondylolisthesis
- Pelvis and sacrum
  - Cancellous bone sclerosis common
- Femoral neck
  - Compression stress fracture
    - Lower medial femoral neck: Cortex and cancellous bone sclerotic, rarely progress to complete break
  - Distraction stress fracture
    - Upper femoral neck: Start as hairline fractures, may progress to complete break
- Tibia
  - Anterior midshaft
    - Distraction fracture; hairline fracture may progress to complete fracture
  - Posterior superior metadiaphysis
    - Compression fracture causing cortical thickening and cancellous sclerosis; heals with rest
  - Inferior metadiaphysis
    - Cancellous bone sclerosis
- Tarsals
  - Sclerotic bands of cancellous bone sclerosis

CT Findings
- Best modality for showing pars interarticularis stress fractures
- Demonstrates: Hairline fractures, areas of intracortical radiolucency, subperiosteal new bone

Nuclear Medicine Findings
- Bone scanning: Sensitivity ≈100%
  - Intense cortical uptake
  - Abnormal in 6-72 hours
  - Multiple areas may be seen
- Pars interarticularis stress fracture
  - Fracture has increased uptake: Scan becomes normal when lesion progresses to chronic phase of spondylolysis

Other Modality Findings
- MR: Sensitivity ≈100%
  - T1WI and T2WI: Areas of marrow hypointensity due to edema, hemorrhage
  - IR, FSE, FS: Areas of marrow hyperintensity against dark background of suppressed fat

Imaging Recommendations
- Best imaging tool: Bone scan or MR when radiographs normal
- Protocol advice
  - Radiography → bone scan → MR
  - CT: Use for high-risk locations such as femoral neck, or when fracture not shown by MR

DIFFERENTIAL DIAGNOSIS

Bone tumor
- Cortical destruction
- Soft tissue mass outside bone

Osteoid osteoma
- Sclerosis with lucent nidus
- Night pain relieved by aspirin

Brodie abscess
- Sclerosis with lucent nidus

Shinsplints (medial tibial stress syndrome)
- MR with fat suppression
  - High signal along medial posterior surface of tibia (traction periostitis)

STRESS FRACTURE

- High signal in longitudinally oriented region of bone marrow within medial part of tibial diaphysis (microdamage and repair)

PATHOLOGY

General Features
- Etiology
  - Microdamage with subsequent repair is normal response of stressed bone
    - Stress fractures result when microdamage rate exceeds repair rate
    - Runners shin pain → fewer kilometers run per week → restoration of microdamage-microrepair equilibrium
- Epidemiology
  - Sports medicine practice
    - Up to 10% of cases are stress fractures
  - Running most frequent cause of stress fractures
  - Track & field: Accounts for 64% of stress fractures in females, 50% in males
  - Risk factors
    - New, different, or rigorous activity
    - Female
    - Race: Relative risk ratio Caucasian: African-American = 2-25:1

Microscopic Features
- Cortical or compact bone
  - Microfracture → osteoclasts form resorption cavities adjacent to osteons → cavities coalescence → stress fracture
    - Bone loss (resorption cavity formation) maximal at 3 weeks
    - Bone reconstruction (filling resorption cavities with lamellar bone) maximal at 90 days
    - Bone loss at greater rate than bone reconstruction → stress fracture
    - Microfractures and stress fractures → periosteal stimulation → subperiosteal new bone formation
- Cancellous or spongy bone
  - Trabecular microfractures → microcallus → sclerotic cancellous bone

CLINICAL ISSUES

Presentation
- Most common signs/symptoms
  - Pain, swelling, warmth, discoloration
  - Palpable periosteal thickening
- Other signs/symptoms
  - Bone percussion → pain
  - Pars interarticularis fracture: Suspect with back pain for several weeks and pain with spinal extension
  - Pelvic stress fracture: Hopping → groin pain
  - Sacral stress fracture: Buttock pain
- After lower extremity cast removed from fracture, 2nd insufficiency fracture may occur secondary to disuse osteopenia
  - Most common locations: Calcaneus, cuboid, tibia
- Young child with refusal to bear weight may have stress/insufficiency fracture
  - Most common locations: Cuboid, calcaneus, tibia

Demographics
- Gender
  - Females: Stress fracture incidence rate (case rate) track & field: 31%, crew: 8%, basketball: 4%, lacrosse: 3%, soccer: 3%
  - Males: Stress fracture incidence rate track & field: 10%, lacrosse: 4%, crew: 2%, football: 1%

Natural History & Prognosis
- Recurrence rate is high: 10-60%
- Prognosis poorer: Anterior tibial and tarsal navicular fractures

Treatment
- Prevention paramount
  - Gradual, deliberate increase in new activity
  - Activity reduction promptly when pain occurs
- Combination of reduced activity, rest, immobilization, casting, internal fixation
  - Compression fractures
    - Reduced activity and rest
  - Tension fractures
    - Internal fixation likely
- Pars interarticularis stress fracture
  - Boston brace or warm-n-form orthosis
  - No bracing with activity modification
  - Majority result in non-union, but can return to full athletic activity except weight-lifting

SELECTED REFERENCES

1. Ahovuo JA et al: Fatigue stress fractures of the sacrum: diagnosis with MR imaging. Eur Radiol. 14(3):500-5, 2004
2. Aoki Y et al: Magnetic resonance imaging in stress fractures and shin splints. Clin Orthop Relat Res. (421):260-7, 2004
3. Lehman RA Jr et al: Tension-sided femoral neck stress fracture in a skeletally immature patient. A case report. J Bone Joint Surg Am. 86-A(6):1292-5, 2004
4. Ogden JA et al: Sever's injury: a stress fracture of the immature calcaneal metaphysis. J Pediatr Orthop. 24(5):488-92, 2004
5. Patterson SP et al: Fatigue fracture of the sacrum in an adolescent. Pediatr Radiol. 34(8):633-5, 2004
6. Biedert R et al: Stress fractures of the medial great toe sesamoids in athletes. Foot Ankle Int. 24(2):137-41, 2003
7. Iwamoto J et al: Stress fractures in athletes: review of 196 cases. J Orthop Sci. 8(3):273-8, 2003
8. Parr TJ et al: Overuse injuries of the olecranon in adolescents. Orthopedics. 26(11):1143-6, 2003
9. Ishibashi Y et al: Comparison of scintigraphy and magnetic resonance imaging for stress injuries of bone. Clin J Sport Med. 12(2):79-84, 2002
10. Kraft DE: Low back pain in the adolescent athlete. Pediatr Clin North Am. 49(3):643-53, 2002
11. Shabat S et al: Stress fractures of the medial malleolus--review of the literature and report of a 15-year-old elite gymnast. Foot Ankle Int. 23(7):647-50, 2002
12. Bennell KL et al: Epidemiology and site specificity of stress fractures. Clin Sports Med. 16(2):179-96, 1997
13. Anderson MW et al: Stress fractures. Radiology. 199(1):1-12, 1996

STRESS FRACTURE

IMAGE GALLERY

Variant

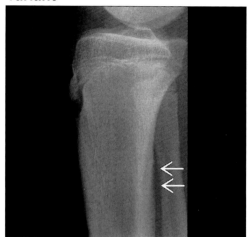
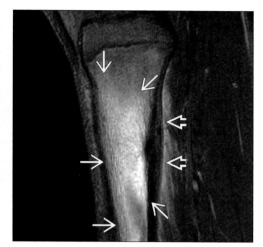

(Left) Lateral radiograph shows area of decreased density (arrows) in a 14 year old's tibia. *(Right)* Sagittal T2 TSE FS MR shows hyperintense marrow edema (arrows) in same patient. Periosteum is elevated (open arrows). Fracture is not seen although presumed present.

Typical

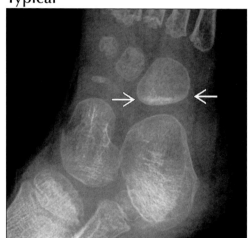
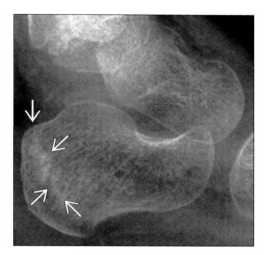

(Left) Oblique radiograph shows healing stress fracture of cuboid as a band of increased density (arrows) in a 3 year old. *(Right)* Lateral radiograph shows healing stress fracture of calcaneus (arrows) as a band of increased density in another 3 year old.

Typical

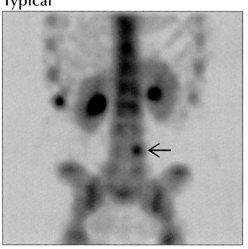
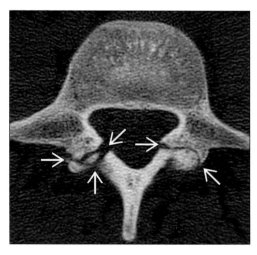

(Left) Anteroposterior SPECT shows increased activity (arrow) in the left L4 lamina of a 19 year old. *(Right)* Axial NECT shows bilateral stress fractures (arrows) of pars interarticularis in same patient.

SUPRACONDYLAR FRACTURE

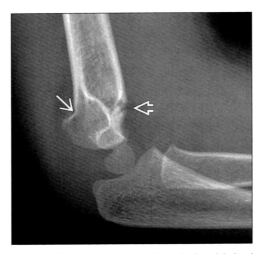

Lateral radiograph shows capitellum displaced behind anterior humeral line. The humerus metaphyseal cortex is buckled (arrow) posteriorly and interrupted anteriorly (open arrow).

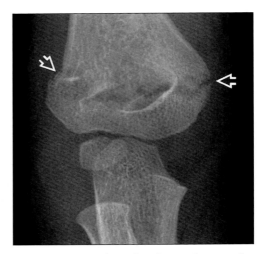

Anteroposterior radiograph shows fracture line (between arrows) traversing supracondylar humeral metaphysis in same child.

TERMINOLOGY

Abbreviations and Synonyms
- Gartland fracture

Definitions
- Transverse fracture of distal humerus from a bending force in hyperextension
- Often due to fall on outstretched arm

IMAGING FINDINGS

General Features
- Best diagnostic clue
  - Radiographs
    - Positive fat pad sign
    - Transverse metaphyseal lucency (fracture line)
    - Mid-capitellum not crossed by anterior humeral line
  - Linear decreased signal intensity surrounded by edema on PD FSE/T2WI of supracondylar humerus
- Location
  - Thin distal humerus at risk between olecranon and coronoid fossae
  - Extraarticular in children
- Size: Involves entire distal humerus above condylar epiphyses
- Morphology
  - Plastic deformity of distal humerus
  - Posterior angulation/displacement usually
  - Fracture line angles from anterior distal to posterior proximal

Radiographic Findings
- Radiography
  - Fracture line in metaphysis on anteroposterior (AP) or angled AP view
  - Fracture line may not be visible in up to 25%
  - Positive fat pad sign on lateral view
  - Anterior humeral line projects anterior to middle third of capitellum in 94%
    - Anterior humeral line: Line that is drawn along anterior cortex of humerus normally bisects the capitellum

CT Findings
- NECT: Linear lucencies in distal humeral metaphysis indicating fracture
- CTA: CT angiography to assess vascular injury

MR Findings
- T1WI
  - Decreased marrow signal indicating bone edema
  - Low signal line indicating fracture line
    - +/- Fragment rotation/displacement on sagittal views

DDx: Supracondylar Fracture

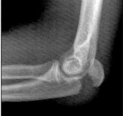
Olecranon Fracture

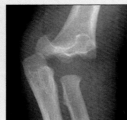
Fracture-Dislocation

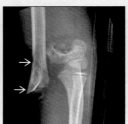
Open Fracture

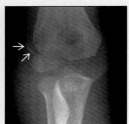
Lateral Condyle

SUPRACONDYLAR FRACTURE

Key Facts

Terminology
- Gartland fracture
- Transverse fracture of distal humerus from a bending force in hyperextension

Imaging Findings
- Mid-capitellum not crossed by anterior humeral line
- Fracture line in metaphysis on anteroposterior (AP) or angled AP view
- Fracture line may not be visible in up to 25%
- Positive fat pad sign on lateral view
- Anterior humeral line projects anterior to middle third of capitellum in 94%

Top Differential Diagnoses
- Lateral condylar fracture

Pathology
- Extension injury more common (95% of cases) than flexion type
- Type I: Nondisplaced fracture (30%)
- Type II: Displaced but intact posterior cortex (24%)
- Type III: Displaced plus complete cortical disruption (45%)

Clinical Issues
- Clinical Profile: Normal, active child

Diagnostic Checklist
- Presence of other fractures, especially olecranon and medial epicondyle
- Associated vascular and neural injuries

  - Low signal joint effusion
- T2WI
  - Increased marrow signal indicating edema
  - FS PD FSE: Visualization improved by using FS
  - High signal joint effusion
    - +/- Periarticular extension of fluid with capsular rupture and vascular injury
  - Low signal fracture lines surrounded by edema
- STIR
  - Very sensitive for bony injury shown as high signal areas in marrow space
  - Especially useful at mid and low-field
- T2* GRE
  - Thin slice capability useful for detailed analysis of fragment and adjacent soft tissues
  - Susceptibility decreases utility for detection of edema in bone

Imaging Recommendations
- Best imaging tool: Radiographs only needed imaging in most cases

DIFFERENTIAL DIAGNOSIS

Lateral condylar fracture
- Fall on an outstretched hand, with impaction of radial head
- Varus stress with elbow flexed/supinated, avulsion by common extensor action
- 17% of distal humerus fractures
- Common in age 5-10 years (peak = 6 years)

Other distal humerus fractures
- Medial epicondyle
  - Varus force on extended arm
- Medial condyle
  - Uncommon
  - Avulsion with forced varus and direct impact on flexed elbow
- T-condylar and lateral epicondyle fractures
  - Less common distal humerus fractures
  - T-condylar = supracondylar with intraarticular extension

Olecranon fracture
- Fall on a flexed, supinated forearm
- Olecranon epiphysis fuses at 16-18 years
- Direct trauma
- Throwing injury (pitchers)

Valgus injury
- Throwing activities
- Includes trabecular injury
- +/- Bone trabecular injury of the capitellum
- +/- Medial collateral ligament (MCL) tear

Capitellum osteochondritis dissecans
- Necrosis of the bone followed by healing response and reossification
- 12-16 year age group (after ossification of capitellum)
- 20% bilateral
- Chronic valgus stress with lateral impaction seen in gymnasts and adolescent pitchers
- Panner's disease (age 7-10 years) as an osteochondrosis

Posterior dislocation
- Ulna and radius displaced proximally
- +/- Extensor tendon tear
- +/- Fractures
  - Coronoid, radial head, posterior capitellum
- Lateral ulnar collateral ligament (LUCL) tear common
- LUCL tear, posterolateral rotating instability (PLRI) predisposing
- Supracondylar fracture associated

PATHOLOGY

General Features
- General path comments
  - Extension injury more common (95% of cases) than flexion type
  - Is extraarticular in children but may be intraarticular in adults

SUPRACONDYLAR FRACTURE

- Brachial artery and median nerve are vulnerable to traction over angulated fracture fragment
- Etiology
  - Hyperextension form - fall onto extended forearm
  - Flexion type - fall onto point of elbow
- Epidemiology
  - Accounts for about 60% of pediatric elbow fractures
  - Rare in adults (< 3%)
  - Common in nondominant side (1.5:1)
- Associated abnormalities
  - Other elbow fractures, esp. olecranon and medial condylar
  - Distal radial fracture (5-6%)
  - Olecranon avulsion fracture
  - Medial condyle impaction
  - Traction injuries to brachial artery (0.5%) and anterior interosseous branch of median nerve (4%)
  - Median neuropathy

Gross Pathologic & Surgical Features
- Oblique transverse fracture through thin aspect of distal humerus between medial and lateral pillars
- Failure of anterior cortex (tensile side)
- Plastic deformity of posterior cortex (compression side)
- Posterior rotation +/- varus malalignment

Microscopic Features
- Disruption of cortex and trabeculae
- Hemorrhage with cellular infiltrate ranging from osteoblasts and osteoclasts to inflammatory cells
  - Infiltrate contains osteoblasts, osteoclasts, and inflammatory cells
  - Depends on fracture age

Staging, Grading or Classification Criteria
- Flexion or extension fracture (extension in 96% of fractures)
- Based on classification of Gartland (for extension injuries)
  - Type I: Nondisplaced fracture (30%)
  - Type II: Displaced but intact posterior cortex (24%)
  - Type III: Displaced plus complete cortical disruption (45%)

CLINICAL ISSUES

Presentation
- Most common signs/symptoms
  - Pain and loss of function
  - Swelling and discoloration
  - Decreased distal pulse
- Clinical Profile: Normal, active child

Demographics
- Age
  - Common in children < 10 years old
  - Median age of incidence = 6 years
  - Only when seen in non-ambulatory infants are such fractures suggestive of abuse
- Gender: M > F

Natural History & Prognosis
- Return of function in over 90%
- Temporary nerve impairment in 10-16% but most recover
- Return of range of motion may take a year
- Neurovascular injuries in displaced supracondylar fractures
  - Anterior interosseous branch of median nerve
  - Radial nerve
  - Brachial artery
- Use of crossed pins may increase incidence of nerve injury
- Olecranon osteotomy reduces functional outcome compared to triceps splitting approach to open reduction with internal fixation (ORIF)

Treatment
- Conservative
  - Type I, splinting in 90 degrees flexion
- Surgical
  - Type II and III = percutaneous lateral pin fixation or ORIF with cross pinning
    - ORIF may be needed in up to 20%
- Complications
  - Failure of reduction
  - Vascular injury (rare)
  - Median nerve injury (traumatic and iatrogenic – up to 5%)
  - Volkmann's contracture secondary to unrecognized untreated acute vascular injury
  - Cubitus varus most common complication (Baumann angle 2-5 degrees greater than unaffected side)
  - Loss of function

DIAGNOSTIC CHECKLIST

Consider
- Presence of other fractures, especially olecranon and medial epicondyle
- Associated vascular and neural injuries

SELECTED REFERENCES

1. Gosens T et al: Neurovascular complications and functional outcome in displaced supracondylar fractures of the humerus in children. Injury .34(4):267-73, 2003
2. O'Driscoll SW et al: Difficult elbow fractures. Pearls and pitfalls. Instr Course Lect. 52:113-34, 2003
3. Cheng JC et al: Epidemiological features of supracondylar fractures of the humerus in Chinese children. J Pediatr Orthop B. 10(1):63-7, 2001
4. Skaggs DL et al: Operative treatment of supracondylar fractures of the humerus in children. The consequences of pin placement. J Bone Joint Surg Am. 83-A(5):735-40, 2001
5. McKee MD et al: Functional outcome after open supracondylar fractures of the humerus. The effect of the surgical approach. J Bone Joint Surg Br. 82(5):646-51, 2000
6. O'Hara LJ et al: Displaced supracondylar fractures of the humerus in children. Audit changes practice. J Bone Joint Surg Br. 82(2):204-10, 2000
7. Sonin A et al: Fractures of the elbow and forearm. Semin Musculoskelet Radiol. 4(2):171-91, 2000

SUPRACONDYLAR FRACTURE

IMAGE GALLERY

Typical

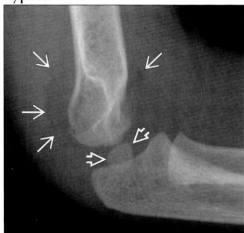
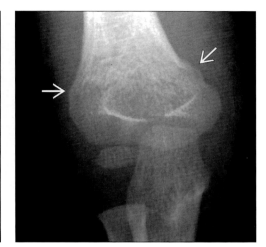

(Left) Lateral radiograph shows anterior and posterior fat pad signs *(arrows)*. Capitellum *(open arrows)* is displaced posterior to anterior humoral line. *(Right)* Anteroposterior radiograph shows subtle buckling of metaphyseal cortex *(arrows)* due to supracondylar fracture in same child.

Typical

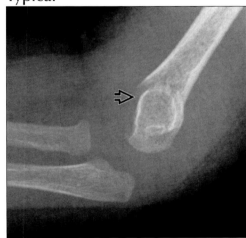
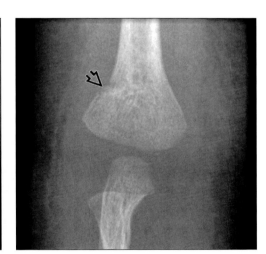

(Left) Lateral radiograph shows interruption of anterior metaphyseal cortex *(arrow)* and posterior rotation of distal humerus in abused 5 month old baby. *(Right)* Anteroposterior radiograph shows cortical interruption *(arrow)* of lateral metaphysis in same baby.

Typical

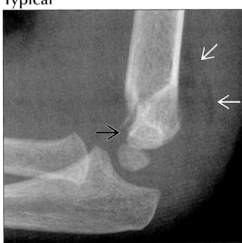
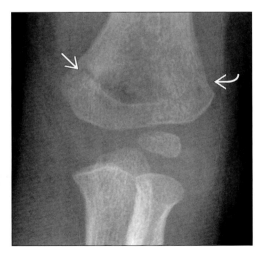

(Left) Lateral radiograph shows an elevated posterior fat pad *(white arrows)* and an anterior cortical interruption *(black arrow)*. Capitellum is displaced posterior to anterior humeral line. *(Right)* Anteroposterior radiograph shows medial fracture line *(arrow)* and lateral cortical angulation *(curved arrow)* in same patient.

TODDLER'S FRACTURES

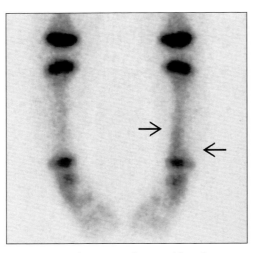

Anteroposterior bone scan shows toddler's fracture as increased uptake (arrows) in the distal left tibia of a 17 month toddler who refuses to walk.

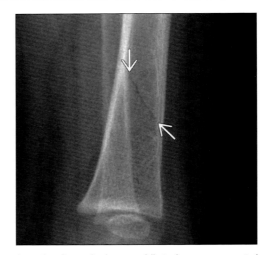

Lateral radiograph shows toddler's fracture as a spiral fracture (arrows) of tibia in same child.

TERMINOLOGY

Definitions
- A clinically subtle lower extremity fracture in a toddler or young child that results in refusal to bear weight, gait disturbance, or inability to walk
- Most common sites for a toddler's fracture are midshaft of tibia, proximal tibia, cuboid, and calcaneus

IMAGING FINDINGS

General Features
- Best diagnostic clue: Hairline spiral fracture of tibia or sclerotic band in a tarsal bone
- Location
  - Tibia
    - Toddler's fracture, type 1: Twisting of foot on leg → spiral fracture, usually in distal third
    - Toddler's fracture, type 2: Knee hyperextension → upper tibial metadiaphysis distraction fracture of posterior cortex and compression of anterior cortex
    - Type 2 may be due to child abuse: Consider possibility if seen in non-ambulatory child
    - Buckle fracture: Distal metaphysis
  - Fibula
    - Distal metadiaphysis
  - Calcaneus
    - Near apophysis (vertical) or along base (horizontal)
  - Talus
    - Neck and body
  - Cuboid
    - Near calcaneus head
  - Metatarsals
    - Shafts and bases
- Size: Usually subtle

Radiographic Findings
- Radiography
  - Overview
    - Normality or only subtle soft tissue swelling may be present in first 7-10 days after injury
    - Periosteal reaction and callus appear eventually (except in fibular plastic-bowing fractures) in tibia, fibula, and metatarsals after 10-14 days
    - Sclerotic bands due to trabecular microcallus appear during healing in metatarsals, tarsals, or tibia
    - Plastic bowing fractures may heal without callus or periosteal reaction
    - Often initial radiographs may be normal and sclerosis or callus formation seen on follow-up radiographs

DDx: Lesions Causing Leg Pain

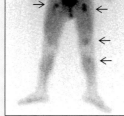
Neuroblastoma

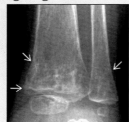
Leukemia

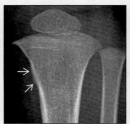
Osteomyelitis

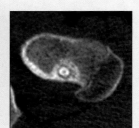
Osteoid Osteoma

TODDLER'S FRACTURES

Key Facts

Terminology
- A clinically subtle lower extremity fracture in a toddler or young child that results in refusal to bear weight, gait disturbance, or inability to walk

Imaging Findings
- Best diagnostic clue: Hairline spiral fracture of tibia or sclerotic band in a tarsal bone
- Type 1 tibial fracture: Spiral hairline fracture often better seen on oblique views
- Type 2 tibial fracture: Buckling of anterior cortex, deepening of tibial tubercle notch, anterior tilt of epiphyseal plate, transverse fracture of posterior cortex
- Bone scan highly sensitive
- > 50% of bone-scan leg abnormalities in children ≤ 5 years are in tarsal bones

Clinical Issues
- Tibia spiral fracture: Gently twisting foot with knee stable (→ tibial torsion) causes pain
- Tarsal fracture: Direct pressure painful
- Metatarsal fracture: Pain when squeezing metatarsals, or when applying axial pressure from each toe towards heel
- Age: 9 months to 5 years

Diagnostic Checklist
- Normal-side comparison views when subtle plastic bowing or buckle fractures suspected

---

- Tibia
  - Type 1 tibial fracture: Spiral hairline fracture often better seen on oblique views
  - Soft-tissue swelling frequent
  - Cortical sclerosis and periosteal reaction eventually
  - Type 2 tibial fracture: Buckling of anterior cortex, deepening of tibial tubercle notch, anterior tilt of epiphyseal plate, transverse fracture of posterior cortex
  - May appear as lucent line or sclerotic band
- Fibula
  - Plastic-bowing and buckle fractures
- Tarsals
  - Cortical: Cortical interruption or buckle fractures
  - Cancellous: Trabecular interruption or compression fractures
- Calcaneus
  - Vertical sclerotic band parallel to apophysis of calcaneus in subcortical marrow space
  - Horizontal sclerotic band parallel to base of calcaneus
  - Similar lesion may occur after cast removed for other fracture and activity resumed
- Cuboid
  - Sclerotic band in subcortical marrow parallel to most proximal cortex
  - Similar lesion may occur after cast removed for other fracture and activity resumed
- Metatarsals
  - Buckle or corner fracture of first metatarsal due to jumping
  - Metatarsal buckle fractures may be multiple

CT Findings
- NECT
  - Intravenous contrast not necessary
  - Thin collimation (1.25 or 2.5 mm)
  - Reconstructed sagittal and coronal images may be helpful in identifying fracture line
  - Often best to include both extremities in field of view for contralateral comparison
  - Abnormal areas of sclerosis or lucency may be way more obvious with comparison side present
  - May be used to demonstrate fracture when tumor or osteomyelitis are other possibilities
  - May show lucent line of fracture
  - If subacute, may show surrounding sclerotic band, cortical thickening or periosteal reaction

Nuclear Medicine Findings
- Bone Scan
  - Bone scan highly sensitive
    - Become positive in 1-2 days
    - Useful for demonstrating all the various toddler's fractures
  - Wide field of view
  - Anesthesia not needed
  - > 50% of bone-scan leg abnormalities in children ≤ 5 years are in tarsal bones

Other Modality Findings
- MR
  - T1WI: Marrow edema and hemorrhage are hypointense
  - T2WI: Marrow edema and hemorrhage are hyperintense
  - Fracture seen as hypointense linear structure with marked surrounding soft tissue and marrow edema
  - No associated soft tissue mass

Imaging Recommendations
- Best imaging tool
  - Radiographs initially, bone scan if radiographs normal
  - Also consider repeat radiographs in 10-14 days if persistent unexplained symptoms
  - CT for evaluation/further characterization of sclerotic lesions
- Protocol advice
  - CT
    - Consider including contralateral leg in field of view for comparison
    - Thin collimation
    - Sagittal and coronal reformats of axial data

TODDLER'S FRACTURES

DIFFERENTIAL DIAGNOSIS

Osteomyelitis
- Most common in children < 5 years of age
  - Femur, tibia, fibular frequently involved
- If chronic, may present with sclerosis but will not typically be linear
- May have sequestrum or sinus tract

Osteoid osteoma
- Area of sclerosis and cortical thickening
- Central lucent nidus (round) rather than linear lucency

Leukemia and neuroblastoma
- First sign of skeletal involvement may be refusal to walk
- Horizontal lucent line in metaphysis
- Typically wider and more poorly defined compared with stress fracture

Septic arthritis
- Most commonly in the hip joint
- Age peak during infancy

Toxic synovitis of the hip
- Occurs most commonly < 10 years of age

Juvenile rheumatoid arthritis
- Peak age of onset 1-3 years of age
- Commonly affects knee and hip

Child abuse
- Very uncommon for abuse to mimic a toddler's fracture

PATHOLOGY

General Features
- Etiology
  - Compression
    - Tarsal and metatarsal fractures
    - Plastic-bowing fractures of long bones
    - Jumping from a height may → first metatarsal corner or buckle fracture (bunk-bed fracture)
  - Torsion
    - Tibial type 1 spiral fracture
  - Bending
    - Tibial buckle fracture
    - Fibular buckle and plastic bowing fractures
  - Forceful hyperextension of knee
    - Tibial type 2 distraction-compression fracture
  - Forceful foot dorsiflexion
    - Talus neck fracture caused by tibial impingement
  - Forceful foot plantarflexion
    - Cuboid compression fracture
- Epidemiology
  - Toddler's type 1 fractures are youngest part of a spectrum of childhood accidental spiral tibial fractures occurring in children age 1-8 years
    - Mean age 4 years to 3 months
    - M:F = 69:31
    - Left:Right = 45.5:54.5

CLINICAL ISSUES

Presentation
- Most common signs/symptoms
  - Refusal to walk or bear weight
  - Physical examination
    - Tibia spiral fracture: Gently twisting foot with knee stable (→ tibial torsion) causes pain
    - Tarsal fracture: Direct pressure painful
    - Metatarsal fracture: Pain when squeezing metatarsals, or when applying axial pressure from each toe towards heel

Demographics
- Age: 9 months to 5 years

Natural History & Prognosis
- Rapid healing without deformity
  - Theoretical exception could be persistent anterior angulation of tibial epiphysis in tibial type 2 fractures

Treatment
- Options range from no treatment to long-leg cast

DIAGNOSTIC CHECKLIST

Consider
- Normal-side comparison views when subtle plastic bowing or buckle fractures suspected

Image Interpretation Pearls
- Toddler who refrains from bearing weight will commonly have toddler's fracture involving tibia or tarsal bones

SELECTED REFERENCES

1. Swischuk LE et al: Frequently missed fractures in children (value of comparative views). Emerg Radiol. 11(1):22-8, 2004
2. Connolly LP et al: Skeletal scintigraphy in the multimodality assessment of young children with acute skeletal symptoms. Clin Nucl Med. 28(9):746-54, 2003
3. Donnelly LF: Toddler's fracture of the fibula. AJR. 175:922, 2000
4. Kleinman PK: Occult hyperextension "toddler's" fracture by Swischuk, et al. Pediatr Radiol. 29(9):720, 1999
5. Mellick LB et al: Childhood accidental spiral tibial (CAST) fractures. Pediatr Emerg Care. 15(5):307-9, 1999
6. Swischuk LE et al: Upper tibial hyperextension fractures in infants: another occult toddler's fracture. Pediatr Radiol. 29(1):6-9, 1999
7. John SD et al: Expanding the concept of the toddler's fracture. Radiographics. 17(2):367-76, 1997
8. Schindler A et al: Occult fracture of the calcaneus in toddlers. J Pediatr Orthop. 16(2):201-5, 1996
9. Blumberg K et al: The toddler's cuboid fracture. Radiology. 179:93-4, 1991
10. Neumann L: Acute plastic bowing fractures of both the tibia and the fibula in a child. Injury. 21(2):122-3, 1990
11. Dunbar JS et al: Obscure tibial fractures of infants - the toddler's fracture. J Can Assoc Radiol 15:136-44, 1964

TODDLER'S FRACTURES

IMAGE GALLERY

Typical

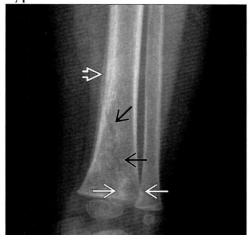
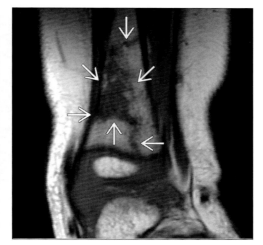

(Left) Anteroposterior radiograph shows healing tibial spiral fracture (black arrows) with cancellous bone sclerosis and periosteal reaction (open arrow). MR done to evaluate possible juxta-epiphyseal lesion (white arrows). (Right) Coronal T1WI shows irregular marrow hypointensity (arrows) due to fracture edema in same patient. No juxta-epiphyseal lesion was present.

Typical

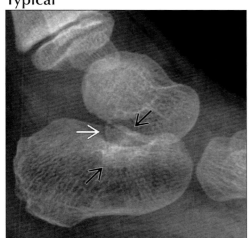
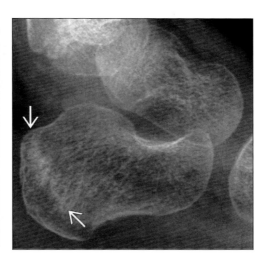

(Left) Lateral radiograph in 4 year old child shows a vertical fracture line (white arrow) in calcaneus with adjacent trabecular sclerosis (black arrows). (Right) Lateral radiograph shows band of trabecular sclerosis (arrows) due to formation of trabecular microcallus in calcaneus of a 3 year old child.

Typical

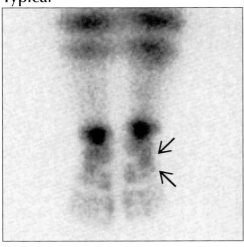
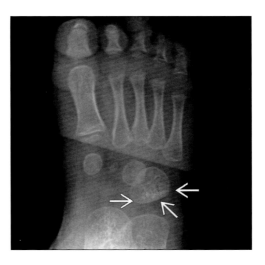

(Left) Anteroposterior bone scan shows subtle increased uptake (arrows) in the region of the cuboid in a 2 year old child. (Right) Anteroposterior radiograph in same child shows sclerotic band (arrows) in cuboid due to a healing fracture.

MEDIAL EPICONDYLE AVULSION

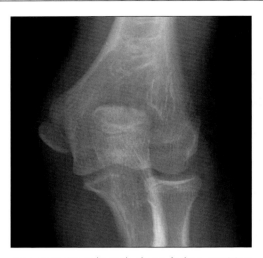
Anteroposterior radiograph shows findings suspicious for an acute avulsion injury of the medial epicondyle (ME), with soft tissue swelling.

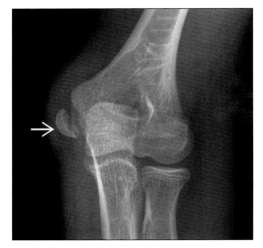
Oblique radiograph in the same patient shows widening of the physis & avulsion of the ME (arrow) to better extent with associated soft tissue swelling.

TERMINOLOGY

Abbreviations and Synonyms
- Medial epicondylar (ME) avulsion, medial epicondylitis (apophysitis), little leaguer's elbow, pitcher's elbow, golfer's elbow, medial tennis elbow

Definitions
- Acute injury
  - Medial epicondylar avulsion
- Chronic stress injury: Golfer's elbow, pitcher's elbow, little leaguer's elbow, medial tennis elbow
  - Degeneration of the common flexor tendon secondary to overload caused by chronic valgus stress

IMAGING FINDINGS

General Features
- Best diagnostic clue: Displaced medial epicondyle ossification center in the acute injury
- Location
  - Medial elbow
  - +/- Entrapped between olecranon & trochlea after elbow dislocation
- Size: Displacement > 5 mm, surgical open reduction
- Morphology
  - Ossification pattern on radiographs
    - Capitellum 1st: 1-2 years old
    - Medial epicondyle: 4-7 years old
    - Trochlea: 8 years
    - Lateral epicondyle: 10-11 years
    - Radial head: 3-6 years
    - Olecranon: 6-12 years
  - Should see medial epicondyle on AP radiograph if trochlea is identified
    - Helps to exclude an entrapped medial epicondyle, can simulate the trochlear ossification center
  - Medial epicondyle apophysis fuses with medial condyle by 18-20 years old
    - Does not contribute to longitudinal growth

Radiographic Findings
- Radiography
  - Displacement of the medial epicondyle in acute injuries
  - Enlargement, sclerosis, fragmentation, widened physis in chronic repetitive injuries
  - Unreliable fat pad sign
    - Older children > 2 year old, medial epicondyle becomes extracapsular
    - May be positive if there are other fractures
    - +/- In elbow dislocation, depends on if the capsule is disrupted

DDx: Spectrum Of Radiographic Findings In Adolescent Pitchers

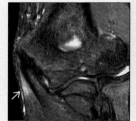
Palmaris Longus Strain

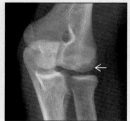
Capitellar OCD

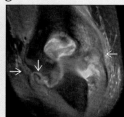
MCL Tear

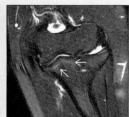
Olecranon Stress Injury

MEDIAL EPICONDYLE AVULSION

Key Facts

Terminology
- Medial epicondylar (ME) avulsion, medial epicondylitis (apophysitis), little leaguer's elbow, pitcher's elbow, golfer's elbow, medial tennis elbow
- Acute injury
- Medial epicondylar avulsion
- Chronic stress injury: Golfer's elbow, pitcher's elbow, little leaguer's elbow, medial tennis elbow
- Degeneration of the common flexor tendon secondary to overload caused by chronic valgus stress

Imaging Findings
- Should see medial epicondyle on AP radiograph if trochlea is identified
- Helps to exclude an entrapped medial epicondyle, can simulate the trochlear ossification center
- AP & lateral radiographs to exclude an acute avulsion
- T1, FS PD FSE (best), FS T2 FSE &/or STIR for ligament/tendon evaluation

Pathology
- Medial epicondyle avulsion; incidence of up to 50% in elbow dislocations
- Ulnar nerve injury in dislocation (25-50%)
- Trapped medial epicondyle in the elbow joint following dislocation (up to 20%)

Diagnostic Checklist
- Should see medial epicondyle when trochlear ossification center is identified
- Displaced medial epicondyle can simulate the trochlear ossification center

---

  - Prior to ossification center appearing radiographically
    - Flake of bone from metaphysis
    - Localized medial soft tissue swelling
    - Joint effusion

MR Findings
- T2WI
  - Medial tension overload
    - Increased signal intensity within the common flexor tendon origin at the medial epicondyle
    - Thickened tendon
  - Hyperintense water signal intensity within the tendon in the case of a partial tear or complete tears
    - FS T2WI FSE or STIR images demonstrate the increased signal to best advantage
    - Hyperintense signal within the common flexor muscle belly in the case of muscle strain
    - Avulsion of medial epicondyle in skeletally immature individuals
    - Strains & tears of the ulnar collateral ligament
  - Ulnar neuritis
    - Hyperintense T2WI signal & thickening of the ulnar nerve usually within the cubital tunnel
  - Lateral compression
    - Osteochondral injuries of the humeral capitellum
    - Hyperintense signal in capitellum on T2 weighted images
    - May see chondromalacia & underlying bone marrow edema or cysts
    - Loose bodies may be present
  - Hyperintense signal in the medial epicondyle in little leaguer's elbow
    - Often associated tendon strain
- STIR: Hyperintense signal in strain & tears
- T2* GRE: Widened & irregular physis in chronic injuries

Ultrasonographic Findings
- Grayscale Ultrasound: To assess displacement prior to ossification center appearing radiographically

Imaging Recommendations
- Best imaging tool
  - AP & lateral radiographs 1st
    - If still questionable 10-15° oblique view for acute avulsion
    - Avulsed fragment usually displaces inferiorly
- Protocol advice
  - AP & lateral radiographs to exclude an acute avulsion
  - T1, FS PD FSE (best), FS T2 FSE &/or STIR for ligament/tendon evaluation

DIFFERENTIAL DIAGNOSIS

Medial collateral ligament injury
- Valgus extension, overload injury
- Tear: Disruption of continuous linear hypointense signal
  - Best imaging sequence: FS PD FSE
  - Partial tears: "T" sign
- Strain: Continuous linear hypointense signal

Flexor or pronator muscle injury/strain
- Common in throwing athlete

Olecranon stress injury
- Common in throwing athlete
- Valgus stress injury
- Marrow edema with olecranon T2WI or STIR

Capitellar osteochondritis dissecans
- 12-17 year old
- Lateral elbow pain, diffuse elbow pain worsens with activity
- Valgus stress

Ulnar neuritis
- Hyperintense T2WI signal & thickening of the ulnar nerve usually within the cubital tunnel

Flexor or pronator muscle strain/tear
- Medial elbow pain

MEDIAL EPICONDYLE AVULSION

- Throwing athlete

Loose bodies
- Acute or repetitive injury

PATHOLOGY

General Features
- Etiology
  - Chronic injury
    - Overuse syndrome found in athletes participating in throwing sports
    - Due to repeated valgus stress causing tendon degeneration
    - Strain → tendinosis → tear
  - Children
    - In children the injury is often to the medial epicondyle itself manifesting as a stress fracture or avulsion of the epicondyle
  - Mechanism for avulsion
    - Forceful contraction of the pronator & flexor muscle groups of the forearm
    - Fall on an outstretched arm with the elbow flexed & hand extended
    - Posterior/lateral elbow dislocation (50-55%)
- Epidemiology: Avulsion: 10% of all elbow fractures
- Associated abnormalities
  - Medial epicondyle avulsion; incidence of up to 50% in elbow dislocations
    - Ulnar nerve injury in dislocation (25-50%)
  - Trapped medial epicondyle in the elbow joint following dislocation (up to 20%)

Gross Pathologic & Surgical Features
- Thickening of the tendon, +/- macroscopic partial tearing or through-and-through tearing
- Avulsed epicondyle in the case of some children
- May include tear of the ulnar collateral ligament

Microscopic Features
- Microscopic tendon degeneration with macroscopic partial or complete tear surrounded by hemorrhage and inflammation

CLINICAL ISSUES

Presentation
- Most common signs/symptoms: Elbow pain
- Other signs/symptoms
  - Palpable freely mobile medial epicondyle
  - Crepitus
  - Athlete participating in throwing sports with onset of medial elbow pain
  - Medial epicondylar pain, increased by valgus stress to elbow (little leaguer's elbow)

Demographics
- Age
  - Avulsion injury: 9-14 year old
  - Older children, near skeletal maturity tend to injury tendons/ligaments similar to adults
- Gender: M > F = 4:1

Natural History & Prognosis
- Good prognosis
- If nonunion occurs may lead to instability

Treatment
- Medial epicondyle avulsion, acute injury
  - Minimally displaced: Immobilization
  - > 5 mm open reduction & pin fixation
  - Surgery for valgus instability
- Chronic tension stress injury
  - Physical therapy and steroid injection with decrease in physical activity
  - Tendon release
  - Tendon repair

DIAGNOSTIC CHECKLIST

Image Interpretation Pearls
- Should see medial epicondyle when trochlear ossification center is identified
  - Displaced medial epicondyle can simulate the trochlear ossification center

SELECTED REFERENCES

1. Kijowski R et al: Radiography of the elbow for evaluation of patients with osteochondritis dissecans of the capitellum. Skeletal Radiol. 34(5):266-71, 2005
2. Kijowski R et al: Magnetic resonance imaging of the elbow. Part I: normal anatomy, imaging technique, and osseous abnormalities. Skeletal Radiol. 33(12):685-97, 2004
3. Williams RJ 3rd et al: Medial collateral ligament tears in the throwing athlete. Instr Course Lect. 53:579-86, 2004
4. Ahmad CS et al: Valgus extension overload syndrome and stress injury of the olecranon. Clin Sports Med. 23(4):665-76, x, 2004
5. Cain EL Jr et al: Elbow injuries in throwing athletes: a current concepts review. Am J Sports Med. 31(4):621-35, 2003
6. Parr TJ et al: Overuse injuries of the olecranon in adolescents. Orthopedics. 26(11):1143-6, 2003
7. Klingele KE et al: Little league elbow: valgus overload injury in the paediatric athlete. Sports Med. 32(15):1005-15, 2002
8. Gilchrist AD et al: Valgus instability of the elbow due to medial epicondyle nonunion: treatment by fragment excision and ligament repair--a report of 5 cases. J Shoulder Elbow Surg. 11(5):493-7, 2002
9. Chen FS et al: Medial elbow problems in the overhead-throwing athlete. J Am Acad Orthop Surg. 9(2):99-113, 2001
10. Kocher MS et al: Upper extremity injuries in the paediatric athlete. Sports Med. 30(2):117-35, 2000
11. Ciccotti MG: Epicondylitis in the athlete. Instr Course Lect. 48:375-81, 1999
12. Fritz RC: MR imaging of sports injuries of the elbow. Magn Reson Imaging Clin N Am, 7(1):51-72, viii, 1999
13. Fowles JV et al: Elbow dislocation with avulsion of the medial humeral epicondyle. J Bone Joint Surg Br. 72(1):102-4, 1990
14. Harrison RB et al: Radiographic clues to fractures of the unossified medial humeral condyle in young children. Skeletal Radiol. 11(3):209-12, 1984
15. Loomer RL: Elbow injuries in athletes. Can J Appl Sport Sci. 7(3):164-6, 1982

MEDIAL EPICONDYLE AVULSION

IMAGE GALLERY

Typical

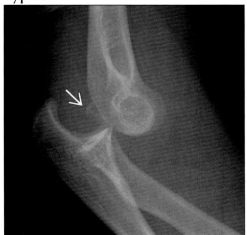
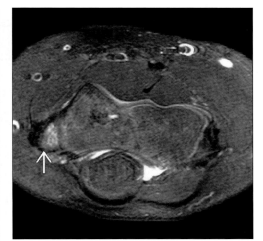

(Left) Lateral radiograph shows an elbow dislocation & an avulsed medial epicondyle (elbow). On subsequent post reduction images this fragment was not entrapped. *(Right)* Axial T2WI MR shows hyperintense signal within the medial epicondyle (arrow) most consistent with medial epicondylitis (apophysitis).

Typical

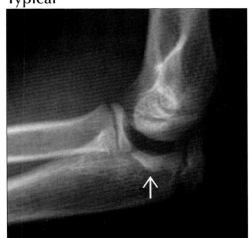
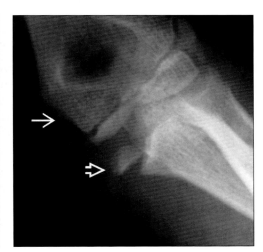

(Left) Lateral radiograph shows a double density over the olecranon (arrow), entrapped avulsed medial epicondyle. *(Right)* Anteroposterior radiograph in the same child shows absence of the normal location of the medial epiphyseal ossification center (arrow) while the trochlea is ossified. The entrapped fragment is seen within the mildly widened medial elbow joint (open arrow).

Typical

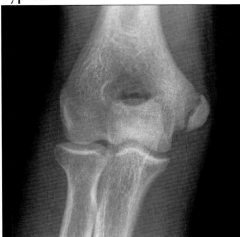
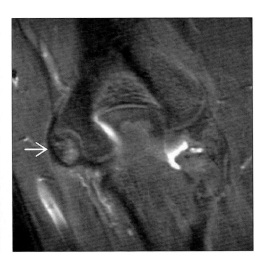

(Left) Anteroposterior radiograph shows a mildly sclerotic medial epicondyle with irregularity & widening of the adjacent physis, medial epicondylitis in this pitcher with chronic recurrent elbow pain. *(Right)* Coronal T2WI MR shows mild hyperintense signal within the medial epicondyle (arrow), epicondylitis in this pitcher with symptomatic medial elbow pain.

OSGOOD-SCHLATTER LESION

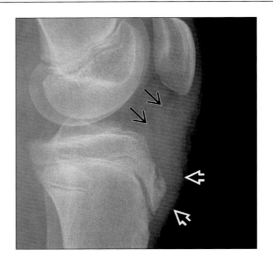

Lateral radiograph shows an indistinct outline of patellar tendon. Edema (arrows) extends into infrapatellar fat pad. Tibial tubercle fragmentation and edema (open arrows) is present.

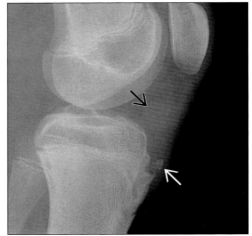

Lateral radiograph shows ossicle avulsed from the tibial tubercle (white arrow). Edema extends into infrapatellar fat pad (black arrow) and patellar tendon.

TERMINOLOGY

Abbreviations and Synonyms
- Osgood-Schlatter disease (OSD), tibial osteochondrosis

Definitions
- Traction apophysitis of patellar tendon insertion on tibial tubercle

IMAGING FINDINGS

General Features
- Best diagnostic clue
  - Radiographs: Tibial tubercle fragmentation with overlying soft tissue edema
  - Acute: Increased signal intensity on FS PD images
    - Within and around the distal patellar tendon at its insertion on tibial tubercle
    - Variable amounts of fluid within surrounding infrapatellar bursa
  - Deep infrapatellar bursa can normally contain a small amount of fluid and should not be confused with OSD
- Location: Tibial tubercle apophysis and distal patellar tendon
- Size: Tibial tubercle and patellar tendon of normal size or enlarged
- Morphology
  - +/- Hypertrophy of tibial tubercle
  - +/- Distension of deep and/or superficial infrapatellar bursa
  - +/- Thickening of the distal patellar tendon
  - +/- Fragmentation of the tibial tubercle

Radiographic Findings
- Radiography
  - Greater than 4 mm soft tissue swelling over the anterior proximal surface of tibia
    - Soft tissue swelling is key to radiographic diagnosis as fragmentation and ossicles can be seen in normal patients
  - Thickening and indistinctness of inferior patellar tendon
  - Ossicle at tibial tubercle in 30-50% of cases
  - +/- Fragmentation of tubercle
    - Fragmentation can also be seen in normal patients
  - Hypertrophy of the tibial tubercle on lateral view

CT Findings
- NECT
  - Not typically used for diagnosis of OSD
  - Hypertrophic tibial tubercle
  - +/- Fragmentation of ossific nucleus, on sagittal reconstruction views
  - Sagittal and 3D reconstruction helpful

DDx: Tendon Orgin-Insertion Abnormalities

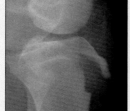

Tubercle Avulsion

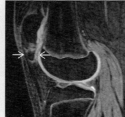

SLJ Disease

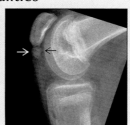

SLJ Disease

OSGOOD-SCHLATTER LESION

Key Facts

Terminology
- Traction apophysitis of patellar tendon insertion on tibial tubercle

Imaging Findings
- Greater than 4 mm soft tissue swelling over the anterior proximal surface of tibia
- Soft tissue swelling is key to radiographic diagnosis as fragmentation and ossicles can be seen in normal patients
- Thickening and indistinctness of inferior patellar tendon
- Ossicle at tibial tubercle in 30-50% of cases
- High signal edema in tibial tubercle, inferior patellar tendon, and surrounding soft tissues including Hoffa's fat pad and anterior to tubercle
- Diagnosis often made clinically
- MR findings of OSD may be seen if MRI of knee obtained for nonspecific knee pain

Top Differential Diagnoses
- Isolated deep or superficial infrapatellar bursitis
- Patellar tendonitis
- Sinding-Larsen-Johansson disease (SLJ disease)

Clinical Issues
- Most common signs/symptoms: Insidious onset of low-grade ache localized to tibial tubercle associated with physical activity

Diagnostic Checklist
- Hypertrophied, edematous tibial tubercle on FS PD FSE key for diagnosis

MR Findings
- T1WI
  - Hypertrophy and/or fragmentation of tibial tubercle
  - Fragmentation of ossific nucleus with a discrete ossicle
  - Heterotopic ossification within the distal patellar tendon
- T2WI
  - High signal edema in tibial tubercle, inferior patellar tendon, and surrounding soft tissues including Hoffa's fat pad and anterior to tubercle
  - Distension of the deep and/or superficial infrapatellar bursae indicating reactive bursitis
  - FS PD FSE and T2* GRE are most sensitive sequences
    - Signal increase is variable: From intermediate to hyperintense (subchondral edema of tibial tubercle)
    - Thickening of the distal patellar tendon with increase in signal intensity
- Diagnosis often made clinically
  - MR findings of OSD may be seen if MRI of knee obtained for nonspecific knee pain

Nuclear Medicine Findings
- Bone Scan: Positive in cases of tubercle apophysitis

Imaging Recommendations
- Best imaging tool
  - Usually clinical diagnosis
  - Radiographs can be used to document fragmentation and overlying soft tissue swelling
  - Edema and tendon tears are identified on FS PD FSE, T2* GRE or STIR images
- Protocol advice: FS PD FSE in sagittal and axial plane

DIFFERENTIAL DIAGNOSIS

Isolated deep or superficial infrapatellar bursitis
- Adults with kneeling occupations
  - Older age group compared to OSD
- Fluid-signal intensity on T2WI

Patellar tendonitis
- Jumper's knee
- Same age group and similar circumstances as OSD
- May be differentiated by MRI in many cases

Sinding-Larsen-Johansson disease (SLJ disease)
- Traction apophysitis of inferior pole of patella
- Irregular and sometimes fragmented appearance of inferior patella
  - Bony avulsion
  - Soft tissue calcification/ossification
  - Elongation of inferior pole of patella
- Indistinctness of superior patellar tendon (rather than inferior as in OSD)
- Painful region at patellar level, above tibial tubercle

PATHOLOGY

General Features
- General path comments: Traction apophysitis
- Etiology
  - Repetitive microtraction trauma
    - Anterior tibial tubercle
    - During formation of secondary ossification center
  - Multiple submaximal avulsion fractures of patellar tendon insertion caused by traction microtrauma
    - Occurs particularly during eccentric contractions of strong extensor mechanism
    - Common in jumping sports: Basketball and volleyball – boys; gymnastics, soccer, other jumping sports - girls
- Associated abnormalities: Patellar tendon tears (partial tears) in some cases
- Distribution: Young active patients

Gross Pathologic & Surgical Features
- Thickened, indurated patellar tendon
- Multiple ossific bodies may be present within the tendon or about the tubercle

OSGOOD-SCHLATTER LESION

Microscopic Features
- Focal tendon collagen degeneration
- Tendon microtears
- Influx of inflammatory cells in surrounding soft tissues
- Bursal synovial hypertrophy and inflammatory infiltrate
- Heterotopic bone formation and/or fragmentation
- Three normal histologic zones within immature tibial tubercle
  - Proximal: Columnar cartilage
  - Midzone: Fibrocartilage
  - Distal: Fibrous tissue blending with tibial perichondrium
- Physiologic epiphysiodesis of tibial tubercle starts proximally and extends centrifugally and distally

CLINICAL ISSUES

Presentation
- Most common signs/symptoms: Insidious onset of low-grade ache localized to tibial tubercle associated with physical activity
- Clinical Profile
  - Young active patient with anterior knee pain
  - Bilateral 20-30%
  - Symptoms occur during rapid growth period as tibial tubercle is maturing
  - Aggravated by acceleration/deceleration, direct blows
  - Tubercle prominence often bilateral although symptoms are usually unilateral
  - +/- Tenderness also around patella and patellar tendon
  - Quadriceps atrophy
  - Extensor lag
  - Resisted knee extension causes pain
  - Tightness
    - Quadriceps
    - Hamstrings
    - Gastrocnemius
    - Iliotibial band

Demographics
- Age
  - Typically occurs at onset of adolescent growth spurt
    - Boys: 10-15 years old
    - Girls: 8-13 years old
- Gender: M > F

Natural History & Prognosis
- Usually self-limited
- Patellar tendinitis and bursitis are common sources of pain independent of fracture healing
- Residual hypertrophy of the tibial tubercle or fragmentation
- Ossification within the patellar tendon
- Prognosis excellent
- Post-surgical prognosis improved in older child near skeletal maturity

Treatment
- Conservative
  - Rest from offending activity
  - Exercises to restore strength and flexibility of extensor mechanism
  - Non-steroidal anti-inflammatory medication
- Surgical
  - For recalcitrant cases
  - For those patients with ossification around the tibial tubercle or within the patellar tendon
  - Tuberosity debulking
  - Linear osteotomy with excision of the tuberosity
  - Bone plug placement: Less common
  - Tuberosity drilling: Less common
- Complications: Excision before skeletal maturity can result in
  - Residual prominence of the tubercle
  - Decreased range of motion
  - Genu recurvatum deformity
    - Due to premature fusion of the tubercle

DIAGNOSTIC CHECKLIST

Consider
- Uncomplicated patellar tendonitis in absence of tuberosity changes

Image Interpretation Pearls
- Hypertrophied, edematous tibial tubercle on FS PD FSE key for diagnosis

SELECTED REFERENCES
1. Adirim TA et al: Overview of injuries in the young athlete. Sports Med. 33(1):75-81, 2003
2. Delee J et al: Orthopaedic Sports Medicine. Hip and Pelvis. vol 1. 2nd ed. Philadelphia PA, Saunders, 25:1443-80, 2003
3. Olivieri I et al: Enthesitis of spondylarthritis can masquerade as Osgood-Schlatter disease by radiographic findings. Arthritis Rheum. 49(1):147-8, 2003
4. Duri ZA et al: The immature athlete. Clin Sports Med. 21(3):461-82, 2002
5. Hirano A et al: Magnetic resonance imaging of Osgood-Schlatter disease. The course of the disease. Skeletal Radiol. 31(6):334-42, 2002
6. Orava S et al: Results of surgical treatment of unresolved Osgood-Schlatter lesion. Ann Chir Gynaecol. 89(4):298-302, 2000
7. de Inocencio J: Musculoskeletal pain in primary pediatric care: Analysis of 1000 consecutive general pediatric clinic visits. Pediatrics. 102(6):E63, 1998
8. Nowinski RJ et al: Hyphenated history: Osgood-Schlatter disease. Am J Orthop. 27(8):584-5, 1998
9. Aparicio G et al: Radiologic study of patellar height in Osgood-Schlatter disease. J Pediatr Orthop. 17(1):63-6, 1997
10. McCarroll JR et al: Anterior cruciate ligament reconstruction in athletes with an ossicle associated with Osgood-Schlatter's disease. Arthroscopy. 12(5):556-60, 1996

OSGOOD-SCHLATTER LESION

IMAGE GALLERY

Typical

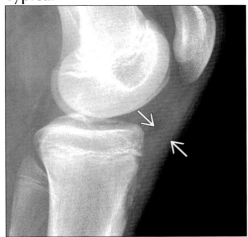
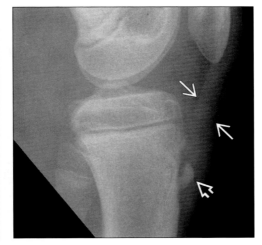

(Left) Lateral radiograph shows tibial tubercle is fragmented. Lower part of the patellar tendon is swollen (arrows) and its outline is indistinct. *(Right)* Lateral radiograph shows bone fragment (open arrow) almost separate from tubercle. Lower patellar tendon is swollen (arrows) and its anterior outline is indistinct.

Typical

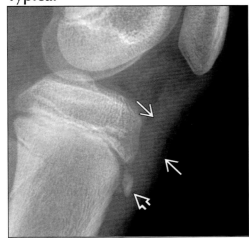
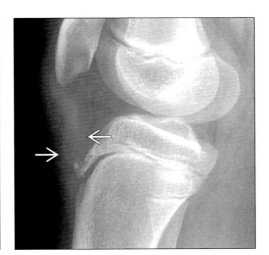

(Left) Lateral radiograph shows the lower 2/3 of the patellar tendon is swollen (arrows). A separate, perhaps avulsed, ossicle (open arrow) is part of tibial tubercle. *(Right)* Lateral radiograph shows lower part of the patellar tendon is swollen (arrows) and its outlines are indistinct. Some fragmentation of tibial tubercle is seen.

Typical

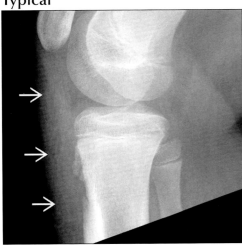
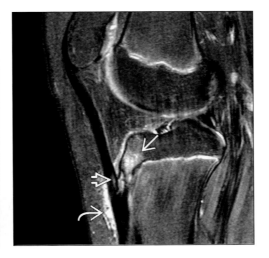

(Left) Lateral radiograph shows the outline of the patellar tendon is indistinct and the subcutaneous tissue anterior to the patellar tendon is edematous (arrows). *(Right)* Sagittal T2 TSE MR shows edema of subcutaneous tissue over patellar tendon (curved arrow), within the tendon (open arrow), and in tibial tubercle bone marrow (arrow).

CHRONIC FOREIGN BODY

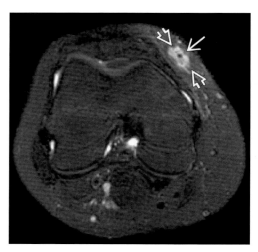

Axial T2WI MR shows area of high signal inflammatory change (open arrows) with square low signal area (arrow) in the center consistent with foreign body.

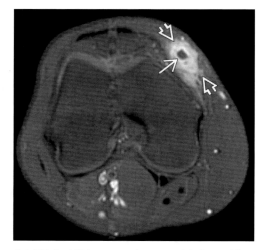

Axial T1 C+ MR in same patient as on left shows diffuse enhancement of inflammatory changes (open arrows) and low signal structure (arrow) in center consistent with foreign body.

TERMINOLOGY

Abbreviations and Synonyms
- Foreign body (FB) granuloma
- Chronic FB

Definitions
- Chronic foreign bodies may incite surrounding inflammation/granulation tissue and present as soft tissue mass
- May present well after the traumatic event that introduced the foreign body is forgotten

IMAGING FINDINGS

General Features
- Best diagnostic clue: Soft tissue mass on MR with central low signal focus
- Location
  o Introduced foreign bodies from minor trauma will most often be confined to the subcutaneous tissues
  o Tend to occur in areas prone to be injured
    ▪ Plantar aspect of feet: From children walking barefoot
    ▪ Anterior aspect over knee/shin: From falling on knee/shin
    ▪ Hands: From falling on outstretched arm
    ▪ Elbow: From falling on elbow
    ▪ Buttocks: From falling on buttocks

Radiographic Findings
- Radiography
  o In most cases, foreign body is not radiopaque and mass will appear as nonspecific soft tissue mass/fullness
  o May see radiopaque foreign body (approximately 3% of foreign bodies)
  o May see findings of associated osteomyelitis
  o Glass as a foreign body
    ▪ Most glass is radiopaque: One study took multiple pieces of glass from all different sources and placed in meat and radiographed
    ▪ Almost all types of glass were radiopaque
    ▪ Concept that only leaded glass is radiopqaue is incorrect

CT Findings
- Not typically used for identification of foreign bodies in soft tissues
- Orbit is an exception
  o If object penetrating orbit is wooden (such as a stick), wood typically appears as low attenuation (high air content) on CT examinations

DDx: Soft Tissue Mass

Fat Necrosis | *Osteosarcoma* | *ST Sarcoma* | *Agr Fibromatosis*

CHRONIC FOREIGN BODY

Key Facts

Terminology
- Chronic foreign bodies may incite surrounding inflammation/granulation tissue and present as soft tissue mass
- May present well after the traumatic event that introduced the foreign body is forgotten

Imaging Findings
- Introduced foreign bodies from minor trauma will most often be confined to the subcutaneous tissues
- Tend to occur in areas prone to be injured
- Plantar aspect of feet: From children walking barefoot
- Anterior aspect over knee/shin: From falling on knee/shin
- Hands: From falling on outstretched arm
- Elbow: From falling on elbow
- Buttocks: From falling on buttocks
- May see radiopaque foreign body (approximately 3% of foreign bodies)
- Ultrasound may identify chronic foreign or acute foreign bodies in subcutaneous tissues
- If geographic focus of low signal identified in middle of high T2WI soft tissue mass in subcutaneous tissue, think chronic foreign body

Top Differential Diagnoses
- Soft tissue malignancy
- Soft tissue mass from primary bone tumor
- Post traumatic fat necrosis
- Hemangioma
- Vascular malformation

Pathology
- Granulomatous reaction surrounding foreign body

MR Findings
- May appear as nonspecific soft tissue mass (high in T2 weighted signal)
- Surrounding inflammation may enhance diffusely
- May have poorly-defined edema in adjacent soft tissues
  - Will appear as high T2 weighted signal
- Clues to foreign body as etiology
  - Low signal focus in central portion of soft tissue mass
  - Focus is low in signal on all sequences for most foreign bodies
    - Glass, plastic, metal, wood
  - May see metal artifact
  - Focus has non-anatomic, geographic shape (square, triangular)
  - Abnormal signal tract noted from skin surface into soft tissue lesion

Ultrasonographic Findings
- Grayscale Ultrasound
  - Ultrasound may identify chronic foreign or acute foreign bodies in subcutaneous tissues
  - Most foreign bodies appear as hyperechoic areas
  - Often surrounding area of hypoechogenicity related to surrounding edema/granulation tissue formation
  - If ultrasound performed after attempt made to remove foreign body, ultrasound exam can be difficult
    - Gas introduced into wound can obscure visualization
    - Echoes caused by introduced gas can mimic foreign body
    - Suggest ultrasound evaluation prior to attempted removal of foreign body
  - Ultrasound guidance can be utilized in an attempt to guide removal of foreign bodies

Nuclear Medicine Findings
- Bone Scan
  - Areas of soft tissue inflammation from foreign body may appear as hot on soft tissue phase of bone scan
  - Bone scan not modality of choice to work-up potential foreign body but may be obtained in setting of cellulitis and possible osteomyelitis

Imaging Recommendations
- Best imaging tool
  - Radiography
  - MRI to work up nonspecific soft tissue mass
    - If geographic focus of low signal identified in middle of high T2WI soft tissue mass in subcutaneous tissue, think chronic foreign body
- If findings on MR questionable for chronic foreign body, radiographs may be helpful to demonstrate radiopaque foreign body

DIFFERENTIAL DIAGNOSIS

Soft tissue malignancy
- Findings of foreign body absent
- More common in areas not prone to foreign bodies (proximal to mid extremities)
- Soft tissue malignancies uncommonly confined to subcutaneous tissues
- May not be able to differentiate foreign body from soft tissue malignancy in some cases

Soft tissue mass from primary bone tumor
- Underlying bone involvement
  - Cortical destruction
  - Periosteal reaction
  - Bone marrow edema
- Soft tissue mass extending from abnormal bone

Post traumatic fat necrosis
- Another entity that can occur after trauma and presents long after trauma is forgotten
- With traumatic injury, there is laceration of the subcutaneous fat and associated hematoma
- As that hematoma and injured fat begin to scar, scar tissue may present as firm palpable mass
- Typically occurs in similar areas as FB: Areas prone to injury

CHRONIC FOREIGN BODY

- Particularly anterior to tibia (shin) and buttocks
- At MR imaging, plaque-like area of high T2WI signal confined to subcutaneous tissues typically anterior to tibia
  - Area may enhance with gadolinium
  - Stellate area of low signal on T1 weighted images surrounded by high signal fat
  - No dominant, geographic mass identified

Hemangioma
- Discrete mass with diffuse enhancement
- Prominent draining veins and feeding arteries
  - Appear as flow voids on most imaging sequences
  - Are bright in signal on gradient echo sequences indicating high flow

Vascular malformation
- Venous malformation
  - Serpiginous tangle of abnormal veins that demonstrate high T2WI signal, contrast-enhancement, and no evidence of high flow on gradient echo images
- Lymphatic malformation
  - Multicystic mass without enhancement of cyst contents but can have septal enhancement

PATHOLOGY

General Features
- General path comments
  - During play, children often fall and injure areas such as the knee, elbow, shin, and buttocks
  - During such trauma, foreign bodies such as glass, plastic, or wood may be introduced into the subcutaneous tissues
  - Introduction of such foreign bodies may go unnoticed
  - Chronic presence of foreign body induces inflammatory reaction
  - Pyogenic infection and chronic granulomatous formation may be introduced
  - Granulomatous reaction may enlarge over time and present as firm palpable mass
  - At time of presentation, history of introducing trauma may be long forgotten

Microscopic Features
- Granulomatous reaction surrounding foreign body

CLINICAL ISSUES

Presentation
- Most common signs/symptoms
  - Most commonly presents as a firm soft tissue mass
    - Typically painless
    - Presentation of mass may occur well after traumatic incident that introduced the foreign body
    - Often no specific traumatic incident is recalled
- Other signs/symptoms
  - Less commonly, may present with signs/symptoms of inflammation
  - Skin may be red, inflamed over area of foreign body
  - Sinus tract may develop to skin

Demographics
- Age
  - May occur in children of any age
  - Typically does not occur in nonambulatory infants
- Gender: More common in boys

Natural History & Prognosis
- Progressive enlargement of granulomatous mass if foreign body does not spontaneously work its way to surface or surgical removal

Treatment
- Surgical removal of foreign body
- Ultrasound guidance may be helpful in removal of the foreign body
  - If ultrasound is to be utilized, it should be used before exploration of wound and introduction of gas into wound
  - Gas may obscure or mimic areas of foreign body: Shadowing echogenicity

SELECTED REFERENCES

1. Laor T: MR imaging of soft tissue tumors and tumor-like lesions. Pediatr Radiol. 34(1):24-37, 2004
2. Lin CJ et al: A foreign body embedded in the mobile tongue masquerading as a neoplasm. Eur Arch Otorhinolaryngol. 260(5):277-9, 2003
3. Siegel MJ: Magnetic resonance imaging of musculoskeletal soft tissue masses. Radiol Clin North Am. 39(4):701-20, 2001
4. Rohde V et al: Foreign body granuloma mimicking a benign intraspinal tumour. Br J Neurosurg. 13(4):417-9, 1999
5. Donnelly LF et al: The multiple presentations of foreign bodies in children. AJR. 170:471-7, 1998
6. Korneich L et al: Preoperative localization of a foreign body by magnetic resonance imaging. Eur J Radiol. 27:13-7, 1998
7. Karcnik TJ et al: Foreign body granuloma simulating solid neoplasm on MR. Clin Imaging. 21(4):269-72, 1997
8. Tsai TS et al: Fat necrosis after trauma: a benign cause of palpable lumps in children. AJR Am J Roentgenol. 169(6):1623-6, 1997
9. Bissett GS 3rd: MR imaging of soft-tissue masses in children. Magn Reson Imaging Clin N Am. 4(4):697-719, 1996
10. Jelinek J et al: MR imaging of soft-tissue masses. Mass-like lesions that simulate neoplasms. Magn Reson Imaging Clin N Am. 3(4):727-41, 1995
11. Sundaram M et al: MR imaging of benign soft-tissue masses. Magn Reson Imaging Clin N Am. 3(4):609-27, 1995
12. Ezaki T et al: Foreign-body granuloma mimicking an extrahepatically growing liver tumor: report of a case. Surg Today. 24(9):829-32, 1994
13. Ferguson PC et al: Foreign-body abscesses presenting as soft-tissue tumours: two case reports. Can J Surg. 37(6):503-7, 1994
14. Varma DG et al: Magnetic resonance imaging appearance of foreign body granulomas of the upper arms. Clin Imaging. 18(1):39-42, 1994
15. Oikarinen KS et al: Visibility of foreign bodies in soft tissue in plain radiography, computed tomography, magnetic resonance imaging, and ultrasound. An invitro study. Int J Oral Maxillofac Surg. 22:119-24, 1993

CHRONIC FOREIGN BODY

IMAGE GALLERY

Typical

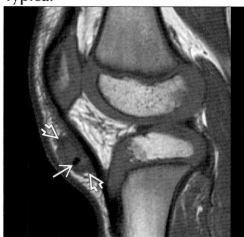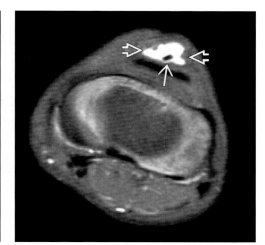

(Left) Sagittal T1WI MR shows soft tissue mass *(open arrows)* anterior to patellar tendon with central low signal area *(arrow)* consistent with foreign body. *(Right)* Axial PD/Intermediate MR in same patient shows high signal area *(open arrows)* with central low signal area *(arrow)*.

Typical

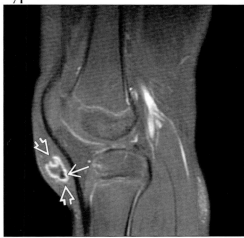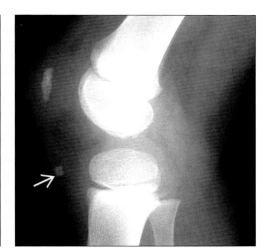

(Left) Sagittal T1 C+ MR shows ring enhancement in region of mass *(open arrows)*. Again noted is the low attenuation structure in center *(arrow)*. *(Right)* Lateral radiograph obtained after MRI because of suspicion of foreign body shows radiopaque foreign body *(arrow)* (later shown to be piece of glass).

Variant

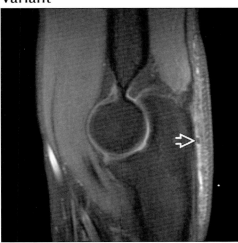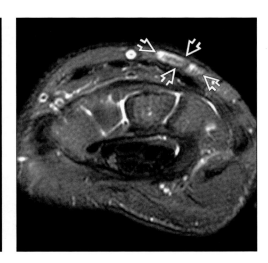

(Left) Sagittal T2WI MR shows soft tissue edema posterior to elbow with low signal area *(arrow)* in deep subcutaneous tissues. *(Right)* Axial T2WI MR shows area of high signal in dorsum of hand. No area of foreign body is identified at imaging. Resection showed foreign body with surrounding inflammation.

OSTEOMYELITIS

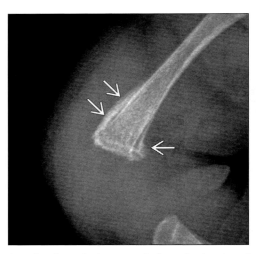

Lateral radiograph shows newly formed subperiosteal new bone (arrows) surrounding the femoral metaphysis of a 7 week old baby.

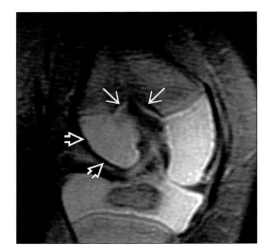

Coronal FSE PD T2 MR shows absent distal femoral ossification center and tenting (arrows) of tethered, centrally obliterated physis 4 months later. Undergrowth of lateral condyle (open arrows).

TERMINOLOGY

Definitions
- Bone and bone marrow inflammation usually due to an infectious agent: Bacterial mostly; fungal, viral, parasitic occasionally

IMAGING FINDINGS

General Features
- Best diagnostic clue: Aggressive destructive lesion in metaphysis of child < 5 years old
- Location
  - Long-bone metaphyses 70% (femur > tibia > humerus > fibula), short bones 6%, pelvis 5%, spine 2%
  - Calvaria
    - Potts puffy tumor of scalp: subgaleal abscess forms over osteomyelitis; usually due to frontal sinusitis
    - Infected cephalohematoma
  - Mandible
    - Primary chronic osteomyelitis: Nonsuppurative, noninfectious
    - Actinomycosis
  - Cervical spine
    - Adenoidectomy a cause of osteomyelitis
  - Pelvis: Symptoms mimic urinary tract infection, septic hip, acute abdomen, radiculitis
  - Calcaneus
    - Puncture through sole: Inferior cortex, Pseudomonas (P) aeruginosa
    - Hematogenous: Posterior half near apophysis
  - Great toe
    - Stubbing → hyperflexion → distal phalanx physeal distraction fracture → nail bed disruption → distal phalanx osteomyelitis

Radiographic Findings
- Radiography
  - Absence of findings does not exclude osteomyelitis
  - Earliest finding: Soft tissue swelling next to bone
  - Displacement or obliteration of fat planes
  - Bony destruction visible 7-14 days (or longer) after onset
    - Vague lucency → permeation → destruction
  - Periosteal reaction seen at 7-10 days
  - Chronic osteomyelitis: Sclerosis or mixed sclerotic/lucent; lucent tract extending through cortex; sequestrum (radiodense)

CT Findings
- NECT
  - CT: Bone destruction, intra-medullary gas and fat-fluid level, periosteal reaction, sequestrum, involucrum

DDx: Osteolytic Lesions

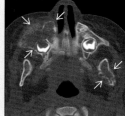
Neuroblastoma

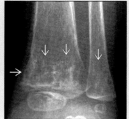
Leukemia

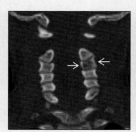
LCH

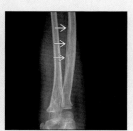
Ewing

OSTEOMYELITIS

Key Facts

Imaging Findings
- Best diagnostic clue: Aggressive destructive lesion in metaphysis of child < 5 years old
- Long-bone metaphyses 70% (femur > tibia > humerus > fibula), short bones 6%, pelvis 5%, spine 2%
- Pelvis: Symptoms mimic urinary tract infection, septic hip, acute abdomen, radiculitis
- Earliest finding: Soft tissue swelling next to bone
- CT: Bone destruction, intra-medullary gas and fat-fluid level, periosteal reaction, sequestrum, involucrum
- Well-defined areas that do not enhance with gadolinium: Suspect necrosis or abscess formation
- Grayscale Ultrasound: Excludes/includes pyarthrosis, shows soft tissue swelling, also periosteal thickening, hyperemia and elevation due to subperiosteal abscess
- Bone Scan: Positive 24-72 hours, demonstrates multiple sites
- Best imaging tool: MR best choice when abscess recognition will dictate need for surgery

Pathology
- Tendency to occur in metaphyses or metaphyseal equivalents (bone next to cartilage, e.g., calcaneal apophysis and acetabulum)
- Staphyloccus (S) aureus commonest (43%), then β-hemolytic streptococcus (S) (10%) and S. pneumoniae (10%)

Clinical Issues
- Incidence 1-3:1,000 in neonatal intensive care

  - CT: Increased attenuation of involved marrow
- CECT: Rim-enhancement of intra- and extra-osseous abscesses
- Bony destruction/sclerosis
- Surrounding soft-tissue swelling
- CT may be performed to better delineate bony changes
  - Lucent tract through cortex
  - Bony sequestrum

MR Findings
- T1WI: Marrow edema: Hypointense signal
- T2WI
  - Marrow edema: Hyperintense signal
  - Cellulitis and sinus tracts: Hyperintense signal
  - Extramedullary fat-fluid level
    - Cortical perforation allows marrow fat to leak outside bone
- STIR: Marrow edema: Hyperintense signal
- T1 C+
  - Enhancement: Marrow and periosteal inflammation
  - Abscess: Peripheral enhancement/central nonenhancement
- Usually large areas of surrounding edema in soft tissue/marrow
- Well-defined areas that do not enhance with gadolinium: Suspect necrosis or abscess formation

Ultrasonographic Findings
- Grayscale Ultrasound: Excludes/includes pyarthrosis, shows soft tissue swelling, also periosteal thickening, hyperemia and elevation due to subperiosteal abscess

Nuclear Medicine Findings
- Bone Scan
  - Increased uptake in angiographic, blood-pool, and delayed phases; sensitivity 82%
    - Central photopenia if intraosseous infarct or abscess
  - Bone Scan: Positive 24-72 hours, demonstrates multiple sites

Other Modality Findings
- Brodie abscess
  - Intramedullary, lytic on CT, target appearance on MR, geographic destruction, well-defined edges, marginal sclerosis, no bone enlargement
  - Metadiaphysis of tubular bones: 63% lower extremities

Imaging Recommendations
- Best imaging tool: MR best choice when abscess recognition will dictate need for surgery
- Protocol advice: T1, T2 FS, STIR, T1 C+
- If suspicious of focal area based on symptoms or radiographic findings: MRI
- If area of involvement not clear or multiple areas suspected: Bone scintigraphy
- If further evaluating sclerotic bone lesion: CT

DIFFERENTIAL DIAGNOSIS

Permeative bone lesion in child < 5 years
- Osteomyelitis
- Langerhans cell histiocytosis (LCH)
- Neuroblastoma metastasis

Permeative bone lesion in child > 5 years
- Ewing sarcoma
- Lymphoma or leukemia
- Osteomyelitis
- Langerhans cell histiocytosis

PATHOLOGY

General Features
- General path comments
  - Tendency to occur in metaphyses or metaphyseal equivalents (bone next to cartilage, e.g., calcaneal apophysis and acetabulum)
    - Thought related to rich but slow-moving blood supply to these regions
- Etiology

OSTEOMYELITIS

- Staphyloccus (S) aureus commonest (43%), then β-hemolytic streptococcus (S) (10%) and S. pneumoniae (10%)
  - Penetrating trauma: P. aeruginosa
  - Sickle cell disease: Salmonella
- SAPHO syndrome: Synovitis, acne, pustulosis, hyperostosis, osteitis
  - Recurrent multifocal osteomyelitis of long-bone metaphyses and medial clavicles
- CRMO: Chronic recurrent multifocal osteomyelitis
  - Non-pyogenic, unknown cause, prolonged or recurrent course, children and adolescents
- Epidemiology
  - 1/5,000 children < 13 years in USA; 1:800 - 1:10,000 elsewhere
  - Three routes of infection: Hematogenous, contiguous, direct implantation
  - Neonates at highest risk
    - Immature host-defense system
    - Transphyseal sinusoids connect metaphyseal and epiphyseal blood vessels allowing metaphyseal-epiphyseal infection spread: Increased incidence of epiphyseal damage
    - Newborn intensive care babies: Umbilical catheter a risk factor
    - Most common: S. aureus, β streptococcus, Candida (C) albicans

Gross Pathologic & Surgical Features
- Inflammation: Inflammatory cellular response
  - Myelitis
    - Involvement of fat and hematopoietic tissue
    - Abscess if ischemia (increased intraosseous pressure), infarct, necrosis, and liquefaction
  - Osteitis
    - Involvement of cortical and trabecular bone
    - If bone necrosis and resorption: Cortex porous/fenestrated exposing subperiosteal space to infection
    - Sequestrum if large volume necrotic; subsequently extruded, surgically removed, or dissolved by osteoclasts
  - Periostitis
    - Subperiosteal abscess
    - Periosteal elevation: Cortical bone infarct due to interrupted blood supply
    - Subperiosteal new bone formation

CLINICAL ISSUES

Presentation
- Most common signs/symptoms: Fever, pain, tenderness
- Neonatal osteomyelitis
  - Nonspecific: Lethargy, irritability, poor feeding, unstable temperature
  - Specific: Limited movement or discomfort with movement, tenderness, pseudoparalysis, swelling, warmth, erythema
  - Hematogenous origin
  - Commonest: Humerus, femur, tibia, fibula
  - Accompanying septic arthritis frequent

- Because of young age, presentation typically nonspecific and diagnosis delayed
- May present with fever of unknown origin, sepsis, chronic irritability
- Sickle cell disease: Osteomyelitis frequently due to salmonella as well as S. aureus
- Erythrocyte sedimentation rate elevated in vast majority

Demographics
- Age
  - Primarily a disease of infants and young children
    - 1/3 cases occur before 2 years of age
    - 1/2 cases occur before 5 years of age
  - Incidence 1-3:1,000 in neonatal intensive care
  - Vertebral osteomyelitis: Age 8-20 years
  - Vertebral diskitis: Age < 5 years

Natural History & Prognosis
- Neonatal osteomyelitis: 40% have later extremity shortening/deformity due to physeal injury
- Adjacent septic arthritis common when age < 1

Treatment
- Identify infectious agent: Imaging-guided needle aspiration or open surgical biopsy
- Antibiotics, pain management
- Surgery/intervention
  - Abscess (intra-osseous, subperiosteal, parosteal) drainage, sequestrectomy, management of sinus tracts and pathological fractures

SELECTED REFERENCES

1. Saigal G et al: Imaging of osteomyelitis with special reference to children. Semin Musculoskelet Radiol. 8(3):255-65, 2004
2. Earwaker JW et al: SAPHO: syndrome or concept? Imaging findings. Skeletal Radiol. 32(6):311-27, 2003
3. Hui CL et al: Extramedullary fat fluid level on MRI as a specific sign for osteomyelitis. Australas Radiol. 47(4):443-6, 2003
4. Ibia EO et al: Group A beta-hemolytic streptococcal osteomyelitis in children. Pediatrics. 112(1 Pt 1):e22-6, 2003
5. Studler U et al: Widening of the greater trochanteric physis in the immature skeleton: a radiographic sign of femoral osteomyelitis (2003:6b). Eur Radiol. 13(9):2238-40, 2003
6. Kleinman PK: A regional approach to osteomyelitis of the lower extremities in children. Radiol Clin North Am. 40(5):1033-59, 2002
7. McPherson DM: Osteomyelitis in the neonate. Neonatal Netw. 21(1):9-22, 2002
8. Oudjhane K et al: Imaging of osteomyelitis in children. Radiol Clin North Am. 39(2):251-66, 2001
9. Gylys-Morin VM: MR imaging of pediatric musculoskeletal inflammatory and infectious disorders. Magn Reson Imaging Clin N Am. 6(3):537-59, 1998
10. Lopes TD et al: Quantitative analysis of the plain radiographic appearance of Brodie's abscess. Invest Radiol. 32(1):51-8, 1997
11. Nelson JD: Acute osteomyelitis in children. Infect Dis Clin North Am. 4(3):513-22, 1990

OSTEOMYELITIS

IMAGE GALLERY

Typical

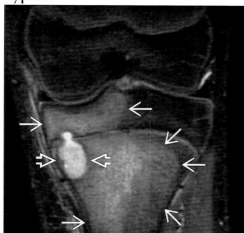
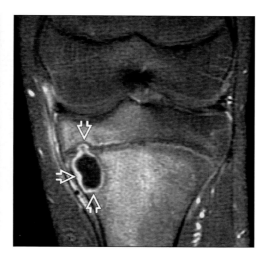

(Left) Coronal STIR MR showing Brodie abscess (open arrows) crossing physis into epiphysis with extensive marrow edema (arrows). *(Right)* Coronal T1 C+ MR shows Brodie abscess with a well defined rim of enhancement (open arrows) and extensive marrow edema in the same child.

Typical

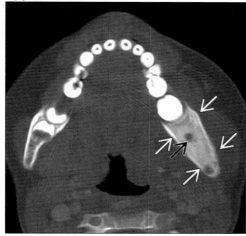
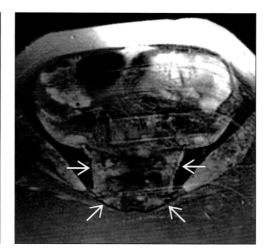

(Left) Axial CECT shows mandible (white arrows) with medullary expansion and sclerosis in a child with chronic actinomycosis osteomyelitis. Mandibular canal (black arrow) is enlarged and indistinct. *(Right)* Axial FSE T2 MR shows increased signal of the entire sacrum (arrows) due to osteomyelitis. Hypointense iliac bone marrow signal due to iron deposition in sickle cell disease.

Typical

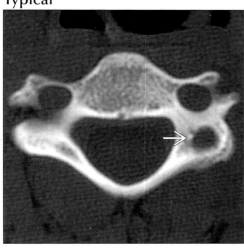
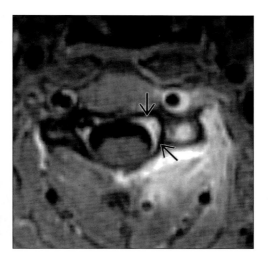

(Left) Axial NECT shows bone destruction (arrow) due to osteomyelitis in the lateral mass of a cervical vertebra. *(Right)* Axial T1 FS C+ MR shows intense enhancement within the lesion and surrounding tissues including the epidural space (arrows) in same patient.

SYPHILIS, MUSCULOSKELETAL

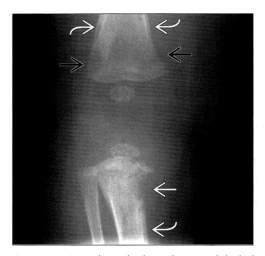

Anteroposterior radiograph shows large medial tibial metaphyseal defect representing Wimberger sign (white arrow), incomplete metaphyseal band (black arrows), and periosteal reaction (curved arrows).

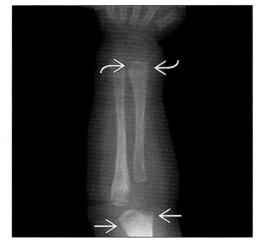

Anteroposterior radiograph shows metaphyseal band in distal radius (curved arrows) with destruction of medial radial cortex. A metaphyseal band is present in the distal humerus (arrows).

TERMINOLOGY

Abbreviations and Synonyms
- "The Great Imitator": Sir William Osler

Definitions
- Congenital syphilis
  - Congenital syphilis: Transplacental transmission to fetus of Treponema pallidum (T. pallidum) from mother with untreated or recently treated primary or secondary syphilis and spirochetemia
- Acquired syphilis
  - Acquired syphilis: Occurrence of syphilis via sexual transmission; an abusive situation in children and adolescents
  - Rare exception: Infection from a contagious maternal mucosal oral or genital lesion at birth

IMAGING FINDINGS

General Features
- Best diagnostic clue
  - Wimberger sign: Deep erosive destruction of medial upper tibial metaphyses
    - Sequestra occasionally contained within region of destruction
  - Other conditions that cause Wimberger sign: Osteomyelitis, hyperparathyroidism, infantile fibromatosis
- Location: Syphilitic osteochondritis affects tibia > femur > humerus

Radiographic Findings
- Long bones
  - Osteochondritis → moth-eaten, serrated metaphyses
    - Tibia (44%) > femur (20%) > humerus (10%)
    - Wimberger sign seen in 20%
    - Metaphyseal lucent bands; may be very distinct and striking
  - Periostitis
  - Pathological fractures, frequently multiple → pseudoparalysis because of pain
  - Symptomatic infants: Long bones abnormal in 90%
  - Asymptomatic infants: Long bones abnormal in 20%
- Short bones
  - Periostitis most common
- Skull
  - Multiple lytic calvarial lesions with irregular margins
- Chest
  - Hazy increased density due to pneumonia alba

Ultrasonographic Findings
- Nephropathy, hepatitis, hepatomegaly, splenomegaly, ascites

DDx: Diseases With Abnormal Metaphyses

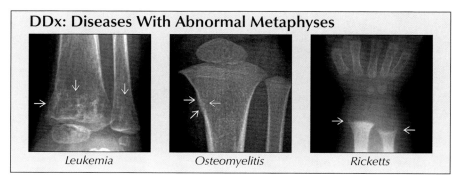

Leukemia   Osteomyelitis   Ricketts

SYPHILIS, MUSCULOSKELETAL

Key Facts

Terminology
- Congenital syphilis: Transplacental transmission to fetus of Treponema pallidum (T. pallidum) from mother with untreated or recently treated primary or secondary syphilis and spirochetemia
- Acquired syphilis: Occurrence of syphilis via sexual transmission; an abusive situation in children and adolescents

Imaging Findings
- Wimberger sign: Deep erosive destruction of medial upper tibial metaphyses
- Osteochondritis → moth-eaten, serrated metaphyses

Pathology
- Mother with untreated syphilis in primary or secondary stage has near-100% chance of infecting her newborn
- Children investigated for sexual abuse: Incidence of syphilis 0.3-0.8:1,000
- Incidence of congenital syphilis: 10:100,000 live births in USA

Diagnostic Checklist
- Consider congenital syphilis when baby has symmetrical osteitis and periosteal reaction
- Consider congenital syphilis as well as child abuse in infant with multiple pathologic fractures

DIFFERENTIAL DIAGNOSIS

Bacterial osteomyelitis
- Usually monostotic

Leukemia
- Symmetrical metaphyseal lucent bands
- Osteopenia and periosteal reaction
- Hemogram abnormal

Neuroblastoma
- Widespread bone metastases tend to be asymmetrical

Ricketts
- Osteopenia, widened physis, loss of zone of provisional calcification, metaphyseal cupping and fraying
  - Renal osteodystrophy: Metaphyseal cortical bone resorption in tibia may resemble a Wimberger sign

Scurvy (vitamin C deficiency)
- Metaphyseal lucent bands adjacent to thickened zones of provisional calcification
- Subperiosteal hemorrhage → subperiosteal new bone formation covering enlarged subperiosteal space
- Occurs at 6 months to 2 years usually

Infantile hypophosphatasia
- Osteopenia, periosteal reaction, fractures

Infantile cortical hyperostosis (Caffey disease)
- Periosteal reaction of mandible, clavicle, ulna, other long bones, ilia, ribs, skull

Weismann-Netter syndrome: Anterior bowing of lower legs with dwarfism
- Tibia and fibular bowing may start as early as 1 year
  - Also femoral bowing, coxa and genu vara, genu square pelvis, horizontal sacrum, radio-ulnar and humeral bowing, rib abnormalities, mental retardation, dural calcification

PATHOLOGY

General Features
- Etiology
  - Mother with untreated syphilis in primary or secondary stage has near-100% chance of infecting her newborn
  - Infant's bone abnormalities present usually only when maternal VDRL titers positive at > 1:4 dilution
  - Children investigated for sexual abuse: Incidence of syphilis 0.3-0.8:1,000
- Epidemiology
  - Incidence of congenital syphilis: 10:100,000 live births in USA
  - Parents more likely to be African-American, Hispanic, low socio-economic status, cocaine users
  - Additional risk factors: Maternal age less than 30 years, maternal treatment for syphilis within 30 days of delivery, and absent or inadequate prenatal care
  - Associated with stillbirth, neonatal death, and premature delivery
- Laboratory tests for syphilis
  - Direct visualization
    - Dark-field microscopy
    - Direct fluorescent antibody test for T. pallidum
  - Treponemal tests
    - TPHA: T. pallidum hemagglutinin assay
    - FTA-ABS: Fluorescent treponemal antibody absorbed
    - PCR: polymerase chain reaction → detection of T. pallidum DNA
  - Nontreponemal tests
    - VDRL: Venereal Disease Research Laboratories titre
    - RPR: Rapid plasma reagin titre

CLINICAL ISSUES

Presentation
- Most common signs/symptoms: Fever, irritability, failure to thrive
- Other signs/symptoms

SYPHILIS, MUSCULOSKELETAL

- Congenital syphilis
- Onset at age 0-2 years in early type; onset at age 2-≈30 years late type
- Early-onset congenital syphilis
  - Rhinorrhea, sometimes bloody
  - Anemia, thrombocytopenia, leukopenia, leukocytosis
  - Maculopapular rash on hands and feet
  - Fissures around the mucous membranes of mouth, nares, and anus (rhagades)
  - Pseudoparalysis: Refusal to move a painful extremity; paralysis is flaccid, bilateral, and symmetric; incidence is 23%
  - Syphilitic glomerulonephritis → nephrotic syndrome
  - Hepatitis → extensive hepatic calcifications
  - Pneumonia alba
  - Pulmonary abscess
  - Ulceration and stenosis of terminal ileum → rectal bleeding, intestinal atresia, meconium ileus, syphilitic pancreatitis → pancreatic exocrine insufficiency
  - Gumma: Intra-abdominal, pituitary → hypopituitarism
- Late-onset congenital syphilis
  - Pathognomonic: Interstitial keratitis, mulberry molars, Hutchinson (notched) second-dentition incisors
  - Hutchinson's triad: Hutchinson teeth, interstitial keratitis, deafness
  - Interstitial keratitis: Most common late finding, usually appears close to puberty
  - Bone changes: Fontal bossing, saddle nose, maxillary hypoplasia, hard palate perforation, sabre tibia
  - Clutton's joints: Symmetrical painless joint effusions, usually involving knees
  - Gummatous periostitis
  - Aseptic meningitis
- Acquired syphilis
  - Chancre → adenopathy → rash, condylomata, mucous patches with red border
  - Interstitial keratitis not seen
  - Uveitis and chorioretinitis do occur
  - Gummatous periostitis

Treatment
- Prevention of transmission through early prenatal care and treatment of seropositive mothers is effective
- Intravenous penicillin
- If abuse, remove child to safe environment

DIAGNOSTIC CHECKLIST

Image Interpretation Pearls
- Consider congenital syphilis when baby has symmetrical osteitis and periosteal reaction
- Consider congenital syphilis as well as child abuse in infant with multiple pathologic fractures
- "Routine" radiography of long bones of babies as part of evaluation of suspected congenital syphilis not useful
- Even if abnormal, findings do no change syphilis management

SELECTED REFERENCES

1. Bell C et al: Pulmonary abscesses in congenital syphilis. Arch Pathol Lab Med. 126(4):484-6, 2002
2. Busby G et al: Value of routine long bone radiographs in management of babies with a positive VDRL at the Mount Hope Women's Hospital. West Indian Med J. 51(4):225-7, 2002
3. Nolt D et al: Survival with hypopituitarism from congenital syphilis. Pediatrics. 109(4):e63, 2002
4. Coimbra AV et al: Weismann-Netter-Stuhl syndrome: first Brazilian case reports. Joint Bone Spine. 67(6):539-43, 2000
5. Ajayi NA et al: Intestinal ulceration, obstruction, and haemorrhage in congenital syphilis. Pediatr Surg Int. 15(5-6):391-3, 1999
6. Christian CW et al: Preschoolers with syphilis. Pediatrics. 103(1):E4, 1999
7. Moyer VA et al: Contribution of long-bone radiographs to the management of congenital syphilis in the newborn infant. Arch Pediatr Adolesc Med. 152(4):353-7, 1998
8. Ghadouane M et al: Skeletal lesions in early congenital syphilis (a review of 86 cases). Rev Rhum Engl Ed. 62(6):433-7, 1995
9. Herman TE: Extensive hepatic calcification secondary to fulminant neonatal syphilitic hepatitis. Pediatr Radiol. 25(2):120-2, 1995
10. Lim HK et al: Congenital syphilis mimicking child abuse. Pediatr Radiol. 25(7):560-1, 1995
11. Shah AM et al: Late onset congenital syphilis. Indian Pediatr. 32(7):795-8, 1995
12. Starling SP: Syphilis in infants and young children. Pediatr Ann. 23(7):334-40, 1994

SYPHILIS, MUSCULOSKELETAL

IMAGE GALLERY

Typical

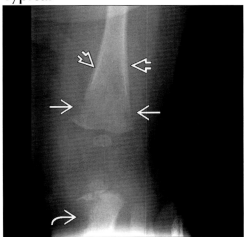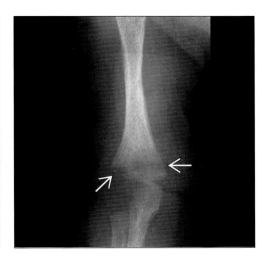

(Left) Anteroposterior radiograph shows Wimberger sign (curved arrow), femoral metaphyseal cortical destruction (arrows), and periosteal reaction (open arrows). *(Right)* Anteroposterior radiograph shows metaphyseal lucent band in the distal humerus. Marginal bone destruction (arrows) is present.

Typical

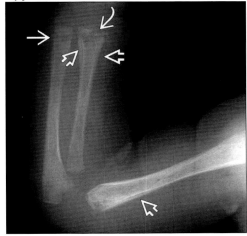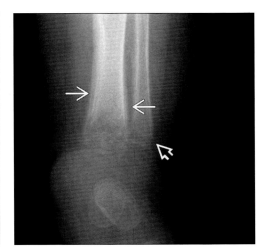

(Left) Anteroposterior radiograph shows ulnar metaphyseal lucent band (arrow), radial metaphysis destructive lesion (curved arrow), and periosteal reaction (open arrows). *(Right)* Anteroposterior radiograph shows a fracture (open arrow) through the metaphyseal lucent line in the distal fibula and periostitis (arrows) around the tibial metaphysis.

Typical

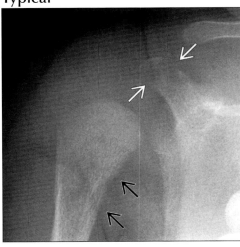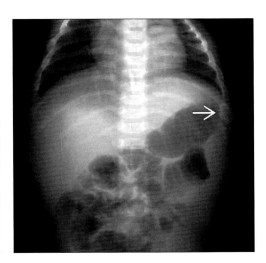

(Left) Anteroposterior radiograph shows a fracture (white arrows) of the acromion process and medial metaphyseal cortical osteolysis (black arrows) of the upper humerus in an abused child with congenital syphilis. *(Right)* Anteroposterior radiograph shows shows two rib fractures (arrow) and syphilitic hepatosplenomegaly in the same patient.

INFANTILE HEMANGIOMA, MUSCULOSKELETAL

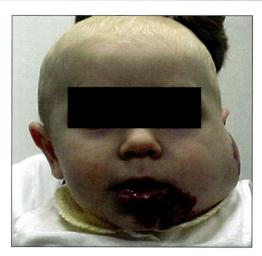

Clinical photograph shows skin manifestations of hemangioma and associated underlying soft tissue mass.

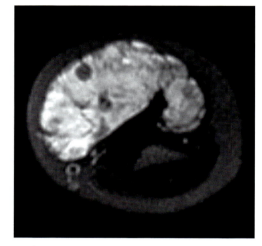

Axial T2WI MR shows lobulated high signal mass with diffuse enhancement in the subcutaneous tissues anterior to elbow.

TERMINOLOGY

Abbreviations and Synonyms
- Capillary hemangioma, infantile hemangioma

Definitions
- Hemangioma: Cellular proliferation of endothelial cells, true neoplasm
  - Two stage process of growth (proliferation) and regression
  - Small or absent at birth, rapid growth over first several months of life, involution over months to years
  - Most common tumor of childhood (12% of infants)
- Vascular malformations: (In contrast) not true neoplasms
  - Present at birth and enlarge proportionally to child
  - Do not involute and remain throughout life
  - Subcategorized based on types of channels: Lymphatic, capillary, venous, arteriovenous, and mixed malformations

IMAGING FINDINGS

General Features
- Location
  - Head and neck (60%)
  - Trunk (25%)
  - Extremities (15%)
- General imaging features
  - Discrete, well-defined, lobulated mass
  - Diffuse enhancement
  - Homogeneous in appearance
  - High flow vessels both within and adjacent to mass
  - Decreased size and fatty replacement during involutional phase

Radiographic Findings
- Radiography: Soft tissue mass

CT Findings
- Not typically used for diagnosis of suspected hemangioma in extremities but may be obtained in work-up of mediastinal mass or head and neck lesions
- Discrete, lobulated mass with prominent draining veins
- Diffuse enhancement

MR Findings
- Discrete lobulated mass
- Hyperintense on T2 weighted images
- Isointense to muscle on T1 weighted images
- Prominent draining veins seen as both central and peripheral vascular structures
  - Seen as flow voids
  - May show high flow on GRE images

DDx: Soft Tissue Masses

Venous Malf | Lymphatic Malf | AVM | Sarcoma

INFANTILE HEMANGIOMA, MUSCULOSKELETAL

Key Facts

Terminology
- Hemangioma: Cellular proliferation of endothelial cells, true neoplasm
- Two stage process of growth (proliferation) and regression
- Small or absent at birth, rapid growth over first several months of life, involution over months to years
- Most common tumor of childhood (12% of infants)

Imaging Findings
- Head and neck (60%)
- Trunk (25%)
- Extremities (15%)
- General imaging features
- Discrete, well-defined, lobulated mass
- Diffuse enhancement
- Homogeneous in appearance
- High flow vessels both within and adjacent to mass
- Decreased size and fatty replacement during involutional phase

Clinical Issues
- Often present as asymptomatic mass
- May present with findings of complications: Fissure formation, ulceration and bleeding, compression of vital structures, Kasabach-Merritt syndrome
- Typically absent or small at birth: Often not noticed (60% not seen at birth)
- Rapid growth during proliferative phase: 3-9 months
- Slow involution: 18 months-10 years
- Most hemangiomas require no therapy or imaging
- Initial treatment is systemic steroids

- Diffuse enhancement with gadolinium
- Involuting hemangioma may demonstrate components of fat signal

Ultrasonographic Findings
- Lobulated, well-defined mass
- Variable echogenicity
- Often confined to subcutaneous tissues
- Increased color Doppler flow
  - High vessel density (> 5 vessels/cm2)
- Sensitivity of 84%, specificity 98%

Angiographic Findings
- Conventional
  - Only performed if embolization being considered for refractory complications, such as heart failure
  - Well-circumscribed mass or masses
  - Intense, persistent tissue staining

Imaging Recommendations
- Most hemangiomas can be diagnosed on basis of physical appearance and temporal growth history and imaging not necessary
- Imaging used if diagnosis or extent of disease in question
- MRI is the imaging test of choice
- MR protocols should include
  - T1 weighted images
  - T2 weighted fat-saturated images
  - Post-gadolinium T1 weighted images
  - Gradient echo imaging sequences: To determine the presence or absence of high (arterial) flow through the lesions
    - Important because high flow lesions typically treated with transarterial embolization and low flow lesions treated with percutaneous sclerosis

DIFFERENTIAL DIAGNOSIS

Venous malformation
- Multiple serpentine channels that appear high in signal on T2 images
- Enhancement in channels
- No high signal on gradient echo images
- Phleboliths
- Present at birth, growth proportionally to child
- No regression

Arteriovenous malformation (AVM)
- Tangle of vessels
- No focal mass associated
- High flow on gradient echo images

Lymphatic malformation
- Multiple cysts of various sizes that are high T2 signal and may show peripheral but not diffuse enhancement
- Present at birth

Soft tissue sarcoma (fibrosarcoma, rhabdomyosarcoma)
- If mass does not meet both clinical and MR criteria for one of the above lesions, sarcoma should be considered and biopsy performed
- In young children, the most common malignancy confused with hemangioma is congenital fibrosarcoma

PATHOLOGY

General Features
- General path comments
  - Cellular proliferation of endothelial cells
  - True neoplasm
  - Mass of proliferative, hyperplastic endothelial cells that form syncytial masses
  - During proliferative phase, high expression of angiogenic factors
  - Increased mast cells
- Genetics
  - Majority sporadic
  - Rare association with chromosome 5q31-q33
- Etiology: Clonal expansion of angioblasts with high expression of growth factors/angiogenesis markers
- Epidemiology

INFANTILE HEMANGIOMA, MUSCULOSKELETAL

- Most common tumor of childhood
- Occur in 12% of children
- Higher incidence in twins and premature infants (29%)
- Associated abnormalities: PHACE syndrome [posterior fossa mass, hemangioma, arterial abnormalities (stenosis, aneurysm), cardiovascular (aortic coarctation, cardiac anomalies), eye abnormalities] also supraumbilical median raphe

CLINICAL ISSUES

Presentation
- Most common signs/symptoms
  - Often present as asymptomatic mass
    - When dermal involvement (most common): Strawberry appearing mass
    - When deep to skin: Skin often has bluish tint due to draining veins
- Other signs/symptoms
  - During proliferative phase, high flow may cause: Bruit, pulsatility, and warmth
  - May present with findings of complications: Fissure formation, ulceration and bleeding, compression of vital structures, Kasabach-Merritt syndrome
  - Multiple cutaneous hemangiomas may be associated with visceral hemangioma
  - "Beard" distribution on face associated with subglottic hemangioma (may cause stridor)

Demographics
- Age
  - Typically absent or small at birth: Often not noticed (60% not seen at birth)
  - Rapid growth during proliferative phase: 3-9 months
  - Slow involution: 18 months-10 years
  - 50% involution by 5 years of age
- Gender: M:F = 3:1
- Ethnicity: More common in Caucasians, uncommon in African-Americans, Asians

Natural History & Prognosis
- Potential complications
  - Kasabach-Merritt syndrome (consumptive coagulopathy associated with hemangioma)
    - More common with kaposiform hemangioendothelioma subtype
    - Often respond poorly to steroids
  - Compression of vital structures (airway, orbit)
  - Fissure formation, ulceration, bleeding
  - Psychological issues (when on face, particularly nose)
  - Heart failure

Treatment
- Most hemangiomas require no therapy or imaging
  - Therapy reserved for hemangiomas with or with the potential of complications
- Initial treatment is systemic steroids
  - 30% respond dramatically
  - Another 40% have some response
  - Side effects: Irritability, weight gain, cushingoid appearance, growth delay, hypertension, diabetes, gastroesophageal reflux, infections
- Other therapies: Direct steroid injection, interferon, surgical removal, embolization, laser therapy for skin involvement

DIAGNOSTIC CHECKLIST

Consider
- If imaging appearance, temporal history, or findings on physical exam are atypical, exclude other lesions

SELECTED REFERENCES

1. Gampper TJ et al: Vascular anomalies: hemangiomas. Plast Reconstr Surg. 110(2):572-85; quiz 586; discussion 587-8, 2002
2. Konez O et al: Magnetic resonance of vascular anomalies. Magn Reson Imaging Clin N Am. 10(2):363-88, vii, 2002
3. Donnelly LF et al: Centennial dissertation. Vascular malformations and hemangiomas: a practical approach in a multidisciplinary clinic. AJR. 174:597-608, 2000
4. Donnelly LF et al: Vascular malformations and hemangiomas: a practical approach in a multidisciplinary clinic. AJR Am J Roentgenol. 174(3):597-608, 2000
5. Donnelly LF et al: Marked acute tissue swelling following percutaneous sclerosis of low-flow vascular malformations: a predictor of both prolonged recovery and therapeutic effect. Pediatr Radiol. 30(6):415-9, 2000
6. Fordham LA et al: Imaging of congenital vascular and lymphatic anomalies of the head and neck. Neuroimaging Clin N Am. 10(1):117-36, viii, 2000
7. Mulliken JB et al: Vascular anomalies. Curr Probl Surg. 37(8):517-84, 2000
8. Donnelly LF et al: Combined sonographic and fluoroscopic guidance: a modified technique for percutaneous sclerosis of low-flow vascular malformations. AJR Am J Roentgenol. 173(3):655-7, 1999
9. Dubois J et al: Imaging and therapeutic approach of hemangiomas and vascular malformations in the pediatric age group. Pediatr Radiol. 29(12):879-93, 1999
10. Robertson RL et al: Head and neck vascular anomalies of childhood. Neuroimaging Clin N Am. 9(1):115-32, 1999
11. Dubois J et al: Imaging of hemangiomas and vascular malformations in children. Acad Radiol. 5(5):390-400, 1998
12. Laor T et al: Congenital anomalies and vascular birthmarks of the lower extremities. Magn Reson Imaging Clin N Am. 6(3):497-519, 1998
13. Laor T et al: Magnetic resonance venography of congenital vascular malformations of the extremities. Pediatr Radiol. 26(6):371-80, 1996
14. Barnes PD et al: Hemangiomas and vascular malformations of the head and neck: MR characterization. AJNR Am J Neuroradiol. 15(1):193-5, 1994
15. Wahrman JE et al: Hemangiomas. Pediatr Rev. 15(7):266-71, 1994
16. Meyer JS et al: Biological classification of soft-tissue vascular anomalies: MR correlation. AJR. 157:559-64, 1991
17. Smith MB et al: Differentiation and treatment of hemangiomas and arteriovenous malformations. J La State Med Soc. 141(6):41-3, 1989
18. Mulliken JB et al: Hemangiomas and vascular malformations in infants and children: a classification based on endothelial characteristics. Plast Reconstr Surg. 69:412-22, 1982

INFANTILE HEMANGIOMA, MUSCULOSKELETAL

IMAGE GALLERY

Typical

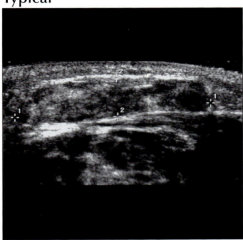
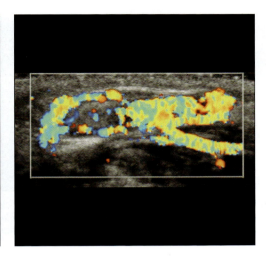

(Left) Ultrasound shows well-defined lobulated mass with markedly increased Doppler flow. *(Right)* Color Doppler ultrasound in same patient shows well-defined lobulated mass to have markedly increased Doppler flow.

Typical

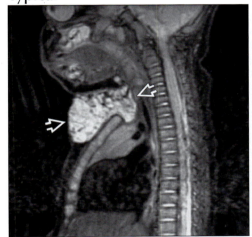
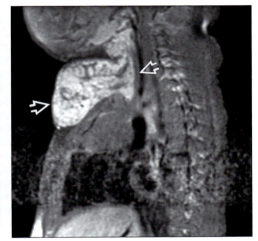

(Left) Sagittal T2WI MR shows large, well-circumscribed mass (arrows) in anterior neck/chest wall with multiple flow voids within the mass. *(Right)* Sagittal T1 C+ MR in same patient shows mass (arrows) to diffusely enhance with contrast. There are some septations and vessels that do not enhance.

Typical

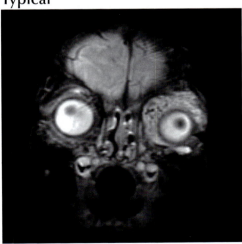
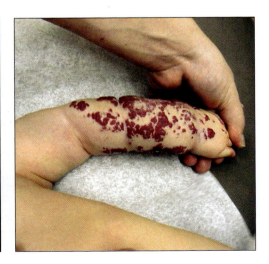

(Left) Coronal STIR MR shows lobulated, well-defined mass in orbit with high T2W signal and flow voids. *(Right)* Clinical photograph shows skin manifestation of hemangioma with strawberry appearance.

VENOUS MALFORMATIONS

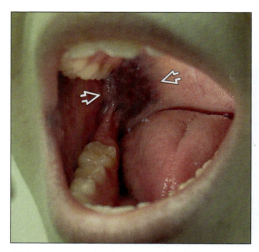

Clinical photograph shows venous malformation as bluish area (arrows) of mucous membrane.

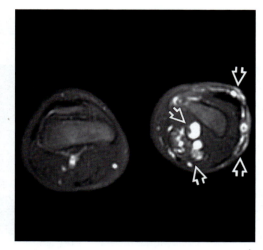

Axial T2WI MR shows venous malformation of left lower extremity as multiple high signal serpentine areas (arrows). Right leg is normal.

TERMINOLOGY

Abbreviations and Synonyms
- Venous malformation (VM)
- Misnamed as: Cavernous hemangioma, phlebangioma

Definitions
- Vascular malformation: Congenital malformation that is not true neoplasm, (hemangiomas are)
  - Present at birth and enlarge proportional to child
  - Do not involute and remain throughout life unless treated
  - Subcategorized based on types of channels: Venous, lymphatic, capillary, arteriovenous, and mixed
  - Venous malformation are subtype of vascular malformation
- Venous malformation: Dysplasias of small and large venous channels
  - Most common symptomatic vascular malformation
  - May be focal mass or diffuse abnormality of extremity venous structures (multiple varicosities)

IMAGING FINDINGS

General Features
- Best diagnostic clue: Tangle of serpentine channels with slow venous flow
- Location
  - Head and neck (40%)
  - Extremities (40%)
  - Trunk (20%)
- General Imaging Features
  - Multilocular or septated mass
  - Serpentine channels are characteristic pattern
  - Channels and "cystic" areas enhance diffusely
  - May have associated nonvascular hamartomatous connective tissue component
    - Some of the connective tissue stromal areas between channels may not enhance diffusely
    - May contain fat
  - May be associated with muscular atrophy
  - Bone involvement uncommon
  - Often lesions do not respect tissue/fascial planes and may involve multiple tissue types: Muscles, subcutaneous tissues
  - Channels contain slow moving venous blood
    - No evidence of rapid flow in channels

Radiographic Findings
- Radiography
  - Soft tissue mass
  - Bones typically normal - involvement rare
    - Gorham-Stout syndrome: Disappearing bone disease from involvement with venous malformations

DDx: Soft Tissue Mass

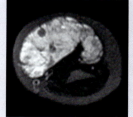
Hemangioma

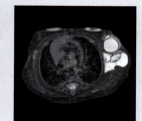
Lymphatic Malf

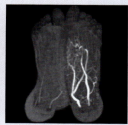
AVM

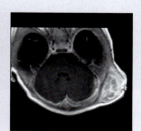
Sarcoma

VENOUS MALFORMATIONS

Key Facts

Terminology
- Vascular malformation: Congenital malformation that is not true neoplasm, (hemangiomas are)
- Present at birth and enlarge proportional to child
- Do not involute and remain throughout life unless treated
- Subcategorized based on types of channels: Venous, lymphatic, capillary, arteriovenous, and mixed
- Venous malformation are subtype of vascular malformation
- Venous malformation: Dysplasias of small and large venous channels
- Most common symptomatic vascular malformation
- May be focal mass or diffuse abnormality of extremity venous structures (multiple varicosities)

Imaging Findings
- Multilocular or septated mass
- Serpentine channels are characteristic pattern
- Channels and "cystic" areas enhance diffusely
- May have associated nonvascular hamartomatous connective tissue component
- Some of the connective tissue stromal areas between channels may not enhance diffusely
- May contain fat
- May be associated with muscular atrophy
- Bone involvement uncommon
- Often lesions do not respect tissue/fascial planes and may involve multiple tissue types: Muscles, subcutaneous tissues
- Channels contain slow moving venous blood
- No evidence of rapid flow in channels

  - May see calcified phleboliths

Fluoroscopic Findings
- Direct cannulation and injection of contrast shows multiple channels and lakes of venous structures that directly communicate with veins
- Used for imaging guidance for percutaneous sclerosis

CT Findings
- Not typically utilized in work-up of venous malformations
- Soft tissue mass with multiple channels that diffusely enhance
- Calcified phleboliths may be present

MR Findings
- T1WI
  - Soft tissue mass intermediate in signal
  - Phleboliths may appear dark in signal
  - Acute thrombus in venous channels may be high or low in signal depending up age
- T2WI: Venous channels high in signal
- T2* GRE: No evidence of high flow in vessels
- T1 C+
  - Venous channels and excess draining veins will diffusely enhance
  - Surrounding connective tissue stoma may not enhance

Ultrasonographic Findings
- Grayscale Ultrasound
  - Mixed echogenic lesion
  - Tangles of hypoechoic tubular structures
  - Serpentine structures
  - Phleboliths: Shadowing echogenic area
- Color Doppler: No evidence of arterial flow
- Pulsed Doppler: No evidence of arterial wave forms in lesion or draining veins
- Power Doppler: No evidence of arterial flow
- Ultrasound may be utilized for several indications
  - Guidance of interventional procedures particularly percutaneous sclerosis
  - Diagnostic characterization of a soft tissue mass

Angiographic Findings
- Conventional
  - Not required
  - Normal findings

Imaging Recommendations
- MRI is the imaging test of choice for making diagnosis and evaluating extent of disease
- MR protocols should include
  - T1 weighted images
  - T2 weighted fat-saturated images
  - Post-gadolinium T1 weighted images
  - Gradient echo imaging sequences: To determine the presence or absence of high (arterial) flow through the lesions
    - Important because high flow lesions typically treated with transarterial embolization and low flow lesions treated with percutaneous sclerosis

DIFFERENTIAL DIAGNOSIS

Hemangioma
- Exhibit cellular proliferation
- Small or absent at birth, rapid growth during infancy, involution during childhood
- Lobulated mass that shows diffuse, high T2 signal and diffuse enhancement
- May be prominent draining veins that appear as flow voids (low signal)

High-flow vascular malformation
- Tangle of vessels/no soft tissue mass
- High flow on gradient echo images

Lymphatic malformation
- Multiple cysts of various sizes that are high T2 signal and may show peripheral but not diffuse enhancement

VENOUS MALFORMATIONS

Soft tissue sarcoma (MRI)
- If mass does not meet both clinical and MR criteria for one of the above lesions, sarcoma should be considered and biopsy performed

PATHOLOGY

General Features
- General path comments
  - VM are dysplasias of small and large venous channels
  - Do not have a component of high arterial flow
  - Lesions may be mixed with both venous and lymphatic components
    - This is not uncommon
  - Soft, compressible, non-pulsatile mass
- Associated abnormalities
  - Blue rubber bleb nevus syndrome
    - Venous malformations seen in skin, gastrointestinal, and musculoskeletal systems
  - Maffucci syndrome
    - Venous malformations seen in association with multiple enchondromatosis
  - Klippel-Trenaunay syndrome
    - Capillary-lymphaticovenous malformation of lower extremity
    - Dermal capillary stain with lymphatic vesicles
    - Varicosities of superficial veins
    - Anomalies and occasionally absence of deep venous system
    - Bony overgrowth of involved extremity

CLINICAL ISSUES

Presentation
- Most common signs/symptoms
  - Often present with pain
  - May present as symptomatic mass
- Other signs/symptoms
  - Decreased range of motion, deformity
  - Lesion may be visible on physical examination if skin is involved
  - May appear as soft tissue mass: Sometimes with bluish hue
  - Patients often have increasing symptoms in late childhood or early adulthood
  - Hormonal influences may cause rapid growth during teenage years in girls
  - Enlarge when the limb is dependent or Valsalva maneuver
  - Decompress with elevation or compression

Demographics
- Age
  - Most commonly diagnosed at birth
  - May be discovered at any age - growth with child
  - May enlarge suddenly secondary to hemorrhage, thrombosis, hormonal changes
  - Pain may become an increasing problem during puberty

Natural History & Prognosis
- Prognosis related to whether lesion focal or diffusely infiltrating
- Often is a life-time problem with treatment aimed at reducing symptoms rather than eliminating disease

Treatment
- Aspirin to treat and prevent thrombosis
- Elastic compression garments
- Percutaneous sclerosis
  - Direct injection with ethanol or other sclerosing agent under fluoroscopic/ultrasound guidance
  - Performed under general anesthesia
  - Complete relief of pain in 20%
  - Partial or temporary relief of pain in 60%
  - No relief of pain in 20%
  - Complications in 10-15%
  - Potential complications include: Skin necrosis, nerve damage, extremity swelling (requiring steroids), muscle atrophy, deep vein thrombosis, pulmonary embolism, disseminated intravascular coagulation, death
- Surgical resection with or without percutaneous sclerosis

SELECTED REFERENCES

1. Konez O et al: Magnetic resonance of vascular anomalies. Magn Reson Imaging Clin N Am. 10(2):363-88, vii, 2002
2. Donnelly LF et al: Marked acute tissue swelling following percutaneous sclerosis of low-flow vascular malformations: a predictor of both prolonged recovery and therapeutic effect. Pediatr Radiol. 30(6):415-9, 2000
3. Donnelly LF et al: Vascular malformations and hemangiomas: a practical approach in a multidisciplinary clinic. AJR Am J Roentgenol. 174(3):597-608, 2000
4. Fordham LA et al: Imaging of congenital vascular and lymphatic anomalies of the head and neck. Neuroimaging Clin N Am. 10(1):117-36, viii, 2000
5. Mulliken JB et al: Vascular anomalies. Curr Probl Surg. 37(8):517-84, 2000
6. Donnelly LF et al: Combined sonographic and fluoroscopic guidance: a modified technique for percutaneous sclerosis of low-flow vascular malformations. AJR Am J Roentgenol. 173(3):655-7, 1999
7. Dubois J et al: Imaging and therapeutic approach of hemangiomas and vascular malformations in the pediatric age group. Pediatr Radiol. 29(12):879-93, 1999
8. Robertson RL et al: Head and neck vascular anomalies of childhood. Neuroimaging Clin N Am. 9(1):115-32, 1999
9. Dubois J et al: Imaging of hemangiomas and vascular malformations in children. Acad Radiol. 5(5):390-400, 1998
10. Laor T et al: Congenital anomalies and vascular birthmarks of the lower extremities. Magn Reson Imaging Clin N Am. 6(3):497-519, 1998
11. Laor T et al: Magnetic resonance venography of congenital vascular malformations of the extremities. Pediatr Radiol. 26(6):371-80, 1996
12. Barnes PD et al: Hemangiomas and vascular malformations of the head and neck: MR characterization. AJNR Am J Neuroradiol. 15(1):193-5, 1994
13. Wahrman JE et al: Hemangiomas. Pediatr Rev. 15(7):266-71, 1994
14. Meyer JS et al: Biological classification of soft-tissue vascular anomalies: MR correlation. AJR. 157:559-64, 1991

VENOUS MALFORMATIONS

IMAGE GALLERY

Typical

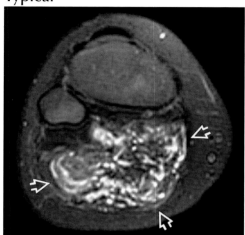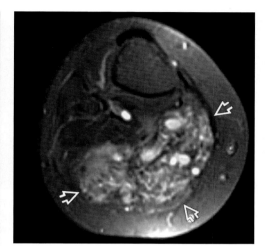

(Left) Axial T2WI MR shows focal mass (arrows) involving musculature posterior to knee with serpentine areas of high signal. *(Right)* Axial T1 C+ MR in same patient as on left shows focal mass (arrows) with enhancement of serpentine areas.

Typical

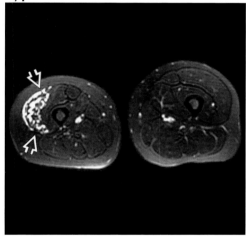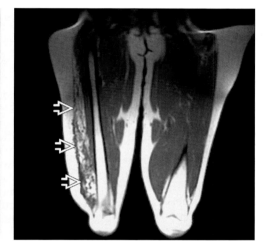

(Left) Axial T2WI MR shows focal mass (arrows) in the right vastus lateralis with serpentine areas of high signal. *(Right)* Coronal T1WI MR in same patient shows superior to inferior extent of lesion (arrows) which contains fat in hamartomatous stroma.

Typical

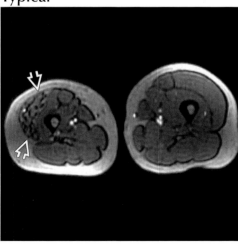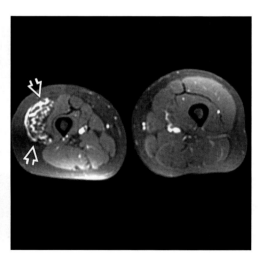

(Left) Axial T2* GRE MR in same patient shows no evidence of high flow in the lesion (arrows). Note atrophy of all of ipsilateral muscles compared to contralateral thigh. *(Right)* Axial T1 C+ MR in same patient shows enhancement of serpentine channels in mass (arrows). Again note diffuse muscle atrophy on ipsilateral side.

LYMPHATIC MALFORMATION

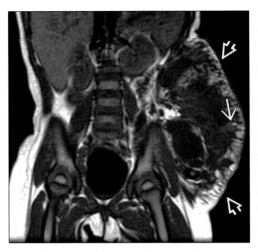

Coronal T1WI MR shows multicystic fluid-signal mass (open arrows). Note several cysts have high signal related to hemorrhage (arrow). Note hamartomatous fat in lesion.

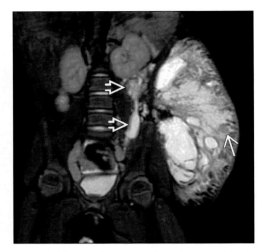

Coronal STIR MR in same patient shows multicystic fluid-signal mass. Most cysts have high signal but some have low signal (arrow). Note extension into abdominal cavity (open arrows).

TERMINOLOGY

Abbreviations and Synonyms
- Cystic hygroma: When involves the head and neck
- Lymphatic malformation (LM)
- Incorrect terminology: Lymphangioma - not a neoplasm

Definitions
- Vascular malformation: Congenital malformation that is not true neoplasm (hemangiomas are)
  - Present at birth and enlarge proportional to child
  - Do not involute without intervention and remain throughout life
  - Subcategorized based on type of channels: Lymphatic, venous, capillary, arteriovenous, and mixed
  - Lymphatic malformations are subtype of vascular malformation
- Lymphatic malformation
  - Dysplastic collection of lymph-containing cystic structures lined by endothelium
  - Usually macrocystic, may be microcystic
  - May enlarge rapidly related to hemorrhage, inflammation
  - One of the more common causes of soft tissue masses in head and neck of infants

IMAGING FINDINGS

General Features
- Best diagnostic clue: Multicystic mass most commonly in neck/axilla
- Location
  - Head and neck (70%)
  - Axilla (20%)
  - Others trunk, extremities, mesentery, retroperitoneum, pelvis (10%)
- General Imaging Features
  - Multicystic mass
  - Smooth and well-defined
  - Size and number of cysts highly variable
  - Septal enhancement of cysts may be present but no enhancement of central portions
  - Hamartomatous connective tissue often surrounds cysts
    - May contain abnormal amounts of fat
  - Content of cysts variable in imaging appearance due to hemorrhage or proteinaceous fluid
  - Most typically involve soft tissues
  - Often lesions do not respect tissue/fascial planes and may involve multiple tissue types: Muscles, subcutaneous tissues
  - Bone involvement uncommon
  - There may be atrophy of involved muscular structures

DDx: Soft Tissue Mass

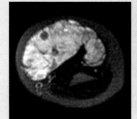
Hemangioma

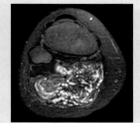
Venous Malf

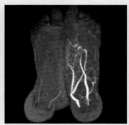
AVM

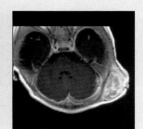
Sarcoma

LYMPHATIC MALFORMATION

Key Facts

Terminology
- Dysplastic collection of lymph-containing cystic structures lined by endothelium
- Usually macrocystic, may be microcystic
- May enlarge rapidly related to hemorrhage, inflammation
- One of the more common causes of soft tissue masses in head and neck of infants

Imaging Findings
- Multicystic mass
- Smooth and well-defined
- Size and number of cysts highly variable
- Septal enhancement of cysts may be present but no enhancement of central portions
- Content of cysts variable in imaging appearance due to hemorrhage or proteinaceous fluid

- Most typically involve soft tissues
- Often lesions do not respect tissue/fascial planes and may involve multiple tissue types: Muscles, subcutaneous tissues
- Bone involvement uncommon
- There may be atrophy of involved muscular structures
- No evidence of increased flow in lesions

Clinical Issues
- Most common signs/symptoms: Soft, pliable, soft tissue mass
- Identified at birth in 65% of cases
- 90% present prior to 2 years of age
- Primary treatment of lymphatic malformations is either surgical resection or percutaneous sclerosis

○ No evidence of increased flow in lesions
○ No evidence of flow voids
○ Microcystic lesions are uncommon and may be rather homogeneous with diffuse enhancement

Radiographic Findings
- Radiography: Soft tissue mass

Fluoroscopic Findings
- Injection of contrast utilized during imaging guidance for percutaneous sclerosis
- Contrast fills single or multiple communicating cysts

CT Findings
- Typically, multilocular low attenuation mass
- Enhancement of septae with contrast
- Content of cysts may be bright or have fluid/fluid levels related to hemorrhage or proteinaceous fluid

MR Findings
- T1WI
  ○ Multilocular cystic mass with cyst content most typically isointense to muscle
  ○ Cyst content variable due to hemorrhage or proteinaceous fluid
    ▪ May be high in signal
    ▪ May show fluid-fluid levels
  ○ No evidence of abnormal number of flow void vessels
- T2WI: Cyst content typically high in signal but variable
- T2* GRE: No evidence of high flow vessels
- T1 C+
  ○ Enhancement of cystic septae and intervening connective tissue
  ○ No enhancement in central portions of cysts

Ultrasonographic Findings
- Grayscale Ultrasound: Multilocular cystic mass
- Color Doppler
  ○ No flow identified in cysts
  ○ Flow may be identified in septae between cysts

Imaging Recommendations
- MRI is the imaging test of choice for making diagnosis and evaluating extent of disease
- MR protocols should include
  ○ T1 weighted images
  ○ T2 weighted fat saturated images
  ○ Post-gadolinium T1 weighted images
  ○ Gradient echo imaging sequences: To determine the presence or absence of high (arterial) flow through the lesions
    ▪ Important because high flow lesions typically treated with transarterial embolization and low flow lesions treated with percutaneous sclerosis

DIFFERENTIAL DIAGNOSIS

Hemangioma
- Exhibits cellular proliferation
- Small or absent at birth, rapid growth during infancy, involution during childhood
- Lobulated mass that shows diffuse high T2 signal and diffuse enhancement
- May be prominent draining veins that appear as flow voids (low signal)

Venous malformation
- Multiple serpentine channels that appear high in signal on T2 images and may show enhancement in channels but not diffusely
- No high signal on gradient echo images
- Phleboliths

Arteriovenous malformation (AVM)
- Tangle of vessels, no soft tissue mass
- High flow on gradient echo images

Soft tissue sarcoma
- If mass does not meet both clinical and MR criteria for one of the above lesions, sarcoma should be considered and biopsy performed

LYMPHATIC MALFORMATION

PATHOLOGY

General Features
- General path comments
  - Dysplastic collection of lymph-containing cystic structures lined by endothelium
  - May be macro or microcystic
  - Microcystic may have a more solid appearance
  - Related to maldevelopment of the cervical-facial lymphatic system
  - May be mixed with both lymphatic and venous components
- Associated abnormalities
  - Turner syndrome
  - Noonan syndrome
  - Multiple pterygium syndrome
  - Trisomy 21, 13, and 18
  - Klippel-Trenaunay syndrome
    - Capillary-lymphaticovenous malformation of lower extremity
    - Dermal capillary stain with lymphatic vesicles
    - Varicosities of superficial veins
    - Anomalies and occasionally absence of deep venous system
    - Bony overgrowth of involved extremity

CLINICAL ISSUES

Presentation
- Most common signs/symptoms: Soft, pliable, soft tissue mass
- Other signs/symptoms
  - May present as diffuse limb enlargement
  - Superficial vesicles representing extensions of deeper lymphatics may be seen in the skin
  - Often, however, overlying skin normal
  - Usually non-painful at presentation unless present with rapid enlargement due to hemorrhage/inflammation
  - May compress airway or other vital structures

Demographics
- Age
  - Identified at birth in 65% of cases
  - 90% present prior to 2 years of age
  - May present late when increase rapidly in size related to hemorrhage or viral illness

Natural History & Prognosis
- Recurrence may occur
- Small, focal lesions have excellent prognosis
- Large, infiltrating lesions have more poor prognosis

Treatment
- Primary treatment of lymphatic malformations is either surgical resection or percutaneous sclerosis
  - If lesions involve critical tissues/neurovascular bundles: May treat with percutaneous sclerosis
  - Sometimes combination sclerosis/surgical resection performed
- Percutaneous sclerosis
  - Direct injection of ethanol or other sclerotic agent (Ethibloc, 50% dextrose, bleomycin, OK-432, triamcinolone)
  - Procedure with ultrasound/fluoro guidance
  - Performed under general anesthesia
  - Drain may be left in place to help collapse cyst after sclerosing agent utilized
  - Decrease in size in 80% of cases
  - Complications in 10-15%, major complications uncommon
  - Potential complications: Skin necrosis, nerve damage, extremity swelling (requiring steroids), muscle atrophy, disseminated intravascular coagulation
  - Full results of sclerosis may take months to manifest
    - Process of inflammation and clot formation, followed by scarring and decrease in volume
    - Marked soft tissue swelling right after procedure
    - May take multiple staged procedures to treat lesion
- Conservative supportive therapies
  - Compression garments
  - Pneumatic pumps

SELECTED REFERENCES

1. Konez O et al: Magnetic resonance of vascular anomalies. Magn Reson Imaging Clin N Am. 10(2):363-88, vii, 2002
2. Donnelly LF et al: Vascular malformations and hemangiomas: a practical approach in a multidisciplinary clinic. AJR Am J Roentgenol. 174(3):597-608, 2000
3. Donnelly LF et al: Marked acute tissue swelling following percutaneous sclerosis of low-flow vascular malformations: a predictor of both prolonged recovery and therapeutic effect. Pediatr Radiol. 30(6):415-9, 2000
4. Fordham LA et al: Imaging of congenital vascular and lymphatic anomalies of the head and neck. Neuroimaging Clin N Am. 10(1):117-36, viii, 2000
5. Mulliken JB et al: Vascular anomalies. Curr Probl Surg. 37(8):517-84, 2000
6. Donnelly LF et al: Combined sonographic and fluoroscopic guidance: a modified technique for percutaneous sclerosis of low-flow vascular malformations. AJR Am J Roentgenol. 173(3):655-7, 1999
7. Dubois J et al: Imaging and therapeutic approach of hemangiomas and vascular malformations in the pediatric age group. Pediatr Radiol. 29(12):879-93, 1999
8. Robertson RL et al: Head and neck vascular anomalies of childhood. Neuroimaging Clin N Am. 9(1):115-32, 1999
9. Dubois J et al: Imaging of hemangiomas and vascular malformations in children. Acad Radiol. 5(5):390-400, 1998
10. Laor T et al: Congenital anomalies and vascular birthmarks of the lower extremities. Magn Reson Imaging Clin N Am. 6(3):497-519, 1998
11. Laor T et al: Magnetic resonance venography of congenital vascular malformations of the extremities. Pediatr Radiol. 26(6):371-80, 1996
12. Barnes PD et al: Hemangiomas and vascular malformations of the head and neck: MR characterization. AJNR Am J Neuroradiol. 15(1):193-5, 1994
13. Meyer JS et al: Biological classification of soft-tissue vascular anomalies: MR correlation. AJR. 157:559-64, 1991
14. Mulliken JB et al: Hemangiomas and vascular malformations in infants and children: a classification based on endothelial characteristics. Plast Reconstr Surg. 69:412-22, 1982

LYMPHATIC MALFORMATION

IMAGE GALLERY

Typical

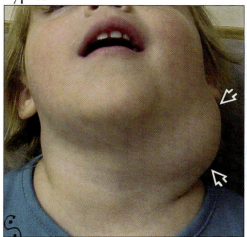
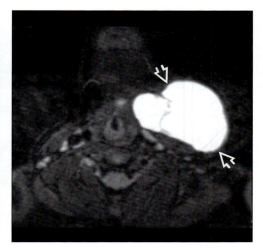

(Left) Clinical photograph shows soft tissue mass (arrows) in left neck. *(Right)* Axial T2WI MR in same patient as on left shows large, high signal, cystic structure (arrows) with septation.

Typical

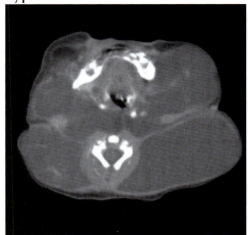
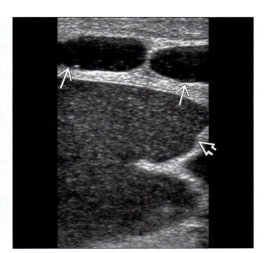

(Left) Axial CECT in neonate shows extensive multicystic fluid-filled mass throughout cervical region. Entire neck is abnormal bilaterally. *(Right)* Ultrasound shows multicystic fluid-filled mass. Content of cysts is variable. Two smaller cysts (arrows) demonstrate relatively anechoic fluid and larger cyst (open arrow) more echogenic fluid.

Typical

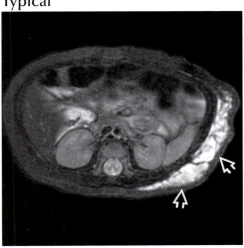
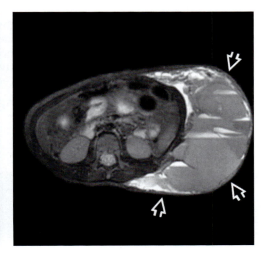

(Left) Axial T2WI MR shows multicystic fluid-signal mass that rapidly increased in size during viral illness. Initial study shows high signal, multiseptated mass (arrows) in left flank. *(Right)* Axial T2WI MR obtained one month later after rapid growth shows marked enlargement of mass (arrows) that now contain multiple fluid-fluid levels suggestive of interval hemorrhage/inflammation.

ARTERIOVENOUS MALFORMATION

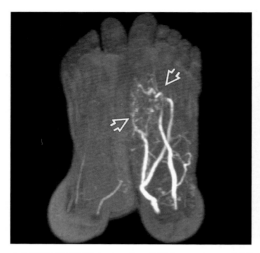

Axial T2* GRE MR depicted on MIP image shows AVM of the left foot as abnormal tangle of high flow vessels (arrows) with prominent arterial vessels feeding the lesion. Note relatively sparse contralateral vessels.

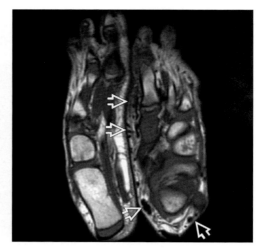

Axial T1WI MR in same patient shows multiple, asymmetric signal voids (arrows).

TERMINOLOGY

Abbreviations and Synonyms
- Arteriovenous (AV) malformation
- Arteriovenous malformation (AVM)
- High flow vascular malformation

Definitions
- Vascular malformation: Congenital malformation that is not a true neoplasm (hemangiomas are)
  - Present at birth and enlarge proportional to child
  - Do not involute without intervention and remain throughout life
  - Subcategorized based on type of channels: Arteriovenous, lymphatic, venous, capillary, or mixed
  - Arteriovenous malformations are subtype of vascular malformations
- Arteriovenous malformation: Congenital lesion with abnormal direct connection between arterial and venous structures
  - Bypassing capillary bed
  - Tangle of vessels without discrete soft tissue mass
  - High flow within vessels
  - Much less common than venous malformation, lymphatic malformation, or hemangioma

IMAGING FINDINGS

General Features
- Best diagnostic clue: Tangle of abnormal vessels without associated soft tissue mass
- Location: Occur in any location
- General Imaging Features
  - Abnormal tangle of blood vessels
  - Prominent draining veins
  - High flow demonstrated in involved vessels (arterialization of veins)
  - The lesions may have surrounding connective tissue stroma
    - May contain fatty components
  - No associated soft tissue mass
  - May have surrounding edema
  - Are often focal but may be diffuse involving a large part of an extremity

Radiographic Findings
- Radiography
  - Soft tissue mass may be present
  - Rarely, bone involvement may be shown as destructive mass
  - Bone overgrowth may be present

MR Findings
- T1WI

DDx: Soft Tissue Lesion

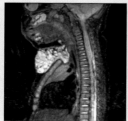

Hemangioma

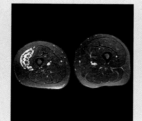

Venous Malf

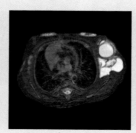

Lymphatic Malf

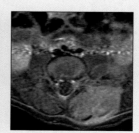

Sarcoma

ARTERIOVENOUS MALFORMATION

Key Facts

Terminology
- Vascular malformation: Congenital malformation that is not a true neoplasm (hemangiomas are)
- Present at birth and enlarge proportional to child
- Do not involute without intervention and remain throughout life
- Subcategorized based on type of channels: Arteriovenous, lymphatic, venous, capillary, or mixed
- Arteriovenous malformations are subtype of vascular malformations
- Arteriovenous malformation: Congenital lesion with abnormal direct connection between arterial and venous structures
- Bypassing capillary bed
- Much less common than venous malformation, lymphatic malformation, or hemangioma

Imaging Findings
- Abnormal tangle of blood vessels
- Prominent draining veins
- High flow demonstrated in involved vessels (arterialization of veins)
- The lesions may have surrounding connective tissue stroma
- May contain fatty components
- No associated soft tissue mass
- May have surrounding edema

Clinical Issues
- Transarterial embolization
- Coaxial systems used to achieve cannulation of subselective arteries
- Embolization materials include: Coils, Gelfoam particles, ethanol

---

  - Tangle of abnormal vessels
  - Flow void in multiple vessels
- T2WI
  - Flow void in multiple vessels
  - Absence of discrete soft tissue mass
  - May be high signal in surrounding tissues related to edema
- T2* GRE: Multiple vessels showing high signal indicative of rapid flow
- T1 C+: Intense contrast-enhancement of multiple vessels
- MRA
  - Demonstration of nidus of abnormal vessels
  - Feeding arterial structures
    - Helpful for pre-embolization planning
  - Draining venous structures
  - Enlarged draining veins typically much larger than feeding arteries

Ultrasonographic Findings
- Grayscale Ultrasound
  - Heterogeneous lesions
  - Multiple abnormal tangle of tubular structures
  - Large feeding arterial and exiting venous structures
  - No defined soft tissue mass
- Color Doppler
  - High vessel density
  - Multiple vessels in abnormal tangle
  - Afferent arteries and efferent veins
- Pulsed Doppler
  - High systolic flow
  - Arteriovenous shunting
  - Arterial wave forms in venous structures (pulsatile flow)

Echocardiographic Findings
- May show findings of congestive heart failure

Angiographic Findings
- Essential for planning and performing embolization therapy
- Dilatation of feeding arterial structures
- Early venous opacification from arteriovenous shunting
- Large draining efferent veins
- Typically there are numerous feeding arterial structures
  - Often more feeding vessels become apparent after embolization of the originally identified feeding arteries

Imaging Recommendations
- Best imaging tool
  - MR or Doppler ultrasound for diagnosis
  - Arteriography and transarterial embolization for therapy

DIFFERENTIAL DIAGNOSIS

Hemangioma
- Exhibits cellular proliferation
- During proliferative phase, will show high flow vessels
- Demonstrates discrete soft tissue mass, unlike AVM
- Small or absent at birth
- Rapid growth during infancy
- Involution during childhood

Venous malformation
- Multiple serpentine channels that appear high in signal on T2WIs
- Channels show enhancement
- No high signal seen on gradient echo images to suggest high flow
- Phleboliths

Lymphatic malformation
- Multiple cysts of various sizes that are high T2W signal and may show peripheral but not diffuse enhancement
- No abnormal flow voids

Soft tissue sarcoma
- If soft tissue mass is identified, the lesion is not a simple AVM

ARTERIOVENOUS MALFORMATION

- If lesion does not appear as classic hemangioma, other soft tissue masses such as sarcoma should be suspected

Arteriovenous fistula
- Direct communication between artery and vein
- No evidence of abnormal tangle of dysplastic vessels

PATHOLOGY

General Features
- General path comments
  - Direct connection between arterial and venous system that bypasses capillary bed
  - The connections are lined with endothelial cells
- Epidemiology: Much less common than other lesions such as venous and lymphatic malformations as well as hemangiomas

CLINICAL ISSUES

Presentation
- Most common signs/symptoms: Pulsatile mass
- Other signs/symptoms
  - Thrill, bruit, hyperthermia
  - Skeletal overgrowth
  - Trophic changes
  - Pain
  - Bleeding from ulceration
  - Congestive heart failure
  - Steal phenomenon
  - Ulceration and bleeding
  - Embolism
  - May enlarge rapidly related to hemorrhage, thrombosis
  - Leg length (or limb) discrepancy - from bony overgrowth of affected limb

Demographics
- Age
  - May present at any time during childhood or sometimes in adulthood
  - May be exacerbated and present during puberty or pregnancy
  - Large shunting lesions typically present earlier: Often soon after birth
- Gender: M = F

Treatment
- Transarterial embolization
  - Performed under general anesthesia
  - Coaxial systems used to achieve cannulation of subselective arteries
  - Embolization materials include: Coils, Gelfoam particles, ethanol
  - Very important to embolize very distal feeding branches as proximal embolization may preclude access to more distal branches that may become recanalized from other sources
  - After embolization of each feeding artery, repeat angiogram is performed to identify other feeding vessels
    - Typically there are multiple feeding vessels
  - Ultrasound with Doppler directly over lesion during procedure may be helpful in evaluating for cessation of flow and thrombosis of nidus
  - If arterial feeders not accessible, direct puncture of feeding arteries may be attempted under ultrasound guidance
- Surgical excision
  - Usually attempted in conjunction with embolization to decrease flow and minimize hemorrhage
- Conservative management
  - Compression garments

DIAGNOSTIC CHECKLIST

Image Interpretation Pearls
- Tangle of high flow vessels without associated soft tissue mass = arteriovenous malformation
- If soft tissue mass present, think hemangioma or vascular malignancy

SELECTED REFERENCES

1. Gampper TJ et al: Vascular anomalies: hemangiomas. Plast Reconstr Surg. 110(2):572-85; quiz 586; discussion 587-8, 2002
2. Konez O et al: Magnetic resonance of vascular anomalies. Magn Reson Imaging Clin N Am. 10(2):363-88, vii, 2002
3. Donnelly LF et al: Marked acute tissue swelling following percutaneous sclerosis of low-flow vascular malformations: a predictor of both prolonged recovery and therapeutic effect. Pediatr Radiol. 30(6):415-9, 2000
4. Donnelly LF et al: Vascular malformations and hemangiomas: a practical approach in a multidisciplinary clinic. AJR Am J Roentgenol. 174(3):597-608, 2000
5. Fordham LA et al: Imaging of congenital vascular and lymphatic anomalies of the head and neck. Neuroimaging Clin N Am. 10(1):117-36, viii, 2000
6. Mulliken JB et al: Vascular anomalies. Curr Probl Surg. 37(8):517-84, 2000
7. Donnelly LF et al: Combined sonographic and fluoroscopic guidance: a modified technique for percutaneous sclerosis of low-flow vascular malformations. AJR Am J Roentgenol. 173(3):655-7, 1999
8. Dubois J et al: Imaging and therapeutic approach of hemangiomas and vascular malformations in the pediatric age group. Pediatr Radiol. 29(12):879-93, 1999
9. Robertson RL et al: Head and neck vascular anomalies of childhood. Neuroimaging Clin N Am. 9(1):115-32, 1999
10. Dubois J et al: Imaging of hemangiomas and vascular malformations in children. Acad Radiol. 5(5):390-400, 1998
11. Laor T et al: Congenital anomalies and vascular birthmarks of the lower extremities. Magn Reson Imaging Clin N Am. 6(3):497-519, 1998
12. Laor T et al: Magnetic resonance venography of congenital vascular malformations of the extremities. Pediatr Radiol. 26(6):371-80, 1996
13. Barnes PD et al: Hemangiomas and vascular malformations of the head and neck: MR characterization. AJNR Am J Neuroradiol. 15(1):193-5, 1994
14. Wahrman JE et al: Hemangiomas. Pediatr Rev. 15(7):266-71, 1994
15. Smith MB et al: Differentiation and treatment of hemangiomas and arteriovenous malformations. J La State Med Soc. 141(6):41-3, 1989

ARTERIOVENOUS MALFORMATION

IMAGE GALLERY

Typical

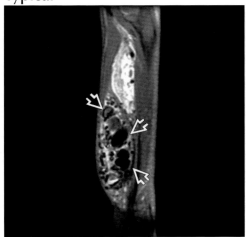
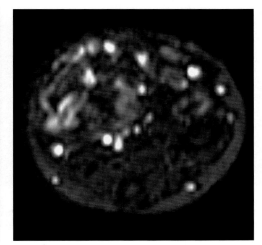

(Left) Sagittal T1 C+ MR of forearm shows multiple signal voids with surrounding enhancing hamartomatous connective tissue and edema. The larger vessels (arrows) are the dilated efferent veins. *(Right)* Axial T2* GRE MR in same patient shows signal in multiple vessels consistent with high arterial flow in AVM.

Typical

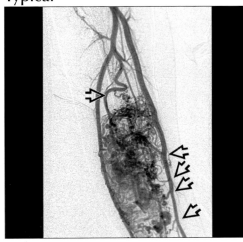
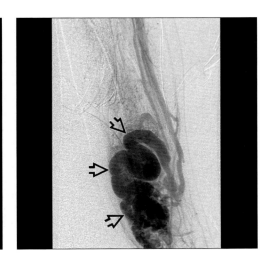

(Left) Angiography (early arterial phase) in same patient shows AVM as abnormal tangle of vessels with multiple feeding arteries (arrows). *(Right)* Angiography (in venous phase) in same patient shows massively enlarged draining veins (arrows). Multiple embolizations were performed eventually followed by surgical resection.

Variant

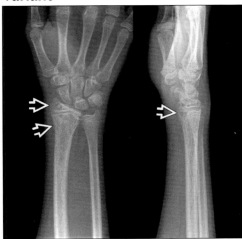
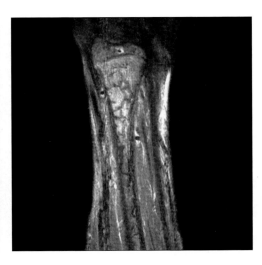

(Left) Radiograph shows abnormal mottled lucency (arrows) in distal epiphysis and metaphysis of radius. *(Right)* Coronal T2WI MR in same patient shows abnormal signal in distal radius with multiple serpentine flow voids consistent with vessels. Gradient echo (not shown) showed high flow consistent with AVM.

AGGRESSIVE FIBROMATOSIS

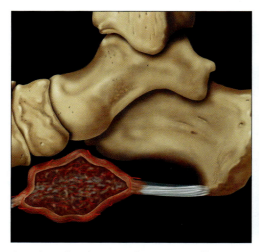

Sagittal graphic shows a soft tissue mass, fibromatosis (red) along the plantar aspect of the foot.

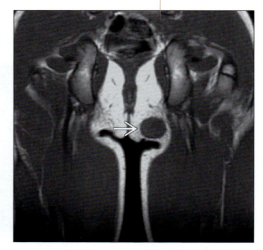

Coronal T1WI MR shows a discrete well-defined homogeneous mass isointense to muscle within the medial subcutaneous fat of the left hip (arrow) in this patient with aggressive fibromatosis.

TERMINOLOGY

Abbreviations and Synonyms
- Aggressive fibromatosis, extraabdominal desmoid tumor, musculoaponeurotic fibromatosis

Definitions
- Group of benign disorders with fibrous growth, tendency to infiltrate adjacent tissues, recurs & lacks metastatic disease

IMAGING FINDINGS

General Features
- Location
  - Superficial
    - Plantar, palmar, penile fibromatosis
  - Deep: Intra-abdominal & extra-abdominal
    - Extra-abdominal fibromatosis = extra-abdominal desmoid
    - Slow insidious growth over weeks to months prior to presentation for evaluation
    - Involves superficial fasciae, deep tendons, aponeuroses, muscles
    - Extremity (70%): Shoulder, upper arm, thigh, neck, pelvis, abdomen, forearm
    - Multicentric 10-15%
    - Intra-abdominal: Abdominal wall & mesenteric
  - Infantile fibromatosis
- Size
  - Superficial type up to 5 cm
  - Deep type usually < 10 cm but can be quite large up to 20 cm (especially in Gardner syndrome)
- Fibromatosis
  - Aggressive fibromatosis
    - = Infantile fibromatosis, extra-abdominal desmoid tumor, musculoaponeurotic fibromatosis
    - 1st & 2nd decade
    - +/- Multifocal
    - Erosions or bowing of bones
    - Nodular (more common in adults) or infiltrative (children) patterns
  - Myofibromatosis
    - Most common in infancy, infancy → adults
    - ↑ Size & number to 1 year of age then can regress
    - 3 types: Solitary, multicentric with or without visceral involvement
    - Bones, muscle, subcutaneous tissue, viscera
    - +/- Calcifications
    - May have a target appearance on MR or US (center mildly hyperintense on T1 & nonenhancing)
    - Osteolytic; sharply defined (metaphyseal > diaphyseal)
  - Fibromatosis colli

DDx: Soft Tissue Masses

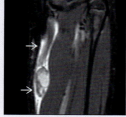

Synovial Sarcoma

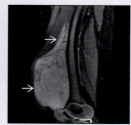

Rhabdomyosarcoma

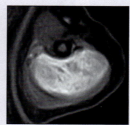

Infantile Fibrosarcoma

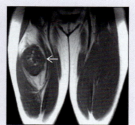

Venous Malformation

AGGRESSIVE FIBROMATOSIS

Key Facts

Terminology
- Aggressive fibromatosis, extraabdominal desmoid tumor, musculoaponeurotic fibromatosis
- Group of benign disorders with fibrous growth, tendency to infiltrate adjacent tissues, recurs & lacks metastatic disease

Imaging Findings
- Typical: Hypointense to muscle
- Can be isointense to muscle
- Typical: Hyperintense with areas of hypointense signal regions (fibrous components)
- Hypo → hyperintense signal compared to skeletal muscle
- Depends on the cellular compared to collagen components
- The more cellular the more hyperintense signal

Pathology
- Epidemiology: 2-4/1,000,000 per year

Clinical Issues
- Firm poorly-circumscribed slowly growing mass
- Tends to extend beyond palpable limits
- 20-40 years (peak age: 23 years)
- Infantile fibromatosis typical < 2 years, rarely > 5 years old
- Recurrence in 65%

Diagnostic Checklist
- Can mimic other soft tissue sarcomas (fibrosarcomas) especially if infiltrating, but lack metastatic potential

---

- 2-4 weeks old at presentation, often history of breech presentation, instrumentation, & primiparous birth
- Enlargement of the sternocleidomastoid muscle
- Diagnosis most commonly made upon physical exam, sometimes on ultrasound, rarely need CT or MR to make diagnosis
- No recurrence, self limiting, spontaneously resolves, resolves with physical therapy, rarely surgery needed
  - Congenital infantile fibrosarcoma
    - Congenital, histologic diagnosis is difficult, +/- metastatic disease (truncal > extremity)
    - < 5 year old, typically presents < 2 years of age, commonly neonatal
    - Can erode adjacent bone
    - Heterogeneous enhancement
    - Better prognosis than adults
  - Adult fibrosarcoma
    - Teenagers → adults
    - Can contain calcifications or ossification
    - Higher cellularity, more mitoses, increased nuclear pleomorphism, +/- metastases compared to fibromatosis
  - Fibrous hamartoma of infancy
    - Neonates → young children (typically 1st two years of life, ¼ congenital)
    - Subcutaneous or reticular dermis, 0.5 → 4 cm
    - Axilla, shoulders, inguinal region, & chest wall most common location
    - Excision usually curative, excellent prognosis
    - MR: Varying amounts of fibrous & fatty tissue
  - Angiofibroma
    - Adolescent males, peak age 15 years old
    - Clinical triad: Nasopharyngeal mass, nasal obstruction & epistaxis
    - Typical: Pterygopalatine fossa & sphenopalatine foramen expansion
    - Homogeneous enhancement, high vascularity
    - Recurs up to 60%
  - Hyaline fibromatosis
    - Autosomal recessive
    - Joint contractures, lytic bone lesions, gingival hyperplasia, papulonodular skin lesions
    - Infantile form can involve multiple organs
  - Venous malformation
    - Calcifications on conventional radiographs low flow lesion with phleboliths &/or thrombi with diffuse enhancement on MR

Radiographic Findings
- Radiography
  - Soft tissue mass
  - +/- Periosteal reaction, cortical destruction, scalloping or erosions

CT Findings
- NECT
  - Soft tissue mass hyperdense to muscle
  - If close proximity to bone: Erosion, cortical destruction, periosteal reaction, bowing
  - +/- Adjacent osseous changes
- CECT: Intense contrast-enhancement

MR Findings
- T1WI
  - Typical: Hypointense to muscle
  - Can be isointense to muscle
- T2WI
  - Typical: Hyperintense with areas of hypointense signal regions (fibrous components)
  - Heterogeneous
  - Hypo → hyperintense signal compared to skeletal muscle
  - Depends on the cellular compared to collagen components
    - The more cellular the more hyperintense signal
- T1 C+: Intense enhancement
- Poorly defined
  - Invasion of fat & muscle

Ultrasonographic Findings
- Grayscale Ultrasound: Nonspecific soft tissue mass, variable echogenicity, smooth well defined margins

AGGRESSIVE FIBROMATOSIS

DIFFERENTIAL DIAGNOSIS

Malignant fibrous histiocytoma (MFH)
- Arises in deep soft tissues
- Calcifications

Synovial sarcoma
- In close proximity to joint
- Amorphous calcifications

Rhabdomyosarcoma
- +/- Necrotic or hemorrhagic foci
- Hyperintense T2WI signal
- Metastases

Fibrosarcoma
- Mimics adult & congenital infantile types
- Metastases
- +/- Necrotic or hemorrhagic foci
- Hyperintense T2WI signal

Venous malformation
- Calcifications on conventional radiographs, low flow lesion with phleboliths &/or thrombi with diffuse enhancement on MR

PATHOLOGY

General Features
- General path comments
  - Fibrous tissue proliferation with varying amounts of collagen
  - Locally aggressive infiltrative behavior & recurrences
  - Incapable of metastasizing & self limited
- Etiology: Unknown, but genetic, hormonal, trauma etiologies have been suggested
- Epidemiology: 2-4/1,000,000 per year
- Associated abnormalities
  - Familial: Gardner syndrome associated with intra-abdominal mesenteric fibromatosis
  - Trisomies 7, 8, 14, 20

Gross Pathologic & Surgical Features
- Firm, gray-white mass, streaky scar-like cross section
- May appear well-circumscribed but microscopically have ill-defined borders

Microscopic Features
- Proliferation of uniform fibroblastic cells
  - Accompanied & separated by dense collagenous stroma, sparse mitoses, lacks nuclear pleomorphism
  - Resembling hypertrophic scar tissue

CLINICAL ISSUES

Presentation
- Most common signs/symptoms
  - Firm poorly-circumscribed slowly growing mass
  - Tends to extend beyond palpable limits
  - Flexion contractions
  - +/- Tenderness (related to nerve compression or infiltration)
  - 10% are multifocal

Demographics
- Age
  - 20-40 years (peak age: 23 years)
  - Infantile fibromatosis typical < 2 years, rarely > 5 years old
- Ethnicity: More common in Caucasians

Natural History & Prognosis
- Recurrence in 65%
  - Tend to recur along surgical margin
- Younger patients have a higher recurrence rate

Treatment
- Surgical excision with wide margins
  - 31-50% recurrence
  - 71-90% recurrence with incomplete excision
- Anti-estrogen (Tamoxifen) therapy
- Nonsteroidal therapy
- Radiation therapy in recurrent, partially or unresectable lesions
- Amputations (occasional) for palliative repeated recurrences & nonresponsive to adjuvant therapy

DIAGNOSTIC CHECKLIST

Consider
- Can mimic other soft tissue sarcomas (fibrosarcomas) especially if infiltrating, but lack metastatic potential

Image Interpretation Pearls
- Often contains regions of ↓ signal on MR T1WI & T2WI images

SELECTED REFERENCES

1. Kingston CA et al: Imaging of desmoid fibromatosis in pediatric patients. AJR Am J Roentgenol. 178(1):191-9, 2002
2. Sorensen A et al: Treatment of aggressive fibromatosis: a retrospective study of 72 patients followed for 1-27 years. Acta Orthop Scand. 73(2):213-9, 2002
3. Netscher DT et al: Infantile myofibromatosis: case report of a solitary hand lesion with emphasis on differential diagnosis and management. Ann Plast Surg. 46(1):62-7, 2001
4. Ahn JM et al: Infantile fibromatosis in childhood: findings on MR imaging and pathologic correlation. Clin Radiol. 55(1):19-24, 2000
5. Mehrotra AK et al: Fibromatoses of the extremities: clinicopathologic study of 36 cases. J Surg Oncol. 74(4):291-6, 2000
6. Eich GF et al: Fibrous tumours in children: imaging features of a heterogeneous group of disorders. Pediatr Radiol. 28(7):500-9, 1998
7. Hartman TE et al: MR imaging of extraabdominal desmoids: differentiation from other neoplasms. AJR Am J Roentgenol. 158(3):581-5, 1992
8. Liu P et al: MRI of fibromatosis: With pathologic correlation. Pediatr Radiol. 22:587-9, 1992
9. O'Keefe F et al: Magnetic resonance imaging in aggressive fibromatosis. Clin Radiol. 42(3):170-3, 1990
10. Hudson TM et al: Aggressive fibromatosis: evaluation by computed tomography and angiography. Radiology. 150(2):495-501, 1984

AGGRESSIVE FIBROMATOSIS

IMAGE GALLERY

Typical

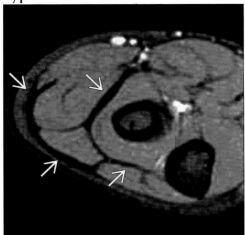
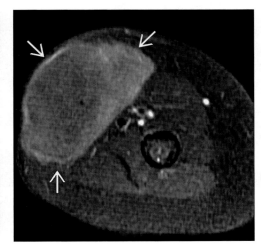

(Left) Axial PD/Intermediate MR shows markedly hypointense diffusely infiltrating mass in multiple muscle-fascial plane in the forearm (arrows) in this child with aggressive fibromatosis. *(Right)* Axial T1 C+ MR shows a large enhancing mass in the subcutaneous soft tissue (arrows), in this patient with aggressive fibromatosis.

Typical

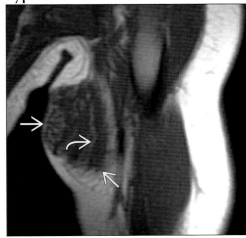
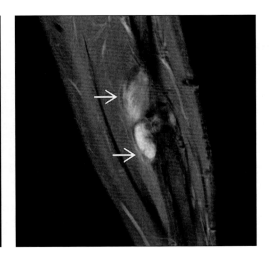

(Left) Coronal T1WI MR shows a mass (arrows) in the upper arm with characteristic internal fat stranding (curved arrow) of an infantile myofibromatosis. *(Right)* Coronal T1 C+ MR shows an enhancing mass (arrows) surrounding the forearm bone graft, consistent with recurrent aggressive fibromatosis.

Typical

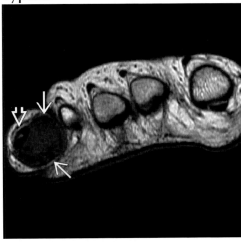
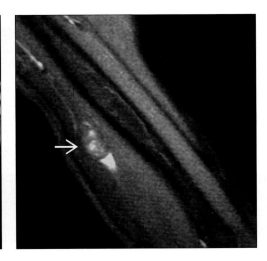

(Left) Coronal T1WI MR shows a hypointense foot mass (arrows) within the plantar soft tissue of the middle phalanx of the 5th digit with flattening of the plantar margin & remodeling of the middle phalanx (open arrow) in this patient with aggressive fibromatosis. *(Right)* Sagittal STIR MR shows a heterogeneously hyperintense mass (arrow) in this patient with aggressive fibromatosis.

RHABDOMYOSARCOMA, MUSCULOSKELETAL

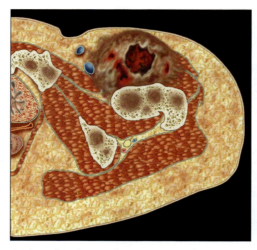

Axial graphic shows a heterogeneous soft tissue mass anterior to the left hip. Areas of hemorrhage are shown in red. Note multifocal osseous metastatic disease (in brown).

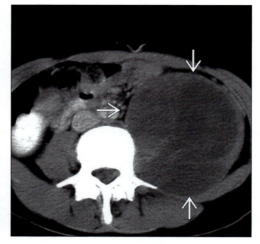

Axial CECT shows massive enlargement & replacement of the left psoas muscle by a hypodense RMS (arrows).

TERMINOLOGY

Abbreviations and Synonyms
- Alveolar rhabdomyosarcoma, embryonal rhabdomyosarcoma, rhabdomyosarcoma (RMS)

Definitions
- Mesenchymal sarcoma arising from "rhabdomyoblasts" (primitive muscle cell), lacks normal differentiation into skeletal muscle

IMAGING FINDINGS

General Features
- Best diagnostic clue: Large heterogeneous soft tissue mass
- Location
  ○ Head & neck: 28-40%
    ▪ Nasopharynx, sinuses, orbit (7%)
  ○ Genitourinary: 20%
    ▪ Prostate, bladder, vagina, paratesticular
  ○ Extremities: 15-20%
  ○ Truncal: 11%
  ○ Retroperitoneal: 6%
- Size: Depends on location & histology
- Morphology
  ○ Can occur anywhere in the body
  ○ 5-10% of childhood malignant solid tumors
  ○ 70%: < 10 year old at initial presentation
  ○ Embryonal RMS (60-70% of childhood RMS)
    ▪ Resembles skeletal muscles in 6-8 week fetus
    ▪ Most common type in < 15 year olds
    ▪ Genitourinary or head & neck
  ○ Alveolar RMS (20% of RMS)
    ▪ Resembles skeletal muscle in a 10 week fetus
    ▪ Adolescents
    ▪ Extremity, trunk & perianal/perirectal
  ○ Botryoid RMS (10% of RMS)
    ▪ Subtype of embryonal RMS (sarcoma botryoides)
    ▪ Vagina, bladder, biliary tree & nasopharynx
    ▪ Typical: Grape-like polyploid masses or clusters
  ○ Pleomorphic RMS
    ▪ 30-50 year olds, rarely in children

Radiographic Findings
- Soft tissue mass similar to muscle on radiographs
- 1/4 have adjacent bone destruction

CT Findings
- NECT
  ○ Difficult to separate from & isodense to skeletal muscle
  ○ Can have hemorrhage & adjacent osseous destruction
- CECT: Enhances heterogeneously

DDx: Soft Tissue Masses

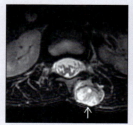
Extraosseous Ewing

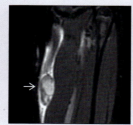
Synovial Cell Sarcoma

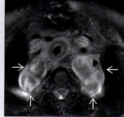
NF

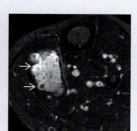
Venous Malformation

RHABDOMYOSARCOMA, MUSCULOSKELETAL

Key Facts

Terminology
- Mesenchymal sarcoma arising from "rhabdomyoblasts" (primitive muscle cell), lacks normal differentiation into skeletal muscle

Imaging Findings
- Head & neck: 28-40%
- Extremities: 15-20%
- Can occur anywhere in the body
- 5-10% of childhood malignant solid tumors
- 70%: < 10 year old at initial presentation
- Embryonal RMS (60-70% of childhood RMS)
- Alveolar RMS (20% of RMS)

Top Differential Diagnoses
- Other sarcomas
- Neuroblastoma (NBL)
- Vascular malformation & hemangiomas
- Hematoma

Pathology
- Embryonal: Loss of genomic material from chromosome 11
- Alveolar: Translocation chromosome 1 or 2 & 13
- Epidemiology: 4-6 cases/1,000,000 a year

Clinical Issues
- 2 Age peaks: 2-6 & 14-18 year old
- Embryonal: < 15 years old (head & neck, GU)
- Alveolar: 14-18 Years old (extremity, paratesticular, & truncal)

Diagnostic Checklist
- Unexplained hematoma in an extremity, need to exclude an underlying sarcoma

MR Findings
- T1WI: Typical: Similar signal to skeletal muscle
- T2WI
  - Typical: Hyperintense to skeletal muscle
  - Heterogeneous & can have areas of hemorrhage
- T1 C+
  - Typical: Enhances heterogeneously
  - Prominent vascularity

Angiographic Findings
- Hypervascular mass

Nuclear Medicine Findings
- PET
  - Intense FDG uptake by the soft tissue tumor
  - Helpful for differentiating post therapeutic change from recurrent of residual RMS
- Bone scan for skeletal metastases

Imaging Recommendations
- Best imaging tool: MR (C+/-)
- Protocol advice: T1, FS T2WI, STIR, T1 C+ MR

DIFFERENTIAL DIAGNOSIS

Other sarcomas
- Synovial cell sarcoma
  - Calcifications in 1/3, can appear nonaggressive
  - Not intra-articular, but near joint
- Primitive peripheral neuroectodermal tumor & extraosseous Ewing sarcoma
  - Small round blue cell tumor, no calcifications, heterogeneous enhancement on MR & CECT
  - Nonspecific soft tissue mass: Looks like RMS
- Fibrosarcoma
  - Present at birth = congenital-infantile fibrosarcoma, mostly a tumor of adults
- Myxoid liposarcoma & malignant fibrous histiocytoma (MFH)

Neurofibroma (NF) or malignant peripheral nerve sheath tumor
- Most common in Neurofibromatosis type 1
- Loss of target appearance: Atypical neurofibroma or sarcoma degeneration
- Also consider malignant degeneration: Mass becomes painful or ↑ in size

Neuroblastoma (NBL)
- Predominates in ages 1-5 year olds, most commonly adrenal origin & along the sympathetic chain, calcifications in majority
- ↑ Catecholamines & vasoactive intestinal polypeptides (VIP)
- Unusual metastatic disease to skeletal muscle

Vascular malformation & hemangiomas
- Venous malformation: +/- Phleboliths, slow flow lesion with enhancement
- Hemangiomas: Present at birth, rapid proliferative stage followed by a slower involutional stage, high flow lesion with diffuse enhancement

Hematoma
- Trauma history usual; consider underlying sarcoma if spontaneous bleed without trauma

PATHOLOGY

General Features
- Genetics
  - Embryonal: Loss of genomic material from chromosome 11
  - Alveolar: Translocation chromosome 1 or 2 & 13
    - Translocation t(2;13) (q35;q14), results in PAX3-FKHR fusion gene (55%)
    - Translocation t(1;13)(p36;q14), results in PAX7-FKHR fusion gene (22%)
    - Better prognosis in PAX7-FKHR than PAX3-FKHR (more invasive)

RHABDOMYOSARCOMA, MUSCULOSKELETAL

- Etiology: Primitive mesenchymal cell, "rhabdomyoblast" fails to differentiate into skeletal muscle
- Epidemiology: 4-6 cases/1,000,000 a year
- Associated abnormalities: Increased in neurofibromatosis, Li-Fraumeni syndrome (familial cluster of RMS & osteogenic sarcoma) & Beckwith-Wiedemann

Gross Pathologic & Surgical Features
- Variable: Infiltrative → pseudocapsule

Microscopic Features
- Embryonal RMS: Primitive cells with dense spindle shaped cells with hyperchromatic nuclei & cytoplasmic processes, strap cell appearance
- Alveolar RMS: Large oval cells separated into nests "alveoli" separated by fibrous septa
- Central cells are necrotic & loosely arranged with the peripheral cells arranged into well organized "picket fence" appearance
- Immunohistochemical staining: MyoD1, myoglobin, myogenin, actin & desmin

Staging, Grading or Classification Criteria
- Classification for malignant musculoskeletal tumors
  - Stage IA: Low grade, intracompartmental
  - Stage IB: Low grade, extracompartmental
  - Stage IIA: High grade, intracompartmental
  - Stage IIB: High grade, extracompartmental
  - Stage III: Metastases
- TNM
  - T1: Confined to site of origin
  - T2: Extension beyond site of origin
  - N0: No lymph nodes clinically
  - N1: Lymph nodes clinically involved
  - M0: No distant metastases
  - M1: Distant metastases
- Stage I: Favorable sites, any disease, any nodal (LN) (orbit, GU (not bladder or prostate), or head & neck)
- Stage II: Unfavorable sites, but small, (-) LN (extremity, bladder, prostate or parameningeal)
- Stage III: Unfavorable sites, small or large, but (+) LN
- Stage IV: Distant metastases

CLINICAL ISSUES

Presentation
- Most common signs/symptoms: Local swelling or palpable soft tissue mass
- Other signs/symptoms: < 1/2 Pain, symptoms depend on location

Demographics
- Age
  - 2 Age peaks: 2-6 & 14-18 year old
    - Embryonal: < 15 years old (head & neck, GU)
    - Alveolar: 14-18 Years old (extremity, paratesticular, & truncal)
- Gender: Overall M > F (1.5:1), extremity: M < F (0.8:1), GU: M > F (3:1)

Natural History & Prognosis
- Tumor expression of p-glycoprotein gene: More likely multidrug resistance
- Prognosis depends on
  - Site of tumor
    - Orbit & non-parameningeal more favorable
    - Extremity poorer prognosis: ↑ incidence of alveolar RMS, often lymph node (LN) (+), more often metastases at presentation
  - Size: < 5 cm more favorable
  - LN involvement: No nodes > regional nodes > metastatic disease (poorest prognosis)
  - Histologic type: (Embryonal RMS > alveolar RMS)
    - Alveolar RMS typically ↓ prognosis than embryonal RMS, related to older age, extremity location & more commonly distant metastases at presentation
    - Alveolar ↓ prognosis < 1 year old & > 10 years old
  - Age: Younger better prognosis
  - DNA component
    - Hyperdiploid (embryonal RMS) better than diploid or tetraploid (alveolar RMS)
  - Amount of disease after surgical resection
    - No disease: 90%, microscopic residual disease: 80% & gross disease: 70% 5 year survivals
- Metastatic disease: (20%) lung, bone marrow, lymph nodes
  - Parameningeal disease in paranasal sinuses, middle ear, mastoid, nasal cavity

Treatment
- Wide surgical excision
- Adjuvant & neoadjuvant chemotherapy & radiation
- Sometimes amputation for disease control

DIAGNOSTIC CHECKLIST

Consider
- Unexplained hematoma in an extremity, need to exclude an underlying sarcoma

SELECTED REFERENCES

1. Sebire NJ et al: Myogenin and MyoD1 expression in paediatric rhabdomyosarcomas. J Clin Pathol. 56(6):412-6, 2003
2. Sorensen PH et al: PAX3-FKHR and PAX7-FKHR gene fusions are prognostic indicators in alveolar rhabdomyosarcoma: a report from the children's oncology group. J Clin Oncol. 20(11):2672-9, 2002
3. McCarville MB et al: Rhabdomyosarcoma in pediatric patients: the good, the bad, and the unusual. AJR Am J Roentgenol. 176(6):1563-9, 2001
4. Kransdorf MJ et al: Imaging of soft tissue tumors, 1st ed. Philadelphia PA, W.B. Saunders, 226-33, 1997
5. Newton WA Jr et al: Classification of rhabdomyosarcomas and related sarcomas. Pathologic aspects and proposal for a new classification--an Intergroup Rhabdomyosarcoma Study. Cancer. 76(6):1073-85, 1995
6. Tsokos M et al: Rhabdomyosarcoma. A new classification scheme related to prognosis. Arch Pathol Lab Med. 116(8):847-55, 1992

RHABDOMYOSARCOMA, MUSCULOSKELETAL

IMAGE GALLERY

Typical

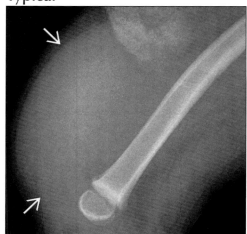
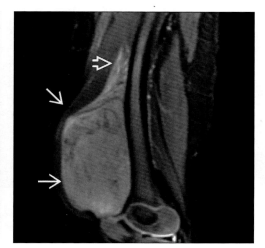

(Left) Lateral radiograph shows massive soft tissue mass in the mid & lower anterior thigh *(arrows)* with mild saucerization of the outer anterior femoral cortex. *(Right)* Sagittal STIR MR image of the same 2 year old patient shows heterogeneous hyperintense mass *(arrows)* within the thigh with a tail of mass extending proximally *(open arrow)*, embryonal RMS.

Variant

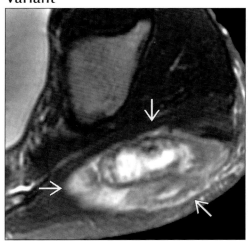
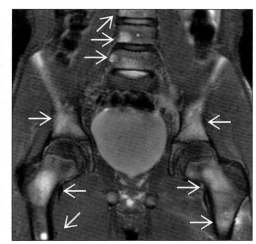

(Left) Axial T2WI MR shows a left gluteal heterogeneous, predominantly hyperintense mass *(arrows)*. *(Right)* Coronal STIR MR in the same patient at presentation shows findings of a stage IV tumor with multifocal scattered hyperintense osseous metastatic deposits *(arrows)* within the lower lumbar spine, pelvis & femurs.

Typical

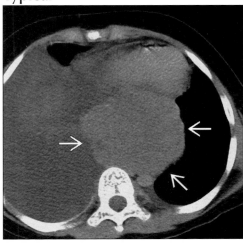
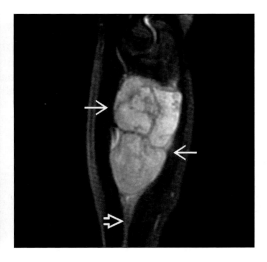

(Left) Axial NECT of the chest shows a large soft tissue mass within the posterior mediastinum *(arrows)* & a large pleural effusion. *(Right)* Sagittal T2WI MR of the forearm shows a lobulated hyperintense mass *(arrows)* with tumor or peritumoral edema extending in a distal tail *(open arrow)*.

EWING SARCOMA

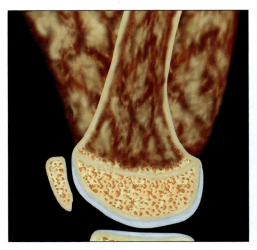

Sagittal graphic shows tumor replacement of the femoral metadiaphysis marrow cavity with a large soft tissue mass shown in brown.

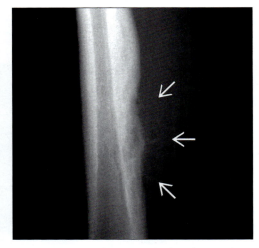

Anteroposterior radiograph of the femur shows diaphyseal cortical thickening & aggressive periosteal reaction (arrows).

TERMINOLOGY

Abbreviations and Synonyms
- Closely related to primitive neuroectodermal tumor (PNET) of bone
- Ewing sarcoma, Ewing tumor, malignant primary bone tumor

Definitions
- Aggressive, small, round, blue cell tumor that typically arises in bone

IMAGING FINDINGS

General Features
- Best diagnostic clue
  - Classic imaging appearance
    - Central, diaphyseal, lytic, lamellated "onion skin" or permeated periosteal reaction
    - Child during second decade of life
  - Lesions most often involve metadiaphysis (more common than diaphyseal)
  - Radiographic appearance variable
- Location
  - Upper/lower extremities > pelvis > ribs (can occur in any bone & soft tissue)
    - Pelvic girdle or long tubular bones: 70-75%
    - Lower extremity: 50%
    - Ribs: 7%
    - Metaphyseal & diaphyseal: 94%
  - Greater propensity for flat bones (scapula, pelvis) than other primary bone malignancies
  - Flat bones typically involved in older children (> 10 years old) than seen with long bone
- Size: > 5 cm
- Morphology
  - Most common during second decade of life
  - Exceedingly rare before 5 years of age
  - If diaphyseal tend to be central, if metaphysis tend to be eccentric
  - However, diaphyseal involvement more common than with other bone malignancies
  - Rarely, may have extraosseous Ewing sarcoma arising in soft tissues rather than from bone
    - Appears as nonspecific soft tissue mass
- Metastatic disease
  - Other sites of bone
  - Lung: 15-30% at presentation

Radiographic Findings
- Radiography
  - Highly aggressive appearance
  - Lucent ill-defined intramedullary lesion, poorly marginated

DDx: Ewing Sarcoma

| Osteomyelitis | NBL Metastasis | LCH | Osteosarcoma |

EWING SARCOMA

Key Facts

Terminology
- Closely related to primitive neuroectodermal tumor (PNET) of bone
- Ewing sarcoma, Ewing tumor, malignant primary bone tumor
- Aggressive, small, round, blue cell tumor that typically arises in bone

Imaging Findings
- Classic imaging appearance
- Central, diaphyseal, lytic, lamellated "onion skin" or permeated periosteal reaction
- Most common during second decade of life
- Exceedingly rare before 5 years of age
- Metastatic disease
- Other sites of bone
- Lung: 15-30% at presentation
- MR modality of choice for depicting extent of local disease

Top Differential Diagnoses
- Osteomyelitis
- Osteosarcoma
- Metastatic neuroblastoma (NBL)
- Langerhans cell histiocytosis (LCH)

Clinical Issues
- Presents with pain & swelling
- Tenderness/palpable mass
- May be associated with systemic symptoms/signs: Leukocytosis, fever, anemia, elevated sedimentation rate (1/3)
- Mimics osteomyelitis

- Permeative or moth eaten appearance from cortical destruction
  - Infiltration of tumor through the haversian canals of the cortical bone
- Cortical thickening, violation or rarely saucerization
- Aggressive periosteal reaction
  - Spiculated
  - Lamellated "onion skin"
  - "Sun burst" or "hair standing on end"; periosteal reaction laid down along Sharpey fibers (attach periosteum to underlying cortical bone) in an attempt to wall off tumor
  - Codman triangle; elevation of new bone along the margin of periosteal reaction
- No ossified tumor matrix, can be sclerotic in flat bones
- Pathologic fracture
- Associated soft tissue mass
  - Disproportionately larger than the amount of bone destruction
- Ewing may appear as very sclerotic lesion in up to 15% of cases
  - When sclerosis present, confined to bone; unlike osteosarcoma
  - 1/3 reactive sclerosis

CT Findings
- NECT: Depicts the aggressive periosteal reaction, soft tissue & intramedullary components
- May be helpful in demonstrating bony destruction, particularly in complex anatomic areas (pelvis, head & neck)
  - CT > MRI in determining cortical bone destruction
- Chest CT for pulmonary metastasis

MR Findings
- T1WI: ↓ To intermediate signal compared to fatty marrow
- T2WI: ↑ Signal compared to skeletal muscle
- STIR: ↑ Signal of the tumor & peritumoral edema
- T1 C+
  - Heterogeneous enhancement
  - Baseline for post chemotherapy MR in determining response to therapy
- MR modality of choice for depicting extent of local disease
- Destructive mass arising from bone typically with associated soft tissue mass
- Dynamic enhanced MR
  - Tumor response to chemotherapy
  - Intramedullary extent verses marrow edema

Nuclear Medicine Findings
- Bone Scan
  - Intense uptake
  - Used for evaluation of metastatic bone disease
- PET
  - 2-[fluorine 18]-fluoro-e-deoxyglucose (FDG)
    - Monitoring response to therapy & metastatic disease
    - Differentiates tumor recurrence from surgical or therapy response
    - Possible predictor of outcome
- Gallium-67 Scan: Monitoring response to therapy
- Thallium 201
  - Monitoring response to therapy
  - Can overestimate tumor viability

Imaging Recommendations
- Best imaging tool: MRI for local evaluation
- Protocol advice: Joint to joint marrow sequence for extent of disease (T1 or STIR) then smaller field of view: FS T2WI MR, STIR, T1 C+

DIFFERENTIAL DIAGNOSIS

Osteomyelitis
- More common in children < 5 years
- Can have very aggressive imaging appearance
- More rapid rate of progression after onset of symptoms (by 2 weeks on radiographs)
  - Ewing slower course (destructive changes usually evident at 6-12 weeks)

EWING SARCOMA

Osteosarcoma
- Osteoid tumor matrix in 90%
- More commonly involves metaphysis

Metastatic neuroblastoma (NBL)
- More common in children < 3 years of age

Langerhans cell histiocytosis (LCH)
- Can have very aggressive appearance
- Rapid rate of radiographic appearance after onset of symptoms (1-2 weeks), can also disappear rapidly ("Tempo phenomenon")

PATHOLOGY

General Features
- General path comments
  - Aggressive, small, round, blue cell tumor
  - Similar to primitive neuroectodermal tumor
- Genetics: Translocation chromosome q24 & q12 of chromosome 11 & 22 resulting in a fusion gene (EWS/FLI1) expression of chimeric protein (90% cases)

Gross Pathologic & Surgical Features
- Grayish white tumors with areas of necrosis, hemorrhage
- Aggressive spread: Along marrow cavity, through cortex, beyond periosteum

Microscopic Features
- Highly cellular, sheets of cells, little stroma
- Small, round, blue cell tumor
- Electron microscopy shows no neurosecretory granules (in contrast to true PNET)

Staging, Grading or Classification Criteria
- Enneking staging system for malignant musculoskeletal tumors
  - Stage IA: Low grade, intracompartmental
  - Stage IB: Low grade, extracompartmental
  - Stage IIA: High grade, intracompartmental
  - Stage IIB: High grade, extracompartmental
  - Stage III: Distant metastasis

CLINICAL ISSUES

Presentation
- Most common signs/symptoms
  - Presents with pain & swelling
  - Tenderness/palpable mass
- Other signs/symptoms
  - May be associated with systemic symptoms/signs: Leukocytosis, fever, anemia, elevated sedimentation rate (1/3)
    - Mimics osteomyelitis
    - More commonly has metastatic disease
  - Pathologic fracture (up to 15%)

Demographics
- Age
  - Second most common primary bone malignancy in children after osteosarcoma
  - 5-25 years, peak 10-15 year olds
  - Exceedingly rare before 5 years of age
- Gender: M > F (1.5-2:1)
- Ethnicity: Caucasians: 95%, African-Americans (2%)

Natural History & Prognosis
- 5 year survival rate related to stage at diagnosis
  - 70% when disease localized
  - 30% when metastatic disease
- Poorer prognosis when presenting
  - Metastatic disease: 15-30% at presentation
  - Larger tumor volume
  - Pelvic location
- Survival better for lesions of extremities than those of axial skeleton
  - Pelvic lesions tend to be larger at presentation

Treatment
- Chemotherapy
  - Vincristine, cyclophosphamide, doxorubicin or actinomycin D
- Resection of primary tumor
- Limb salvage procedures

DIAGNOSTIC CHECKLIST

Consider
- FDG PET in determining residual/recurrent tumor from therapeutic changes

Image Interpretation Pearls
- Sometimes mimics osteomyelitis on imaging, clinically & laboratory

SELECTED REFERENCES

1. Schuetze SM et al: Use of positron emission tomography in localized extremity soft tissue sarcoma treated with neoadjuvant chemotherapy. Cancer. 103(2):339-48, 2005
2. Kutluk MT et al: Treatment results and prognostic factors in Ewing sarcoma. Pediatr Hematol Oncol. 21(7):597-610, 2004
3. Hawkins DS et al: Evaluation of chemotherapy response in pediatric bone sarcomas by [F-18]-fluorodeoxy-D-glucose positron emission tomography. Cancer. 94(12):3277-84, 2002
4. Lang P et al: Musculoskeletal neoplasm: perineoplastic edema versus tumor on dynamic postcontrast MR images with spatial mapping of instantaneous enhancement rates. Radiology. 197(3):831-9, 1995
5. Eggli KD et al: Ewing's sarcoma. Radiol Clin North Am. 31:325-37, 1993
6. Reinus WR et al: Prognostic features of Ewing sarcoma on plain radiograph and computed tomography scan after initial treatment. A Pediatric Oncology Groups study (8246). Cancer 72:2503-10, 1993
7. Erlemann R et al: Musculoskeletal neoplasms: static and dynamic Gd-DTPA--enhanced MR imaging. Radiology. 171(3):767-73, 1989
8. Rud NP et al: Extraosseous Ewing's sarcoma. A study of 42 cases. Cancer. 64(7):1548-53, 1989
9. Reinus WR et al: Radiology of Ewing's sarcoma; intergroup Ewing's Sarcoma Study (IESS). RadioGraphics. 4:929-44, 1984
10. Lombardi F et al: Ewing's sarcoma: an approach to radiological diagnosis. Tumori. 65(3):389-99, 1979

EWING SARCOMA

IMAGE GALLERY

Typical

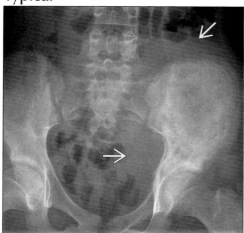
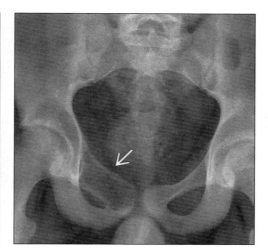

(Left) Anteroposterior radiograph shows large soft tissue mass *(arrows)*, periosteal reaction with a mixed lytic & sclerotic replacement of the left iliac wing. This patient had lung metastases at presentation. *(Right)* Anteroposterior radiograph of the pelvis shows bone expansion & permeative appearance of the right pubic ramus *(arrow)*. In children, involvement of flat bones is common in Ewing sarcoma, but uncommon in other primary bone tumors.

Typical

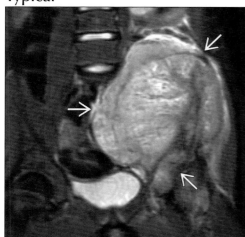
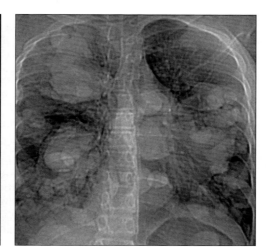

(Left) Coronal STIR MR shows very large hyperintense mass *(arrows)*. *(Right)* Frontal scout image in the same patient from a NECT shows innumerable metastases throughout the lungs. This is more commonly seen at presentation in patients with larger masses & central location.

Typical

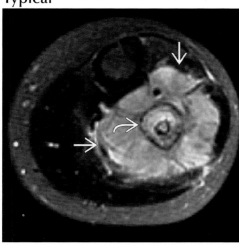
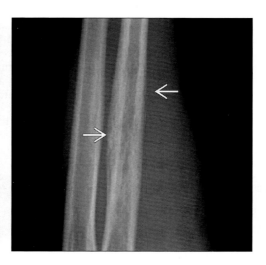

(Left) Axial T2WI MR shows expansion of the proximal fibula *(curved arrow)* with permeative appearance of the underlying bone & a large hyperintense soft tissue mass *(arrows)*. Notice the typical disproportionate size of the soft tissue mass to the amount of bone destruction. *(Right)* Anteroposterior radiograph shows a poorly defined radial diaphyseal lesion with aggressive periosteal reaction & permeative bone destruction *(arrows)*.

OSTEOSARCOMA

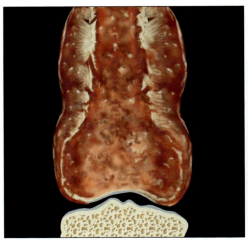

Coronal graphic image shows a permeative mass replacing the marrow space extending into the adjacent soft tissues.

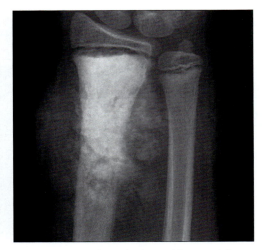

Anteroposterior radiograph shows diffuse medullary & cortical bone destruction with associated aggressive periosteal reaction. Cloud-like osteoid matrix is seen within the soft tissue mass.

TERMINOLOGY

Abbreviations and Synonyms
- Osteogenic sarcoma (OGS), conventional osteosarcoma

Definitions
- Malignant tumor with ability to produce osteoid directly from neoplastic cells

IMAGING FINDINGS

General Features
- Best diagnostic clue: Aggressive bone lesion with new bone formation
- Location
  - 55-80% around knee
    - Femur: 40% (75% distal)
    - Tibia: 20% (80% proximal)
  - Humerus: 10%
  - Metaphysis long bones (90%), diaphysis: 10%
  - Extension into epiphysis (75%)
  - Flat bones, vertebral bodies (20%)
- Most common malignant primary bone tumor in children/young adults
- Second most common primary malignant bone tumor
- New bone formation: Sclerotic (cloud-like) density that is seen outside of expected area of normal bone
  - Seen in 90% of cases
- Appearance depends upon degree of new bone formation and degree of bone destruction
  - Bone destruction: Poorly-defined lucent areas with cortical destruction with aggressive periosteal reaction
  - Bone production: Will appear as sclerotic density

Radiographic Findings
- Radiography
  - Primary osseous osteosarcoma (95%)
  - Conventional osteosarcoma (75-85% of all OGS)
    - Arises from medullary cavity
    - Poorly-defined, intramedullary mass, extends through cortex
    - Moth-eaten bone destruction
    - Aggressive periosteal reaction: Codman triangle, sunburst
    - Indistinct borders with wide zone of transition
    - Cloud-like soft tissue mass (90%)
  - Telangiectatic osteosarcoma (< 5%)
    - Very malignant, possible worse prognosis
    - Purely lytic lesion, geographic, blow-out appearance
    - Cystic cavities filled with blood/necrosis
    - Fluid levels (may mimic ABC)

DDx: Osteosarcoma

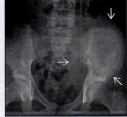
Ewing Sarcoma

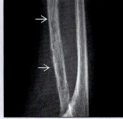
Osteomyelitis

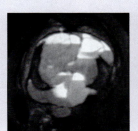
ABC

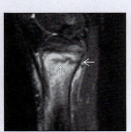
Stress Fracture

OSTEOSARCOMA

Key Facts

Terminology
- Osteogenic sarcoma (OGS), conventional osteosarcoma

Imaging Findings
- 55-80% around knee
- New bone formation: Sclerotic (cloud-like) density that is seen outside of expected area of normal bone
- Conventional osteosarcoma (75-85% of all OGS)
- Important to image entire involved bone to detect skip lesions
- To determine extent of tumor within bone marrow & soft tissue, relationship to vessels and nerves
- Telangiectatic OGS can have fluid/fluid levels (90%) similar to an ABC
- Telangiectatic OGS: Look for enhancing mass or peripheral nodule enhancement on MR or CECT

Top Differential Diagnoses
- Ewing sarcoma
- Stress fracture
- Aneurysmal bone cyst (ABC)
- Important to distinguish from telangiectatic OGS
- Osteomyelitis
- Myositis ossificans

Clinical Issues
- Most common signs/symptoms: Pain, development of soft tissue swelling or mass, fever
- Pulmonary metastases common, can cause pneumothorax (calcifying)
- Bimodal age: 10-30 years, > 60 years old
- Most common: 10-15 years of age
- Gender: M ≥ F, 3:2 to 2:1

- Multicentric osteosarcoma (1%)
  - Synchronous osteoblastic osteosarcoma at multiple sites (usually symmetric)
  - Exclusively in children (5-10 years)
  - Extremely poor prognosis
- Periosteal osteosarcoma (1%)
  - Usually no medullary involvement, diaphyseal
  - Intermediate to high grade
  - 85-95%: Femur + tibia; 5-10%: Ulna + humerus
  - Attached to underlying cortex at origin with thickening, scalloping or saucerization of underlying cortex
- Parosteal osteosarcoma (3%)
  - Low grade osteosarcoma, better prognosis than conventional OGS
  - Age: 20-50 years (older than conventional OGS)
  - Metaphyseal, distal posterior femur
  - No medullary involvement
- Secondary osteosarcoma (5%)
  - Arises in association with preexisting lesion of bone such as Paget disease, prior radiation, dedifferentiated chondrosarcoma, or bone infarct

MR Findings
- T1WI
  - Low signal intensity: Mineralized tumor
  - Low-intermediate signal intensity: Solid, non-mineralized tumor
- T2WI
  - Low signal intensity: Mineralized tumor
  - High signal intensity: Non-mineralized tumor, soft tissue mass
- STIR: Or T1 in depicting marrow extent, joint to joint imaging
- Important to image entire involved bone to detect skip lesions
- To determine extent of tumor within bone marrow & soft tissue, relationship to vessels and nerves
- Dynamic MR may be helpful distinguishing tumor verses marrow edema
- Telangiectatic OGS can have fluid/fluid levels (90%) similar to an ABC
- Telangiectatic OGS: Look for enhancing mass or peripheral nodule enhancement on MR or CECT

Nuclear Medicine Findings
- Bone Scan
  - Intense uptake
  - For staging: Detection of skip lesions, metastases
- PET
  - Intense activity
  - Differentiating viable tumor from post therapeutic change

Imaging Recommendations
- Best imaging tool
  - Radiograph 1st in evaluation of bone tumor: Diagnostic
  - CT of chest for metastatic disease
  - Bone scan for skeletal metastases
  - MRI for therapy planning & guiding biopsy
- Protocol advice
  - Joint to joint to determine marrow extent: T1 or STIR (STIR can overestimate marrow disease)
  - FS T2WI MR, STIR & T1 C+ of the tumor

DIFFERENTIAL DIAGNOSIS

Ewing sarcoma
- Diaphysis of long bones, large soft tissue mass
- No matrix or osteoid production

Stress fracture
- NECT or MR: No trabecular bone destruction
- NECT or MR: Sclerosis, trabecular or cortical fracture line +/- callus

Aneurysmal bone cyst (ABC)
- Important to distinguish from telangiectatic OGS
- No soft tissue mass or nodular enhancement
- Thin septal enhancement: "honeycomb" appearance
- Fluid-fluid levels in cystic cavities, differ in signal intensity related to different stages of blood products

OSTEOSARCOMA

Osteomyelitis
- No osteoid or bone production
- Chronic osteomyelitis: Can be mixed sclerotic & lucent regions

Myositis ossificans
- Calcified, subacute to chronic hematoma
- Calcifications seen as densities in periphery of lesions (calcified borders) in contrast to intralesional cloudy calcification seen with osteosarcoma

PATHOLOGY

General Features
- Epidemiology: 400-600 children per year

Gross Pathologic & Surgical Features
- White-tan, firm, gritty mass with foci of hemorrhage and necrosis
- Penetration of cortex with often large extraosseous tumor mass
- Periosteal reaction visible as lamellae of new bone at periphery of lesion

Microscopic Features
- Highly pleomorphic, spindle-shaped tumor cells producing different forms of osteoid
- Three histologic subtypes depending on sarcomatous component: Osteoblastic, chondroblastic, fibroblastic osteosarcoma

Staging, Grading or Classification Criteria
- Enneking staging system for malignant musculoskeletal tumors
  - Stage IA: Low grade, intracompartmental
  - Stage IB: Low grade extracompartmental
  - Stage IIA: High grade, intracompartmental
  - Stage IIB: High grade, extracompartmental
  - Stage III: Distant metastasis

CLINICAL ISSUES

Presentation
- Most common signs/symptoms: Pain, development of soft tissue swelling or mass, fever
- Clinical Profile
  - Pathologic fracture: Up to 20%
  - Pulmonary metastases common, can cause pneumothorax (calcifying)
    - Other metastases: Lymph nodes, liver, brain & bone (uncommon)
  - Increased alkaline phosphatase (2-3X normal): More likely to have lung metastasis
  - Lactate dehydrogenase: Higher in metastatic disease at presentation

Demographics
- Age
  - Bimodal age: 10-30 years, > 60 years old
  - Most common: 10-15 years of age
- Gender: M ≥ F, 3:2 to 2:1

Natural History & Prognosis
- Predisposing conditions: Hereditary retinoblastoma, previous radiation
- Prognosis depends on
  - Age, sex, tumor volume, site & classification
  - Best predictor: Degree of necrosis following chemotherapy
- Lung metastases & skip lesion have a worse prognosis

Treatment
- Adjuvant and neoadjuvant chemotherapy and surgical resection
- Limb salvage procedures (used in 80% of cases)
- 5 year survival has increased to 77%

DIAGNOSTIC CHECKLIST

Consider
- Telangiectatic OGS if fluid-fluid levels & an enhancing nodule or mass (more than thin septal enhancement) on CT or MR

Image Interpretation Pearls
- Image joint for extent & therapy planning, don't miss skip or metastatic lesions

SELECTED REFERENCES

1. Bacci G et al: Prognostic significance of serum lactate dehydrogenase in osteosarcoma of the extremity: experience at Rizzoli on 1421 patients treated over the last 30 years. Tumori. 90(5):478-84, 2004
2. Kaste SC et al: Tumor size as a predictor of outcome in pediatric non-metastatic osteosarcoma of the extremity. Pediatr Blood Cancer. 43(7):723-8, 2004
3. Sajadi KR et al: The incidence and prognosis of osteosarcoma skip metastases. Clin Orthop Relat Res. (426):92-6, 2004
4. Wilkins RM et al: Superior survival in treatment of primary nonmetastatic pediatric osteosarcoma of the extremity. Ann Surg Oncol. 10(5):498-507, 2003
5. Bredella MA et al: Value of FDG positron emission tomography in conjunction with MR imaging for evaluating therapy response in patients with musculoskeletal sarcomas. AJR Am J Roentgenol. 179(5):1145-50, 2002
6. Reddick WE et al: Dynamic magnetic resonance imaging of regional contrast access as an additional prognostic factor in pediatric osteosarcoma. Cancer. 91(12):2230-7, 2001
7. Onikul E et al: Accuracy of MR imaging for estimating intraosseous extent of osteosarcoma. AJR Am J Roentgenol. 167(5):1211-5, 1996
8. Lang P et al: Musculoskeletal neoplasm: perineoplastic edema versus tumor on dynamic postcontrast MR images with spatial mapping of instantaneous enhancement rates. Radiology. 197(3):831-9, 1995
9. Rosenberg ZS et al: Osteosarcoma: Subtle, rare, and misleading plain film features. AJR Am J Roentgenol. 165:1209-14, 1995
10. Mervak TR et al: Telangiectatic osteosarcoma. Clin Orthop. 270:135-9, 1991
11. Erlemann R et al: Musculoskeletal neoplasms: static and dynamic Gd-DTPA--enhanced MR imaging. Radiology. 171(3):767-73, 1989

OSTEOSARCOMA

IMAGE GALLERY

Typical

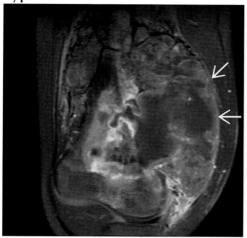
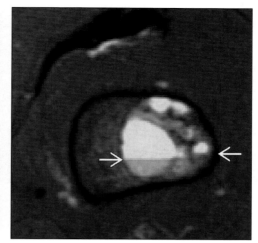

(Left) Coronal T1 C+ MR shows hypointense signal consistent with the mineralized portion *(arrows)* of the large osteogenic sarcoma. Spotty enhancement is seen within the medullary canal & within the soft tissues. *(Right)* Axial T2WI MR shows multiple fluid-fluid levels *(arrows)* without marrow edema. More proximal images show bone destruction, in this patient with a telangiectatic osteosarcoma.

Typical

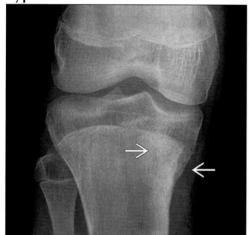
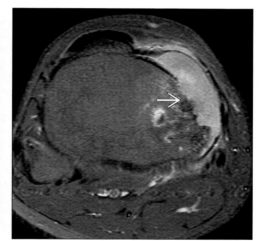

(Left) Anteroposterior radiograph in this sickle cell patient shows a mixed lytic & sclerotic lesion in the medial tibial metaphysis *(arrows)* with cortical destruction. *(Right)* Axial T1 C+ MR image in the same patient shows cortical destruction *(arrow)* with a hyperintense soft tissue mass extending into the medial soft tissues. This was a fibroblastic osteogenic sarcoma.

Typical

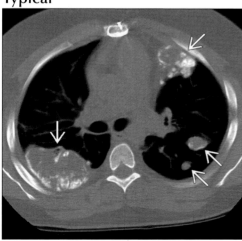
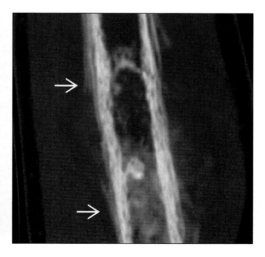

(Left) Axial CECT shows pleural & parenchymal ossifying lung metastases *(arrows)* in this patient with a large pelvis osteogenic sarcoma. *(Right)* Coronal reconstructed NECT image shows permeative destruction of the cortex with Codman triangles *(arrows)*.

LEUKEMIA, MUSCULOSKELETAL

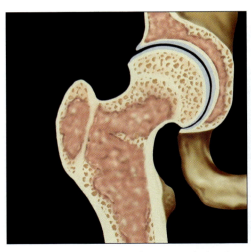

Coronal graphic shows replacement of the bone marrow by leukemia infiltrate.

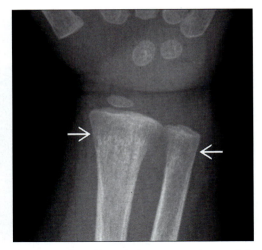

Anteroposterior radiograph shows permeative osteolytic changes of the distal metaphyses of the radius & ulna (arrows).

TERMINOLOGY

Abbreviations and Synonyms
- Acute lymphocytic leukemia (ALL), acute myelogenous leukemia (AML), granulocytic sarcoma, myeloblastoma, chloroma, chronic myelogenous leukemia (CML), chronic lymphocytic leukemia (CLL)

Definitions
- Malignancy of hematopoietic stem cell with diffuse infiltration or replacement of the bone marrow by malignant cells

IMAGING FINDINGS

General Features
- Location
  - Children: Long bones
    - Femur > humerus > pelvis > spine > tibia
  - Adults: Axial skeleton
- Morphology: Permeative to moth eaten osseous destruction

Radiographic Findings
- Radiography
  - Diffuse osteopenia of spine & long bones
    - Often normal
    - Coarse trabeculae
    - Multiple flattened, collapsed or biconcave vertebrae
  - "Leukemic lines" (40-53% in ALL)
    - Transverse, radiolucent metaphyseal bands involving large joints
    - Horizontal bands in vertebral bodies
    - Dense metaphyseal bands post therapy
    - Stress of disease or leukemic infiltration
  - Focal bone destruction
    - Multiple well-defined osteolytic lesions
    - Moth eaten or permeative appearance
    - Sutural widening or diastasis with prominent convolutional markings of skull
  - Periostitis of long bones
    - Periosteal reaction (1/4)
    - Smooth, lamellated or sunburst
    - Subperiosteal infiltration by malignant cells through the haversian canals
    - Subperiosteal hemorrhage
  - Sclerosis
    - Typically myelogenous leukemia
  - Pathologic fracture
    - Usually metaphyseal
    - Can simulate nonaccidental trauma
  - Chloroma (granulocytic sarcoma)
    - Extramedullary mass with granulocytic precursor cells

DDx: Permeative Destructive Bone Lesions

Osteomyelitis | Congenital Syphilis | LCH | Lymphoma

LEKEMIA, MUSCULOSKELETAL

Key Facts

Terminology
- Acute lymphocytic leukemia (ALL), acute myelogenous leukemia (AML), granulocytic sarcoma, myeloblastoma, chloroma, chronic myelogenous leukemia (CML), chronic lymphocytic leukemia (CLL)
- Malignancy of hematopoietic stem cell with diffuse infiltration or replacement of the bone marrow by malignant cells

Imaging Findings
- Children: Long bones
- Adults: Axial skeleton
- T1WI: Hypointense leukemic infiltrate replacing high signal intensity marrow fat
- T2WI: Hyperintense increased marrow signal
- STIR: Hyperintense signal of leukemic marrow
- T1, FS T2 FSE, or STIR, +/- FS T1 C+

Top Differential Diagnoses
- Metastatic neuroblastoma (NB)
- Langerhans cell histiocytosis (LCH)
- Osteomyelitis
- Congenital syphilis
- Lymphoma
- Ewing sarcoma

Pathology
- ALL most common form in children
- Leading cause of malignancy & death in < 15 year old

Clinical Issues
- Gender: M > F
- Ethnicity: Caucasians most common

- Typically AML; occasionally seen in myelodysplastic or myeloproliferative disorders
- Concurrent to onset of leukemia, during remission or relapse
- Most commonly head & neck, soft tissue or bony mass
- Can simulate meningioma or epidural hematoma
- Associated with translocation (8;21)
- CT or MR to differentiate from hematoma or abscess
- Poor prognosis

CT Findings
- NECT
  - Permeative bone destruction
  - Soft tissue or bony mass of chloroma

MR Findings
- T1WI: Hypointense leukemic infiltrate replacing high signal intensity marrow fat
- T2WI: Hyperintense increased marrow signal
- STIR: Hyperintense signal of leukemic marrow

Nuclear Medicine Findings
- Bone Scan
  - Increased radiotracer uptake in tumor
  - May underestimate disease
- PET
  - Potential role
    - Detecting extramedullary disease
    - Monitoring post therapeutic response of lesions

Imaging Recommendations
- Best imaging tool
  - MR
    - When radiographs are normal
    - Depicting extent of disease
    - Differentiating abscess, hematoma from chloroma
- Protocol advice
  - T1, FS T2 FSE, or STIR, +/- FS T1 C+
  - Whole body STIR

DIFFERENTIAL DIAGNOSIS

Metastatic neuroblastoma (NB)
- Bone involvement similar to leukemia
  - Metaphyseal bands
  - Moth eaten bone destruction (also consider other metastatic disease)
- Hair-on-end appearance of skull

Langerhans cell histiocytosis (LCH)
- Lytic lesion
- Periosteal reaction
- Soft tissue mass

Osteomyelitis
- Symptoms similar to leukemia
- Periosteal reaction, bone destruction, soft tissue extension similar to leukemia
- Acute or chronic recurrent multifocal osteomyelitis

Congenital syphilis
- Hepatosplenomegaly, lymphadenopathy, anemia, skin rash
- Younger at presentation
- Metaphyseal lucent bands (stress vs. infection) to lytic metaphyseal serrations
- Wimberger sign: Focal destruction of the medial proximal tibial metaphysis

Lymphoma
- Mostly solitary, occasionally multifocal
- Soft tissue mass greater than amount of bone destruction
- Older age group

Ewing sarcoma
- No metaphyseal lucent lines
- Typical: Aggressive periosteal reaction & bone destruction
- Large soft tissue mass

LEUKEMIA, MUSCULOSKELETAL

PATHOLOGY

General Features
- General path comments
  - Classified
    - Basis of cell maturity: Acute (blasts) or chronic (more mature cells)
    - Basis of cell type: Lymphocytic or myelogenous form
  - Clinical & radiographic signs of bone marrow involvement typically in children with acute leukemia
- Genetics
  - ↑ ALL in Down syndrome & chromosomal translocations
  - CML translocation chromosome 9 & 22, Philadelphia chromosome
- Etiology: Arises from primitive stem cell either de-novo or from preexisting preleukemic state
- Epidemiology
  - ALL most common form in children
  - Leading cause of malignancy & death in < 15 year old
  - ALL: (75%), AML: (10-15%), CML: (5%)
- Associated abnormalities: Myelodysplastic syndrome (1/3 develop AML)

Gross Pathologic & Surgical Features
- Hyperemic/hemorrhagic bone marrow with destruction of bony trabeculae or osteosclerosis
- Areas of bone infarction

Microscopic Features
- Acute: Infiltration of bone marrow by poorly-differentiated blast cells
  - ALL
    - Pattern-less sheets of small blue cells
  - AML
    - Wright's stain or Giemsa preparation of lysosomal cytoplasmic structure = Auer rods (diagnostic)
- Chronic: Mature leukocyte infiltration
  - CML
    - Mature granulocyte with normal lymphocyte count, Philadelphia chromosome
  - CLL
    - Mature lymphocytes

CLINICAL ISSUES

Presentation
- Most common signs/symptoms
  - Sharp, localized, recurrent paraarticular arthralgias (in 75%)
  - Fatigue (anemia)
  - Fever +/- infection
  - Bleeding
- Other signs/symptoms
  - Joint effusion
  - Elevated erthrocyte sedimentation rate
  - May be confused with
    - Rheumatic fever, rheumatoid arthritis & osteomyelitis
  - Hepatosplenomegaly, lymphadenopathy
  - Avascular necrosis in patient on steroids

Demographics
- Age
  - ALL: Peak 2-10 years
  - AML: Peak > 65 years, but accounts for 15-20% of childhood leukemias
  - CML: Peak: 30-50 years
  - CLL: Median age 60 years
- Gender: M > F
- Ethnicity: Caucasians most common

Natural History & Prognosis
- ALL
  - Complete remission in > 90%
  - 50-80% disease free 5 year survival with treatment
- AML
  - 60-80% remission
  - 10-30% disease free 5 year survival with treatment

Treatment
- Chemotherapy, combined chemotherapy & radiation
- Intrathecal chemotherapy for CNS disease
- Granulocyte colony-stimulating factor (G-CSF)
- Bone marrow transplant
- Steroids

SELECTED REFERENCES

1. Gassas A et al: A basic classification and a comprehensive examination of pediatric myeloproliferative syndromes. J Pediatr Hematol Oncol. 27(4):192-6, 2005
2. Ozkaynak MF et al: Randomized comparison of antibiotics with and without granulocyte colony-stimulating factor in children with chemotherapy-induced febrile neutropenia: A report from the Children's Oncology Group. Pediatr Blood Cancer. 2005
3. Saracco P et al: Steroid withdrawal syndrome during steroid tapering in childhood acute lymphoblastic leukemia: a controlled study comparing prednisone versus dexamethasone in induction phase. J Pediatr Hematol Oncol. 27(3):141-4, 2005
4. Rubnitz JE et al: Death during induction therapy and first remission of acute leukemia in childhood: the St. Jude experience. Cancer. 101(7):1677-84, 2004
5. Kuenzle K et al: Detection of extramedullary infiltrates in acute myelogenous leukemia with whole-body positron emission tomography and 2-deoxy-2-[18F]-fluoro-D-glucose. Mol Imaging Biol. 4(2):179-83, 2002
6. Gallagher DJ et al: Orthopedic manifestations of acute pediatric leukemia. Orthop Clin North Am. 27:635-44, 1996
7. Heinrich SD et al: The prognostic significance of the skeletal manifestations of acute lymphoblastic leukemia of childhood. J Pediatr Orthop. 14:105-11, 1994
8. Oestreich AE: Imaging of the skeleton and soft tissues in children. Curr Opin Radiol. 4:55-61, 1992
9. Romaniuk CS: Case report: granulocytic sarcoma (chloroma) presenting as a cerebellopontine angle mass. Clin Radiol. 45(4):284-5, 1992
10. Kao SC et al: Intracranial granulocytic sarcoma (chloroma): MR findings. J Comput Assist Tomogr. 11(6):938-41, 1987
11. Meis JM et al: Granulocytic sarcoma in nonleukemic patients. Cancer. 58(12):2697-709, 1986

LEUKEMIA, MUSCULOSKELETAL

IMAGE GALLERY

Typical

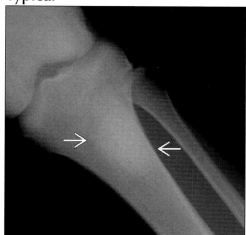
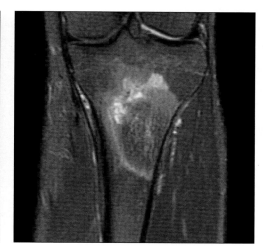

(Left) Anteroposterior radiograph shows diffuse sclerosis of the proximal tibia, clinically & radiographically mistaken for chronic osteomyelitis *(arrows)*. *(Right)* Coronal T2WI MR in the same patient shows heterogeneous hyperintense (edema) surrounding hypointense signal (sclerosis) within the tibia corresponding to the radiographic abnormality, granulocytic sarcoma (leukemia) by biopsy.

Variant

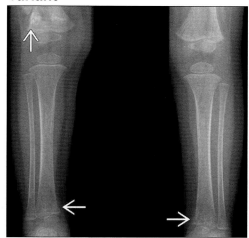
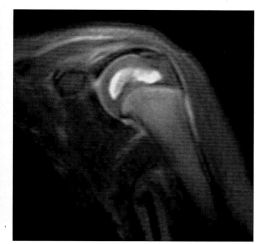

(Left) Anteroposterior radiograph of each leg shows pathologic fractures of the femoral, tibial, & fibular metaphyses *(arrows)*, permeative osteolytic changes of the underlying bone. This initially was mistaken for nonaccidental trauma. *(Right)* Coronal T2WI MR shows hyperintense epiphyseal signal replacing the normal fatty marrow, in this patient with leukemia.

Typical

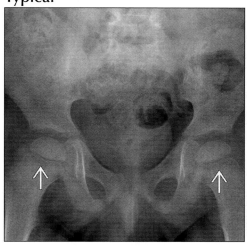
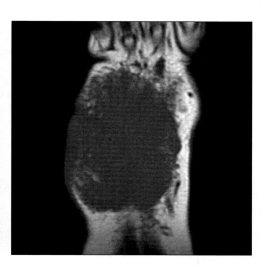

(Left) Anteroposterior radiograph shows subtle transverse radiolucent lines in the proximal femur, leukemic lines *(arrows)*. *(Right)* Coronal T1WI MR shows large hypointense soft tissue mass in the distal wrist, chloroma.

LANGERHANS CELL HISTIOCYTOSIS

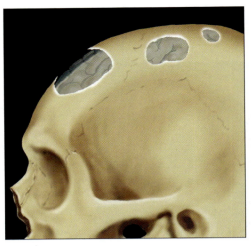

Drawing shows multiple skull lesions with well-defined borders.

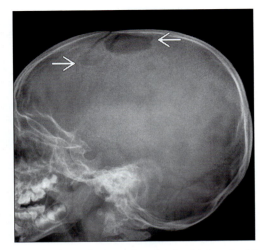

Lateral radiograph shows 2 well-defined lytic calvarial lesions without a sclerotic margin (arrows).

TERMINOLOGY

Abbreviations and Synonyms
- Langerhans cell histiocytosis (LCH), histiocytosis X, eosinophilic granuloma (EG), Hand-Schüller-Christian disease, Letterer-Siwe disease

Definitions
- Idiopathic group of disorders that can manifest as focal, localized or systemic disease

IMAGING FINDINGS

General Features
- Best diagnostic clue: Well-defined lytic beveled skull lesion without sclerotic rim
- Location
  - Monostotic involvement: 50-75%
  - Multifocal involvement: 10-20%
  - Common sites of involvement in decreasing order of frequency: Skull, mandible, ribs (expansile lesion), femur, pelvis, spine
- Morphology
  - Radiographic appearance of skeletal involvement of LCH extremely variable
    - Lucent or sclerotic, permeative or geographic, well-defined sclerotic or poorly-defined borders

Radiographic Findings
- Radiography
  - Skull (50%)
    - Well-defined lytic lesion without sclerotic rim
    - "Beveled" edges: Greater involvement of the inner than the outer table
    - Sclerotic rim during healing phase
    - Coalescence of lesions, geographic skull
    - Button sequestrum
    - Soft tissue mass overlying lytic lesion
    - Floating tooth: Lesion in alveolar portion of mandible
  - Appendicular skeleton
    - Variable appearance
    - Lesions respect joint space/growth plate
  - Spine
    - Vertebra plana: Complete collapse of vertebral body
  - Pelvis
    - Involved in young children

CT Findings
- NECT
  - Extent of cortical & soft tissue involvement
  - Skull: Beveled lytic skull lesion, temporal bone destruction

DDx: Lytic Bone Lesions

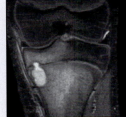
Brodie Abscess

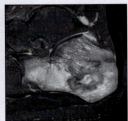
Lymphoma

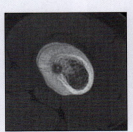
Osteoid Osteoma

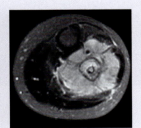
Ewing Sarcoma

LANGERHANS CELL HISTIOCYTOSIS

Key Facts

Imaging Findings
- Best diagnostic clue: Well-defined lytic beveled skull lesion without sclerotic rim

Top Differential Diagnoses
- Osteomyelitis
- Metastatic neuroblastoma (NB)
- Leukemia
- Ewing sarcoma

Pathology
- Letterer-Siwe (acute disseminated form): 10%
- Hand-Schüller-Christian (chronic disseminated form): 20%
- Eosinophilic granuloma (isolated bone or lung involvement): 70%
- < 1% of biopsied primary bone tumors

Clinical Issues
- Localized bone pain, tenderness
- Fever, elevated sedimentation rate, leukocytosis
- Age: 0-30 years, mean age: 5-10 years
- Gender: M:F = 2:1
- Spontaneous regression within 3 months up to 2 years
- Conservative: Immobilization brace
- Vertebral plana; partial or complete return of vertebral body height

Diagnostic Checklist
- When multifocal bone lesions always consider LCH, metastatic disease & infection
- Many bone scans are falsely negative, addition of skeletal survey or total body MR to assess extent to disease

---

  - Long bones: Endosteal scalloping, permeative, periosteal reaction (most common lamellated), widened medullary canal, cortical thinning, intracortical tunneling
  - Guide biopsies, especially spine

MR Findings
- T1WI: Hypointense signal intensity replacing marrow fat
- T2WI: Hyperintense signal intensity, focal lesion surrounded by ill-defined marrow & soft tissue edema
- STIR
  - Hyperintense signal intensity
  - Whole body STIR to assess for multifocal disease
- T1 C+: Marked enhancement
- Destructive lesion with surrounding edema

Nuclear Medicine Findings
- Bone Scan
  - Lesions may demonstrate decreased tracer uptake sometimes with surrounding halo of increased uptake surrounding area
    - Particularly in skull lesions
  - Most lesions increased tracer uptake
  - Lesions may not be detected with scintigraphy alone, false negative
    - Important to obtain radiographic survey to evaluate for multiple lesions

Imaging Recommendations
- Best imaging tool: Radiographs, MRI
- Protocol advice
  - MR: T1, FS T2 FSE, or STIR, +/- FS T1 C+
  - Whole body STIR MR
- Initial lesion often identified with radiography
- Radiographic skeletal survey with or without bone scintigraphy obtained to identify other bony lesions
- Chest radiograph or CT to evaluate for pulmonary involvement
  - Lung: High resolution imaging; nodules → honeycombing
  - Recurrent pneumothorax

DIFFERENTIAL DIAGNOSIS

Osteomyelitis
- Similar symptoms
- Moth eaten appearance
- Periosteal reaction & soft tissue extension can be similar

Metastatic neuroblastoma (NB)
- Metaphyseal bands or lytic metaphyseal permeative lesions

Leukemia
- Metaphyseal bands or lytic metaphyseal permeative to moth eaten lesions
- Collapsed vertebral body, vertebral plana

Ewing sarcoma
- Permeative bone destruction
- Aggressive periosteal reaction (can be lamellated), typical large soft tissue mass
- Progression of tumor
  - LCH: "Tempo phenomenon" rapid progression & disappearance of lesion

Lymphoma
- Older age group
- Mostly solitary, occasionally multifocal

Congenital syphilis
- Can sometimes be confused with acute disseminated disease
- Hepatosplenomegaly, lymphadenopathy, skin rash, lytic bone lesions
- Wimberger sign: Focal destruction proximal medial tibia

Other benign, malignant & metastatic diseases
- Osteoid osteoma, osteoblastoma, chondroblastoma, giant cell, metastatic rhabdomyosarcoma

LANGERHANS CELL HISTIOCYTOSIS

PATHOLOGY

General Features
- General path comments
  - Group of disorders involving abnormal proliferation of Langerhans cell histiocytes in organs of reticuloendothelial system (RES)
  - Letterer-Siwe (acute disseminated form): 10%
    - Occurs in children < 1 year of age
    - Acute onset of hepatosplenomegaly, rash, lymphadenopathy, marrow failure, pulmonary involvement
    - Skeletal involvement may be absent
  - Hand-Schüller-Christian (chronic disseminated form): 20%
    - Chronic form of systemic LCH
    - Most have skeletal involvement
    - Hepatosplenomegaly, diabetes insipidus, exophthalmos, dermatitis, growth retardation
  - Eosinophilic granuloma (isolated bone or lung involvement): 70%
    - Most common 10-14 years of age
- Etiology: Unclear whether process is inflammatory or neoplastic
- Epidemiology
  - < 1% of biopsied primary bone tumors
  - Incidence: 0.05-0.5 per 100,000 children per year in the US

Gross Pathologic & Surgical Features
- Yellow, gray, or brown tumor mass with hemorrhagic areas

Microscopic Features
- Proliferation of Langerhans cells → produce prostaglandin, causes bone resorption
- Infiltrate of histiocytes, eosinophils, lymphocytes, neutrophils, plasma cells +/- bone necrosis

CLINICAL ISSUES

Presentation
- Most common signs/symptoms
  - Localized bone pain, tenderness
  - Soft tissue swelling
- Other signs/symptoms
  - Skin rash
  - Soft tissue mass, exophthalmos
  - Pathologic fracture
  - Systemic: Hepatosplenomegaly, lymphadenopathy, skin rash, punctate calcifications in enlarged thymus
  - Draining otitis externa, acute mastoiditis, gingivitis
- Clinical Profile
  - Fever, elevated sedimentation rate, leukocytosis
  - Peripheral eosinophilia

Demographics
- Age: 0-30 years, mean age: 5-10 years
- Gender: M:F = 2:1
- Ethnicity: More common in Caucasians

Natural History & Prognosis
- Eosinophilic granuloma has best prognosis
  - Spontaneous regression within 3 months up to 2 years
- Chronic disseminated disease (Hand-Schüller-Christian), typically spontaneous remission, but fatal in up to 15%
- Acute disseminated disease (Letterer-Siwe) worse prognosis, often resulting in death (up to 3/4)
- Lung involvement (older age group 20-40 year olds)
  - Worsened by smoking

Treatment
- Observation
- Conservative: Immobilization brace
  - Vertebral plana; partial or complete return of vertebral body height
- Excision & curettage, chemotherapy

DIAGNOSTIC CHECKLIST

Consider
- When multifocal bone lesions always consider LCH, metastatic disease & infection

Image Interpretation Pearls
- Many bone scans are falsely negative, addition of skeletal survey or total body MR to assess extent to disease

SELECTED REFERENCES

1. Garg S et al: Langerhans cell histiocytosis of the spine in children. Long-term follow-up. J Bone Joint Surg Am. 86-A(8):1740-50, 2004
2. Laffan EE et al: Whole-body magnetic resonance imaging: a useful additional sequence in paediatric imaging. Pediatr Radiol. 34(6):472-80, 2004
3. Schmidt S et al: Extra-osseous involvement of Langerhans' cell histiocytosis in children. Pediatr Radiol. 34(4):313-21, 2004
4. Kilborn TN et al: Paediatric manifestations of Langerhans cell histiocytosis: A review of the clinical and radiological findings. Clin Radiol. 58:269-78, 2003
5. Arico M et al: Clinical aspects of Langerhans cell histiocytosis. Hematol Oncol Clin North Am. 12:247-58, 1998
6. Broadbent V et al: Current therapy for Langerhans cell histiocytosis. Hematol Oncol Clin North Am. 12:327-38, 1998
7. Greenspan A et al: Differential diagnosis of tumors and tumor-like lesions of bones and joints. 1st ed. Philadelphia PA, Lippincott-Raven, 247-55, 1998
8. Lieberman PH et al: Langerhans cell (eosinophilic) granulomatosis. A clinicopathologic study encompassing 50 years. Am J Surg Pathol. 20:519-52, 1996
9. Fisher AJ et al: Quantitative analysis of the plain radiographic appearance of eosinophilic granuloma. Invest Radiol. 30:466-73, 1995
10. Kilpatrick SE et al: Langerhans cell histiocytosis (histiocytosis X) of bone. A clinicopathologic analysis of 263 pediatric and adult cases. Cancer 76:2471-84, 1995
11. Beltran J et al: Eosinophilic granuloma: MRI manifestations. Skeletal Radiol. 22:157-61, 1993
12. David R et al: Radiologic features of eosinophilic granuloma of bone. Am J Roentgenol. 153:1021-6, 1989

LANGERHANS CELL HISTIOCYTOSIS

IMAGE GALLERY

Typical

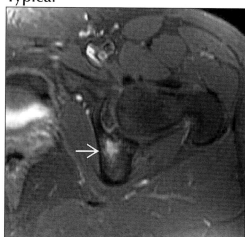
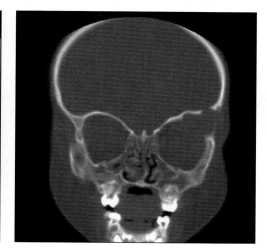

(Left) Axial T1 C+ MR shows focal enhancement (arrow) of the left posterior acetabulum, LCH lesion in this patient with left hip pain. *(Right)* Coronal NECT reformat image shows destructive lytic lesion involving the left lateral orbit & skull base in this patient with long-standing LCH & exophthalmos.

Typical

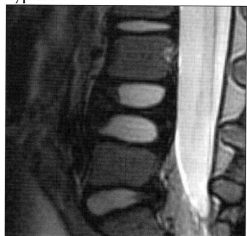
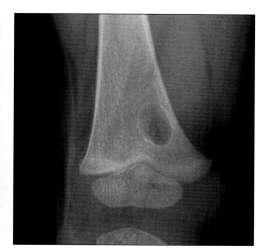

(Left) Sagittal T2WI MR shows dramatic vertebra plana of the L4 vertebral body with preservation of the posterior elements. Notice the lack of disc space involvement. *(Right)* Anteroposterior radiograph shows a well-defined lytic femoral lesion. Notice the sclerotic margin, typically indicating healing phase of LCH.

Typical

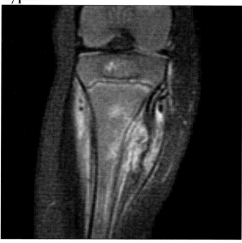
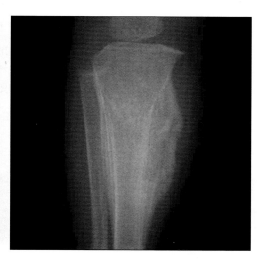

(Left) Coronal T2WI MR shows diffuse ill-defined hyperintense signal (marrow edema) in the tibia with a large subperiosteal component & dramatic thickened periosteal reaction. *(Right)* Anteroposterior radiograph in the same patient shows dramatic periosteal reaction (cloaking) & ossification around the proximal tibia.

FIBROXANTHOMA

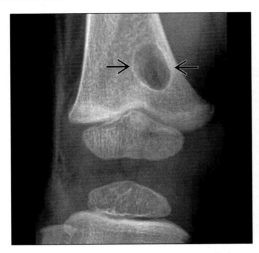

Anteroposterior radiograph shows an oval lesion (arrows) in femoral metaphysis. Lesion has a thin, sclerotic margin.

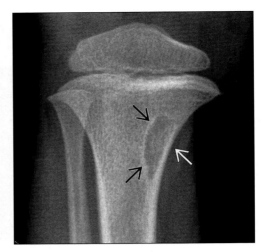

Anteroposterior radiograph shows an elongated lesion (arrows) in tibial metaphysis. Elongation is parallel to long axis of tibia. Margin is thin and sclerotic.

TERMINOLOGY

Abbreviations and Synonyms
- Metaphyseal fibrous defect, benign fibrous histiocytoma, nonossifying fibroma, fibrous cortical defect, benign cortical defect

Definitions
- Benign asymptomatic hamartomatous lesion of children
- Term "fibroxanthoma" includes
  - Nonossifying fibroma (NOF)
  - Fibrous cortical defect (FCD)

IMAGING FINDINGS

General Features
- Best diagnostic clue: Well-defined, expansile, eccentric, lytic lesion with scalloped or smooth sclerotic margins in metaphysis of long bone
- Location
  - Metaphysis of long bone: 90%
    - Close to growth plate
    - Distance from growth plate increases with age
  - Tibia: 43%
  - Femur: 38%
  - Fibula: 8%
  - Less common in upper extremity: 8%
    - Humerus: 5%
  - Multifocal: 50%
- Size: 0.5-7 cm
- Morphology: Eccentric cortex-based lytic lesion

Radiographic Findings
- Radiography
  - Eccentric, cortical lytic lesion with thin scalloped or smooth sclerotic margins
  - Fibroxanthoma may be called FCD if < 2 cm (usually intracortical)
  - Fibroxanthoma may be called NOF when > 2 cm (begins to balloon into medullary cavity)
    - Can extend into or primarily involve medullary cavity
  - Outward expansion of overlying cortex
  - Cortex may be thinned but is intact
  - No matrix calcification
  - Trabeculation may be present in periphery of lesion
  - Increased mineralization in healing stages
    - Begins at diaphyseal end and progresses toward growth plate
  - Long axis of lesion parallel to long axis of bone

CT Findings
- NECT
  - Well-defined lytic lesion with surrounding sclerosis

DDx: Lesions Thinning Bone Cortex

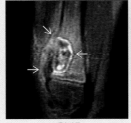
CMF

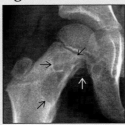
ABC

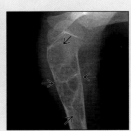
UBC

FIBROXANTHOMA

Key Facts

Imaging Findings
- Best diagnostic clue: Well-defined, expansile, eccentric, lytic lesion with scalloped or smooth sclerotic margins in metaphysis of long bone
- Metaphysis of long bone: 90%
- Fibroxanthoma may be called FCD if < 2 cm (usually intracortical)
- Fibroxanthoma may be called NOF when > 2 cm (begins to balloon into medullary cavity)
- Radiographs diagnostic

Top Differential Diagnoses
- Cortical desmoid
- Aneurysmal bone cyst (ABC)
- Unicameral bone cyst (UBC)
- Fibrous dysplasia
- Chondromyxoid fibroma (CMF)

Pathology
- Most common fibrous lesion of bone
- Occurs in 20-30% of normal population during 1st and 2nd decades of life

Clinical Issues
- Most common signs/symptoms: Usually asymptomatic and identified incidentally
- May cause pain, pathologic fracture
- Benign lesion, no malignant transformation
- Spontaneous regression
- Usually does not require treatment
- Curettage with bone grafting of larger lesions at risk for fracture

Diagnostic Checklist
- No need to biopsy if appearance typical

- Attenuation slightly higher than normal bone marrow
- No soft tissue mass
- CECT: Enhancement

MR Findings
- T1WI
  - Low signal intensity
  - Peripheral hypointense rim (reactive sclerosis)
- T2WI
  - Low to high signal intensity
  - Septations
  - Peripheral hypointense rim (reactive sclerosis)
  - No soft tissue mass
- T1 C+: Enhancement

Ultrasonographic Findings
- Color Doppler
  - Cortical indentation
  - Tissue hypoechoic
  - Blood vessels at periphery and within lesion

Nuclear Medicine Findings
- Bone Scan
  - Active lesions have increased radiotracer uptake
    - Uptake less during involution

Imaging Recommendations
- Best imaging tool
  - Radiographs diagnostic
    - Usually no other imaging needed
- Protocol advice
  - Radiographs
  - CT helpful in showing medullary involvement and pathologic fractures
  - CT for pre-operative planning
  - Larger lesions require radiographic follow-up to assess progression and fracture risk
    - Radiographs every 4-6 months

DIFFERENTIAL DIAGNOSIS

Cortical desmoid
- At tendon insertion
- Typically posterior distal femur

Aneurysmal bone cyst (ABC)
- Marked expansion of affected bone
- CT/MR: Fluid-fluid levels
- Periosteal new bone formation

Unicameral bone cyst (UBC)
- Centrally located
- "Fallen fragment" sign in case of fracture

Fibrous dysplasia
- Expansile medullary lesion
- Ground glass appearance of matrix

Chondromyxoid fibroma (CMF)
- Geographic pattern of bone destruction
- Periosteal new bone formation
- May be intra-cortical

PATHOLOGY

General Features
- General path comments
  - Non-neoplastic process that occurs in the juxtaphyseal metaphysis of long bones
  - NOF results from growth of FCD that has expanded into medullary cavity
- Genetics
  - Neurofibromatosis, type 1 (NF1)
    - Multifocal fibroxanthoma of long bones
    - May be bilateral and symmetric
  - Jaffe-Campanacci syndrome (may be subset of NF1)
    - Multifocal fibroxanthoma with extraskeletal manifestations in children
    - Cafe-au-lait spots
    - Mental retardation
    - Hypogonadism, cryptorchidism

FIBROXANTHOMA

- Congenital cardiovascular defects
- Etiology
  - Developmental defect arising in trabeculae of tubular bones
    - Migrates toward diaphysis as bone grows
  - May be result of periosteal injury
- Epidemiology
  - Most common fibrous lesion of bone
  - Occurs in 20-30% of normal population during 1st and 2nd decades of life
  - FCD: 30-40% of children develop one or more lesions
  - NOF: 2% of biopsied primary bone tumors
- Associated abnormalities: Simultaneous contiguous osteosarcoma very rare

Gross Pathologic & Surgical Features
- Eccentric, cortically based lesion with well-demarcated and scalloped or smooth inner boundary
- Fibrous, fleshy tissue with shades of grey and yellow
  - Color dependent on relative proportions of fibrous tissue and foamy histiocytes
- Cystic changes, hemorrhage, necrosis in larger lesion with pathologic fracture
- Involuted lesions: Replacement of fibrous component by cholesterol

Microscopic Features
- NOF and FCD are histologically identical
- Bundles of spindle-shaped fibroblasts, scattered multinucleated giant cells, and foamy histiocytes
- Foam cells more common in older lesions
- Hemosiderin pigment in stromal cells
- Arranged in storiform pattern (star-like arrangement of cells and fibers)
- Periosteum thickened

Staging, Grading or Classification Criteria
- Surgical staging for benign musculoskeletal tumors
  - Stage 1: Latent
  - Stage 2: Active
  - Stage 3: Aggressive

CLINICAL ISSUES

Presentation
- Most common signs/symptoms: Usually asymptomatic and identified incidentally
- Clinical Profile
  - During adolescence fibroxanthoma represents active stage 2 lesion
  - May cause pain, pathologic fracture
    - Increased risk of pathologic fracture if lesion is larger than 3.3 cm or involves > 50% of weight bearing bone
  - Very rare: Hypophosphatemic vitamin D resistant rickets, osteomalacia
    - Tumor may secrete substance that increases renal tubular resorption of phosphorus

Demographics
- Age
  - 2-20 years, peak: 10-15 years
  - Not seen after age 30 years
- Gender: M:F = 2:1

Natural History & Prognosis
- Benign lesion, no malignant transformation
- Presents during childhood, disappears in late adolescence
- Spontaneous regression
  - Involution over 2-4 years
- Heals by membranous ossification
- Bone island in adult may be residue of incompletely involuted fibroxanthoma

Treatment
- Usually does not require treatment
  - If lesion involves > 50% of transverse diameter of bone, increased risk of fracture
- Curettage with bone grafting of larger lesions at risk for fracture
  - Risk of growth disturbance from injury to growth plate
- Casting after pathologic fracture to avoid injury to physis during surgery
  - Lesion may heal after fracture

DIAGNOSTIC CHECKLIST

Consider
- No need to biopsy if appearance typical

SELECTED REFERENCES

1. Colby RS et al: Is Jaffe-Campanacci syndrome just a manifestation of neurofibromatosis type 1? Am J Med Genet A. 123(1):60-3, 2003
2. Loberant N et al: Gray-scale and Doppler characteristics of fibrous cortical defects in a child. J Clin Ultrasound. 31(7):369-74, 2003
3. Yanagawa T et al: The natural history of disappearing bone tumours and tumour-like conditions. Clin Radiol. 56(11):877-86, 2001
4. Smith SE et al: Primary musculoskeletal neoplasms of fibrous origin. Semin Musculoskel Radiol. 4:73-88, 2000
5. Suginoshita T et al: Case report: natural development of osteosarcoma from precancerous lesion. Anticancer Res. 20(1B):511-4, 2000
6. Dorfman HD et al: Bone tumors. 1st ed. St. Louis MO, Mosby. 205-15, 1998
7. Greenspan A et al: Differential diagnosis of tumors and tumor-like lesions of bones and joints. 1st ed. Philadelphia PA, Lippincott-Raven, 492-514, 1998
8. Friedland JA et al: Quantitative analysis of the plain radiographic appearance of nonossifying fibroma. Invest Radiol. 30:474-9, 1995
9. Park HR et al: Chondromyxoid fibroma of the femur: a case report with intra-cortical location. J Korean Med Sci. 10(1):51-6, 1995
10. Araki Y et al: MRI of fibrous cortical defect of the femur. Radiat Med. 12:93-8, 1994
11. Hudson TM et al: Fibrous lesions of bone. Radiol Clin North Am. 31:279-97, 1993
12. Unni KK et al: Fibrous and fibrohistiocytic lesions of bone. Semin Orthop. 6:177-86, 1991
13. Kransdorf MJ et al: MR appearance of fibroxanthoma. J Comput Assist Tomogr. 12:612-5, 1988

FIBROXANTHOMA

IMAGE GALLERY

Typical

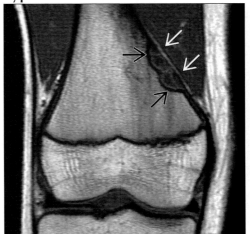 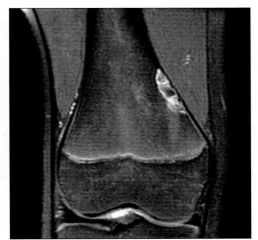

(Left) Coronal T1WI MR shows hypointense lesion (white arrows) and its deep hypointense, thin margin (black arrows). *(Right)* Coronal FSE T2 MR shows same lesion's heterogeneous hyperintense signal.

Typical

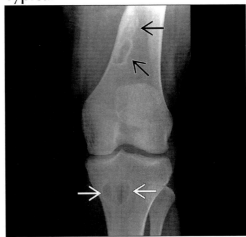 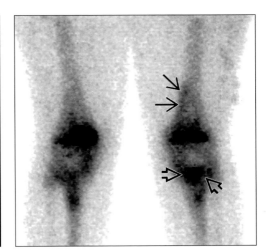

(Left) Anteroposterior radiograph shows shows fibroxanthomas in the femur (black arrows) and tibia (white arrows). *(Right)* Anteroposterior bone scan of same patient shows Tc-99m methylene diphosphonate (MDP) is taken up by both femoral (arrows) and tibial (open arrows) fibroxanthomas.

Typical

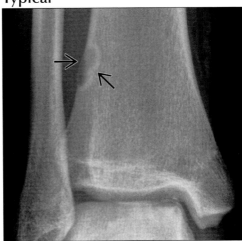 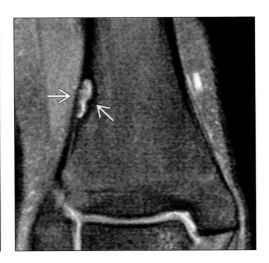

(Left) Anteroposterior radiograph shows small fibroxanthoma (arrows) in tibial metadiaphysis. It is elongated parallel to longitudinal axis of tibia and has a thin, sclerotic margin. *(Right)* Coronal PD T2 FSE FS MR in same patient shows hyperintense lesion (arrows) surrounded by thin, hypointense margin.

OSTEOID OSTEOMA

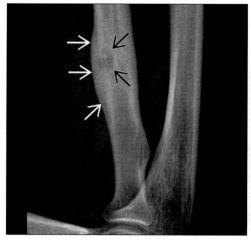

Lateral radiograph shows dense subperiosteal new bone (white arrows) over lucent cortical nidus (black arrows) in the radius of a 14 year old.

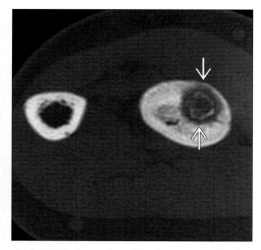

Axial NECT shows the nidus (arrows) made of 2 concentric areas of hypoattenuation enclosing a narrow hyperattenuated ring in same patient.

TERMINOLOGY

Definitions
- Benign lesion characterized by < 2 cm nidus of osteoid/woven bone in vascular tissue

IMAGING FINDINGS

General Features
- Best diagnostic clue: Well-defined lytic to sclerotic lesion with surrounding sclerosis
- Location
  - Metaphysis/diaphysis of long bones: 65-80%
    - Femur, tibia: 53-60%
  - Phalanges of hands and feet: 21%
  - Spine: 9%
    - Posterior elements: 90%
    - Vertebral body: 10%
  - Cortical: 70-80%
    - Long bone diaphysis
  - Cancellous: 25%
    - Femoral neck, hands and feet
    - Often intraarticular
  - Intraarticular/periarticular: 10%
    - Subchondral, subsynovial, intracortical, etc.
  - Subperiosteal: Rare
  - Extremely rare in skull and facial bones

- Size: Nidus: < 1.5-2 cm
- Morphology
  - Lucent nidus with marked surrounding periosteal reaction
    - Multicentric: < 20 cases reported in literature
    - Elongated: Resembled string of 3 beads in one case

Radiographic Findings
- Radiography
  - Cortical lesion
    - Radiolucent central nidus < 1.5 cm with surrounding dense sclerosis
    - Periosteal reaction may be present
  - Cancellous/intraarticular lesion
    - Mild reactive sclerosis
    - Associated periostitis away from lesion
    - Joint effusion, synovitis
  - Subperiosteal lesion
    - Round soft tissue mass adjacent to cortex
    - Surrounding reactive changes usually absent
  - Atypical in children < 5 years
    - Limb overgrowth if located near physis
    - Contour deformity: Tibia valgus, cortical bulge mimicking osteocartilaginous exostosis
    - Nidus elliptical rather than round

CT Findings
- NECT

DDx: Lucent Bone Lesions

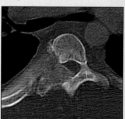
Osteoblastoma

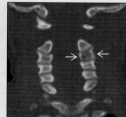
LCH

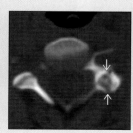
LCH

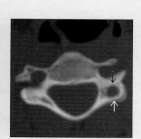
Osteomyelitis

OSTEOID OSTEOMA

Key Facts

Imaging Findings
- Best diagnostic clue: Well-defined lytic to sclerotic lesion with surrounding sclerosis

Top Differential Diagnoses
- Osteomyelitis (Brodie abscess)
- Langerhans-cell histiocytosis (LCH)
- Stress fracture
- Osteoblastoma
- Osteoma

Pathology
- Nidus has limited growth potential
- 4% of primary bone tumors
- 12% of benign bone tumors

Clinical Issues
- Most common signs/symptoms: Local pain worse at night, decreased by salicylates in less than 30 minutes (75%)
- Local swelling and point tenderness
- Spinal involvement: Painful scoliosis with concavity of curvature toward side of lesion
- No malignant potential
- No growth progression
- Can regress spontaneously
- Surgical en-block resection of nidus curative if nidus completely removed
- Percutaneous removal (CT guided)
- Percutaneous radio-frequency ablation (CT guided)
- Medical management: Nonsteroidal antiinflammatory drugs

- o Small, well-defined, round/oval nidus surrounded by sclerosis
- o Use thin sections (1-2 mm)

MR Findings
- T1WI: Nidus isointense to muscle
- T2WI: Radiolucent areas of nidus: Intermediate to high signal intensity
- T1 C+
  - o Dynamic imaging: Peak enhancement during arterial phase, early partial washout
    - Slower, progressive enhancement of adjacent bone marrow
- Low signal on all pulse sequences if nidus is completely mineralized
- May have extensive bone marrow edema which can obscure nidus
- Can show synovitis and joint effusion with intraarticular lesion

Ultrasonographic Findings
- Color Doppler
  - o Increased vascularity of nidus
  - o Can be used to localize lesion for biopsy

Angiographic Findings
- Intense blush of nidus during early arterial phase that persists during venous phase

Nuclear Medicine Findings
- Bone Scan
  - o Increased uptake
  - o Double density sign: Small focus of increased activity (nidus) surrounded by larger area of less intense activity (reactive sclerosis)
- PET: Can be used to detect osteoid osteoma in anatomically complex areas (posterior elements of spine)

Imaging Recommendations
- Best imaging tool: CT study of choice for identifying nidus
- Protocol advice: MRI in difficult cases to evaluate for joint effusion, synovitis

DIFFERENTIAL DIAGNOSIS

Osteomyelitis (Brodie abscess)
- Linear, serpentine tract, extends away from abscess cavity
- Cortical destruction

Langerhans-cell histiocytosis (LCH)
- Adjacent osteosclerosis rare
- Often polyostotic

Stress fracture
- Radiolucency more linear and perpendicular to cortex (rather than parallel)

Osteoblastoma
- Larger (> 2-2.5 cm)
- Progresses, no regression

Osteoma
- Cold on bone scan
- No periosteal reaction
- No nidus

PATHOLOGY

General Features
- General path comments
  - o Benign tumor consisting of osteoblastic mass (nidus) surrounded by zone of reactive sclerosis
    - Zone of sclerosis not integral part of tumor, represents secondary reversible change
    - Nidus has limited growth potential
  - o Prostaglandin E2 elevated 100-1000 times within nidus (likely cause of pain and vasodilatation)
  - o Tumor can regress spontaneously, possibly secondary to infarction
- Etiology
  - o Unknown: May be inflammatory, traumatic, vascular, viral
  - o Benign, highly vascular osteoblastic proliferation
- Epidemiology

OSTEOID OSTEOMA

- 4% of primary bone tumors
- 12% of benign bone tumors

Gross Pathologic & Surgical Features
- Nidus: Red/tan mass of gritty osseous tissue
- Easily separated from surrounding reactive bone
- Less than 1 cm in greatest dimension

Microscopic Features
- Nidus composed of osteoid tissue or mineralized, immature, woven bone
- Osteoid matrix and bone form trabeculae
  - Surrounded by highly vascular, fibrous stroma with osteoblastic and osteoclastic activity
- Sclerosis surrounding lesion composed of dense bone
- Adjacent synovium may be thickened and infiltrated with inflammatory cells and lymphoid follicles
  - Lymphofollicular synovitis; can simulate rheumatoid arthritis

Staging, Grading or Classification Criteria
- Surgical staging system for benign musculoskeletal tumors
  - Stage 1: Latent
  - Stage 2: Active
  - Stage 3: Aggressive

CLINICAL ISSUES

Presentation
- Most common signs/symptoms: Local pain worse at night, decreased by salicylates in less than 30 minutes (75%)
- Clinical Profile
  - Local swelling and point tenderness
  - Pain exacerbated by alcohol
  - Average duration of symptoms: 3 years
  - Spinal involvement: Painful scoliosis with concavity of curvature toward side of lesion
    - Idiopathic scoliosis: Never painful
    - Scoliosis improves/resolves if nidus is resected within 15 months after diagnosis
    - Neurologic abnormalities in 6% of patients with spine involvement
  - Intraarticular lesion
    - Pain, synovitis, effusion
    - Contracture: Decreased range of motion
  - Elevated urinary excretion of major prostacyclin metabolite (2,3-dinor-6-keto-PGF 1 α)
    - Returns to normal after removal of nidus

Demographics
- Age: 10-35 years
- Gender: M:F = 2-3:1
- Ethnicity: Rare in African-Americans

Natural History & Prognosis
- No malignant potential
- No growth progression
- Can regress spontaneously
- Regression of active stage 2 lesion to latent stage 1 lesion: 3 years (average)

Treatment
- Surgical en-block resection of nidus curative if nidus completely removed
  - Recurrence due to incomplete resection of nidus
  - Tetracycline and radionuclide labeling for lesion location at surgery
- Percutaneous removal (CT guided)
- Percutaneous radio-frequency ablation (CT guided)
  - Under general or spinal anesthesia
- Percutaneous thermocoagulation (CT guided)
- Medical management: Nonsteroidal antiinflammatory drugs
  - Can induce permanent relief of symptoms and regression of nidus

DIAGNOSTIC CHECKLIST

Consider
- Consider medical management as initial treatment since lesions can regress spontaneously
- Image guided therapy often more successful than surgical resection

SELECTED REFERENCES

1. Marinelli A et al: Osteoid osteoma simulating an osteocartilaginous exostosis. Skeletal Radiol. 33(3):181-5, 2004
2. Szendroi M et al: Intraarticular osteoid osteoma: clinical features, imaging results, and comparison with extraarticular localization. J Rheumatol. 31(5):957-64, 2004
3. Chiou YY et al: "Beaded" osteoid osteoma: a possible transition between solitary and multicentric tumor. Skeletal Radiol. 32(7):412-5, 2003
4. DeFriend DE et al: Percutaneous laser photocoagulation of osteoid osteoma under CT guidance. Clin Radiol. 58:222-6, 2003
5. Liu PT et al: Imaging of osteoid osteoma with dynamic gadolinium-enhanced MR imaging. Radiology. 227:691-700, 2003
6. Dorfman HD et al: Bone tumors. 1st ed. St. Louis MO, Mosby. 85-103, 1998
7. Greenspan A et al: Differential diagnosis of tumors and tumor-like lesions of bones and joints. 1st ed. Philadelphia PA, Lippencott-Raven, 36-46, 1998
8. Assoun J et al: Osteoid osteoma: MR imaging versus CT. Radiology. 191:217-23, 1994
9. Bilchik T et al: Osteoid osteoma: The role of radionuclide bone imaging, conventional radiography and computed tomography in its management. J Nucl Med. 33:269-71, 1992
10. Cassar-Pullicino VN et al: Intra-articular osteoid osteoma. Clin Radiol. 45:153-60, 1992
11. Greco F et al: Prostaglandins in osteoid osteoma. Int Orthop. 15:35-7, 1991
12. Azouz EM et al: Osteoid osteoma and osteoblastoma of the spine in children. Report of 22 cases with brief literature review. Pediatr Radiol. 16:25-31, 1986
13. Cohen MD et al: Osteoid osteoma: 95 cases and a review of the literature. Semin Arthritis Rheum. 12:265-81, 1983

OSTEOID OSTEOMA

IMAGE GALLERY

Typical

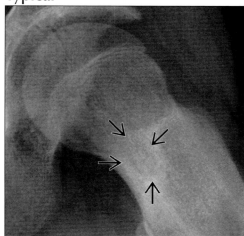
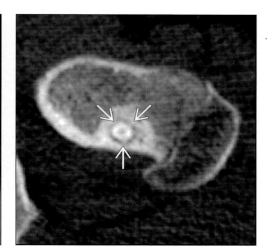

(Left) Frog-lateral radiograph shows a lucent nidus (arrows) in the femoral neck of a 12 year old. *(Right)* Axial NECT in same child shows nidus (arrows) with bull's eye arrangement of layers of increased and decreased attenuation.

Typical

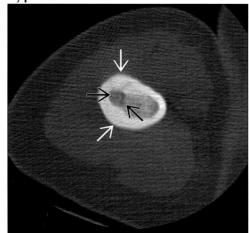
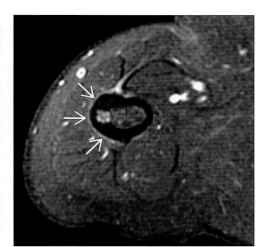

(Left) Axial NECT shows hypoattenuated nidus (black arrows) surrounded by subperiosteal new bone (white arrows) in humerus of a 16 year old. *(Right)* Axial T1 C+ MR shows enhancement of nidus and adjacent periosteum (arrows) in same patient.

Typical

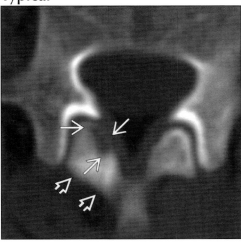
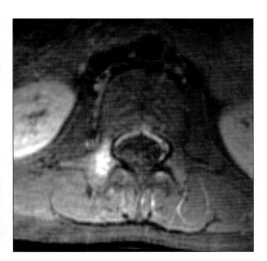

(Left) Axial NECT shows increased attenuation of lamina (open arrows) posterior to nidus (arrows) in L2 lamina of a 10 year old. *(Right)* Axial T1 C+ MR shows enhancement of lamina, transverse process, and pedicle in same patient.

DEVELOPMENTAL DYSPLASIA OF THE HIP

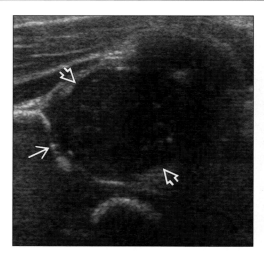

Coronal ultrasound shows normal, Graf type I hip. Femoral head (open arrows) is covered by > 50% by acetabular roof (arrow) and alpha angle is > 60 degrees (superior to left).

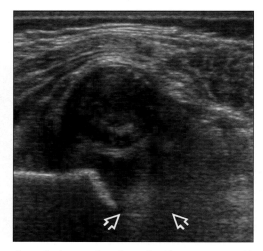

Coronal ultrasound performed with patient in Pavlik harness shows dislocated femoral head positioned superficial/lateral and superior to acetabular fossa (arrows). This is a Graf type 3 hip.

TERMINOLOGY

Abbreviations and Synonyms
- Developmental dysplasia of the hip (DDH), congenital dysplasia of hip (CDH), congenital hip dislocation

Definitions
- Abnormal position of the femoral head relative to the acetabulum which results in abnormal growth of both components of the hip
- More common in breech babies, fetuses with oligohydramnios
- Much more common in girls than boys
- Ligamentous laxity contributes to DDH

IMAGING FINDINGS

General Features
- Best diagnostic clue: Abnormal position or shape of femoral head, delayed ossification of the femoral head
- Location: On radiographs and ultrasound, the femur is superolaterally displaced from the acetabulum
- Size: Look for asymmetry of femoral head ossification center

Radiographic Findings
- Radiography
  - Several lines are used to assess hip location and acetabular morphology
  - Horizontal line of Hilgenreiner connects the superior aspect of the triradiate cartilage bilaterally
  - A perpendicular, vertical line, Perkins line, is then drawn from the superior lateral rim of the acetabulum through the line of Hilgenreiner
  - Perkins line should intersect the medial femoral metaphysis or the femoral head should project in the inferior medial quadrant created by these lines; the femoral head usually ossifies by 2-3 months
  - The angle of the acetabular roof can also be measured and should be less than 30 degrees in the neonate and decrease as the hip matures
  - Shenton line is drawn along the undersurface of the femoral trochanter and extends to the superior aspect of the obturator foramen
    - Normally, represents a contiguous arc
    - If noncontiguous, suspicious for DDH

CT Findings
- NECT
  - Limited CT scans are sometimes performed to confirm hip position after open surgical reduction
  - Low mA setting and judicious slice selection help limit radiation dose in these young patients

DDx: Other Neonatal Hip Conditions

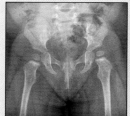
Coxa Valga

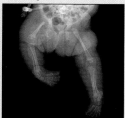
PFFD

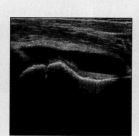
Hip Effusion

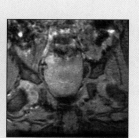
Post Septic Hip Left

DEVELOPMENTAL DYSPLASIA OF THE HIP

Key Facts

Terminology
- Developmental dysplasia of the hip (DDH), congenital dysplasia of hip (CDH), congenital hip dislocation
- Abnormal position of the femoral head relative to the acetabulum which results in abnormal growth of both components of the hip

Imaging Findings
- Best diagnostic clue: Abnormal position or shape of femoral head, delayed ossification of the femoral head

Top Differential Diagnoses
- Cerebral palsy, congenital coxa valga, neuromuscular disease
- Proximal focal femoral deficiency (PFFD)

Pathology
- Modified Graf staging of DDH
- Type 1
- Mature, normal hip
- Type 2a
- "Physiologic immaturity" at < 3 months
- Type 2b
- Still immature at age > 3 months
- Type 2c
- "Critical" hip, subluxed, unstable hip
- Type 3
- Hip has eccentric head, is dislocated
- Type 4
- Severe dysplasia, inverted labrum

MR Findings
- MRI used only in difficult cases, casted patients, and to assess post-op appearance

Ultrasonographic Findings
- Grayscale Ultrasound
  - Sonography is able to directly visualize the cartilaginous components of the hip, determine the position of the femoral head, depth of the acetabulum, and evaluate dynamic instability
  - The method of hip sonography developed by Graf and Harke evaluates acetabular morphology, angle of the acetabular roof (alpha angle), coverage of the femoral head, and dynamic subluxation during stress maneuvers
  - The combined static (anatomic) exam and dynamic (physiologic stress) exam is now the standard of care
- Color Doppler
  - Reported to be helpful in assessing femoral head perfusion, especially in patients being treated in Pavlik harness
  - Not generally part of the standard hip ultrasound exam

Non-Vascular Interventions
- Arthrogram: Arthrography is occasionally performed intra-operatively

Other Modality Findings
- Occasionally CT or MR scans are performed to assess hip position in casted patients post-operatively

Imaging Recommendations
- Best imaging tool
  - Ultrasound is modality of choice for infants up to 4-5 months old
  - Once the proximal femoral epiphysis ossifies, sonography becomes more difficult
    - The femoral head ossification center blocks the ultrasound beam, limiting evaluation of the acetabulum
    - Radiographs then become mainstay of imaging
- Protocol advice
  - Careful ultrasound technique is mandatory
  - The optimal coronal plane through the center of the hip should include
    - A straight segment of the iliac wing
    - The femoral head at maximal diameter
    - The triradiate cartilage between ossified acetabular roof and ischium
    - The greater trochanter and femoral neck should be visible
    - The fovea within the femoral head may be visible

DIFFERENTIAL DIAGNOSIS

Cerebral palsy, congenital coxa valga, neuromuscular disease
- In these disorders abnormal muscular tension causes subluxation/abnormal alignment, rather than ligamentous laxity and bone deficiency

Pyogenic arthritis of infancy
- Joint aspiration and clinical signs of infection distinguish this entity

Proximal focal femoral deficiency (PFFD)
- PFFD is a rare birth defect characterized by lack of development of the upper end of the femur

PATHOLOGY

General Features
- General path comments
  - Lax, dislocatable, or unstable hip joint felt to be due to
    - Ligamentous laxity - effects of maternal hormones
    - Deficient acetabular fossa and steep acetabular roof
    - Deficient femoral head or head-neck angulation
    - Interposition of connective or fibrous tissue between the femoral head and acetabulum
  - Embryology-anatomy

DEVELOPMENTAL DYSPLASIA OF THE HIP

- The cartilaginous components on both sides of the hip joint require the close apposition of the other to develop properly
- Genetics: More common in Caucasians than African-Americans
- Epidemiology: Incidence 1 in 200 births

Staging, Grading or Classification Criteria
- Modified Graf staging of DDH
- Acetabular roof angle (alpha) is important in staging scheme
- Degree of "coverage" of femoral head is not strictly part of Graf original staging, but is important
- Type 1
  - Mature, normal hip
  - Acetabular roof covers > 50% of head
  - Alpha angle > 60 degrees
- Type 2a
  - "Physiologic immaturity" at < 3 months
  - Acetabular roof covers < 50% of head
  - Alpha angle between 50-59 degrees
- Type 2b
  - Still immature at age > 3 months
  - Acetabular roof covers < 50% of head
  - Alpha angle between 50-59 degrees
- Type 2c
  - "Critical" hip, subluxed, unstable hip
  - Alpha angle 43-49 degrees
- Type 3
  - Hip has eccentric head, is dislocated
  - Alpha angle < 43 degrees
- Type 4
  - Severe dysplasia, inverted labrum
  - Alpha angle < 43 degrees

CLINICAL ISSUES

Presentation
- Most common signs/symptoms
  - Asymmetric skin or gluteal folds
  - Leg length discrepancy
  - Palpable click or clunk during stress maneuvers: Ortolani & Barlow
- Other signs/symptoms: Delayed ambulation or limp in toddlers

Demographics
- Gender: M:F = 1:5-8

Natural History & Prognosis
- If untreated abnormal stress on hip can cause long term disability, limb shortening, decreased range of motion, degenerative changes, avascular necrosis
- Excellent when diagnosed and treated early (harness or splint)
- Delayed diagnosis or treatment can result in irreversible dysplasia requiring iliac osteotomy/shelving procedure
- Some patients may eventually require hip replacement

Treatment
- Pavlik harness to flex, abduct, and externally rotate the hip(s)
- Occasionally surgical hip reduction and casting is required
- Salter osteotomy, steele triple osteotomy, Pemberton or Chiari procedure, femoral osteotomy: Typical surgical procedures performed

SELECTED REFERENCES

1. Dorn U et al: Ultrasound for screening developmental dysplasia of the hip: a European perspective. Curr Opin Pediatr. 17(1):30-3, 2005
2. Kayser R et al: Proximal focal femoral deficiency--a rare entity in the sonographic differential diagnosis of developmental dysplasia of the hip. J Pediatr. 146(1):141, 2005
3. Papavasiliou VA et al: Surgical treatment of developmental dysplasia of the hip in the periadolescent period. J Orthop Sci. 10(1):15-21, 2005
4. Roovers EA et al: Effectiveness of ultrasound screening for developmental dysplasia of the hip. Arch Dis Child Fetal Neonatal Ed. 90(1):F25-30, 2005
5. Albinana J et al: Acetabular dysplasia after treatment for developmental dysplasia of the hip. Implications for secondary procedures. 86(6):876-86, 2004
6. Domzalski M et al: Avascular necrosis after surgical treatment for development dysplasia of the hip. Int Orthop. 28(2):65-8, 2004
7. Ferzli JE et al: Anterior axial ultrasound in monitoring infants with Pavlik harness. Eur Radiol. 14(1):73-7, 2004
8. Ito H et al: Chiari pelvic osteotomy for advanced osteoarthritis in patients with hip dysplasia. J Bone Joint Surg Am. 86-A(7):1439-45, 2004
9. Kamath SU et al: Does developmental dysplasia of the hip cause a delay in walking? J Pediatr Orthop. 24(3):265, 2004
10. Trousdale RT: Acetabular osteotomy: indications and results. Clin Orthop Relat Res. (429):182-7, 2004
11. Ucar DH et al: Treatment of developmental dysplasia of the hip with Pavlik harness: prospective study in Graf type IIc or more severe hips. J Pediatr Orthop B. 13(2):70-4, 2004
12. American Institute of Ultrasound in Medicine: AIUM Practice Guideline for the performance of the ultrasound examination for detection of developmental dysplasia of the hip. J Ultrasound Med. 22(10):1131-6, 2003
13. Bohm P et al: Salter's innominate osteotomy for hip dysplasia in adolescents and young adults: results in 58 patients (69 osteotomies) at 4-12 years. Acta Orthop Scand. 74(3):277-86, 2003
14. Dezateux C et al: Performance, treatment pathways, and effects of alternative policy options for screening for developmental dysplasia of the hip in the United Kingdom. Arch Dis Child. 88(9):753-9, 2003
15. Mubarak SJ et al: Pavlik: the man and his method. J Pediatr Orthop. 23(3):342-6, 2003
16. Roovers EA et al: Ultrasonographic screening for developmental dysplasia of the hip in infants. Reproducibility of assessments made by radiographers. 85(5):726-30, 2003
17. Babcock DS et al: Developmental dysplasia of the hip. American College of Radiology. ACR Appropriateness Criteria. Radiology. 215 Suppl:819-27, 2000
18. Graf R et al: Advantages and disadvantages of various access routes in sonographic diagnosis of dysplasia and luxation in the infant hip. J Pediatr Orthop B. 6(4):248-52, 1997

DEVELOPMENTAL DYSPLASIA OF THE HIP

IMAGE GALLERY

Typical

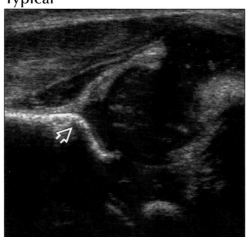
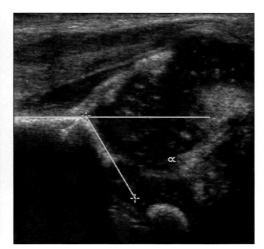

(Left) Coronal ultrasound shows a Graf type 2a hip, with mild rounding of the acetabular roof margin laterally *(arrow)*, alpha angle between 50 and 60 degrees, and adequate coverage of femoral head. *(Right)* Coronal ultrasound shows lines measuring the alpha angle in the same patient who is less than 3 months of age and has physiologic immaturity of the hips.

Typical

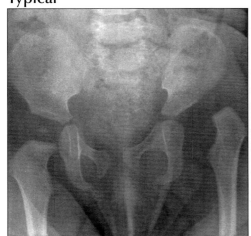
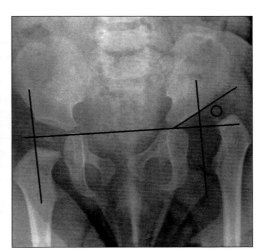

(Left) Anteroposterior radiograph shows dislocated left hip and delayed/absent ossification center of the left femoral head in this 5 month old infant. *(Right)* Anteroposterior radiograph shows the horizontal line of Hilgenreiner. The vertical line is Perkins line and the acetabular roof angle is drawn on the left. The circle estimates the position of the unossified left femoral head.

Typical

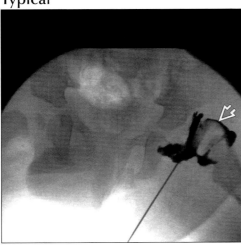
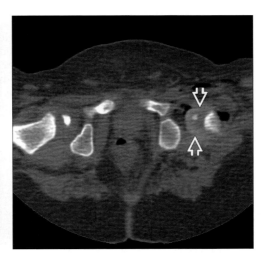

(Left) Anteroposterior radiograph taken during left hip arthrogram shows iodinated contrast outlining cartilaginous, dislocated left femoral head *(arrow)*. Note shallow left acetabulum compared to right. *(Right)* Axial NECT shows relocation of the left femoral head post-operatively *(arrows)* in the same patient. Note gas in the left hip joint and disparate size of the acetabula.

PROXIMAL FOCAL FEMORAL DEFICIENCY

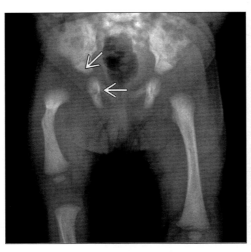

Anteroposterior radiograph shows Aitken class A or B PFFD on right in a five day old. Right acetabulum (arrows) well formed. Musculature of right leg hypoplastic, & leg tapers from hip downward.

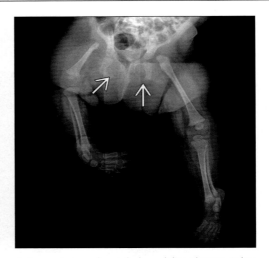

Anteroposterior radiograph shows bilateral PFFD. Aitken class D on right and C on left. Acetabula and femoral heads absent; severe right femoral shortening. Obturator foramina enlarged (arrows).

TERMINOLOGY

Abbreviations and Synonyms
- Proximal femoral focal deficiency (PFFD)

Definitions
- PFFD is a malformation in which complete growth and development of upper femur fails to occur
- PFFD encompasses a spectrum ranging from mere mild shortening and varus deformity of an otherwise normal femur to severe handicap of absent femur except for condyles accompanied by acetabular aplasia, thigh muscular hypoplasia and dysplasia, and short lower extremity

IMAGING FINDINGS

General Features
- Best diagnostic clue: Short femur with dysmorphic or absent head and neck

Radiographic Findings
- Radiography
  o Pelvis
    ▪ Obturator foramen: Enlarged
    ▪ Acetabulum: Supra-acetabular bump of Court, horizontal or dysplastic roof
    ▪ When femoral head fixed in acetabulum, concurrence of supra-acetabular bump, enlarged obturator foramen, horizontal acetabular roof, and pencil-pointing of upper end of detached distal femur common
  o Femur
    ▪ Short femur; delayed appearance or non-appearance of femoral capital ossification center (average age of appearance in PFFD 25 months)
    ▪ Misshapen femoral head and neck, coxa varum
    ▪ Upper end of disconnected distal femur: Either bulbous or pencil-pointed

MR Findings
- MR
  o Shows cartilage structure of acetabulum and upper femur in infants to assist prognosis and treatment planning
  o Presence or absence of an unossified femoral head and neck, and connection (or absence of connection) between femoral head and shaft can be identified
  o Hip joint space is incompletely formed when femoral head is fixed in acetabulum
  o Sartorius muscle is enlarged, which may explain the flexion, abduction, and external rotation of hip

DDx: Short Femur

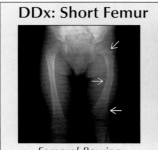

Femoral Bowing

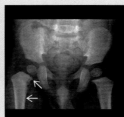

Coxa Varum

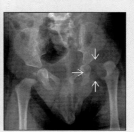

DDH

PROXIMAL FOCAL FEMORAL DEFICIENCY

Key Facts

Imaging Findings
- Shows cartilage structure of acetabulum and upper femur in infants to assist prognosis and treatment planning
- Presence or absence of an unossified femoral head and neck, and connection (or absence of connection) between femoral head and shaft can be identified
- Useful for prenatal diagnosis; and in infants to identify femoral head

Pathology
- Incidence: 1:52,000 births
- Ipsilateral fibular hemimelia (absence) in ≈50% (suspect when lateral malleolus absent)
- Milder dysplasia (70%): Aitken classes A and B (femoral head is present within acetabulum)
- More severe dysplasia (30%): Aitken classes C and D (no femoral head, and acetabulum is either severely dysplastic or absent)

Clinical Issues
- Treatment is highly individualized; including (when PFFD unilateral) a prosthesis, limb lengthening, hip reconstruction, and foot amputation

Diagnostic Checklist
- If radiographs show a normal acetabulum at birth, normal cartilaginous femoral head is likely

---

- Aitken class A: Hip external rotators are larger and abductors are smaller than normal; obturator externus muscle is straight
- Aitken class B-C: Obturator externus muscle is L-shaped

Ultrasonographic Findings
- Useful for prenatal diagnosis; and in infants to identify femoral head
- Assist in Aitken/Anton classification
- Assess mobility of femoral head within the acetabulum (PFFD can be misdiagnosed as Graf type 4 hip dysplasia)

Other Modality Findings
- Arthrography: Used to assess whether femoral head is mobile or fixed within acetabulum, and to gauge size and shape of femoral head
  - Caution: Femoral head can appear fixed to acetabulum when a distal bone discontinuity is present

Imaging Recommendations
- Best imaging tool: Radiography followed by MRI

DIFFERENTIAL DIAGNOSIS

Congenital short femur
- No specific abnormalities of head, neck, shaft

Congenital coxa vara
- Head, neck, and shaft otherwise normal

Developmental dysplasia of hip (DDH)
- Graf type 4

Traumatic femoral capital epiphysiolysis in newborn
- Pain plus edema of inguinal crease and upper thigh

PATHOLOGY

General Features
- Genetics: Several familial cases are in literature; no known genetic cause
- Etiology
  - Embryology
    - Developmental insult resulting in PFFD occurs at 4-6 weeks during limb-bud formation, growth, and differentiation
    - Acetabulum and proximal femur develop from a common anlage in embryo
    - 4 weeks, lower limb buds are formed
    - 5 weeks, individual muscles of legs begin to form
    - 6 weeks, skeletal cartilage begins to form
    - 7 weeks, acetabulum begins to take shape
    - 9 weeks, cleft forms between femur and acetabulum to form hip joint, whose shape is fully formed
- Epidemiology
  - Incidence: 1:52,000 births
  - Maternal thalidomide is a cause of PFFD
  - Bilateral PFFD in 10-15%, often Aitken class D
- Associated abnormalities
  - Ipsilateral fibular hemimelia (absence) in ≈50% (suspect when lateral malleolus absent)
  - Knee often unstable and may dislocate
  - Absent or hypoplastic cruciate ligaments and menisci
  - Ball-and-socket ankle, clubfoot, talocalcaneal and tarsal coalition, decreased number of foot rays
  - Rare: Brain atrophy, caudal regression syndrome, cleft palate, congenital heart disease, facial anomalies, femoral-fibula-ulna complex (FFU), Hirschsprung disease, maternal diabetes, Pierre-Robin anomaly, spinal deformities, syndactyly

Gross Pathologic & Surgical Features
- Varying degrees of connection of femoral head and remainder of femur
  - Osteocartilaginous connection

PROXIMAL FOCAL FEMORAL DEFICIENCY

- ○ Discontinuity: No bone connection (called "pseudarthrosis" in some reports)
  - Subtrochanteric (27%), femoral neck (15%), both subtrochanteric and femoral neck (4%)
- ○ Most common: Single discontinuity located below trochanteric region
- ○ Discontinuity may eventually fill in with bone in Aitken type A PFFD, but always residual severe varus deformity and short femur
  - Discontinuity does not heal in Aitken type B
- A bulbous bony tuft, perhaps apophysis of greater trochanter, forms at superior tip of disconnected distal femur in Aitken types B and C
  - ○ The tip of the disconnected distal femur is pointed (pencil-pointed) in Aitken type D; there is no bony tuft

Microscopic Features
- Failure of organization of proliferative hypertrophic chondrocytes into longitudinal columns
- Disorganized vascular invasion with honeycomb rather than columnar pattern of primary trabeculae

Staging, Grading or Classification Criteria
- At least 8 classification schemes; two simplest offer good correlation between radiographic appearance and complexity of orthopedic management to secure best functional result
  - ○ Aitken classification (1968)
    - Class A (38%): Femoral head present and acetabulum normal; all parts of femur connected by bone; subtrochanteric varus common
    - Class B (32%): Femoral head present within acetabulum and acetabulum adequate or moderately dysplastic; bone does not connect femoral head and shaft
    - Class C (17%): Femoral head absent or represented by an ossicle; acetabulum severely dysplastic
    - Class D (13%): Both femoral head and acetabulum absent; distal femoral segment shortened and deformed; obturator foramen of pelvis enlarged
  - ○ Anton classification (1999)
    - Milder dysplasia (70%): Aitken classes A and B (femoral head is present within acetabulum)
    - More severe dysplasia (30%): Aitken classes C and D (no femoral head, and acetabulum is either severely dysplastic or absent)

CLINICAL ISSUES

Presentation
- Most common signs/symptoms
  - ○ Characteristic short, bulky thigh that tapers towards the knee, producing a "ship's funnel" appearance
  - ○ Hip is held in flexion, abduction, and external rotation
  - ○ Thigh muscles, especially abductors, hypoplastic
- Other signs/symptoms
  - ○ Flexion contractures and instability of hip and knee are common
  - ○ Limb-length shortening of 35-50%

Demographics
- Gender: M:F = 2:1

Treatment
- Biomechanical problems
  - ○ Hip instability, malrotation of thigh with flexed knee, poor development of proximal musculature, short limbs
- Treatment is highly individualized; including (when PFFD unilateral) a prosthesis, limb lengthening, hip reconstruction, and foot amputation
- Bilateral PFFD: Most ambulate well on shortened legs
  - ○ Usually not treated surgically unless severe foot deformities
  - ○ Children get about at home without prostheses; prostheses used in social settings to achieve stature closer to that of peers

DIAGNOSTIC CHECKLIST

Image Interpretation Pearls
- If radiographs show a normal acetabulum at birth, normal cartilaginous femoral head is likely

SELECTED REFERENCES

1. Kayser R et al: Proximal focal femoral deficiency--a rare entity in the sonographic differential diagnosis of developmental dysplasia of the hip. J Pediatr. 146(1):141, 2005
2. Anton CG et al: Proximal Femoral Focal Deficiency(PFFD): More Than An Abnormal Hip. Semin Musculoskelet Radiol. 3(3):215-226, 1999
3. Fordham LA et al: Fibular Hemimelia: More Than Just An Absent Bone. Semin Musculoskelet Radiol. 3(3):227-238, 1999
4. Court C et al: Radiological study of severe proximal femoral focal deficiency. J Pediatr Orthop. 17(4):520-4, 1997
5. Goddard NJ et al: Natural history and treatment of instability of the hip in proximal femoral focal deficiency. J Pediatr Orthop B. 4(2):145-9, 1995
6. Bryant DD 3rd et al: Proximal femoral focal deficiency: evaluation and management. Orthopedics. 14(7):775-84, 1991.
7. Pirani S et al: Soft tissue anatomy of proximal femoral focal deficiency. J Pediatr Orthop. 11(5):563-70, 1991
8. Boden SD et al: Proximal femoral focal deficiency. Evidence for a defect in proliferation and maturation of chondrocytes. J Bone Joint Surg Am. 71(8):1119-29, 1989
9. Hillmann JS et al: Proximal femoral focal deficiency: radiologic analysis of 49 cases. Radiology. 165(3):769-73, 1987
10. Hamanishi C: Congenital short femur. Clinical, genetic and epidemiological comparison of the naturally occurring condition with that caused by thalidomide. J Bone Joint Surg Br. 62(3):307-20, 1980
11. Towbin R et al: Neonatal traumatic proximal femoral epiphysiolysis. Pediatrics. 63(3):456-9, 1979
12. Aitken GT. Proximal femoral focal deficiency: Definition, classification, and management . In Aitken GT, (ed): Proximal Femoral Focal Deficiency, A Congenital Anomaly: A Symposium. Washington D.C.: National Academy of Sciences. 1-22, 1968

PROXIMAL FOCAL FEMORAL DEFICIENCY

IMAGE GALLERY

Typical

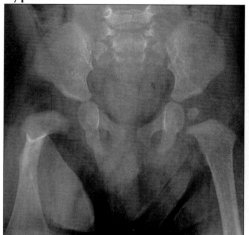
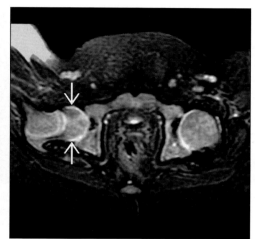

(Left) Anteroposterior radiograph shows Aitken class A or B PFFD on right in five-month old. Acetabulum well formed but status of femoral head (delayed ossification-center appearance) not apparent. *(Right)* Axial FSE T2 MR of the same patient shows well-formed right femoral head (arrows) although it is smaller than left femoral head. Femoral neck is intact. Aitken classification becomes type A.

Typical

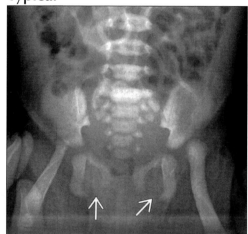
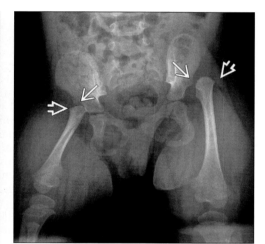

(Left) Anteroposterior radiograph shows bilateral PFFD, Aitken type D on right (severe femoral shortening) and type C or D on left in newborn. Acetabulae absent. Obturator foramina enlarged (arrows). *(Right)* Anteroposterior radiograph of same patient at 1.5 years shows tufted appearance of both upper femurs (open arrows) and supra-acetabular bumps (arrows). Obturator foramina remain large.

Typical

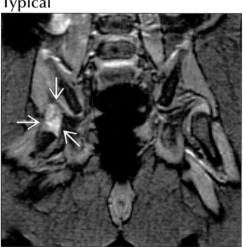
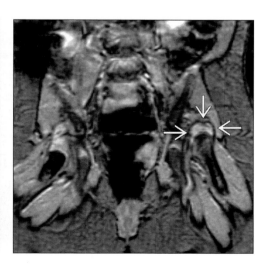

(Left) Coronal MPGR MR in same child at 7 months shows that right femur is capped by a cartilage cylinder (arrows). *(Right)* Coronal MPGR MR in same child shows that left femur is capped by a hemispherical cartilage structure (arrows).

LEGG-CALVE-PERTHES DISEASE

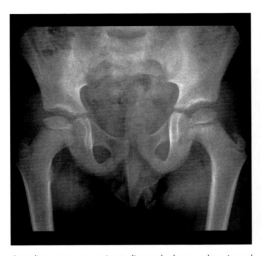

Standing anteroposterior radiograph shows sclerosis and flattening of right femoral capital epiphysis in a 6 year old. Inferomedial joint space is widened, and acetabular roof is demineralized.

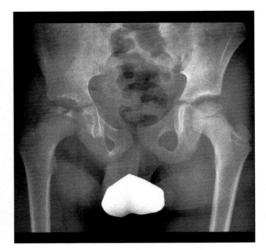

Standing anteroposterior radiograph shows epiphyseal fragmentation and further volume loss 12 months later in the same child. Right acetabulum and femoral metadiaphysis are osteopenic.

TERMINOLOGY

Abbreviations and Synonyms
- Legg-Perthes or Perthes disease, avascular necrosis (AVN) of proximal femoral epiphysis, osteochondritis coxae juvenilis, coxa plana

Definitions
- An osteochondrosis due to AVN of capital femoral epiphysis

IMAGING FINDINGS

General Features
- Best diagnostic clue: Fragmentation and flattening of sclerotic capital epiphysis
- Size: Variable size from peripheral irregularity of epiphyseal ossification center to complete replacement of normal marrow fat
- Morphology
  o Early: Epiphysis variably fragmented and flattened
  o Late: Coxa plana, coxa magna

Radiographic Findings
- Radiography
  o Fragmentation and flattening of sclerotic capital epiphysis
  o Subchondral fracture (lucency) of epiphysis
  o Metaphyseal irregularity, osteopenia, cystic/pseudocystic changes
  o Joint space (inferomedial) widening, intact subchondral plate
  o Retarded bone age
  o Waldenström's radiographic staging
    ▪ Initial stage: Increased head-socket distance, subchondral plate thinning, dense epiphysis
    ▪ Fragmentation stage: Subchondral fracture, inhomogeneous dense epiphysis, metaphyseal cysts/pseudocysts
    ▪ Reparative stage: Removal of sclerotic bone and replacement with normal bone, epiphysis more homogeneous
    ▪ Growth stage: Approaches final femoral shape
    ▪ Definite stage: Final shape: Congruent vs. incongruent hip joint

MR Findings
- T1WI
  o Hypointense intraarticular effusion
  o Hypointense irregularity along periphery of ossific nucleus
  o Linear hypointensity traversing femoral ossification center in early stages

DDx: Abnormalities Of Femoral Epiphysis

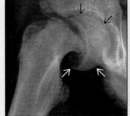
SCFE

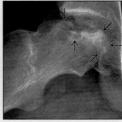
Gaucher Disease

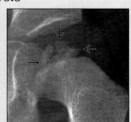
Meyer Dysplasia

LEGG-CALVE-PERTHES DISEASE

Key Facts

Imaging Findings
- Best diagnostic clue: Fragmentation and flattening of sclerotic capital epiphysis
- Size: Variable size from peripheral irregularity of epiphyseal ossification center to complete replacement of normal marrow fat
- Late: Coxa plana, coxa magna
- Hypointense epiphyseal marrow center on T1 and T2WI

Top Differential Diagnoses
- Toxic synovitis
- Septic hip
- Juvenile chronic arthritis
- Juvenile osteonecrosis

Pathology
- Insufficiency of capital epiphyseal blood supply with physis acting as a barrier
- Ischemia may be arterial or venous
- 15-20% with bilateral involvement

Clinical Issues
- Most common signs/symptoms: Limp due to groin, thigh or referred knee pain
- 3-12 years
- Median: 7 years
- Gender: M:F = 4-5:1

Diagnostic Checklist
- Use coronal T1WI to detect subtle peripheral or linear areas of epiphyseal marrow hypointensity

---

- Revascularization of necrotic epiphysis: Replacement of hypointense focus with marrow fat signal intensity
- T2WI
  - FS PD or T2 FSE images to assess articular cartilage thickness, chondral irregularities
  - Physeal cartilage ± hyperintense on T2WI (in early stage disease)
  - Loss of femoral head containment in acetabulum
    - Intermediate signal hypertrophied synovium in iliopsoas recess
    - Thickening of intermediate signal epiphyseal cartilage
  - Hyperintense joint effusion
- Hypointense epiphyseal marrow center on T1 and T2WI
- Sagittal T1 and T2WI also useful to display acetabular and femoral head cartilage

Nuclear Medicine Findings
- Bone scintigraphy
  - Early decrease secondary to interruption of blood supply
  - Increased uptake late: With revascularization

Imaging Recommendations
- Best imaging tool: MR for early detection of epiphyseal ossification center irregularity
- Protocol advice
  - Coronal: T1, FS PD FSE, T2*
  - Axial: T1, PD, FS PD FSE
  - Sagittal: FS PD FSE

DIFFERENTIAL DIAGNOSIS

Toxic synovitis
- Self-limiting acute synovitis (3-10 days), usually in boys < 4 years; improves in < 5 days with bedrest and anti-inflammatory medications
- Significant effusion, capsular distension

Septic hip
- Acutely ill, fever, leukocytosis
- Hips held in flexion, abduction and external rotation vs. hip adduction in Legg-Calve-Perthes disease
- Joint effusion, ± joint debris, ± reactive marrow edema

Juvenile chronic arthritis
- Limp, hip pain, thigh atrophy, fever, rash, positive antinuclear antibody
- Epiphyseal erosions

Juvenile osteonecrosis
- AVN due to known cause: Sickle cell anemia, thalassemia, coagulopathy, after hip dislocation

Slipped capital femoral epiphysis (SCFE)
- Posterior-inferior displacement of proximal femoral epiphysis
- Pain, limp, limited internal rotation and abduction

Meyer dysplasia
- Age 2-4 years; mostly boys; bilateral 60%; asymptomatic

Osteoid osteoma
- Local pain worse at night, decreased by salicylates
- Local swelling, point tenderness
- Extensive marrow edema on FS PD FSE or STIR

PATHOLOGY

General Features
- Etiology
  - Insufficiency of capital epiphyseal blood supply with physis acting as a barrier
  - Infarction: Causes trabecular fracture with decreased epiphyseal height
  - Ischemia may be arterial or venous
- Epidemiology
  - 15-20% with bilateral involvement
  - 1:1,200 < 15 years old

LEGG-CALVE-PERTHES DISEASE

Gross Pathologic & Surgical Features
- Initial stage
  - Necrosis of epiphyseal bone and marrow; vascular invasion of necrotic bone
  - Epiphyseal cartilage hypertrophy; articular cartilage overgrowth
- Fragmentation
  - Necrotic bone resorbed
  - Metaphyseal cysts/pseudocysts containing cartilage
  - Cartilage hypertrophy
- Reparative
  - Complete replacement of necrotic bone

Microscopic Features
- Epiphyseal cartilage
  - Disordered collagen, fibrosis
  - Increased proteoglycan concentration
  - Decrease in structural glycoproteins
- Infarction
  - Necrosis of epiphyseal bone and marrow
  - New blood vessels invade
  - Resorption of necrotic bone, new bone formation

Staging, Grading or Classification Criteria
- Catterall classification: Based on extent of epiphyseal involvement
  - Group I: < ¼ epiphysis involved
  - Group II : < ½ epiphysis involved
  - Group III: Most of epiphysis involved
  - Group IV: All epiphysis involved
  - Risk factors: Lateral subluxation, Gage's sign (radiolucent V in lateral epiphysis), horizontal physis
- Salter-Thompson scheme: Based on extent and location of subchondral fracture
  - A: Fracture < 50% span of epiphysis
  - B: Fracture > 50% span of epiphysis
- Herring system: Based on lateral pillar (LP) involvement (LP = the 5-30% of epiphysis lateral to vertical fragmentation line)
  - A: LP uninvolved
  - B: < 50% LP loss of height
  - B/C border group: Narrow LP >50% original height; poorly ossified LP with at least 50% original height, or LP exactly 50% that is depressed relative to central pillar
  - C: > 50% LP loss of height

CLINICAL ISSUES

Presentation
- Most common signs/symptoms: Limp due to groin, thigh or referred knee pain
- Clinical Profile
  - No specific history of trauma
  - Decreased range of motion (internal rotation, abduction), painful gait, muscle atrophy

Demographics
- Age
  - 3-12 years
  - Median: 7 years
- Gender: M:F = 4-5:1

Natural History & Prognosis
- Limb length inequality and thigh atrophy if poor result
- Younger age of presentation: Prognosis better
  - > 8 years old at onset: Prognosis worse
- Classification of outcome when skeleton mature
  - Mose classification: Evaluates sphericity of femoral head
    - Arthritis more likely when femoral head more that 2 mm out of round
    - Coxa plana, coxa magna
- > 20% epiphyseal extrusion from acetabulum or > 50% capital epiphysis involvement: Prognosis poor

Treatment
- Conservative
  - Bed rest + abduction stretching & bracing
  - 50% improve with no treatment
- Surgical
  - Femoral/pelvic osteotomies to contain hip

DIAGNOSTIC CHECKLIST

Consider
- Use coronal T1WI to detect subtle peripheral or linear areas of epiphyseal marrow hypointensity

SELECTED REFERENCES

1. Rowe SM et al: Dysplasia epiphysealis capitis femoris: meyer dysplasia. J Pediatr Orthop. 25(1):18-21, 2005
2. Herring JA et al: Legg-Calve-Perthes disease. Part I: Classification of radiographs with use of the modified lateral pillar and Stulberg classifications. J Bone Joint Surg Am. 86-A(10):2103-20, 2004
3. Cho TJ et al: Femoral head deformity in Catterall groups III and IV Legg-Calve-Perthes disease: Magnetic resonance imaging analysis in coronal and sagittal planes. J Pediatr Orthop. 22(5):601-6, 2002
4. Fitzgerald RH et al: Orthopaedics. Legg-Calvé-Perthes. St. Louis MO, Mosby, Sect 9 (9-19):1420-32, 2002
5. De Sanctis N et al: Legg-Calve-Perthes disease by MRI. Part II: Pathomorphologenesis and new classification. J Pediatr Orthop. 20(4):463-70, 2000
6. De Sanctis N et al: Prognostic evaluation of Legg-Calve-Perthes disease by MRI. Part I: The role of physeal involvement. J Pediatr Orthop. 20(4):455-62, 2000
7. Gabriel H et al: MR imaging of hip disorders. Radiographics. 14:763-81, 1994
8. Bos CFA et al: Sequential magnetic resonance imaging in Perthes' disease. J Bone Joint Surg. 73:219-24, 1991
9. Egund N et al: Legg-Calve-Perthes disease: Imaging with MR. Radiology. 179:89-92, 1991
10. Rush BH et al: Legg-Calve-Perthes disease: Detection of cartilaginous and synovial changes with MR imaging. Radiology. 167:473-6, 1988
11. Thompson GH et al: Legg-Calve-Perthes disease: Current concepts and controversies. Orthop Clin North Am. 18:617, 1987
12. Toby EB et al: Magnetic resonance imaging of pediatric hip disorders. J Pediatr Orthop. 5:665-71, 1985

LEGG-CALVE-PERTHES DISEASE

IMAGE GALLERY

Typical

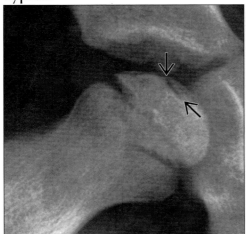
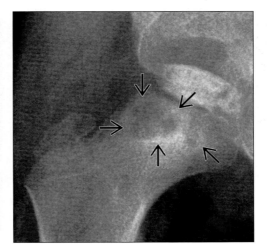

(Left) Frog-lateral radiograph shows a subchondral fracture line (arrows) in slightly sclerotic epiphysis. *(Right)* Anteroposterior radiograph shows femoral neck cysts or pseudocysts (arrows) beneath sclerotic and compressed capital epiphysis.

Typical

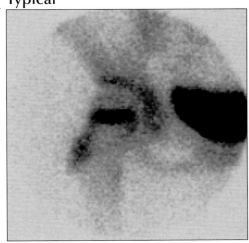
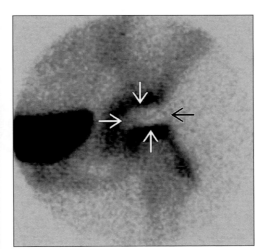

(Left) Anteroposterior pinhole bone scan shows normal perfusion of the right capital femoral epiphysis. The intense physeal uptake is normal. *(Right)* Anteroposterior pinhole bone scan shows cold defect in lateral 2/3rds of left capital epiphysis (arrows outline entire epiphysis) in same child.

Typical

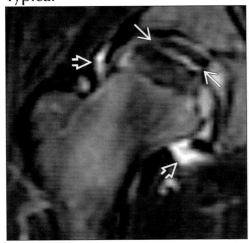
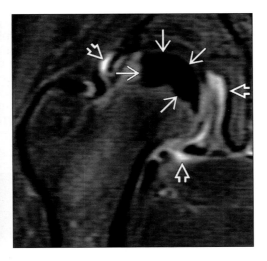

(Left) Coronal FSE T2 MR shows the hyperintense signals of a subchondral fracture (arrows) and hip-joint synovitis (open arrows). *(Right)* Coronal T1 C+ MR shows non-perfusion of most capital-epiphysis marrow (arrows) in same child. Synovial enhancement (open arrows) due to synovitis.

SLIPPED CAPITAL FEMORAL EPIPHYSIS

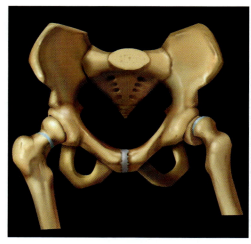

Graphic shows left capital femoral epiphysis that has slipped posteriorly and medially relative to the metaphysis.

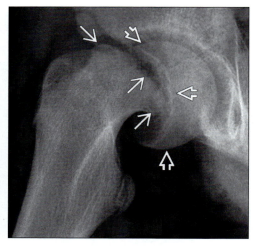

Frog-lateral radiograph shows moderately severe SCFE with epiphysis (open arrows) displaced posteriorly more than 1/3 of its diameter on metaphysis (arrows).

TERMINOLOGY

Abbreviations and Synonyms
- Slipped capital femoral epiphysis (SCFE) pronounced "Skiffie"

Definitions
- Salter-Harris type-1 femoral capital physis fracture due to repetitive stress of weight-bearing
  - This definition does not include traumatic Salter-Harris type-1 fracture of the hip because etiology and management are different

IMAGING FINDINGS

General Features
- Best diagnostic clue: Posterior displacement of femoral capital epiphysis relative to metaphysis on frog-leg lateral view
- Location
  - Bilateral: Incidence varies widely in literature reports
    - Bilateral eventually in 18-100%
    - Bilateral manifest SCFE at initial presentation: 9-18%
    - Opposite-side SCFE occurs usually within 24 months of the first occurrence
- Morphology: Capital femoral epiphysis slips posteriorly and medially relative to metaphysis

Radiographic Findings
- Radiography
  - Widening of capital femoral physis
    - May occur before slip recognizable ("pre-slip")
  - Medial displacement of capital epiphysis relative to metaphysis
    - This is seen on anteroposterior radiograph
    - Capital epiphysis drops toward or below Klein's line (a line drawn along top of the femoral neck and continued towards acetabulum; line ordinarily crosses a small portion of capital femoral ossification center)
  - Posterior displacement of capital epiphysis relative to metaphysis
    - Seen on frog-lateral radiograph as medial displacement of epiphysis relative to metaphysis; ≈ 90° external rotation of femur on frog-lateral means that what is really posterior displacement of epiphysis looks like medial displacement on radiograph
    - Seen on cross-table lateral radiograph with 25° flexion as true posterior displacement of epiphysis
    - This displacement may be visible before abnormalities can be seen on anteroposterior radiograph

DDx: Diseases Causing Painful Hip

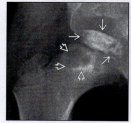

Legg-Calve-Perthes

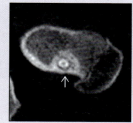

Osteoid Osteoma

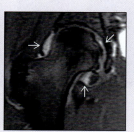

Synovitis

SLIPPED CAPITAL FEMORAL EPIPHYSIS

Key Facts

Terminology
- Salter-Harris type-1 femoral capital physis fracture due to repetitive stress of weight-bearing

Imaging Findings
- Bilateral eventually in 18-100%
- Opposite-side SCFE occurs usually within 24 months of the first occurrence
- Morphology: Capital femoral epiphysis slips posteriorly and medially relative to metaphysis
- Capital epiphysis drops toward or below Klein's line (a line drawn along top of the femoral neck and continued towards acetabulum; line ordinarily crosses a small portion of capital femoral ossification center)

- MR: Physeal widening is a constant feature, hyperintensity is inconstant; MR is more sensitive than radiography; physeal widening can be seen on MR before apparent on radiographs

Pathology
- Epidemiology: Incidence: 0.7 to 3.4:100,000

Clinical Issues
- Pain primarily in hip, groin, or proximal thigh in 85%; distal thigh or knee pain in 15%
- Age: Girls: Range 8-15 years, average 11-12 years; boys: range 10-17 years, average 13-14 years
- Premature osteoarthritis: Develops during adulthood in 1/4-1/3 patients (SCFE may be the most common cause of degenerative joint disease in middle life)

- ○ Metaphysis: Scalloping, irregularity, sclerosis, and posterior beaking
- ○ Staging of radiographic findings
  - Mild → moderate → severe: Displacement of ossification center by < 1/3 → 1/3 - 2/3 → > 2/3 metaphyseal diameter

CT Findings
- Physeal widening
- Metaphyseal scalloping and beaking

MR Findings
- MR: Physeal widening is a constant feature, hyperintensity is inconstant; MR is more sensitive than radiography; physeal widening can be seen on MR before apparent on radiographs
- Marrow edema and synovitis is inconstant

Nuclear Medicine Findings
- Bone Scan
  - ○ Chondrolysis: Increased uptake on both acetabular and femoral sides of hip joint due to associated synovitis
  - ○ Avascular necrosis: Decreased uptake in femoral epiphysis

Imaging Recommendations
- Best imaging tool
  - ○ Anteroposterior and frog-lateral radiographs of both hips; frog-lateral view is obtained with femurs abducted and rotated externally
    - Be careful not to use force to secure frog-lateral position; there is a possibility of increasing slip by applying pressure
  - ○ Cross-table lateral radiograph with hip joint flexed 25° very sensitive for detecting posterior slipping
- Protocol advice: Normal radiographs do not exclude SCFE

DIFFERENTIAL DIAGNOSIS

Legg-Calve-Perthes disease
- Younger age group: 5-8 years; presents as irritable hip with subsequent sclerosis and collapse of capital ossification center
- Hairline epiphyseal fracture
- Marrow edema and synovitis

Hip joint inflammation
- Non-infectious synovitis, rheumatoid arthritis, infectious synovitis with or without osteomyelitis caused by a variety of agents ranging from Staphylococcus aureus to Mycobacterium tuberculosis

Osteoid osteoma
- Pain, worse at night, relieved by aspirin

Irritable hip
- Limp, pain, and limited range of hip motion; imaging studies are normal; self-limited (diagnosis by exclusion)

Traumatic SCFE
- Unequivocal history of trauma in adolescence
- Newborns: A rare occurrence, almost always associated with difficult breech delivery; hip flexed, abducted, externally rotated; pain plus edema of inguinal crease and upper thigh (diagnosis made by ultrasound or arthrography)

PATHOLOGY

General Features
- General path comments: SCFE is unique because it has no parallel in other bones and its occurrence is limited to narrow age range of puberty
- Epidemiology: Incidence: 0.7 to 3.4:100,000

Microscopic Features
- Fracture occurs in zone of hypertrophic chondrocytes

SLIPPED CAPITAL FEMORAL EPIPHYSIS

- Anterior tear in periosteum with moderate and severe slips

CLINICAL ISSUES

Presentation
- Most common signs/symptoms
  - Limp, pain, or limitation of hip motion while walking or running
    - Pain primarily in hip, groin, or proximal thigh in 85%; distal thigh or knee pain in 15%
- Other signs/symptoms
  - Staging of clinical presentations
    - Acute onset: Sudden onset and progression of symptoms (duration less than three weeks)
    - Chronic onset: Gradual onset and progression of symptoms (duration greater than three weeks)
    - Acute on chronic onset: Gradual onset and progression of symptoms suddenly becomes worse; most frequent presentation
    - Stable versus unstable SCFE: Stable if the child can bear weight and unstable if child unable to bear weight even with crutches
  - Limited range of motion
    - Loss of internal rotation or fixed external rotation
    - Leg-length shortening

Demographics
- Age: Girls: Range 8-15 years, average 11-12 years; boys: range 10-17 years, average 13-14 years
- Gender: M:F = 2.5:1
- Ethnicity: Slightly more common in African-Americans than in Caucasians or Hispanics
- Predisposing factors
  - Obesity is currently most significant factor
  - Adolescent growth spurt
  - Endocrine: Primary hypothyroidism, pituitary dysfunction, growth-hormone deficiency, hypogonadism (small testes)
  - Renal rickets, radiation therapy, chemotherapy
  - Prior developmental dysplasia of hip
  - Down syndrome

Natural History & Prognosis
- Premature osteoarthritis: Develops during adulthood in 1/4-1/3 patients (SCFE may be the most common cause of degenerative joint disease in middle life)
  - "Pistol grip" deformity of upper femur, leg-length shortening
- Outcome directly related to severity of slip
- Prognosis poorer when SCFE unstable at time of diagnosis

Treatment
- Surgical insertion of pins or screws to immobilize epiphysis on physeal plate in situ, i.e., without attempting reduction
  - Surgical complications
    - Chondrolysis (10%): Hip-joint space narrowing, pain, limited range of motion; may be accompanying synovitis; SCFE is commonest cause (chondrolysis may also occur after Spica cast immobilization, hip-joint trauma, infectious and non-infectious arthritis)
    - Avascular necrosis (1%): Causes persistent pain and limitation of motion; diagnosis confirmed by bone scan; incidence increased when there has been open reduction with fixation, or when multiple pins cross the superolateral quadrant of the capital femoral ossification center (interfering with blood supply)
    - Pin or screw penetration of hip joint or extrusion: Diagnosed by radiography

DIAGNOSTIC CHECKLIST

Image Interpretation Pearls
- Be cautious when using opposite asymptomatic hip as a normal control for radiographic evaluation of painful one
  - Quite possible that opposite side has unrecognized SCFE

SELECTED REFERENCES

1. Billing L et al: Slipped capital femoral epiphysis. The mechanical function of the periosteum: new aspects and theory including bilaterality. Acta Radiol Suppl. (431):1-27, 2004
2. Bosch P et al: Slipped capital femoral epiphysis in patients with Down syndrome. J Pediatr Orthop. 24(3):271-7, 2004
3. Kuhn JP et al: Caffey's Pediatric Diagnostic Imaging. 10th edition. 2277-9, 2004
4. Billing L et al: Reliable X-ray diagnosis of slipped capital femoral epiphysis by combining the conventional and a new simplified geometrical method. Pediatr Radiol. 32(6):423-30, 2002
5. Kennedy JG et al: Osteonecrosis of the femoral head associated with slipped capital femoral epiphysis. J Pediatr Orthop. 21(2):189-93, 2001
6. Matava MJ et al: Knee pain as the initial symptom of slipped capital femoral epiphysis: an analysis of initial presentation and treatment. J Pediatr Orthop. 19(4):455-60, 1999
7. Hansson G et al: Long-term results after nailing in situ of slipped upper femoral epiphysis. A 30-year follow-up of 59 hips. J Bone Joint Surg Br. 80(1):70-7, 1998
8. Umans H et al: Slipped capital femoral epiphysis: a physeal lesion diagnosed by MRI, with radiographic and CT correlation. Skeletal Radiol. 27(3):139-44, 1998
9. Boles CA et al: Slipped capital femoral epiphysis. Radiographics. 17(4):809-23, 1997
10. Jerre R et al: Bilaterality in slipped capital femoral epiphysis: importance of a reliable radiographic method. J Pediatr Orthop B. 5(2):80-4, 1996
11. Lubicky JP: Chondrolysis and avascular necrosis: complications of slipped capital femoral epiphysis. J Pediatr Orthop B. 5(3):162-7, 1996
12. Warner WC Jr et al: Chondrolysis after slipped capital femoral epiphysis. J Pediatr Orthop B. 5(3):168-72, 1996
13. Maffulli N et al: Common skeletal injuries in young athletes. Sports Med. 19(2):137-49, 1995
14. Towbin R et al: Neonatal traumatic proximal femoral epiphysiolysis. Pediatrics. 63(3):456-9, 1979

SLIPPED CAPITAL FEMORAL EPIPHYSIS

IMAGE GALLERY

Typical

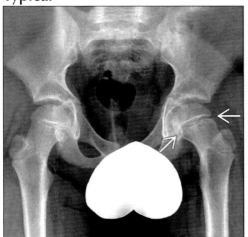
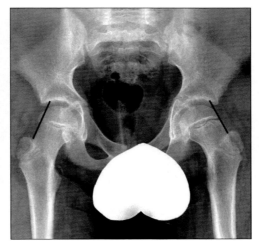

(Left) Anteroposterior radiograph shows widening (arrows) of the capital femoral physis on the left. *(Right)* Anteroposterior radiograph of same patient with Klein's lines superimposed upon superior borders of femoral necks shows that left capital epiphysis has slipped medially several millimeters in comparison to normal right side.

Typical

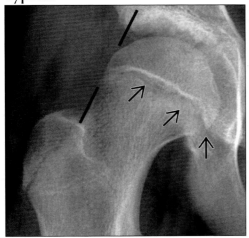
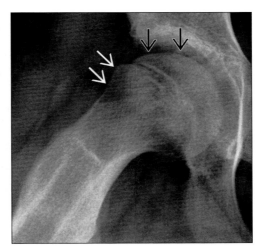

(Left) Anteroposterior radiograph shows medial displacement of capital epiphysis relative to Klein's line (deliberately interrupted) and widening of the medial 3/4ths of the physis (arrows). *(Right)* Frog-lateral radiograph shows mild SCFE with slight posterior displacement of the capital ossification center (black arrows) relative to the metaphysis (white arrows) in the same patient.

Typical

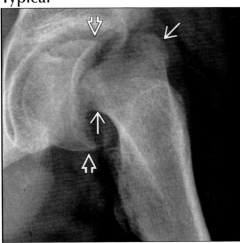
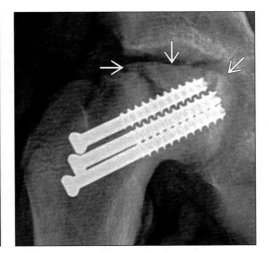

(Left) Frog-lateral radiograph shows moderate SCFE with capital ossification center (open arrows) rotated posteriorly more than 1/3 the width of metaphysis (arrows). *(Right)* Anteroposterior radiograph shows flattening and sclerosis of the femoral head (arrows) due to avascular necrosis following insertion of screws.

ACHONDROPLASIA

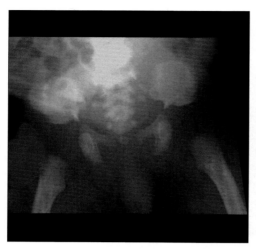

Anteroposterior radiograph shows squared ilia, whose height is decreased, and horizontal acetabular roofs in a newborn. The shape of the upper femurs resembles an ice cream scoop.

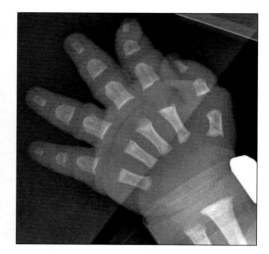

Anteroposterior radiograph shows a "trident hand" variant in a newborn. The fingers are of approximately equal length and diverge from one another in two pairs and the thumb.

TERMINOLOGY

Definitions
- Achondroplasia is a short-stature skeletal dysplasia caused by mutation of fibroblast growth factor receptor-3 gene
- Achondroplasia group of dysplasias has many common features including 4p 16.3 gene map locus
  - Thanatophoric dysplasia
    - Commonest lethal bone dysplasia: Lungs cannot ventilate due to short ribs; micromelia
  - Achondroplasia
    - Commonest nonlethal bone dysplasia: Large cranium; small face and chest; short limbs
  - Hypochondroplasia
    - Usually not recognized until children > 2 years old
    - Severe forms overlap with achondroplasia
    - Narrow interpediculate distance in lumbar spine
    - Fibular overgrowth
- Rhizomelic (root-limb) shortening
  - Femur and humerus are relatively shorter than distal bones
  - Seen with achondroplasia and thanatophoric dysplasia
- Mesomelic (mid-limb) shortening: Rare
  - Radius-ulna and tibia-fibula are relatively shortest
  - Seen in fetal face syndrome and variants of mesomelic dysplasia
- Acromelic (end-limb) shortening
  - Hand and foot bones are relatively shortest
  - Seen in asphyxiating thoracic dystrophy and chondroectodermal dysplasia
- Micromelic (small-limb) shortening: Severe shortening, rare
  - Seen in micromelic dwarfism and Thalidomide syndrome

IMAGING FINDINGS

Radiographic Findings
- Radiography
  - Skull, face and brain
    - Calvaria enlarged with frontal bossing, megalencephaly
    - Skull base small with narrow foramen magnum
    - Petrous pyramids closer to midline than normal
    - Basal angle low: 85°-120°; steep clivus
    - Basilar impression
    - Narrow jugular foramina may cause hydrocephalus via venous hypertension
    - Short petrous carotid canals
    - Mastoids underpneumatized
    - Mid-face hypoplasia, dental crowding
    - Choanal atresia: Occasional
  - Spine

DDx: Dwarfism With Slow Growth Of Enchondral Bone

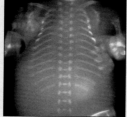

Hmzgs Achndrplsia

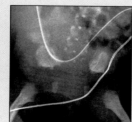

Thanatophoric Dyspl

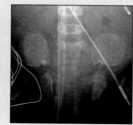

Ellis Van Creveld

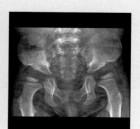

Morquio Disease

ACHONDROPLASIA

Key Facts

Terminology
- Achondroplasia is a short-stature skeletal dysplasia caused by mutation of fibroblast growth factor receptor-3 gene
- Usually not recognized until children > 2 years old
- Rhizomelic (root-limb) shortening

Imaging Findings
- Calvaria enlarged with frontal bossing, megalencephaly
- Skull base small with narrow foramen magnum
- Narrow jugular foramina may cause hydrocephalus via venous hypertension
- Interpediculate distances get progressively smaller lower in lumbar spine (this is opposite of normal)
- Thoraco-lumbar gibbus or kyphosis in infancy
- Increased lumbar lordosis after infancy
- Short wide iliac bones with horizontal acetabular roofs and rounded iliac crests at top (tombstone or elephant-ear appearance)
- Trident hand: 3 forks; thumb, digits 2 & 3, digits 4 & 5
- Lower femoral epiphysis cone or chevron shaped
- Bowlegs: Genu varum
- Fibula longer than tibia

Pathology
- 80% of cases are new mutations
- Vertebral bodies and skull base: Impaired endochondral growth results in stenosis of foramen magnum and spinal canal
- Heterozygous achondroplasia: Incidence is 1:10,000-30,000 live births
- Cervicomedullary decompression surgery in 17%

- Spinal canal stenosis seen as short pedicles on lateral view and decreased interpediculate distances on AP view
- Interpediculate distances get progressively smaller lower in lumbar spine (this is opposite of normal)
- Vertebral bodies: Short, flat, bullet-shaped in early life; concave posterior surface (scalloping); decreased height of vertebral bodies makes disk spaces look relatively large
- Transverse processes short
- Thoraco-lumbar gibbus or kyphosis in infancy
- Increased lumbar lordosis after infancy
- Cervical instability
- Chest
  - Short ribs and sternum
  - Cup-shaped anterior rib ends
  - Clavicles: Musk ox horn shape, relatively long
- Pelvis
  - Short wide iliac bones with horizontal acetabular roofs and rounded iliac crests at top (tombstone or elephant-ear appearance)
  - Champagne glass shaped inner margin
  - Sacrosciatic notch small
- Upper extremity
  - Rhizomelic shortening: Humerus barely longer than ulna
  - Outward lateral bulging of humerus at deltoid insertion
  - Concave medial distal radial metaphysis
  - Hand: Retarded bone age
  - Metacarpals and phalanges short, stubby
  - Trident hand: 3 forks; thumb, digits 2 & 3, digits 4 & 5
  - Appears trident-like because there is gap between digits 3 & 4
- Lower extremity
  - Rhizomelic shortening: Femur barely longer than tibia
  - Femoral necks short
  - Hemispheric femoral head
  - Ice cream scoop shape of the upper femurs in infants
- Flared (widened) metaphyses capped by large epiphyses
- Diaphyseal widths normal but seem wide because bones short
- Lower femoral epiphysis cone or chevron shaped
- Bowlegs: Genu varum
- Upper tibial metaphysis concave
- Delayed ossification of tibial epiphysis
- Fibula longer than tibia
- Ankle valgus due to bowlegs with medial talar tilt
- Posteroinferior calcaneal pseudospurs before ossification of the calcaneal apophysis

Ultrasonographic Findings
- Grayscale Ultrasound: Prenatal studies are normal on early scans, with long-bone shortening seen after 22 weeks gestation

Other Modality Findings
- MR: Herniated nucleus pulposus
- CT: Ventricular enlargement frequent

DIFFERENTIAL DIAGNOSIS

Hypochondroplasia
- Mild form of short-limbed dwarfism
- Often not clinically apparent until 2 years old
- Macrocephaly and frontal bossing
- Hands and feet broad and stubby
- Midface hypoplasia
- Foramen magnum small
- Lumbar spine: Decreased interpediculate distance
- Vertebral bodies: Platyspondyly and posterior scalloping

Pseudo-Achondroplasia
- Normal face

Metatropic dysplasia
- Dumbell femurs, caudal appendage (tail)

ACHONDROPLASIA

Other conditions with enchondral slowing
- For example: Homozygous achondroplasia (Hmzgs Achndrplsia), thanatophoric dysplasia, Ellis van Creveld syndrome, Morquio disease

PATHOLOGY

General Features
- Genetics
  - Defect on chromosome 4p
    - Fibroblast growth factor receptor-3 gene (FGFR3) mutation
    - Prenatal diagnosis by amniocentesis or chorionic villus sampling
  - Autosomal dominant
  - Heterozygous: Common
  - Homozygous: Rare, lethal
  - 80% of cases are new mutations
- Etiology
  - Decreased rate of endochondral ossification
    - Vertebral bodies and skull base: Impaired endochondral growth results in stenosis of foramen magnum and spinal canal
  - Associated with advanced paternal age
- Epidemiology
  - Heterozygous achondroplasia: Incidence is 1:10,000-30,000 live births
  - Otitis media in 90% during first 2 years
    - Ventilation tubes inserted in 80% sometime during life
    - Conductive hearing loss in 40%
  - Cervicomedullary decompression surgery in 17%
  - Tibial bowing in 42%
    - Tibial osteotomy in 22%

Microscopic Features
- Histology of epiphyseal and growth plate cartilage is normal

CLINICAL ISSUES

Presentation
- Most common signs/symptoms
  - Face is characteristic with midface hypoplasia, saddle nose and frontal bossing
  - Rhizomelic limb-shortening
  - Elbow extension is limited
  - Trident hand
  - Dorsilumbar gibbus or kyphosis
  - Lumbar lordosis exaggerated
    - Buttocks prominent and abdomen protuberant after walking begins
  - Delayed gross and fine motor milestones; hypotonia
- Cardiorespiratory and sleep dysfunction
  - Mild midface hypoplasia and relative adenotonsillar hypertrophy: Treat with tonsillectomy and adenoidectomy
  - Upper airway obstruction and jugular foramen stenosis: Treat with shunt and nocturnal continuous positive airway pressure
  - Upper airway obstruction associated with hypoglossal canal stenosis: Treat with multiple schemes including foramen magnum decompression

Demographics
- Age: Obesity common and disabling in older children

Natural History & Prognosis
- Normal lifespan and intelligence
- Increased incidence of orthopedic and neurologic complications
  - Cervical instability in infancy
  - Basilar impression, Chiari 1, syringomyelia
  - 7% risk of sudden death due to cervicomedullary compression: Suspect with central hypopnea, small foramen magnum, and leg hyperreflexia
  - Spinal stenosis
  - Leg bowing

Treatment
- Treatment available for most of complications
  - Urgent to treat cranio-cervical junction stenosis to prevent sudden death

SELECTED REFERENCES

1. Haga N: Management of disabilities associated with achondroplasia. J Orthop Sci. 9(1):103-7, 2004
2. Oestreich AE: The acrophysis: a unifying concept for understanding enchondral bone growth and its disorders. II. Abnormal growth. Skeletal Radiol. 33(3):119-28, 2004
3. Hill V et al: Experiences at the time of diagnosis of parents who have a child with a bone dysplasia resulting in short stature. Am J Med Genet. 122A(2):100-7, 2003
4. Cheema JI et al: Radiographic characteristics of lower-extremity bowing in children. Radiographics. 23(4):871-80, 2003
5. Cohen MM Jr: Some chondrodysplasias with short limbs: molecular perspectives. Am J Med Genet. 112(3):304-13, 2002
6. Stanley G et al: Observations on the cause of bowlegs in achondroplasia. J Pediatr Orthop. 22(1):112-6, 2002
7. Thomeer RT et al: Surgical treatment of lumbar stenosis in achondroplasia. J Neurosurg Spine. 96(3):292-7, 2002
8. Prinster C et al: Diagnosis of hypochondroplasia: the role of radiological interpretation. Pediatr Radiol. 31(3):203-8, 2001
9. Keiper GL Jr et al: Achondroplasia and cervicomedullary compression: prospective evaluation and surgical treatment. Pediatr Neurosurg. 31(2):78-83, 1999
10. Lemyre E et al: Bone dysplasia series. Achondroplasia, hypochondroplasia and thanatophoric dysplasia: review and update. Can Assoc Radiol J. 50(3):185-97, 1999
11. Cohen MM Jr: Achondroplasia, hypochondroplasia and thanatophoric dysplasia: clinically related skeletal dysplasias that are also related at the molecular level. Int J Oral Maxillofac Surg. 27(6):451-5, 1998
12. Tasker RC et al: Distinct patterns of respiratory difficulty in young children with achondroplasia: a clinical, sleep, and lung function study. Arch Dis Child. 79(2):99-108, 1998
13. Levin TL et al: Lumbar gibbus in storage diseases and bone dysplasias. Pediatr Radiol. 27(4):289-94, 1997
14. Shohat M et al: Hearing loss and temporal bone structure in achondroplasia. Am J Med Genet. 45(5):548-51, 1993
15. Wong VC et al: Basilar impression in a child with hypochondroplasia. Pediatr Neurol. 7(1):62-4, 1991
16. Hammerschlag W et al: Cervical instability in an achondroplastic infant. J Pediatr Orthop. 8(4):481-4, 1988

ACHONDROPLASIA

IMAGE GALLERY

Typical

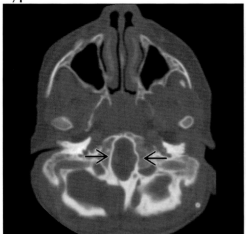
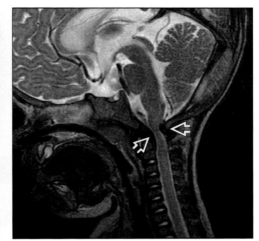

(Left) Axial NECT shows narrow foramen magnum *(arrows)*. *(Right)* Sagittal T2WI FS MR shows narrow foramen magnum and compression of medulla and upper cervical spine *(arrows)*. Middle and lower cervical spinal canal stenotic with little room for CSF. Clivus steep.

Typical

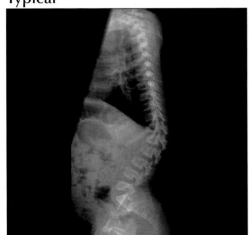
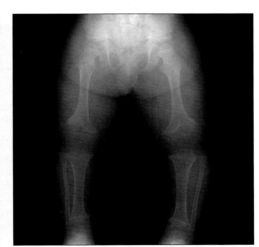

(Left) Lateral radiograph shows lower dorsal gibbus, exaggerated lumbar lordosis, and L2 beaking. *(Right)* Anteroposterior radiograph shows horizontal acetabular roofs, narrow sacro-sciatic notches, short femoral necks, metaphyseal flaring, cone- or chevron-shaped epiphyses, and long fibulae.

Typical

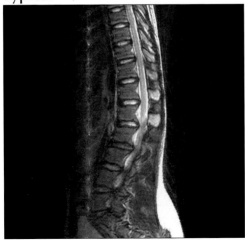
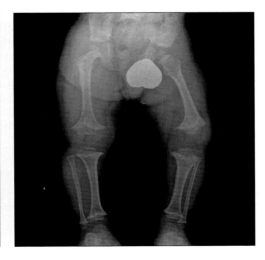

(Left) Sagittal T2WI MR shows stenosis of spinal canal and posterior scalloping of vertebral bodies. Lumbar lordosis is exaggerated. *(Right)* Anteroposterior radiograph shows genu varum, cone- or chevron-shaped distal femoral epiphyses, and long fibulae.

MUCOPOLYSACCHARIDOSES (MPS)

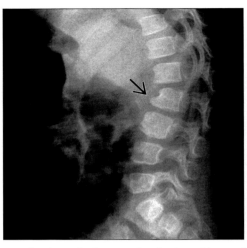

Lateral radiograph shows a dorsolumbar gibbus and vertebral beaking (arrow) of L2.

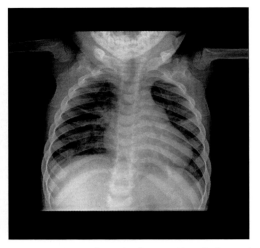

Anteroposterior radiograph shows widened ribs and humeral neck varus (hatched-shaped humerus). Scapulae are elevated.

TERMINOLOGY

Abbreviations and Synonyms
- Mucopolysaccharidoses (MPS), Gargoylism (politically incorrect)
- MPS 1-H: Hurler syndrome
- MPS 1-S: Scheie syndrome
- MPS 1-H/S: Hurler/Scheie syndrome
- MPS 2: Hunter syndrome
- MPS 3: Sanfilippo syndrome
- MPS 4: Morquio syndrome
- MPS 5: Nonexistent, now classified as MPS 1-S
- MPS 6: Maroteaux-Lamy syndrome
- MPS 7: Sly syndrome or β-glucuronidase deficiency
- MPS 8: Nonexistent
- MPS 9: Hyaluronidase deficiency

Definitions
- Mucopolysaccharidoses: Heterogenous group of lysosomal storage diseases caused by deficiency of enzymes that degrade glycosaminoglycans (formerly called mucopolysaccharides)
- Dysostosis Multiplex Group: Includes all storage diseases that result in a skeletal dysplasia
  - Mucopolysaccharidoses (MPS), mucolipidoses, others (Gaucher disease, Niemann-Pick disease, gangliosidosis, fucosidosis, mannosidosis, sialidosis)
  - Dysostosis Multiplex (DM): Constellation of bone-dysplasia features seen variably in MPS

IMAGING FINDINGS

General Features
- Best diagnostic clue: Dorsolumbar gibbus with vertebral beaking

Radiographic Findings
- Radiography
  - Key radiographic findings
    - Dorsolumbar gibbus with anteriorly beaked vertebral bodies
    - Wide ribs with oar-shape
    - Short and thick clavicles
    - Characteristic pelvic appearance: Ilia small and tapered, steep acetabular roof, coxa valga
    - Pointed proximal metacarpals

Other Modality Findings
- MPS 1-H, Hurler syndrome: Severe DM
  - Central nervous system: White-matter low attenuation, delayed myelination, T2 white matter hyperintensity, enlarged Virchow-Robin spaces and cysts, sulcal enlargement, ventriculomegaly, dural thickening → craniocervical junction spinal cord compression

DDx: Abnormal Metaphyses & Epiphyses

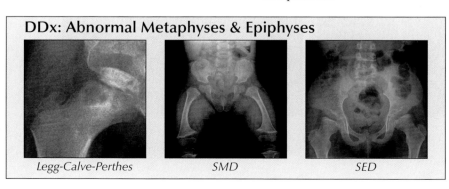

Legg-Calve-Perthes   SMD   SED

MUCOPOLYSACCHARIDOSES (MPS)

Key Facts

Imaging Findings
- Key radiographic findings
- Dorsolumbar gibbus with anteriorly beaked vertebral bodies
- Wide ribs with oar-shape
- Short and thick clavicles
- Characteristic pelvic appearance: Ilia small and tapered, steep acetabular roof, coxa valga
- Pointed proximal metacarpals
- Central nervous system: White-matter low attenuation, delayed myelination, T2 white matter hyperintensity, enlarged Virchow-Robin spaces and cysts, sulcal enlargement, ventriculomegaly, dural thickening → craniocervical junction spinal cord compression

Pathology
- All MPS have a known autosomal recessive (except MPS-2, which is X-linked recessive) genetic abnormality causing an enzymatic deficiency
- Intracellular accumulation of partially degraded glycosaminoglycans

Clinical Issues
- 45% parents of MPS-1 children: First clue was change in child's appearance
- Brain: Regression of speech and learning skills → mental retardation (not in MPS 4 & 6), behavior problems, hyperactivity
- Prevention of CNS damage: Perinatal screening → earliest possible treatment
- Bone marrow transplantation (BMT)

- o Skull and face: Macrocranium, dolichocephaly or early closure sagittal and lambdoid sutures, thickened skull base, enlarged J-shaped sella, mandibular condyles flat or concave, temporomandibular joint ankylosis, underpneumatized mastoids, dentigerous cysts, macroglossia, calcified stylohyoid ligament
- o Spine: Hypoplastic dens with C1/2 subluxation, C3/4 subluxation, dorsolumbar gibbus, beaked vertebral bodies
- o Chest and shoulders: Trachea narrow, ribs wide and oar-shaped, clavicles short and thick, scapulae elevated with dysmorphic glenoid fossae
- o Arms: Humeral neck varus (hatchet-shaped humerus), wide humeral midshaft, distal radius and ulnar physes tilt toward each other, carpals small and irregular, wide metacarpals and proximal and middle phalanges, pointed proximal ends of metacarpals 2-5
- o Pelvis and hips: Ilia small and taper inferiorly, acetabular roofs steep, femoral head subluxation, coxa valga
- o Cardiovascular: Cardiomyopathy, aorta and other arteries narrow, mitral and aortic stenosis
- MPS 1-S, Scheie syndrome
  - o Mild DM
- MPS 1-H/S, Hurler-Scheie syndrome
  - o Mild-to-moderate DM
- MPS 2, Hunter syndrome
  - o Mild-to-severe DM
- MPS 3A-D, Sanfilippo syndrome
  - o Mild or absent DM
  - o Attenuated (mild) form: Mental retardation without DM
- MPS 4A-B, Morquio syndrome
  - o Type A: Severe DM
    - Odontoid small or absent
    - Trachea: Narrow, soft, may collapse during neck flexion
    - Pectus carinatum
    - Femoral head: Aseptic necrosis
  - o Type B: Moderate DM
- MPS 6, Maroteaux-Lamy syndrome
  - o Mild-to-severe DM
- MPS 7, Sly syndrome
  - o Mild-to-severe DM
    - Femoral head: Aseptic necrosis
- MPS 9, hyaluronidase deficiency
  - o Mild DM: Only 1 case known

Imaging Recommendations
- Best imaging tool: Skeletal radiographs, brain MR

DIFFERENTIAL DIAGNOSIS

Legg-Calve-Perthes disease
- Ideopathic avascular necrosis (AVN) of femoral head
- No clinical or lab features of MPS; no imaging signs of DM

Spondyloepiphyseal dysplasia (SED)
- No clinical or lab features of MPS
- Findings are within spine and epiphysis

Multiple epiphyseal dysplasia
- No clinical or lab features of MPS
- Findings are within epiphysis

Spondylometaphyseal dysplasia (SMD)
- No clinical or lab features of MPS
- Findings are within spine and metaphysis

PATHOLOGY

General Features
- Genetics
  - o All MPS have a known autosomal recessive (except MPS-2, which is X-linked recessive) genetic abnormality causing an enzymatic deficiency
    - A few females with MPS-2: Autosomal X-chromosomal translocation and non-random X-chromosome inactivation
    - Subsequent pregnancy: 25% risk of MPS
  - o MPS 1H/S: 74 MPS mutations reported to date

MUCOPOLYSACCHARIDOSES (MPS)

- Epidemiology
  - Combined prevalence of all MPS types in Australia is 1:22,500
  - 1:100,000 live births: MPS-1H, MPS-4A
  - 0.6:100,000 live births: MPS-2
  - 1:200,000 live births: MPS-3
  - 1:500,000 live births: MPS-1H/S
  - Extremely rare: MPS-7

Microscopic Features
- Intracellular accumulation of partially degraded glycosaminoglycans

CLINICAL ISSUES

Presentation
- Most common signs/symptoms
  - 45% parents of MPS-1 children: First clue was change in child's appearance
  - Brain: Regression of speech and learning skills → mental retardation (not in MPS 4 & 6), behavior problems, hyperactivity
  - Head and face: Large head, coarse hair with hirsutism, coarse facial features, proptosis, corneal opacification and glaucoma, photophobia, rhinitis, recurrent otitis media, progressive hearing loss, flared nostrils, protruding tongue
  - Neck: Adenotonsillar enlargement, snoring, sleep apnea, tracheobronchomalacia
  - Spine and chest: Thoracolumbar gibbus, spondylolisthesis in adults with MPS-3, pectus carinatum
  - Respiratory: Frequent pneumonia
  - Cardiovascular: Valvular thickening, stenosis, insufficiency; cardiomyopathy, congestive heart failure
  - Abdomen: Protuberant due to hepatosplenomegaly, umbilical/inguinal hernia, intestinal pseudo-obstruction, idiopathic diarrhea
  - General: Short stature (except MPS-1S), flexion contractures (claw hand), thick skin, carpal tunnel syndrome
  - Hydrops fetalis, intrauterine growth acceleration with advanced bone age: MPS-7
  - General anesthesia: Risk increased due to difficult intubation due to redundant supraglottic tissue, smaller airway, and unstable C1/C2 joints in MPS 1, 2, 4, 6, 7

Demographics
- Age
  - Clinical onset before 1 year: MPS-7
  - Clinical onset 1-2 years: MPS-1H, MPS-1H/S
  - Clinical onset 1-3 years: MPS-4A
  - Clinical onset 2-4 years: MPS-2, MPS-6
  - Clinical onset 2-6 years: MPS-3
  - Radiographic onset: May be at birth

Natural History & Prognosis
- Life span without treatment: MPS-1 < 10 years, MPS-2 ≈ 15 years
- Normal life span: MPS-1S

Treatment
- Prevention of CNS damage: Perinatal screening → earliest possible treatment
  - Lysosomal enzyme assay
    - Prenatal: Cells cultured from amniotic fluid or chorionic villus biopsy
    - Postnatal: assay of serum, leukocytes, cultured fibroblasts
- Bone marrow transplantation (BMT)
  - Early BMT beneficial: MPS-1H (but does not arrest bone dysplasia), MPS-6
    - Best done when < 2 years old and no CNS disease
  - BMT not beneficial: MPS-2, MPS-3
    - Fails to arrest encephalopathy
- Enzyme replacement therapy: MPS-1, perhaps MPS-2 and MPS-6
  - Shortcoming: Enzymes introduced intravenously do not cross blood-brain barrier
- Surgery
  - Hydrocephalus: ventriculoperitoneal shunt
  - Corneal opacity: Corneal transplant
  - Spine: C1/C2 stabilization, craniocervical junction decompression, fusion of progressive kyphosis
  - Airway obstruction or eustachian tube obstruction: tonsillectomy and adenoidectomy
  - Valvular heart disease: Valve replacement
  - Carpal tunnel decompression
  - Hernia repair

SELECTED REFERENCES
1. Muenzer J et al: Advances in the treatment of mucopolysaccharidosis type I. N Engl J Med. 350(19):1932-4, 2004
2. Muenzer J: The mucopolysaccharidoses: a heterogeneous group of disorders with variable pediatric presentations. J Pediatr. 144(5 Suppl):S27-34, 2004
3. Kachur E et al: Mucopolysaccharidoses and spinal cord compression: case report and review of the literature with implications of bone marrow transplantation. Neurosurgery. 47(1):223-8; discussion 228-9, 2000
4. Currarino G et al: Congenital glenoid dysplasia. Pediatr Radiol. 28(1):30-7, 1998
5. Tokieda K et al: Intrauterine growth acceleration in the case of a severe form of mucopolysaccharidosis type VII. J Perinat Med. 26(3):235-9, 1998
6. Taybi H et al: Radiology of Syndromes, Metabolic Disorders, and Skeletal Dysplasias. 4th Ed. Mosby, St. Louis, 1996
7. Wraith JE: The mucopolysaccharidoses: a clinical review and guide to management. Arch Dis Child. 72(3):263-7, 1995
8. Eggli KD et al: The mucopolysaccharidoses and related conditions. Semin Roentgenol. 21(4):275-94, 1986

MUCOPOLYSACCHARIDOSES (MPS)

IMAGE GALLERY

Typical

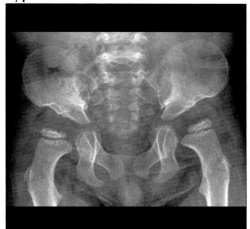 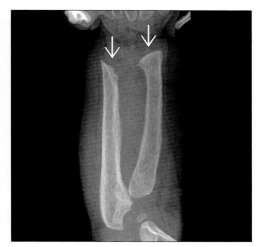

(Left) Anteroposterior radiograph shows characteristic pelvis: Small ilia which taper inferiorly, steep acetabuli, and coxa valga. *(Right)* Anteroposterior radiograph shows that distal radial and ulnar physes tilt toward each other (arrows).

Typical

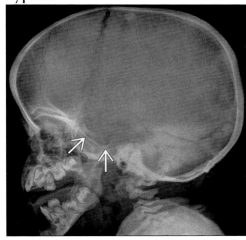 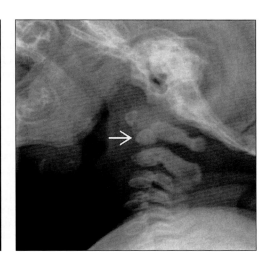

(Left) Lateral radiograph shows macrocranium, dolichocephaly, unaerated mastoids, and a large, J-shaped sella turcica (arrows). *(Right)* Lateral radiograph shows hypoplastic odontoid process (arrow).

Typical

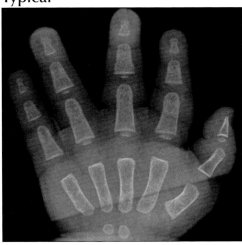 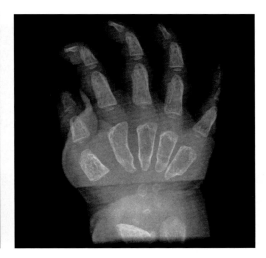

(Left) Anteroposterior radiograph shows a trident hand. The three prongs of trident are digits 5 & 4, digits 3 & 2, and the thumb. Fixed separation of digits 3 & 4 causes the trident. *(Right)* Anteroposterior radiograph shows claw hand with small, irregular carpals; widened metacarpals, proximal phalanges, and middle phalanges. Note the pointed proximal ends of metacarpals 2-5.

OSTEOGENESIS IMPERFECTA (OI)

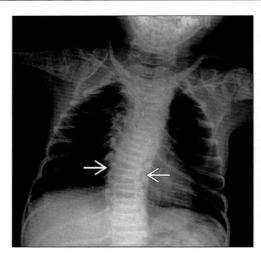

Anteroposterior radiograph in 11 year old child shows osteopenia, gracile distorted ribs, bowed clavicles, overtubulated humeri, scoliosis, and platyspondyly (arrows).

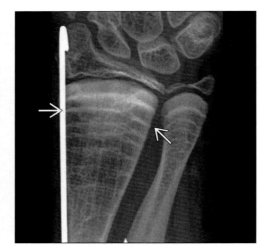

Anteroposterior radiograph shows multiple thin sclerotic metaphyseal bands (arrows) parallel to the physis marking cycles of biphosphonate therapy in an 11 year old.

TERMINOLOGY

Abbreviations and Synonyms
- Osteogenesis imperfecta (OI), van der Hoeve - de Kleyn syndrome, fragilitas osseum

Definitions
- OI is a disorder in which bone mass and strength are decreased, and other connective tissue abnormalities occur
- Sillence classification scheme modified by Rauch and Glorieux below based on clinical assessment is widely used, but shortcoming is that various types overlap and prognosis so variable
- OI type 1: Mild, not deforming
  - Sclerae: Blue in most
  - Fractures: Spectrum of none (in 10%) → numerous; less common after puberty
  - Stature: Usually normal; mild scoliosis and kyphosis in 20% of adults
  - Dentinogenesis imperfecta: May be present
- OI type 2: Perinatal lethal
  - Sclerae: Blue
  - Myriad of prenatal fractures
  - Death due to intra-cranial hemorrhage, pulmonary hypoplasia and multiple rib fractures → respiratory failure
    - Some may survive few weeks
- OI type 3: Deformation severe
  - Triangular face due to relative macrocranium and under-developed facial bones
  - Sclerae: Grey
  - Kyphoscoliosis, chest deformity, bowed bones, short stature
  - Stature: Short
  - Usually wheelchair-bound
- OI type 4: Deformation moderate
  - Sclerae: White
  - Bowing of long bones, vertebral fractures
  - Dentinogenesis imperfecta: In some but not all
  - Stature: Short
  - Walk with braces or crutches
- OI type 5: Deformation moderate
  - Sclerae: White
  - Stature: Short
  - Dentinogenesis imperfecta: Absent
  - Calcified radio-ulnar interosseous membrane → radial head dislocation
  - Hyperplastic callus formation
- OI type 6: Deformation moderate to severe
  - Sclerae: White
  - Stature: Moderately short
  - Defined on basis of bone histology: ↑ osteoid in bone and "fish-scale" pattern of lamellation in compact bone
- OI type 7: Deformation moderate

DDx: Diseases Causing Bowed Bones

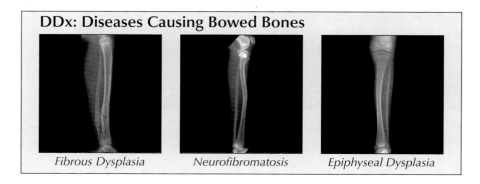

Fibrous Dysplasia | Neurofibromatosis | Epiphyseal Dysplasia

OSTEOGENESIS IMPERFECTA (OI)

Key Facts

Imaging Findings
- Best diagnostic clue: Fractures in thin, over-tubulated bones
- After bisphosphonate therapy: Multiple thin sclerotic metaphyseal bands paralleling growth plates and corresponding to number of treatments
- MR: Useful in evaluation of basilar impression

Pathology
- Negative collagen type 1 study doesn't exclude OI
- OI type 1: Incidence 1:30,000 live births
- OI type 2: Recurrence risk in subsequent siblings is 2-6%; due to mosaicism in one parent
- OI type 3: Incidence 1:70,000

Clinical Issues
- Hearing loss is usually not significant in childhood, but subtle audiometric abnormalities are present in many children and adolescents
- Type 3: Premature death associated with cardiorespiratory complications and pulmonary hypertension due to kyphoscoliosis in 2/3rds patients
- Biphosphonate: ↑ Bone cortical mass, ↓ chronic bone pain, ↑ sense of well-being

Diagnostic Checklist
- Radiographic features of OI are distributed differently in various types

---

- Stature: Mild shortening
- Sclerae: White
- Dentinogenesis imperfecta: Absent
- Humeri and femurs: Short, coxa vara

IMAGING FINDINGS

General Features
- Best diagnostic clue: Fractures in thin, over-tubulated bones
- Location
  - Skull
    - Macrocranium
    - Frontal bossing, wide fontanelles and sutures
    - Multiple wormian bones: 10 or more
    - Basilar impression or invagination
  - Spine
    - Kyphoscoliosis, biconcave or flattened vertebral bodies, compression fractures
    - Spondylolisthesis due to pedicle elongation
  - Chest
    - Thorax deformity → respiratory insufficiency, mitral valve prolapse, aortic dilatation, mitral and aortic insufficiency
    - Sternum-manubrium bowing (convex outward)
  - Pelvis and hips
    - Coxa vara, protrusio acetabuli
  - Long bones
    - Thin cortex, diaphyseal over-tubulation (thin, gracile), "popcorn" calcifications in metaphyses especially knee and ankle resolve in adolescence (common in type 3, also seen in types 1 and 4), bowing, hyperplastic callus formation plus radio-ulnar interosseous membrane calcification → radial head dislocation in type 5
    - Simultaneous bilateral tibial tubercle avulsion fractures, bilateral olecranon apophysis fractures
    - After bisphosphonate therapy: Multiple thin sclerotic metaphyseal bands paralleling growth plates and corresponding to number of treatments
  - Feet
    - Flatfoot and skewfoot (forefoot adduction, heel valgus, navicular abduction on talus)

Radiographic Findings
- Radiography
  - Multiple fractures
  - Multiple Wormian bones
  - Osteopenia
  - "Popcorn epiphyses" in type 3

CT Findings
- NECT
  - Useful for defining structural problems in axial skeleton
    - Basilar invagination
    - Temporal bone: Otic capsule abnormalities resembling otospongiosis; stapes crura fractures and footplate fixation
    - Pedicle elongation in spondylolisthesis

Other Modality Findings
- MR: Useful in evaluation of basilar impression

DIFFERENTIAL DIAGNOSIS

Diseases that cause bone-bowing
- Neurofibromatosis type 1, fibrous dysplasia, hyperparathyroidism, hyperphosphatasia, rickets, many bone dysplasias

Diseases with fragile bones
- Bruck syndrome
  - Fragile bones with congenital joint contractures
- Osteoporosis-pseudoglioma syndrome
  - Fragile bones with congenital blindness due to vitreous hyperplasia, cataracts, and glaucoma
- Cole-Carpenter syndrome
  - Fragile bones with cranial synostosis and ocular proptosis
- Idiopathic juvenile osteoporosis
  - No extraskeletal abnormalities

OSTEOGENESIS IMPERFECTA (OI)

Hyperplastic callus formation
- Osteomyelitis, myositis ossificans, stress fracture, osteochondroma, and osteosarcoma (extremely rare)

Child-abuse
- Broken bones accompanied by retinal hemorrhage, intracranial evidence of injury, and bruises
- No Wormian bones, osteopenia

PATHOLOGY

General Features
- Genetics
  - OI type 1: Premature stop codon in COL1A1
  - OI types 2-4: Glycine substitutions in COL1A1 or COL1A2
  - OI types 5-7: Unknown
  - Screening for OI biochemical abnormalities
    - Cultured skin fibroblasts: Assess amount and structure of type 1 procollagen molecules; a positive collagen type 1 study confirms diagnosis of OI
    - Leukocyte DNA: Coding region of the COL1A1 and COL1A2 genes is screened for mutations
    - Both of these approaches are thought to detect almost 90% of all collagen type 1 mutations
    - Negative collagen type 1 study doesn't exclude OI
    - Negative result leaves open possibility that either a collagen type 1 mutation is present but was not detected, or that child has a form of the disorder (OI types 5-7) that is not associated with collagen type 1 mutations
- Epidemiology
  - OI type 1: Incidence 1:30,000 live births
  - OI type 2: Recurrence risk in subsequent siblings is 2-6%; due to mosaicism in one parent
  - OI type 3: Incidence 1:70,000
  - OI type 7: Occurs within community of Native Americans in Northern Quebec, Canada

Microscopic Features
- Formation of lamellae in osteons
  - Lamellae are thin and irregular; have a mesh-like pattern in type 5 and a fish-scale pattern in type 6
- Thin bone cortex; marrow trabeculae thinned and fewer

CLINICAL ISSUES

Presentation
- Other signs/symptoms
  - Severity of OI (mild → severe)
    - Type 1 < 4 < 6 < 7 < 3 < 2
- Head
  - Internal carotid artery stenosis
  - Brainstem and cranial nerve compression due to basilar invagination
    - Basilar invagination present when odontoid tip ≥ 7 mm above McGregor line (hard palate to lowest point on the occipital squamosa)
    - Risk factor may be early sitting
- Hearing loss is usually not significant in childhood, but subtle audiometric abnormalities are present in many children and adolescents
- Face
  - Triangular face: Relative macrocranium and under-developed facial bones
  - Blue sclerae
    - Sign not valuable in infancy because may be a finding in healthy babies
  - Dentinogenesis imperfecta
    - Apt to be more clinically evident in primary teeth than in secondary
- Abdomen: ↑ Incidence hernias
- Ligaments and skin: Hyperlax ligaments and thin skin

Natural History & Prognosis
- Type 2: Fatal
- Type 3: Premature death associated with cardiorespiratory complications and pulmonary hypertension due to kyphoscoliosis in 2/3rds patients

Treatment
- Physical therapy, rehabilitation, orthopedic surgery, and obesity-prevention
- Biphosphonate: ↑ Bone cortical mass, ↓ chronic bone pain, ↑ sense of well-being

DIAGNOSTIC CHECKLIST

Image Interpretation Pearls
- Radiographic features of OI are distributed differently in various types
- It is not possible to classify OI by radiographic appearance alone
- Family history, clinical features, histological findings, collagen analysis, and genetic screening all contribute to classification

SELECTED REFERENCES

1. Plotkin H: Syndromes with congenital brittle bones. BMC Pediatr. 4(1):16, 2004
2. Rauch F et al: Osteogenesis imperfecta. Lancet. 363(9418):1377-85, 2004
3. Tamborlane JW et al: Osteogenesis imperfecta presenting as simultaneous bilateral tibial tubercle avulsion fractures in a child: a case report. J Pediatr Orthop. 24(6):620-2, 2004
4. Albayram S et al: Abnormalities in the cerebral arterial system in osteogenesis imperfecta. AJNR Am J Neuroradiol. 24(4):748-50, 2003
5. Grissom LE et al: Radiographic features of bisphosphonate therapy in pediatric patients. Pediatr Radiol. 33(4):226-9, 2003
6. Zeitlin L et al: Modern approach to children with osteogenesis imperfecta. J Pediatr Orthop B. 12(2):77-87, 2003
7. Basu PS et al: Spondylolisthesis in osteogenesis imperfecta due to pedicle elongation: report of two cases. Spine. 26(21):E506-9, 2001
8. Ablin DS: Osteogenesis imperfecta: a review. Can Assoc Radiol J. 49(2):110-23, 1998
9. Herman TE et al: Inherited diseases of bone density in children. Radiol Clin North Am. 29(1):149-64, 1991

OSTEOGENESIS IMPERFECTA (OI)

IMAGE GALLERY

Typical

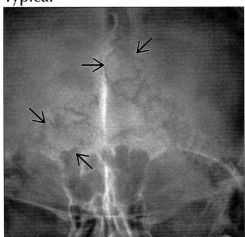 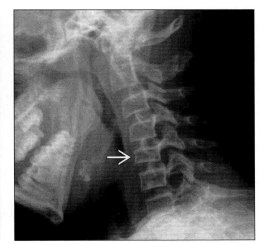

(Left) Postero-anterior radiograph shows multiple Wormian bones (arrows) in lambdoid suture. *(Right)* Lateral radiograph shows compression fracture (arrow) of C5 in a 13 year old. Sclerotic margins of vertebral bodies, a result of dense bone created during biphosphonate therapy.

Typical

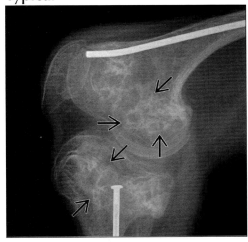 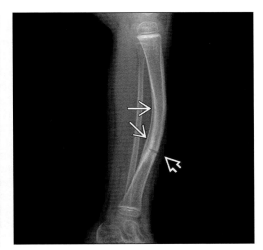

(Left) Lateral radiograph shows "popcorn" calcifications (arrows) in the distal femur and proximal tibia of a 16 year old. *(Right)* Lateral radiograph shows tibial bowing, periosteal reaction (arrows), and an insufficiency fracture (open arrow), which is a stress fracture of abnormal bone.

Typical

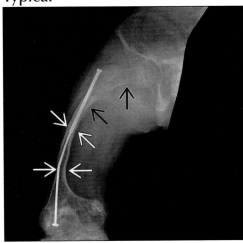 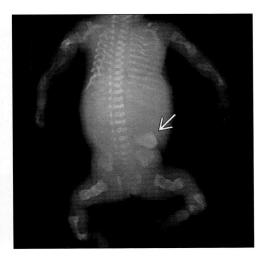

(Left) Anteroposterior radiograph shows coxa vara (black arrows) and overtubulation (white arrows) of the femoral diaphysis. *(Right)* Anteroposterior radiograph shows accordioned femurs, beaded ribs due to multiple fractures, angular bowing of tibias, and flat vertebrae in a 22 week fetus with OI type 2. Umbilical cord stump (arrow) above pelvis.

OSTEOPETROSIS

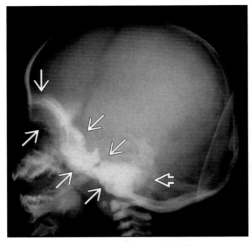

Lateral radiograph shows sclerosis of skull base (arrows) and mastoids (open arrow).

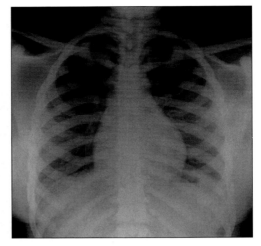

Posteroanterior radiograph shows dense and widened ribs, dense clavicles with diminished marrow space, and mild scoliosis.

TERMINOLOGY

Abbreviations and Synonyms
- Marble bone disease, Albers-Schonberg disease

Definitions
- Heterogenous group of genetic disorders characterized by increased bone density due to impaired bone resorption by osteoclasts
  - Osteopetrosis, autosomal dominant, type 1, online Mendelian Inheritance in Man (OMIM) 607634
    - Universal osteosclerosis, but sclerosis of cranial vault is marked while spine is almost unaffected
  - Osteopetrosis, autosomal dominant, type 2, OMIM 166600
    - Universal osteosclerosis, but sclerosis predominantly involves spine, pelvis, and skull base
  - Osteopetrosis, autosomal recessive, OMIM 259700; also called malignant infantile osteopetrosis
    - Macrocephaly, progressive deafness and blindness, hepatosplenomegaly, and severe anemia beginning in fetal life or early infancy
  - Osteopetrosis, mild autosomal recessive form, OMIM 259710
    - Mandibular prognathism, genu valgum, anemia, hepatosplenomegaly, and tendency for fractures and mandibular osteomyelitis

IMAGING FINDINGS

General Features
- Location
  - Skull, brain, and face
    - Macrocranium
    - Ventriculomegaly, tonsillar herniation, dural venous stenosis
    - Thick, dense skull base and/or calvaria
    - Neural: Narrowed neural foramina including foramen magnum
    - Vascular: Narrowed carotid canal, foramina transversarium, jugular foramen
    - Paranasal sinuses underdeveloped or absent, choanal stenosis, proptosis
    - Ocular hypertelorism
    - Mandible: Short body, wide ramus, frequent site of osteomyelitis
    - Teeth: Retention of deciduous teeth, increased incidence of caries and dental abscesses, ankylosis of cementum to bone
  - Axial skeleton and spinal cord
    - Cervical spine: Compression myopathy
    - Vertebrae: Bone-within-bone appearance, sclerotic borders of vertebral bodies resembling a picture frame, osteomyelitis
    - Spinal cord: Syringomyelia
    - Costochondral junctions: Widening

DDx: Bone Dysplasias

Achondroplasia | Epiphysis Dysplasia | Spondylodysplasia

OSTEOPETROSIS

Key Facts

Terminology
- Heterogenous group of genetic disorders characterized by increased bone density due to impaired bone resorption by osteoclasts

Imaging Findings
- Neural: Narrowed neural foramina including foramen magnum
- Paranasal sinuses underdeveloped or absent, choanal stenosis, proptosis
- Ocular hypertelorism
- Teeth: Retention of deciduous teeth, increased incidence of caries and dental abscesses, ankylosis of cementum to bone
- Vertebrae: Bone-within-bone appearance, sclerotic borders of vertebral bodies resembling a picture frame, osteomyelitis
- Pelvis: Bone-within-bone appearance
- Metaphyseal widening/flaring caused by defective tubular remodeling (Erlenmeyer-flask or club-like deformity)
- Fractures: Pathologic if due to mild trauma, and insufficiency-type if due to repetitive stress; usually heal well
- Paradoxical superimposed rickets secondary to low serum calcium from sequestration of calcium in bone

Clinical Issues
- Neurologic: Cranial nerve palsies involving optic, trigeminal, facial, acoustic, and other cranial nerves
- Death in severe forms due to bone-marrow failure → anemia, thrombocytopenia, and infection

---

- Ribs: Widening
- Pelvis: Bone-within-bone appearance
- Appendicular skeleton
  - Dense skeleton: May be generalized or with alternate radiolucent bands in metaphyses
  - Metaphyseal widening/flaring caused by defective tubular remodeling (Erlenmeyer-flask or club-like deformity)
  - Rickets
  - Coxa vara
  - Osteomyelitis
  - Bowing of long bones
  - Fractures: Pathologic if due to mild trauma, and insufficiency-type if due to repetitive stress; usually heal well
- Osteopetrorickets
  - Paradoxical superimposed rickets secondary to low serum calcium from sequestration of calcium in bone
  - Metaphyseal widening, cupping, and fraying of rickets superimposed over findings of osteopetrosis

CT Findings
- Vascular and neural foramen narrowing

MR Findings
- Absence of bone marrow
  - Extramedullary hematopoiesis
- Carpal tunnel compression
- Ventriculomegaly, tonsillar herniation, dural venous stenosis

Ultrasonographic Findings
- Prenatal: Macrocephaly, hydrocephalus, fractures

Angiographic Findings
- Carotid canal, foramen transversarium, jugular foramen stenosis

Nuclear Medicine Findings
- Increased uptake at bone ends

DIFFERENTIAL DIAGNOSIS

Anhidrotic ectodermal dysplasia, with immunodeficiency, osteopetrosis, and lymphedema OMIM 300301
- In infants born of mothers with mild incontinentia pigmenti

Biphonsphonate-induced osteopetrosis
- Metaphyses: Undertubulated, dense transverse bands
- Marginal sclerosis: Epiphyses and vertebral bodies
- Bone scan: ↑ Metaphyseal uptake

Chronic renal failure
- Vertebral bodies: Sclerosis of upper and lower thirds (rugger jersey)
- Other bones: Osteopenia with patchy osteosclerosis, cortical erosions (due to secondary hyperparathyroidism), metaphyseal sclerotic bands, rickets

Craniodiaphyseal dysplasia, OMIM 218300
- Severe osteopetrosis, wide long- and short-bone diaphyses with thick cortices

Craniometaphyseal dysplasia, autosomal dominant OMIM 123000
- Craniofacial sclerosis with narrowing of cranial-nerve foramina, mild early Erlenmeyer-flask flaring of metaphyses
- Spine not involved

Dysosteosclerosis OMIM 224300
- Osteosclerosis, platyspondyly, short stature, tendency to fracture

Osteopetrosis with renal tubular acidosis, OMIM 259730
- Carbonic anhydrase II deficiency
  - Osteopetrosis is severe
  - Brain calcifications (marble brain disease)

OSTEOPETROSIS

Osteopathia striata with cranial sclerosis OMIM 166500
- Craniofacial sclerosis with narrowing of cranial-nerve foramina
- Longitudinal striations of osteosclerosis in long bones

Osteosclerotic bone dysplasia, lethal, OMIM 259775
- Osteosclerosis, microcephaly, exophthalmos, hypoplastic nose and mid-face, and cleft palate.
- Fatal in fetus or newborn

Pycnodysostosis OMIM 265800
- Separated sutures and persistent anterior fontanelle, near-zero mandibular angle, phalangeal tuft resorption
- Short stature, nail hypoplasia

Pyle disease OMIM 265900
- Skull only mildly sclerotic: This distinguishes bone dysplasia from craniometaphyseal dysplasia in which cranial sclerosis is conspicuous
  - Erlenmeyer-flask flaring of metaphyses

Sclerosteosis OMIM 269500, also called cortical hyperostosis with syndactyly
- Similar to Van Buchem hyperostosis corticalis generalisata, but with a squared appearance of the mandible and cutaneous syndactyly

Van Buchem hyperostosis corticalis generalisata OMIM 239100
- Generalized osteosclerosis beginning at puberty occasionally leading to cranial nerve deficits

Van Buchem disease, type 2 OMIM 607636
- Autosomal dominant inheritance, in contrast to Van Buchem disease OMIM 239100

PATHOLOGY

General Features
- Genetics: Genetic abnormalities in 3 of 4 kinds of osteopetrosis have been mapped to specific loci; the locus for mild autosomal recessive form (OMIM 259710) has not been reported

Gross Pathologic & Surgical Features
- Narrowing and fibrosis of marrow cavities

Microscopic Features
- Diminished resorption of enchondral cartilage
- Increased numbers of osteoclasts

CLINICAL ISSUES

Presentation
- Other signs/symptoms
  - Infancy
    - Anemia or pancytopenia
    - Hepatomegaly (due to extramedullary hematopoiesis) and jaundice
    - Obstructive sleep apnea
    - Rickets
    - Early death
  - Childhood
    - Neurologic: Cranial nerve palsies involving optic, trigeminal, facial, acoustic, and other cranial nerves
    - Macrocephaly
    - Anemia
    - Renal tubular acidosis, rickets, hypophosphatemia, elevated acid phosphatase
    - Rickets
  - Adulthood
    - May be asymptomatic
    - Short stature
    - Bone pain
    - Osteomyelitis and dental abscess
    - Carpal tunnel syndrome
    - Periodontal disease
    - Tumors: Non-Hodgkin lymphoma, leukemia, bronchogenic carcinoma
  - Rickets: Results from the inability to maintain normal calcium-phosphorus balance in extracellular fluid
  - Enzymes: Serum creatine kinase brain isoenzyme and acid phosphatase elevated in osteopetrosis

Natural History & Prognosis
- Death in severe forms due to bone-marrow failure → anemia, thrombocytopenia, and infection

Treatment
- Bone marrow transplantation
  - Addresses both bone-marrow failure and underlying metabolic abnormality
  - Perform before foraminal narrowing → cranial neuropathy, if possible
- Gamma interferon, erythropoietin, vitamin D helpful in some

SELECTED REFERENCES
1. Online Mendelian Inheritance in Man. Johns Hopkins University. http://www.ncbi.nlm.nih.gov/entrez/query.fcgi?db=OMIM
2. Tolar J et al: Osteopetrosis. N Engl J Med. 351(27):2839-49, 2004
3. Kuhn JP et al: Caffey's Pediatric Diagnostic Imaging. 10th ed. Mosby, Philadelphia. 2253, 2167-2173, 2245-2248, 2003
4. Kulkarni ML et al: Rickets in osteopetrosis--a paradoxical association. Indian Pediatr. 40(6):561-5, 2003
5. Whyte MP et al: Bisphosphonate-induced osteopetrosis. N Engl J Med. 349(5):457-63, 2003
6. Steward CG: Neurological aspects of osteopetrosis. Neuropathol Appl Neurobiol. 29(2):87-97, 2003
7. Taybi, H et al: Radiology of Syndromes, Metabolic Disorders, and Skeletal Dysplasias. 4th ed. Mosby. 886-891, 1995
8. Herman TE et al: Inherited diseases of bone density in children. Radiol Clin North Am. 29(1):149-64, 1991

OSTEOPETROSIS

IMAGE GALLERY

Typical

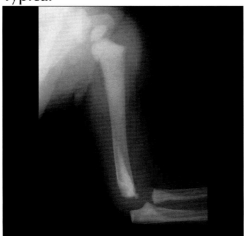
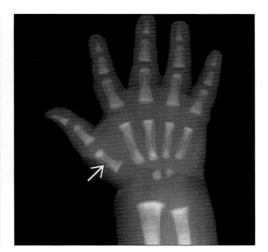

(Left) Lateral radiograph shows increased density of humerus, radius, and ulna. *(Right)* Posteroanterior radiograph shows increased density of all bones. Note bone-in-bone appearance in metacarpals (arrow) and phalanges.

Typical

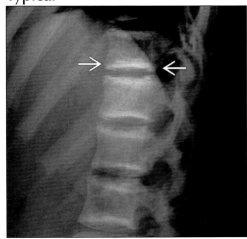
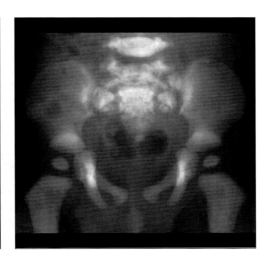

(Left) Lateral radiograph shows bands (arrows) of increased density next to end plates within vertebral bodies. *(Right)* Anteroposterior radiograph shows dense spine, pelvis, and femurs. Femoral marrow space almost entirely absent.

Typical

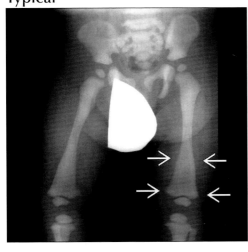
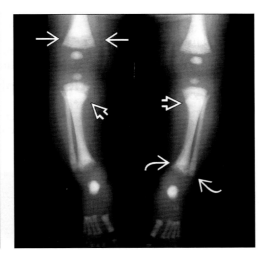

(Left) Anteroposterior radiograph shows undertubulation (arrows) of lower femoral metaphyses (Erlenmeyer flask deformity). *(Right)* Anteroposterior radiograph shows dense bones with metaphyseal banding (arrows), metaphyseal undertubulation (open arrows) and metaphyseal fraying due to rickets (curved arrows).

JUVENILE RHEUMATOID ARTHRITIS

- Sacroiliitis, enthesitis (uncommon in JRA)

Pigmented villonodular synovitis (PVNS)
- Monoarticular, hemosiderin deposition

Synovial chondromatosis or osteochondromatosis (SOC)
- Multiple intraarticular bodies +/- ossified, typically monoarticular & large joints
- Sometimes confused with loose or rice bodies

Hemophilic arthropathy
- Usually clinical or family history
- Repetitive hemorrhage into joints with hemosiderin deposition, radiodense joint effusion on radiographs
- Knee, elbow, ankle, may involve multiple joints

Infectious or septic arthritis
- Septic
  - Majority are monoarticular, commonly from adjacent osteomyelitis
  - Staphylococcus aureus most common
- Acute rheumatic fever, Lyme disease, viral, fungal, or reactive

Transient synovitis
- Self-limited, typical 3-6 year old, diagnosis of exclusion
- Normal radiographs cannot exclude

Leukemia
- Can present with arthritis symptoms (arthralgias & pain)

Post-traumatic
- Trauma history

PATHOLOGY

General Features
- Etiology
  - Unknown
  - Linked to infection: Influenza virus, parvovirus B19
  - Trauma, immunologic, stress, familial (case reports)
- Epidemiology: 10-15 cases/100,000
- Associated abnormalities: HLA associations

Microscopic Features
- Synovial villous hypertrophy & hyperplasia with inflammatory infiltration +/- rice bodies composed of fibrous tissue

CLINICAL ISSUES

Presentation
- Most common signs/symptoms
  - Fatigue
  - Morning stiffness
- Other signs/symptoms
  - Weight loss, growth failure
  - Systemic
    - Daily spiking fevers to 39° C ≥ 2 weeks duration (sometimes several times per day) with temperature returning to normal in between + an arthritis of ≥ 1 joint
    - Evanescent rash
    - Extra-articular disease: Lymphadenopathy, pericarditis, hepatosplenomegaly, muscle tenderness, leukocytosis

Demographics
- Age: Peak: 1-3 years (largest peak) & 8-10 years (smaller peak)
- Gender: M < F overall, systemic M = F
- Laboratory
  - Erythrocyte sedimentation rate (ESR)
    - To assess active disease, monitor therapy
    - Often normal in oligoarthritis
  - C-Reactive protein
    - More reliable
  - Antinuclear antibodies (ANA)
    - Highest in children with both oligoarthritis & uveitis
    - (+) In up to 1/4 of children with JRA, helpful in distinguishing from lupus (SLE)
  - RF
    - Rarely (+) in children < 7 years old & 85% are (-)
    - Not as useful as ANA
- Complications
  - Avascular necrosis (steroids), flexion contractures, uveitis, secondary osteoarthritis from cartilage destruction, osteoporotic insufficiency fractures, amyloidosis
  - Systemic: Macrophage activation syndrome, pericarditis

Natural History & Prognosis
- Predictors of physical disability
  - ↑ ESR, extensive & symmetric arthritis, (+) IgM RF, DRB1*08, DRB1*01, HLA-B27 in combination with DRB1*08, early onset & female

Treatment
- Nonsteroidal anti-inflammatory drugs (NSAIDs), methotrexate, tumor necrosis factor inhibitor, anticytokine therapy

SELECTED REFERENCES

1. Silverman E et al: Leflunomide or methotrexate for juvenile rheumatoid arthritis. N Engl J Med. 352(16):1655-66, 2005
2. McGhee JL et al: Clinical utility of antinuclear antibody tests in children. BMC Pediatr. 4(1):13, 2004
3. Prahalad S: Genetics of juvenile idiopathic arthritis: an update. Curr Opin Rheumatol. 16(5):588-94, 2004
4. Flato B et al: Prognostic factors in juvenile rheumatoid arthritis: a case-control study revealing early predictors and outcome after 14.9 years. J Rheumatol. 30(2):386-93, 2003
5. Ramanan AV et al: Macrophage activation syndrome following initiation of etanercept in a child with systemic onset juvenile rheumatoid arthritis. J Rheumatol. 30(2):401-3, 2003
6. Cassidy JT et al: A study of classification criteria for a diagnosis of juvenile rheumatoid arthritis. Arthritis Rheum. 29(2):274-81, 1986

JUVENILE RHEUMATOID ARTHRITIS

IMAGE GALLERY

Typical

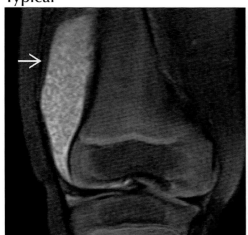
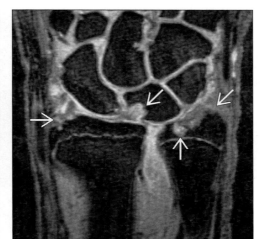

(Left) Coronal T2WI MR shows complex hyperintense knee joint effusion containing hypointense rice bodies (arrow). *(Right)* Coronal 3D GE image shows diffuse hyperintense erosions throughout the wrist (arrows).

Typical

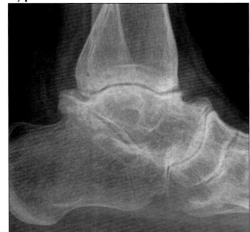
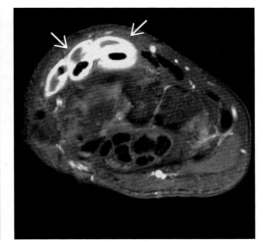

(Left) Lateral radiograph shows degenerative arthritis changes (from long-standing JRA); diffuse joint space narrowing, large spurs & flattening of the talar dome. *(Right)* Axial T1 C+ MR shows diffuse intense enhancement surrounding the extensor pollicis longus, extensor carpi radialis brevis & longus tendons, tenosynovitis (arrows).

Typical

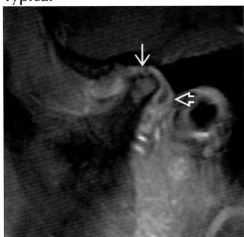
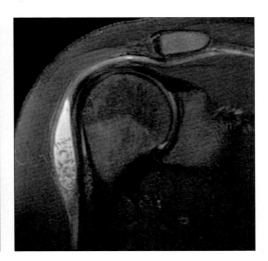

(Left) Sagittal T1WI MR shows moderate effusion with surrounding enhancement, synovitis (open arrow) of the right TMJ. Notice the irregular contour of the mandibular condyle, erosive disease (arrow). *(Right)* Coronal T2WI MR shows subdeltoid hyperintense bursa effusion containing hypointense rice bodies.

DERMATOMYOSITIS

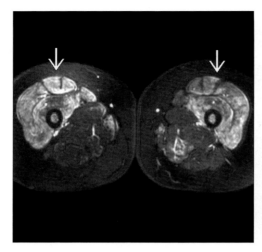

Axial T2WI MR shows typical changes of DM with hyperintense intramuscular signal with a predilection for the anterior compartment musculature (arrows).

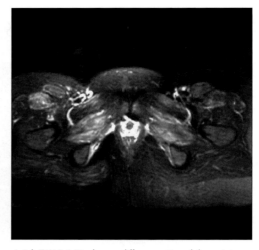

Axial T2WI MR shows diffuse scattered hyperintense signal changes within the pelvic musculature.

TERMINOLOGY

Abbreviations and Synonyms
- Dermatomyositis (DM), juvenile dermatomyositis, idiopathic inflammatory myopathy, dermatomyositis sine myositis, amyopathic DM

Definitions
- Idiopathic inflammatory myopathy with diffuse nonsuppurative inflammation of striated muscle and skin

IMAGING FINDINGS

General Features
- Best diagnostic clue: Hyperintense T2WI MR signal, bilateral symmetric anterior compartment thigh muscles and pelvis
- Location
  o Proximal musculature, thigh > pelvis > upper extremities
    ▪ Anterior compartment thigh: Vastus lateralis & vastus intermedius muscles most common
  o Can involve pharyngeal striated muscles leading to dysphagia
- Morphology
  o 5 major criteria for diagnosis of juvenile DM
    ▪ Symmetric proximal muscle weakness
    ▪ Characteristic changes on muscle biopsy
    ▪ ↑ Muscle enzymes in serum [creatine kinase (CK), aldolase, aspartate aminotransferase (AST), lactate dehydrogenase (LDH)]
    ▪ Electromyographic abnormality of myopathy & denervation
    ▪ Characteristic skin rash
  o Idiopathic myopathies
    ▪ Dermatomyositis = skin + muscle involvement
    ▪ Polymyositis; mostly muscle involvement
    ▪ Inclusion body myositis (most common in the older age, > 50 year olds), more refractory to treatment with immunosuppression
  o Amyopathic DM: Skin involvement without myopathy
    ▪ MR suggested to exclude subclinical muscle involvement
  o Anti-Jo-1 higher frequency in
    ▪ Interstitial lung disease
    ▪ Polyarthritis
    ▪ Raynaud phenomenon
    ▪ "Mechanic hand"
  o MR imaging
    ▪ Guide biopsy, monitor therapy, determine extent of disease
    ▪ Aid in clinical dilemma of differentiating steroid myopathy from persistent DM

DDx: Intramuscular Edema

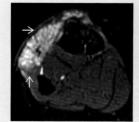

Denervation

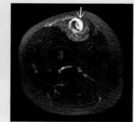

Muscle Injury

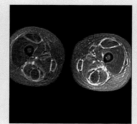

Eosinophilic Fasciitis

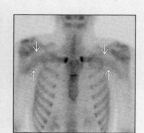

Rhabdomyolysis

DERMATOMYOSITIS

Key Facts

Terminology
- Idiopathic inflammatory myopathy with diffuse nonsuppurative inflammation of striated muscle and skin

Imaging Findings
- Best diagnostic clue: Hyperintense T2WI MR signal, bilateral symmetric anterior compartment thigh muscles and pelvis
- Proximal musculature, thigh > pelvis > upper extremities
- 5 major criteria for diagnosis of juvenile DM
- Symmetric proximal muscle weakness
- Characteristic changes on muscle biopsy
- ↑ Muscle enzymes in serum [creatine kinase (CK), aldolase, aspartate aminotransferase (AST), lactate dehydrogenase (LDH)]
- Electromyographic abnormality of myopathy & denervation
- Characteristic skin rash

Top Differential Diagnoses
- Eosinophilic fasciitis
- Infectious myositis
- Muscle injuries
- Subacute muscle denervation
- Radiation therapy

Pathology
- Epidemiology: 5/1,000,000

Clinical Issues
- Peak: 40-50s
- Children: 5-14 years old

Radiographic Findings
- Muscle, fascial or subcutaneous calcifications
- Muscular atrophy, osteoporosis

Fluoroscopic Findings
- Upper GI: Esophageal dysmotility

CT Findings
- Soft tissue calcifications (25-50%)
  - Develops 6 months to years after onset of disease, usually periarticular
  - Punctate to sheet-like
- High resolution NECT of Lung
  - Interstitial lung disease, ↓ lung volumes

MR Findings
- Hyperintense T2WI signal
  - Intramuscular (predominant), perimuscular, subcutaneous
- Anterior compartment of thighs & pelvis most common
- Fatty infiltration over months → years
- Abnormalities will enhance on post gadolinium images but not more sensitive than FS T2WI and usually not needed

Imaging Recommendations
- Best imaging tool: MRI: FS T2WI FSE or STIR

DIFFERENTIAL DIAGNOSIS

Eosinophilic fasciitis
- Hyperintense signal T2WI MR & enhancement within the fascia (predominant) & adjacent muscle, +/- fascial thickening on T1WI MR
- Peripheral eosinophilia, hypergammabulinemia, ↑ ESR & scleroderma-like skin changes

Infectious myositis
- Suppurative, +/- abscess (bacterial infection)
- (-) Abscess (viral)

Muscle injuries
- Contusion → hematoma or musculotendinous junction injuries
- Myositis ossificans
- History of trauma (usual), not symmetrical muscular distribution

Subacute muscle denervation
- MR findings can be delayed up to 4 weeks following denervation
- Can lead to fatty infiltration of the muscle if innervation is not restored

Radiation therapy
- History of radiation therapy
- Well-delineated, sharp margin of edema within radiation field

Polymyositis
- Imaging appearance & clinically overlaps DM
- Lacks characteristic skin rash
- Involves skeletal muscle only
- Less association with malignancy
- Older age group; questionable occurrence in children

Rhabdomyolysis
- Many etiologies: Traumatic verses atraumatic (including systemic diseases, drug reactions)
- Myoglobinuria

Other
- Compartment syndromes, necrotizing fasciitis, connective tissue diseases

PATHOLOGY

General Features
- Etiology
  - Idiopathic; HLA (DR3 & B8), coxsackievirus B, immune complex
  - Autoimmune disorder (possibly cell mediated)
  - Anti-nuclear antibodies

DERMATOMYOSITIS

- Antibodies to tRNA synthetases (most common; Anti-Jo-1)
- Anti-Mi-2: Specific but not sensitive (25% DM)
• Epidemiology: 5/1,000,000
• Associated abnormalities: Mixed connective tissue disease (overlap syndrome)

Microscopic Features
• Skeletal muscle: Inflammatory infiltrates with intrafiber edema, atrophy, necrosis with degeneration & regeneration of variable sized muscle fibers leading to fibrous proliferation with fatty infiltration

CLINICAL ISSUES

Presentation
• Most common signs/symptoms: Proximal muscle weakness +/- tenderness, easily fatigued
• Other signs/symptoms
  - Contracture with atrophy
  - Rash: (Heliotrope rash & Gottron papules are classic)
    - May precede (usual), occur during or after muscle weakness symptoms present
    - Heliotrope rash: Violaceous to dusky erythematous symmetrical periorbital rash
    - Gottron papules: Metacarpal-phalangeal, proximal interphalangeal, or distal interphalangeal joints; elevated violaceous papules on elbows, knees & feet
    - Periungual telangiectasis, scaly alopecia, ulcers
    - Photosensitive rash
    - Erythematous malar area rash & V of chest
  - Subcutaneous & periorbital edema
  - Arthralgias & arthritis
  - Fever, fatigue &/or weight loss
  - Raynaud phenomenon
  - Extra-articular manifestations
    - Pericarditis, pulmonary fibrosis
    - Dysphagia, GI symptoms & ulceration
  - Soft tissue calcifications (more commonly in children)
  - Pregnancy can worsen symptoms
  - Laboratory
    - ↑ Erythrocyte sedimentation rate (ESR)
    - ↑ CK (most sensitive & specific), LDH, AST, aldolase
    - Negative lupus band test

Demographics
• Age
  - Any age, bimodal distribution
    - Peak: 40-50s
    - Children: 5-14 years old
• Gender: M < F; 1:2
• Ethnicity: African-American > Caucasians

Natural History & Prognosis
• Poorer prognosis for juvenile DM
  - Late onset of therapy
  - Steroid dose too ↓ (initially)
  - Recalcitrant disease
  - Pharyngeal involvement
• Associated with malignancy (much more common in adults)
  - Older age at onset (> 45 years old)
  - Male
  - Ovarian, breast, pancreatic, gastric, colorectal, lung & lymphoma
• Mortality up to 10%

Treatment
• Complications
  - Calcinosis, contractures, avascular necrosis (AVN) (steroids)
• Corticosteroids
• Immunosuppression
  - Methotrexate
  - Azathioprine
• Intravenous immunoglobulins (IVIg)
• Antimalarials (hydroxychloroquine sulfate)
• Probenecid (for calcinosis)

DIAGNOSTIC CHECKLIST

Image Interpretation Pearls
• Hyperintense T2WI or STIR within the anterior thigh muscles +/- subcutaneous fat edema
• Include proximal & distal joints for AVN on follow-up studies

SELECTED REFERENCES
1. Moulton SJ et al: Eosinophilic fasciitis: spectrum of MRI findings. AJR Am J Roentgenol. 184(3):975-8, 2005
2. Antonioli CM et al: Dermatomyositis associated with lymphoproliferative disorder of NK cells and occult small cell lung carcinoma. Clin Rheumatol. 23(3):239-41, 2004
3. Danko K et al: Long-term survival of patients with idiopathic inflammatory myopathies according to clinical features: a longitudinal study of 162 cases. Medicine (Baltimore). 83(1):35-42, 2004
4. Ertekin C et al: Oropharyngeal dysphagia in polymyositis/dermatomyositis. Clin Neurol Neurosurg. 107(1):32-7, 2004
5. Fathi M et al: Interstitial lung disease, a common manifestation of newly diagnosed polymyositis and dermatomyositis. Ann Rheum Dis. 63(3):297-301, 2004
6. Amato AA et al: Treatment of idiopathic inflammatory myopathies. Curr Opin Neurol. 16(5):569-75, 2003
7. Mastaglia FL et al: Inflammatory myopathies: clinical, diagnostic and therapeutic aspects. Muscle Nerve. 27(4):407-25, 2003
8. Mendez EP et al: US incidence of juvenile dermatomyositis, 1995-1998: results from the National Institute of Arthritis and Musculoskeletal and Skin Diseases Registry. Arthritis Rheum. 49(3):300-5, 2003
9. Miller FW et al: Diagnostic criteria for polymyositis and dermatomyositis. Lancet. 362(9397):1762-3; author reply 1763, 2003
10. Oddis CV: Idiopathic inflammatory myopathies: a treatment update. Curr Rheumatol Rep. 5(6):431-6, 2003
11. May DA et al: Abnormal signal intensity in skeletal muscle at MR imaging: patterns, pearls, and pitfalls. Radiographics. 20 Spec No:S295-315, 2000
12. Bohan A et al: Polymyositis and dermatomyositis (second of two parts). N Engl J Med. 292(8):403-7, 1975
13. Bohan A et al: Polymyositis and dermatomyositis (first of two parts). N Engl J Med. 292(7):344-7, 1975

DERMATOMYOSITIS

IMAGE GALLERY

Typical

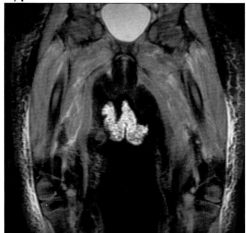
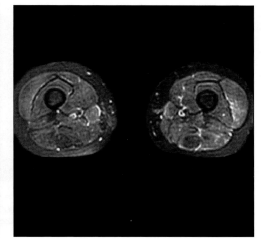

(Left) Coronal STIR MR shows diffuse hyperintense signal both in the subcutaneous soft tissue & all visible pelvic & thigh musculature. *(Right)* Axial T2WI MR shows abnormal hyperintense signal within all muscles of the bilateral anterior & posterior thigh compartments.

Variant

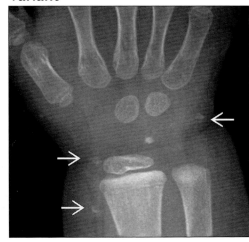
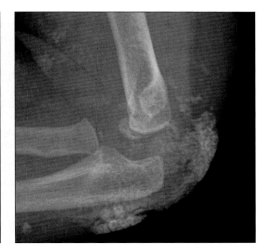

(Left) Anteroposterior radiograph shows multifocal punctate calcification in the wrist in this patient with DM. *(Right)* Lateral radiograph shows diffuse periarticular & subcutaneous calcifications around the elbow in this patient several years after initial presentation of DM.

Variant

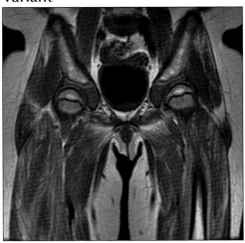
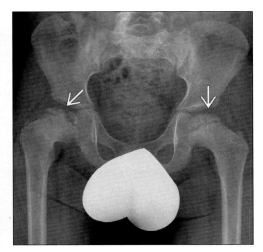

(Left) Coronal T1WI MR shows hyperintense signal within the pelvic & thigh musculature, consistent with fatty infiltration from long standing DM. *(Right)* Anteroposterior radiograph shows fragmentation of both femoral heads (arrows), AVN from long term steroid therapy treating DM.

CLUB FOOT (TALIPES EQUINOVARUS)

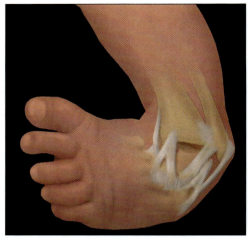

Anteroposterior graphic shows a club foot with equinus, inversion, and some forefoot adduction.

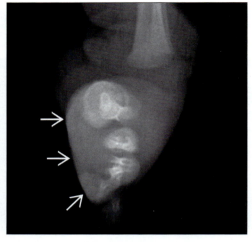

Anteroposterior oblique radiograph shows almost 90 degree inversion (arrows) of plantar aspect of foot relative to long axis of tibia in a 5 day old baby.

TERMINOLOGY

Abbreviations and Synonyms
- Talipes equinovarus
- Talipes
  - From Latin "talus," ankle and "pes," foot; has come to be the first word for club foot by common usage

Definitions
- Plantarflexion of calcaneus relative to tibia (equinus), inversion of hindfoot (varus), forefoot adduction (varus also)

IMAGING FINDINGS

Radiographic Findings
- Radiography
  - Angles measured on weightbearing images
  - Talocalcaneal angle normally 20-40° in anteroposterior (AP) view
    - Decreased in club foot: 10-0° typical (hindfoot varus)
  - Talocalcaneal angle normally 35-50° in lateral view
    - Decreased in club foot: 20 to -10° typical
  - Talo-first metatarsal angle normally 0-15° in AP view
    - Increased in club foot: 20-40° typical (forefoot varus)
  - Talus: Lateral rotation within ankle joint
  - Calcaneus: Medial rotation, equinus
  - Talo-navicular joint: Medial subluxation of navicular
  - Calcaneo-cuboid: Medial subluxation of cuboid

CT Findings
- NECT
  - Shaded surface reconstruction valuable in older child
    - Not useful in babies, whose foot bones are mostly cartilage

MR Findings
- Club feet may require multiplanar reconstruction to best show tibio-talar, talocalcaneal, talonavicular, and calcaneocuboid joints in their anatomic planes while simulating weightbearing
- T1WI: Joint spaces
- T2WI: Cartilage
- STIR: Joint spaces, distinguishing cartilage from adjacent soft tissue

Ultrasonographic Findings
- Grayscale Ultrasound
  - Prenatal
    - Most club feet recognized before birth
    - Club foot forms in first trimester
    - Fetus foot short, plantarflexed, and bent medially
  - Postnatal

DDx: Deformed Feet

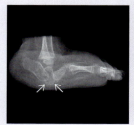

Vertical Talus

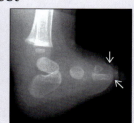

Amniotic Band

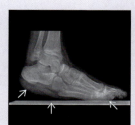

Rockerbottom

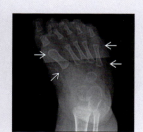

Metatarsus Adductus

CLUB FOOT (TALIPES EQUINOVARUS)

Key Facts

Terminology
- Plantarflexion of calcaneus relative to tibia (equinus), inversion of hindfoot (varus), forefoot adduction (varus also)

Imaging Findings
- Talus: Lateral rotation within ankle joint
- Calcaneus: Medial rotation, equinus
- Talo-navicular joint: Medial subluxation of navicular
- Calcaneo-cuboid: Medial subluxation of cuboid
- Anterior tibial artery hypoplastic or absent in 85% severe club feet; just 2 reports of absent posterior tibial artery
- Protocol advice: Radiographs taken in most "anatomical" or corrected position possible; forced dorsiflexion of foot partially overcomes equinus

Pathology
- Family history of club foot in 24%
- Monozygotic twins: 33% risk of both affected
- Dizygotic twins: 3% risk of both affected

Clinical Issues
- Gender: M:F = 2.5:1
- Ethnicity: 0.4-0.5:1000 in Chinese, 0.9-1.2:1000 in Caucasians, 6-7:1000 in Polynesians
- Mild lower leg asymmetry with age with unilateral club foot after treatment: Foot shortened average of 1.6 cm, calf circumference 2.5 cm less, leg length 0.6 cm less at end of childhood

---

- Search for occult spinal dysraphism
- Assess position of calcaneus relative to tibia, status of anterior tibial artery

Angiographic Findings
- Anterior tibial artery hypoplastic or absent in 85% severe club feet; just 2 reports of absent posterior tibial artery

Imaging Recommendations
- Best imaging tool: Plain radiographs
- Protocol advice: Radiographs taken in most "anatomical" or corrected position possible; forced dorsiflexion of foot partially overcomes equinus

DIFFERENTIAL DIAGNOSIS

Metatarsus adductus
- Forefoot varus without other findings of club foot

Congenital vertical talus
- Talus head faces convex sole, equinus heel, dorsiflexed forefoot, navicular not anterior to anterior talus on plantar flexion

Rockerbottom foot
- Rockerbottom: Foot foreshortened and convex, like "Persian slipper"
- May be associated with club foot repair
- 70% bilateral
- Frequently associated with trisomy 18

Amniotic band syndrome
- Varies from simple ring constrictions to major craniofacial and visceral defects

Vertical calcaneus in myelodysplasia
- Decreased knee extension with heel ulceration; forefoot cannot contact floor

Congenital diastasis of inferior tibiofibular joint
- Talus dome superiorly displaced between tibial and fibular metaphyses

PATHOLOGY

General Features
- Genetics
  ○ Family history of club foot in 24%
  ○ Siblings: 30x increased risk
    ▪ Monozygotic twins: 33% risk of both affected
    ▪ Dizygotic twins: 3% risk of both affected
- Etiology
  ○ Fetal akinesia deformation sequence
    ▪ Arthrogryposis and amyoplasia, Pena Shokeir syndrome, type 1
  ○ Intrauterine growth retardation, polyhydramnios, oligohydramnios (renal hypoplasia), after amniocentesis during 77-90 days gestation
  ○ Spinal dysraphism, sacral agenesis
  ○ Fetal muscle disease: Myotonic dystrophy

Microscopic Features
- Type 1 to type 2 muscle fiber ratio: Increased from 1:2 (normal) to 7:1

Staging, Grading or Classification Criteria
- Idiopathic congenital; 50% bilateral
- Teratologic
  ○ Myelodysplasia, arthrogryposis and amyoplasia
- Syndromic
  ○ Diastrophic dysplasia, Larsen syndrome, craniocarpotarsal dysplasia (Freeman-Sheldon syndrome), Wolf-Hirschhorn syndrome, Antley-Bixler syndrome
- Acquired
  ○ Cerebral palsy (CP): Onset after birth, often > 5 years
  ○ Present in 22% hemiplegic, 8% diplegic, 8% quadriplegic CP

CLUB FOOT (TALIPES EQUINOVARUS)

CLINICAL ISSUES

Presentation
- Most common signs/symptoms
  - Hindfoot: Varus and equinus
  - Forefoot: Adduction
  - Undergrowth: Foot bones, tibia and fibula, calf muscles
  - Stiffness: Ankle and foot
- In association with other anomalies
  - Amniotic bands, myelodysplasia, developmental hip dysplasia
  - Diastrophic dysplasia, Larsen syndrome, craniocarpotarsal dysplasia (Freeman-Sheldon syndrome), Wolf-Hirschhorn syndrome, Antley-Bixler syndrome
- Myelodysplastic club foot
  - Occurs in all levels of paraplegia, but commoner when motor function ↓ L4 absent
  - May recur after treatment
  - Charcot joint (neuropathic destruction) may occur
- Trisomy 18
  - Club foot in 23%, rockerbottom in 10%
- Trisomy 21
  - Club foot usually bilateral

Demographics
- Gender: M:F = 2.5:1
- Ethnicity: 0.4-0.5:1000 in Chinese, 0.9-1.2:1000 in Caucasians, 6-7:1000 in Polynesians

Natural History & Prognosis
- Mild lower leg asymmetry with age with unilateral club foot after treatment: Foot shortened average of 1.6 cm, calf circumference 2.5 cm less, leg length 0.6 cm less at end of childhood

Treatment
- Idiopathic club foot
  - Nonsurgical at first: Birth to 3-12 months
    - Ponsetti method: Manipulation and weekly casting; 78% excellent or good results; correct forefoot adduction and heel varus first, equinus last
    - French method: Physiotherapy, taping, and passive motion daily for 2 months tapered to 3x a week for 6 months; good results in 63%
    - Kite and Lovell technique; lengthwise stretching of foot, then cast foot with pressure to move talus medially and navicular laterally; correct forefoot adduction and heel varus first, equinus last
    - Botulinum toxin injection to relax muscles and permit stretching
  - Dennis-Brown and Thompson dynamic splinting
    - Bar width of infant's shoulders with baby shoes attached
    - Shoes permit progressive external rotation of feet
    - Infant's kicking and leg movement stretches contracted tissues reducing deformity; 60% corrected without surgery
  - Surgical: After 3-12 months if needed
    - Combination of soft tissue releases, osteotomies, tendon transfers
    - Medial plantar release: Abductor hallucis, flexor hallucis, flexor hallucis longus, peroneus longus tendons released; relaxing incisions of calcaneocuboid and medial talocalcaneal joint capsules; division of posterior tibial tendon slips to cuneiforms and bases of metatarsals 2-4
    - Posterior release: Z-plasty of Achilles tendon; relaxing incision of posterior and lateral talocalcaneal and ankle joint; calcaneofibular and posterior talofibular ligaments divided
    - Lateral release: Rotates calcaneus outward relative to talus; talonavicular and calcaneocuboid capsulotomies; lateral portion of talocalcaneal interosseous ligament cut
    - Reduction and internal fixation: Desired reduced position of talonavicular, calcaneocuboid, and subtalar joints maintained with pins
    - Triple arthrodesis: In older children (average 8.4 years) with persistent severe hindfoot deformities → 68% excellent or good results
- Myelodysplastic club foot
  - Treatment goal: Braceable plantigrade foot that is free of pain and ulceration
  - Charcot arthropathy: Immediate immobilization and no weight bearing when suspected (erythema, swelling) and radiographs still normal
- Surgical complications
  - Wound dehiscence, neurovascular injury; talus and navicular avascular necrosis
  - Forefoot adduction
  - Cavovarus deformity
    - Treatment: Anterior tibial tendon transfer
  - Rockerbottom foot
    - Treatment is surgical

SELECTED REFERENCES

1. Choi IH et al: Congenital diastasis of the inferior tibiofibular joint: report of three additional cases treated by the Ilizarov method and literature review. J Pediatr Orthop. 24(3):304-11, 2004
2. Noonan KJ et al: Nonsurgical management of idiopathic clubfoot. J Am Acad Orthop Surg. 11(6):392-402, 2003
3. Bernstein RM: Arthrogryposis and amyoplasia. J Am Acad Orthop Surg. 10(6):417-24, 2002
4. Cummings RJ et al: Congenital clubfoot. Instr Course Lect. 51:385-400, 2002
5. Harty MP: Imaging of pediatric foot disorders. Radiol Clin North Am. 39(4):733-48, 2001
6. Tredwell SJ et al: Review of the effect of early amniocentesis on foot deformity in the neonate. J Pediatr Orthop. 21(5):636-41, 2001
7. Greene WB: Cerebral palsy. Evaluation and management of equinus and equinovarus deformities. Foot Ankle Clin. 5(2):265-80, 2000
8. Noonan KJ et al: Care of the pediatric foot in myelodysplasia. Foot Ankle Clin. 5(2):281-304, vi, 2000
9. Tachdjian, MO: Clinical Pediatric Orthopedics. Ed 1. Appleton & Lange, Stamford CT. 12-24, 1997
10. Quillin SP et al: Absent posterior tibial artery associated with clubfoot deformity: an unusual variant. J Vasc Interv Radiol. 5(3):497-9, 1994
11. Galindo MJ Jr et al: Triple arthrodesis in young children: a salvage procedure after failed releases in severely affected feet. Foot Ankle. 7(6):319-25, 1987

CLUB FOOT (TALIPES EQUINOVARUS)

IMAGE GALLERY

Typical

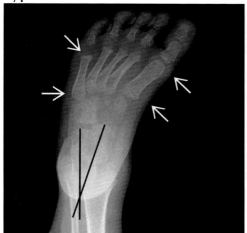
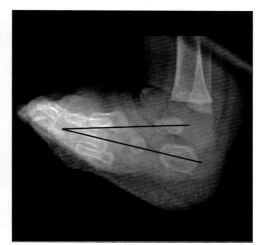

(Left) Anteroposterior radiograph shows forefoot adduction (arrows) and hindfoot varus in the same child. Talocalcaneal angle is slightly decreased at 18 degrees. *(Right)* Lateral radiograph shows a decreased talo-calcaneal angle of 20 degrees in a 5 month old baby.

Typical

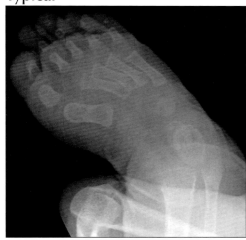
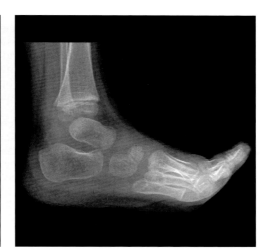

(Left) Anteroposterior radiograph shows marked forefoot adduction in same child as above right. *(Right)* Lateral radiograph with maximum dorsiflexion shows that hindfoot dorsiflexion is decreased in a 12 year old.

Typical

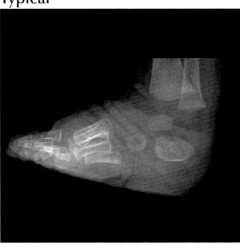
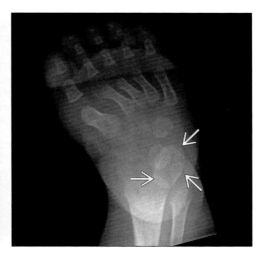

(Left) Lateral radiograph shows a decreased talo-calcaneal angle and limited dorsiflexion of hindfoot in a five month old child. *(Right)* Anteroposterior radiograph shows rotated calcaneus (arrows) causing hindfoot varus in same child. There is forefoot adduction.

VACTERL ASSOCIATION

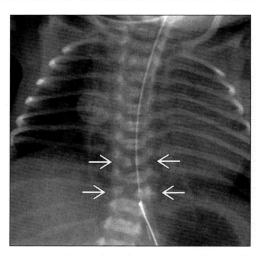

Anteroposterior radiograph shows newborn with VACTERL including heart disease. The low thoracic scoliosis is accompanied by sagittal clefts (arrows) of T8 and T10.

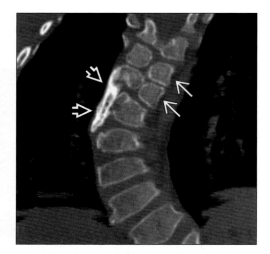

Coronal NECT shows child with VACTERL and scoliosis associated with T5/6 hemivertebrae (arrows) and a bony bar (open arrows) just below.

TERMINOLOGY

Abbreviations and Synonyms
- VATER, VACTER, VACTEL association, TREACLE, ARTICLE, ARTICLE V, axial mesodermal dysplasia spectrum

Definitions
- Non-random association of anomalies involving multiple organ systems except brain: (V)ertebral/vascular, (A)nal/auricular, (C)ardiac, (T)racheoesophageal fistula, (E)sophageal atresia, (R)enal/radial/rib, (L)imb
  - Clubfoot and congenital hip dislocation are excluded if these are only limb anomalies
- Diagnosis of VACTERL association: When 3 of these malformations are present

IMAGING FINDINGS

General Features
- Best diagnostic clue: Vertebral anomalies in presence of other malformations

Radiographic Findings
- Radiography
  - Vertebral anomalies
    - Hemivertebrae, cleft vertebrae, block vertebrae, hypersegmentation, vertebral bars, caudal regression, kyphosis, scoliosis
  - Head and neck
    - Choanal atresia
    - Cleft lip/palate
    - Auricular defects
  - Chest
    - Congenital heart disease: Many diverse types; ventricular septal defect (30%), patent ductus arteriosus (26%), atrial septal defect (20%)
    - Esophageal atresia, tracheo-esophageal fistula (19-25% such infants have VACTERL association)
    - Lung agenesis
    - Horseshoe lung (both lungs fused posteriorly by isthmus of lung parenchyma)
    - Ectopic bronchus
  - Abdomen and pelvis
    - Microgastria
    - Duodenal atresia, malrotation, Meckel diverticulum
    - Anal anomalies: Imperforate anus with or without fistula
    - Urogenital anomalies: Renal agenesis is commonest (bilateral in ≈13%); also, multicystic dysplasia, horseshoe kidney, ectopia, hydronephrosis, persistent urachus, cryptorchidism, vaginal atresia

DDx: Lesions Pointing Toward VACTERL Dx

Rib/Spine Fusion *Sacral Agenesis* *Absent Radius*

VACTERL ASSOCIATION

Key Facts

Terminology
- Non-random association of anomalies involving multiple organ systems except brain: (V)ertebral/vascular, (A)nal/auricular, (C)ardiac, (T)racheoesophageal fistula, (E)sophageal atresia, (R)enal/radial/rib, (L)imb
- Diagnosis of VACTERL association: When 3 of these malformations are present

Imaging Findings
- Best diagnostic clue: Vertebral anomalies in presence of other malformations
- Congenital heart disease: Many diverse types; ventricular septal defect (30%), patent ductus arteriosus (26%), atrial septal defect (20%)
- Esophageal atresia, tracheo-esophageal fistula (19-25% such infants have VACTERL association)

- Vertebrae: Vertebral fusion, hemivertebrae, butterfly vertebrae, segmentation defects, partially or completely absent sacrum, caudal regression
- Actively seek other components of VACTERL association when one or two are known to be present

Pathology
- Concurrence of 3 or more specific VACTERL anomalies 95 times more frequent than would be expected by chance

Diagnostic Checklist
- Think of the VACTERL association when vertebral anomalies exist in a child with other known malformations

---

- Inguinal hernia
- Axial skeleton
  - Vertebrae: Vertebral fusion, hemivertebrae, butterfly vertebrae, segmentation defects, partially or completely absent sacrum, caudal regression
  - Ribs: Fusion, bifid, hypoplasia, and supernumerary/cervical (28% children with such rib anomalies have VACTERL association)
  - Spine: Scoliosis, kyphosis
- Limbs or Extremities
  - Radial ray: Dysplastic or absent radius, radioulnar synostosis, thumb hypoplasia, radial polydactyly, absent scaphoid, radial artery hypoplasia
  - Hands: Polydactyly, syndactyly
  - Absence or hypoplasia: Humerus, radius, femur, tibia, fibula
  - Reduction deformities (34%) and polydactyly (20%) are commonest
- Genitourinary systems
  - Multicystic dysplasia, agenesis, hydronephrosis, ectopia, persistent urachus

Ultrasonographic Findings
- Prenatal ultrasound: May suggest diagnosis

Angiographic Findings
- Radial artery: Hypoplasia

Imaging Recommendations
- Actively seek other components of VACTERL association when one or two are known to be present

DIFFERENTIAL DIAGNOSIS

Trisomy 13
- Microcephaly, holoprosencephaly, microphthalmia
- Ribs absent or small, polydactyly

Trisomy 18
- Clenched fist, microcephaly, micrognathia, rocker-bottom feet
- 95% lethal in first year

PHAVER syndrome
- Syndrome of limb (P)terygia, congenital (H)eart anomalies, (V)ertebral defects, (E)ar anomalies, and (R)adial defects

Others syndromes with findings overlapping VACTERL
- Holt-Oram (heart-hand syndrome)
  - Cardiac conduction defect with or without inter-atrial/ventricular septal defect; thumb, wrist, and forearm abnormalities
- Thrombocytopenia absent-radius syndrome
- Pseudothalidomide syndrome
  - Microcephaly, double-cleft palate and lip, face hemangiomas, corneal vascularization, phocomelia
- Jarcho-Levin syndrome
  - Multiple vertebral fusions → short trunk, rib malformations, respiratory insufficiency
- VACTERL-H (VACTERL) and (H)ydrocephalus
  - Severe mental retardation; poor prognosis

PATHOLOGY

General Features
- Genetics: Associated with trisomies 13 and 18, cri du chat syndrome
- Etiology
  - Abnormal mesodermal development before 35th fetal day
  - Risk factors: Maternal diabetes, prenatal lead exposure
- Epidemiology
  - Incidence of VACTERL association: 1.6:10,000 live births
    - Tendency to occur more often in Caucasian boys
    - Prematurity: Approximately one third
    - Stillborn: 12%
  - Frequency of anomalies in VACTERL
    - Cardiac 77%
    - Renal 72%
    - Anal 63%

VACTERL ASSOCIATION

- Radial ray 58%
- Tracheoesophageal 40% (19-25% of children with esophageal atresia with or without tracheoesophageal atresia have VACTERL association)
- Vertebral 37%
  - Concurrence of 2 specific VACTERL anomalies 11 times more frequent than would be expected by chance
    - Reasonable to consider that these children belong to VACTERL continuum
  - Concurrence of 3 or more specific VACTERL anomalies 95 times more frequent than would be expected by chance
  - VACTERL children: 72% have 3 specific VACTERL anomalies, 24% have 4, 8% have 5
    - Most common 3-anomaly combinations: Cardiac-renal-limb and cardiac-renal-anal
    - Most common 5-anomaly combination: Cardiac-renal-limb-anal-tracheoesophageal fistula
- Associated abnormalities
  - Cleft palate 18%
  - Neural tube defect 10%
  - Diaphragmatic hernia 8%
  - Omphalocele 6%
  - Exstrophy of cloaca
  - Cystic adenoid malformation of lung
  - MURCS association (Mu)llerian hypoplasia/aplasia, (R)enal agenesis and (C)ervicothoracic (S)omite dysplasia
  - Syrenomelia
  - Goldenhar syndrome: Occulo-auricular-vertebral spectrum
  - Zellweger syndrome: Imperfect myelination of nerve tracts, microgyria, abnormal skull, craniofacial malformations, glaucoma, seizures, cataracts, mental and growth retardation, calcific deposits in long bones, hypospadias, renal cysts, hepatomegaly, hyperbilirubinemia, extramedullary hematopoiesis and cardiac defects due to decreased peroxisomes in many tissues
  - Meckel syndrome: Lethal malformation complex characterized by occipital encephalocele, microcephaly, microphthalmia, abnormal facies, cleft palate, cataracts, polydactyly, congenital heart defect, genital anomalies, and polycystic degeneration of kidneys, liver, and pancreas

CLINICAL ISSUES

Presentation
- Other signs/symptoms
  - Prenatal
    - Polyhydramnios: Often present when esophageal atresia
    - Single umbilical artery

Natural History & Prognosis
- Mortality (not due to any specific defect, such as heart disease)
  - 28% neonatal mortality
  - 48% mortality in first year
- Intelligence usually normal

Treatment
- If prenatal diagnosis: Delivery at tertiary care facility

DIAGNOSTIC CHECKLIST

Image Interpretation Pearls
- Think of the VACTERL association when vertebral anomalies exist in a child with other known malformations

SELECTED REFERENCES

1. Haller JO et al: Tracheoesophageal fistula (H-type) in neonates with imperforate anus and the VATER association. Pediatr Radiol. 34(1):83-5, 2004
2. Wattanasirichaigoon D et al: Rib defects in patterns of multiple malformations: a retrospective review and phenotypic analysis of 47 cases. Am J Med Genet. 122A(1):63-9, 2003
3. Evans JA et al: Tibial agenesis with radial ray and cardiovascular defects. Clin Dysmorphol. 11(3):163-9, 2002
4. Spruijt L et al: VATER--tibia aplasia association: report on two patients. Clin Dysmorphol. 11(4):283-7, 2002
5. Wales PW et al: Horseshoe lung in association with other foregut anomalies: what is the significance? J Pediatr Surg. 37(8):1205-7, 2002
6. Kallen K et al: VATER non-random association of congenital malformations: study based on data from four malformation registers. Am J Med Genet. 101(1):26-32, 2001
7. Rittler M et al: VACTERL association, epidemiologic definition and delineation. Am J Med Genet. 63(4):529-36, 1996
8. Torfs CP et al: Population-based study of tracheoesophageal fistula and esophageal atresia. Teratology. 52(4):220-32, 1995
9. James HE et al: Distal spinal cord pathology in the VATER association. J Pediatr Surg. 29(11):1501-3, 1994
10. Corsello G et al: VATER/VACTERL association: clinical variability and expanding phenotype including laryngeal stenosis. Am J Med Genet. 44(6):813-5, 1992
11. Obregon MG et al: Horseshoe lung: an additional component of the Vater association. Pediatr Radiol. 22(2):158, 1992
12. Wulfsberg EA et al: Vertebral hypersegmentation in a case of the VATER association. Am J Med Genet. 42(6):766-70, 1992
13. Bass J: Radial artery hypoplasia: a further association with the VATER syndrome? J Urol. 146(3):824-5, 1991
14. Levine F et al: VACTERL association with high prenatal lead exposure: similarities to animal models of lead teratogenicity. Pediatrics. 87(3):390-2, 1991
15. Chittmittrapap S et al: Oesophageal atresia and associated anomalies. Arch Dis Child. 64(3):364-8, 1989
16. Fernbach SK et al: The expanded spectrum of limb anomalies in the VATER association. Pediatr Radiol. 18(3):215-20, 1988
17. Knowles S et al: Pulmonary agenesis as part of the VACTERL sequence. Arch Dis Child. 63(7 Spec No):723-6, 1988
18. Touloukian RJ et al: High proximal pouch esophageal atresia with vertebral, rib, and sternal anomalies: an additional component to the VATER association. J Pediatr Surg. 23(1 Pt 2):76-9, 1988
19. Treble NJ: Congenital absence of the scaphoid in the "VATER" association. J Hand Surg [Br]. 10(2):251-2, 1985

VACTERL ASSOCIATION

IMAGE GALLERY

Typical

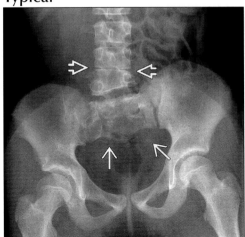
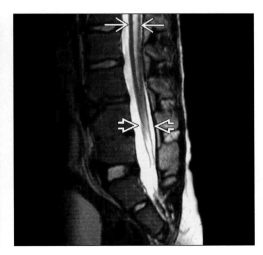

(Left) Anteroposterior radiograph shows 13 year old with VACTERL, partial sacral agenesis (arrows), and fusion of 2 lower lumbar vertebrae (open arrows). *(Right)* Sagittal T2WI MR shows syringomyelia (arrows), and a low spinal cord (open arrows) at the L4 or L5 level in same patient.

Typical

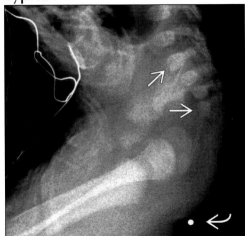
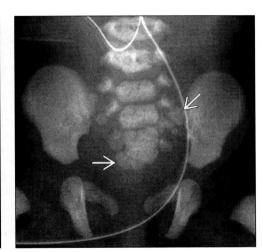

(Left) Lateral radiograph shows newborn with VACTERL and an imperforate anus; a lead shot (curved arrow) is seen in the anal dimple. Partial sacral agenesis; only the superior 4 vertebral bodies (arrows) have formed. *(Right)* Anteroposterior radiograph shows newborn with VACTERL. The sacrum curves to the right accompanied by anomalous asymmetric ossification centers (arrows) on both sides.

Typical

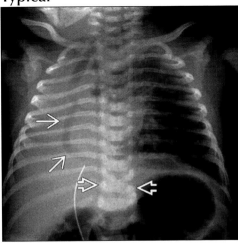
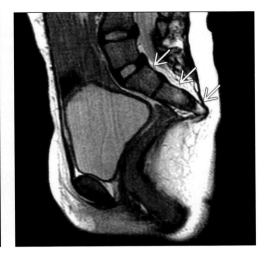

(Left) Anteroposterior radiograph shows newborn with VACTERL including right-lung agenesis, tracheo-esophageal fistula with air in esophagus (arrows), and malformed thoracic vertebrae (open arrows). *(Right)* Sagittal FSE T2 MR shows child with VACTERL and partial sacral agenesis with only 3 sacral segments (arrows).

TARSAL COALITION

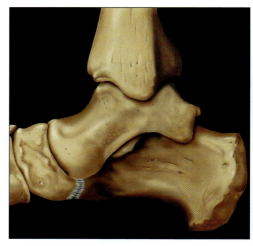

Lateral graphic shows calcaneonavicular nonosseous coalition.

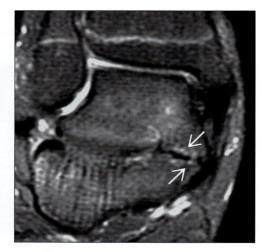

Coronal T2WI MR shows irregularity, narrowing & mild reactive subchondral edema (arrows) of the talocalcaneal joint, consistent with a nonosseous coalition.

TERMINOLOGY

Abbreviations and Synonyms
- Tarsal fusion, coalitions

Definitions
- Congenital or acquired abnormal fusion of the tarsal bones
  - This fusion may be osseous, cartilaginous or a fibrous union

IMAGING FINDINGS

General Features
- Best diagnostic clue: Visualized close apposition or fusion of the middle facet of the talocalcaneal joint or anterodorsal calcaneus to navicular
- Location
  - Calcaneonavicular
  - Talocalcaneal
  - Uncommon: Talonavicular and calcaneocuboid
- Morphology
  - Synostosis = ossific bar
  - Synchondrosis = cartilaginous bar
  - Syndesmosis = fibrous union

Radiographic Findings
- Radiography
  - Calcaneonavicular coalition
    - 45° internal oblique view (Sloman view)
    - Ossific bar connecting calcaneus to navicular
    - Irregularity, sclerosis or narrowing of the calcaneonavicular space (fibrous or cartilaginous coalition)
    - "Anteater nose" sign = elongation of the anterosuperior calcaneus on lateral view
    - Broadening of the medial aspect of the anterosuperior calcaneus in close apposition to the navicular
    - +/- Hypoplastic talar head
    - Radiography typically diagnostic, other imaging not needed
  - Talocalcaneal coalition
    - Harris-Beath (axial) & lateral views
    - Difficult to see coalition, CT often needed
    - Most common middle facet, less common involvement of anterior or posterior facets
    - Talar beak: Impaired subtalar motion → periosteal elevation at insertion of talocalcaneal ligament → cycles of osseous repair → beak (not specific for coalition)
    - Rounding of lateral talar process
    - Middle facet inapparent on lateral view

DDx: Limited Subtalar Motion & Pain

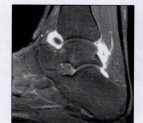
JRA

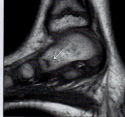
Talar Fracture

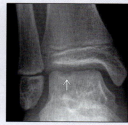
OCD

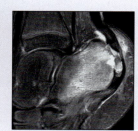
Osteomyelitis

TARSAL COALITION

Key Facts

Terminology
- Congenital or acquired abnormal fusion of the tarsal bones

Imaging Findings
- Calcaneonavicular coalition
- "Anteater nose" sign = elongation of the anterosuperior calcaneus on lateral view
- Talocalcaneal coalition
- C sign: Continuous uninterrupted line formed by medial talar dome & sustentaculum tali on lateral view (50%) (sign of flat feet)

Top Differential Diagnoses
- Subtalar fractures
- Osteomyelitis
- Osteochondritis dissecans (OCD)
- Juvenile rheumatoid arthritis (JRA)
- Tumor

Pathology
- Congenital failure of segmentation & differentiation of primitive mesenchyme
- Acquired: Trauma, infection, arthritis or surgery
- 1% incidence
- 90% of all coalitions are talocalcaneal or calcaneonavicular

Diagnostic Checklist
- Talocalcaneal coalition: Coronal NECT or MRI
- Calcaneonavicular coalition: 45° internal oblique radiograph

---

- "Ball in socket" ankle joint: Concave surfaces of tibia & fibula, domed talus (convex proximal margin), uncommon & nonspecific sign
- C sign: Continuous uninterrupted line formed by medial talar dome & sustentaculum tali on lateral view (50%) (sign of flat feet)
- Narrowing of posterior subtalar joint
- Normal middle & posterior facets are parallel to each other on Harris-Beath view, slants inferomedially in fibrous or cartilaginous coalition (bar in ossific coalition)
- CT Findings
  - NECT
  - Either direct axial & coronal images or multislice scanners with axial & coronal reformation (+/- sagittal reformations)
  - Calcaneonavicular coalition
    - Joint space narrowing or reactive sclerosis
    - Widening of the medial aspect of the anterosuperior calcaneus
    - +/- Bony bridge
    - Best seen on axial plane
  - Talocalcaneal coalition
    - Ossific bar (best on coronal images)
    - Downward (or horizontal orientation) sloping sustentaculum along middle facet (normally slopes upward medially)
    - Reactive subchondral sclerosis, narrowing, cystic & hypertrophic changes of talocalcaneal joint (especially middle facet)
    - +/- Broadening or hypoplasia of sustentaculum

MR Findings
- T1WI
  - Calcaneonavicular coalition
    - Sagittal & axial images best for detecting coalition
    - Narrowing of calcaneonavicular space
    - Hypointense reactive changes
  - Talocalcaneal coalition
    - Coronal image best for detecting coalition
    - Osseous: Bar with marrow signal connection
    - Fibrous & cartilaginous: Hypointense signal connection with hypointense subchondral marrow changes
    - +/- Talar beaking
    - Talar neck concavity
- T2WI
  - Ossific: Bone marrow contiguity across either talocalcaneal or calcaneonavicular coalition
  - Cartilaginous: Hyperintense fluid signal connection with reactive hyperintense subchondral bone marrow edema
  - Fibrous: Intermediate signal connection with reactive hyperintense subchondral bone marrow edema
  - Cartilaginous & fibrous: Decreased joint space

Imaging Recommendations
- Best imaging tool
  - NECT or 3 plane MRI: Talocalcaneal coalition
  - 45° oblique view: Calcaneonavicular coalition
- Protocol advice
  - Multislice NECT: Axial 2.5 mm reconstruct at 1.25 mm, coronal reformation (+/- sagittal)
  - NECT (spiral CT): Direct 3 mm axial or coronal planes, 3 mm reconstructions with pitch 1.5
  - MRI: Coronal & sagittal; T1, FS PD/T2 FSE +/- STIR (fibrous coalitions)

DIFFERENTIAL DIAGNOSIS

Subtalar fractures
- Talar fractures
- Calcaneal fractures

Osteomyelitis
- Marrow hyperintensity, +/- erosion or sinus tract
- Pain, fever, erythema; ↑ C-reactive protein, sedimentation rate & white blood cells (WBC)

Osteochondritis dissecans (OCD)
- Talar dome
- Mostly adolescents, M > F

TARSAL COALITION

- Most common location: Lateral aspect of medial femoral condyle

Juvenile rheumatoid arthritis (JRA)
- Pannus formation joints on ankle & foot with +/- cartilage or osseous erosions
- Reactive marrow edema
- +/- Tenosynovitis

Tumor
- Chondroblastoma
- Bone cyst

PATHOLOGY

General Features
- Genetics: Autosomal dominance with high penetrance
- Etiology
  - Congenital failure of segmentation & differentiation of primitive mesenchyme
  - Acquired: Trauma, infection, arthritis or surgery
- Epidemiology
  - 1% incidence
  - 90% of all coalitions are talocalcaneal or calcaneonavicular
    - Talocalcaneal slightly more common
  - Bilateral: 25-50%
  - Other tarsal coalitions are uncommon
- Associated abnormalities
  - Apert
  - Hand-foot-uterus syndrome
  - Proximal focal femoral deficiency
  - Hereditary symphalangism

Gross Pathologic & Surgical Features
- Osseous
- Fibrous
- Cartilaginous

CLINICAL ISSUES

Presentation
- Most common signs/symptoms: Pain & stiffness with limited subtalar motion
- Other signs/symptoms
  - Commonly asymptomatic, discovered after imaging for trauma
  - Pes planus + heel valgus
  - Flattening of the medial arch
  - Pain with activity
  - Peroneal spastic flatfoot
    - Rigid valgus deformity, pain & peroneal muscle spasm
    - Tarsal coalition is the most common cause
    - Other causes: Fracture, arthritis & some tumors

Demographics
- Age
  - Calcaneonavicular (8-12 years) earlier due to earlier ossification
  - Talocalcaneal (12-16 years)
  - Fibrous coalition at birth, ossifies 2nd decade
- Gender: M > F

Natural History & Prognosis
- Coalitions at birth may be fibrous or cartilaginous and later ossify
- Symptoms more severe when coalition ossifies
- Decreased hindfoot motion makes child prone to ankle sprains
- Commonly discovered after imaging for ankle injuries

Treatment
- Conservative: (1st)
  - Nonsteroidal antiinflammatory medication, steroids, trial of casting, orthotics & physical therapy
- Surgical
  - Calcaneonavicular: Resection of bony bridge with extensor digitorum brevis interposition
  - Talocalcaneal: Resection of middle facet bony bridge with fat interposition
  - If excision fails or severe degenerative disease: Fusion or triple arthrodesis

DIAGNOSTIC CHECKLIST

Consider
- Talocalcaneal coalition: Coronal NECT or MRI
- Calcaneonavicular coalition: 45° internal oblique radiograph

SELECTED REFERENCES

1. Crim JR et al: Radiographic diagnosis of tarsal coalition. AJR Am J Roentgenol. 182(2):323-8, 2004
2. Bohne WH: Tarsal coalition. Curr Opin Pediatr. 13(1):29-35, 2001
3. Brown RR et al: The C sign: more specific for flatfoot deformity than subtalar coalition. Skeletal Radiol. 30(2):84-7, 2001
4. Blakemore LC et al: The rigid flatfoot. Tarsal coalitions. Clin Podiatr Med Surg. 17(3):531-55, 2000
5. Newman JS et al: Congenital tarsal coalition: multimodality evaluation with emphasis on CT and MR imaging. Radiographics. 20(2):321-32; quiz 526-7, 532, 2000
6. Varner KE et al: Tarsal coalition in adults. Foot Ankle Int. 21(8):669-72, 2000
7. Gessner AJ et al: Tarsal Coalition in Pediatric Patients. Semin Musculoskelet Radiol. 3(3):239-246, 1999
8. Sakellariou A et al: Tarsal coalition. Orthopedics. 22(11):1066-73; discussion 1073-4; quiz 10, 1999
9. Emery KH et al: Tarsal coalition: a blinded comparison of MRI and CT. Pediatr Radiol. 28(8):612-6, 1998
10. Vincent KA: Tarsal coalition and painful flatfoot. J Am Acad Orthop Surg. 6(5):274-81, 1998
11. Kulik SA Jr et al: Tarsal coalition. Foot Ankle Int. 17(5):286-96, 1996
12. Laor T et al: MR imaging in congenital lower limb deformities. Pediatr Radiol. 26(6):381-7, 1996
13. Lateur LM et al: Subtalar coalition: diagnosis with the C sign on lateral radiographs of the ankle. Radiology. 193(3):847-51, 1994
14. Pfeiffer WH et al: Clinical results after tarsal tunnel decompression. J Bone Joint Surg Am. 76(8):1222-30, 1994
15. Oestreich AE et al: The "anteater nose": a direct sign of calcaneonavicular coalition on the lateral radiograph. J Pediatr Orthop. 7(6):709-11, 1987

TARSAL COALITION

IMAGE GALLERY

Typical

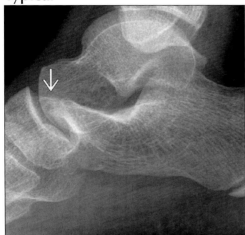 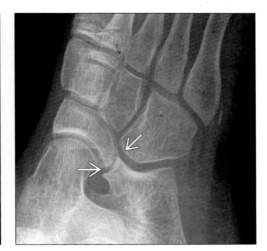

(Left) Lateral radiograph shows elongation of the anterior dorsal calcaneus, typical example of an "anteater nose" sign of calcaneonavicular coalition (arrow). *(Right)* Oblique radiograph shows a calcaneonavicular nonosseous coalition (arrows) with narrowing, sclerosis and subchondral cyst formation.

Typical

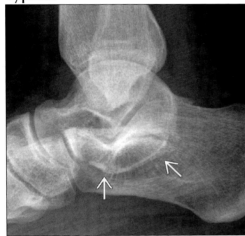 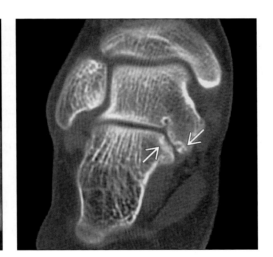

(Left) Lateral radiograph shows typical complete or continuous "C sign" (arrows) of a talocalcaneal coalition. The "C sign" is formed by the medial talar dome & the posteroinferior sustentaculum. *(Right)* Coronal NECT shows nonosseous talocalcaneal coalition (arrows) with joint space narrowing, irregularity, cystic subchondral changes & downward sloping of the sustentaculum tali.

Typical

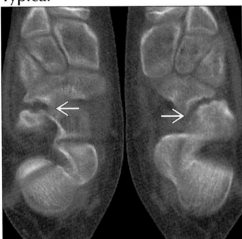 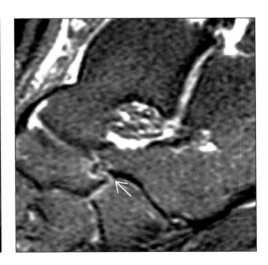

(Left) Axial NECT shows typical example of bilateral nonosseous calcaneonavicular coalition with irregularity, narrowing & sclerosis (arrows). *(Right)* Sagittal PD/Intermediate MR shows typical findings of a calcaneonavicular nonosseous coalition with narrowing, irregularity of the joint with subchondral reactive marrow edema (arrow).

DISCOID MENISCUS

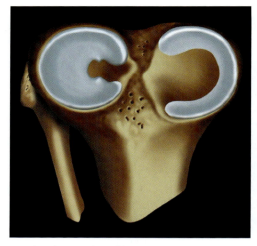

Graphic shows a discoid lateral meniscus with minimal resorption of the central portion of the meniscus & greater than 50% coverage of the lateral tibial plateau.

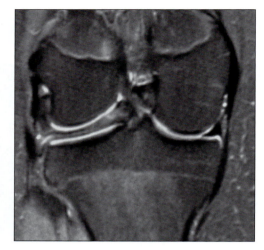

Coronal PD/Intermediate MR shows discoid lateral meniscus with degeneration, evident by hyperintense signal. The inner margin does not taper normally & extends into the intercondylar notch.

TERMINOLOGY

Definitions
- Large, congenitally dysplastic meniscus with loss of the normal semi-lunar shape
- Due to deficiency of the normal meniscal attachments

IMAGING FINDINGS

General Features
- Best diagnostic clue
  - Continuity of the anterior and posterior horns on ≥ 3 MR consecutive sagittal images (4-5 mm slices)
    - \> 50% coverage of the lateral tibial plateau on images
    - Loss of the normal semilunar morphology
- Location
  - Lateral >> medial discoid meniscus; (7:1)
  - Sometimes bilateral
- Size
  - ≥ 2 mm in height greater than medial meniscus
  - \> 13 mm in cross section
    - Normal: 5-13 mm from the capsular margin to the free edge on a central coronal image
- Morphology: Large or pancake-like meniscus

Radiographic Findings
- Radiography
  - Discoid lateral meniscus
    - High fibular head
    - Hypoplastic femoral condyle
    - Hypoplastic lateral tibial spine
    - Widened tibiofemoral joint space
    - Cupping of the lateral tibial plateau

MR Findings
- T1WI
  - Meniscal size > 13 mm in cross section is consistent
  - Normal hypointense meniscus: 5-13 mm from capsular margin to free edge on a central coronal image
  - Continuous body, continuity of the anterior and posterior horns ≥ 3 consecutive sagittal images (4-5 mm thick images)
  - Prominent ligament of Wrisberg
  - Does not taper medially
- T2WI
  - Normal meniscus is hypointense
  - Intrameniscal signal, intermediate to hyperintense signal on conventional spin echo (CSE) PD, FS PD FSE, or T2* GRE
    - Difficult to determine if intrameniscal signal indicates a tear, mucoid degeneration, or cyst
    - Extensive signal abnormality can reflect a tear

DDx: Cause Of Knee Locking

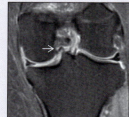
Bucket-Handle Tear

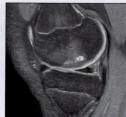
OCD

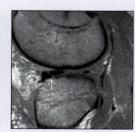
Flipped Meniscus

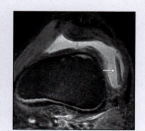
Loose Body

DISCOID MENISCUS

Key Facts

Terminology
- Large, congenitally dysplastic meniscus with loss of the normal semi-lunar shape

Imaging Findings
- Continuity of the anterior and posterior horns on ≥ 3 MR consecutive sagittal images (4-5 mm slices)
- > 50% coverage of the lateral tibial plateau on images
- Lateral > > medial discoid meniscus; (7:1)
- ≥ 2 mm in height greater than medial meniscus
- > 13 mm in cross section

Top Differential Diagnoses
- Flipped meniscus
- Bucket-handle tear
- Loose bodies
- Osteochondritis dissecans (OCD)

Pathology
- Failure of fetal discoid form to involute
- Derived from mesenchyme that is initially disc shaped then forms semilunar shape
- 1.5-4.5% discoid lateral meniscus

Clinical Issues
- Often asymptomatic in children (most common)
- Patients often present with pain, clicking and snapping

Diagnostic Checklist
- Sagittal images: 3 or more consecutive images bowtie configuration maintained, think discoid meniscus

---

- Unusual tears can happen: Double radial tear
- PD/Intermediate
  - Hypointense slab-like shaped meniscus
  - Frequently demonstrates meniscal tear or intrameniscal tear seen as increased signal intensity on short TE images within the substance of the meniscus (intrameniscal tear) or extending to an articular surface (tear)
- T2* GRE
  - Hyperintense signal
    - Mucinous degeneration
    - Intrameniscal cyst
    - Tears; (horizontal tears most common)
    - Tears are seen as hyperintense signal on PD, T2, T2* GRE
  - More prone to more complex tears
  - Complete discoid meniscus has "pancake" appearance
    - Extending from the intercondylar notch to the periphery of the compartment
- MR arthrography
  - May have a role in distinguishing meniscal tear from intrameniscal tear
  - If contrast extends into meniscus = tear
  - If contrast does not enter meniscus = intrameniscal tear, cyst or degeneration

Imaging Recommendations
- Best imaging tool: MRI sagittal images with confirmation on coronal data sets
- Protocol advice
  - Detect tears in discoid meniscus
    - CSE PD, FS PD FSE & T2* GRE

DIFFERENTIAL DIAGNOSIS

Vacuum phenomenon
- Typically in the hyperextended knee
- Decreased signal intensity in the joint between the weightbearing surfaces
- Rarely homogeneous like a discoid meniscus

Flipped meniscus
- Meniscus is torn in this situation giving abnormal morphology to the "donor site" where portions of the meniscus are missing, thus allowing distinction from the discoid meniscus
- "Double anterior horn sign"
  - Usually posterior horn flipped anteriorly
- < 2 bowties on consecutive sagittal images (5 mm slices)
  - ≥ 3 bowties on consecutive sagittal images in discoid meniscus

Bucket-handle tear
- Longitudinal vertical peripheral tear with displacement of a meniscal fragment into the intercondylar notch
- "Double posterior cruciate ligament (PCL) sign"
  - Displaced meniscal fragment anterior to the PCL creating 2 PCLs
- Foreshortened, truncated & abnormal sized meniscus on sagittal images
- < 2 bowties on consecutive sagittal images (5 mm slices)
  - ≥ 3 bowties on consecutive sagittal images in discoid meniscus

Loose bodies
- Cartilage and/or bone
- Often trauma history

Osteochondritis dissecans (OCD)
- Most common lateral aspect of the medial femoral condyle
- Traumatic history: 50%
- Stable
  - May have considerable subchondral edema
  - No fluid undercutting fragment
- Unstable
  - Loose body
  - Fluid insinuating beneath fragment = unstable OCD
  - Large size: > 1 cm in size
  - Large cystic areas beneath OCD lesions

DISCOID MENISCUS

PATHOLOGY

General Features
- General path comments: Pancake or large meniscus which may demonstrate intrameniscal degeneration or meniscal tear
- Etiology
  - Deficient normal meniscal attachments
  - Failure of fetal discoid form to involute
    - Derived from mesenchyme that is initially disc shaped then forms semilunar shape
- Epidemiology
  - 1.5-4.5% discoid lateral meniscus
    - Japan: 15%
  - 0.1-0.6% discoid medial meniscus

Gross Pathologic & Surgical Features
- Pancake or large, otherwise normal-appearing meniscus in the medial or lateral compartment
  - Lateral:Medial = 7:1
- Wrisberg-ligament type discoid meniscus lacks posterior meniscotibial attachment

Microscopic Features
- Microscopically normal meniscus
  - Meniscus may demonstrate mucoid degeneration &/or tear

Staging, Grading or Classification Criteria
- Watanabe classification
  - Complete discoid meniscus (stable)
    - Extending into the intercondylar notch on coronal images
  - Incomplete (stable)
    - Partially extends to the intercondylar notch on coronal images
  - Wrisberg-ligament type (unstable)
    - Lacks posterolateral meniscal-tibial attachment
    - Hypermobile

CLINICAL ISSUES

Presentation
- Most common signs/symptoms
  - Often asymptomatic in children (most common)
  - Symptomatic even without tears
  - Patients often present with pain, clicking and snapping
  - Locking is a common presentation in children
  - "Giving way"
  - Effusion
- Symptoms may not develop until adolescents or young adulthood
- Snapping knee syndrome
  - Snap in flexion & extension
  - < 10 year old
  - Wrisberg type
  - Virtually pathognomic for discoid lateral meniscus
- Bilateral: 25-50%

Demographics
- Age
  - Children asymptomatic
    - If symptomatic < 10 years old, "snapping knee" most common
    - Uncommonly symptomatic < 10 years old
    - Adolescence: Variable symptoms
  - Adults usually symptomatic
    - Peak incidence for injury
    - Female: 2nd decade
    - Male: 30s
- Gender: M > F
- Ethnicity: Higher incidence in Asians

Natural History & Prognosis
- When a discoid meniscus is present: More prone to be torn

Treatment
- Conservative 1st
- Partial meniscectomy with saucerization
- Partial resection of discoid portion back to a more normal shaped meniscus

DIAGNOSTIC CHECKLIST

Consider
- Displaced meniscal tear as a differential diagnosis for the same common symptoms

Image Interpretation Pearls
- Sagittal images: 3 or more consecutive images bowtie configuration maintained, think discoid meniscus
- Slab-like shape with meniscus non-tapering into the intercondylar notch
- Commonly torn

SELECTED REFERENCES

1. Youm T et al: Discoid lateral meniscus: evaluation and treatment. Am J Orthop. 33(5):234-8, 2004
2. Chiang H et al: Discoid lateral meniscus: clinical manifestations and arthroscopic treatment. J Formos Med Assoc. 102(1):17-22, 2003
3. Bin SI et al: Correlation between type of discoid lateral menisci and tear pattern. Knee Surg Sports Traumatol Arthrosc. 10(4):218-22, 2002
4. Ahn JH et al: Discoid lateral meniscus in children: clinical manifestations and morphology. J Pediatr Orthop. 21(6):812-6, 2001
5. Choi NH et al: Medial and lateral discoid meniscus in the same knee. Arthroscopy. 17(2):E9, 2001
6. Rohren EM et al: Discoid lateral meniscus and the frequency of meniscal tears. Skeletal Radiol. 30(6):316-20, 2001
7. Araki Y et al: MR imaging of meniscal tears with discoid lateral meniscus. Eur J Radiol. 27(2):153-60, 1998
8. Connolly B et al: Discoid meniscus in children: magnetic resonance imaging characteristics. Can Assoc Radiol J. 47(5):347-54, 1996
9. Auge WK 2nd et al: Bilateral discoid medial menisci with extensive intrasubstance cleavage tears: MRI and arthroscopic correlation. Arthroscopy. 10(3):313-8, 1994
10. Silverman JM et al: Discoid menisci of the knee: MR imaging appearance. Radiology. 173(2):351-4, 1989

DISCOID MENISCUS

IMAGE GALLERY

Typical

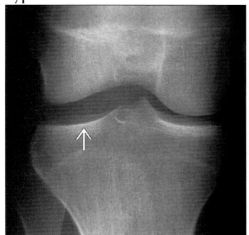
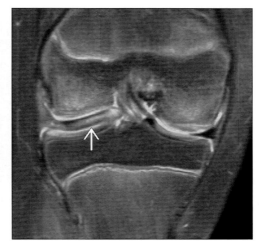

(Left) Anteroposterior radiograph shows widening of the lateral joint compartment (arrow). *(Right)* Coronal PD/Intermediate MR shows discoid lateral meniscus (arrow) occupying the lateral compartment. The meniscus lacks inner tapering margin with extension into intercondylar notch. Diffuse hyperintense signal within the meniscus is consistent with degeneration and a tear.

Typical

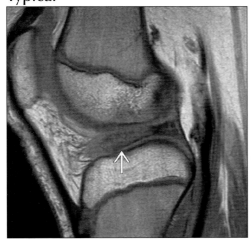
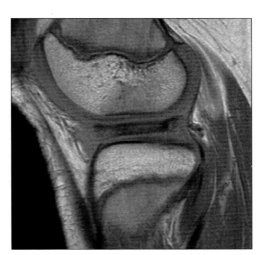

(Left) Sagittal CSE PD image shows abnormal intermediate signal within the discoid meniscus (arrow), consistent with degeneration. A complex tear was identified on other imaging sequences. *(Right)* Sagittal CSE PD image shows discoid lateral meniscus. Meniscus bowtie is continuous with the anterior & posterior horns on multiple sagittal images, characteristic.

Typical

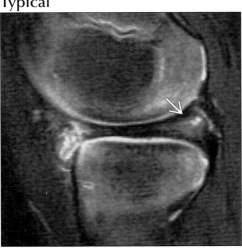
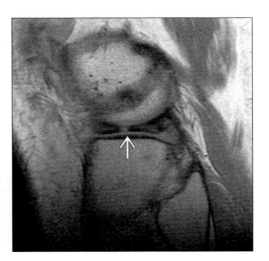

(Left) Sagittal PD/Intermediate MR shows degenerated & torn discoid lateral meniscus (arrow). *(Right)* Sagittal CSE PD image shows a degenerative discoid lateral meniscus. Hyperintense signal (arrow) is consistent with a tear. Meniscal bowties were identified on 3 consecutive images.

DISTAL FEMORAL METAPHYSEAL IRREGULARITY

  - Periosteal involvement
- MR
  - Periosteal, soft tissue involvement

Fibroxanthoma
- Identical to or overlaps DFMI in some cases
- Radiographs
  - Elongated in long axis of femur
  - Margin: Thin, sclerotic
- MR
  - T1 C+
    - Lesion enhances
  - T1WI
    - Lesion hypointense
  - T2WI
    - Lesion varies from hypointense to hyperintense

Non-ossifying fibroma
- Radiographs
  - Sclerotic border
  - Eccentric
  - Metaphyseal
- MR
  - T1WI: Lesions hypointense with even more hypointense margin (sclerotic border) at base
  - T2WI: Lesions intensity variable; hypointense margin at base

Leukemia
- Radiographs
  - Polyostotic metaphyseal abnormalities
  - Metaphyseal lucent band: Band horizontally oriented

Metaphyseal corner fracture
- Corner or bucket handle appearance
- Associated with child abuse in infants, much younger than DMFI

PATHOLOGY

General Features
- Etiology
  - Avulsion injury
    - At medial gastrocnemius heads origin or distal adductor magnus musculotendinous insertion

Microscopic Features
- Reactive process rather than neoplastic
  - Composed of cartilage, fibrous vascular tissue, fibrin
    - Cellular components: Chronic inflammatory cells, giant cells, osteoclasts
- Cellular appearance of healing process may mimic malignancy
- Histology on needle biopsy may lead to inappropriate amputation
- A "don't touch" lesion
- Avoid unnecessary biopsy

CLINICAL ISSUES

Presentation
- Most common signs/symptoms
  - Asymptomatic usually
    - Local pain an uncommon presentation

Demographics
- Age
  - Pediatric (immature-skeleton) population
    - Age range: 3-17 years; most common 10-15 years
  - Population including all ages
    - Age range 4-64 years; average age 34 years
- Gender: M:F = 1.4-3:1

Natural History & Prognosis
- Often disappears after epiphyseal closure

Treatment
- None
- Recognize lesion as variation not in need of biopsy
- Avoid unnecessary biopsy

SELECTED REFERENCES

1. Nakatani T et al: Periosteal osteoblastoma of the distal femur. Skeletal Radiol. 33(2):107-11, 2004
2. Verdonk PC et al: Distal femoral cortical irregularity in a 13-year old boy. A case report. Acta Orthop Belg. 69(4):377-81, 2003
3. Nawata K et al: Anomalies of ossification in the posterolateral femoral condyle: assessment by MRI. Pediatr Radiol. 29(10):781-4, 1999
4. Posch TJ et al: Marrow MR signal abnormality associated with bilateral avulsive cortical irregularities in a gymnast. Skeletal Radiol. 27(9):511-4, 1998
5. Suh JS et al: MR appearance of distal femoral cortical irregularity (cortical desmoid). J Comput Assist Tomogr. 20(2):328-32, 1996
6. Yamazaki T et al: MR findings of avulsive cortical irregularity of the distal femur. Skeletal Radiol. 24(1):43-6, 1995
7. Craigen MA et al: Symptomatic cortical irregularities of the distal femur simulating malignancy. J Bone Joint Surg Br. 76(5):814-7, 1994
8. Velchik MG et al: Bone scintigraphy: differentiating benign cortical irregularity of the distal femur from malignancy. J Nucl Med. 25(1):72-4, 1984
9. Resnick D et al: Distal femoral cortical defects, irregularities, and excavations. Radiology. 143(2):345-54, 1982
10. Kreis WR et al: Irregularity of the distal femoral metaphysis simulating malignancy: case report. J Bone Joint Surg Am. 59(6):38, 1977
11. Bufkin WJ: The avulsive cortical irregularity. Am J Roentgenol Radium Ther Nucl Med. 112(3):487-92, 1971
12. Brower AC et al: Histological nature of the cortical irregularity of the medial posterior distal femoral metaphysis in children. Radiology. 99(2):389-92, 1971
13. Schreiber SN et al: Irregularity of distal medial femoral epiphysis (Caffey). Direct observation at surgery four years later. N Y State J Med. 70(23):2921-2, 1970

DISTAL FEMORAL METAPHYSEAL IRREGULARITY

IMAGE GALLERY

Typical

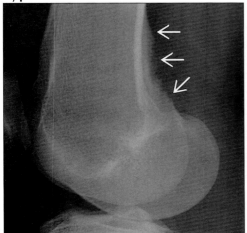
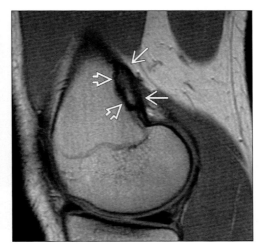

(Left) Lateral radiograph shows DFMI (arrows) in a 17 year old girl. *(Right)* Sagittal PD FSE MR in same patient shows hypointense periosteum (arrows) within the DFMI. A dark line (open arrows) represents thickened cortex at DFMI base.

Typical

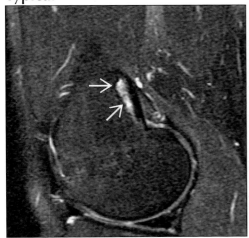
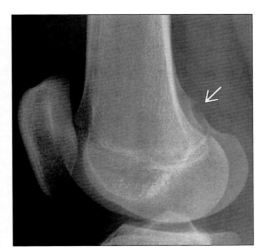

(Left) Sagittal T2 TSE FS MR in same patient shows central portion of DFMI to show hyperintense signal (arrows). *(Right)* Lateral radiograph shows a small DFMI (arrow) in a 14 year old girl.

Typical

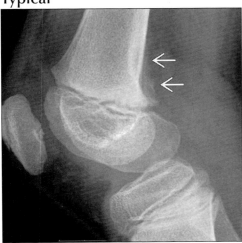
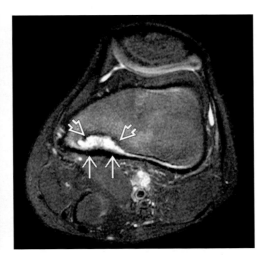

(Left) Lateral radiograph shows a DFMI with irregular, spiculated margins (arrows) in a 10 year old girl. The appearance can be deceivingly aggressive in appearance. *(Right)* Axial T2 TSE FS MR in same patient shows hyperintense signal of tissue (arrows) within same patient's DFMI. A hypointense margin (open arrows) is at lesion's base.

RICKETS

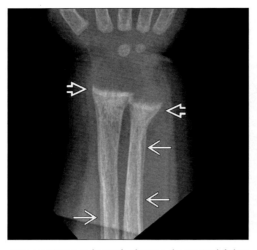

Anteroposterior radiograph shows subperiosteal failure of bone calcification (arrows) and metaphyseal cupping and splaying (open arrows) in a 12 month old with nutritional rickets.

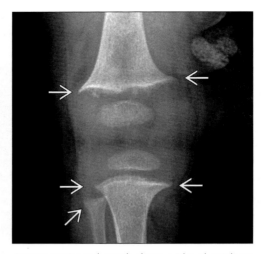

Anteroposterior radiograph shows widened epiphyses and splayed metaphyses (arrows) around knee joint in a 10 month old with nutritional rickets.

TERMINOLOGY

Abbreviations and Synonyms
- English disease

Definitions
- Rickets is failure of mineralization of osteoid and newly-formed bone in child's skeleton
- Causes of rickets in children younger than six months
  - Hypophosphatasia
    - Hypophosphatemia/hypocalcemia is cause of rickets in severe osteopetrosis
  - Prematurity
    - Radiologic rickets in 55% with birth weight < 1000 gm
  - Primary hyperparathyroidism
  - Prenatal factors
    - Maternal hyperparathyroidism
    - Maternal vitamin D deficiency
    - Maternal renal insufficiency
- Causes of rickets in children older than six months
  - Nutritional rickets: Simple vitamin D deficiency due to lack of vitamin D in diet or inadequate exposure to sunlight is most common cause; calcium deficiency a cause in Turkey and in both tropical and subtropical Africa (rare elsewhere)
  - Liver disease: Impaired 25-hydroxyvitamin D formation: Also, unconjugated bilirubin → interference with osteoblast function
    - Chronic liver disease: Extrahepatic biliary atresia, total parenteral nutrition, tyrosinemia
    - Anticonvulsant therapy: Phenytoin and phenobarbital activate P-450 cytochrome oxidase → accelerated conversion of 25-hydroxyvitamin D to inactive metabolites
  - Malabsorption: Binding with malabsorbed fatty acids → impaired calcium and vitamin D absorption
    - Celiac disease
    - Inflammatory bowel disease
    - Pancreatic insufficiency
  - Renal tubular insufficiency: Various impairments of renal tubular resorption of phosphate and 1-alpha-hydroxylation of 25-hydroxyvitamin D
    - Vitamin D resistant rickets (familial hypophosphatemic rickets or x-linked hypophosphatemic rickets); most frequent cause of renal-tubular insufficiency rickets
    - Vitamin D dependent (pseudodeficiency rickets); due to defective 1-alpha-hydroxylation in renal proximal tubule or end-organ resistance to vitamin D
    - Fanconi syndrome (nephrotic-glucosuric dwarfism with hypophosphatemic rickets)

DDx: Epiphysometaphyseal Lucent Lesions

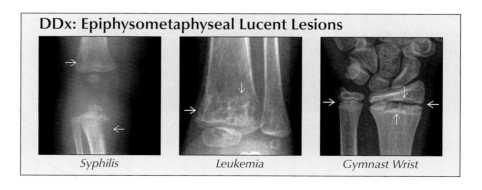

Syphilis   *Leukemia*   *Gymnast Wrist*

RICKETS

Key Facts

Terminology
- Nutritional rickets: Simple vitamin D deficiency due to lack of vitamin D in diet or inadequate exposure to sunlight is most common cause; calcium deficiency a cause in Turkey and in both tropical and subtropical Africa (rare elsewhere)

Imaging Findings
- Best diagnostic clue: Widened long-bone physes with cupped, splayed, and frayed metaphyses
- Healing: Increased density in zone of provisional calcification seen after treatment in 2-3 weeks with nutritional rickets and 2-3 months with renal rickets

Top Differential Diagnoses
- Leukemia
- Congenital syphilis

- Gymnast wrist

Pathology
- Normal bone development depends upon ready availability of calcium, phosphorus, and vitamin D
- Rickets: Calcification of cartilage and osteoid does not occur → widening of the zone of provisional calcification, which is perceived as physeal widening on radiographs
- Rickets: Metaphyseal widening and cupping caused by stress at sites of ligament attachments, splaying of cartilage cells peripherally, and microfracturing of primary spongiosa by protrusion of physeal cartilage

Clinical Issues
- Most cases of rickets respond to vitamin D therapy and, if necessary, calcium supplementation

---

- Lowe (oculocerebrorenal syndrome); cataracts, glaucoma, severe mental retardation
- Cystine storage disease
- Oncogenic rickets: Paraneoplastic syndrome that has been reported with non-ossifying fibroma, hemangiopericytoma, osteoblastoma, and linear sebaceous nevus syndrome
- Ifosfamide renal-tubule toxicity: Side affect of an alkylating agent used to treat malignancy
- Chronic renal disease: Renal osteodystrophy a combination of rickets and secondary hyperparathyroidism
  - Impaired glomerular function → phosphorus retention → hypocalcemia
  - Tubular dysfunction → impaired synthesis of 1,25-dihydroxyvitamin D → hypocalcemia
  - Hypocalcemia → hyperparathyroidism
  - Seen in pyelonephritis, polycystic kidney disease, chronic glomerulonephritis, renal tubular acidosis

IMAGING FINDINGS

General Features
- Best diagnostic clue: Widened long-bone physes with cupped, splayed, and frayed metaphyses

Radiographic Findings
- Skull and face
  - Postural molding
  - Frontal bossing
  - Premature fusion of sagittal suture
  - Delayed eruption of teeth, enamel hypoplasia
- Axial skeleton
  - Costo-chondral junctions: Cupping of rib ends, widening of rib epiphyseal cartilage (rachitic rosary)
  - Spine: Scoliosis, biconcave vertebral bodies
  - Pelvis: Tri-radiate appearance due to inward migration of sacrum and acetabula; causes dystocia in adulthood
- Appendicular skeleton
  - Epiphyses: Outline of ossification centers is indistinct
  - Physes: Widening and irregularity
  - Metaphyses: Fraying, splaying, and widening
  - Diaphyses: Bowing, osteopenia, sub-periosteal lucent lines, tunneling, fractures
    - Bowdler spurs: Radial, ulnar, and fibular transverse bone spurs underneath cutaneous dimples in hypophosphatasia
  - Bowing: Most common in femur and tibia
    - Severe in neonatal hypophosphatasia
  - Hip: Coxa vara, protrusio acetabuli
  - Knees: Genu valgum or varum
  - Osteoporosis: Profound in neonatal hypophosphatasia
  - Periosteal reaction: Due either to occult fracture or accumulation of unmineralized osteoid under periosteum (tunneling)
- Soft tissues
  - Late development of calcification in joint capsules, ligaments, and tendon insertions in vitamin D resistant rickets
  - Nephrocalcinosis in hypophosphatasia
- Renal osteodystrophy
  - Subperiosteal bone resorption
    - Best seen in lamina dura of teeth, distal clavicle, distal radius and ulna, middle phalanges of hands, medial femoral neck, and upper medial proximal tibia (mimics Wimberger sign seen in congenital syphilis)
  - Outer bone cortex unsharp and hazy
  - Endosteal bone resorption → lacy pattern of inner cortex (cortical tunneling)
  - Increased risk for slipped capital femoral epiphysis
  - Brown tumors of hyperparathyroidism
- Healing rickets after vitamin D therapy
  - Healing: Increased density in zone of provisional calcification seen after treatment in 2-3 weeks with nutritional rickets and 2-3 months with renal rickets

MR Findings
- Widened physes with increased T2 signal
  - Physeal width 2.5-3.0 mm in rickets (normal range 0.9-1.9 mm)
- Absent zone of provisional calcification

RICKETS

Ultrasonographic Findings
- Nephrocalcinosis: Monitor kidneys, especially in hypophosphatasia

DIFFERENTIAL DIAGNOSIS

Leukemia
- Metaphyseal lucent bands mimic epiphyseal widening

Congenital syphilis
- Metaphyseal lucent bands due to syphilitic osteitis mimic epiphyseal widening
- Focal destruction of upper medial tibial metaphysis cortex mimics cortical bone resorption seen in renal osteodystrophy

Gymnast wrist
- Widening of the distal radial and ulnar physes due to repetitive stress

PATHOLOGY

General Features
- Etiology
  - Normal bone development depends upon ready availability of calcium, phosphorus, and vitamin D
    - Rickets is a consequence of decreased availability of these substances
  - Calcium
    - Essential for formation of hydroxyapatite crystals
  - Phosphorus
    - Essential for formation of hydroxyapatite crystals
  - Vitamin D
    - Promotes absorption of calcium from intestine
    - Promotes calcium resorption in renal proximal tubules
    - Regulates apoptosis of chondrocytes, mineralization of cartilage matrix, and metaphyseal angiogenesis
- Epidemiology
  - African-American children: Skin melanin pigment absorbs ultraviolet radiation; African-Americans need more sunlight exposure to achieve adequate vitamin D production
  - Rickets may be caused by dietary calcium deficiency in Turkey and in both tropical and subtropical Africa

Microscopic Features
- Physis consists of four zones of cartilage
  - Resting cartilage cells
  - Proliferating cartilage cells
  - Hypertrophic columns of cartilage cells
  - Provisional calcification of cartilage matrix
    - First 3 zones are radiolucent; 4th zone's density similar to that of spongy bone
- Metaphyseal spongiosa adjacent to zone of provisional calcification: Cartilage matrix replaced by osteoid, followed by remodeling and calcification → spongy bone occupying marrow cavity
- Rickets: Calcification of cartilage and osteoid does not occur → widening of the zone of provisional calcification, which is perceived as physeal widening on radiographs
  - Diminished calcification of cartilage matrix, continued osteoid production by osteoblasts, and diminished resorption of osteoid because of impaired osteoclast function
- Rickets: Metaphyseal widening and cupping caused by stress at sites of ligament attachments, splaying of cartilage cells peripherally, and microfracturing of primary spongiosa by protrusion of physeal cartilage

CLINICAL ISSUES

Presentation
- Most common signs/symptoms
  - Upper and lower extremities
    - Short stature
    - Bow legs and (uncommonly) knock knees
    - Swelling of wrists, knees, and ankles
  - Skull
    - Craniotabes (soft skull bones that can be easily indented), frontal bossing
    - Delayed closure of anterior fontanelle
  - Torso
    - Scoliosis, accentuated lumbar lordosis
    - Rickets rosary: Expanded costo-chondral junctions
    - Harrison's sulcus deformity of soft rib cage, caused by inward diaphragmatic pull
  - Seizures due to hypocalcemia

Treatment
- Most cases of rickets respond to vitamin D therapy and, if necessary, calcium supplementation

SELECTED REFERENCES
1. Kulkarni ML et al: Rickets in osteopetrosis--a paradoxical association. Indian Pediatr. 40(6):561-5, 2003
2. Wharton B et al: Rickets. Lancet. 362(9393):1389-400, 2003
3. Mughal Z: Rickets in childhood. Semin Musculoskelet Radiol. 6(3):183-90, 2002
4. States LJ: Imaging of metabolic bone disease and marrow disorders in children. Radiol Clin North Am. 39(4):749-72, 2001
5. Ecklund K et al: Rickets on MR images. Pediatr Radiol. 29(9):673-5, 1999
6. Backstrom MC et al: Metabolic bone disease of prematurity. Ann Med. 28(4):275-82, 1996
7. Lee DY et al: Acquired vitamin D-resistant rickets caused by aggressive osteoblastoma in the pelvis: a case report with ten years' follow-up and review of the literature. J Pediatr Orthop. 14(6):793-8, 1994
8. Herman TE et al: Inherited diseases of bone density in children. Radiol Clin North Am. 29(1):149-64, 1991
9. Oestreich AE et al: Prominent transverse (Bowdler) bone spurs as a diagnostic clue in a case of neonatal hypophosphatasia without metaphyseal irregularity. Pediatr Radiol. 19(5):341-2, 1989

RICKETS

IMAGE GALLERY

Typical

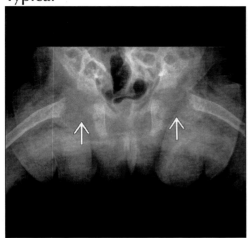
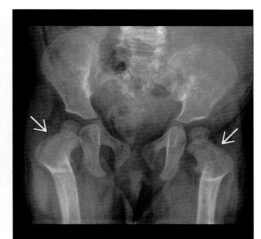

(Left) Frog-lateral radiograph shows pelvic osteopenia and unossified femoral necks *(arrows)* in a nine month old child with renal rickets. *(Right)* Anteroposterior radiograph shows deformed femoral necks *(arrows)*, greater trochanters, and lesser trochanters 12 months later in same child.

Typical

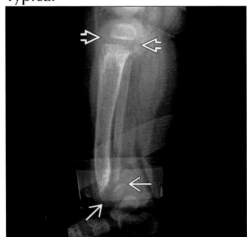
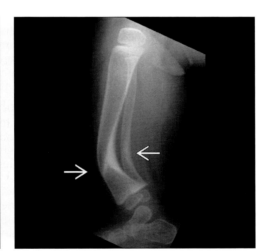

(Left) Lateral radiograph shows epiphysiodesis-like deformity *(arrows)* of the distal tibia and fibula in a nine month old with renal rickets. Proximal tibial physis is wide *(open arrows)*. *(Right)* Lateral radiograph of same child nine months later shows angular bowing *(arrows)* of the tibia and fibula and healing of rickets.

Typical

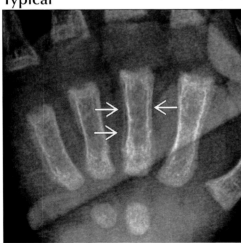
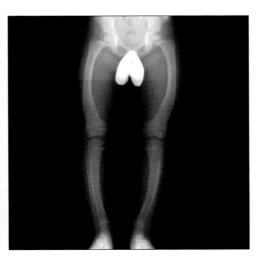

(Left) Posteroanterior radiograph shows cortical subperiosteal resorption and tunneling *(arrows)* in metacarpals due to secondary hyperparathyroidism in 10 month old with severe nutritional rickets. *(Right)* Anteroposterior radiograph shows bowed femurs and tibias with mild bowlegs in a 6.5 year old with hypophosphatemic rickets.

FIBROMATOSIS COLLI

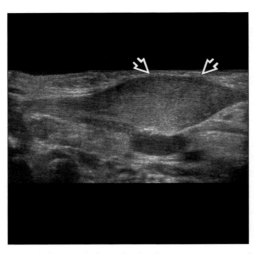

Sagittal ultrasound shows focal enlargement (arrows) of the sternocleidomastoid muscle which is mildly increased in echotexture. Note fusiform thickening without extension outside the muscle belly.

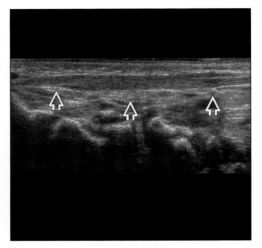

Sagittal ultrasound shows normal contralateral side in the same patient. Note the uniform thickness of the sternocleidomastoid muscle along its entire length (arrows).

TERMINOLOGY

Abbreviations and Synonyms
- Sternocleidomastoid pseudotumor, sternocleidomastoid tumor of infancy (SCTI), congenital muscular torticollis, neonatal torticollis

Definitions
- Most common cervical "mass" of infancy; benign fibrosis of sternocleidomastoid; postulated to be due to birth trauma or peripartum injury
- Torticollis (AKA: Wry neck) is a persistent twisting of the neck such that the ear on the affected side is positioned lower and more midline than normal

IMAGING FINDINGS

General Features
- Best diagnostic clue
  - Focal thickening and fibrosis of sternal or clavicular head of sternocleidomastoid muscle (SCM)
  - Process is entirely intra-muscular, without local invasion or inflammatory changes
- Location
  - Middle or lower third of SCM muscle belly
  - Sternal and clavicular muscle bundles equally often affected
- Size
  - 1-3 cm in length
  - May increase in size in first 2-3 months of life
- Morphology: Thickening of muscle that blends with normal muscle above and below and lacks surrounding inflammatory changes or adenopathy

Radiographic Findings
- Occasionally cervical spine films are obtained to exclude bony abnormality causing torticollis
  - Hemivertebrae or omovertebral bones are congenital anomalies that are not equivalent to fibromatosis colli
- May see nonspecific soft tissue fullness or "mass"
- Virtually never calcifies
  - If calcium is seen, consider neuroblastoma and teratoma

CT Findings
- Nonenhancing focal thickening of sternocleidomastoid muscle
- Axial or coronal imaging optimal for showing both SCM, side to side comparison
- No associated adenopathy or regional inflammatory changes

MR Findings
- T1WI
  - Fusiform enlargement of affected SCM

DDx: Differential Considerations

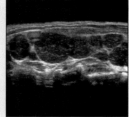
Cervical Adenopathy

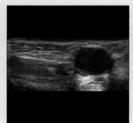
Thyroglossal Duct Cyst

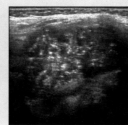
Neuroblastoma

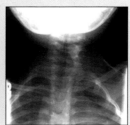
Omovertebral Bone

FIBROMATOSIS COLLI

Key Facts

Terminology
- Sternocleidomastoid pseudotumor, sternocleidomastoid tumor of infancy (SCTI), congenital muscular torticollis, neonatal torticollis
- Most common cervical "mass" of infancy; benign fibrosis of sternocleidomastoid; postulated to be due to birth trauma or peripartum injury

Imaging Findings
- Focal thickening and fibrosis of sternal or clavicular head of sternocleidomastoid muscle (SCM)
- Middle or lower third of SCM muscle belly
- Morphology: Thickening of muscle that blends with normal muscle above and below and lacks surrounding inflammatory changes or adenopathy
- Subtle alteration of echotexture and muscular enlargement within the sternal or clavicular head of the SCM
- Affected sternocleidomastoid is shorter and thicker than the contralateral side

Top Differential Diagnoses
- Cervical lymphadenopathy
- Congenital neuroblastoma
- Rhabdomyosarcoma
- Branchial cleft and cervical arch anomalies

Clinical Issues
- Painless palpable mass and torticollis
- Self-limited, usually resolves completely by 6 months of age

---

- Variable signal intensity
  - Usually isointense-hypointense to normal muscle
- T2WI
  - Variable signal intensity
    - Zones of hypointensity at maximal enhancement
    - Hypointense zones probably due to evolving fibrosis
    - Hyperintense to isointense to other muscles elsewhere within affected muscle
- T1 C+: Affected muscle enhances heterogeneously
- Affected sternocleidomastoid is shorter and thicker than the contralateral side

Ultrasonographic Findings
- Grayscale Ultrasound
  - Subtle alteration of echotexture and muscular enlargement within the sternal or clavicular head of the SCM
    - Hypoechoic mass, hyperechoic mass, and mixed echotexture have all been described in fibromatosis colli
  - Affected sternocleidomastoid is shorter and thicker than the contralateral side
    - Comparison with asymptomatic side is useful
    - Extended field of view imaging to show entire length of SCM is useful
  - Fascial planes surrounding the sternocleidomastoid are preserved
  - No associated adenopathy, edema, or fluid collection
  - Lack of extra-muscular involvement excludes other differential diagnoses
- Color Doppler
  - Variable hyperemia in acute phase
  - May see diminished blood-flow in quiescent, fibrotic phase

Imaging Recommendations
- Best imaging tool
  - Ultrasound is modality of choice when imaging is required
  - Often diagnosed clinically without imaging
  - MRI reserved for atypical cases
  - Intracranial (in rhabdomyosarcoma) and intraspinal (in neuroblastoma) extension are best imaged with MRI
  - CT is best modality for showing bony erosion, destruction, remodeling, or congenital scoliosis
- Protocol advice
  - regardless of modality of imaging, absence of the following findings suggests fibromatosis colli
    - Involvement of tissues outside the sternocleidomastoid muscle
    - Associated lymphadenopathy
    - Airway compression
    - Vascular encasement
    - Bone involvement
    - Intracranial/intraspinal extension
    - Other neck masses

DIFFERENTIAL DIAGNOSIS

Cervical lymphadenopathy
- Nodes are usually easily recognizable, though when enlarged and confluent may appear mass-like
- Adenopathy more likely to have lobulated contour than smooth, spindle shape of SCTI

Congenital neuroblastoma
- This tumor would originate along the sympathetic nerves in the neck outside the sternocleidomastoid muscle
- Growth may be invasive or more benign in appearance, insinuating between adjacent structures
- Look for calcification, intraspinal extension, and bony erosion

Rhabdomyosarcoma
- Typically enhancing, more vascular than adjacent muscle and has invasive growth pattern
- Look for vascular encasement and intracranial extension

Branchial cleft and cervical arch anomalies
- More often cystic than solid and arise adjacent to sternocleidomastoid rather than within the muscle

Infantile desmoid fibromatosis of the sternocleidomastoid muscle
- Infiltrative, aggressive growth pattern is different from SCTI
- Local recurrence common after resection of infantile fibromatosis lesions

Cervical extension of mediastinal thymus
- Look for contiguity with mediastinal thymic tissue
- Sonographically thymus has characteristic "dot and dash" appearance

Cervical teratoma
- Typically contain calcification, are often large, and present with airway or feeding difficulties

Spinal fusion anomalies
- Cervical scoliosis due to hemivertebra, fused vertebra, bony bar, omovertebral body, etc. (can cause torticollis)

PATHOLOGY

General Features
- Genetics: No genetic predisposition
- Etiology: Uncertain: Probably due to perinatal injury, partial muscle tear or intramuscular hematoma
- Epidemiology: Present in 0.4% of live births

Gross Pathologic & Surgical Features
- Seldom resected
- Fine needle aspirates more common than excisional specimens
- Firm, spindle shaped thickening of muscle, without transmuscular inflammation

Microscopic Features
- Cytologic features of fibromatosis are bland-appearing fibroblasts and degenerative atrophic skeletal muscle in a clean background
- Collagen is always present
- Occasional muscle giant cells, bland, bare nuclei, and parallel clusters of fibroblasts

CLINICAL ISSUES

Presentation
- Most common signs/symptoms
  - Painless palpable mass and torticollis
  - Contralateral occipital flattening (plagiocephaly) is common
  - History of breech presentation and "difficult" vaginal birth are common, but not mandatory
- Other signs/symptoms: If severe or persistent, limited range of motion in the neck and facial asymmetry can result

Demographics
- Age
  - Newborn infants
  - Classically noticed at less than 8 weeks of age, but may worsen in first 2-3 months of life
- Gender: Males slightly more often affected than females
- Right side affected more often than left
- Breech presentation associated

Natural History & Prognosis
- Self-limited, usually resolves completely by 6 months of age
- Occasional cases recur or flare during periods of rapid somatic growth

Treatment
- Physical therapy to encourage full range of motion, "stretch" the sternocleidomastoid muscle
- 90% full recovery with conservative treatment/physiotherapy
- Surgery only indicated in unusual cases when craniofacial asymmetry or refractory torticollis persists after one year

SELECTED REFERENCES
1. Ekinci S et al: Infantile fibromatosis of the sternocleidomastoid muscle mimicking muscular torticollis. J Pediatr Surg. 39(9):1424-5, 2004
2. Parikh SN et al: Magnetic resonance imaging in the evaluation of infantile torticollis. Orthopedics. 27(5):509-15, 2004
3. Sharma S et al: Fibromatosis colli in infants. A cytologic study of eight cases. Acta Cytol. 47(3):359-62, 2003
4. Robbin MR et al: Imaging of musculoskeletal fibromatosis. Radiographics. 21(3):585-600, 2001
5. Toma PL et al: Paediatric ultrasound. II. Other applications. Eur Radiol. 11(12):2369-98, 2001
6. Jaber MR et al: Sternocleidomastoid tumor of infancy: two cases of an interesting entity. Int J Pediatr Otorhinolaryngol. 47(3):269-74, 1999
7. Ablin DS et al: Ultrasound and MR imaging of fibromatosis colli (sternomastoid tumor of infancy). Pediatr Radiol. 28(4):230-3, 1998
8. Bedi DG et al: Fibromatosis colli of infancy: variability of sonographic appearance. J Clin Ultrasound. 26(7):345-8, 1998
9. Eich GF et al: Fibrous tumours in children: imaging features of a heterogeneous group of disorders. Pediatr Radiol. 28(7):500-9, 1998
10. Garant M et al: Aggressive fibromatosis of the neck: MR findings. AJNR Am J Neuroradiol. 18(8):1429-31, 1997
11. Snitzer EL et al: Magnetic resonance imaging appearance of fibromatosis colli. Magn Reson Imaging. 15(7):869-71, 1997
12. Vazquez E et al: US, CT, and MR imaging of neck lesions in children. Radiographics. 15(1):105-22, 1995
13. Glasier CM et al: High resolution ultrasound characterization of soft tissue masses in children. Pediatr Radiol. 17(3):233-7, 1987
14. Kraus R et al: Sonography of neck masses in children. AJR Am J Roentgenol. 146(3):609-13, 1986

FIBROMATOSIS COLLI

IMAGE GALLERY

Typical

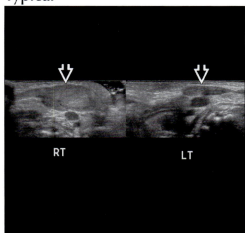 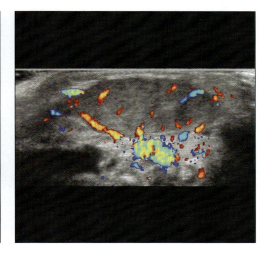

(Left) Transverse ultrasound comparing the two sides of the neck in a patient with fibromatosis colli. The SCM (arrows) is focally enlarged and mildly heterogeneous in echotexture on the right, and normal on the left. *(Right)* Transverse color Doppler ultrasound in the same patient shows normal to mildly decreased blood-flow within the enlarged muscle belly, suggesting healing phase of fibromatosis colli.

Typical

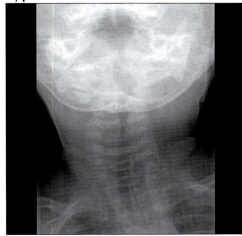 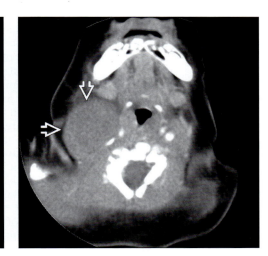

(Left) Anteroposterior radiograph shows twisted position of the neck in a patient with torticollis. The bones are normal; the airway is not compromised, and the soft tissues on the left are thickened. *(Right)* Axial CECT shows well-defined "mass" of thickened sternocleidomastoid muscle on the right (arrows) in a patient with fibromatosis colli. Note the lack of local invasion, inflammatory change and adenopathy.

Typical

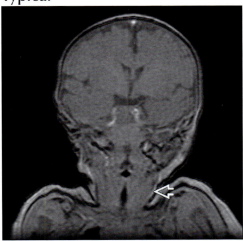 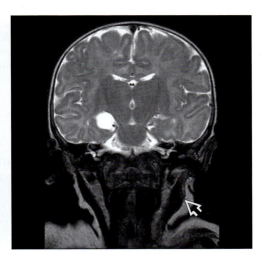

(Left) Coronal PD/Intermediate MR shows minimal thickening of the left SCM (arrow) compared to the right in a 14 month old with persistent torticollis who was scanned to exclude mass, given his persistent symptoms. *(Right)* Coronal T2WI MR shows focal thickening but normal signal intensity in the left SCM (arrow) in a patient with fibromatosis colli. This patient also had MRI for atypical clinical symptoms.

OSTEOCHONDRITIS DISSECANS

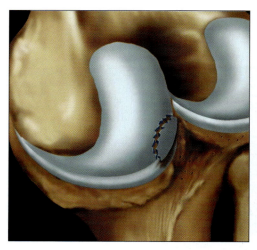

Coronal oblique graphic shows an osteochondral lesion of the lateral aspect of the medial femoral condyle (MFC). This is typical of OCD.

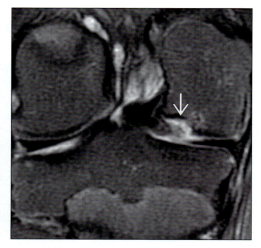

Coronal T2WI MR shows partially detached unstable lesion of the MFC with an overlying cartilage breach & fluid partially surrounding the OCD fragment (arrow).

TERMINOLOGY

Abbreviations and Synonyms
- Osteochondritis dissecans (OCD)

Definitions
- Osteochondrosis characterized by necrosis of bone followed by reossification & healing

IMAGING FINDINGS

General Features
- Best diagnostic clue: Osteochondral lesion within the lateral aspect of the medial femoral condyle (MFC) +/- loose fragment in a young adolescent athlete
- Location
  - Usually affects the lateral aspect of the MFC but can also affect the weight bearing surface of the lateral femoral condyle (LFC), tibia or patella
  - Much less commonly seen in elbow, ankle or hip
  - Rare in shoulder or wrist
- Size: Osteochondral fragment of variable size either contiguous with the donor site or detached from it
- Morphology: Joint cartilage + bone creating a crescent/oval osteochondral fragment
- Usually a lesion of adolescence often seen in athletes
- Osteochondral abnormalities including a stable or unstable fragment characterize the disease on MR imaging
- Predictors of instability on MR include
  - > 1 cm size
  - Displacement fragment or loose body
  - Fluid or arthrographic contrast between the fragment & parent bone
  - Cystic areas within the donor site
  - Enhancement of granulation tissue on post-gadolinium images between the donor site & fragment
- Additional signs of instability on radiographs
  - Larger than 0.8 cm² in area
  - Sclerotic margin > 3 mm
- Predictor of stability
  - Continuity of fragment with the parent bone without high signal intensity interface

Radiographic Findings
- Radiography
  - AP, lateral, axial (sunrise or merchant) views are suggested
  - Lucent subchondral lesion surrounded by a sclerotic margin

DDx: Osteochondral Signal Abnormalities & Variants

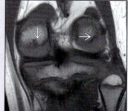
Normal Ossification

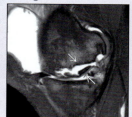
AVN

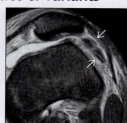
Osteochondral Fx

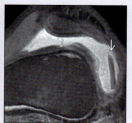
Delamination Injury

OSTEOCHONDRITIS DISSECANS

Key Facts

Terminology
- Osteochondritis dissecans (OCD)
- Osteochondrosis characterized by necrosis of bone followed by reossification & healing

Imaging Findings
- Predictors of instability on MR include
- > 1 cm size
- Displacement fragment or loose body
- Fluid or arthrographic contrast between the fragment & parent bone
- Cystic areas within the donor site
- Enhancement of granulation tissue on post-gadolinium images between the donor site & fragment
- Predictor of stability
- Continuity of fragment with the parent bone without high signal intensity interface
- MR arthrography: Improves visualization of fluid across articular cartilage surface thus helping determine whether the lesion is stable or unstable

Top Differential Diagnoses
- Normal irregular distal femoral epiphyseal ossification
- Avascular necrosis
- Osteochondral fracture or injury

Pathology
- MFC in 70-85%

Clinical Issues
- Gender: M > F = 3:1

- May demonstrate an area of sclerosis or fragmentation typically affecting the lateral aspect of the medial femoral condyle with or without a loose fragment

CT Findings
- NECT
  - CT arthrography
    - Contrast between OCD lesion & parent bone = instability
    - Loose bodies

MR Findings
- T1WI
  - Hypointense in fragment
  - +/- Hypointense subchondral marrow edema
- T2WI
  - Variable hyperintense signal, edema in the osteochondral fragment & adjacent marrow
  - The overlying defects in the articular cartilage are best appreciated on FS PD/T2WI FSE or stir images
  - FS PD/T2WI images may demonstrate direct extension of subchondral fluid indicating instability
  - +/- Hyperintense subchondral cysts
  - +/- Hyperintense synovium or joint fluid
- MR arthrography with intra-articular gadolinium
  - Contrast between OCD fragment & parent bone = unstable fragment
  - Loose bodies
- Chondral fragments are best seen on fat-saturated fast spin echo images
- All pulse sequences may demonstrate loose osteochondral fragments

Nuclear Medicine Findings
- Bone Scan: Focal significant accumulation of radioisotope on 3 phase bone scan can be a predictor of a loose body

Imaging Recommendations
- Best imaging tool: MRI or MR arthrography
- Protocol advice
  - AP, lateral, sunrise or merchant radiographs 1st
  - FS PD/T2WI FSE sagittal, coronal +/- axial (depending on location of OCD)
  - STIR, 3D GE cartilage sequence
  - Cartilage fragments: FS PD FSE
- MR arthrography: Improves visualization of fluid across articular cartilage surface thus helping determine whether the lesion is stable or unstable

DIFFERENTIAL DIAGNOSIS

Normal irregular distal femoral epiphyseal ossification
- More posteriorly in the femoral condyles than OCD
- Asymptomatic
- Most commonly lateral condyle
- Typical: No hyperintense T2WI signal changes in adjacent bone marrow

Avascular necrosis
- History of steroid therapy, lupus, sickle cell disease or other predisposing condition

Osteochondral fracture or injury
- Trauma history
- Different location than typical OCD lesions

Stress or insufficiency fracture
- Sclerotic band
- Not usually in subchondral location

PATHOLOGY

General Features
- General path comments
  - Unstable lesions
    - Large size (typically > 1 cm)
    - Cyst-like lesion beneath the osteochondrotic lesion
    - Contains loose granulation tissue
  - Loose fragment

OSTEOCHONDRITIS DISSECANS

- Fluid insinuating beneath the fragment at arthrography
- Loose body formation and residual deformity often present
- Etiology
  - Unknown, idiopathic
  - Repetitive microtrauma &/or ischemia
  - A predisposing trauma history is found in approximately 50%

Gross Pathologic & Surgical Features
- Necrotic desiccated bone fragment in unstable lesions
- Lateral aspect of MFC OCD usually extend to the intercondylar notch
- MFC in 70-85%
  - Lateral aspect of MFC: 55-60%
- LFC: 10-20%
- Patella: 5%
- Bilateral: 25-33%

Microscopic Features
- Osteonecrosis with variable amounts of healing

Staging, Grading or Classification Criteria
- Based on arthroscopic findings
- Stage 1: The lesion is 1 to 3 cm in size with intact articular cartilage
- Stage 2: Articular cartilage defect without a loose body
- Stage 3: Partially detached osteochondral fragments with or without fibrous tissue interposition
- Stage 4: Loose body formation

CLINICAL ISSUES

Presentation
- Most common signs/symptoms: Pain aggravated by exercise
- Other signs/symptoms
  - Can be asymptomatic
  - Swelling, pain over lesion
  - Clicking, catching or grinding
  - Locking
    - Must increase suspicion of unstable OCD

Demographics
- Age
  - Primarily affects male patients 10 to 20 years of age
  - Often seen in athletes
- Gender: M > F = 3:1

Natural History & Prognosis
- Usually spontaneous healing
- Unstable lesions rarely spontaneously heal
- Higher rate of spontaneous healing in children < 12 years old than adults
- Lesions along the weight bearing area of the condyle tend to not heal as readily

Treatment
- Stable lesions
  - Rest
    - Physical therapy
  - Splinting
  - NSAIDs
- Unstable lesions
  - Abrasion chondroplasty or chondral resurfacing
  - Drilling
  - Microfracture
  - Osteochondral autografts (OATS) or allografts
  - Chondrocyte implantation

DIAGNOSTIC CHECKLIST

Consider
- Osteochondral lesion involving the lateral aspect of MFC

Image Interpretation Pearls
- MR helpful in differentiating normal irregular ossification of the femoral condyle verses OCD in the knee

SELECTED REFERENCES

1. Cepero S et al: Osteochondritis of the femoral condyles in children and adolescents: our experience over the last 28 years. J Pediatr Orthop B. 14(1):24-9, 2005
2. Agung M et al: Osteochondritis dissecans of the talus treated by the transplantation of tissue-engineered cartilage. Arthroscopy. 20(10):1075-80, 2004
3. Flynn JM et al: Osteochondritis dissecans of the knee. J Pediatr Orthop. 24(4):434-43, 2004
4. Kobayashi T et al: Surgical fixation of massive osteochondritis dissecans lesion using cylindrical osteochondral plugs. Arthroscopy. 20(9):981-6, 2004
5. Nakagawa T et al: Internal fixation for osteochondritis dissecans of the knee. Knee Surg Sports Traumatol Arthrosc. 2004
6. Nixon AJ et al: Arthroscopic reattachment of osteochondritis dissecans lesions using resorbable polydioxanone pins. Equine Vet J. 36(5):376-83, 2004
7. Wright RW et al: Osteochondritis dissecans of the knee: long-term results of excision of the fragment. Clin Orthop Relat Res. (424):239-43, 2004
8. Boutin RD et al: MR imaging features of osteochondritis dissecans of the femoral sulcus. AJR Am J Roentgenol. 180(3):641-5, 2003
9. Letts M et al: Osteochondritis dissecans of the talus in children. J Pediatr Orthop. 23(5):617-25, 2003
10. Pill SG et al: Role of magnetic resonance imaging and clinical criteria in predicting successful nonoperative treatment of osteochondritis dissecans in children. J Pediatr Orthop. 23(1):102-8, 2003
11. Roach R: Osteochondral lesions of the talus. J Am Podiatr Med Assoc. 93(4):307-11, 2003
12. Robertson W et al: Osteochondritis dissecans of the knee in children. Curr Opin Pediatr. 15(1):38-44, 2003
13. Wall E et al: Juvenile osteochondritis dissecans. Orthop Clin North Am. 34(3):341-53, 2003
14. Long G et al: Magnetic resonance imaging of injuries in the child athlete. Clin Radiol. 54(12):781-91, 1999
15. Sales de Gauzy JC et al: Natural course of osteochondritis dissecans in children. J Pediatr Orthop B. 8(1):26-8, 1999
16. Cahill BR: Osteochondritis Dissecans of the Knee: Treatment of Juvenile and Adult Forms. J Am Acad Orthop Surg. 3(4) 237-47, 1995

OSTEOCHONDRITIS DISSECANS

IMAGE GALLERY

Typical

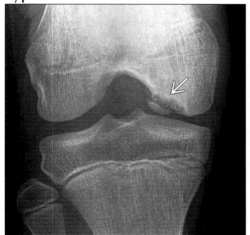
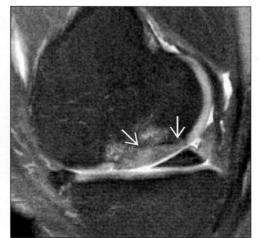

(Left) Radiograph tunnel view shows fragmentation & sclerosis of the adjacent MFC consistent with an OCD lesion *(arrow)*. This was a stable lesion on MR. *(Right)* Sagittal T2WI MR shows a stable, (despite > 1 cm in size) mildly hyperintense OCD lesion *(arrows)* with surrounding edema of the MFC. Note the intact overlying cartilage without fluid undermining the fragment.

Typical

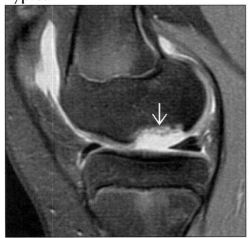
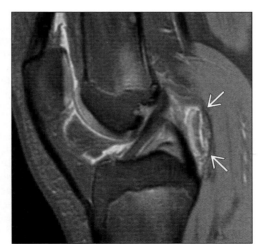

(Left) Sagittal PD/Intermediate MR shows an large hole (osteochondral defect) in the MFC *(arrow)* replaced by fluid. This is consistent with an unstable OCD & displaced fragment. *(Right)* Sagittal PD/Intermediate MR in the same patient shows the large displaced osteochondral fragment *(arrows)* posterior to the PCL.

Variant

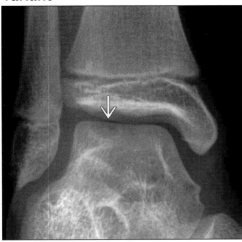
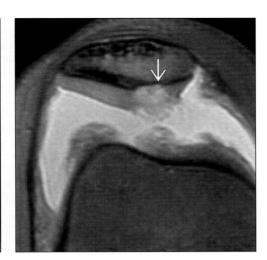

(Left) Anteroposterior radiograph shows a lucent lesion in the lateral talar dome *(arrow)* with a minimal sclerotic margin, consistent with a OCD lesion. *(Right)* Axial PD/Intermediate MR shows hyperintense signal, an OCD lesion *(arrow)* at the apex of the patellar cartilage.

SICKLE CELL ANEMIA, BONE

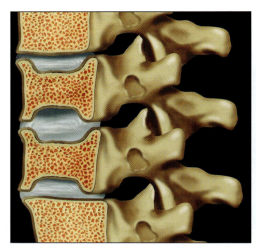

Lateral graphic shows the "H" shape of vertebral bodies caused by depression of the central parts of vertebral end plates.

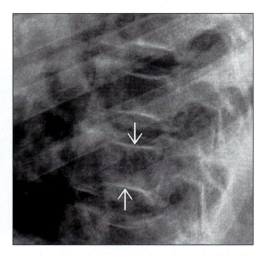

Lateral radiograph shows H-shaped vertebral bodies due to movement of the central part of the vertebral end plates (arrows) away from the intervertebral disks

TERMINOLOGY

Definitions
- Sickle cell (SS) disease
  - Homozygous sickle cell disease: Anemia severe
- Sickle cell (SC) disease
  - Sickle cell - hemoglobin C disease: Anemia mild
- SS-α thalassemia
  - Sickle cell - α thalassemia: Anemia severe
- SS-β thalassemia
  - Sickle cell - β thalassemia: Anemia mild-to-severe
- Sickle cell trait
  - Heterozygous carrier of gene

IMAGING FINDINGS

General Features
- Best diagnostic clue
  - H-shaped vertebrae
  - Bone marrow infarction
  - Sclerotic bone in marrow cavity

Radiographic Findings
- Radiography
  - Skull and face
    - Widening of diploic space with hair-on-end appearance
    - Mandible: Coarse marrow trabeculae; avascular necrosis of condyle
    - Bone infarctions causing areas of lucency or sclerosis
    - Temporal bone: Extramedullary hematopoiesis in middle ear
    - Orbital wall infarction with proptosis (orbital compression syndrome)
  - Spine
    - Depressed vertebral end plates: Bodies H-shaped if central depression is symmetric
    - Vertebral infarction with decreased height: Adjacent vertebra may show compensatory enlargement (tower vertebra)
    - Thoracic kyphosis and lumbar lordosis, osteopenia
    - Extramedullary hematopoiesis mass in spinal canal
  - Chest
    - Rib infarction: Can be part of the acute chest syndrome (chest pain, dyspnea, cough with new pulmonary consolidation)
    - Ribs and sternum: Bone infarctions causing areas of lucency or sclerosis within bone
    - Extramedullary hematopoiesis: Posterior mediastinum
  - Pelvis
    - Osteomyelitis, osteitis pubis, protrusio acetabuli
  - Extremities

DDx: Narrow Vertebral Bodies

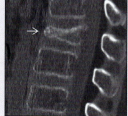

Steroid Use

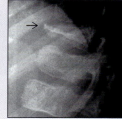

Leukemia

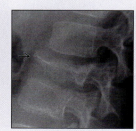

LCH Vertebra Plana

SICKLE CELL ANEMIA, BONE

Key Facts

Imaging Findings
- Widening of diploic space with hair-on-end appearance
- Rib infarction: Can be part of the acute chest syndrome (chest pain, dyspnea, cough with new pulmonary consolidation)
- Diametaphyseal infarction: Areas within bone of lucency or sclerosis after healing (months)
- Epiphyseal infarction commonest in humerus and femoral heads: Partial or complete epiphyseal necrosis
- Osteomyelitis: Most common in femur, tibia, humerus
- Dactylitis (hand-foot syndrome): Bone infarcts of phalanges and metacarpals/metatarsals of hands and feet usually at age 6-24 months
- Diffusely low signal of bone marrow on T1WI: Hematopoietic marrow instead of fatty marrow, transfusion hemosiderosis
- Bone marrow infarction: Photopenic defect initially on bone scan, may become photon-intense with healing and revascularization
- Infarction much more common than osteomyelitis

Pathology
- Incidence: 1 in 500-650 African-Americans

Clinical Issues
- Ethnicity: Majority of cases in African-Americans; also occurs in people of Spanish, Mediterranean, Turkish, Arabian Peninsula, and Indian subcontinent descent

---

- Diametaphyseal infarction: Areas within bone of lucency or sclerosis after healing (months)
- Epiphyseal infarction commonest in humerus and femoral heads: Partial or complete epiphyseal necrosis
- Osteomyelitis: Most common in femur, tibia, humerus
- Dactylitis (hand-foot syndrome): Bone infarcts of phalanges and metacarpals/metatarsals of hands and feet usually at age 6-24 months
- Dactylitis: Just soft tissue edema seen initially; then subperiosteal new bone formation and mottled cortical rarefaction visible
- Coarse trabecular pattern of spongiosa
- Cone-shaped epiphyses of metacarpals and phalanges
- Erosive disease of calcaneus: Superior cortex poorly-defined
- Retarded bone age
- IVP: Nephromegaly, renal papillary necrosis, focal cortical hypertrophy

MR Findings
- T1WI
  - Diffusely low signal of bone marrow on T1WI: Hematopoietic marrow instead of fatty marrow, transfusion hemosiderosis
  - Acute marrow infarction: Isointense or slightly hyperintense
- T2WI
  - Diffusely low signal of bone marrow: Hematopoietic marrow instead of fatty marrow, transfusion hemosiderosis
  - Acute marrow infarction: Focal hyperintense area
- T1 C+
  - Areas of avascular necrosis and acute marrow infarction do not enhance
  - Healing marrow infarcts may show intense marginal enhancement
  - Areas of osteomyelitis enhance
  - Difficult often to differentiate between osteomyelitis and infarction

Ultrasonographic Findings
- Grayscale Ultrasound: Nephromegaly

Nuclear Medicine Findings
- Bone Scan
  - Symmetric, marked expansion of hematopoietic marrow involving femur, calvaria, small bones of hand and feet
  - Bone marrow infarction: Photopenic defect initially on bone scan, may become photon-intense with healing and revascularization
  - Bone infarction vs. osteomyelitis
    - Infarction: Tc99m methylene diphosphonate (MDP) bone scan shows ↑ activity; Tc99m sulfur colloid marrow scan shows ↓ activity
    - Osteomyelitis: Tc99m MDP bone scan shows ↑ activity; Tc99m sulfur colloid marrow scan shows normal activity
    - Osteomyelitis: Ga67 citrate scan shows ↑ activity
    - Infarction much more common than osteomyelitis

DIFFERENTIAL DIAGNOSIS

Thalassemia
- Changes due to expansion of bone marrow are the same as in sickle cell disease, but exaggerated
- H-shaped vertebra
- Hair-on-end skull diploe
- Avascular necrosis less common than in sickle cell anemia
- Paravertebral masses: Extramedullary hematopoiesis

Familial hemolytic anemia (hereditary spherocytosis)
- Skull: Slight diploic widening
- Gallstones

Pyruvate kinase deficiency
- Wide diploic space, gallstones

SICKLE CELL ANEMIA, BONE

Glucose-6-phosphate dehydrogenase deficiency
- Bone changes absent

Sickle cell trait (heterozygous carrier)
- Marrow infarction is rare

Vertebral compression: Langerhans cell histiocytosis (LCH), leukemia, steroids
- Osteopenia or osteolysis

PATHOLOGY

General Features
- Genetics
  - Gene located on the short arm of chromosome 11
    - Homozygous: Sickle cell anemia always occurs
    - Heterozygous: Events such as bone infarction occur rarely
- Etiology
  - Normal human hemoglobin molecule contains 4 globin chains: 2 α and 2 β chains
    - In sickle cell disease, β chains are abnormal and the 2 β chains twist around each other (polymerization) causing rigid hemoglobin molecules and RBC (red blood cell) distortion
    - RBC distortion exaggerated with hypoxemia causing sickling (banana-shaped RBCs)
    - Sickled cells are short-lived (hemolytic anemia) and block small vessels (infarction)
- Epidemiology
  - Incidence: 1 in 500-650 African-Americans
  - Incidence: 1 in 2000 Hispanics coming from the Caribbean, Central America, South America
  - Stroke in 11% before 20 years old
  - Painful crisis in 50% by age 5
    - Most common cause of hospitalization; acute chest syndrome is the second most common cause
  - Percent of all bone infarcts found in individual bones: Femur 16%, tibia 15%, humerus 13%, spine 11%, radius 10%, ulna 8%, pelvis 8%, others 19%
  - 50-70% have gallstones by adulthood

Microscopic Features
- Normally, red or cellular marrow converts to yellow or fatty marrow during childhood
  - Begins in distal arms and legs
  - Red marrow residua persist in adult vertebrae, sternum, pelvis, ribs
- Cellular marrow persists in adults with sickle cell disease

CLINICAL ISSUES

Presentation
- Most common signs/symptoms: Pain due to vaso-occlusive crisis involving any organ, most commonly bone
- Painful chest and abdominal crises begin at 2-3 years of age; may be accompanied by bone infarctions
- Hemolytic anemia: Jaundice, gallstones
- Marrow, liver, pancreas hemosiderosis due to multiple transfusions
- Splenomegaly at first, then splenic atrophy
- Skeletal pain due to bone marrow infarction, osteomyelitis
- Osteomyelitis: Salmonella twice as common as Staphylococcus
- ASPEN syndrome: (A)ssociation of (S)S disease, (P)riapism, (E)xchange transfusion, and (N)eurologic events
- Autosplenectomy by progressive infarction

Demographics
- Ethnicity: Majority of cases in African-Americans; also occurs in people of Spanish, Mediterranean, Turkish, Arabian Peninsula, and Indian subcontinent descent

Natural History & Prognosis
- Mean survival 42 years
- Acute chest syndrome is the commonest cause of death

Treatment
- Sickle cell crisis: Oxygen, hydration, pain management, blood transfusion
  - High-dose methylprednisolone can reduce duration of pain
- Prophylactic penicillin, pneumococcal and H influenza vaccines to prevent infection

SELECTED REFERENCES
1. Kim SK et al: Natural history and distribution of bone and bone marrow infarction in sickle hemoglobinopathies. J Nucl Med. 43(7):896-900, 2002
2. Lonergan GJ et al: Sickle cell anemia. Radiographics. 21(4):971-94, 2001
3. Naran AD et al: Sickle cell disease with orbital infarction and epidural hematoma. Pediatr Radiol. 31(4):257-9, 2001
4. Rucknagel DL: The role of rib infarcts in the acute chest syndrome of sickle cell diseases. Pediatr Pathol Mol Med. 20(2):137-54, 2001
5. Skaggs DL et al: Differentiation between bone infarction and acute osteomyelitis in children with sickle-cell disease with use of sequential radionuclide bone-marrow and bone scans. J Bone Joint Surg Am. 83-A(12):1810-3, 2001
6. Umans H et al: The diagnostic role of gadolinium enhanced MRI in distinguishing between acute medullary bone infarct and osteomyelitis. Magn Reson Imaging. 18(3):255-62, 2000
7. Marlow TJ et al: "Tower vertebra": a new observation in sickle cell disease. Skeletal Radiol. 27(4):195-8, 1998
8. Howlett DC et al: The role of CT and MR in imaging the complications of sickle cell disease. Clin Radiol. 52(11):821-9, 1997
9. Gelfand MJ et al: Simultaneous occurrence of rib infarction and pulmonary infiltrates in sickle cell disease patients with acute chest syndrome. J Nucl Med. 34(4):614-8, 1993
10. el-Sabbagh AM et al: Avascular necrosis of temporomandibular joint in sickle cell disease. Clin Rheumatol. 8(3):393-7, 1989
11. Rao VM et al: Femoral head avascular necrosis in sickle cell anemia: MR characteristics. Magn Reson Imaging. 6:661-7, 1988

SICKLE CELL ANEMIA, BONE

IMAGE GALLERY

Typical

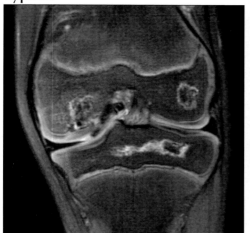
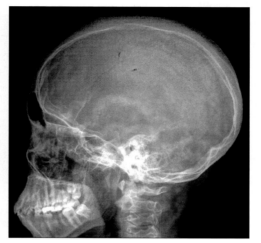

(Left) Coronal T2WI MR shows bone infarcts in femoral and tibial epiphyses. Infarcts have hypointense centers and hyperintense margins. *(Right)* Lateral radiograph shows widened diploic space and thinned outer table of the calvaria in the frontal and parietal bones of a 16 year old.

Typical

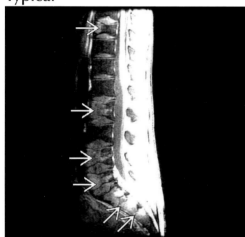
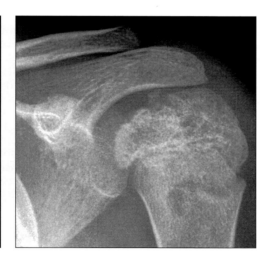

(Left) Sagittal T1WI MR shows increased signal in several thoracic and lumbar vertebrae and sacrum (arrows) due to bone marrow infarctions. *(Right)* Anteroposterior radiograph shows fragmentation and sclerosis of the medial third of humeral head ossification center due to bone infarction.

Typical

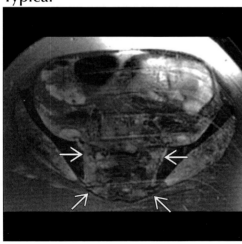
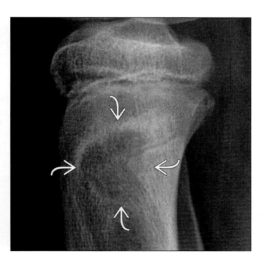

(Left) Axial T2WI MR shows increased signal of the entire sacrum (arrows) due to osteomyelitis. The signal of iliac bones is hypointense due to iron deposition. *(Right)* Lateral radiograph shows a healing tibial metaphysis bone infarct with a lucent center and sclerotic margins (arrows).

SCOLIOSIS

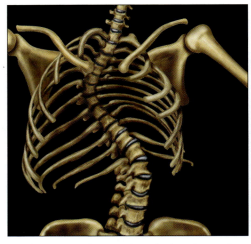

Graphic image shows S-shaped idiopathic scoliotic curve.

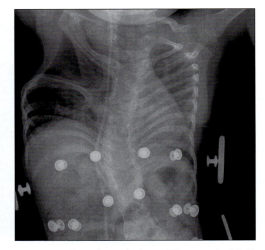

Anteroposterior radiograph shows diffuse vertebral & rib anomalies throughout the entire spine in this patient with a congenital scoliosis.

TERMINOLOGY

Abbreviations and Synonyms
- Scoliosis, idiopathic scoliosis, neuromuscular scoliosis, congenital scoliosis

Definitions
- Presence of lateral curvature(s) in the spine of over 10°, often associated with vertebral rotation
- 2 types
  o Flexible: Nonstructural; corrects with lateral bending
  o Structural: Rigid; does not demonstrate complete correction with lateral bending
- Idiopathic
  o Most common; 70-85% of all scoliosis
  o Infantile: < 3 years of age
    ▪ Typically develops 1st 6 months of life
    ▪ 1/4 associated with hip dysplasia
    ▪ Typical: Convex left thoracic curve (70%)
  o Juvenile: 4 to 9 years
    ▪ Typical: Convex right thoracic curve, progressive with growth
  o Adolescent: > 10 years
    ▪ Most common type; typical: Convex right S-shaped thoracic curve
    ▪ Compensatory left convex lumbar, ↑ rapidly with growth spurts
  o Most idiopathic scoliosis is not associated with underlying cause
    ▪ However, underlying anomalies can cause similar curves: Syringohydromyelia, Chiari I, cord neoplasm, disc disease
- Congenital
  o Result of vertebral anomalies; most common hemivertebrae (45%)
  o Typical: Thoracic or thoracolumbar curve
  o Occult spinal abnormality (15-40%)
  o Progressive scoliosis (3/4)
  o Image with MR
    ▪ Progressive curve (> 10°/year) or surgery planned
  o Associated with
    ▪ Spinal dysraphism: Lipoma, diastematomyelia, syringohydromyelia, tethered cord
    ▪ Genitourinary anomalies (6%), cardiac anomalies (15%), rib anomalies
- Neuromuscular
  o Cerebral palsy (CP), poliomyelitis, muscular dystrophy, syringohydromyelia, cord neoplasm
- Posttraumatic or inflammatory
  o Juvenile rheumatoid arthritis, tuberculosis, radiation therapy
- Dysplasias
  o Neurofibromatosis, Marfan syndrome, Ehlers-Danlos syndrome
- Neoplasm: Osteoid osteoma

DDx: Scoliosis

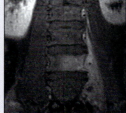

Osteomyelitis

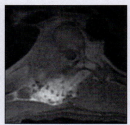

Osteosarcoma

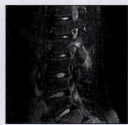

Osteoid Osteoma

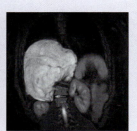

Ganglioneuroma

SCOLIOSIS

Key Facts

Terminology
- Presence of lateral curvature(s) in the spine of over 10°, often associated with vertebral rotation
- Idiopathic
- Most common; 70-85% of all scoliosis
- Congenital
- Neuromuscular
- Posttraumatic or inflammatory
- Dysplasias
- Neoplasm: Osteoid osteoma

Imaging Findings
- Helical with coronal, sagittal & 3D reconstruction for surgical planning
- Indications for MRI
- Congenital scoliosis
- Juvenile onset: 4-9 years
- Convex left thoracic or thoracolumbar curve
- Rapid progression of the curve (> 1 degree per month)
- Pain, headache, or neurological signs (cutaneous abdominal reflex) and symptoms (weakness, paresthesia, ataxia)

Pathology
- Epidemiology: 0.2-0.5% of the population in US

Clinical Issues
- Usually asymptomatic
- Rod or wire breakage, slippage of hook, infection, spondylolysis, superior mesenteric artery syndrome, pseudoarthrosis
- Fractured rod indicates failure of fusion
- Respiratory compromise

- Imaging evaluation depends on the cause of scoliosis
  - Initial erect anteroposterior from chin to greater trochanter
    - Posteroanterior on follow-up (less breast radiation) with gonadal & breast shielding
  - Lateral if clinical concern of excessive kyphosis or lordosis
  - Lateral bending films to assess the degree of mobility
  - Cobb method of measuring scoliosis angle
    - Perpendiculars to a line along the upper endplate of the upper vertebral body of the curve & a line along the lower endplate of the lower vertebral body of the curve
    - If endplates not seen use pedicles
    - Same vertebral bodies for follow-up measurements
- Left wrist/hand bone age film to assess amount of potential growth remaining in patient
- Iliac crests on the scoliosis study also provide clue to skeletal maturation
  - Iliac crest divided into 4 quadrants; Risser grade according to ossification of the iliac apophysis
  - Risser 0 no ossification; Risser I only lateral 1/4 ossified → to Risser IV all 4 quadrants ossified, Risser V fused iliac apophysis to ileum
  - At skeletal maturity scoliosis is unlikely to progress, unless > 40-50°

IMAGING FINDINGS

General Features
- Best diagnostic clue: Lateral curvature(s) in the spine
- Location: Classic imaging appearance: S-shaped curvature of the spine

Radiographic Findings
- Radiography
  - Idiopathic
    - Prevalence of typical curvature: Convex right thoracic curve > right thoracic & left lumbar > right thoracolumbar > right lumbar
    - Atypical curves: Convex left thoracic curve, left thoracolumbar, left cervical, left cervicothoracic
    - Vertebral rotation, L5 spondylolysis may be present
  - Congenital
    - Failure of vertebral formation (wedge vertebra, hemivertebra)
    - Failure of segmentation (pedicle bar, block vertebra)
    - Combination
  - Neuromuscular
    - Single long curve
  - Neurofibromatosis
    - Most lack distinctive diagnostic features
    - Classic: High thoracic acute curvature, kyphosis, rib anomalies, posterior vertebral scalloping

CT Findings
- NECT
  - Helical with coronal, sagittal & 3D reconstruction for surgical planning
  - Evaluates congenital vertebral anomalies
  - Assess spine for pseudoarthrosis following spinal fusion surgery

MR Findings
- T1WI: Coronal T1WI to evaluate vertebral anomalies
- Indications for MRI
  - Congenital scoliosis
  - Juvenile onset: 4-9 years
  - Convex left thoracic or thoracolumbar curve
  - Rapid progression of the curve (> 1 degree per month)
  - Pain, headache, or neurological signs (cutaneous abdominal reflex) and symptoms (weakness, paresthesia, ataxia)

Nuclear Medicine Findings
- Bone Scan: SPECT imaging for pseudoarthrosis following spinal fusion surgery

Imaging Recommendations
- Best imaging tool
  - Initial standing frontal & lateral scoliosis radiographs

SCOLIOSIS

- CT & MRI
- Protocol advice
  - T1, PDWI, T2WI or STIR
  - Helical NECT with sagittal & coronal reformats

DIFFERENTIAL DIAGNOSIS

Various other causes for scoliosis
- Differentiated by clinical history, plain film findings, and supplemented by MRI

Scoliosis
- Osteoid osteoma
  - Painful scoliosis
  - Typical: Pedicle or lamina
  - Ipsilateral to the convex side of the curve
- Inflammation, infection or tumor
  - Osteomyelitis, appendicitis, paraspinal mass or abscess, osteosarcoma
  - Painful scoliosis
- Limb length discrepancy
  - Convex curve ipsilateral to the shorter lower extremity
- Post-radiation
  - History of radiation, fatty replaced vertebral bodies

PATHOLOGY

General Features
- General path comments: Scoliosis represents a developmental anomaly of the spine
- Genetics: Autosomal dominant transmittance in idiopathic scoliosis, strongly familial (80%)
- Etiology: Majority are idiopathic
- Epidemiology: 0.2-0.5% of the population in US

CLINICAL ISSUES

Presentation
- Most common signs/symptoms
  - Usually asymptomatic
  - Pain from progressive curvature or degenerative disc & facet disease
  - Idiopathic scoliosis usually detected during physical exam

Demographics
- Age
  - Idiopathic
    - Infantile: Typically 1st 6 months; juvenile: 4-10 years; adolescent: 10 years to skeletal maturity
- Gender
  - Idiopathic: Female predilection (7 to 9:1)
  - Girls tend to progress more than boys in idiopathic scoliosis

Natural History & Prognosis
- Curvature less than 30 degrees will not progress when skeletally mature
- Worsening curvature in 25% of the cases
  - During adolescent growth spurts
  - Curves greater than 40 to 50 degrees after skeletal maturity
  - Cardiopulmonary complications from severe scoliosis
- Excellent prognosis with proper follow-up and treatment

Treatment
- Options, risks, complications
  - Rod or wire breakage, slippage of hook, infection, spondylolysis, superior mesenteric artery syndrome, pseudoarthrosis
    - Fractured rod indicates failure of fusion
  - Respiratory compromise
- Idiopathic
  - Observe < 20°
  - Brace (orthotics)
    - Unless < 10 years old at presentation, typically progressive
  - Electrical stimulation
  - Segmental fusion with pedicle screw fixation, thorascopic instrumentation & fusion
  - Anterior or posterior fusion with instrumentation in skeletally mature patients with > 40 degrees of curvature
- Congenital
  - Observation
  - Surgical: When progressive curve
    - In situ fusion, orthotic rarely helpful, anterior & posterior epiphysiodesis, hemivertebrae resection, reconstructive osteotomies
- Neuromuscular
  - Typical: Anterior & posterior spinal fusion

DIAGNOSTIC CHECKLIST

Image Interpretation Pearls
- Levoscoliosis or painful scoliosis, MR to exclude spinal pathology

SELECTED REFERENCES

1. Hedequist D et al: Congenital scoliosis. J Am Acad Orthop Surg. 12(4):266-75, 2004
2. Christodoulou A et al: Idiopathic scoliosis. Segmental fusion with transpedicular screws. Stud Health Technol Inform. 91:433-7, 2002
3. Goldberg CJ et al: The natural history of early onset scoliosis. Stud Health Technol Inform. 91:68-70, 2002
4. Vitale MG et al: Orthopaedic manifestations of neurofibromatosis in children: an update. Clin Orthop Relat Res. (401):107-18, 2002
5. Mohanty S et al: Patterns of presentation of congenital scoliosis. J Orthop Surg (Hong Kong). 8(2):33-37, 2000
6. Maiocco B et al: Adolescent idiopathic scoliosis and the presence of spinal cord abnormalities: Preoperative magnetic resonance imaging analysis. Spine. 22:2537-41, 1997
7. Barnes PD et al: Atypical idiopathic scoliosis: MR imaging evaluation. Radiology. 186:247-53, 1993
8. Nokes SR et al: Childhood scoliosis: MR imaging. Radiology. 164:791-7, 1987
9. McMaster MJ: Occult intraspinal anomalies and congenital scoliosis. J Bone Joint Surg Am. 66(4):588-601, 1984

SCOLIOSIS

IMAGE GALLERY

Typical

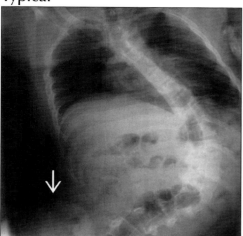
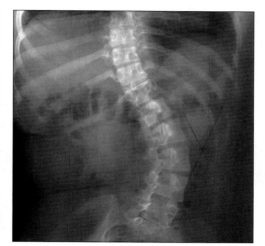

(Left) Anteroposterior radiograph shows a single long C-shaped of the thoracolumbar spine, neuromuscular scoliosis. Notice the associated pelvic obliquity (arrow) which is a typical finding in this patient with CP. *(Right)* Anteroposterior radiograph shows a long C-shaped neuromuscular scoliosis of the lumbar spine with pelvic obliquity & vertebral body rotation in this patient with poliomyelitis.

Typical

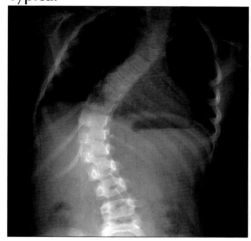
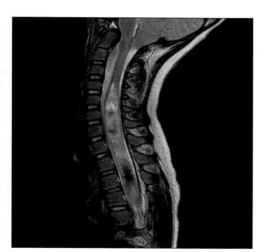

(Left) Anteroposterior radiograph shows an idiopathic scoliosis, a long dextroscoliosis of the thoracolumbar spine. *(Right)* Sagittal T2WI MR image in the same patient shows a large syringohydromyelia, that extended to approximately T10 (not on this image). Patient was imaged due to a rapidly progressive scoliosis & planning surgery.

Typical

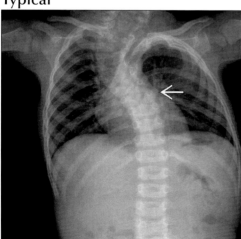
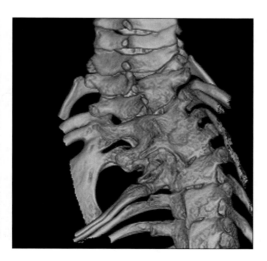

(Left) Anteroposterior radiograph shows numerous lower cervical & upper thoracic vertebral anomalies in this patient with congenital scoliosis. Notice the hemivertebra at the apex of the curve (arrow). *(Right)* 3D reformat image NECT for surgical planning shows numerous rib & vertebral segmentation anomalies in the upper thoracic spine in this congenital scoliosis.

SPONDYLOLYSIS

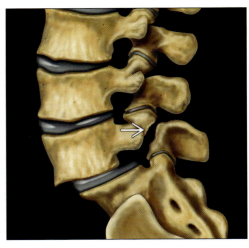

Sagittal graphic shows a separated defect within the pars interarticularis, spondylolysis at L5 (arrow) with anterior slippage, spondylolisthesis of L5 on S1.

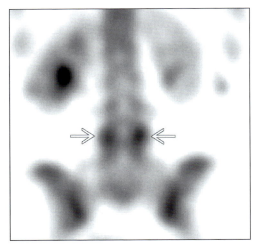

Coronal SPECT image from a bone scan shows intense uptake of tracer in the bilateral L4 posterior elements (arrows), healing bilateral spondylolysis.

TERMINOLOGY

Abbreviations and Synonyms
- Lysis, isthmic spondylolysis

Definitions
- Spondylolysis: Defects or breaks in the pars interarticularis thought to result from repetitive stress injury
- Spondylolisthesis: Anterior slipping of vertebral body above spondylolysis in relationship to vertebral body below spondylolysis

IMAGING FINDINGS

General Features
- Best diagnostic clue
  - Elongation of the spinal canal at the level of the pars defects on axial MR imaging
  - Classic imaging appearance: Discontinuity in the neck of the "Scotty dog" on oblique views of the lumbar spine
- Location
  - L5: 85%
  - L4: 15%
  - Rare elsewhere
  - Cervical spine usually congenital
- Morphology: Horizontal orientation on axial images
- Other key facts
  - 10-15% unilateral defects
    - Unilateral healing or union of a defect that was initially bilateral

Radiographic Findings
- Radiography
  - Anteroposterior, lateral & oblique radiographs for evaluation
  - Oblique film is most sensitive radiograph
  - Break in the neck of the "Scotty dog" as the pars interarticularis defect on oblique views of the standing lumbar spine
  - Anterolisthesis

CT Findings
- NECT
  - Discontinuous or "incomplete ring" sign on axial imaging
    - May simulate "extra" or double facet joints
  - Sometimes confused with a facet joint
    - Spondylolysis is located above the normal facet joint
    - Facet joint is smooth while spondylolysis typically is irregular or fragmented with sclerosis
    - More coronal in orientation compared to the facet joint

DDx: Spectrum Of Radiographic Findings In Back Pain

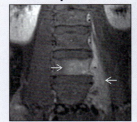
Osteomyelitis

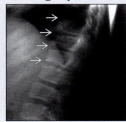
Scheuermann Disease

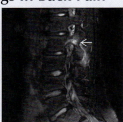
Osteoid Osteoma

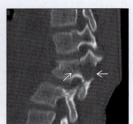
Chance Fracture

SPONDYLOLYSIS

Key Facts

Terminology
- Lysis, isthmic spondylolysis
- Spondylolysis: Defects or breaks in the pars interarticularis thought to result from repetitive stress injury
- Spondylolisthesis: Anterior slipping of vertebral body above spondylolysis in relationship to vertebral body below spondylolysis

Imaging Findings
- Elongation of the spinal canal at the level of the pars defects on axial MR imaging
- Classic imaging appearance: Discontinuity in the neck of the "Scotty dog" on oblique views of the lumbar spine
- L5: 85%
- L4: 15%
- Rare elsewhere
- Cervical spine usually congenital
- Intense focal uptake in the posterior elements unilaterally or bilaterally
- SPECT imaging helpful for diagnosis
- Triangular pattern of uptake on sagittal images

Pathology
- 4.4% at age 6
- 6% in adults
- Prevalence of 5-7% in the general population
- Higher incidence in competitive athletes, especially males
- Spondylolisthesis (50%)

Clinical Issues
- Age: 10-20 year old

○ Sagittal or oblique sagittal reformatted imaging vital in assessment
○ Linear lucency or defect in the pars interarticularis
○ Fragmentation of the pars interarticularis
○ Spondylolisthesis & foraminal narrowing on sagittal reformatted images
○ May be insensitive to early stress injury (edema with microtrabecular fracture)
○ Secondary finding of sclerosis &/or hypertrophy of contralateral pedicle & lamina
○ Anterolisthesis

MR Findings
- T1WI
  ○ Hypointense signal in pars interarticularis
  ○ Discontinuity (best sagittal images)
- T2WI
  ○ Hyperintense signal in pars interarticularis (marrow edema)
  ○ Hypointense signal in pars interarticularis (reactive sclerosis)
- Elongation of the spinal canal at the level of the pars defects
- More horizontal configuration of the affected neural foramina on sagittal imaging
- Loss of fat surrounding the exiting nerve roots
- Decreased disc height
- MR
  ○ Sensitivity: 57-86%
  ○ Specificity: 81-82%
  ○ Positive predictive value: 14-18%
  ○ Negative predictive value: 97-99%

Nuclear Medicine Findings
- Bone Scan
  ○ Intense focal uptake in the posterior elements unilaterally or bilaterally
  ○ SPECT imaging helpful for diagnosis
    ▪ Triangular pattern of uptake on sagittal images
  ○ Remote or healed may be occult (normal)

Imaging Recommendations
- Best imaging tool: Helical NECT with sagittal reformats
- Protocol advice
  ○ Radiographs 1st (best obliques), if normal consider nuclear medicine bone scan
  ○ Thin section helical NECT with sagittal reformats

DIFFERENTIAL DIAGNOSIS

Spectrum of radiologic findings in back pain
- Musculoskeletal
  ○ Normal (muscular)
  ○ Scoliosis, fracture (trauma history), osteoporotic compression fractures (usually known systemic disease &/or steroids)
  ○ Scheuermann disease
    ▪ Results in abnormal kyphosis (> 40 °), wedged vertebral body, irregularity of endplates (3 or more contiguous levels), Schmorl nodes, narrowing of intervertebral disc spaces, scoliosis
- Infection
  ○ Discitis, osteomyelitis, sacroiliitis, paraspinal inflammation/abscess, pyelonephritis, pelvic inflammatory disease
- Tumor
  ○ Osteoid osteoma, osteoblastoma, Langerhans cell histiocytosis, leukemia, lymphoma, metastatic disease, neurofibroma
- Inflammatory
  ○ Ankylosing spondylitis, psoriatic arthritis, Reiter disease, inflammatory bowel disease
- Miscellaneous
  ○ Sickle cell, syrinx

PATHOLOGY

General Features
- Genetics
  ○ Predisposing familial conditions to spondylolysis

SPONDYLOLYSIS

- Marfan syndrome
- Osteogenesis imperfecta
- Osteopetrosis
- Inherited traits
- Etiology
  - Repetitive exposure to simultaneous forces of muscle contraction, gravity, and rotational force
  - Participation in gymnastics, weight lifting, wrestling, and football at a young age
  - Repeated micro-fractures of the pars interarticularis
- Epidemiology
  - 4.4% at age 6
  - 6% in adults
  - Prevalence of 5-7% in the general population
  - Higher incidence in competitive athletes, especially males
- Associated abnormalities
  - Spondylolisthesis (50%)
  - Scoliosis
  - Scheuermann disease

Staging, Grading or Classification Criteria
- Grades of spondylolisthesis
  - Grade 1 spondylolisthesis
    - Superior vertebral body subluxed by up to one-fourth of a vertebral body
  - Grade 2
    - Subluxation by one-fourth to one half a vertebral body
  - Grade 3
    - Subluxation by half to three-fourths of a vertebral body
  - Grade 4
    - Subluxation by greater than three-fourths width of a vertebral body

CLINICAL ISSUES

Presentation
- Most common signs/symptoms: Asymptomatic (80%)
- Other signs/symptoms
  - Tight hamstring muscles
    - Waddling gait secondary to tight hamstring muscles
- Back spasms or radiating pain
- Chronic low back pain in older children and adults
- Back pain exacerbated by rigorous activities
- Radiculopathy & cauda equina syndrome in spondylolysis with high grade spondylolisthesis

Demographics
- Age: 10-20 year old
- Gender: M > F = 2-4:1
- Ethnicity: Eskimos

Natural History & Prognosis
- Little progression with horizontal sacrum
  - Lumbosacral angle > or = 100 degrees
- Disease progression with vertical sacrum
  - Lumbosacral angle < 100 degrees
- Conservative measures in patients with < 50% slips
  - Two-thirds success rate of symptomatic relief
- Posterolateral fusion in patients with > 50% slips
  - 60-70% solid fusion rate
  - 10-12% complication rate of neurological deficit following fusion
- Complications
  - Radiculopathy, nerve root pinching or impingement
  - Spinal stenosis & cauda equina syndrome
    - Usually results from a significant spondylolisthesis
  - Degenerative disc disease

Treatment
- Nonsteroidal anti-inflammatory drugs (NSAIDs)
- Analgesics
- Physical therapy
- Hyperintense T2WI signal within pars interarticularis
  - May reflect a stress injury, not yet fracture
  - Brace therapy
- Conservative therapy in spondylolysis patients with grade 1 or 2 spondylolisthesis
  - Back brace treatment
  - Modification of activity
- Surgical interventions in symptomatic spondylolysis patients with any degree of spondylolisthesis or patients who fail conservative therapy
  - Gradual traction in hyperextension
  - Cast immobilization
  - Posterolateral fusion

DIAGNOSTIC CHECKLIST

Consider
- Stress injury or early spondylolysis when typical bone scan findings with lack of radiographic changes on radiographs or NECT

Image Interpretation Pearls
- Sagittal or oblique sagittal NECT reformats & sagittal MR images, most important plane for diagnosis
- Identify a complete ring at each & every lumbar level on axial NECT imaging

SELECTED REFERENCES

1. Cohen E et al: Magnetic resonance imaging in diagnosis and follow-up of impending spondylolysis in children and adolescents: early treatment may prevent pars defects. J Pediatr Orthop B. 14(2):63-7, 2005
2. McTimoney CA et al: Current evaluation and management of spondylolysis and spondylolisthesis. Curr Sports Med Rep. 2(1):41-6, 2003
3. Standaert CJ: Spondylolysis in the adolescent athlete. Clin J Sport Med. 12(2):119-22, 2002
4. Van der Wall H et al: Distinguishing scintigraphic features of spondylolysis. J Pediatr Orthop. 22(3):308-11, 2002
5. Logroscino G et al: Spondylolysis and spondylolisthesis in the pediatric and adolescent population. Childs Nerv Syst. 17(11):644-55, 2001
6. Ulmer J et al: MR Imaging of Lumbar Spondylolysis: The Importance of Ancillary Observations. AJR. 169:233-9, 1997
7. Blanda J et al: Defects of pars interarticularis in athletes: a protocol for nonoperative treatment. J Spinal Disord. 6(5):406-11, 1993
8. Reynolds R: Spondylolysis and Spondylolisthesis. Seminars in Spine Surgery. 4:235-47, 1992

SPONDYLOLYSIS

IMAGE GALLERY

Typical

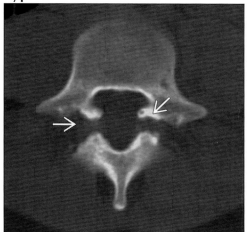
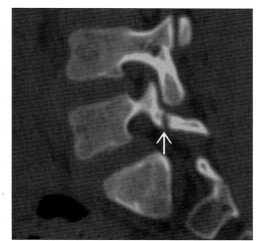

(Left) Axial NECT image from an abdominal study shows an incomplete ring with bilateral fragmented & distracted pars interarticularis defects (arrows), spondylolysis at L5 in this asymptomatic patient. *(Right)* Sagittal reformat image in the same patient shows linear lucency through the right pars interarticularis at L5 (arrow), spondylolysis in this patient with back pain.

Typical

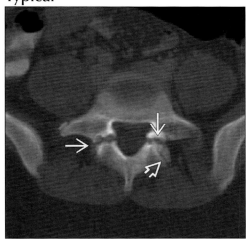
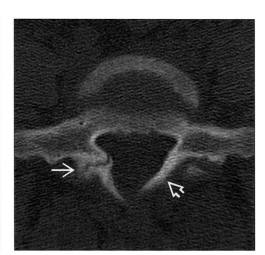

(Left) Axial CECT shows bilateral spondylolysis; an incomplete ring, double facet on the left, elongation of the spinal canal with fractures of the bilateral pars interarticularis at L5 (arrows). Notice the coronal orientation verses the facet joint (open arrow). *(Right)* Axial NECT image shows lucency & callus of the right pars interarticularis (open arrow). Notice the mild reactive sclerosis of the contralateral pars interarticularis & lamina from stress injury (arrow).

Typical

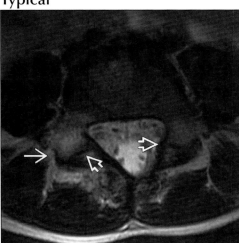
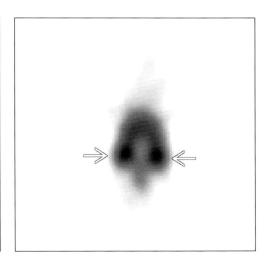

(Left) Axial T2WI MR shows focal hyperintense marrow signal, edema within the right pedicle & lamina at L5 (arrow). Bilateral bands of hypointense signal (open arrows) within the pars interarticularis, spondylolysis. The lack of edema on the left is consistent with a healing defect. *(Right)* Axial SPECT image from a bone scan shows intense tracer uptake in the bilateral L4 pars interarticularis (arrows), healing spondylolysis.

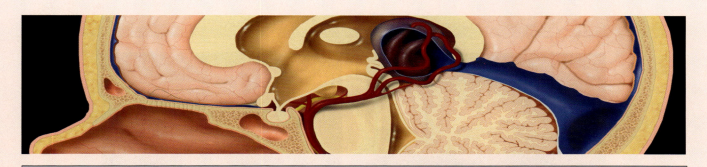

SECTION 7: Neuro

Introduction and Overview

Neuro	7-2

Congenital Malformations

The Dandy Walker Malformation	7-6
Chiari I	7-10
Chiari II with Myelomeningocele	7-14
Encephaloceles	7-18
Holoprosencephaly	7-22
Callosal Dysgenesis	7-26
Hemimegalencephaly	7-30
Schizencephaly	7-34
Occult Spinal Dysraphism	7-38
Diastematomyelia	7-42

Neurocutaneous Syndromes

Neurofibromatosis Type 1	7-46
Tuberous Sclerosis	7-50

Inflammation and Infection

TORCH Infections	7-54
Brain Abscess	7-58
Acute Disseminated Encephalomyelitis	7-62

Metabolic Disease

The Leukodystrophies	7-66
Mitochondrial Encephalopathies	7-70

Trauma

Atlanto-Axial Injuries	7-74
Child Abuse, Brain	7-78

Cysts and Cyst-Like Lesions

Colloid Cyst	7-82
Arachnoid Cyst	7-86
Dermoid and Epidermoid Cysts	7-90

Neoplasms

Pilocytic Astrocytoma	7-94
Medulloblastoma	7-98
Ependymoma	7-102
Brainstem Glioma	7-106
Craniopharyngioma	7-110
Germinoma, Brain	7-114
Choroid Plexus Papilloma	7-118
Spinal Cord Astrocytoma	7-122

Vascular Abnormalities

Germinal Matrix Hemorrhage	7-126
Hypoxic Ischemic Encephalopathy	7-130
Childhood Stroke	7-134
Vein of Galen Aneurysmal Malformation	7-138

Miscellaneous

Normal Myelination	7-142
Hydrocephalus	7-146

Head and Neck Lesions

Nasal Dermal Sinus	7-150
Choanal Atresia	7-154
Otic Capsule Dysplasias	7-158
Aural Atresia	7-162
First Branchial Apparatus Anomalies	7-166
Second Branchial Apparatus Anomalies	7-170
Third Branchial Apparatus Anomalies	7-174
Fourth Branchial Apparatus Anomalies	7-178
Congenital Cholesteatoma	7-182
Acquired Cholesteatoma	7-186
Orbital Cellulitis	7-190
Retinoblastoma	7-194
Juvenile Nasopharyngeal Angiofibroma	7-198
Vascular Malformations, Head and Neck	7-202
Rhabdomyosarcoma, Peds Head and Neck	7-206
Infantile Hemangioma, Head and Neck	7-210

NEURO

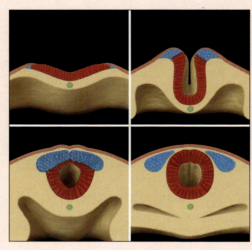

These 4 images show progressive stages of neural tube development, with formation and infolding of neural plate (red), ventral notochord (green), and lateral migration of neural crest (blue).

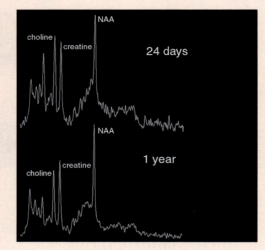

Normal MRS in the white matter at 24 days of life and 1 year shows relative decreases in choline, and an increase in NAA, reflecting proliferation and maturation of neurons.

Terminology

Abbreviations
- CNS: Central nervous system
- CSF: Cerebrospinal fluid
- SAS: Subarachnoid space
- SAH: Subarachnoid hemorrhage
- MRS: MR spectroscopy
- NAA: N-acetyl-aspartate
- IVH: Intraventricular hemorrhage
- ACA: Anterior cerebral artery
- MCA: Middle cerebral artery
- PCA: Posterior cerebral artery
- NF1: Neurofibromatosis type 1
- TS: Tuberous sclerosis
- JNA: Juvenile nasal angiofibroma
- TGD: Thyroglossal duct

Definitions
- Congenital malformations
  o Malformations of brain and spine development are frequently encountered in pediatric neuroimaging
  o Can be very intimidating ⇒ confusing vocabulary, complex embryologic concepts
  o Can be grossly divided into problems with neural tube closure/conformation and problems with cellular proliferation and organization
- Neurocutaneous syndromes
  o The two most commonly encountered phakomatoses are NF1 and TS
  o These conditions present with a wide range of neuroimaging manifestations and provide a constant challenge for imaging and diagnosis
- Inflammation and infection
  o Chronic inflammatory and demyelinating processes are more common in adults
  o Acute pyogenic or destructive lesions are more commonly encountered in children
  o Vertical (in utero) transmission of infection remains a significant cause of morbidity
- Metabolic disease
  o Rapidly broadening category of conditions, due to increasing understanding of human genetic code
  o Two major groups are presented ⇒ leukodystrophies and mitochondrial encephalopathies
    ▪ These encompass a large percentage of the metabolic brain disease that a pediatric neuroimager is likely to encounter in practice
- Trauma
  o Most traumatic brain and spine lesions are similar in their appearance in both children and adults
  o Atlanto-axial injuries are relatively unique to pediatrics and require specific understanding for proper assessment
  o Neurologic injury from child abuse is the #1 cause of mortality in children < 2
- Cysts & cyst-like lesions
  o As a group, colloid cysts, arachnoid cysts, and dermoid/epidermoid inclusion cysts are much more frequently encountered in children
- Neoplasms
  o Brain tumors are the leading cause of cancer deaths in children, and the most common solid tumors encountered
  o They are a much more heterogeneous group of lesions than brain tumors in adults
- Vascular abnormalities
  o Under-recognized and under-appreciated cause of neurologic morbidity and mortality in children
- Miscellaneous
  o Hydrocephalus and disorders of CSF hydrodynamics are a major source of morbidity in children
  o Understanding of normal myelination is key to the diagnosis of leukodystrophies and other metabolic conditions
- Head & neck lesions
  o Congenital lesions of the head and neck are much more frequently encountered in pediatric neuroimaging than in adults
  o Retinoblastoma, rhabdomyosarcoma, and JNA are almost exclusively seen in pediatric populations

NEURO

The Pediatric Neuroradiologist As Consultant

- 15 years ago the majority of pediatric neuroimaging studies were ordered by emergency physicians or neuroscience specialists
  - Neurosurgery
  - Neurology
  - Otorhinolaryngology
  - Orthopedic surgery
- Radiologist had a limited role in guiding further evaluation and clinical follow-up
- Today the majority of pediatric neuroimaging studies are ordered by pediatricians and other primary care physicians
  - The pediatric radiologist has a responsibility to ensure appropriate patient evaluation and disposition
- Can suggest most appropriate modality for investigation of clinical symptoms, incorporating knowledge of radiation and sedation risks into decision
  - The pediatric radiologist/neuroradiologist can be a valuable source of neuroscience information for the primary care physician
    - The radiologist often has more experience/familiarity with infrequently encountered neuropathology
    - Can relate experience with prior similar cases or patterns of practice of referring specialists
- The pediatric neuroradiologist may be directly consulted for endovascular therapy
  - Arteriovenous malformation embolization, aneurysm occlusion, tumor embolization, bone biopsy, sclerotherapy

- Capillary hemangioma and vascular malformations are common lesions that are being treated more aggressively and successfully

Imaging Modalities

Radiography
- Radiographs have a limited role in pediatric neuroradiology
  - Documentation/localization of skull fractures, shunts, coils, clips
  - Evaluation of premature craniosynostosis
    - Some benefit in screening, largely replaced by 3D CT

Ultrasound
- Primarily used in neonate and young infant
  - Excellent for monitoring/screening of neonatal IVH, spinal cord tethering
  - No harmful bioeffects
- Limited use for brain or spine in children > 6-9 months

Computed Tomography
- Major benefits are high resolution, wide availability, specificity
- Speed and versatility have been dramatically augmented by helical and multidetector technology
- Radiation exposure is major limiting factor

MR
- Favored tool for diagnosis of most pediatric neuropathology
- Expense, time, and the need for sedation are largest hurdles
- MR safety and implanted device compatibility are becoming greater concerns
  - More children have MR-incompatible devices
  - Well-documented MR safety policies and procedures need to be established, maintained, and followed
- MR environment is hostile to neonates, especially premature
  - MR-compatible incubators can make imaging much less noxious
    - Full monitoring/support capability, temperature control, reduced noise

MRS
- MR spectroscopy has broad applications in pediatric neuroradiology
- NAA reflects neuronal integrity
  - Obliterated in astrocytomas (no neuronal component in tumor)
- Choline reflects degree of cellular turnover
  - Rapidly growing tumor will elevate choline dramatically
- Myo-inositol reflects reactive white matter changes
  - Often elevated in dysplastic lesions or inflammatory processes
- Lactate is elevated in ischemia
  - Reflects anaerobic metabolism
- Single voxel (4-8 cubic centimeters) acquisitions provide most accurate differentiation of metabolite resonances
- Multivoxel acquisition allows some differentiation of metabolite distribution over sampled region

Nuclear Medicine
- Functional and physiologic studies are becoming more clinically applied
- Utility increases when combined with CT or MR (i.e. PET-CT)

Catheter Angiography
- Complication rate is extremely low in children
- Most radiologists have very limited experience in pediatric neuroangiography
- Excellent image quality of MRA and CTA in children severely limits the clinical indications for diagnostic catheter angiography
  - Diagnostic-only studies typically limited to suspected small vessel angiopathy (CNS vasculitis), pre-operative evaluation of vascular lesions, or post-therapy studies

NEURO

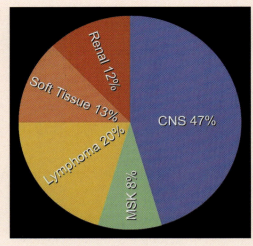

Pie chart shows the percentage of various categories of solid neoplasms in children under 14, with CNS lesions comprising nearly half; they also are the leading cause of cancer death.

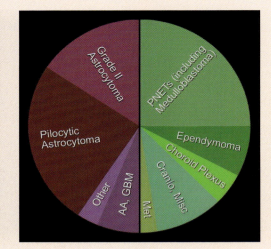

Pie chart shows distribution of tumor types among pediatric CNS neoplasms. Although various astrocytomas account for nearly half, the variety of pathology is much greater than in adults.

Radiation Safety

Radiation Exposure And CT

- Exposure to significant amounts of radiation is known to increase the risk of developing cancer later in life
  - This risk is significantly greater in children than adults
  - The risk is greatest in children under 2 years of age
- Indications for neuroimaging in children have broadened considerably in the past decade
  - Accordingly, the number of CT exams performed in children has markedly increased
  - Recent technologic advances have made CT more useful, efficient, and accessible for imaging children
- Pediatric neuroradiologists are obligated to take steps to ensure that radiation exposure is minimized without compromising exam quality
  - Exam techniques should be adjusted for age, size, and exam type to minimize exposure
    - Infant head CT requires much less technique than teenage spine CT
    - Exams evaluating for shunt malfunction require less technique than exams evaluating for acute stroke
  - Recommendations should be made for exams without ionizing radiation (MR, US) when more appropriate
  - Number and timing of follow-up exams should be judiciously allocated

Sedation

Strategies For Reducing Sedation

- Use of distraction devices such as headphones and video goggles can dramatically reduce the number of cases requiring sedation
  - Children who "fail" to hold still with these devices will still need to be sedated, either at the same setting or later
- Motion-insensitive sequences can achieve high-quality images with significant patient motion
  - Single-shot images requiring 1 second or less per slice
    - Significant reduction in signal to noise and contrast resolution
    - Differing signal characteristics than spin-echo sequences
  - Sequences that fill k-space in a rotational fashion to reduce motion artifact
    - Limited sequence types and scan angles
    - Longer acquisition than comparable fast spin-echo sequences
- Alternative imaging modalities
  - CT with helical acquisition more readily tolerated
  - US in infants < 9 months

Caveats In Reducing Sedation

- Use of CT instead of MR increases risk of radiation exposure
- CT or US may not be as sensitive or appropriate as MR for indication
- The neuroradiologist may feel pressured to "make do" with sub-optimal exam quality in order to avoid sedation

Related References

1. Grant PE et al: Application of new MR techniques in pediatric patients. Magn Reson Imaging Clin N Am. 11(3):493-522, 2003
2. Care M: Imaging in suspected child abuse: what to expect and what to order. Pediatr Ann. 31(10):651-9, 2002
3. Hedlund GL: Neuroradiology of the central nervous system in childhood. Neurol Clin. 20(4):965-81, vi, 2002
4. Hunter JV et al: MR spectroscopy in pediatric neuroradiology. Magn Reson Imaging Clin N Am. 9(1):165-89, ix, 2001
5. Raybaud C et al: Neuroimaging of epilepsy in children. Magn Reson Imaging Clin N Am. 9(1):121-47, viii, 2001
6. Tortori-Donati P et al: Magnetic resonance imaging of spinal dysraphism. Top Magn Reson Imaging. 12(6):375-409, 2001
7. Barkovich AJ: Concepts of myelin and myelination in neuroradiology. AJNR Am J Neuroradiol. 21(6):1099-109, 2000

NEURO

IMAGE GALLERY

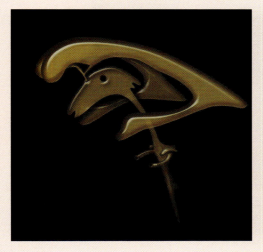
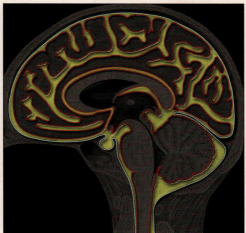

(Left) Oblique graphic of the ventricular system. The ventricles act as a type of lymphatic system for the CNS, maintaining homeostasis of interstitial fluid and providing humoral communication. *(Right)* Axial graphic of the subarachnoid space (SAS). CSF has net movement from ventricles into the SAS; it is actively transported from there into the dural sinuses by the arachnoid granulations.

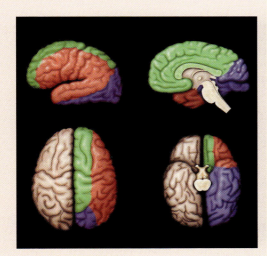
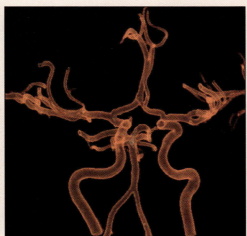

(Left) Graphic shows major intracranial arterial territories. Note that ACA distribution (green) is paramedian, MCA (red) has a classic wedge, and PCA (blue) has significant supply to the temporal lobe. *(Right)* Coronal oblique transparent 3D reconstruction of a routine pediatric MRA. High cardiac output and smooth vessel morphology allow for exquisite non-invasive vascular imaging in children.

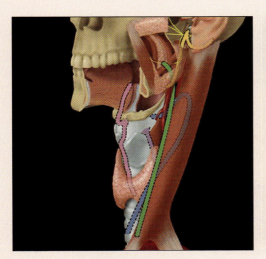
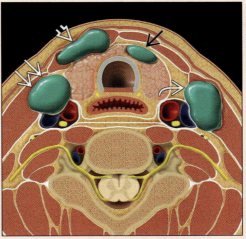

(Left) Sagittal oblique graphic shows course of migration and potential locations of 1st (yellow), second (green), third (blue), and fourth (purple) branchial cleft anomalies, and also TGD (pink). *(Right)* Axial graphic of characteristic locations of congenital cystic lesions of the neck. White arrows ⇒ 2nd/3rd BCC, open arrow ⇒ TGD cyst, black arrow ⇒ 4th BCC, curved arrow ⇒ thymic cyst.

THE DANDY WALKER MALFORMATION

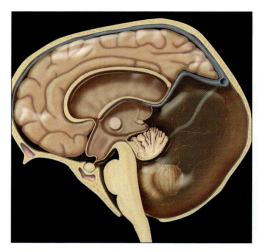

Sagittal graphic of the Dandy Walker malformation with hydrocephalus, showing marked enlargement of the posterior fossa by dorsal expansion of the fourth ventricle, elevating the tentorium.

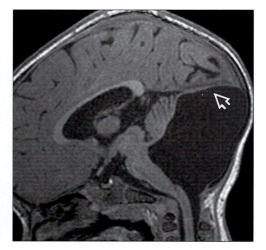

Sagittal T1WI MR shows characteristic features of classic Dandy Walker malformation, with enlarged posterior fossa, elevated tentorium (arrow), expansion of fourth ventricle, and hypoplastic vermis.

TERMINOLOGY

Abbreviations and Synonyms
- Dandy Walker malformation (DWM), Dandy Walker spectrum (DWS); Dandy Walker complex (DWC); Dandy Walker variant (DWV), Dandy Walker continuum

Definitions
- First described by Walter Dandy and Kenneth Blackfan in 1914
  - Ascribed to obstruction of 4th ventricular foramina ⇒ incorrect
- Three criteria established for "classic" malformation
  - Enlarged posterior fossa with upward displacement of tentorium ⇒ "torcular-lambdoid inversion"
  - Severe vermian hypoplasia or agenesis
  - Cystic dilatation of 4th ventricle ⇒ does not communicate with sub-arachnoid space (SAS)
- Dandy Walker variant
  - Term used by various authors to categorize similar malformations that don't meet all three criteria
    - Vermian hypoplasia and cyst without enlarged posterior fossa
    - Incomplete vermian agenesis
    - Cases where cyst communicates with subarachnoid space
- Dandy Walker complex, Dandy Walker spectrum
  - All-encompassing terms that include DWM, DWV, and sometimes mega cisterna magna and Blake pouch cyst
  - Recognize overlap of findings and places them on a continuum of anomalies

IMAGING FINDINGS

General Features
- Best diagnostic clue: Expanded posterior fossa with little or no vermis
- Location: Posterior fossa
- Size: If posterior fossa is not enlarged it is not a classic DWM
- Morphology
  - Residual vermian tissue bean-shaped
  - Rotated superiorly by cyst

Radiographic Findings
- Radiography
  - Enlarged calvaria, particularly posterior fossa
  - Transverse sinus grooves elevated above lambda

CT Findings
- NECT
  - Cyst communicates with 4th ventricle, displaces cerebellar hemispheres anterolaterally
  - Occipital bone may appear scalloped, remodeled

DDx: Congenital Cerebellar Malformations

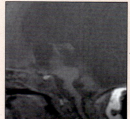
Walker-Warburg

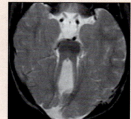
Joubert

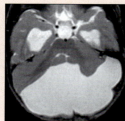
Arachnoid Cyst

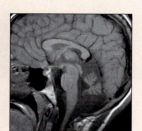
Hypoplasia

THE DANDY WALKER MALFORMATION

Key Facts

Terminology
- First described by Walter Dandy and Kenneth Blackfan in 1914
- Three criteria established for "classic" malformation
- Enlarged posterior fossa with upward displacement of tentorium ⇒ "torcular-lambdoid inversion"
- Severe vermian hypoplasia or agenesis
- Cystic dilatation of 4th ventricle ⇒ does not communicate with sub-arachnoid space (SAS)
- Dandy Walker variant
- Term used by various authors to categorize similar malformations that don't meet all three criteria

Pathology
- Epidemiology: 1:25,000-30,000 births
- 2/3 have associated central nervous system (CNS) anomalies
- Associated anomalies have greatest impact on prognosis/outcome
- Dandy Walker spectrum ⇒ includes essentially all cystic malformations except arachnoid cyst

Clinical Issues
- Most common signs/symptoms: Macrocephaly, hydrocephalus (> 80%)
- Age: 80% diagnosed by 1 y
- Intelligence normal in 35 to 50%

Diagnostic Checklist
- Thin sagittal views in T1-, T2WI crucial for delineation, diagnosis
- Identification of associated anomalies and degree of cerebellar hypoplasia more important than classification of malformation

MR Findings
- T1WI
  - 4th ventricle opens dorsally to large cyst
  - Cyst wall difficult to discern
  - Cyst contents isointense to cerebrospinal fluid (CSF)
- T2WI: Vermian remnant rotated up, over cyst
- FLAIR: May see slight difference in signal between cyst and SAS
- DWI: May see slightly restricted diffusion in cyst
- MRV
  - Elevated torcular Herophili
  - "Inverted Y" appearance of confluence on frontal projection

Ultrasonographic Findings
- Grayscale Ultrasound: Fetal diagnosis of DWM and DWV possible

Angiographic Findings
- Absent posterior inferior cerebellar arteries

Non-Vascular Interventions
- Cisternography
  - Used to differentiate mega cisterna magna from arachnoid cyst
  - Can assess patency of ventricular system in DWM prior to shunting

Imaging Recommendations
- Best imaging tool: MR best characterizes severity, associated anomalies
- Protocol advice
  - Thin sagittal T1 and T2
  - Thin coronal T1 for supratentorial abnormalities

DIFFERENTIAL DIAGNOSIS

Mega cisterna magna
- No clear definition of when a large cisterna magna becomes "mega"
- No malformation of the vermis
- No compression of the 4th ventricle
- Can sometimes extend over hemispheres and under tentorium
- Fills immediately with intrathecal contrast agents

Retrocerebellar arachnoid cyst
- Does not enlarge 4th ventricle
  - Elevates vermis and compresses ventricle
- Not traversed by falx cerebelli
- Does not fill immediately with intrathecal contrast

Walker-Warburg syndrome
- Autosomal recessive
- Type II lissencephaly with retinal and cerebellar malformations
- Inferior vermian hypoplasia
- "Striking cobra" morphology of brainstem

Chiari IV
- Severe cerebellar hypoplasia

Joubert anomaly
- Episodic hyperpnea, oculomotor apraxia, retinal dystrophy
- 4th ventricle has "bat-wing" shape
- Midbrain has shape of "molar tooth"

Rhombencephalosynapsis
- Congenital fusion of cerebellar hemispheres in midline
- Vermian agenesis

Cerebellar hypoplasia
- Feature of multiple syndromes
  - Olivopontocerebellar degeneration
  - Spinocerebellar ataxia
  - Carbohydrate deficient glycoprotein syndrome type 1a

PATHOLOGY

General Features
- General path comments

CHIARI I

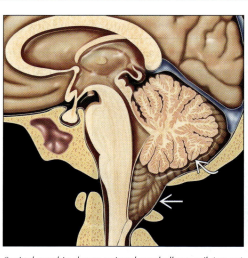

Sagittal graphic shows pointed cerebellar tonsil (arrow) displaced inferiorly through the foramen magnum, with a normal vermis (curved arrow) and no downward mass effect on posterior fossa.

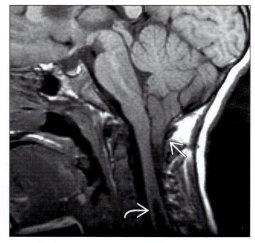

Sagittal T1WI MR shows abnormally pointed cerebellar tonsils (arrow) projecting 1.5 cm below the plane of the foramen magnum. Note syrinx in mid-cervical cord (curved arrow).

TERMINOLOGY

Abbreviations and Synonyms
- Chiari type I malformation (Ch 1); cerebellar (CBLL) tonsil ectopia

Definitions
- Caudal protrusion of pointed CBLL tonsils below foramen magnum (FM)

IMAGING FINDINGS

General Features
- Best diagnostic clue
  - Low-lying, pointed (not rounded), "peg-like" CBLL tonsils
  - Effacement of normal cerebrospinal fluid (CSF) spaces at FM
- Location
  - Position of tonsil tips typically measured from "opisthion-basion" (O-B) line
  - Position of tonsils not as important as abnormal morphology or degree of CSF effacement
- Size
  - Do not rely on measurement of tonsil position alone
  - Accurate depiction of O-B line problematic
    - Inclusion or exclusion of cortex/periosteum changes position
    - Apparent position of line different on T1 or T2WI
  - Tonsil tips can normally lie 5-6 mm below FM
  - Unless tonsils ≥ 5 mm and/or pointed, probably not Ch 1
- Morphology
  - Normal cerebellar tonsils have rounded inferior margin
  - Pointed, wedge-shaped, or peg-like in Ch 1

Radiographic Findings
- Radiography
  - Osseous anomalies of basi-occiput in up to 50%
    - Short clivus, craniovertebral segmentation/fusion anomalies, dorsally oriented odontoid
    - ↑ Angulation of posteriorly tilted odontoid process (more common in females) ⇒ ↑ symptoms

CT Findings
- NECT
  - Excellent screening modality
    - Can avoid issues of sedation for MR imaging in children with apnea
  - Routine head studies should start at level of C1
    - "Crowded" FM on axial images
    - Effacement of CSF around upper cord on image between C1 ring and occipital condyles
  - Helical scanners easily create sagittal reformats

DDx: Tonsillar Herniation

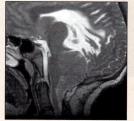
Chiari 2

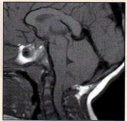
L-P Shunt

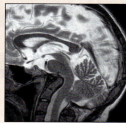
Basilar Invagination

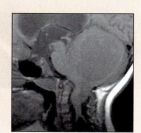
Cerebellar Mass

CHIARI I

Key Facts

Terminology
- Caudal protrusion of pointed CBLL tonsils below foramen magnum (FM)

Imaging Findings
- Low-lying, pointed (not rounded), "peg-like" CBLL tonsils
- Effacement of normal cerebrospinal fluid (CSF) spaces at FM
- Tonsil tips can normally lie 5-6 mm below FM
- Phase-contrast cine MR can show pulsatile systolic tonsillar descent ⇒ "pistoning"
- Intra-operative US after bony decompression and before incising dura
- Best imaging tool: MR brain with thin sagittal views

Pathology
- Crowding at FM compresses obex and effaces subarachnoid space
- CSF in central canal cannot exit superiorly through obex
- CSF in cervical subarachnoid space cannot ascend to be resorbed through arachnoid granulations
- Pistoning motion of tonsils causes "water-hammer" pressure increases in spinal subarachnoid space
- Drives fluid back into central canal of cord ⇒ hydrosyringomyelia

Clinical Issues
- Prevalence of symptoms ↑ if canal diameter < 19 mm, tonsil descent > 10 mm
- Treatment aim = restore normal CSF flow at FM

- CECT: Opacification of posterior inferior cerebellar arteries (PICA) can help more clearly show level of CBLL tonsils

MR Findings
- T1WI
  - Best sequence for showing relationship of tonsils and FM
  - Can show status of obex
  - FLAIR T1 can suppress flow-related signal in CSF
    - Clearer definition of tonsil position
  - Can help distinguish "pre-syrinx" from true syrinx in cervical cord
    - True syrinx contents isointense to CSF
  - Short clivus ⇒ apparent descent of 4th ventricle, medulla
- T2WI
  - Sometimes show tonsil position better than T1WI
    - Complementary sequences
  - Hypointense flow-related artifact in CSF may make tonsil tips difficult to define
  - Displaced tonsils may have abnormally hyperintense signal
    - Indicates encephalomalacia/necrosis
  - Look for upper cervical cord edema, syrinx
    - Signal abnormality without cystic change indicates "pre-syrinx" state
- T1 C+
  - Syrinx associated with Ch 1 will have no associated cord enhancement
  - Tumor or inflammatory syringes typically have regions of enhancement
- MRV
  - May be of benefit in identifying venous anomalies that complicate surgery
  - Dural sinus thrombosis may be a cause of pseudotumor cerebri and tonsillar herniation
- MR Cine
  - Phase-contrast cine MR can show pulsatile systolic tonsillar descent ⇒ "pistoning"
    - May indicate greater likelihood of developing syrinx
  - Can also show obstruction of CSF flow through FM

Ultrasonographic Findings
- Grayscale Ultrasound
  - Intra-operative US after bony decompression and before incising dura
    - Shows if bony decompression alone can resolve pistoning and restore normal CSF flow
    - Shows degree of remaining compression of obex

Non-Vascular Interventions
- Myelography
  - Can show position and motion of CBLL tonsils
  - Cord enlargement implies syrinx (nonspecific)

Imaging Recommendations
- Best imaging tool: MR brain with thin sagittal views
- Protocol advice
  - MR brain +/- CSF flow studies
  - Spine MRI to detect syrinx, tethered cord

DIFFERENTIAL DIAGNOSIS

Acquired tonsillar herniation
- "Push from above"
  - Tonsillar herniation 2° ↑ intracranial pressure (ICP) or mass
    - Posterior fossa tumor, abscess, hematoma, pseudotumor cerebri
- "Pull from below"
  - Lumbar puncture or lumbo-peritoneal (L-P) shunt ⇒ intracranial hypotension
    - "Sagging" brainstem, acquired tonsillar herniation
  - Spontaneous intracranial hypotension
    - Cryptic CSF leak
    - Indium-111 nuclear medicine cisternography for diagnosis

Basilar invagination
- Elevation of FM relative to CBLL

Chiari 2 malformation (Ch 2)
- Virtually 100% associated with neural tube defects (myelomeningocele)

CHIARI II WITH MYELOMENINGOCELE

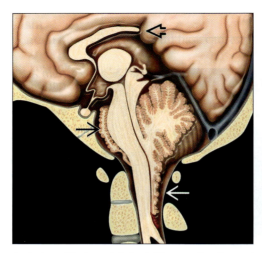

Sagittal graphic shows inferior (white arrow) and ventral (black arrow) herniation of cerebellar tissue due to a small posterior fossa. Open arrow points to the dysmorphic corpus callosum.

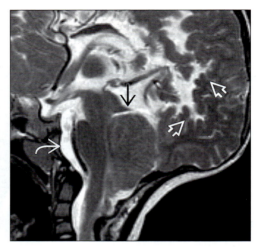

Sagittal T2WI MR shows additional characteristic findings of the Chiari II malformation, with tectal beaking (black arrow), clival scalloping (curved arrow), and stenogyria (open arrows).

TERMINOLOGY

Abbreviations and Synonyms
- Arnold-Chiari malformation (AC2), Chiari type II (Ch 2)

Definitions
- Complex malformation of hindbrain virtually 100% associated with neural tube closure defect (NTD)

IMAGING FINDINGS

General Features
- Best diagnostic clue
  - Presence of myelomeningocele (MMC)
  - Small posterior fossa
  - "Beaked" tectum
- Location
  - NTD is usually lumbar MMC
  - Brain malformation most apparent in posterior fossa
- Size
  - Small posterior fossa
  - NTD typically large
- Morphology
  - Cascade of posterior fossa herniations
    - Vermis (nodulus)
    - Choroid plexus of 4th V

Radiographic Findings
- Radiography
  - "Lacunar" skull (lückenschädel)
    - Thumbprint-like lucencies throughout calvaria
    - Largely resolves by 6 months
    - Not caused by increased pressure or hydrocephalus
  - Widened lumbar canal with posterior element deficiencies at MMC

CT Findings
- NECT
  - Small posterior fossa (PF)
    - Large, funnel-shaped foramen magnum
    - Scalloped posterior margins of petrous pyramids
  - Dural abnormalities
    - Fenestrated/hypoplastic falx ⇒ interdigitated gyri
    - Absent falx cerebelli
  - Colpocephaly
    - Enlargement of atria and occipital horns of lateral ventricles relative to frontal horns
  - Tiny or completely effaced 4th ventricle
  - Pituitary can appear prominent due to shallow sella turcica
  - Valentine heart shape of midbrain
  - Absent posterior elements at NTD

DDx: The Chiari Malformations

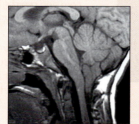
Chiari I

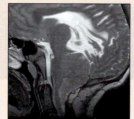
Chiari II

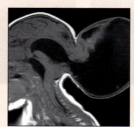
Chiari III

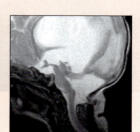
Chiari IV

CHIARI II WITH MYELOMENINGOCELE

Key Facts

Terminology
- Complex malformation of hindbrain virtually 100% associated with neural tube closure defect (NTD)

Imaging Findings
- Presence of myelomeningocele (MMC)
- "Beaked" tectum
- Cascade of posterior fossa herniations
- "Lacunar" skull (lückenschädel)
- Pituitary can appear prominent due to shallow sella turcica
- Cerebellar (CBLL) hemispheres/tonsils "wrap" anteriorly around medulla
- May be complicated by syrinx (20-90%)
- In-utero repair of MMC may reduce hydrocephalus

Pathology
- General path comments: NTD induces malformations of skull, dura, hindbrain, cerebellum, midbrain, posterior cerebrum, spinal cord
- Failure of neural tube closure ⇒ cerebral spinal fluid (CSF) escapes through NTD
- NTD acts as "pop-off" valve for CSF in neural tube ⇒ lack of pressure in vesicle for 4th ventricle
- Reduced CSF pressure ⇒ abnormal mesenchymal development ⇒ small PF, dysgenesis of falx, posterior cerebrum

Diagnostic Checklist
- Increasing symptoms may signal development of syrinx
- Ventricles may become non-compliant over time

MR Findings
- T1WI
  - Small PF ⇒ contents herniate ↓ into cervical canal, shift ↑ through incisura
    - Cerebellar (CBLL) hemispheres/tonsils "wrap" anteriorly around medulla
    - Compressed, elongated, low-lying 4th ventricle
  - Dysgenetic corpus callosum in 90%
  - Midbrain anomalies
    - "Beaked" tectum
    - Large massa intermedia
  - Fetal elongation of cord into lumbar MMC
- T2WI
  - Ventricles
    - Lateral: Pointed anterior horns, colpocephaly
    - 3rd: High-riding with dysgenetic corpus callosum
    - 4th: Elongated, "straw-like" without posterior point (fastigium)
  - Small PF
    - Low-lying tentorium
    - "Cascade" of tissue down, behind medulla
  - Cervical spine
    - Medullary "kink" best seen on T2WI
    - Often compressed against cervical cord
    - Typically at C3 level or lower
  - Lumbar spine
    - Most common location of MMC
    - Uncommonly imaged prior to repair
    - Cord tethered dorsally into open defect
    - May be complicated by syrinx (20-90%)
    - Syrinx can develop after surgical repair
  - Diastematomyelia 5%
- MRA: Small PF and dysgenetic corpus callosum cause unusual configuration of arterial tree
- MRV: Torcular, transverse sinuses extremely low
- Fetal MR
  - Clearly defines level and size of NTD
  - Required prior to fetal surgery
    - In-utero repair of MMC may reduce hydrocephalus

Ultrasonographic Findings
- Grayscale Ultrasound
  - Fetal ultrasound (US)
    - MMC defined as early as 10 weeks on US
    - "Lemon" or "banana" signs in posterior fossa recognized as early as 12 weeks gestation

Imaging Recommendations
- Best imaging tool: MRI brain + spine
- Protocol advice
  - NTD repair typically performed without pre-operative imaging
    - This is changing with increased use of fetal MR and pre-op spine MR
  - Early brain imaging typically with CT
    - Assess degree of hydrocephalus
    - Assess response to ventricular drainage
  - Surveillance Imaging
    - CT to assess for shunt malfunction
    - Shunt assessment CT may be replaced by fast limited MR
    - Spinal MR to assess for development of syrinx or presence of diastematomyelia
    - Brain MR to evaluate degree of brainstem compression if new symptoms develop
    - Brain MR to evaluate for heterotopia if seizures develop

DIFFERENTIAL DIAGNOSIS

Severe, chronic shunted congenital hydrocephalus
- May cause collapsed brain, upward herniated cerebellum, but no spina bifida

Other Chiari malformations
- Chiari I: Pointed and low-lying CBLL tonsils
- Chiari III: Occipital-cervical encephalocele
  - Intracranial features shared with Ch II
- Chiari IV: Severe cerebellar hypoplasia
  - Abandoned terminology

CHIARI II WITH MYELOMENINGOCELE

PATHOLOGY

General Features
- General path comments: NTD induces malformations of skull, dura, hindbrain, cerebellum, midbrain, posterior cerebrum, spinal cord
- Genetics
  - 4-8% risk recurrence if one affected child
  - Menthylene-Tetra-Hydrofolate-Reductase (MTHFR) mutations associated with abnormal folate metabolism
  - MTHFR mutations + folate deficiency ⇒ ↑ risk NTD
  - Decreases in serum folate are seen with anti-epileptic drugs, oral contraceptives, and smoking
- Etiology
  - Embryology
    - Manifests at 4th fetal week
    - Failure of neural tube closure ⇒ cerebral spinal fluid (CSF) escapes through NTD
    - NTD acts as "pop-off" valve for CSF in neural tube ⇒ lack of pressure in vesicle for 4th ventricle
    - Reduced CSF pressure ⇒ abnormal mesenchymal development ⇒ small PF, dysgenesis of falx, posterior cerebrum
  - New studies demonstrate that vimentin is focally upregulated in the ependyma in dysgenetic regions
- Epidemiology
  - 0.44:1,000 births
    - Decreasing with folate replacement
- Associated abnormalities
  - +/- Absent septum pellucidum/fused forniceal columns
  - Gray matter heterotopia
  - Stenogyria: Small and crowded gyri in parietal and occipital lobes
    - Due to disorganization of white matter tracts in posterior cerebrum
    - Best appreciated on sagittal imaging

Gross Pathologic & Surgical Features
- Small and crowded PF with superior and interior herniations
- Multiple dural defects
- Secondary osseous changes
  - Scalloping of clivus and petrous pyramids
  - Lückenschädel

Microscopic Features
- Purkinje cell loss
- Variable sclerosis of herniated tissues

CLINICAL ISSUES

Presentation
- Most common signs/symptoms: MMC grossly apparent at delivery if not diagnosed prenatally
- Other signs/symptoms
  - Macrocrania from hydrocephalus
  - Lower extremity paralysis
  - Bowel and bladder dysfunction

Demographics
- Age
  - Identified in utero or at birth
    - Fetal screening: ↑ α-feto protein
- Gender: Slight female predominance
- Ethnicity
  - ↑ Incidence in British Isles
  - ↑ Incidence in Hispanics

Natural History & Prognosis
- Morbidity from three factors
  - Complications of hydrocephalus and shunt malfunction
  - Renal disease associated with neurogenic bladder
  - Brainstem compression

Treatment
- Folate supplements given to mothers
  - From pre-conception to 6 weeks post conception diminishes risk of MMC
- Primary repair of MMC
- CSF diversion/shunting
- In-utero repair of NTD may lessen severity of brain malformation

DIAGNOSTIC CHECKLIST

Consider
- Increasing symptoms may signal development of syrinx
- Brainstem compression may cause sedation and anesthesia risks

Image Interpretation Pearls
- Ventricles may become non-compliant over time
  - Marked ↑ in pressure with little ↑ in volume
- Don't be surprised by prominent-looking pituitary

SELECTED REFERENCES
1. Mueller D et al: Prospective analysis of self-perceived quality of life before and after posterior fossa decompression in 112 patients with Chiari malformation with or without syringomyelia. Neurosurg Focus. 18(2):ECP2, 2005
2. Sutton LN et al: Fetal surgery for myelomeningocele. Clin Neurosurg. 51:155-62, 2004
3. Aaronson OS et al: Myelomeningocele: prenatal evaluation--comparison between transabdominal US and MR imaging. Radiology. 227(3):839-43, 2003
4. Johnson MP et al: Fetal myelomeningocele repair: short-term clinical outcomes. Am J Obstet Gynecol. 189(2):482-7, 2003
5. McLone DG et al: The Chiari II malformation: cause and impact. Childs Nerv Syst.19(7-8):540-50, 2003
6. Tubbs RS et al: Absence of the falx cerebelli in a Chiari II malformation. Clin Anat. 15(3):193-5, 2002
7. Coley BD: Ultrasound diagnosis of luckenschadel (lacunar skull). Pediatr Radiol. 30(2):82-4, 2000
8. Northrup H et al: Spina bifida & other neural tube defects. Curr Probl Pediatr. 30:313-32, 2000
9. Mutchinick OM et al: High prevalence of the thermolabile methylenetetrahydrofolate reductase variant in Mexico: a country with a very high prevalence of neural tube defects. Mol Genet Metab. 68(4):461-7, 1999
10. Rollins N et al: Coexistent holoprosencephaly and Chiari II malformation. AJNR Am J Neuroradiol. 20(9):1678-81, 1999

CHIARI II WITH MYELOMENINGOCELE

IMAGE GALLERY

Typical

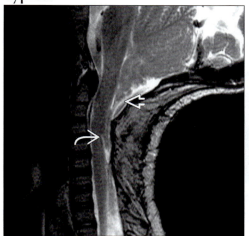
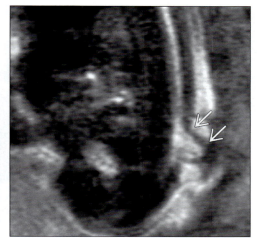

(Left) Sagittal T2WI MR shows inferior herniation of cerebellar tissue *(open arrow)* with clearly defined medullary "kink" *(curved arrow)*. The medullary kink is usually compressed against the cord. *(Right)* Sagittal T2WI MR of 22 week fetus with Ch II shows distal spinal cord projecting through dorsal dysraphic defect at L4 *(arrows)*. Fetal surgery can alter outcome of Ch II malformation.

Typical

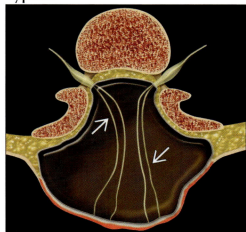
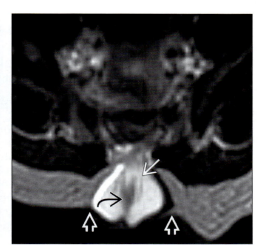

(Left) Axial graphic shows ventral and dorsal nerve roots *(arrows)* traversing myelomeningocele cavity to exit through neural foramina. Posterior border of cavity is the neural placode *(red line)*. *(Right)* Axial T2WI MR through myelomeningocele shows nerve roots *(arrow)* extending anteriorly from placode *(curved arrow)* toward spinal canal. Open arrows show edge of skin defect.

Typical

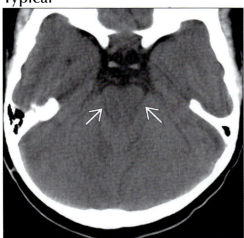
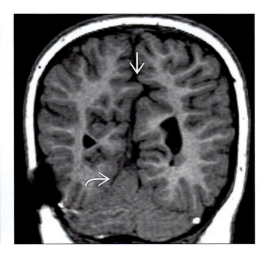

(Left) Axial NECT shows characteristic "valentine heart" shape of midbrain in Ch II, caused by anterior displacement of cerebellar hemispheres compressing dorsolateral margins of midbrain *(arrows)*. *(Right)* Coronal T1WI MR shows interdigitating sulci *(arrow)* due to fenestration of interhemispheric falx, and "towering" cerebellar vermis projecting up through incisura *(curved arrow)*.

ENCEPHALOCELES

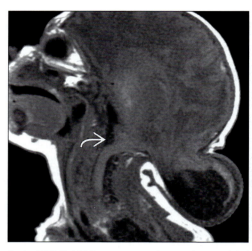

Sagittal T1WI MR in a neonate shows a low occipital encephalocele with herniation of cerebellar and occipital lobe neural tissue into it. Note marked distortion of brainstem (curved arrow).

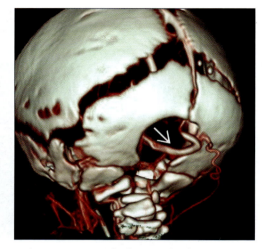

Right posterior view of volume-rendered reconstruction of CTA study in same infant shows displacement of straight sinus and torcular (arrow) into the encephalocele defect.

TERMINOLOGY

Abbreviations and Synonyms
- Cephalocele, meningocele, meningoencephalocele, gliocele

Definitions
- Congenital herniation of one or more intracranial structures through a defect in the skull
  - Meningocele ⇒ herniation of meninges and cerebrospinal fluid (CSF)
  - Meningoencephalocele ⇒ meninges, CSF, and brain
  - Atretic parietal cephalocele (APC) ⇒ meninges, fibrous tissue
  - Gliocele ⇒ CSF-filled glial-lined cyst

IMAGING FINDINGS

General Features
- Best diagnostic clue: Cranial defect with mass projecting through it and distortion of subjacent brain parenchyma
- Location
  - Occipito-cervical (Chiari 3), occipital, parietal, frontal, temporal, fronto-ethmoidal, spheno-maxillary, spheno-orbital, nasopharyngeal, lateral
  - Nearly always midline
- Size: APCs are flat, some lesions are larger than entire cranium

Radiographic Findings
- Radiography: Midline skull defect of variable size

CT Findings
- NECT
  - Distortion of brain morphology
    - Posterior (occipital, occipito-cervical) encephaloceles cause morphology similar to the Chiari 2 malformation
  - Microcephaly
    - Displaced neural tissue reduces volume of intracranial contents
  - Use caution in evaluating the cribriform plate in infants
    - Mostly cartilaginous at birth
    - Does not fully ossify until after 2 years of age
    - Only large defects can be confidently identified
- CTA
  - CTA/CTV single best modality to demonstrate vascular and bony anatomy around defect
    - Ideal for surgical planning
    - Clearly defines relationship of dural sinuses to skull defect
    - Clearly demonstrates displacement of vascular structures into encephalocele

DDx: Nasopharyngeal Masses In Children

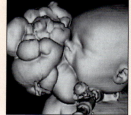
Teratoma

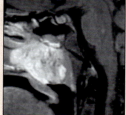
Angiofibroma

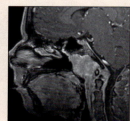
Carcinoma

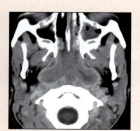
Large Adenoids

ENCEPHALOCELES

Key Facts

Terminology
- Congenital herniation of one or more intracranial structures through a defect in the skull
- Meningocele ⇒ herniation of meninges and cerebrospinal fluid (CSF)
- Meningoencephalocele ⇒ meninges, CSF, and brain
- Atretic parietal cephalocele (APC) ⇒ meninges, fibrous tissue
- Gliocele ⇒ CSF-filled glial-lined cyst

Imaging Findings
- Nearly always midline
- Posterior (occipital, occipito-cervical) encephaloceles cause morphology similar to the Chiari 2 malformation
- Use caution in evaluating the cribriform plate in infants
- CTA/CTV single best modality to demonstrate vascular and bony anatomy around defect
- Clearly demonstrates displacement of vascular structures into encephalocele
- Single best sequence for definition of encephalocele in neonate
- Sagittal thin profile imaging is key
- Best imaging tool: MR and CTA are complementary tools in evaluation of encephaloceles

Pathology
- Occipital lesions are the most common in North America and Europe: 80%
- Fronto-ethmoidal lesions are more common in Southeast Asia (1:5,000 live births)

- Complementary with MR

MR Findings
- T1WI
  - Displacement of neural structures, vessels, ventricles into encephalocele
  - Bony margins may be difficult to resolve
- T2WI
  - Single best sequence for definition of encephalocele in neonate
    - Distinction of neural tissue from CSF and vessels more clear than T1WI
  - Sagittal thin profile imaging is key
  - Distinction of vascular structures from bone may be problematic (both hypointense)
  - APC ⇒ elevation of straight sinus and elongation of supra-vermian cistern
- T2* GRE: Can show hemorrhagic complications of delivery, surgery
- T1 C+: Key for differentiating nasopharyngeal tumors (they enhance) from nasopharyngeal encephaloceles (they don't)
- MRA
  - Can show vascular anatomy, displacement of arteries into encephalocele
  - Sometimes limited in neonate by rapid or turbulent flow, small vessel size
- MRV
  - Can show vascular anatomy, displacement of veins into encephalocele
  - Sometimes limited in neonate by rapid or turbulent flow, small vessel size

Ultrasonographic Findings
- Large lesions characteristically identified in utero
  - Occipito-cervical encephalocele can mimic cystic hygroma
- Further evaluation with fetal MR may be warranted

Non-Vascular Interventions
- Cisternography with CT
  - Sometimes used in inferior-anterior lesions (fronto-ethmoidal, nasopharyngeal) to assess contiguity of sac with subarachnoid space
    - Chance of false-negative if flow is intermittent
    - Need to keep head/face down after instillation of contrast
    - Low volumes of iso-osmolar water soluble agent

Imaging Recommendations
- Best imaging tool: MR and CTA are complementary tools in evaluation of encephaloceles
- Protocol advice
  - Studies may need to be performed in unusual positions in neonates with large lesions who cannot lie supine
    - Volumetric (3D) acquisitions key for sorting out anatomy
  - Thin slice T2WI can define relationship of defect to remaining intracranial contents
  - CTA is ideal for demonstrating relationship of dural sinuses to bony defect
    - Sinus is frequently located right along margin of bone defect
    - Vascular/osseous anatomy more clearly shown than with MRV/MRA

DIFFERENTIAL DIAGNOSIS

Nasal dermoid
- Intracranial involvement in 25%
  - Wide foramen cecum, bifid cristae galli
- MRI: ↓ T1, ↑ T2 signal
- DWI: Restricted diffusion (best sign)

Capillary hemangioma of infancy
- Most common pediatric frontonasal mass, strawberry
- Faint macular stain ("stork bite") ⇒ rapid postnatal growth
- Can also occur along sagittal suture
  - Mimic of APC

ENCEPHALOCELES

Nasal glioma
- "Encephaloceles that have lost their intracranial connection"
- Persistent fibrovascular stalk in 15-20%
- Mixed signal intensity, variable enhancement

Nasopharyngeal neoplasms
- Rhabdomyosarcoma, lymphoma, nasopharyngeal carcinoma
- Juvenile nasopharyngeal angiofibroma, nasopharyngeal teratoma
- Nearly all enhance ⇒ easily distinguished on MR

Orbital neurofibroma and sphenoid defect in NF1
- Mimics orbito-frontal encephalocele
- Pulsatile exophthalmos

Posterior skull/scalp tumors
- Angiosarcoma, osteosarcoma ⇒ enhance strongly, bone destruction
- Dermoids ⇒ more often off-midline

PATHOLOGY

General Features
- General path comments
  - Herniations of meninges, brain, and/or ventricle through a bone defect
  - Occasionally reported with amniotic banding syndrome
  - Embryology-anatomy
    - Disturbed separation of surface ectoderm and neuroectoderm in midline after closure of neural folds (4th gestational week)
- Genetics: High association with midline face and brain anomalies
- Etiology: Unknown
- Epidemiology
  - Occipital lesions are the most common in North America and Europe: 80%
  - Fronto-ethmoidal lesions are more common in Southeast Asia (1:5,000 live births)
    - 1:35,000 live births North America
- Associated abnormalities
  - Parietal, occipital ⇒ Chiari 2, Dandy-Walker, callosal dysgenesis
  - Nasopharyngeal ⇒ 80% callosal dysgenesis
  - Frontal-ethmoidal encephaloceles are on a spectrum of abnormalities that includes nasal dermoids, nasal gliomas, and dermal sinuses

Gross Pathologic & Surgical Features
- Variable amounts of fibrotic, gliotic, dysplastic tissue in sac
- Not enough room in calvaria to "push back" normal appearing tissue

CLINICAL ISSUES

Presentation
- Most common signs/symptoms
  - Occipital, parietal ⇒ clinically obvious mass
  - Fronto-ethmoidal ⇒ nasal stuffiness, nasal mass, nasal pit (dermal sinus)
  - Nasopharyngeal ⇒ nasopharyngeal mass, obligatory mouth-breathing, nasal stuffiness
  - APC ⇒ hairless patch or scab
- Other signs/symptoms
  - Recurrent meningitis
  - Neurologic deficit, seizure, developmental delay (from associated malformation)
- Midline facial features typical: Hypertelorism, broad nasal bridge

Natural History & Prognosis
- Long-term outcome dictated by amount of herniated tissue and presence and severity of other associated intracranial anomalies

Treatment
- Surgery: Combined approach with ENT, plastics and neurosurgery

DIAGNOSTIC CHECKLIST

Consider
- Consider cryptic encephalocele when encountering recurrent meningitis
- Don't forget encephalocele when considering ethmoid mucocele on CT

Image Interpretation Pearls
- Use CTA and MR together for pre-surgical definition of lesions
- Rely on thin T2WI MR for ethmoidal lesions in children ⇒ not enough bone in cribiform plate for CT

SELECTED REFERENCES
1. Bozinov O et al: Surgical closure and reconstruction of a large occipital encephalocele without parenchymal excision. Childs Nerv Syst. 21(2):144-7, 2005
2. Motojima T et al: Recurrent meningitis associated with a petrous apex cephalocele. J Child Neurol. 20(2):168-70, 2005
3. Tubbs RS et al: Parietal cephalocele. Pediatr Neurosurg. 40(1):37-8, 2004
4. Willatt JM et al: Calvarial masses of infants and children. A radiological approach. Clin Radiol. 59(6):474-86, 2004
5. Morimoto K et al: Sphenoid encephalocele without hypothalamic-pituitary and optic nerve dysfunction. Pediatr Neurosurg. 38(3):160-1, 2003
6. Mahapatra AK et al: Anterior encephaloceles: A study of 92 cases. Pediatr Neurosurg. 36(3):113-8, 2002
7. Patterson RJ et al: Atretic parietal cephaloceles revisited: an enlarging clinical and imaging spectrum? AJNR Am J Neuroradiol. 19(4):791-5, 1998

ENCEPHALOCELES

IMAGE GALLERY

Typical

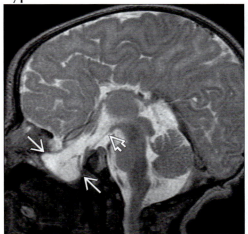
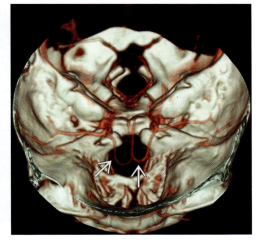

(Left) Sagittal T2WI MR shows a large spheno-ethmoidal encephalocele *(arrows)* passing through a bone defect in front of the anterior clinoids. Optic chiasm is inferiorly displaced *(open arrow)*. *(Right)* Anterior-superior view of a volume-rendered CTA reconstruction in the same infant shows the anterior cerebral arteries *(arrows)* passing through the defect in the planum sphenoidale.

Typical

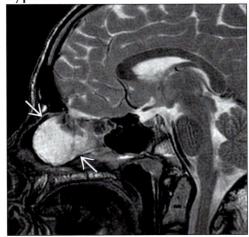
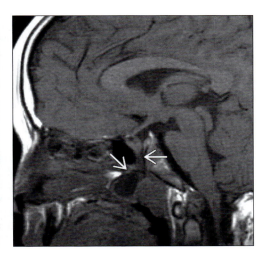

(Left) Sagittal T2WI MR shows a fronto-ethmoidal meningocele *(arrows)* that contained no neural tissue at surgery. The nasal mass was discovered after several episode of meningitis. *(Right)* Sagittal T1WI MR shows a fluid-filled sphenoidal encephalocele *(arrows)* that projects into nasopharynx anterior to adenoidal pad. Pituitary tissue falls into the margins of the defect.

Typical

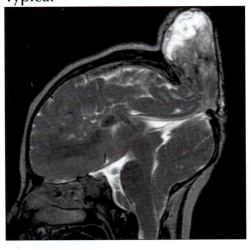
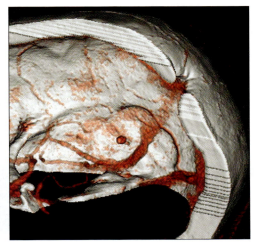

(Left) Sagittal T2WI MR shows large parietal encephalocele with extensive amorphous neural tissue inside it. Note the distortion of the tectum and vermis, reminiscent of the Chiari 2 malformation. *(Right)* Sagittal cut-away view of a 3D-CTA study shows deviation of the straight sinus up to an atretic parietal cephalocele. No intracranial tissue passes beyond the margins of the defect.

HOLOPROSENCEPHALY

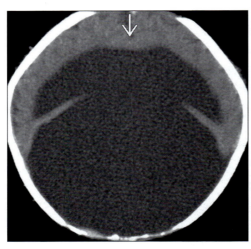

Axial NECT shows characteristic "Amadeus" silhouette of ventricular morphology in alobar holoprosencephaly. Arrow points to contiguous gyrus crossing the midline.

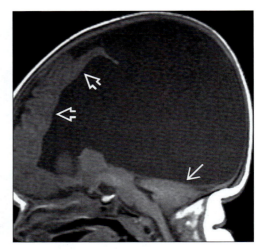

Sagittal T1WI MR in alobar holoprosencephaly shows inferior flattening of tentorium (arrow) and anterior displacement of hemispheric tissue (open arrows) by large monoventricle.

TERMINOLOGY

Abbreviations and Synonyms
- Holoprosencephaly (HPE)

Definitions
- Spectrum of congenital structural forebrain malformations characterized by midline hemisphere fusion
- Result from failure of normal prosencephalic cleavage
- Traditionally divided into alobar, semilobar, and lobar forms, plus midline interhemispheric variant (MIH) or syntelencephaly

IMAGING FINDINGS

General Features
- Best diagnostic clue
  - Alobar HPE ⇒ "pancake" of anterior cerebral tissue
  - Semilobar HPE ⇒ caudate head fusion
  - Lobar HPE ⇒ absent anterior midline falx and fissure, "fading" genu
  - MIH ⇒ sylvian fissures connected across midline over vertex (86%)

Radiographic Findings
- Radiography: Hypotelorism, fused metopic suture or single frontal "plate" of bone, variable degree of microcephaly

CT Findings
- NECT
  - Alobar: Monoventricle, often incompletely covered posteriorly by brain ⇒ dorsal "cyst"
    - "Amadeus" ventricular profile ⇒ resembles silhouette of tricorne hat from popular movie poster
    - Dorsal cyst and monoventricle cause macrocephaly
  - Semilobar: Absent septum pellucidum, partial occipital and temporal horns
  - Lobar: Absent septum pellucidum; formed lateral ventricles including temporal and occipital horns
  - Skull base/vault
    - Cleft palate; variable optic canal hypoplasia
    - Absent or hypoplastic ethmoid sinus, anterior falx (and superior sagittal sinus), crista galli
- CECT
  - Single anterior cerebral artery
  - Dural sinus anomalies

MR Findings
- T1WI

DDx: Large Supratentorial CSF Collections

Hydranencephaly | Schizencephaly | Callosal Agenesis | Hydrocephalus

HOLOPROSENCEPHALY

Key Facts

Terminology
- Spectrum of congenital structural forebrain malformations characterized by midline hemisphere fusion

Imaging Findings
- Alobar HPE ⇒ "pancake" of anterior cerebral tissue
- Semilobar ⇒ posterior corpus callosum present and titled back
- Lobar ⇒ genu of corpus callosum "fades" away

Top Differential Diagnoses
- Severe hydrocephalus
- Open-lip schizencephaly
- Callosal agenesis with interhemispheric cyst
- Hydranencephaly

Pathology
- Mutations affecting signaling genes (e.g., Sonic hedgehog) which regulate neural tube patterning
- Most medial aspects of hemispheres fail to form
- Result ⇒ more lateral structures stay central and fuse to each other

Clinical Issues
- "Face predicts brain": Severe midline anomaly ⇒ severe HPE
- Over-represented in fetal demise, stillbirths

Diagnostic Checklist
- Be sure to distinguish HPE from mimics
- Many have much better prognosis than alobar HPE

- Sagittal imaging
  - Alobar ⇒ tentorium flattened inferiorly, residual cerebral tissue flattened anteriorly
  - Semilobar ⇒ posterior corpus callosum present and titled back
  - Lobar ⇒ genu of corpus callosum "fades" away
  - MIH ⇒ central body of callosum "bitten" away, with dysmorphic gray matter (GM) in defect
- Axial imaging
  - Amadeus ventricle in alobar HPE
  - Small 3rd ventricle from nuclei fusion
  - Crossing sulcus/gyrus resembles schizencephalic clefts in MIH
- T2WI
  - Delayed myelin maturation in classical HPE, but normal in middle hemispheric variant (MIH)
  - Following are variable
    - Degree of frontal lobe hypoplasia, basal nuclei fusion
    - Presence of dorsal cyst (suprapineal recess)
    - Degree of hypoplasia or absence of olfactory nerves (best seen on coronal views)
    - Subcortical heterotopia anterior to interhemispheric fissure and subjacent to shallow frontal sulci
  - Semilobar and lobar HPE are often microcephalic
- DWI: DTI demonstrates absence of corticospinal tracts in alobar HPE
- MRA: Azygous or absent anterior cerebral artery (ACA)
- MRV
  - Absent superior sagittal, inferior sagittal and straight sinuses
  - Cortical veins and deep veins drain directly to torcular

Ultrasonographic Findings
- Grayscale Ultrasound: Diagnosable on fetal ultrasound (and fetal MRI)
- Color Doppler: Absent superior sagittal sinus, variable absence of deep and midline venous structures

Angiographic Findings
- Conventional
  - Azygous or absent ACA
  - Fan-like array of arteries over surface of "pancake"
  - If ACA absent, middle cerebral arteries have more medial course

Imaging Recommendations
- Best imaging tool: MRI
- Protocol advice: Multiplanar MR imaging with special attention to midline structures

DIFFERENTIAL DIAGNOSIS

Severe hydrocephalus
- Macrocephalic (HPE usually microcephalic)
- Consequence of aqueductal stenosis
- PD/Intermediate best to show residual thin mantle of cortex underneath calvaria
- Preservation of falx

Open-lip schizencephaly
- Large and bilateral schizencephaly can mimic semilobar or alobar HPE
- Residual posterior cerebral tissue along falx
- Anterior falx preserved

Callosal agenesis with interhemispheric cyst
- Much better prognosis than alobar HPE
- Displaces cerebral tissue to sides of cranium, not to front

Hydranencephaly
- Obliteration of parenchyma in carotid territory
- Residual cerebral tissue is along top of tentorium (posterior cerebral artery territory)

Other holoprosencephaly spectrum disorders
- Septo-optic dysplasia
- Central incisor syndrome
- Nonspecific midline dysplasias & frontonasal dysplasia, agnathia-otocephaly, anencephaly

HOLOPROSENCEPHALY

PATHOLOGY

General Features
- General path comments
  - Embryology-anatomy
    - Normal prosencephalic cleavage occurs 4-6 wks
- Genetics
  - Cytogenetic abnormality in 50%: Especially trisomy 13; also 18q-, 18p-, 3p, 7-, trisomy 9, 1q15q, 11q12-q13
  - Familial HPE: 5+ implicated genes
    - HPE1 (21q22.3), HPE2 (SIX3 - 2p21), HPE3 (Sonic hedgehog gene - 7q36), HPE4 (TGIF-18p), HPE5 (ZIC2 - 13q32)
- Etiology
  - Mutations affecting signaling genes (e.g., Sonic hedgehog) which regulate neural tube patterning
  - Most medial aspects of hemispheres fail to form
    - Result ⇒ more lateral structures stay central and fuse to each other
- Epidemiology
  - 1 to 1.4 per 10,000 live births
    - Severe lesions often result in spontaneous abortion
- Associated abnormalities
  - Maternal risk factors
    - ETOH, diabetes, retinoic acid
    - Infants of diabetic mothers ⇒ alobar HPE with normal facies
  - Facial anomalies ⇒ central incisor; proboscis; single naris; single nasal bone/absent internasal suture and caudal metopic suture
    - +/- Midline facial clefting; premaxillary agenesis if severe; absent superior lingual frenulum
  - Non-facial/non-CNS anomalies 65%

Gross Pathologic & Surgical Features
- Extreme hypoplasia of neocortex
- Variable degrees of fusion of diencephalon and thalamus/basal ganglia with incorporation into upper brainstem
  - Associated attenuation of anterior recess 3rd ventricle
- Dorsal cyst (especially in association with noncleaved thalamus) felt to represent expansion of partially blocked posterodorsal 3rd ventricle

Staging, Grading or Classification Criteria
- Alobar, semilobar, lobar classification of DeMyer
- MIH described as HPE variant by Barkovich in 1993
- Arrhinencephaly ⇒ absence of olfactory bulbs
  - Associated finding with HPE versus variant
- Septo-optic dysplasia ⇒ more severe cases overlap with HPE in etiology and presentation

CLINICAL ISSUES

Presentation
- Most common signs/symptoms
  - Mentally retarded microcephalic infant with midline facial anomalies, disturbed endocrine function
  - Worst (classic alobar HPE) = cyclopia, proboscis, midline facial clefting, microcephaly
  - Most common "brain plus face" malformation
    - "Face predicts brain": Severe midline anomaly ⇒ severe HPE
    - Function predicted by degree of non-separation of brain structures
- Other signs/symptoms
  - Seizures (50%) and mental retardation: Most severe with cortical malformations
  - Severity of pituitary/hypothalamic malfunction correlates with degree of hypothalamic non-separation

Demographics
- Age: Presentation in infancy (can be diagnosed with fetal US or MRI)
- Gender: M:F = 1.4:1

Natural History & Prognosis
- Over-represented in fetal demise, stillbirths
- Clinical severity relates to degree of hemispheric and deep gray nuclei non-separation

Treatment
- Treat seizures and endocrine dysfunction

DIAGNOSTIC CHECKLIST

Consider
- Be sure to distinguish HPE from mimics
  - Many have much better prognosis than alobar HPE

Image Interpretation Pearls
- Alobar HPE and mimics all displace residual brain
  - Recognize presence of posterior residual or lateral displacement to spot mimics

SELECTED REFERENCES
1. Barkovich AJ: Pediatric Neuroimaging, 4th ed. Lippincott Williams & Wilkins. 364-74, 2005
2. Hayashi M et al: Neuropatholigcal evaluation of the diencephalon, basal ganglia and upper brainstem in alobar holoprosencephaly. Acta Neuropathol. 107(3):190-6, 2004
3. Pulitzer SB et al: Prenatal MR findings of the middle interhemispheric variant of holoprosencephaly. AJNR Am J Neuroradiol. 25(6):1034-6, 2004
4. Barkovich AJ et al: Analysis of the cerebral cortex in HPE with attention to the Sylvian fissures. AJNR. 23:143-50, 2002
5. Blaas HG et al: Brains and faces in holoprosencephaly: Pre- and postnatal description of 30 cases. Ultrasound Obstet Gynecol. 19(1):24-38, 2002
6. Simon EM et al: The middle interhemispheric variant of holoprosencephaly. AJNR. 23(1):151-6, 2002
7. Simon EM et al: The dorsal cyst in holoprosencephaly and the role of the thalamus in its formation. Neuroradiology. 43(9):787-91, 2002

HOLOPROSENCEPHALY

IMAGE GALLERY

Typical

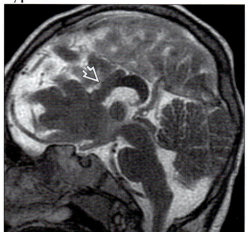 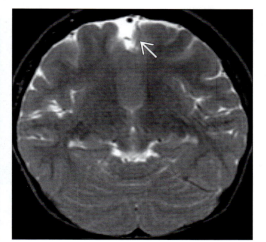

(Left) Sagittal T2WI MR in lobar HPE shows how rostrum, genu, and anterior body of corpus callosum "fade away" (open arrow); this contradicts the usual chronology of callosal dysgenesis. *(Right)* Axial T2WI MR in the same child shows frontal cortex fused across the midline anteriorly, and absence of the interhemispheric falx. Arrow points to the "meandering" anterior cerebral artery.

Typical

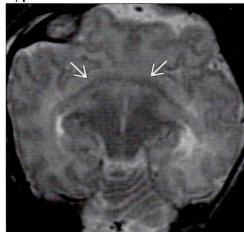 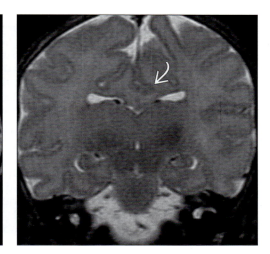

(Left) Axial T2WI MR in an infant with semilobar holoprosencephaly shows prominence of the anterior commissure (arrows). *(Right)* Coronal T2WI MR shows frontal cortex crossing the midline below a partially formed falx (arrow), and fusion of the caudate heads, horizontally deviating the frontal horns.

Variant

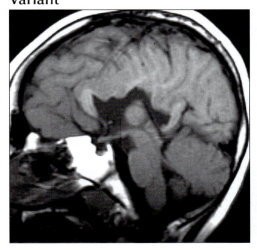 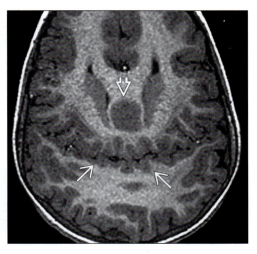

(Left) Sagittal T1WI MR shows the midline interhemispheric variant of HPE, with absence of the body of the corpus callosum and fusion of cortex across the midline defect. *(Right)* Axial T1WI MR shows MIH with contiguous gyri extending across the midline (arrows) from the apex of the sylvian fissures, with a second mass of fused gray matter more anteriorly (open arrow).

CALLOSAL DYSGENESIS

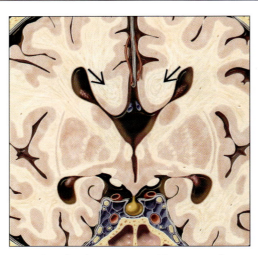

Coronal graphic shows agenesis of the corpus callosum, with bundles of Probst (arrows) separated from frontal horns by everted cingulate gyri.

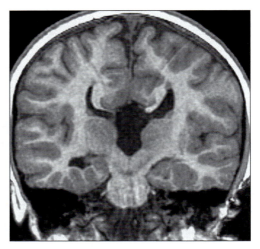

Coronal T1WI MR shows characteristic "Texas Longhorn" configuration of the frontal horns and third ventricle in agenesis of the corpus callosum.

TERMINOLOGY

Abbreviations and Synonyms
- Agenesis of the corpus callosum (CC)

Definitions
- Congenital malformation resulting in hypoplasia or absence of all or part of corpus callosum

IMAGING FINDINGS

General Features
- Best diagnostic clue
  - Axial: Parallel lateral ventricles
  - Coronal: Anterior horns resemble "Viking helmet" or "Texas longhorn"
- Size: CC remnants vary in size, shape
- Morphology
  - CC segments (front to back)
    - Rostrum, genu, body, isthmus, splenium

Radiographic Findings
- Radiography
  - Orbital hypertelorism
  - Rim calcification (Ca++) of midline lipoma

CT Findings
- NECT
  - Lateral ventricles are key to diagnosis
    - Lateral ventricles appear parallel in dysgenesis of CC
    - Colpocephaly (dilated posteriorly)
    - Pointed frontal horns
  - Variable findings
    - Midline cyst or lipoma
- CTA: "Meandering" anterior cerebral arteries (ACAs)

MR Findings
- T1WI
  - Sagittal
    - Radially arrayed gyri up from 3rd ventricle
    - Everted cingulate gyrus, absent cingulate sulcus
    - Hyperintense lipoma (if present)
  - Coronal
    - Longhorn-shaped anterior horns
    - Elongated foramina of Monro
    - "Keyhole" temporal horns & vertical hippocampi
  - Ventriculomegaly seen in type I interhemispheric cyst variant
    - Cyst is a diverticulum of lateral ventricle
    - Mimics alobar holoprosencephaly
- T2WI
  - Colpocephaly
    - Result of loss of normal white matter (WM) architecture in posterior frontal and parietal lobes

DDx: Diminished Corpus Callosum

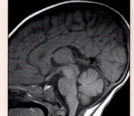
Normal Neonate

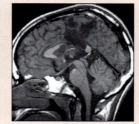
Gunshot Injury

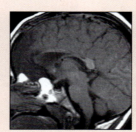
Prior Callosotomy

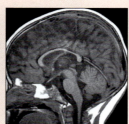
PVL

CALLOSAL DYSGENESIS

Key Facts

Terminology
- Agenesis of the corpus callosum (CC)
- Congenital malformation resulting in hypoplasia or absence of all or part of corpus callosum

Imaging Findings
- CC segments (front to back)
- Rostrum, genu, body, isthmus, splenium
- Lateral ventricles appear parallel in dysgenesis of CC
- Radially arrayed gyri up from 3rd ventricle
- Longhorn-shaped anterior horns
- Ventriculomegaly seen in type I interhemispheric cyst variant
- Mimics alobar holoprosencephaly
- Colpocephaly
- WM tracts more loosely packed with dysgenesis, resulting in relative dilation of trigones
- Probst bundles are densely packed WM tracts running parallel to interhemispheric fissure

Top Differential Diagnoses
- Destruction of callosum
- Immature callosum

Pathology
- Multiple genes contribute to formation of CC
- 0.5-70 per 10,000 live births
- 4% of CNS malformations
- Associated with multiple named syndromes and malformations (50-80%)
- Agenesis with interhemispheric cyst
- Type 1 ⇒ cyst is diverticulum of lateral ventricle
- Type 2 ⇒ multiple interhemispheric cysts, hyperdense/hyperintense to CSF

- Densely packed WM tracts converging into CC account for concave shape of ventricular trigone
- WM tracts more loosely packed with dysgenesis, resulting in relative dilation of trigones
  - Probst bundles are densely packed WM tracts running parallel to interhemispheric fissure
    - Normally would cross through CC
    - Run between cingulate gyrus and ventricles, indenting medial wall of ventricles
    - Slightly hypointense on T2WI, like internal capsule and anterior commissure
- T2* GRE: Calcified rim of lipoma
- MRA
  - ACAs "meander", no CC genu to curve around
  - +/- Azygous ACA
- MRV
  - Occasional midline venous anomalies
    - Persistent falcine sinus common
- DTI
  - Fiber tracts from all brain regions converge on remnant of CC
  - In complete agenesis they form Probst bundles

Ultrasonographic Findings
- Grayscale Ultrasound
  - Coronal
    - Absent CC
    - Trident lateral ventricles
    - Widely spaced lateral ventricles, colpocephaly
  - Sagittal
    - Radially arranged gyri "point to" 3rd ventricle
- Color Doppler: ACAs wander between frontal lobes

Angiographic Findings
- Conventional
  - ACAs don't conform to normal CC shape
  - +/- Azygous ACA

Imaging Recommendations
- Best imaging tool: MR
- Protocol advice: Multiplanar MR (look for additional malformations)

DIFFERENTIAL DIAGNOSIS

Destruction of callosum
- Surgery (callosotomy), trauma
- Periventricular pattern of injury in premature/neonates ⇒ periventricular leukomalacia (PVL)
- Metabolic (Marchiafava-Bignami with necrosis, longitudinal splitting of CC)

Attenuation of callosum
- Hydrocephalus stretches CC and flattens fiber tracts
- Thinning often remains even after successful treatment

Immature callosum
- CC may be difficult to perceive in neonate
  - Look for cingulate gyrus

Malformations with colpocephaly
- Chiari 2, lobar holoprosencephaly
  - Have some degree of dysgenesis of CC

PATHOLOGY

General Features
- General path comments
  - Associated with midline anomalies ⇒ lipoma, dorsal/interhemispheric cysts, inferior vermian hypoplasia
  - Cortical maldevelopment ⇒ heterotopia, schizencephaly, lissencephaly
  - Ocular/spinal/facial anomalies
  - Embryology
    - Groove forms in lamina reuniens around 8 weeks gestation ⇒ sulcus medianus telencephali medii
    - Fills with cellular material from meninx primitiva
    - Material guides axons across the midline
    - Posterior genu and anterior body form first, followed by posterior body, splenium, and finally rostrum
    - Partial agenesis reflects order of development

HEMIMEGALENCEPHALY

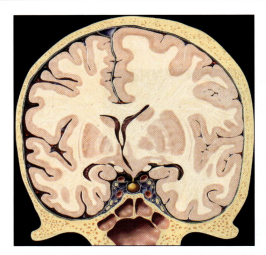

Coronal graphic shows enlargement of entire left hemisphere with thickening of cortical ribbon and broadening of gyri typical of hemimegalencephaly.

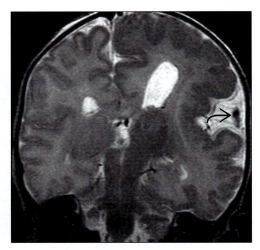

Coronal T2WI MR in an infant with seizures shows left hemisphere hemimegalencephaly. Note ipsilateral ventriculomegaly and large primitive-appearing vein in sylvian fissure (arrow).

TERMINOLOGY

Abbreviations and Synonyms
- Unilateral megalencephaly, focal megalencephaly

Definitions
- Hamartomatous overgrowth of part or all of a hemisphere
- Defect of cellular organization and neuronal migration

IMAGING FINDINGS

General Features
- Best diagnostic clue
  - Enlarged hemisphere with thickened cortical ribbon
  - Large ipsilateral ventricle with abnormally shaped frontal horn
  - Broad featureless gyri with shallow sulci
  - Abnormal primitive veins overlying shallow sulci
- Size: May affect entire hemisphere, or single lobe
- Morphology: Sulci typically shallow, with enlarged gyri

Radiographic Findings
- Radiography
  - Asymmetric calvaria
  - Some associated with ipsilateral hemihypertrophy

CT Findings
- NECT
  - Large cerebral hemisphere with deviation of posterior falx and occipital pole to opposite side
  - Lateral ventricle is large with abnormally shaped frontal horn
  - Thickened cortex with increased attenuation, occasional calcification (Ca++)
- CECT: Large vessels, developmental venous anomalies (DVAs)
- CTA: May show enlarged ipsilateral vessels which are tortuous or bizarre

MR Findings
- T1WI
  - Thick cortex: Pachygyria, polygyria, fused gyri and shallow sulci
  - Gray matter heterotopia scattered throughout hemisphere
  - Rarely affects ipsilateral cerebellum and brainstem
  - Alteration of white matter (WM) signal
    - ↑ Signal ⇒ accelerated myelination, Ca++
    - ↓ Signal ⇒ dysmyelination, hypomyelination
- T2WI
  - Size, signal intensity of affected hemisphere can change
    - Progression of myelination, development of Ca++
    - Volume loss 2° to unremitting seizures

DDx: Enlarged Or Asymmetric Cerebral Hemispheres

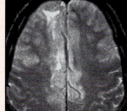
Gliomatosis

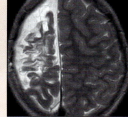
Encephalitis

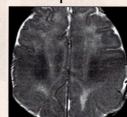
Pachygyria

HEMIMEGALENCEPHALY

Key Facts

Terminology
- Hamartomatous overgrowth of part or all of a hemisphere
- Defect of cellular organization and neuronal migration

Imaging Findings
- Enlarged hemisphere with thickened cortical ribbon
- Large ipsilateral ventricle with abnormally shaped frontal horn
- Some associated with ipsilateral hemihypertrophy
- Size, signal intensity of affected hemisphere can change
- Progression of myelination, development of Ca++
- Volume loss 2° to unremitting seizures
- Gray/white differentiation can be blurred
- Dysplastic cortex often hypointense on T2WI

Pathology
- Abnormal proliferation, migration and differentiation of neurons
- Associated with neurocutaneous and overgrowth syndromes
- Neurons are decreased in number
- Glial cells are increased in number

Clinical Issues
- Hemispherectomy removes seizure focus
- Halts injury to contralateral hemisphere
- Early surgery allows brain plasticity to take over function of resected areas
- Contralateral hemisphere must be normal
- Shunting of post-operative cavity often necessary
- Possible increased risk of hemorrhage into surgical cavity with minor trauma

---

- ○ Gray/white differentiation can be blurred
- ○ Dysplastic cortex often hypointense on T2WI
  - ■ Especially in neonates and infants
- FLAIR: ↑ Signal in WM, poor gray/white definition, reflecting altered myelination
- T2* GRE: Sensitive for Ca++
- DWI: Diffusion tractography can show increased number/density of fiber tracts
- T1 C+
  - ○ Enhancement of DVAs
  - ○ Occasional faint parenchymal enhancement
- MRV: Anomalous venous pattern
- MRS: With seizures, progressive ↓ NAA and ↑ creatine, choline, and myoinositol ⇒ reflects glial proliferation
- Magnetoencephalography (MEG)
  - ○ Somatosensory maps predict severity of cortical lamination defects

Ultrasonographic Findings
- Grayscale Ultrasound
  - ○ Displaced midline and hemispheric overgrowth
    - ■ Diagnosis can be made in fetus and neonate
- Color Doppler
  - ○ +/- Enlarged ipsilateral arteries
  - ○ Frequent dysplastic, primitive venous system

Angiographic Findings
- Conventional
  - ○ +/- High flow shunting to involved side
  - ○ Modified Wada testing can be used to suppress seizures from abnormal hemisphere to unmask contralateral seizure activity

Nuclear Medicine Findings
- PET: Glucose hypometabolism of affected hemisphere in 50%

Imaging Recommendations
- Best imaging tool: Multiplanar MRI
- Protocol advice
  - ○ Image before seizures lead to significant atrophy of involved hemisphere
  - ○ Close analysis of contralateral hemisphere essential

- ■ Contralateral malformations, seizure foci contradiction to hemispherectomy
- ■ Thin slice T1WI to identify heterotopia

DIFFERENTIAL DIAGNOSIS

Disorders of neuronal migration
- Unilateral ⇒ schizencephaly, focal polymicrogyria, focal cortical dysplasia
- Bilateral/diffuse ⇒ agyria/pachygyria, band heterotopia, x-linked subependymal heterotopia

Tuberous sclerosis (TS)
- Lobar or hemispheric hamartomatous overgrowth
  - ○ Both are disorders of cellular proliferation
- Superficial resemblance of balloon cells in hemimegalencephaly and TS
  - ○ But immunohistochemistry and electron microscopic profiles different

Syndromes with disordered migration/organization
- Fukuyama muscular dystrophy
- Muscle-eye-brain disease
- Congenital bilateral perisylvian syndrome

Hemiatrophy
- Rasmussen syndrome: Chronic focal encephalitis
  - ○ Unilateral fronto-temporal atrophy
  - ○ Progressive atrophy, signal change of caudate & putamen

Gliomatosis cerebri
- Low grade glioma diffusely infiltrating multiple lobes
- Rare in children
  - ○ Multifocal glioma is more common in children, higher grade

HEMIMEGALENCEPHALY

PATHOLOGY

General Features
- General path comments
  - Abnormal proliferation, migration and differentiation of neurons
  - Embryologic theories
    - Insult to developing brain leads to development of too many synapses, persistence of supernumerary axons and potential for white matter overgrowth
    - Localized epidermal growth factor (EGF) in cortical neurons and glial cells may lead to excessive proliferation
- Genetics: Associated with some proliferation and hemihypertrophy syndromes
- Epidemiology: Account for ≈ 3% of cortical dysplasias that are diagnosed by imaging
- Associated abnormalities
  - Associated with neurocutaneous and overgrowth syndromes
    - Neurofibromatosis type 1, tuberous sclerosis, Klippel-Trenaunay-Weber, Proteus syndrome
    - Unilateral hypomelanosis of Ito, epidermal nevus syndrome, congenital infiltrating lipomatosis, incontinentia pigmenti

Gross Pathologic & Surgical Features
- Large hemisphere, shallow sulci, fused & disorganized gyri
- Regional polymicrogyria, pachygyria and heterotopia

Microscopic Features
- Giant neurons, loss of horizontal layering of neurons
  - Neurons are decreased in number
- White matter hypertrophy & gliosis
  - Glial cells are increased in number
- Balloon cells ⇒ hypertrophic atypical cells that have variable reactivity for neuronal and glial proteins
  - Contain few lysosomes, microfilaments, microtubules and abundant lipofuscin granules

CLINICAL ISSUES

Presentation
- Most common signs/symptoms
  - Seizures
    - Infantile spasms, focal and generalized
  - Macrocrania
- Other signs/symptoms
  - Developmental delay, hemiparesis
  - Systemic overgrowth syndromes

Demographics
- Age: Usually diagnosed during first year of life

Natural History & Prognosis
- Intractable seizures ⇒ progressive injury to "good" hemisphere
- Hemispherectomy removes seizure focus
  - Halts injury to contralateral hemisphere
  - Early surgery allows brain plasticity to take over function of resected areas

Treatment
- Anticonvulsants often ineffective
- Occasional shunting to control head size and cerebellar displacement
- Surgical hemispherectomy
  - Contralateral hemisphere must be normal
  - Modified hemispherectomy ⇒ resect frontal, temporal, parietal lobes, infarct occipital
  - Reports of endovascular hemispherectomy ⇒ embolization of major arteries to infarct abnormal hemisphere/lobes
  - Shunting of post-operative cavity often necessary
  - Possible increased risk of hemorrhage into surgical cavity with minor trauma

DIAGNOSTIC CHECKLIST

Consider
- Hemihypertrophy syndromes: Remember potential airway compromise, sedation risk

Image Interpretation Pearls
- Serial imaging can show remarkable signal transformation with myelin maturation
- Involved hemisphere may atrophy (effect of chronic seizures)

SELECTED REFERENCES

1. Barkovich AJ: Pediatric Neuroimaging, 4th ed. Lippincott Williams & Wilkins. 337-41, 2005
2. Alfonso I et al: Bilateral decreased oxygenation during focal status epilepticus in a neonate with hemimegalencephaly. J Child Neurol. 19(5):394-6, 2004
3. Broumandi DD et al: Best cases from the AFIP: hemimegalencephaly. Radiographics. 24(3):843-8, 2004
4. Jonas R et al: Cerebral hemispherectomy: hospital course, seizure, developmental, language, and motor outcomes. Neurology. 62(10):1712-21, 2004
5. Devlin AM et al: Clinical outcomes of hemispherectomy for epilepsy in childhood and adolescence. Brain. 126(Pt 3):556-66, 2003
6. Flores-Sarnat L et al: Hemimegalencephaly: Part 2. Neuropathology suggests a disorder of cellular lineage. J Child Neurol. 18(11):776-785, 2003
7. Maher CO et al: Cortical resection for epilepsy in children with linear sebaceous nevus syndrome. Pediatr Neurosurg. 39(3):129-35, 2003
8. Flores-Sarnat L: Hemimegalencephaly: Part 1. Genetic, clinical, and imaging aspects. J Child Neurol, 17(5):373-84, 2002
9. Galluzzi P et al: Hemimegalencephaly in tuberous sclerosis complex. J Child Neurol. 17(9):677-80, 2002
10. Ishibashi H et al: Somatosensory evoked magnetic fields in hemimegalencephaly. Neurol Res. 24(5):459-62, 2002
11. DiRocco F et al. Hemimegalencephaly involving the cerebellum. Pediatr Neurosurg. 35(5):274-6, 2001
12. Hoffmann KT et al: MRI and 18F-flourodeoxyglucose PET in hemimegalencephaly. 42(10):749-752, 2000
13. Hanefeld F et al: Hemimegalencephaly: Localized proton magnetic resonance spectroscopy in vivo. Epilepsia. 36(12):1215-1224, 1995

HEMIMEGALENCEPHALY

IMAGE GALLERY

Typical

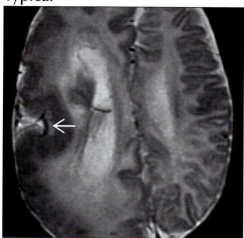
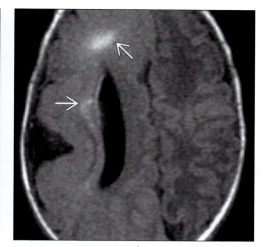

(Left) Axial T2WI MR shows right-sided hemimegalencephaly with thickened cortex lining a shallow sylvian fissure that contains an abnormal blood vessel *(arrow)*. *(Right)* Axial T1WI MR in the same infant shows regions of hyperintense signal *(arrows)* in the white matter of the enlarged hemisphere that may represent dystrophic Ca++, blood, or abnormal myelin.

Typical

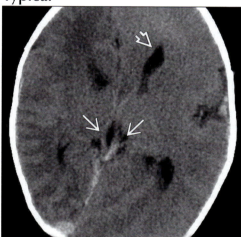
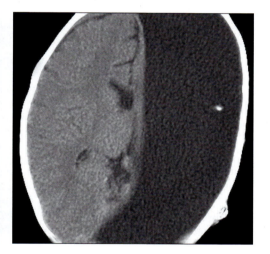

(Left) Axial CECT shows characteristic pointing of frontal horn *(open arrow)* seen in hemimegalencephaly. Note asymmetry of internal cerebral veins *(arrows)*. *(Right)* Axial NECT in the same child after hemispherectomy. Shunting of the post-operative cavity is typically required after surgery, and there may be an increased risk of hemorrhage with minor trauma.

Variant

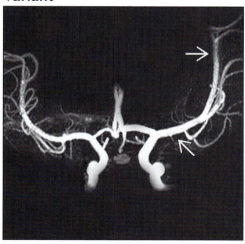
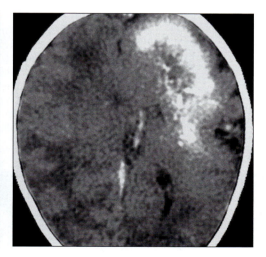

(Left) Coronal MRA child with hemimegalencephaly on the left reveals mild but diffuse enlargement of the ipsilateral carotid circulation, with some elevation of LMCA branches *(arrows)*. *(Right)* Axial NECT shows extensive dystrophic calcification in the frontal lobe of this child with left-sided hemimegalencephaly.

SCHIZENCEPHALY

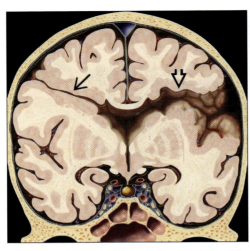

Coronal graphic shows bilateral schizencephalic clefts, closed on the right (arrow), and open on the left (open arrow). Dysplastic GM lining clefts has an irregular morphology.

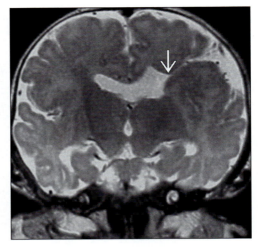

Coronal T2WI MR shows closed-lip schizencephaly on the left, with prominent ventricular dimple (arrow).

TERMINOLOGY

Abbreviations and Synonyms
- Schizencephaly, agenetic porencephaly

Definitions
- Clefts in the brain parenchyma that extend from the cortical surface to the ventricle (pia to ependyma), lined by dysplastic gray matter (GM)

IMAGING FINDINGS

General Features
- Best diagnostic clue
  - Abnormal cleft in hemisphere lined by gray matter
    - Look for dimple in wall of ventricle if cleft is narrow/closed
- Location: Frontal and parietal lobes near central sulcus most common
- Size
  - "Closed-lip" lesions are small, with walls apposed to each other
  - "Open-lip" lesions can be very large, mimicking hydranencephaly
- Morphology
  - Up to half of schizencephalies are bilateral
    - When bilateral, 60% open on both sides, 20% open on only one side
    - When unilateral, 2/3 are open

CT Findings
- NECT
  - Cleft of cerebrospinal fluid (CSF) density
  - GM lining clefts can be slightly hyperdense
  - Dimple on wall of ventricle where cleft intersects it
    - May be best clue for closed-lip lesions
  - Calcifications (Ca++) when associated with cytomegalovirus (CMV)
  - Large open-lip schizencephaly can be associated with expansion/thinning of overlying calvaria
    - Chronic effect of CSF pulsations
    - May require CSF diversion
- CECT: Large, primitive appearing veins near cleft

MR Findings
- T1WI
  - Distinction of GM lining the cleft can be difficult prior to myelination
  - Closed lip ⇒ irregular tract of GM extending from cortical ribbon to ventricle
    - GM lining cleft can appear "cobblestoned" ⇒ dysplastic
    - GM/WM border may be indistinct or irregular
  - Open lip ⇒ "canal" of CSF may be wide and wedge-shaped or have nearly parallel walls

DDx: Cortical Defects And Clefts In The Brain

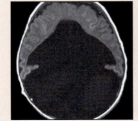
Holoprosencephaly

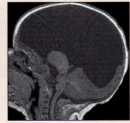
Hydranencephaly

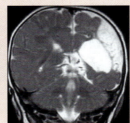
Prenatal Stroke

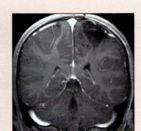
Surgical Cavity

SCHIZENCEPHALY

Key Facts

Terminology
- Clefts in the brain parenchyma that extend from the cortical surface to the ventricle (pia to ependyma), lined by dysplastic gray matter (GM)

Imaging Findings
- Look for dimple in wall of ventricle if cleft is narrow/closed
- Location: Frontal and parietal lobes near central sulcus most common
- Up to half of schizencephalies are bilateral
- Distinction of GM lining the cleft can be difficult prior to myelination

Top Differential Diagnoses
- Encephaloclastic porencephaly
- Holoprosencephaly

Pathology
- Early prenatal insult affecting germinal zone prior to neuronal migration
- Insult can be genetically determined (EMX2 gene), or 2° to infection, trauma, vascular insult
- Absence of the septum pellucidum in 70% of schizencephaly, especially bilateral

Clinical Issues
- Unilateral ⇒ seizures and mild motor deficit ("congenital" hemiparesis)
- Bilateral ⇒ severe developmental delay, paresis, spasticity
- Seizures are reportedly more common in unilateral schizencephaly
- Magnitude of clefts and associated lesions govern severity of impairment

---

- GM lining cleft can be harder to discern in open-lip schizencephaly
- T2WI
  - Infolding of gray matter along transmantle clefts
    - In unmyelinated infant, GM/WM distinction more clear on T2WI
    - Abnormal GM along cleft typically hypointense on T2WI
  - +/- Arachnoid membrane covering cleft, easily ruptured
- FLAIR: Not recommended in children < 1 year due to poor gray-white distinction
- T2* GRE: May show Ca++ if associated with CMV
- T1 C+: Associated developmental venous anomalies (DVAs) well shown with contrast
- MRA
  - MCA candelabra can "fall" into large clefts
  - Displaced along walls of cleft in subarachnoid space, not free within "canal"
- 3D surface rendered MRI
  - Best defines relationship of gyri/sulci to cleft in cerebral mantle
- Functional MR
  - Functional reorganization of the undamaged hemisphere reported

Ultrasonographic Findings
- Grayscale Ultrasound: Diagnosable by fetal ultrasound and fetal MRI; progressive changes have been reported

Angiographic Findings
- Conventional: Middle cerebral artery deficiencies occur, may be difficult to confirm when bilaterally symmetrical

Nuclear Medicine Findings
- PET: Normal or ↑ glucose metabolism and perfusion of wall of cleft (normal gray matter activity)

Imaging Recommendations
- Best imaging tool: MRI
- Protocol advice
  - Prior to myelination ⇒ T2WI
  - After myelination complete ⇒ T1WI
    - Thin slice "volume" acquisitions that allow multiplanar and surface-rendered reformatting

DIFFERENTIAL DIAGNOSIS

Encephaloclastic porencephaly
- Cleft in brain due to insult after neuronal migration complete
- Lined by gliotic WM, not dysplastic GM!

Hydranencephaly
- Destruction of tissue in middle and anterior cerebral artery territory
- May actually be most extreme form of bilateral schizencephaly

Holoprosencephaly
- Open-lip schizencephaly can mimic semilobar holoprosencephaly
- No dysplastic GM lining CSF cavities
- Holoprosencephaly has midline fusion anomalies

Post-operative cavities
- History should suffice

Trans-mantle heterotopia
- May actually represent a form of closed-lip schizencephaly

PATHOLOGY

General Features
- General path comments
  - Insult or inherited mutation lead to same pathologic/imaging features, typically in MCA distribution
    - Intrauterine insults include: Infection (CMV), maternal trauma or toxin exposure
    - Reported with alloimmune thrombocytopenia (acquired, but subsequent pregnancies have same risk of intrauterine damage)

SCHIZENCEPHALY

- ○ Experimental schizencephaly induced by mumps virus
  - ■ Antigen detected in ventricular zone neuroepithelial cells & radial glial fibers ⇒ destruction & disordered migration
- Genetics
  - ○ EMX2 (gene locus 10q26.1) is a regulatory gene with a role in structural patterning of developing forebrain
    - ■ EMX2 is expressed in germinal matrix of developing neocortex
    - ■ Mutations in the homeobox gene EMX2 seen in some cases; particularly type II schizencephaly (bilateral)
- Etiology
  - ○ Early prenatal insult affecting germinal zone prior to neuronal migration
    - ■ "Spot-weld" effect, preventing normal migration and organization
    - ■ Insult can be genetically determined (EMX2 gene), or 2° to infection, trauma, vascular insult
- Epidemiology
  - ○ Bilateral clefts are more commonly reported by pathology
  - ○ Unilateral slightly more commonly reported by imaging
- Associated abnormalities
  - ○ Frontal lobe dysplasia or inferior fusion, partial clefts, loss of WM, ventricular diverticula
  - ○ Hippocampal and callosal anomalies
  - ○ Septo-optic dysplasia (SOD, de Morsier syndrome)
    - ■ Absence of the septum pellucidum in 70% of schizencephaly, especially bilateral
    - ■ Schizencephaly is usually bilateral in SOD
    - ■ Optic nerve hypoplasia in 1/3 of schizencephaly
    - ■ Imaging is not sensitive in detection of optic nerve hypoplasia (≈ 50%)
  - ○ Heterotopia, incomplete heterotopia-lined clefts, and peri-opercular dysplasias commonly associated

Gross Pathologic & Surgical Features

- Transmantle clefts with separated or apposed gray matter lining
- Abnormal cortical array of pachygyria, polymicrogyria, or near normal-sized gyri "dive" into cleft
- Thalami, corticospinal tracts may be atrophied or not formed

Microscopic Features

- Little, if any glial scarring
- Loss of normal laminar architecture
- Pachygyria, polymicrogyria, or heterotopic gray matter

Staging, Grading or Classification Criteria

- Type I (closed-lip): Fused pial-ependymal seam lined by gray matter forms "furrow" in cortex
- Type II (open-lip): Large, gray matter lined, fluid-filled cerebrospinal fluid clefts

CLINICAL ISSUES

Presentation

- Most common signs/symptoms
  - ○ Unilateral ⇒ seizures and mild motor deficit ("congenital" hemiparesis)
  - ○ Bilateral ⇒ severe developmental delay, paresis, spasticity
    - ■ Seizures are reportedly more common in unilateral schizencephaly
- Other signs/symptoms: Microcephaly or plagiocephaly

Natural History & Prognosis

- Magnitude of clefts and associated lesions govern severity of impairment

Treatment

- Treat seizures and hydrocephalus; physiotherapy for motor deficits

DIAGNOSTIC CHECKLIST

Consider

- Image to confirm etiology of "congenital hemiparesis": Perinatal stroke versus unilateral schizencephaly

Image Interpretation Pearls

- Axial and coronal imaging to avoid "in-plane" oversight of closed-lip schizencephaly
  - ○ If plane of imaging is the same as plane of cleft, abnormality easily overlooked
- Lateral ventricle walls should be smooth
  - ○ "Dimple" in wall ⇒ look for closed-lip schizencephaly
  - ○ "Angle" of wall ⇒ consequence of periventricular injury (PVL)
  - ○ "Lump" on wall ⇒ GM heterotopion or subependymal nodule of tuberous sclerosis

SELECTED REFERENCES

1. Guerrini R: Genetic malformations of the cerebral cortex and epilepsy. Epilepsia. 46 Suppl 1:32-7, 2005
2. Cecchi C: Emx2, a gene responsible for cortical development, regionalization and area specification. Gene. 29;291(1-2):1-9, 2002
3. Dale ST et al: Neonatal alloimmune thrombocytopenia: Antenatal and postnatal imaging findings in the pediatric brain. AJNR. 23(9):1457-65, 2002
4. Hayashi N et al: Morphological features and associated anomalies of schizencephaly in the clinical population: Detailed analysis of MR images. Neuroradiology. 44(5):418-427, 2002
5. Vandermeeren Y et al: Functional relevance of abnormal fMRI activation pattern after unilateral schizencephaly. Neuroreport. 13(14):1821-4, 2002
6. Raybaud C et al: Schizencephaly: Correlation between the lobar topography of the cleft(s) and absence of the septum pellucidum. Childs Nerv Syst. 17:217-22, 2001
7. Sato N et al: MR evaluation of the hippocampus in patients with congenital malformations of the brain. AJNR. 22(2):389-93, 2001
8. Takano T et al: Experimental schizencephaly induced by Kilham strain of mumps virus: Pathogenesis of cleft formation. Neuroreport. 10(15):3149-54, 1999

SCHIZENCEPHALY

IMAGE GALLERY

Typical

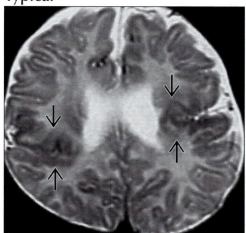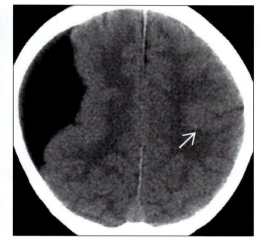

(Left) Axial T2WI MR shows bilateral schizencephalic clefts (arrows) in a neonate. T2WI typically are more sensitive for schizencephaly prior to complete myelination of the white matter. *(Right)* Axial NECT shows broad open-lip schizencephaly on the right and subtle closed-lip schizencephaly on the left (arrow).

Variant

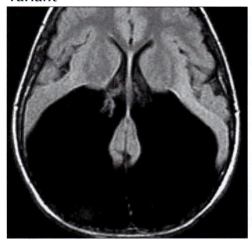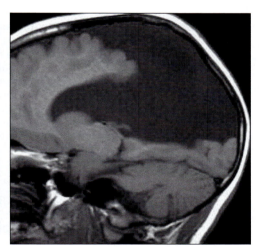

(Left) Axial FLAIR MR shows bilateral open-lip schizencephaly. Large and symmetric lesions like this can mimic terminal hydrocephalus, hydranencephaly, or semi-lobar holoprosencephaly. *(Right)* Sagittal T1WI MR in the same child shows ballooning of ventricles into schizencephalic clefts. Preserved frontal lobes mimics the "shield" hemisphere seen in holoprosencephaly.

Typical

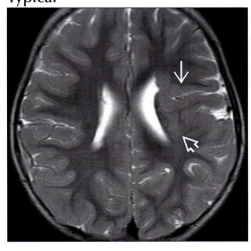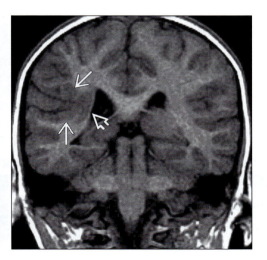

(Left) Axial T2WI MR shows closed-lip schizencephaly on the left (arrow), with adjacent heterotopic GM (open arrow) and characteristic "dimple" of lateral ventricle. *(Right)* Coronal T1WI MR shows a right-sided cleft (arrows) that appears separated from the ventricle by a thin band of white matter (open arrow). Transmantle heterotopia may merely be a variant of schizencephaly.

OCCULT SPINAL DYSRAPHISM

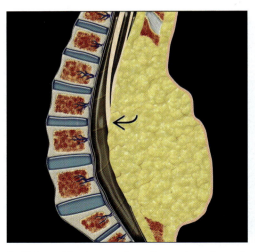

Sagittal graphic shows a large lipomyelomeningocele adherent to a low-lying conus medullaris (arrow).

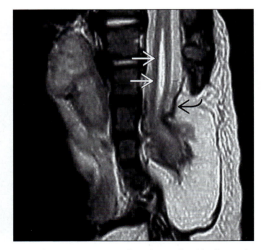

Sagittal T2WI MR in an infant shows distal hydromyelia (white arrows) in association with LPM. Note characteristic hypointense line at posterior margin of neural placode (curved arrow).

TERMINOLOGY

Abbreviations and Synonyms
- Dermal sinus tract (DST, dorsal dermal sinus), lipomyelocele and lipomyelomeningocele (LPM), spinal lipoma, thickened filum terminale, spina bifida occulta
- Tethered cord syndrome (TCS)

Definitions
- Congenital spine malformations characterized by defects in posterior elements but complete or nearly complete skin coverage
  - Lipomyelocele ⇒ congenital malformation characterized by extension of subcutaneous fat into spinal canal where it is adherent to conus/neural placode, tethering it
    - Lipomyelomeningocele has enlargement of theca with bulging of neural placode outside of spinal canal
  - Dermal sinus tract ⇒ sinus tract extending into spinal canal from skin surface, lined by epithelium
  - Spina bifida occulta ⇒ incomplete fusion of posterior elements
    - Radiographic variant that in itself is unimportant
  - Tethered cord ⇒ clinical syndrome (TCS) attributed to increased tension on filum terminale and conus medullaris
    - Cord can be tethered by identifiable masses; lipoma, dermoid, epidermoid
    - Conus is often (but not necessarily) low-lying
    - Filum may appear abnormally thickened, but normal appearing filum can tether cord also
    - Tension on conus can be inferred by demonstration of immobility
  - Spinal lipoma
    - Lipoma completely incorporated into canal
    - Adherent to filum/conus but not contiguous with subcutaneous fat
    - Can cause cord tethering

IMAGING FINDINGS

Radiographic Findings
- Radiography
  - Spina bifida occulta frequently presents with tethering lesions
    - Unhelpful more often than not
  - Scoliosis, vertebral fusion/segmentation anomalies

CT Findings
- NECT: Helical CT with multiplanar and volume rendered reformatting extremely helpful in defining vertebral anomalies associated with dysraphism

DDx: Congenital Spinal Dysraphic Lesions

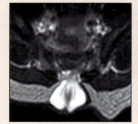

Myelomeningocele

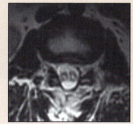

Diastematomyelia

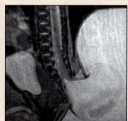

Myelocystocele

OCCULT SPINAL DYSRAPHISM

Key Facts

Terminology
- Congenital spine malformations characterized by defects in posterior elements but complete or nearly complete skin coverage
- Lipomyelocele ⇒ congenital malformation characterized by extension of subcutaneous fat into spinal canal where it is adherent to conus/neural placode, tethering it
- Dermal sinus tract ⇒ sinus tract extending into spinal canal from skin surface, lined by epithelium
- Tethered cord ⇒ clinical syndrome (TCS) attributed to increased tension on filum terminale and conus medullaris
- Filum may appear abnormally thickened, but normal appearing filum can tether cord also

Imaging Findings
- Conus may be better defined on fast spin echo T2WI
- Prone imaging is simplest way to document mobility of conus
- US excellent for evaluation of children less than one year of age

Pathology
- Dimples below the top of gluteal crease end blindly and never enter spinal canal
- Vast majority of sacral dimples require no imaging

Clinical Issues
- LPM and DST require surgery

Diagnostic Checklist
- Tethered cord and re-tethering are clinical diagnoses

MR Findings
- T1WI
  - LPM ⇒ low-lying conus medullaris ("fetal elongation of the conus medullaris"), terminating in fatty mass
    - Fat extends through posterior elements into subcutaneous tissues
    - Cord tethered to dorsal aspect of theca
    - Lipoma asymmetrically located on placode
    - Lipoma "holds" neural tube open, displacing dorsal roots anteriorly
  - Spinal lipoma ⇒ fatty mass adherent to conus or cord
    - Fat does not extend through posterior elements into subcutaneous tissues
    - May be associated with fetal elongation of cord, not always
    - Distal lipomas usually cause cord tethering (TCS)
  - DST ⇒ tract seen as dark band in subcutaneous fat
    - Travels caudally through subcutaneous fat from skin surface
    - Turns cephalad at level of spinous process
    - Slight dimple or "tenting" of dural at site of entry into canal
  - TCS ⇒ ± low-lying conus, thickened filum, terminal lipoma
    - Abnormally low conus = below L2 inferior endplate
    - Myth = conus ascend significantly with growth (little ascension over time)
    - Filum thickness should be ≤ 2 mm at L5
    - Fatty infiltration of filum terminale ⇒ "fibrolipoma"; often incidental and asymptomatic
- T2WI
  - Conus may be better defined on fast spin echo T2WI
  - Dark band of sinus tract easily visible in subcutaneous fat
  - Fast sequences ("single-shot", "HASTE", etc.) can be used to obtain prone images
    - Prone imaging is simplest way to document mobility of conus
    - Conus and proximal filum normally move 1-2 mm anteriorly with prone positioning
    - Scoliosis can prevent normal conus mobility ⇒ "bow-string" effect on cord
- STIR: Excellent for bone and soft tissue edema associated with infectious complications
- T1 C+ FS: Essential in the investigation of possibly infected DST ⇒ enhancement along tract
- MR Cine
  - Phase-contrast cine techniques can show freely moving conus
    - Subjective evaluation, similar to US

Ultrasonographic Findings
- US excellent for evaluation of children less than one year of age
  - Conus and filum clearly seen through cartilaginous spinal elements
  - Conus position and movement can be assessed
- Normal US findings ⇒ no need for further imaging unless symptoms develop/progress

Imaging Recommendations
- Best imaging tool
  - US for screening
  - MR for +US or children over 9-12 months of age
- Protocol advice: Obtain T2WI in supine and prone positions to assess cord mobility

DIFFERENTIAL DIAGNOSIS

Myelomeningocele
- Spinal component of Chiari 2 malformation
- Open neural tube defect with exposed placode

Myelocystocele
- Massive terminal syrinx with ballooning of distal cord/conus through dysraphic defect
- Skin-covered, but hardly occult

Diastematomyelia
- "Spot-weld" between vertebral body and posterior elements
  - Bony, cartilaginous, or fibrous
- Tethers cord if hemicords rejoin

OCCULT SPINAL DYSRAPHISM

Caudal regression syndrome
- Complex of caudal developmental growth abnormalities
- Absent/hypoplastic sacrum and distal spine
- Characteristic "cigar-shaped" conus

Re-tethering
- Surgical repair of dysraphic lesions does not usually bring back cord motion
  - Exception ⇒ may see more motion after lysis of thickened filum; often reverts with time to no mobility, however
- Re-tethering (like tethering) is a clinical diagnosis

PATHOLOGY

General Features
- General path comments
  - Tethering impairs the oxidative metabolism of the cord and stretches the arterioles and venules
    - Possibly leading to syringohydromyelia/myelomalacia
  - Embryology-anatomy
    - Neural tube closes during 3rd and 4th week of gestation with disjunction of neural ectoderm from cutaneous ectoderm
    - The most distal portion of the spinal cord subsequently undergoes retrogressive differentiation
- Etiology
  - LPM ⇒ premature disjunction of cutaneous ectoderm from neural ectoderm, mesenchyme becomes incorporated at closure point of neural tube, differentiates into fat
    - LPM ⇒ mesenchyme remains contiguous with subcutaneous fat
    - Lipoma ⇒ mesenchyme separates from subcutaneous fat
  - DST ⇒ lack of disjunction of cutaneous ectoderm from neural ectoderm at a focal point during neural tube closure
  - TCS ⇒ not enough retrogression leads to thicker than normal filum
- Epidemiology
  - LPM ⇒ 20-56% of occult spinal dysraphism, 20% of skin-covered lumbosacral masses
    - Lipoma ⇒ less common than LPM
  - DST ⇒ rare lesions
    - Low sacral dimples are almost always pilonidal sinus
    - Dimples below the top of gluteal crease end blindly and never enter spinal canal
    - Vast majority of sacral dimples require no imaging
  - TCS ⇒ controversial; incidence dependent upon criteria used for diagnosis
    - Should asymptomatic low-lying conus hypomobility be included?
- Associated abnormalities
  - VACTERL syndrome, anorectal and genitourinary malformations
  - Hydromyelia/syringomyelia can complicate any dysraphic lesion
  - Epidermoid and dermoid cysts can complicate any dysraphic lesion

CLINICAL ISSUES

Presentation
- Most common signs/symptoms
  - TCS ⇒ low back or leg pain
  - LPM ⇒ Urinary bladder dysfunction, urinary tract infection (UTI)
  - DST ⇒ incidentally noticed dimple
    - Purulent discharge indicates infection
- Other signs/symptoms
  - Cutaneous stigmata ⇒ hemangioma, discoloration, fawn tail
  - Lower extremity stiffness, numbness, weakness, and abnormal reflexes
  - Scoliosis and foot deformities, muscle atrophy

Demographics
- Age: Small LPM frequently present in pre-adolescents with recurrent UTI

Treatment
- LPM and DST require surgery
  - Improvement or stabilization of most neurological deficits
  - Untreated will worsen in majority of symptomatic patients
- TCS ⇒ by definition should be symptomatic
  - Surgical untethering associated with relief of symptoms in majority
  - Prophylactic surgery more controversial

DIAGNOSTIC CHECKLIST

Consider
- Most fibrolipomas are incidental findings of no clinical significance
- Tethered cord and re-tethering are clinical diagnoses
  - Can be supported by imaging findings
  - Imaging alone is not enough

Image Interpretation Pearls
- Do prone images first in sedated patients, while effects of sedation are strongest

SELECTED REFERENCES
1. Grossman R et al: Subacute formation of syrinx post-untethering of spinal cord. Pediatr Neurosurg. 40(5):234-7, 2004
2. Guggisberg D et al: Skin markers of occult spinal dysraphism in children: a review of 54 cases. Arch Dermatol. 140(9):1109-15, 2004
3. Hudgins RJ et al: Tethered spinal cord following repair of myelomeningocele. Neurosurg Focus. 16(2):E7, 2004
4. Wehby MC et al: Occult tight filum terminale syndrome: results of surgical untethering. Pediatr Neurosurg. 40(2):51-7; discussion 58, 2004
5. van der Meulen WD et al: Analysis of different treatment modalities of tethered cord syndrome. Childs Nerv Syst. 18(9-10):513-7, 2002

OCCULT SPINAL DYSRAPHISM

IMAGE GALLERY

Typical

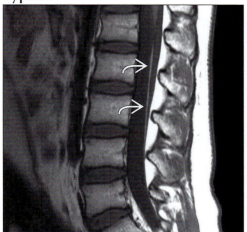
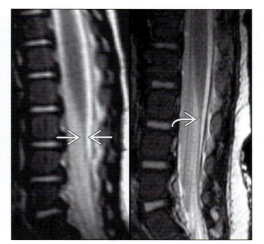

(Left) Sagittal T1WI MR shows hyperintense signal and thickening of filum terminale *(arrows)*, with normal conus position. Most fibrolipomas of the filum are incidental findings. *(Right)* Sagittal T2WI MR prone *(arrows)* and supine *(curved arrow)* show no change in position of the conus. Lack of mobility can support the clinical diagnosis of tethered cord syndrome.

Typical

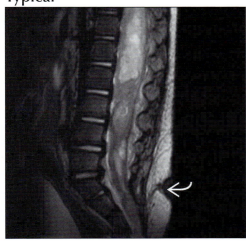
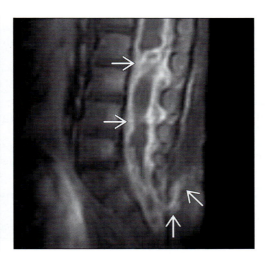

(Left) Sagittal T2WI MR in an infant with purulent drainage from a lumbar dimple shows a dark sinus tract in subcutaneous fat *(arrow)*, and irregular expansion of cord with abnormal signal. *(Right)* Sagittal T1 C+ MR with fat-saturation shows enhancement along tract and into low-lying spinal cord *(arrows)*. Dorsal dermal sinus with intraspinal abscess.

Typical

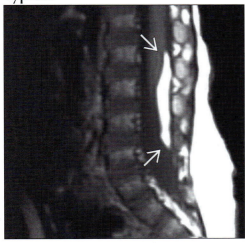
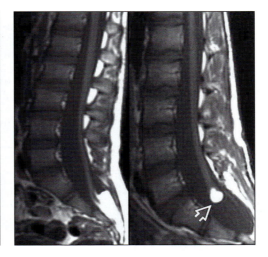

(Left) Sagittal T1WI MR shows spinal lipoma *(arrows)* with low position of conus (L3-4). Most spinal lipomas are associated with some degree of tethering, unlike fibrolipomas of the filum. *(Right)* Sagittal T1WI MR before and after *(arrow)* surgical release of spinal lipoma show retraction of conus/lipoma. Release of tension is usually associated with decrease in neurological symptoms.

DIASTEMATOMYELIA

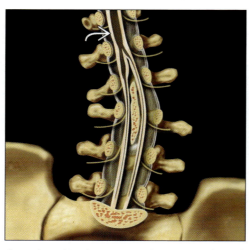

Coronal graphic shows type I diastematomyelia with large osseous spur splitting low-lying spinal cord. Note syringomyelia superior to diastem (curved arrow).

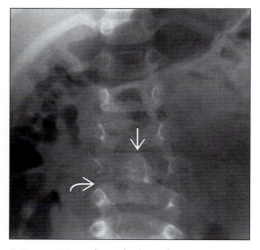

Anteroposterior radiograph shows large osseous spur (arrow). Note widening of canal and fusion anomaly (block vertebra) with next lowest vertebra (curved arrow).

TERMINOLOGY

Abbreviations and Synonyms
- Split cord malformation, "diastem"

Definitions
- Sagittal division of the spinal cord into two hemicords
- In classic diastem, each hemicord has a central canal, ventral nerve root, and dorsal nerve root
- Hemicords are split in the sagittal plane by a fibrous, cartilaginous, or osseous bar

IMAGING FINDINGS

General Features
- Best diagnostic clue
  - Axial MR or US images showing two hemicords
  - Characteristic flaring of cord on sagittal MR
- Location
  - 85% below T8
  - Cervical lesions associated with Klippel-Feil
- Morphology
  - Hemicords reunite below split in majority of diastems
  - Hemicords can stay separate
    - Lesions just above the conus medullaris

Radiographic Findings
- Radiography
  - Osseous spur may be apparent on radiographs
    - < 50%
  - Frequent fusion/segmentation anomalies
  - Scoliosis

CT Findings
- NECT
  - Helical CT excellent for delineating vertebral anomalies and osseous spur
  - Fibrous or cartilaginous spurs can be inapparent

MR Findings
- T1WI
  - Associated syrinx in up to 50% of cases
  - Three dimensional (volumetric) acquisitions can help "straighten" scoliosis
  - Osseous spur may contain fatty marrow ⇒ hyperintense
    - Fibrous spur ⇒ hypointense or isointense
- T2WI
  - Distinction from syrinx easy on sagittal and axial images
    - Axial images clearly demonstrate hemicords
    - Sagittal images show a slight posterior "flare" of cord
  - May show hemicords more clearly than T1WI

DDx: Lesions That Split Or Compress The Spinal Cord

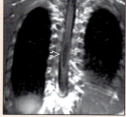
Syrinx

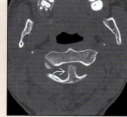
Vertebral Anomaly

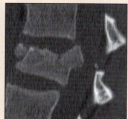
Fracture

DIASTEMATOMYELIA

Key Facts

Terminology
- Split cord malformation, "diastem"
- Sagittal division of the spinal cord into two hemicords
- Hemicords are split in the sagittal plane by a fibrous, cartilaginous, or osseous bar

Imaging Findings
- 85% below T8
- Hemicords reunite below split in majority of diastems
- Osseous spur may be apparent on radiographs
- Helical CT excellent for delineating vertebral anomalies and osseous spur
- Hemicords often better delineated on US than MR in smallest infants
- T2 coronal and axial images demonstrate hemicords

Pathology
- Rare terminal diastem can result in separate conus and filum for each hemicord
- 50% of patients share a dural sac; other 50% demonstrate separate dural tubes
- Congenital splitting of the notochord produces a spectrum of "split notochord syndromes"
- Spur tethers cord if hemicords reunite below (90%)
- Can be tethered by adherent nerve root - "meningocele manque"
- Can have associated thickened filum - need to divide at surgery

Clinical Issues
- Stable or progressive disability if untreated
- Up to 90% of patients stabilize or improve following surgery

---

- Can demonstrate separate dural sacs
  - Distal lesions cause abrupt tapering of conus
    - Resembles nib of fountain pen
  - Fibrous or cartilaginous spur hypointense
  - Fusion anomalies of vertebrae well shown
- Fetal MR
  - May be more sensitive than US for spinal lesions

Ultrasonographic Findings
- High resolution modality in neonates and infants
  - Hemicords often better delineated on US than MR in smallest infants
- Less effective as spine ossifies
- Prenatal diagnosis ⇒ extra posterior echogenic focus

Non-Vascular Interventions
- Myelography
  - CT myelography provided highest resolution of cord and nerve roots
  - Usually not necessary for diagnosis
    - May help with surgical planning by best defining spur and osseous anomalies
    - Can help clearly distinguish single sac in type II lesions

Imaging Recommendations
- Best imaging tool: MRI
- Protocol advice
  - US can be used to screen infants with suspicious cutaneous stigmata
  - MR imaging to investigate positive cases
    - T2 coronal and axial images demonstrate hemicords
    - Axial T2 weighted images optimally demonstrate composition/location of spur, and presence or absence of syrinx
  - Supplement with CT to optimally define spur anatomy if surgical intervention is planned

DIFFERENTIAL DIAGNOSIS

Syringomyelia
- Can mimic diastem on coronal images
- Easily distinguished on sagittal and axial images
- Complicates diastem in 50% of cases

Posterior element anomalies
- Severe impingement from "inverted" spinous process can resemble incomplete diastem spur

Fracture with retropulsed bone
- Easily distinguished by history

Duplicated spinal cord (diplomyelia)
- Exceedingly rare

PATHOLOGY

General Features
- General path comments
  - Strongly associated with other spinal anomalies
  - Cleft almost always completely splits the cord, with a single cord above and below split
    - Rare terminal diastem can result in separate conus and filum for each hemicord
  - 50% of patients share a dural sac; other 50% demonstrate separate dural tubes
- Etiology
  - Embryology
    - Notochord forms in 3rd-4th week gestation
    - Forms between endoderm and ectoderm
    - If connection remains between endoderm and ectoderm, notochord must split or deviate around it
    - Mesoderm is split along with notochord
  - Congenital splitting of the notochord produces a spectrum of "split notochord syndromes"
    - Dorsal enteric fistula/sinus, dorsal enteric cyst/diverticulum
    - Fistulae, cysts, and sinuses represent continued connection between endoderm and ectoderm

NEUROFIBROMATOSIS TYPE 1

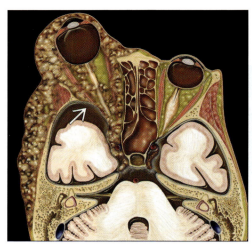

Axial graphic of the orbits shows an infiltrating PNF extending from the cavernous sinus through the orbit into the temporal fossa, with associated "dysplasia" of the sphenoid wing (arrow).

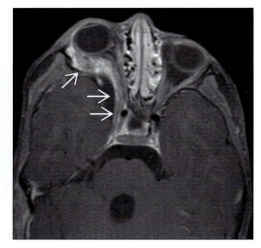

Axial T1 C+ MR with fat-saturation shows proptosis caused by orbital-cavernous PNF with sphenoid wing defect, medial deviation of cavernous sinus and internal carotid artery (arrows).

TERMINOLOGY

Abbreviations and Synonyms
- Neurofibromatosis type 1 (NF1), von Recklinghausen disease

Definitions
- Neurocutaneous disorder (phakomatosis) characterized by
  - Neurofibromas (NF)
  - Dynamic reactive/dysplastic white matter (WM) lesions
  - Cafe-au-lait spots
  - Vascular dysplasias
  - Astrocytomas, primarily of the visual pathways
  - Skeletal dysplastic lesions

IMAGING FINDINGS

General Features
- Best diagnostic clue
  - Hyperintense WM lesions on T2WI
  - Plexiform neurofibromas (PNF)
  - Visual pathway gliomas
- Location
  - WM lesions ⇒ dentate nuclei of cerebellum, globus pallidi, thalami, hippocampi, brainstem
  - PNF ⇒ scalp, along cervical nodal chains, lateral orbit/cavernous sinus
  - Visual pathway gliomas ⇒ intra-orbital optic nerves (ON), chiasm/hypothalamus, rarely optic tracts
- Size
  - WM lesions ⇒ 2-20 mm
  - Visual pathway gliomas ⇒ 3-50 mm
  - PNF ⇒ can be very large
- Morphology
  - WM lesions ⇒ spherical/ovoid, often amorphous
  - Visual pathway glioma ⇒ conform to ON in orbit, can be spherical in chiasm/hypothalamus
    - Buckle ON in orbit ⇒ "dotted i"
  - PNF: Snake-like ropes of tissue, often infiltrating and amorphous

Radiographic Findings
- Radiography
  - Kyphoscoliosis
  - Hypoplastic posterior elements, scalloped vertebrae from dural ectasia, neurofibromas
  - Dysplastic sphenoid wing, ribbon ribs, pseudarthroses

CT Findings
- NECT
  - Bone defects of sphenoid wing and lambdoid suture
  - Enlargement of ON, chiasm, superior orbital fissure

DDx: Neurocutaneous Syndromes

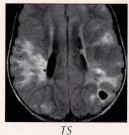
TS

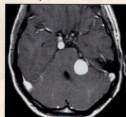
NF2

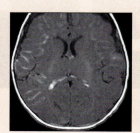
Sturge-Weber

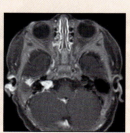
PHACES

NEUROFIBROMATOSIS TYPE 1

Key Facts

Terminology
- Neurofibromas (NF)
- Dynamic reactive/dysplastic white matter (WM) lesions
- Cafe-au-lait spots
- Vascular dysplasias
- Astrocytomas, primarily of the visual pathways
- Skeletal dysplastic lesions

Imaging Findings
- ON gliomas demonstrate moderate enhancement
- Peripheral PNFs have little enhancement
- Poorly-defined hyperintense WM lesions in dentate nuclei of cerebellum, thalamus, GP
- Found in 60-85% of children with NF1
- Diminish with puberty ⇒ gone by adulthood
- Coronal STIR of spine can show extent of lesions
- Cerebellar lesions easier to discern on T2
- Include dedicated imaging of orbits with all brain MRs
- Use MRS to evaluate atypical WM lesions

Pathology
- Sphenoid wing "dysplasia" nearly always associated with PNF of lateral orbit and cavernous sinus
- 1:3000-5000 people have NF1
- WM lesions ⇒ foci of myelin vacuolization

Clinical Issues
- > 30% have learning disabilities

Diagnostic Checklist
- WM lesions may mask underlying infiltrating glioma

  - Helical spine CT can aid in surgical management of scoliosis
- CECT
  - ON gliomas demonstrate moderate enhancement
  - Peripheral PNFs have little enhancement
- CTA
  - Vascular dysplasias, renal artery stenosis, aortic stenosis
  - Moyamoya ⇒ 1° or secondary to radiation therapy (RTx)

MR Findings
- T1WI
  - WM lesions in GP can be hyperintense
  - Enlargement of ON, chiasm
  - PNF ⇒ isointense to brain/cord
- T2WI
  - Poorly-defined hyperintense WM lesions in dentate nuclei of cerebellum, thalamus, GP
    - Found in 60-85% of children with NF1
    - Little or no mass effect
    - Increase in number/size in pre-adolescence
    - Diminish with puberty ⇒ gone by adulthood
  - PNF: "Target" sign (bright with central collagen dot)
- STIR
  - Single best sequence for demonstrating PNF
    - Coronal STIR of spine can show extent of lesions
    - Scoliosis frequently associated with paraspinal neurofibroma along concave margin of curve
- FLAIR
  - Shows WM lesions in GP well
    - Cerebellar lesions easier to discern on T2
- DWI: ↑ ADC values in WM lesions
- T1 C+: PNF and ON glioma have variable enhancement patterns which change over time
- MRA: Moyamoya vascularity
- MRS
  - Can help distinguish WM lesions from infiltrating glioma
    - WM lesion ⇒ elevation of myo-inositol (mI), preserved NAA
    - Glioma ⇒ elevation of choline, ↓ NAA

Angiographic Findings
- Conventional
  - Moyamoya
  - Renal artery stenoses, distal aorta coarctation

Non-Vascular Interventions
- Myelography: Dural ectasia; lateral meningoceles

Imaging Recommendations
- Best imaging tool
  - STIR for PNF
  - T2 and FLAIR for WM lesions
  - T1 C+ with fat-saturation for ON glioma
- Protocol advice
  - Include dedicated imaging of orbits with all brain MRs
  - Include coronal STIR with all spine MRs
  - Use MRS to evaluate atypical WM lesions

DIFFERENTIAL DIAGNOSIS

Other disorders of the NF spectrum
- Mosaic (segmental) NF1 or NF2
- Hereditary spinal NF, familial intestinal NF
- Autosomal dominant café-au-lait spots, autosomal dominant neurofibromas

Neurocutaneous syndromes - phakomatoses
- Tuberous sclerosis (TS)
  - Multiple hamartomas
- Sturge-Weber
  - Retinal, trigeminal, and pial angiomatosis
- Neurofibromatosis type 2 (NF2)
  - Multiple meningiomas and schwannomas
- PHACES
  - Posterior fossa malformations, Hemangiomas, Arterial anomalies, Cardiac anomalies, Eye anomalies, and Sternal clefting
- Von Hippel Lindau disease (VHL)
  - Hemangioblastomas, retinal angiomas, renal cysts and carcinomas

NEUROFIBROMATOSIS TYPE 1

- Multiple others, including ataxia-telangiectasia, neurocutaneous melanosis, incontinentia pigmenti, basal cell nevus syndrome

PATHOLOGY

General Features
- General path comments
  - NF lesions of childhood ⇒ café-au-lait spots, axillary freckling
  - NF lesions of adults ⇒ subcutaneous neurofibromas, Lisch nodules
  - Sphenoid wing "dysplasia" nearly always associated with PNF of lateral orbit and cavernous sinus
    - Tumor remodeling/erosion rather than dysplasia?
- Genetics
  - "NF gene" locus ⇒ long arm of chromosome 17
    - Gene product ⇒ neurofibromin, inactivated in NF1
  - Autosomal dominant; 50% new mutations
  - Variable expression, virtually 100% penetrance
- Etiology
  - Inactivation of neurofibromin allows cell proliferation & tumor development
  - Oligodendrocyte myelin glycoprotein embedded within NF gene
    - May cause myelin dysplasia accounting for WM lesions
- Epidemiology
  - Most common autosomal dominant disorder
  - Most common inherited tumor syndrome
  - 1:3000-5000 people have NF1
- Associated abnormalities: Pheochromocytomas, neurofibrosarcomas, malignant nerve sheath tumors

Gross Pathologic & Surgical Features
- Visual pathway glioma, usually low grade
  - Frank malignancy < 20%
  - Can extend to geniculate bodies & optic radiations
  - Peri-chiasmatic infiltration ⇒ more likely to be aggressive, ↑ frequency precocious puberty
- 1-3% incidence of other astrocytomas
- PNF degeneration to neurofibrosarcoma in 2-12%
- Slight ↑ incidence medulloblastoma/ependymoma
- Lisch nodules (iris hamartomas) in 85% > 10 years old
- Buphthalmos

Microscopic Features
- WM lesions ⇒ foci of myelin vacuolization
- PNF: Schwann cells, perineural fibroblasts, grow along nerve fascicles

Staging, Grading or Classification Criteria
- NF1 if two or more of following
  - 6+ café-au-lait spots, > 5 mm
  - ≥ 2 NF or 1 PNF
  - Axillary/inguinal freckling
  - ON glioma
  - Distinctive bone lesion
  - 1° relative with NF1

CLINICAL ISSUES

Presentation
- Most common signs/symptoms
  - > 95% have skin lesions
  - > 95% have Lisch nodules (adults)
  - ≈ 50% have macrocephaly ⇒ increased WM volume
  - > 30% have learning disabilities
  - ≈ 15% have scoliosis
  - ≈ 15% have visual pathway gliomas
- Other signs/symptoms
  - ≈ 5% have mental retardation
  - ≈ 5% have epilepsy

Demographics
- Age: Café-au-lait spot appear in 1st year of life
- Gender: M = F
- Ethnicity: Risk for ON glioma lower in African-Americans than in Caucasians or Hispanics

Natural History & Prognosis
- NF1 related learning disability 30-60%
  - Associated with WM lesions
- Risk of other CNS tumors ↑ with presence of ON glioma
- ↑ Risk sarcomatous degeneration PNF
- Vascular stenoses: Intra- and extracranial
  - Renal artery stenosis ⇒ hypertension

Treatment
- Clinical observation
- Chemotherapy and radiation therapy for ON gliomas
- Spinal release and fixation for scoliosis
- Debulking surgery for PNF impinging upon airway, alimentary tract
- Angioplasty/surgical grafting for arterial stenoses

DIAGNOSTIC CHECKLIST

Consider
- WM lesions may mask underlying infiltrating glioma
- Remember to look for vascular lesions!

Image Interpretation Pearls
- WM lesions that have mass effect, irregular signal, or atypical location should be viewed with suspicion
  - Consider MRS to investigate further
- Use coronal STIR to assess for spinal and paraspinal NF

SELECTED REFERENCES

1. Tognini G et al: Brain apparent diffusion coefficient evaluation in pediatric patients with neurofibromatosis type 1. J Comput Assist Tomogr. 29(3):298-304, 2005
2. Geldmann R et al: Neurofibromatosis type 1: Motor and cognitive function and T2W MRI hyperintensities. Neurology. 61(12):1725-8, 2003
3. Raininko R et al: Atypical focal non-neoplastic brain changes in neurofibromatosis type 1: Mass effect and contrast enhancement. Neuroradiology. 43(7):586-590, 2001
4. Wilkinson ID et al: Proton MRS of brain lesions in children with neurofibromatosis type 1. Magn Reson Imaging. 19(8):1081-9, 2001

NEUROFIBROMATOSIS TYPE 1

IMAGE GALLERY

Typical

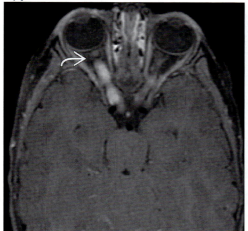
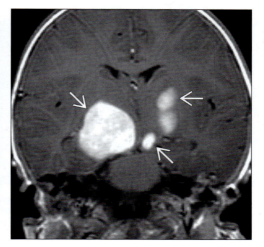

(Left) Axial T1 C+ MR with fat-saturation shows diffuse enlargement and enhancement of optic nerves from bilateral ON glioma. Note buckling of right ON (arrow) ⇒ "dotted I" sign. *(Right)* Coronal T1 C+ MR shows multiple foci of enhancement (arrows) from chiasmatic/hypothalamic glioma. Morbidity is higher in these lesions than in those restricted to the orbit.

Typical

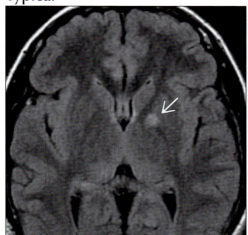
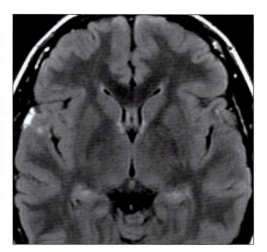

(Left) Axial FLAIR MR shows typical nonspecific WM lesion (arrow) in the left basal ganglia of an 8 year old with NF1. Globus pallidus and cerebellum are the most common locations of these lesions. *(Right)* Axial FLAIR MR in the same patient 3 years later shows near-complete resolution of the previously seen lesion. These signal abnormalities are dynamic, often resolving before adulthood.

Typical

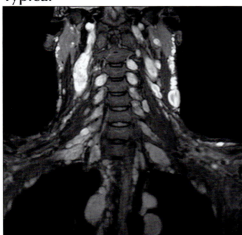
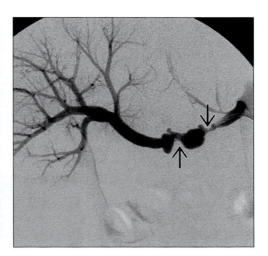

(Left) Coronal STIR MR shows innumerable hyperintense rope-like neurofibromas extending along every nerve root, and paraspinal NFs in the posterior mediastinum. *(Right)* Coronal catheter angiography of the right renal artery in an adolescent with NF1 and hypertension shows severe and irregular renal artery stenoses (arrows).

TUBEROUS SCLEROSIS

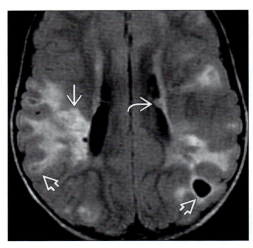

Axial FLAIR MR in a 3 year old shows tubers (open arrows), WM lesions (arrow), and a subependymal nodule (curved arrow). Note the "empty gyrus" in left parietal lobe tuber.

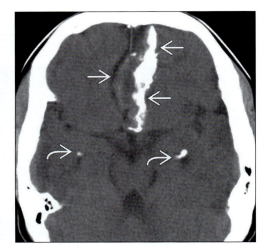

Axial NECT shows Ca++ left frontal lobe in a child with TSC (arrows). These stable hamartomatous lesions can be excised to treat seizures. Curved arrows point to SENs in temporal horns.

TERMINOLOGY

Abbreviations and Synonyms
- Tuberous sclerosis complex (TSC); Bourneville syndrome, Pringle disease, Epiloia

Definitions
- The "original" phakomatosis
  - "Phakoma" first used by Dutch ophthalmologist to describe retinal hamartoma
- Neurocutaneous syndrome - hamartomatosis
  - Hamartomas of multiple organs ⇒ central nervous system (CNS), skin, kidney, bone

IMAGING FINDINGS

General Features
- Best diagnostic clue
  - Cortical/subcortical "tubers"
    - Term refers to potato-like texture observed at gross pathology
  - Subependymal nodules (SENs)
  - Subependymal giant cell astrocytoma (SEGA)
- Location
  - Tubers ⇒ supratentorial > > cerebellum: "Peripheral lesions"
    - Tracts of abnormal white matter (WM) extend from ventricles to tubers
    - Cystic foci in WM ⇒ periventricular cysts
    - Subcortical cystic degeneration in tubers ⇒ "empty gyrus"
  - SEN ⇒ along lateral walls of lateral ventricles: "Central lesions"
    - Body/atrium > > temporal horn
    - SEGA ⇒ enlarging nodule at foramen of Monro
- Morphology
  - Peripheral tubers expand overlying gyrus, triangular
    - 20% have central umbilication
  - SENs irregular and elongated ⇒ "candle drippings" at ventriculography
  - SEGAs become more spherical with increasing size

Radiographic Findings
- Radiography
  - Bone islands (long bones, fingers)
  - Undulating periosteal new bone

CT Findings
- NECT
  - SENs ⇒ calcification (Ca++) increases with time
  - Tubers ⇒ low attenuation subcortical lesion expanding overlying gyrus
    - Some progressive Ca++ over time
  - Hamartomatous lobe ⇒ Ca++ dysplasia/hamartoma of entire lobe (frontal) or hemisphere

DDx: Non-CNS Lesions Of Tuberous Sclerosis

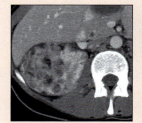

Angiomyolipoma

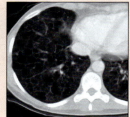

LAM

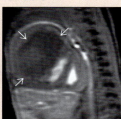

Rhabdomyoma

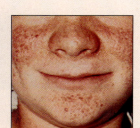

Adenoma Sebaceum

TUBEROUS SCLEROSIS

Key Facts

Terminology
- The "original" phakomatosis
- Hamartomas of multiple organs ⇒ central nervous system (CNS), skin, kidney, bone

Imaging Findings
- Cortical/subcortical "tubers"
- Subependymal nodules (SENs)
- Subependymal giant cell astrocytoma (SEGA)
- Tracts of abnormal white matter (WM) extend from ventricles to tubers
- DWI: ↑ ADC values have been reported in epileptogenic tubers
- 10-15% cortical/subependymal tubers enhance
- MRA: Aneurysms and ectasias occasionally encountered
- ↑ Myo-inositol (mI) in central and peripheral lesions

Top Differential Diagnoses
- TORCH infections that cause periventricular Ca++
- Cortical dysplasia

Pathology
- TSC1 (9q34) encodes "hamartin"
- TSC2 (16p13) encodes "tuberin"
- Tuberin and hamartin combine to form a complex in vivo
- Normally inhibit part of mTOR activity
- RAM ⇒ 40-80% incidence, amenable to embolization
- Cardiac rhabdomyomas ⇒ majority involute spontaneously

Clinical Issues
- Small number of cases have shown SEGA regression with rapamycin therapy

---

- Giant optic drusen
  - Ca++ retinal hamartoma
- CECT
  - Most SENs enhance ⇒ may be masked by Ca++
  - Some peripheral lesions faintly enhance
- CTA: Aneurysms are a less common characteristic of TSC

MR Findings
- T1WI
  - Tubers ⇒ hypointense subcortical lesion expanding overlying gyrus
    - Occasionally hyperintense
  - SENs ⇒ typically slightly hyperintense
    - Best shown on sagittal and coronal images
- T2WI
  - Tubers ⇒ hyperintense
    - More apparent with maturation of normal myelin
- FLAIR
  - Tubers ⇒ hyperintense
    - Empty gyrus and periventricular cysts suppress completely
  - Best sequence for WM tract lesions
- T2* GRE: Helpful to show Ca++ in tubers and SENs
- DWI: ↑ ADC values have been reported in epileptogenic tubers
- T1 C+
  - Best sequence for showing SEN enhancement
    - 30-80% enhance
  - 10-15% cortical/subependymal tubers enhance
- MRA: Aneurysms and ectasias occasionally encountered
- MRS
  - ↑ Myo-inositol (mI) in central and peripheral lesions
  - ↓ NAA with ↑↑ mI in SEN at foramen of Monro = SEGA

Angiographic Findings
- Conventional: Diagnosis/treatment of aneurysms

Nuclear Medicine Findings
- PET
  - Tubers are hypometabolic
  - Epileptogenic tubers show increased uptake of alpha-methyl-tryptophan (AMT)

Imaging Recommendations
- Best imaging tool: MR with contrast
- Protocol advice
  - Use DWI to assess epileptogenic foci
  - Evaluate lesions at foramen of Monro with contrast and MRS
    - Growth or MRS conversion indicate SEGA

DIFFERENTIAL DIAGNOSIS

Non-CNS manifestations of TS
- Renal angiomyolipoma (RAM) ⇒ hamartomatous tumor of kidney
- Lymphangioleiomyomatosis (LAM) ⇒ smooth muscle proliferation in lung interstitium
  - Represents metastatic RAM
- Cardiac rhabdomyoma ⇒ can cause obstruction, arrhythmias
- Adenoma sebaceum ⇒ acne-like subcutaneous hamartoma of face (angiofibroma)
- Ash-leaf spots, shagreen patches, subungual fibroma, dental pits
- Bone islands, periosteal new bone

Infection
- TORCH infections that cause periventricular Ca++
  - Cytomegalovirus (CMV), toxoplasmosis
- Hematogenous spread of infections that cause subcortical lesions
  - Fungus, neurocysticercosis

Neoplasms
- Superficial tumors that can resemble tubers
  - Dysembryoplastic neuroepithelial tumor (DNET), meningioma, meningioangiomatosis
- Intraventricular tumors
  - Choroid plexus tumors, subependymoma, central neurocytoma

TUBEROUS SCLEROSIS

Cortical dysplasia
- Taylor dysplasia, balloon cell dysplasia

X-linked subependymal heterotopia
- Gray matter heterotopia along lateral ventricle margins
- No Ca++ or enhancement

Subcortical ischemia, infarction
- Regions of hyperintense subcortical signal on T2WI and FLAIR
- Restricted diffusion, gyral swelling

PATHOLOGY

General Features
- Genetics
  - Two distinct gene loci
    - TSC1 (9q34) encodes "hamartin"
    - TSC2 (16p13) encodes "tuberin"
    - TSC2 disease is predominant
  - 1/3 familial
    - Autosomal dominant, high penetrance
- Etiology
  - Tuberin and hamartin combine to form a complex in vivo
    - Act together on mTOR (mammalian target of rapamycin)
    - Normally inhibit part of mTOR activity
    - Regulate cell growth and proliferation
  - Mutations prevent them from down-regulating mTOR
  - Affects geminal matrix ⇒ disordered neuronal migration and growth
- Epidemiology: 1:10,000 incidence
- Associated abnormalities
  - RAM ⇒ 40-80% incidence, amenable to embolization
  - Cardiac rhabdomyomas ⇒ majority involute spontaneously

Gross Pathologic & Surgical Features
- Firm cortical masses with umbilication

Microscopic Features
- Balloon cells, giant cells, ectopic neurons
- Myelin loss, vacuolation and gliosis

Staging, Grading or Classification Criteria
- SEGA = WHO grade I
- Diagnostic criteria: Two major or one major + one minor
  - Major: Tuber, SEN, SEGA, cardiac rhabdomyoma, RAM, LAM, adenoma sebaceum, sub-/periungual fibroma, hypomelanotic macules, shagreen patch, retinal hamartoma
  - Minor: WM lesions, dental pits, gingival fibromas, rectal polyps, bone cysts, non-renal hamartoma, retinal achromic patch, confetti skin lesions, multiple renal cysts
- Genetic testing detects mutations in 60-80% of affected individuals

CLINICAL ISSUES

Presentation
- Most common signs/symptoms
  - Classic clinical triad: Adenoma sebaceum, seizures, mental retardation
    - Seen in only 30-40%
  - Infantile spasms ⇒ poorer outcome
  - Autism

Demographics
- Age
  - Rhabdomyomas present prenatally and in infancy
  - CNS lesions present in infancy and childhood
  - Skin lesions present in childhood
  - Renal, lung, and bone lesions present in adulthood

Natural History & Prognosis
- Prognosis dependent upon severity of symptoms (seizures, arrhythmias, renal insufficiency) and success of treatment

Treatment
- Medical anti-seizure therapy, resection of seizure focus
- Resect SEGA if obstructing foramen of Monro
- Rapamycin ⇒ immunosuppressant isolated from fungus found on Easter Island
  - Down-regulates mTOR
  - Small number of cases have shown SEGA regression with rapamycin therapy

DIAGNOSTIC CHECKLIST

Consider
- Remember presentation of non-CNS lesions as patients age

Image Interpretation Pearls
- Don't forget to look for vascular lesions!

SELECTED REFERENCES

1. Karadag D et al: Diffusion tensor imaging in children and adolescents with tuberous sclerosis. Pediatr Radiol. 2005
2. Chan JA et al: Pathogenesis of tuberous sclerosis subependymal giant cell astrocytomas: biallelic inactivation of TSC1 or TSC2 leads to mTOR activation. J Neuropathol Exp Neurol. 63(12):1236-42, 2004
3. Franz DN: Non-neurologic manifestations of tuberous sclerosis complex. J Child Neurol. 19(9):690-8, 2004
4. Bader RS et al: Fetal rhabdomyoma: Prenatal diagnosis, clinical outcome, and incidence of associated tuberous sclerosis complex. J Pediatr. 143(5):620-4, 2003
5. Jansen FE et al: Diffusion-weighted MRI and identification of the epileptogenic tuber in patients with tuberous sclerosis. Arch Neurol. 60(11):1580-4, 2003
6. Jones BV et al: Guglielmi detachable coil embolization of a giant midbasilar aneurysm in a 19-month-old patient. AJNR Am J Neuroradiol. 23(7):1145-8, 2002
7. Cristophe C et al: MRI spectrum of cortical malformations in tuberous sclerosis complex. Brain Dev. 22(8):487-493, 2000

TUBEROUS SCLEROSIS

IMAGE GALLERY

Typical

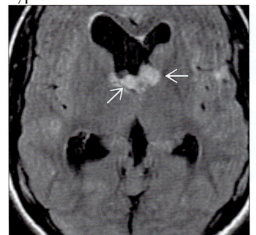
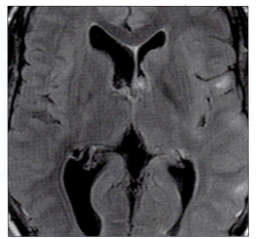

(Left) Axial FLAIR MR shows SEGAs at foramen of Monro (arrows) that had grown over a 1 year period. These tumors become symptomatic when they cause hydrocephalus. *(Right)* Axial FLAIR MR in the same patient 6 months later, after treatment with rapamycin, shows a significant decrease in the size of the tumors.

Typical

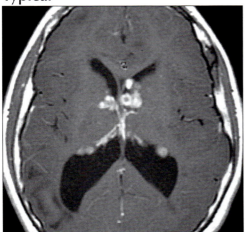
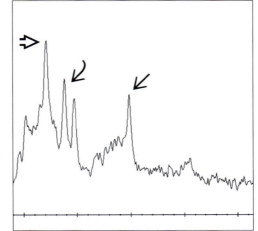

(Left) Axial T1 C+ MR shows multiple enhancing subependymal nodules. Enhancement of SENs is much easier to discern on MR than on CT, and does not in itself indicate transformation to SEGA. *(Right)* MRS shows characteristic short-echo proton spectroscopy profile of a SEGA, with depression of NAA (arrow), elevation of choline (curved arrow) and elevation of myoinositol (open arrow).

Variant

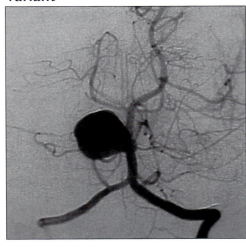
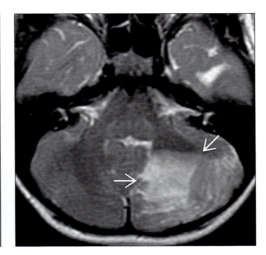

(Left) Anteroposterior catheter angiography with injection in the vertebral artery shows a large mid-basilar aneurysm in a 19 month old. Aneurysms are a known, but uncommon, manifestation of TSC. *(Right)* Axial T2WI MR shows a mass-like tuber in the left cerebellum (arrows) in this 11 year old. Infratentorial lesions are much less common than supratentorial ones.

- o Post-contrast imaging in all three planes
- o MRS and diffusion can help with difficult cases
  - ■ Pulmonary infection, endocarditis, urinary tract infection

BRAIN ABSCESS

- Immunosuppressed patients (chemotherapy, transplant recipients)
  - Penetrating trauma
    - Bone fragments more likely source than metal
    - Post-operative
  - Right-to-left shunts (congenital cardiac malformations, pulmonary arteriovenous fistulas)
    - "Paradoxical" emboli originating in venous system
  - 20-30% have no identifiable source ⇒ cryptogenic
  - Often polymicrobial ⇒ streptococci, staphylococci, anaerobes
    - Neonates ⇒ Citrobacter, Proteus, Pseudomonas, Serratia, Staphylococcus aureus
    - Posttransplant ⇒ Aspergillus, Nocardia, Candida
- Epidemiology: ≈ 2500 cases/year in U.S.

Gross Pathologic & Surgical Features
- Early cerebritis (3-5 days)
  - Unencapsulated mass of leukocytes and edema
    - Scattered foci of necrosis and petechial hemorrhage
- Late cerebritis (4-5 days up to 2 weeks)
  - Necrotic foci coalesce
  - Rim of inflammatory cells, macrophages, granulation tissue, and fibroblasts surrounds necrotic core
  - Surrounding vascular proliferation and vasogenic edema
- Early capsule (begins at around 2 weeks)
  - Well-delineated collagenous capsule
  - Liquefied necrotic core
  - Peripheral gliosis
- Late capsule (weeks to months)
  - Central cavity shrinks
  - Thick wall (collagen, granulation tissue, macrophages, gliosis)

Microscopic Features
- Early cerebritis: Hyperemic tissue with leukocytes, necrotic blood vessels, microorganisms
- Late cerebritis: Progressive necrosis of the neuropil, destruction of leukocytes
- Early capsule: Proliferation of granulation tissue about necrotic core
- Late capsule: Multiple layers of collagen and fibroblasts

CLINICAL ISSUES

Presentation
- Most common signs/symptoms
  - Headache most common symptom (up to 90%)
  - Fever in only 50%
  - Other signs/symptoms: Seizures, altered mental status, focal neurologic deficits
    - ↑ Erythrocyte sedimentation rate (ESR) ⇒ 75%
    - ↑ White blood cell (WBC) count ⇒ 50%

Demographics
- Age
  - May occur at any age
  - 25% occur in patients < 15 years
- Gender: M:F = 2:1

Natural History & Prognosis
- Potentially fatal but treatable lesion
- Prognosis depends on
  - Size of abscess
  - Location of abscess
  - Virulence of infecting organism
  - Systemic condition of patient
- Complications of inadequately or untreated abscesses
  - Intraventricular rupture, ventriculitis (may be fatal)
    - Ventricular debris with irregular fluid level
    - Hydrocephalus
    - Ependymal enhancement typical
  - Meningitis, "daughter" lesions
  - Mass effect, herniation
- Stereotactic surgery + medical therapy have greatly reduced mortality
- Mortality variable, 0-30%

Treatment
- Surgical drainage and/or excision primary therapy
  - May require repeated drainage
  - Re-accumulation of inflammatory fluid/debris after sterilization
- Antibiotics only, if small (< 2.5 cm) or early phase of cerebritis
- Steroids to treat edema and mass effect
- Lumbar puncture (LP) can be hazardous
  - Posterior fossa abscess most common cause of herniation after LP
  - Pathogen often can't be determined

DIAGNOSTIC CHECKLIST

Consider
- Pilocytic astrocytoma can mimic cerebellar abscess
  - Look for associated mastoiditis
- Don't forget aging hematoma
- DWI, MRS helpful in distinguishing abscess from mimics

Image Interpretation Pearls
- Search for local cause such as sinusitis, mastoiditis
- T2 hypointense abscess rim resolves before enhancement in successfully treated patients

SELECTED REFERENCES
1. Gupta RK et al: High Fractional Anisotropy in Brain Abscesses versus Other Cystic Intracranial Lesions. AJNR Am J Neuroradiol. 26(5):1107-14, 2005
2. Unal O et al: Brain abscess drainage by use of MR fluoroscopic guidance. AJNR Am J Neuroradiol. 26(4):839-42, 2005
3. Tsuyuguchi N et al: Evaluation of treatment effects in brain abscess with positron emission tomography: comparison of fluorine-18-fluorodeoxyglucose and carbon-11-methionine. Ann Nucl Med. 17(1):47-51, 2003
4. Lai PH et al: Brain abscess and necrotic brain tumor: discrimination with proton MR spectroscopy and diffusion-weighted imaging. AJNR Am J Neuroradiol. 23(8):1369-77, 2002

BRAIN ABSCESS

IMAGE GALLERY

Typical

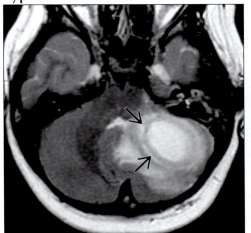
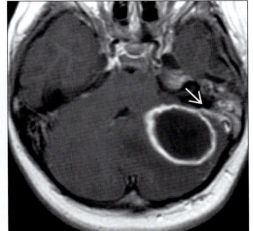

(Left) Axial T2WI MR shows an ovoid mass in the left cerebellar hemisphere with marked surrounding edema. Hypointense signal of capsule *(arrows)* helps distinguish abscess from cystic neoplasm. *(Right)* Axial T1 C+ MR in the same patient shows well-defined enhancing rim of abscess. Note the "tail" of enhancement *(arrow)* that extends to the adjacent inflamed mastoid air cells, the source of the infection.

Typical

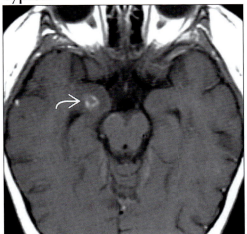
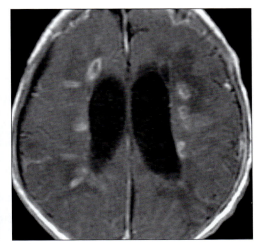

(Left) Axial T1 C+ MR shows a small abscess in the right uncus *(arrow)*. Hematogenous dissemination of infection causing cerebral abscesses is most commonly associated with immunosuppression. *(Right)* Axial T1 C+ MR shows multiple abscesses distributed throughout the cerebral hemispheres. In the immunosuppressed patient the extent of disease can be masked by low neutrophil counts.

Variant

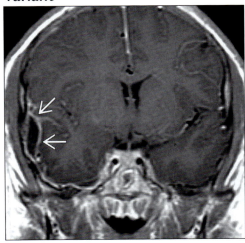
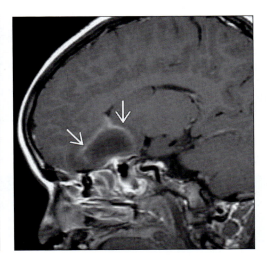

(Left) Coronal T1 C+ MR shows thickened meninges over the right temporal lobe with an extra-axial abscess *(arrows)*. These inflammatory collections can persist long after sterilization of CSF. *(Right)* Sagittal T1 C+ MR shows a frontal abscess *(arrows)* complicating spheno-ethmoid sinusitis. Intra-axial abscess from sinusitis typically arises from retrograde extension along emissary veins.

ACUTE DISSEMINATED ENCEPHALOMYELITIS

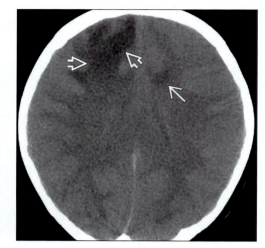

Axial FLAIR MR shows multiple poorly-defined lesions characterized by hyperintense signal (arrows), predominantly in the subcortical white matter, characteristic of ADEM.

Axial NECT shows a tumefactive ADEM lesion in the right frontal lobe (open arrows), with a smaller lesion in the left frontal subcortical white matter (arrow). CT is often normal in ADEM.

TERMINOLOGY

Abbreviations and Synonyms
- Acute disseminated encephalomyelitis (ADEM)

Definitions
- Autoimmune-mediated demyelination
- Affects both brain and spinal cord
- Typically monophasic
  - Multiphasic disseminated encephalomyelitis (MDEM) may actually be variant multiple sclerosis (MS)

IMAGING FINDINGS

General Features
- Best diagnostic clue: Multifocal hyperintense lesions on T2WI and FLAIR 10-14 days after viral infection or vaccination
- Location
  - Brain ⇒ white matter (WM), basal ganglia, some gray matter
    - Cerebrum > cerebellum
  - Spine ⇒ centrally located in cord substance
    - Cervical > thoracic > lumbar
- Size
  - Typically multifocal, small to moderate in size
    - Tumefactive lesions may be large (several cm), with less-than-expected mass effect
- Morphology
  - Amorphous, sometimes spherical or ovoid
    - Less regular in shape than lesions of multiple sclerosis

CT Findings
- NECT
  - Initial CT normal in 40%
  - Low density asymmetric WM lesions
- CECT
  - Typically shows more lesions
  - Multifocal subcortical lesions with mild-to-moderate enhancement

MR Findings
- T1WI: Low signal lesions with minimal mass effect
- T2WI
  - T2 may show hyperintense pontine and brainstem lesions more clearly than FLAIR
    - WM lesions easiest to see on FLAIR
- FLAIR
  - Multifocal FLAIR hyperintensities
    - Range from punctate to mass-like
  - Bilateral but asymmetric
  - Predilection for subcortical white matter
  - Can involve brainstem and posterior fossa
- DWI

DDx: Acquired White Matter Lesions In Children

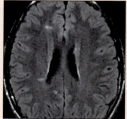
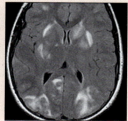
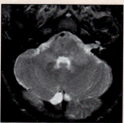
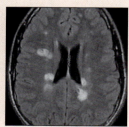

MS | PRES | HLH | Balo

ACUTE DISSEMINATED ENCEPHALOMYELITIS

Key Facts

Terminology
- Acute disseminated encephalomyelitis (ADEM)
- Autoimmune-mediated demyelination
- Affects both brain and spinal cord

Imaging Findings
- Best diagnostic clue: Multifocal hyperintense lesions on T2WI and FLAIR 10-14 days after viral infection or vaccination
- Brain ⇒ white matter (WM), basal ganglia, some gray matter
- Initial CT normal in 40%
- Multifocal subcortical lesions with mild-to-moderate enhancement
- Multifocal FLAIR hyperintensities
- Bilateral but asymmetric
- Predilection for subcortical white matter
- Can involve brainstem and posterior fossa
- Cranial nerve enhancement
- May appear identical to MS

Top Differential Diagnoses
- Multiple sclerosis (MS)
- Histiocytosis syndromes
- Posterior reversible encephalopathy syndrome (PRES)

Clinical Issues
- Multifocal neurological symptoms; 5-14 days after viral illness/immunization
- Usually monophasic, self-limited
- Complete recovery within one month: 50-60%
- Mortality: 10-30%

  - Variably restricted diffusion in acute lesions
    - Some restricted, some not
  - Restricted diffusion can portend worse outcome
    - May indicate lack of reversibility
- T1 C+
  - Punctate enhancement, complete/incomplete ring enhancement, peripheral enhancement
  - Cranial nerve enhancement
- MRS
  - NAA ↓ within lesions
    - Can normalize with resolution of symptoms
  - May see elevation of lactate and choline in acute lesions
- Other sequences
  - Magnetization transfer ratios (MTR) in normal-appearing areas of ADEM patients remain normal
    - MTRs are decreased in normal-appearing areas of patients with MS
  - Mean diffusivity on diffusion tensor imaging (DTI) in normal-appearing areas of ADEM patients remains normal
    - Mean diffusivity is increased in MS

Imaging Recommendations
- Best imaging tool
  - Contrast-enhanced MRI
    - May appear identical to MS
- Protocol advice
  - MRS, DTI, and MTR may provide some insight
  - Most helpful data is history of viral prodrome or vaccination

DIFFERENTIAL DIAGNOSIS

Multiple sclerosis (MS)
- MS is defined by multiple lesions separated by space and time
  - Relapsing-remitting course
- Lesions can be identical to ADEM
- MS lesions often more symmetric than ADEM
- "Multiphasic" or "relapsing" ADEM is likely same entity as MS

Autoimmune-mediated vasculitis
- Multifocal GM/WM lesions
  - Bilateral, usually cortical/subcortical, basal ganglia/thalami
  - Ring-enhancing lesions may mimic infection

Balo concentric sclerosis
- "Variant" of MS characterized by concentric rings of demyelination and preserved myelin
- Initially thought to be uniformly fatal
  - Now known to be self-limited in many instances
- Affects children and young adults

Histiocytosis syndromes
- Langerhans cell histiocytosis (LCH)
  - Cerebellar white matter lesions
  - Bright on T2WI and FLAIR
  - Variably enhancing
  - Rarely supratentorial
- Hemophagocytic lymphohistiocytosis (HLH)
  - Supra-and infratentorial lesions
  - Variably enhancing
  - Associated with parenchymal volume loss

Posterior reversible encephalopathy syndrome (PRES)
- Reversible WM edema induced by hypertension and/or drug effects (cyclosporin)
- Resolves with treatment of hypertension or reduction of offending medication
- Not limited to posterior brain

PATHOLOGY

General Features
- General path comments: Autoimmune mediated demyelination
- Etiology
  - Classically occurs after viral infection or vaccination

ACUTE DISSEMINATED ENCEPHALOMYELITIS

- Specific viral illness: Epstein-Barr, influenza A, mumps, coronavirus
- After exanthematous diseases of childhood (chickenpox, measles)
- Vaccines: Diphtheria, influenza, rabies, smallpox, tetanus, typhoid
  - Can occur spontaneously
    - Subclinical viral prodrome?
- Epidemiology: Most common para/post-infectious disorder
- Associated abnormalities: Acute hemorrhagic leukoencephalopathy variant associated with ulcerative colitis and asthma

Microscopic Features
- Acute myelin breakdown
- Perivenous inflammation; lymphocytic infiltrates
- Relative axonal preservation
- Atypical astrogliosis
- Virus generally not found, unlike viral encephalitides
- Similar to experimental allergic encephalomyelitis, supporting autoimmune-related etiology

Staging, Grading or Classification Criteria
- 4 patterns of disease classified by Tenembaum et al
  - Group A ⇒ lesions < 5 mm
  - Group B ⇒ 1 or more lesions > 5 mm
  - Group C ⇒ bilateral symmetric thalamic disease
  - Group D ⇒ acute hemorrhagic encephalomyelitis

CLINICAL ISSUES

Presentation
- Most common signs/symptoms
  - Usually preceded by prodromal phase: Fever, malaise, myalgia
  - Multifocal neurological symptoms; 5-14 days after viral illness/immunization
    - Initial symptoms: Headache, fever, drowsiness
    - Cranial nerve palsies, seizures, hemiparesis
    - Decreased consciousness (from lethargy to coma)
    - Behavioral changes
- Other signs/symptoms
  - Cerebrospinal fluid often abnormal (↑ leukocytes, ↑ protein)
    - Usually lacks oligoclonal bands

Demographics
- Age: Peak age 3-5 years

Natural History & Prognosis
- Usually monophasic, self-limited
- Variable prognosis
  - Complete recovery within one month: 50-60%
  - Neurologic sequelae (most commonly seizures): 20-30%
  - Mortality: 10-30%
  - Relapses are rare
    - "Relapsing disseminated encephalomyelitis"
    - May not be a separate entity from relapsing-remitting MS
- Varicella and rubella associated ADEM have preferential patterns
  - Rubella-associated ADEM characterized by acute explosive onset, seizures, coma and moderate pyramidal signs
  - Varicella-associated ADEM characterized by cerebellar ataxia and mild pyramidal dysfunction
- Rare manifestations
  - Acute hemorrhagic leukoencephalopathy: 2%
    - Young patients with abrupt symptom onset
    - Fulminant, often ending in death
  - Bilateral striatal necrosis (usually in infants, may be reversible)

Treatment
- Immunomodulatory therapy
  - Steroids
  - Intravenous immunoglobulin
  - Plasmapheresis
- MRI may show prompt regression in response to treatment

DIAGNOSTIC CHECKLIST

Image Interpretation Pearls
- Imaging findings often lag behind symptom onset, resolution
- Distinction from MS dependent upon lack of remittance
- DWI may have some predictive value

SELECTED REFERENCES

1. Axer H et al: Initial DWI and ADC imaging may predict outcome in acute disseminated encephalomyelitis: report of two cases of brain stem encephalitis. J Neurol Neurosurg Psychiatry. 76(7):996-8, 2005
2. Mader I et al: MRI and proton MR spectroscopy in acute disseminated encephalomyelitis. Childs Nerv Syst. 2005
3. Richer LP et al: Neuroimaging features of acute disseminated encephalomyelitis in childhood. Pediatr Neurol. 32(1):30-6, 2005
4. Kuker W et al: Modern MRI tools for the characterization of acute demyelinating lesions: value of chemical shift and diffusion-weighted imaging. Neuroradiology. 46(6):421-6, 2004
5. Leake JA et al: Acute disseminated encephalomyelitis in childhood: epidemiologic, clinical and laboratory features. Pediatr Infect Dis J. 23(8):756-64, 2004
6. Holtmannspotter M et al: A diffusion tensor MRI study of basal ganglia from patients with ADEM. J Neurol Sci. 206(1):27-30, 2003
7. Idrissova ZhR et al: Acute disseminated encephalomyelitis in children: clinical features and HLA-DR linkage. Eur J Neurol. 10(5):537-46, 2003
8. Inglese M et al: Magnetization transfer and diffusion tensor MR imaging of acute disseminated encephalomyelitis. AJNR Am J Neuroradiol. 23(2):267-72, 2002
9. Tenembaum S: Acute disseminated encephalomyelitis: A long-term follow-up study of 84 pediatric patients. Neurology. 59(8):1224-31, 2002
10. Straussberg R et al: Improvement of atypical acute disseminated encephalomyelitis with steroids and intravenous immunoglobulins. Pediatr Neurol. 24(2):139-43, 2001
11. Dale RC et al: Acute disseminated encephalomyelitis, multiphasic disseminated encephalomyelitis and multiple sclerosis in children. Brain. 12:2407-22, 2000

ACUTE DISSEMINATED ENCEPHALOMYELITIS

IMAGE GALLERY

Typical

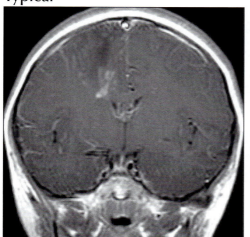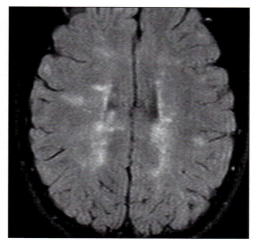

(Left) Coronal T1 C+ MR shows irregular enhancement of a large ADEM lesion in the right frontal lobe. Patterns of enhancement in ADEM are variable, ranging from diffuse to ring-enhancing. *(Right)* Axial FLAIR MR shows multiple hyperintense lesions of ADEM in a 9 year old. FLAIR imaging is sensitive for hemisphere WM lesions, but T2WI may show brainstem lesions to better advantage.

Typical

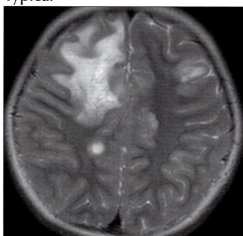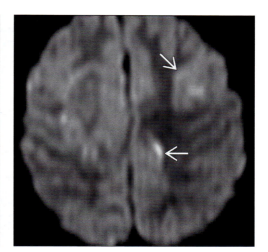

(Left) Axial T2WI MR shows irregularity of signal in a large ADEM lesion. Tumefactive lesions can mimic neoplasm, especially if the history of recent viral illness or vaccination is not known. *(Right)* Axial DWI MR shows some restricted diffusion in smaller left hemisphere lesions (arrows), with irregular diffusion in large right frontal lesion. DWI may have predictive value in ADEM.

Typical

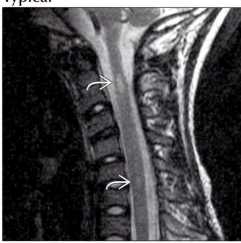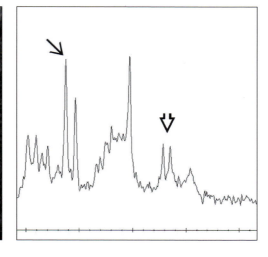

(Left) Sagittal T2WI MR of the cervical spine shows ADEM lesions (arrows) centrally located in the cord. MS lesions are more typically seen in the dorsal one-third of the cord substance. *(Right)* MRS of an ADEM lesions shows elevation of choline (arrow), and a lipid/lactate doublet (open arrow). The latter reflects necrosis, and may portend lack of reversibility of the lesion.

THE LEUKODYSTROPHIES

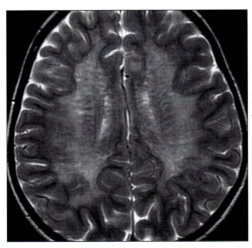

Axial T2WI MR shows characteristic "tigroid" appearance of WM in metachromatic leukodystrophy, caused by relative preservation of myelin in perivascular regions.

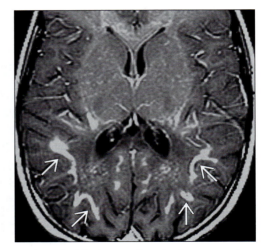

Axial T1 C+ MR shows a line of enhancement along zone of active inflammation in classic X-linked adrenoleukodystrophy (arrows). Contrast can be very helpful in imaging of leukodystrophies.

TERMINOLOGY

Abbreviations and Synonyms
- Adrenoleukodystrophies (ALD), metachromatic leukodystrophy (MLD), Pelizaeus-Merzbacher disease (PMD), Alexander disease, Canavan disease, Krabbe disease (globoid cell leukodystrophy, GLD)

Definitions
- Group of disorders characterized by a defect in production or maintenance of myelin
- Effects on white matter (WM) can be put into three categories
  ○ Dysmyelination: Formation of abnormal myelin
    ▪ Typically results in demyelination
  ○ Demyelination: Destruction of myelin
  ○ Hypomyelination: Failure to form myelin
- Caused by inherited enzyme deficiencies
  ○ Lysosomal or peroxisomal enzymes
- Also caused by mutations in genes for WM structural proteins

IMAGING FINDINGS

General Features
- Best diagnostic clue
  ○ Abnormal signal in WM, usually diffuse and symmetric
  ○ Failure to achieve myelination milestones
- Location
  ○ Cerebral WM > cerebellar WM
    ▪ Exception ⇒ GLD can have early cerebellar WM involvement
    ▪ Exception ⇒ Alexander disease has abnormal signal and enhancement in dentate nuclei
  ○ Some leukodystrophies have characteristic distributions

CT Findings
- NECT
  ○ Decreased WM attenuation
  ○ Megalencephaly in Canavan and Alexander disease
  ○ Increased density in basal ganglia early in GLD
    ▪ Globoid cell accumulation with calcifications
  ○ Most progress to atrophy in later stages of disease

MR Findings
- T1WI
  ○ Best sequence for hypomyelination (PMD)
  ○ Dysmyelination and demyelination may have ↓ signal in WM
  ○ ↑ Signal of periventricular rim in Alexander disease
- T2WI
  ○ MLD
    ▪ ↑ Signal in hemispheric WM

DDx: The Leukodystrophies

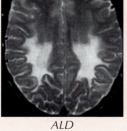
ALD

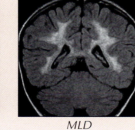
MLD

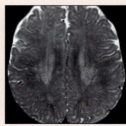
GLD (Krabbe)

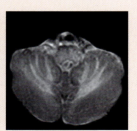
Canavan

THE LEUKODYSTROPHIES

Key Facts

Terminology
- Group of disorders characterized by a defect in production or maintenance of myelin
- Caused by inherited enzyme deficiencies
- Also caused by mutations in genes for WM structural proteins

Imaging Findings
- Abnormal signal in WM, usually diffuse and symmetric
- Failure to achieve myelination milestones
- Some have characteristic enhancement patterns
- Findings on MRS generally reflect neuronal loss and increased cellular turnover

Top Differential Diagnoses
- Metachromatic leukodystrophy
- Krabbe disease (globoid leukodystrophy)
- X-linked adrenoleukodystrophy
- Canavan disease
- Alexander disease
- Pelizaeus-Merzbacher disease

Pathology
- MLD ⇒ accumulation of sulfatide
- ALD ⇒ accumulation of long-chain fatty acids
- GLD ⇒ accumulation of psychosine and cerebroside
- Alexander disease ⇒ excess Rosenthal fibers in white matter
- Canavan disease ⇒ accumulation of NAA

- Early sparing of subcortical U-fibers
- Early sparing of perivascular WM ("tigroid pattern")
- Late involvement of U-fibers, corpus callosum, descending pyramidal tracts, internal capsules
  - ALD
    - Characteristic early involvement of parietal periventricular WM
    - Inner (deep) zone of hyperintensity ⇒ astrogliosis
    - Intermediate zone of hypointensity ⇒ active inflammation
    - Outer zone of hyperintensity ⇒ demyelination
  - GLD
    - ↑ Signal in periventricular WM, pyramidal tracts, cerebellar WM
    - Patchy at first, coalescing with progression
    - Enlarged optic nerves
  - Alexander disease
    - ↑ Signal in frontal WM, thalami, brainstem structures
    - ↓ Signal of periventricular rim
  - Canavan disease
    - ↑ Signal in occipital WM early, progressing to entire brain
    - Early sparing of U-fibers, basal ganglia, corpus callosum
- FLAIR
  - Best sequence for demyelination in children > 2
  - Can be difficult to assess WM signal in children < 2
- DWI
  - Some processes increase diffusion after destruction of myelin
    - ALD ⇒ increased diffusion and ↑ ADC
    - GLD ⇒ increased diffusion and ↑ ADC
    - Alexander disease ⇒ increased diffusion and loss of anisotropy
  - Some restrict diffusion with dysmyelination and demyelination
    - MLD ⇒ restricted diffusion and ↓ ADC
    - Canavan disease ⇒ restricted diffusion and ↓ ADC
  - PMD ⇒ maintained anisotropy despite absence of myelination
- T1 C+
  - Some have characteristic enhancement patterns
    - ALD ⇒ zone of active inflammation
    - GLD ⇒ lumbar nerve roots
    - Alexander disease ⇒ ventricular lining, periventricular rim, frontal WM, optic chiasm, fornix, basal ganglia, thalamus, dentate nucleus, brainstem structures
- MRS
  - Findings on MRS generally reflect neuronal loss and increased cellular turnover
  - Alexander disease ⇒ , ↑↑ myo-inositol (mI), ±↑ choline (Cho), ± ↓ N-acetylaspartic acid (NAA)
  - MLD ⇒ ↑ Cho, ↑ mI
  - ALD ⇒ ↑ Cho, ↑ mI; ↓↓ NAA indicates irreversible neuronal loss
  - GLD ⇒ ↑ Cho, ↑ mI, ↓ NAA
  - Canavan has ↑ NAA, one of the only conditions where this is found

Imaging Recommendations
- Best imaging tool: Contrast-enhanced MR with MRS
- Protocol advice: MRS: Sample abnormal and normal-appearing WM

DIFFERENTIAL DIAGNOSIS

Metachromatic leukodystrophy
- Absent/deficient lysosomal enzyme arylsulfatase-A (ARSA)

Krabbe disease (globoid leukodystrophy)
- Absent/deficient lysosomal enzyme galactosylceramidase I

X-linked adrenoleukodystrophy
- Absent/deficient peroxisomal enzyme acyl-CoA synthetase
  - Loss of function of the peroxisomal transporter ABCD1
- Milder, adult-onset form ⇒ adrenomyeloneuropathy

THE LEUKODYSTROPHIES

- Neonatal ALD is not a sub-type, but a different peroxisomal disorder

Canavan disease
- Absence/deficiency of aspartoacyclase

Alexander disease
- Mutations in gene for glial fibrillary acidic protein (GFAP)

Pelizaeus-Merzbacher disease
- Mutations of gene encoding for myelin proteolipid protein (PLP)
- Lack of myelination without myelin destruction
- Cerebellum may be markedly atrophic

Refsum disease
- Absent/deficient peroxisomal enzyme phytanic acid 2-hydroxylase
- Causes both encephalopathy and peripheral neuropathy
- Imaging abnormalities may not be apparent until 4th decade

PATHOLOGY

General Features
- General path comments
  - MLD ⇒ accumulation of sulfatide
  - ALD ⇒ accumulation of long-chain fatty acids
  - GLD ⇒ accumulation of psychosine and cerebroside
  - Alexander disease ⇒ excess Rosenthal fibers in white matter
  - Canavan disease ⇒ accumulation of NAA
- Genetics
  - MLD ⇒ ARSA gene located at 22q13.31
  - ALD ⇒ defect in gene at Xq28
    - Classic "X-linked adrenoleukodystrophy"
  - GLD ⇒ defect in GALC gene on chromosome 14
  - Alexander disease ⇒ mutations in gene for GFAP on chromosome 17q21
  - Canavan disease ⇒ defect in aspartoacyclase gene on chromosome 17
  - PMD ⇒ PLP gene at Xq21-q22
- Epidemiology
  - Rare diseases that can be increased in incidence in closed communities
    - Typical incidences < 1:100,000
    - Improved detection of milder manifestations with genetic screening has resulted in apparent increases in incidence
  - MLD ↑ In Habbanite Jewish (1:75 live births) and Navajo Indians (1:2,500 live births)
  - Canavan disease ↑↑ in Ashkenazi Jewish population
  - ALD more common in Japan (incidence 1:30,000 to 50,000 boys)
- Associated abnormalities
  - Symptomatic gallbladder disease in MLD
  - Adrenal insufficiency in ALD

Staging, Grading or Classification Criteria
- Classifications based upon severity and age of onset, usually reflecting amount of residual enzymatic activity
  - MLD ⇒ connatal, late infantile, early juvenile, late juvenile
  - ALD ⇒ classic X-linked ALD, adrenomyeloneuropathy
  - GLD ⇒ infantile onset most common, juvenile and adult-onset have been reported
  - Alexander disease ⇒ neonatal, infantile, juvenile, adult-onset
  - PMD ⇒ spastic paraplegia type 2, complicated spastic paraplegia type 2, PMD

CLINICAL ISSUES

Presentation
- Most common signs/symptoms
  - MLD ⇒ gait disturbance, behavioral problems
  - ALD ⇒ cognitive decline, progressive neurologic deterioration
  - GLD ⇒ hyperirritable infant with decreased reflexes
  - Alexander disease ⇒ megalencephaly and developmental delay
  - Canavan disease ⇒ macrocrania and seizures, developmental delay
  - PMD ⇒ nystagmus, poor head control, spasticity, ataxia

Natural History & Prognosis
- Severely affected children typically have progressive neurologic deterioration and death in childhood
- With more sophisticated genetic testing, milder forms are being discovered, with prolonged/normal lifespan

Treatment
- Bone marrow and stem cell transplantation may arrest progress of ALD, MLD, GLD
- Gene therapy may have benefit if diagnosis made early enough

DIAGNOSTIC CHECKLIST

Image Interpretation Pearls
- Contrast-enhanced MR and MRS are key tools in diagnosis

SELECTED REFERENCES
1. Brockmann K et al: Cerebral proton magnetic resonance spectroscopy in infantile Alexander disease. J Neurol. 250(3):300-6, 2003
2. Brockmann K et al: Proton MRS profile of cerebral metabolic abnormalities in Krabbe disease. Neurology. 60(5):819-25, 2003
3. Engelbrecht V et al: Diffusion-weighted MR imaging in the brain in children: findings in the normal brain and in the brain with WM diseases. Radiology. 222(2):410-8, 2002

THE LEUKODYSTROPHIES

IMAGE GALLERY

Typical

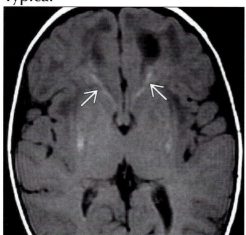 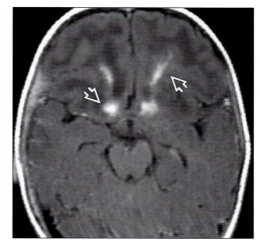

(Left) Axial T1WI MR without contrast shows regions of hypointense signal in frontal WM in a child with Alexander disease. There is a rim of hyperintensity along the frontal horns *(arrows)*. *(Right)* Post-contrast T1WI in the same child shows prominent enhancement in the immediate periventricular region *(arrows)*. Patterns of enhancement can help distinguish various leukodystrophies.

Typical

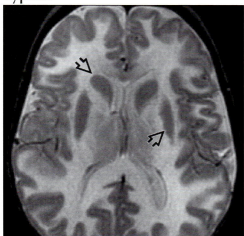 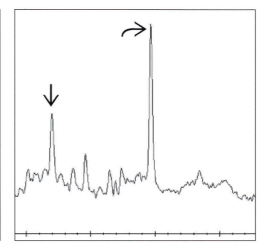

(Left) Axial T2WI MR in an infant with Canavan disease shows marked hyperintense signal and swelling throughout the WM, leaving the corpus striatum as "islands" of tissue centrally *(arrows)*. *(Right)* MRS in the same child shows a marked elevation of NAA *(curved arrow)*, pathognomonic for Canavan disease. Myoinositol *(arrow)* is mildly elevated. Excess NAA is also excreted in the urine.

Typical

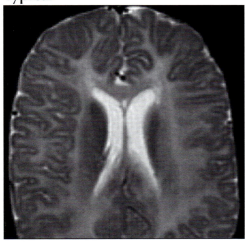 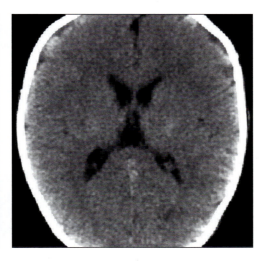

(Left) Axial T2WI MR in a 13 year old with Pelizaeus-Merzbacher disease shows absence of normal hypointense WM signal. This degree of myelination would be appropriate for a 6-8 month old. *(Right)* Axial NECT in an infant with Krabbe disease (GLD) shows faint hyperintensity (presumed Ca++) in the lateral thalamic nuclei. CT may be more sensitive than MR early in the course of GLD.

MITOCHONDRIAL ENCEPHALOPATHIES

Axial T2WI MR shows "salt-and-pepper" pattern of abnormal signal in the putamina in an infant with LS. LS is a clinical syndrome caused by a variety of respiratory chain enzyme defects.

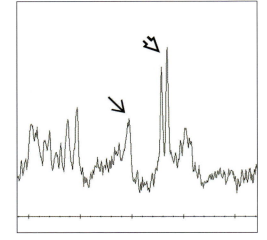

MRS in the same infant shows a large lipid-lactate doublet (open arrow), with reduction of NAA (arrow). Detection of elevated lactate supports the diagnosis of MEM, but is not specific.

TERMINOLOGY

Abbreviations and Synonyms
- Mitochondrial encephalomyelopathies (MEMs)
  - Subacute necrotizing encephalomyelopathy or Leigh syndrome (LS)
  - Pantothenate Kinase-Associated Neurodegeneration (PKAN), or Hallervorden-Spatz syndrome
  - Glutaric Acidurias, type I (GA-1) and type 2 (GA-2)
  - MELAS (myopathy, encephalopathy, lactic acidosis, and stroke-like episodes)
  - Kearns-Sayre syndrome (KSS), ophthalmoplegia
  - Menkes disease (trichopoliodystrophy), Alpers disease, Friedreich ataxia

Definitions
- Genetically based disorders of mitochondrial function resulting in progressive or intermittent brain injury
- Characteristically due to deficiencies/defects of enzymes affecting the respiratory (electron-transport) chain, Krebs cycle, and/or other components of energy production by mitochondria
- Other entities can be included in this categorization; these are the ones most commonly encountered in children

IMAGING FINDINGS

General Features
- Best diagnostic clue
  - MEMs have a broad range of imaging appearances, characterized by regions of brain destruction, volume loss, and/or mineralization
  - They typically affect both gray and white matter
  - Most disorders of mitochondrial function will cause lesions in the basal ganglia
    - Typically bilateral and symmetric
  - MELAS causes peripheral stroke-like lesions
- Location
  - Variable
    - Most common in basal ganglia (BG), brainstem, thalami, dentate nuclei
    - Less commonly diffuse white matter (WM), peripheral cortex, cerebellum
- Size: Focal/diffuse atrophy is characteristic of GA-1, Menkes
- Morphology
  - BG lesions often conform to original shape of nuclei
  - Edema/swelling characteristic of acute lesions; volume loss characteristic of late disease

CT Findings
- NECT
  - Focal hypodensities

DDx: Basal Ganglia Lesions In Children

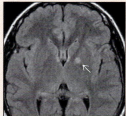 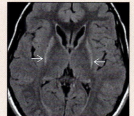 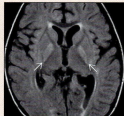 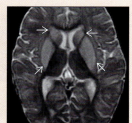

| NF1 | Huntington | Near-Drowning | CMV Encephalitis |

THE LEUKODYSTROPHIES

IMAGE GALLERY

Typical

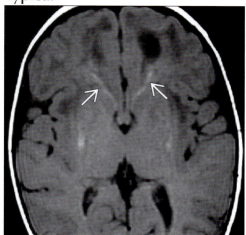
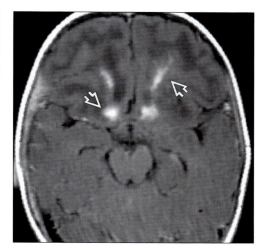

(Left) Axial T1WI MR without contrast shows regions of hypointense signal in frontal WM in a child with Alexander disease. There is a rim of hyperintensity along the frontal horns (arrows). *(Right)* Post-contrast T1WI in the same child shows prominent enhancement in the immediate periventricular region (arrows). Patterns of enhancement can help distinguish various leukodystrophies.

Typical

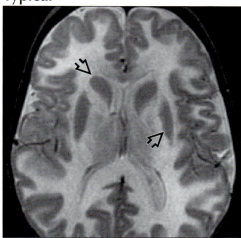
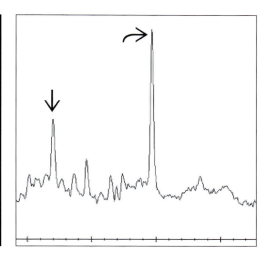

(Left) Axial T2WI MR in an infant with Canavan disease shows marked hyperintense signal and swelling throughout the WM, leaving the corpus striatum as "islands" of tissue centrally (arrows). *(Right)* MRS in the same child shows a marked elevation of NAA (curved arrow), pathognomonic for Canavan disease. Myoinositol (arrow) is mildly elevated. Excess NAA is also excreted in the urine.

Typical

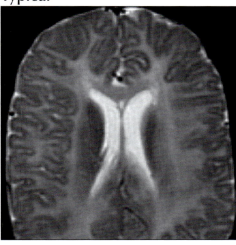
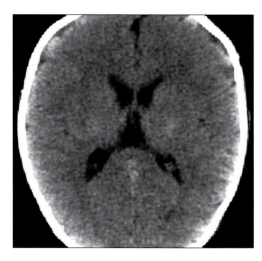

(Left) Axial T2WI MR in a 13 year old with Pelizaeus-Merzbacher disease shows absence of normal hypointense WM signal. This degree of myelination would be appropriate for a 6-8 month old. *(Right)* Axial NECT in an infant with Krabbe disease (GLD) shows faint hyperintensity (presumed Ca++) in the lateral thalamic nuclei. CT may be more sensitive than MR early in the course of GLD.

MITOCHONDRIAL ENCEPHALOPATHIES

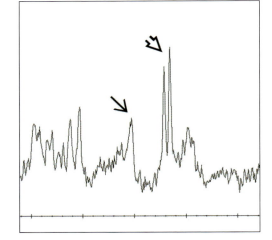

Axial T2WI MR shows "salt-and-pepper" pattern of abnormal signal in the putamina in an infant with LS. LS is a clinical syndrome caused by a variety of respiratory chain enzyme defects.

MRS in the same infant shows a large lipid-lactate doublet (open arrow), with reduction of NAA (arrow). Detection of elevated lactate supports the diagnosis of MEM, but is not specific.

TERMINOLOGY

Abbreviations and Synonyms
- Mitochondrial encephalomyelopathies (MEMs)
  - Subacute necrotizing encephalomyelopathy or Leigh syndrome (LS)
  - Pantothenate Kinase-Associated Neurodegeneration (PKAN), or Hallervorden-Spatz syndrome
  - Glutaric Acidurias, type I (GA-1) and type 2 (GA-2)
  - MELAS (myopathy, encephalopathy, lactic acidosis, and stroke-like episodes)
  - Kearns-Sayre syndrome (KSS), ophthalmoplegia
  - Menkes disease (trichopoliodystrophy), Alpers disease, Friedreich ataxia

Definitions
- Genetically based disorders of mitochondrial function resulting in progressive or intermittent brain injury
- Characteristically due to deficiencies/defects of enzymes affecting the respiratory (electron-transport) chain, Krebs cycle, and/or other components of energy production by mitochondria
- Other entities can be included in this categorization; these are the ones most commonly encountered in children

IMAGING FINDINGS

General Features
- Best diagnostic clue
  - MEMs have a broad range of imaging appearances, characterized by regions of brain destruction, volume loss, and/or mineralization
  - They typically affect both gray and white matter
  - Most disorders of mitochondrial function will cause lesions in the basal ganglia
    - Typically bilateral and symmetric
  - MELAS causes peripheral stroke-like lesions
- Location
  - Variable
    - Most common in basal ganglia (BG), brainstem, thalami, dentate nuclei
    - Less commonly diffuse white matter (WM), peripheral cortex, cerebellum
- Size: Focal/diffuse atrophy is characteristic of GA-1, Menkes
- Morphology
  - BG lesions often conform to original shape of nuclei
  - Edema/swelling characteristic of acute lesions; volume loss characteristic of late disease

CT Findings
- NECT
  - Focal hypodensities

DDx: Basal Ganglia Lesions In Children

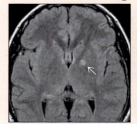
NF1

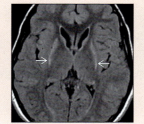
Huntington

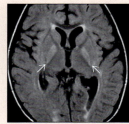
Near-Drowning

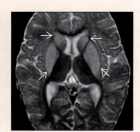
CMV Encephalitis

MITOCHONDRIAL ENCEPHALOPATHIES

Key Facts

Terminology
- Genetically based disorders of mitochondrial function resulting in progressive or intermittent brain injury
- Characteristically due to deficiencies/defects of enzymes affecting the respiratory (electron-transport) chain, Krebs cycle, and/or other components of energy production by mitochondria

Imaging Findings
- MEMs have a broad range of imaging appearances, characterized by regions of brain destruction, volume loss, and/or mineralization
- Most disorders of mitochondrial function will cause lesions in the basal ganglia
- Subdural collections in GA-1 mimic subdural hematomas from child abuse
- PKAN causes characteristic T2 hypointensity in globus pallidus (GP)
- LS typically causes a speckled pattern in deep nuclei
- Detection of lactate characteristic of MEMs
- Absence of lactate does not exclude diagnosis, however

Pathology
- As a group, MEMs are relatively common ≈ 1:8,500

Diagnostic Checklist
- Think of MEMs when encountering an atypical presentation of stroke, severe encephalitis, or seizure
- Don't forget to consider MEMs when an infant presents with subdurals
- Can also have retinal hemorrhages!

- Increased density can be seen in BG in PKAN, KSS
  - May reflect dystrophic calcification (Ca++)
- Diffuse decreased density of WM
- GA-1, Menkes ⇒ volume loss with subdural collections
  - Subdural collections in GA-1 mimic subdural hematomas from child abuse
  - Collections are typically hyperintense relative to CSF

MR Findings
- T1WI
  - Hypointense lesions
    - Foci of hyperintensity may reflect Ca++, blood products, myelin breakdown (rare)
  - Friedreich ataxia ⇒ cerebellar, spinal atrophy
- T2WI
  - MEMs typically cause hyperintense lesions on T2WI and FLAIR
  - PKAN causes characteristic T2 hypointensity in globus pallidus (GP)
    - Due to excess and premature iron deposition
    - Central area of hyperintensity reflects gliosis
    - Combination of hypo- and hyper-intensity lesions ⇒ "eye of the tiger" sign
  - LS typically causes a speckled pattern in deep nuclei
    - Sparing (islands of preserved signal) around vessels?
- DWI
  - MEMs may or may not cause foci of restricted diffusion
    - DWI is not reliable for detection or exclusion of MEMs
- MRS
  - Detection of lactate characteristic of MEMs
    - Absence of lactate does not exclude diagnosis, however
    - May only be elevated during acute crises
  - Chronic lesions typically have ↓ NAA

Nuclear Medicine Findings
- PET: GA-1: ↓ Glucose uptake in BG, thalami, insula, and temporal opercular cortex

Imaging Recommendations
- Best imaging tool: MR is modality of choice in investigation of suspected metabolic disease of any sort
- Protocol advice
  - MRS can be helpful, although often nonspecific
  - ↑ Lactate and restricted diffusion can be clue to true etiology

DIFFERENTIAL DIAGNOSIS

Perinatal asphyxia
- Central pattern of injury affects ventrolateral thalamus and basal ganglia
  - T2 signal abnormalities can be difficult to identify in the unmyelinated brain
    - First echo (PD/intermediate) very helpful
  - T1 hyperintensity seen acutely ⇒ myelin breakdown/clumping?

Kernicterus
- T2 prolongation in GP, subthalamic nuclei, hippocampi
- ↓ NAA on MRS

Near drowning
- History generally definitive
- High lactate implies poorer prognosis

Juvenile Huntington disease
- Symmetric T2 prolongation in putamina
- Caudate atrophy presents later

Neurofibromatosis type 1
- Signal abnormalities in basal ganglia most common brain manifestation
- Evolve/resolve over time

Encephalitis
- Viral encephalidites can cause symmetric basal ganglia T2 prolongation

MITOCHONDRIAL ENCEPHALOPATHIES

- Acute disseminated encephalomyelitis can affect basal ganglia, mimic MELAS/MERRF

Wilson disease
- Disorder of copper metabolism
- Signal changes in basal ganglia most often secondary to hepatic failure
  - T2 changes evident in older children, teens

PATHOLOGY

General Features
- General path comments
  - Main role of mitochondria ⇒ production of ATP for cell energy
    - Mitochondria contain their own DNA, inherited from mother
  - Most MEMs can be caused by variable number of mutations affecting structure/function of mitochondrial-based enzymes
  - Broad phenotypic presentation due to varied distribution of mitochondria throughout various cell types
- Genetics
  - LS ⇒ group of disorders caused by defective terminal oxidative metabolism
    - Defects in pyruvate dehydrogenase complex ⇒ X-linked
    - Cytochrome oxidase (COX) deficiency (respiratory chain complex IV) ⇒ SURF1 gene on chromosome 9
    - Several others genes and enzyme complexes affected
  - PKAN ("classic" form) ⇒ defects on chromosome 22p12.3-13 (PKAN2 gene)
  - MELAS ⇒ mitochondrial DNA defects (tRNA gene)
  - GA-1 ⇒ deficiency of glutaryl-coenzyme A dehydrogenase; gene on chromosome 19p13.2
  - Friedreich ataxia ⇒ chromosome 9q13
    - Mutations of frataxin ⇒ causes deficiency of respiratory chain complexes I-III
  - Menkes ⇒ X-linked, Xq12-q13.3
  - Alpers ⇒ mutations of mitochondrial DNA polymerase gamma subunits
- Etiology: Most pronounced effects are on striated muscle and deep cerebral nuclei ⇒ presumed highest ATP demand
- Epidemiology
  - As a group, MEMs are relatively common ≈ 1:8,500
  - LS is most common mitochondrial disease in children
- Associated abnormalities
  - KSS ⇒ ophthalmoplegia, heart block, retinitis pigmentosa
  - Alpers ⇒ micronodular cirrhosis
  - Menkes ⇒ brittle sparse hair ("kinky" hair disease), osteoporosis
  - Friedreich ataxia ⇒ hypertrophic cardiomyopathy, diabetes

CLINICAL ISSUES

Presentation
- Most common signs/symptoms
  - Psychomotor delay/regression, hypotonia
  - Stroke-like episodes, episodic paresis
  - Metabolic stressors (e.g., infection) may unmask disease or cause deterioration
- Other signs/symptoms
  - Ataxia, ophthalmoplegia, ptosis, vomiting, swallowing and respiratory difficulties, dystonia
  - Seizure, peripheral neuropathy

Demographics
- Age
  - Majority have clinical symptoms in infancy
  - MELAS usually presents in teens
  - Age at onset and severity correlates with degree of enzyme deficit
- Gender: X-linked entities almost exclusively male

Natural History & Prognosis
- LS ⇒ progressive neurodegeneration leading to respiratory failure and death in childhood
- PKAN ⇒ non-uniform progression, 11 year life expectancy after diagnosis
- GA-1 ⇒ progressive atrophy with severe dystonia
- MELAS ⇒ progressive course with episodic insults
- KSS, Friedreich ataxia ⇒ significant morbidity from cardiac effects

Treatment
- In general, MEMs are treated supportively and symptomatically

DIAGNOSTIC CHECKLIST

Image Interpretation Pearls
- Think of MEMs when encountering an atypical presentation of stroke, severe encephalitis, or seizure
- Don't forget to consider MEMs when an infant presents with subdurals
  - Can also have retinal hemorrhages!

SELECTED REFERENCES
1. Abe K et al: Comparison of conventional and diffusion-weighted MRI and proton MR spectroscopy in patients with mitochondrial encephalomyopathy, lactic acidosis, and stroke-like events. Neuroradiology. 46(2):113-7, 2004
2. Gago LC et al: Intraretinal hemorrhages and chronic subdural effusions: glutaric aciduria type 1 can be mistaken for shaken baby syndrome. Retina. 23(5):724-6, 2003
3. Rossi A et al: Leigh Syndrome with COX deficiency and SURF1 gene mutations: MR imaging findings. AJNR Am J Neuroradiol. 24(6):1188-91, 2003
4. Schon EA et al: Neuronal degeneration and mitochondrial dysfunction. J Clin Invest. 111:303-12, 2003
5. Twomey EL et al: Neuroimaging findings in glutaric aciduria type 1. Pediatr Radiol. 33(12):823-30, 2003
6. Flemming K et al: MR spectroscopic findings in a case of Alpers-Huttenlocher syndrome. AJNR Am J Neuroradiol. 23(8):1421-3, 2002

MITOCHONDRIAL ENCEPHALOPATHIES

IMAGE GALLERY

Typical

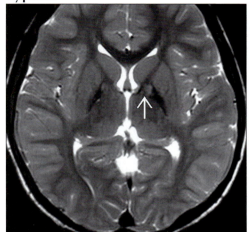
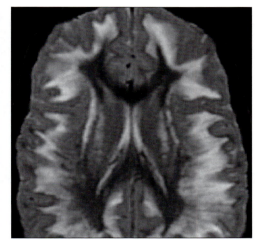

(Left) Axial T2WI MR shows "eye of the tiger" sign in a teenager with PKAN (Hallervorden-Spatz syndrome). Hyperintensity caused by gliosis in central GP *(arrow)* is accentuated by increased iron deposition around it. *(Right)* Axial T2WI MR in Kearns-Sayre syndrome shows diffuse abnormal hyperintense signal in cerebral WM with sparing of the corpus callosum.

Typical

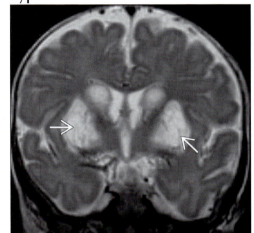
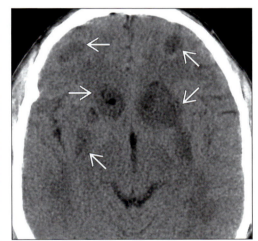

(Left) Coronal T2WI MR in an infant with Leigh syndrome shows linear foci of preserved signal *(arrows)* in abnormal basal ganglia, consistent with sparing around lenticulostriate vessels. *(Right)* Axial NECT in MELAS shows multiple foci of hypodensity in the basal ganglia and frontal lobes *(arrows)*. These "stroke-like" lesions typically do not fit known arterial territories.

Typical

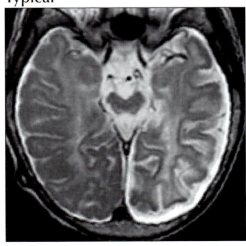
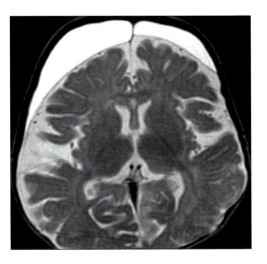

(Left) Axial T2WI MR shows asymmetric volume loss in the temporal and occipital lobes in this child with Menkes syndrome. *(Right)* Axial T2WI MR shows moderate-sized frontal subdural collections in a child with glutaric aciduria type I. MEM presenting with subdural collections can be misdiagnosed as child abuse.

ATLANTO-AXIAL INJURIES

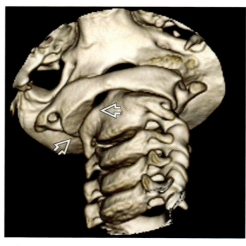

Volume-rendered 3D reconstruction of the cervical spine shows complete uncovering of the atlanto-axial joint on the right (arrows) in this child with rotary dislocation after trauma.

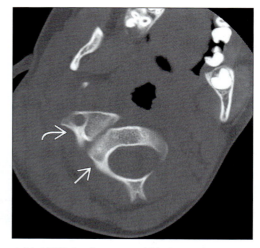

Axial NECT in the same child shows the anterior dislocation of the right lateral mass of C1 (curved arrow) relative to the lateral mass of C2 (arrow). Atlanto-axial rotational dislocation.

TERMINOLOGY

Abbreviations and Synonyms
- Atlanto-occipital dissociation (AOD), atlanto-occipital disruption, atlanto-occipital dislocation, occipitocervical subluxation or dislocation, Jefferson fracture, atlantoaxial dissociation, atlantoaxial rotatory fixation, fixed rotary subluxation, atlantoaxial rotational dislocation

Definitions
- Traumatic injury to the upper cervical region ⇒ occiput to C2
  - Up to 10 times more common in 1st decade than in older children and adults

IMAGING FINDINGS

General Features
- Best diagnostic clue: Abnormal alignment of occiput, C1, or C2 on properly positioned AP and lateral radiographs
- Location: Occiput to C2
- Size
  - Lesions can be obvious on radiographs, or completely inapparent
  - SCIWORA ⇒ Spinal Cord Injury Without Radiographic Abnormality
- Morphology: Relationship of occipital condyles and lateral masses of C1 and C2 should be consistent

Radiographic Findings
- Abnormal asymmetry of lateral atlanto-dental space (LADS)
  - Probably over-emphasized
  - Up to 5 mm asymmetry may be normal
    - Assess range of motion and other views
- Abnormal morphology of C1 "button" on lateral view
  - Becomes less semicircular with rotational injury
  - Anterior joint space more indistinct
- Abnormal distance between occiput and C1
  - Dens to basion distance ≥ 1.4 cm in AOD
    - Most accurate criterion for diagnosis
  - Ratio of basion to posterior ring of C1 distance over opisthion to anterior ring of C1 distance (BC/OA ratio) ≥ 0.9 in AOD
- Lateral displacement of C1 masses on AP view in Jefferson fracture
- Rotation of mandible over upper cervical spine on lateral view
  - Rotation injuries and torticollis
- Anterior subluxation of C1 relative to C2
  - "Button" to dens space increased

DDx: Atlanto-Axial Abnormalities

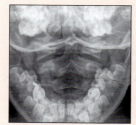

Nl LADS Asymmetry

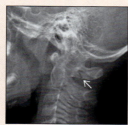

C1 Ring Fracture

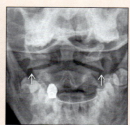

Jefferson Fx

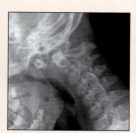

Down Syndrome

ATLANTO-AXIAL INJURIES

Key Facts

Terminology
- Atlanto-occipital dissociation (AOD), atlanto-occipital disruption, atlanto-occipital dislocation, occipitocervical subluxation or dislocation, Jefferson fracture, atlantoaxial dissociation, atlantoaxial rotatory fixation, fixed rotary subluxation, atlantoaxial rotational dislocation
- Traumatic injury to the upper cervical region ⇒ occiput to C2
- Up to 10 times more common in 1st decade than in older children and adults

Imaging Findings
- SCIWORA ⇒ Spinal Cord Injury Without Radiographic Abnormality
- Dens to basion distance ≥ 1.4 cm in AOD
- 10% of craniocervical junction fractures are shown by CT and not radiography
- When performing trauma head CT include C2
- When performing neck CT cover clivus through T1
- When performing MR always include STIR and MRA

Top Differential Diagnoses
- Atlanto-occipital dissociation
- 2-3 times more common in children than adults

Pathology
- Motor vehicle accidents are the most common cause of cervical spine injury in children
- 5% of spinal injuries occur in children
- Higher mortality rate than adults

  ○ Posterior ring of C1 anterior to line drawn from opisthion to posterior margin of C2 ring

CT Findings
- Fractures clearly delineated
  ○ Over 20% of cervical fractures missed by radiography alone
  ○ 10% of craniocervical junction fractures are shown by CT and not radiography
- Sagittal and coronal reformats essential
- Helical with 3D reconstruction ideal for rotational injuries
- "Dynamic CT"
  ○ Axial images through C1-2 in neutral position and with maximal voluntary rotation in each direction
  ○ Measure degree of rotation of C1 relative to C2

MR Findings
- T1WI
  ○ Helpful in identifying blood products
  ○ Fat-sat to differentiate soft tissue blood from fat
- T2WI
  ○ Best sequence for cord edema
    ▪ Axial and sagittal to confirm subtle cases
  ○ Best sequence for ligament integrity
  ○ Coronal T2 for pseudomeningocele
- STIR
  ○ Best sequence for bone and soft tissue edema
  ○ Inherent fat-saturation
    ▪ More reliable than fat-saturation with fast T2WI
- DWI: May have increased sensitivity for cord injury
- MRA
  ○ Key adjunct in cervical spine injuries
  ○ Vertebral artery injury in up to 25% of adults with cervical spine trauma
    ▪ Often clinically occult
- Sagittal imaging key for cord and ligaments

Non-Vascular Interventions
- Myelography: Highest resolution for assessment of nerve root avulsion

Imaging Recommendations
- Best imaging tool
  ○ For bone injury ⇒ helical CT with reformats
  ○ For SCIWORA ⇒ MR of the craniocervical junction (CCJ)
- Protocol advice
  ○ When performing trauma head CT include C2
  ○ When performing neck CT cover clivus through T1
  ○ When performing MR always include STIR and MRA

DIFFERENTIAL DIAGNOSIS

Pseudosubluxation
- Normal anterior translation of C2 relative to C3 in children under 5
- Only significant if posterior ring of C2 translates anterior to line from posterior ring of C1 to posterior ring of C3

Atlanto-occipital dissociation
- Disruption of stabilizing ligaments from occiput to cervical spine
  ○ Tectorial membrane, cruciate ligament, apical ligament, alar ligaments
- Often associated with anterior translation of occiput to C1 (increased BC/OA ratio)
- 2-3 times more common in children than adults
- High mortality rate in the field

Jefferson fracture
- "Burst" fracture of C1
- Axial loading
- Lateral subluxation of lateral masses of C1 relative to C2

Atlantoaxial rotatory fixation
- Fixed rotary subluxation
- Within range of normal rotation, but does not reduce spontaneously or voluntarily
  ○ Little or no trauma antecedent

ATLANTO-AXIAL INJURIES

Atlantoaxial rotational dislocation
- Complete loss of articular contact between lateral masses of C1 and C2
- Injury or disruption of joint capsule

Odontoid fractures
- Much more common in older children and adults
- Type I, II, III based upon level of fracture

Os odontoideum
- Result of fracture through odontoid synchondrosis prior to fusion (5-6 years)
  - Can be a source of instability
  - More common in children with skeletal dysplasias
- Ossiculum terminale ⇒ non-fusion of distal ossification center
  - Smaller and without clinical significance

Ligament instability
- Abnormal laxity of ligaments stabilizing C1-2
- Grisel syndrome ⇒ atlanto-axial instability associated with inflammation in adjacent soft tissues
- Down syndrome ⇒ laxity of transverse ligament
  - 10-20% incidence

Congenital fusion and segmentation anomalies
- C1-occiput, C1-2
- Klippel-Feil

PATHOLOGY

General Features
- Genetics
  - Syndromes associated with ligamentous laxity
    - Down, Morquio, Ehlers-Danlos, Marfan
- Etiology
  - Motor vehicle accidents are the most common cause of cervical spine injury in children
    - Falls are a distant second
- Epidemiology
  - 5% of spinal injuries occur in children
  - 18-21/million population
- Associated abnormalities
  - Higher mortality rate than adults
    - 2.5:1

CLINICAL ISSUES

Presentation
- Most common signs/symptoms
  - AOD
    - Many die prior to reaching medical care
    - Over half in cardiorespiratory arrest
    - As many as 25-30% neurologically intact at presentation
  - Rotational injuries
    - Present with painful torticollis
    - May be delayed presentation after trauma
    - May have little or no trauma antecedent
  - Ligament instability
    - 90% asymptomatic
    - Potential cause of chronic myelopathy
- Other signs/symptoms: Priaprism: Unchecked parasympathetic activity

Demographics
- Age: 0-9 years ⇒ high incidence of upper cervical spine injury compared to adolescents and adults
- Gender
  - M > F in adolescents and teens
  - F ≥ M in first decade

Natural History & Prognosis
- Neurological status at presentation best predictor of outcome
  - Intact or incomplete injury ⇒ likely good outcome
  - Complete loss of function at level of injury ⇒ poor chance of recovery
- Presence of spinal cord hemorrhage ⇒ worse potential for recovery

Treatment
- Support of impaired systemic function
- Stabilization of spine to prevent further injury
  - Standard backboards and collars may worsen malalignment in children under 9 by causing hyperflexion
  - Incorrect collar size: Worsen injury, excessive motion
  - Immobilizing collars: False positive clinical exams
  - Internal or external stabilization devices when condition allows
    - May impair ability to assess with MR
- Identification of extent of injury
  - Combination of clinical and imaging evaluation
- Decompression of lesions causing impingement
- Administration of spinal-injury dose steroids
  - Significant benefit for those presenting with deficit
- Intensive rehabilitation beginning shortly after treatment concludes

DIAGNOSTIC CHECKLIST

Consider
- Remember normal variability of LADS
- Remember pseudosubluxation

SELECTED REFERENCES
1. The Section on Disorders of the Spine and Peripheral Nerves of the American Association of Neurological Surgeons and the CNS: Management of pediatric cervical spine and spinal cord injuries. Neurosurgery. 50(3 Suppl):S85-99, 2002
2. Mirvis SE: How much lateral atlantodental interval asymmetry and atlantoaxial lateral mass asymmetry is acceptable on an open-mouth odontoid radiograph, and when is additional investigation necessary? AJR Am J Roentgenol. 170(4):1106-7, 1998
3. Flanders AE et al: Forecasting motor recovery after cervical spinal cord injury: value of MR imaging. Radiology. 201(3):649-55, 1996
4. Hamilton MG et al: Pediatric spinal injury: review of 174 hospital admissions. J Neurosurg. 77(5):700-4, 1992

ATLANTO-AXIAL INJURIES

IMAGE GALLERY

Typical

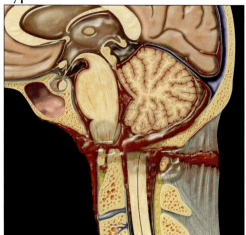
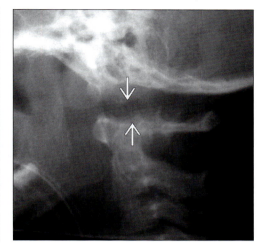

(Left) Lateral graphic shows complete atlanto-occipital dissociation with anterior translation of cranium relative to spine, disruption of cord and ligamentous structures, and extensive hemorrhage. *(Right)* Lateral radiograph shows abnormal widening of the atlanto-occipital articulation (arrows) with only mild anterior translation in this 8 year old with AOD and complete quadriplegia.

Typical

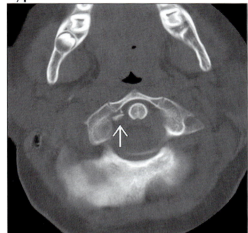
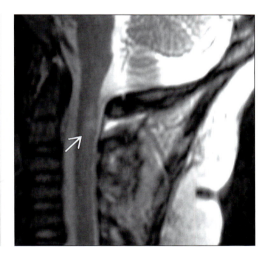

(Left) Axial NECT shows an avulsion fracture from C1 at the site of insertion of the transverse ligament (arrow). Disruption of this ligament can result in atlanto-axial instability. *(Right)* Sagittal T2WI MR in the same child shows abnormal signal in cord (arrow). Cord injury results from direct impact of the ring of C1 and/or secondary vascular compromise.

Typical

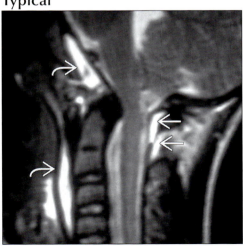
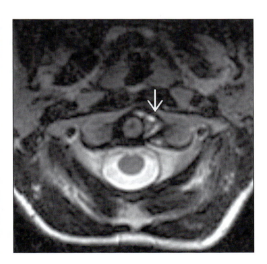

(Left) Sagittal T2WI MR shows disrupted posterior ligaments at C1-2 (arrows), with hematoma around tectorial membrane and in retropharynx (curved arrows) in a child with AOD. *(Right)* Axial T2WI MR shows edema in left atlanto-dental interspace (arrow) from trauma without fracture. MR imaging provides clinically relevant information that is unattainable by other methods.

CHILD ABUSE, BRAIN

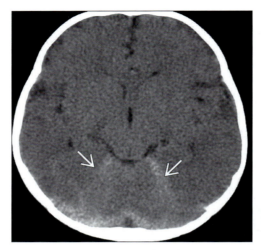

Axial NECT shows poor gray white differentiation and subdural blood along the tentorium (arrows) in a 5 month old with shaking-induced injury.

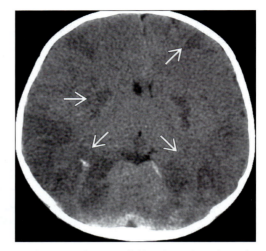

Axial NECT in the same child 12 hours later shows the rapid development of multiple regions of cytotoxic edema (arrows), with effacement of the 3rd ventricle and cisterns.

TERMINOLOGY

Abbreviations and Synonyms
- Nonaccidental trauma (NAT); nonaccidental injury (NAI), shaken-baby syndrome (SBS), battered child syndrome, Caffey-Kempe syndrome
- Rule out parental abuse (ROPA), whiplash shaken infant syndrome, nonaccidental head injury (NAHI), trauma-X
- Multiple alternate titles have been suggested in attempts to minimize accusatory labeling in clinical setting
  - May do more harm than good by causing confusion and hampering communication

Definitions
- Traumatic injury deliberately inflicted on infants and children by adults
  - This discussion centers on cranial injury

IMAGING FINDINGS

General Features
- Best diagnostic clue
  - Multiple brain injuries disproportionally severe relative to proffered history
  - Can be divided into two major groupings
    - Direct impact injury ⇒ result of direct blow to cranium or impact of skull on object
    - Shaking injury ⇒ result of violent to-and-fro motion of head
    - Not exclusive ⇒ shaking injury often compounded by impact
  - Direct impact injury characterized by skull fractures and injury to immediately underlying brain
    - Superficial injury (scalp laceration, swelling) strongly associated
    - High association with other organ injury
  - Shaking injury characterized by diffusely distributed subdural hematomas
    - Imaging characteristics often suggest injuries of differing ages
    - High association with "ischemic" parenchymal injury

Radiographic Findings
- Radiography
  - More sensitive in the detection of skull fractures than standard CT
    - CT is more sensitive and specific for depression and complications of fractures
  - Detection of fractures, a key component in forensic evaluation of suspected child abuse
  - Some fracture patterns are considered more suspicious for child abuse

DDx: Extra-Axial Collections In Children

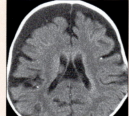
Glutaric Aciduria

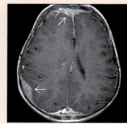
Neuroblastoma

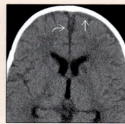
Subdural Empyema

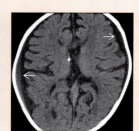
Overshunting

CHILD ABUSE, BRAIN

Key Facts

Terminology
- Traumatic injury deliberately inflicted on infants and children by adults

Imaging Findings
- Multiple brain injuries disproportionally severe relative to proffered history
- Direct impact injury ⇒ result of direct blow to cranium or impact of skull on object
- Shaking injury ⇒ result of violent to-and-fro motion of head
- Not exclusive ⇒ shaking injury often compounded by impact
- More sensitive in the detection of skull fractures than standard CT
- CT is the primary imaging tool in initial evaluation of child abuse

- Parenchymal injury often accompanies shaking injury
- Use PD/Intermediate sequence to detect subtle SDH on MR
- Use DWI to assess parenchymal injury

Pathology
- #1 cause of brain injury death in children < 2

Clinical Issues
- "Killer couch" ⇒ injuries commonly blamed on infant rolling off couch onto floor

Diagnostic Checklist
- Avoid use of vague, oblique, obscuring language in reports
- Avoid temptation to precisely time ICH

- Analysis of abuse and accidental injuries does not support this
- Multiple, compound, diastatic fractures, and fractures crossing sutures imply significant trauma
  - Discordance with suggested history best indicator for child abuse

CT Findings
- NECT
  - CT is the primary imaging tool in initial evaluation of child abuse
  - Sensitive in detection and characterization of fractures
    - Fractures oriented in axial plane may be missed!
  - Very sensitive in the detection and characterization of intracranial hemorrhage (ICH)
  - Subarachnoid hemorrhage (SAH) is common (>50%)
  - Subdural hemorrhage (SDH) is very common
    - Over cerebral convexities, in interhemispheric fissure, overlying tentorium
    - Dominant feature of shaking injury
    - Normal density of subarachnoid space (SAS) stands out next to increased density of SDH
  - Great caution should be exercised if attempting to estimate "age" of ICH
    - Blood loses density based upon multiple factors ⇒ cerebrospinal fluid (CSF) dilution, hematocrit, coagulation status
    - SDHs of same age can have significantly different density
    - Chronic SDHs tend to be uniform in density, slightly greater than CSF in SAH and ventricles
    - Acute SDHs are more likely to be hyperdense
    - However, acute SDH can be hypodense, and focal clots and membranes can cause hyperdensity in chronic SDH
  - Parenchymal injury often accompanies shaking injury
    - Initial CT ⇒ loss of gray-white differentiation, decreased density of supratentorial brain relative to cerebellum
    - Subsequent studies show multiple regions of decreased attenuation, not corresponding to arterial territories
  - Subdural hygromas can develop at 12-26 hours after injury
    - CSF density subdural collections of CSF that leak from SAS
    - Resolve without direct treatment
- CTA
  - Detectable vascular injury relatively uncommon in child abuse
    - Post-traumatic aneurysm, dissection can be demonstrated by CTA

MR Findings
- T1WI
  - Hyperintense hemorrhagic staining of injured cortex
  - Subdurals in posterior fossa clearly shown on sagittal T1WI
- T2WI: Shows loss of cortical ribbon and deep nuclei in neonates
- PD/Intermediate: Possibly most sensitive sequence for detection of small SDH
- T2* GRE: Sensitive for hemorrhagic staining, remote hemorrhage
- DWI: Key sequence for identification of parenchymal insult in shaking injury in acute/subacute stage
- MRA: Proximal vascular correlate (dissection, spasm) rarely shown in association with parenchymal injury
- MRS: Will show ↓ NAA, ↑ lactate in regions of parenchymal injury

Angiographic Findings
- Conventional
  - Post-traumatic pseudoaneurysms occasionally reported
    - Pericallosal artery

Nuclear Medicine Findings
- Bone Scan
  - Can be used to document associated skeletal injury
    - Can miss skull fractures, metaphyseal injuries

CHILD ABUSE, BRAIN

Imaging Recommendations
- Best imaging tool
  - NECT to evaluate brain initially, MR in delayed fashion
  - Radiographs to detect skull fractures (as part of skeletal survey)
- Protocol advice
  - Use PD/Intermediate sequence to detect subtle SDH on MR
  - Use DWI to assess parenchymal injury
  - Consider concomitant spine injury
  - Use MRA or CTA to evaluate suspected pseudoaneurysm

DIFFERENTIAL DIAGNOSIS

Accidental trauma
- Appropriate history for degree of injury

Benign macrocrania
- Self-limited communicating hydrocephalus
- Prominence of extra-axial spaces ⇒ isodense to CSF

Mitochondrial encephalopathies
- Several mitochondrial encephalopathies cause atrophy with subdural collections
- Glutaric acidurias (types I & II), Menkes syndrome
- Rare diseases with pre-existing neurologic symptoms

Overshunting
- "Passive" subdurals can develop from decreased volume associated with CSF shunting

Subdural empyema
- Febrile, sinusitis, meningitis

PATHOLOGY

General Features
- General path comments
  - 85% of fatal child abuse victims have evidence of impact head injury at postmortem examination
  - Cause of death in 80% of fatalities is brain swelling
    - Severe hypoxic ischemic encephalopathy > diffuse axonal injury (DAI)
  - Retinal hemorrhage 70-96% (usually bilateral, always with SDH)
- Etiology
  - Increased vulnerability in infants due to
    - Large head:body ratio + weak neck muscles
    - Developing brain ⇒ less structural integrity prior to myelination, greater susceptibility to injury
- Epidemiology
  - 17-25:100,000 annual incidence
    - Almost certainly under-reported
  - #1 cause of brain injury death in children < 2

CLINICAL ISSUES

Presentation
- Most common signs/symptoms
  - Discordance between stated history & degree of injury
    - Attempt by perpetrator to minimize suspicion
  - "Killer couch" ⇒ injuries commonly blamed on infant rolling off couch onto floor
    - Frequently in infants too young to roll over at all
  - Difficulty breathing, unresponsive
- Other signs/symptoms
  - Poor feeding, vomiting, irritability, seizures, lethargy, coma, apnea
  - Retinal hemorrhage
    - Can be missed on cursory exam
    - Can be seen in glutaric acidurias
- Clinical Profile
  - Perpetrators are most often direct caretakers ⇒ parents, baby-sitters, mother's boyfriend
  - Developmentally delayed, "colicky", premature or low birth weight infants at higher risk
  - Psychosocial stressors and poor coping mechanisms in family environment

Demographics
- Age
  - Majority < 1 year
  - Most common 2-6 months
- Gender: Male > female

Natural History & Prognosis
- High mortality 15-38% (60% if coma at presentation)

Treatment
- Notification of local Child Protection Agency mandated in US/Canada/Australia/some European countries
- Multidisciplinary child abuse & neglect team intervention

DIAGNOSTIC CHECKLIST

Consider
- Avoid use of vague, oblique, obscuring language in reports
  - Can hamper care of child and legal investigation
  - May increase likelihood of interpretation being challenged

Image Interpretation Pearls
- Avoid temptation to precisely time ICH
  - Impossible to precisely state age of bleeding in the absence of "before and after" imaging
  - Reasonable estimates and conclusions are more defensible in court

SELECTED REFERENCES
1. Kleinman PK: Diagnostic Imaging of Child Abuse, 2nd ed. Mosby, pp 285-342, 1998
2. Caffey J: The parent-infant traumatic stress syndrome; (Caffey-Kempe syndrome), (battered babe syndrome). Am J Roentgenol Radium Ther Nucl Med. 114(2):218-29, 1972
3. Silverman FN: Unrecognized trauma in infants, the battered child syndrome, and the syndrome of Ambroise Tardieu. Rigler Lecture. Radiology. 104(2):337-53, 1972

CHILD ABUSE, BRAIN

IMAGE GALLERY

Typical

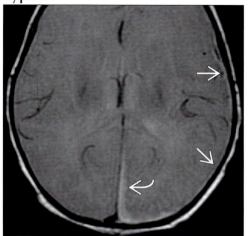
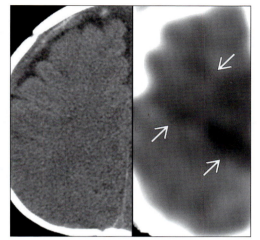

(Left) Axial PD/Intermediate MR shows SDH over left hemisphere. Although blood along falx (curved arrow) would be seen, the small volume laterally (arrows) would be very difficult to detect on CT. (Right) Axial DWI shows region of parenchymal injury (arrows) that is inapparent on NECT through same region. Extent of parenchymal insult has greater impact on prognosis than volume of ICH.

Variant

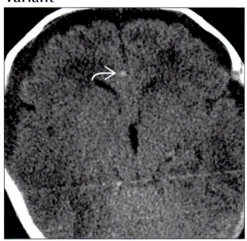
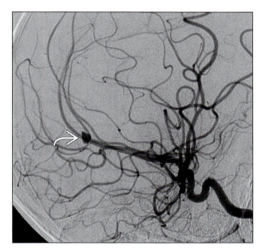

(Left) Axial NECT shows bifrontal SDH and a focus of increased density anterior to corpus callosum (curved arrow) in a 2 month old with shaking injury compounded by direct impact. (Right) Lateral catheter angiography in the same infant shows a post-traumatic pseudoaneurysm at the junction of the pericallosal and callosal-marginal arteries (curved arrow), corresponding to the hyperdensity.

Typical

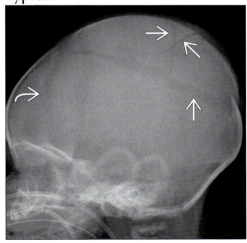
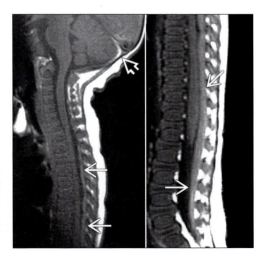

(Left) Lateral radiograph shows multiple fractures (arrows) that cross sutures and are diastatic, accompanied by coronal suture diastasis (curved arrow), from direct-impact injury. (Right) Sagittal T1WI MR of spinal column shows dorsal subdural hematoma (arrows) in a child with shaking injury. Note infratentorial SDH (open arrow). Spine injury is detected in less than 5% of cases.

COLLOID CYST

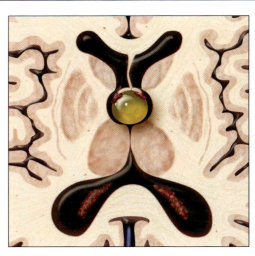

Axial graphic shows characteristic appearance of a colloid cyst, situated just dorsal to the fornix and impinging upon the foramen of Monro on each side.

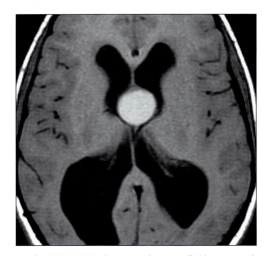

Axial T1WI MR shows a large colloid cyst with hyperintense signal, associated with ventriculomegaly. Not all colloid cysts are hyperintense on T1WI, but this is the most common appearance.

TERMINOLOGY

Abbreviations and Synonyms
- Colloid cyst (CC), paraphyseal cyst

Definitions
- Mucin-containing epithelial-lined cyst at the anterior-superior margin of the third ventricle

IMAGING FINDINGS

General Features
- Best diagnostic clue: Hyperdense midline foramen of Monro mass on NECT
- Location
  - > 99% wedged into foramen of Monro
    - Attached to anterosuperior 3rd ventricular roof
    - Pillars of fornix straddle anterior aspect of cyst
    - Posterior part of frontal horns splayed laterally around cyst
  - < 1% other sites
    - Lateral, 4th ventricles
    - Parenchyma (cerebellum)
    - Extra-axial (prepontine, meninges)
- Size
  - 1-2 mm up to 3 cm
    - Mean size = 15 mm
- Morphology: Usually spherical

CT Findings
- NECT
  - 2/3 hyperdense on CT
  - 1/3 iso/hypodense
  - +/- Hydrocephalus
  - Rarely have hemorrhage, calcification
- CECT
  - Usually doesn't enhance
    - Rare rim-enhancement

MR Findings
- T1WI
  - Signal correlates with cholesterol concentration
    - 2/3 hyperintense on T1WI
    - 1/3 isointense (small CCs may be difficult to see!)
  - May have associated ventriculomegaly
- T2WI
  - Majority isointense to brain on T2WI (small cysts may be difficult to see!)
    - 25% mixed hypointense/hyperintense ("black hole" effect)
    - Fluid-fluid level (uncommon)
- FLAIR
  - Isointense to hyperintense
    - Does not suppress with cerebrospinal fluid (CSF)
- DWI
  - No restricted diffusion

DDx: Frontal Horn And Third Ventricle Masses

Arachnoid Cyst | Fornix Glioma | CPP | SEGA In TS

COLLOID CYST

Key Facts

Terminology
- Mucin-containing epithelial-lined cyst at the anterior-superior margin of the third ventricle

Imaging Findings
- Best diagnostic clue: Hyperdense midline foramen of Monro mass on NECT
- 2/3 hyperdense on CT
- 2/3 hyperintense on T1WI

Top Differential Diagnoses
- CSF flow artifact (MR "pseudocyst")
- Fornix glioma
- Subependymal giant cell astrocytoma (SEGA)
- Choroid plexus cyst
- Neurocysticercosis
- Arachnoid cyst

Pathology
- Derived from embryonic endoderm

Clinical Issues
- Acute foramen of Monro obstruction may lead to rapid onset hydrocephalus, herniation, death
- 40-50% asymptomatic, discovered incidentally
- 8% < 15 y at diagnosis
- Prognosis excellent when diagnosed early and excised

Diagnostic Checklist
- Notify referring MD immediately if CC identified (especially if hydrocephalus is present)
- Trust NECT and findings on T1WI more than T2WI, FLAIR, or DWI
- "Pathology-weighted" sequences can be very insensitive

- DWI of little benefit in evaluation
- T1 C+
  - Usually no enhancement
  - Rare: May show peripheral (rim) enhancement
- MRS
  - Large peak around 2.0 ppm due to "colloid"
    - Mimics normal N-acetyl aspartate peak
  - Small lactate peak

Imaging Recommendations
- Best imaging tool
  - NECT probably most sensitive
    - MR better for surgical planning
- Protocol advice
  - NECT for detection, routine follow-up
    - May be reasonable to just follow asymptomatic cysts < 1 cm without hydrocephalus
  - MR with contrast for pre-operative planning
    - Thin sagittal and coronal imaging through the foramen of Monro

DIFFERENTIAL DIAGNOSIS

CSF flow artifact (MR "pseudocyst")
- Multiplanar technique confirms artifact
- Look for phase artifact

Neoplasm
- Craniopharyngioma
  - 3rd ventricle rare location
  - Usually not wedged into foramen of Monro, fornix
  - Ca++, rim/nodular enhancement common
- Pituitary adenoma
  - Rare in 3rd ventricle
  - Enhances (usually strongly, uniformly)
- Fornix glioma
  - Solid, variably enhancing lesion
  - Infiltrates into parenchyma
- Central neurocytoma
  - Projects into frontal horn from septum pellucidum
  - Rare in children
- Subependymal giant cell astrocytoma (SEGA)
  - Lesion in children with tuberous sclerosis (TS)
  - Solid, lobulated, enhancing mass
- Choroid plexus papilloma (CPP)
  - Rare in 3rd ventricle
  - Tumor of early childhood

Choroid plexus cyst
- Anechoic at ultrasound
- Usually found in infants

Neurocysticercosis
- Multiple lesions within parenchyma and cisterns
- Associated ependymitis or basilar meningitis common
- Ca++ common
- Look for scolex

Arachnoid cyst
- Projecting up from suprasellar cistern
- Doesn't wedge behind fornix
- Follows CSF on FLAIR images

PATHOLOGY

General Features
- General path comments: Gross appearance, location virtually pathognomonic
- Etiology
  - Derived from embryonic endoderm
    - Similar to other foregut-derived cysts (neurenteric, Rathke)
    - Ectopic endodermal elements migrate into velum interpositum
    - Previously thought to be derived from neuroectodermal tissue such as paraphyseal remnants
  - Contents accumulate from mucinous secretions, desquamated epithelial cells
- Epidemiology
  - 0.5-1.0% primary brain tumors
  - 15-20% intraventricular masses
- Associated abnormalities: May result in hydrocephalus

COLLOID CYST

Gross Pathologic & Surgical Features
- Smooth, spherical/ovoid well-delineated cyst
  - Thick gelatinous center, variable viscosity (mucinous or desiccated)
  - Rare ⇒ evidence for recent/remote hemorrhage

Microscopic Features
- Outer wall is a thin fibrous capsule
- Inner lining
  - Simple layer of columnar cells
    - Interspersed goblet cells, scattered ciliated cells
  - Rests on thin connective tissue layer
- Cyst contents
  - Gelatinous ("colloid") material
  - Variable viscosity
  - +/- Necrotic leukocytes, cholesterol clefts
- Immunohistochemistry
  - Individual cells are positive for cytokeratin or epithelial membrane antigen
  - Scattered cells are reactive for Clara cel-specific antigens
- Electron microscopy
  - Resembles mature respiratory epithelium
  - Non-ciliated or tall columnar cells
  - Basal cells contain dense core vesicles

CLINICAL ISSUES

Presentation
- Most common signs/symptoms
  - Headache (50-60%)
  - Acute foramen of Monro obstruction may lead to rapid onset hydrocephalus, herniation, death
  - 40-50% asymptomatic, discovered incidentally
    - 3-, 5-, 10 year incidence of developing cyst-related symptoms ⇒ 0, 0, 8% respectively
- Other signs/symptoms: Nausea, vomiting, memory loss, altered personality, gait disturbance, visual changes

Demographics
- Age
  - Peak = age 40
  - 8% < 15 y at diagnosis
- Gender: M = F

Natural History & Prognosis
- Varies with presence/rate of growth, development of CSF obstruction
- 90% stable or stop enlarging
  - Older age
  - Small cyst
  - No hydrocephalus
  - Hyperdense on NECT, hypointense on T2 weighted MR
- 10% enlarge
  - Younger patients
  - Larger cyst, hydrocephalus
  - Iso/hypodense on NECT, often hyperintense on T2WI
  - May enlarge rapidly, cause coma/death!
- Prognosis excellent when diagnosed early and excised

Treatment
- Most common treatment ⇒ complete surgical resection
  - Image-guided endoscopic approach increasingly common
  - 50% experience short-term memory disturbance (usually resolves)
  - Recurrence rare if resection complete
- Less-favored options
  - Stereotactic aspiration (difficult with extremely viscous/solid cysts)
    - Hyperdensity on CT/hypointensity on T2WI suggest high viscosity and difficulty with percutaneous therapy
  - Ventricular shunting
  - Observation (rare)

DIAGNOSTIC CHECKLIST

Consider
- Notify referring MD immediately if CC identified (especially if hydrocephalus is present)
- Consider CSF flow-artifact
  - Usually most prominent on FLAIR images

Image Interpretation Pearls
- Trust NECT and findings on T1WI more than T2WI, FLAIR, or DWI
  - "Pathology-weighted" sequences can be very insensitive

SELECTED REFERENCES

1. Solaroglu I et al: Transcortical-transventricular approach in colloid cysts of the third ventricle: surgical experience with 26 cases. Neurosurg Rev. 27(2):89-92, 2004
2. Hellwig D et al: Neuroendoscopic treatment for colloid cysts of the third ventricle: the experience of a decade. Neurosurgery. 52(3):525-33; discussion 532-3, 2003
3. Kava MP et al: Colloid cyst of the third ventricle: a cause of sudden death in a child. Indian J Cancer. 40(1):31-3, 2003
4. Peraud A et al: Intraventricular congenital lesions and colloid cysts. Neurosurg Clin N Am. 14(4):607-19, 2003
5. Desai KI et al: Surgical management of colloid cyst of the third ventricle--a study of 105 cases. Surg Neurol. 57(5):295-302; discussion 302-4, 2002
6. Gupta A et al: Intraventricular neurocysticercosis mimicking colloid cyst. Case report. J Neurosurg. 97(1):208-10, 2002
7. Jeffree RL et al: Colloid cyst of the third ventricle: a clinical review of 39 cases. J Clinical Neurosci. 8: 328-31, 2001
8. Armao D et al: Colloid cyst of the third ventricle: imaging-pathologic correlation. AJNR Am J Neuroradiol. 21(8):1470-7, 2000
9. El Khoury C et al: Colloid cysts of the third ventricle: are MR imaging patterns predictive of difficulty with percutaneous treatment? AJNR Am J Neuroradiol. 21(3):489-92, 2000
10. Pollock BE et al: A theory on the natural history of colloid cysts of the third ventricle. Neurosurgery. 46(5):1077-81; discussion 1081-3, 2000

COLLOID CYST

IMAGE GALLERY

Typical

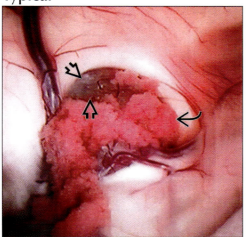
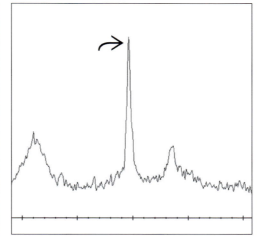

(Left) Intra-operative photograph from endoscopic resection shows the gray colloid cyst (open arrows) displacing choroid plexus (curved arrow) anteriorly in the foramen of Monro. (Right) MRS acquired in the cyst shows a dominant peak at 2.0 ppm (curved arrow); this is near the peak for NAA, but corresponds to the mucinous material filling the cyst, not neural elements.

Typical

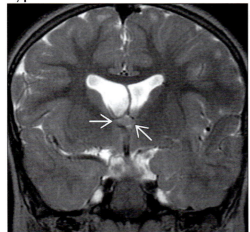
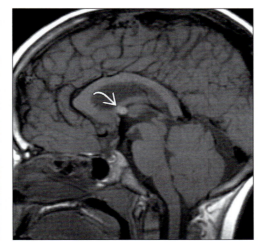

(Left) Coronal T2WI MR shows a small colloid cyst at the anterior-superior aspect of the 3rd ventricle (arrows). Prominent flow void inferior to cyst is from prior 3rd ventriculostomy procedure. (Right) Sagittal T1WI MR in the same child shows the colloid cyst as a focus of hyperintense signal at the foramen of Monro (arrow).

Typical

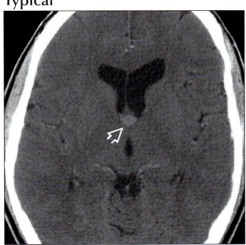
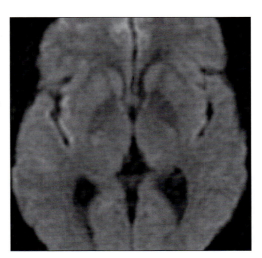

(Left) Axial NECT shows a small colloid cyst just dorsal to the fornix (arrow). It projects slightly to the left of midline, and there is associated enlargement of the left frontal horn. (Right) Axial DWI MR in the same child is notable for the absence of any altered diffusion. CT is often more sensitive than MR for the detection of small colloid cysts.

ARACHNOID CYST

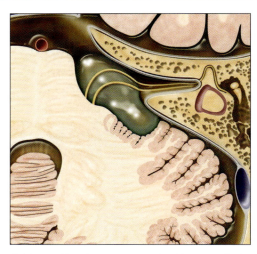
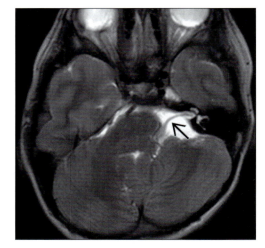

Axial graphic shows an arachnoid cyst of the cerebellopontine angle (CPA) displacing the 7th and 8th cranial nerves superiorly with minimal mass effect upon the adjacent cerebellum.

Axial T2WI MR shows a similar-sized arachnoid cyst in the left CPA. Arrow points to the anteriorly displaced 7th and 8th nerve complex. 75% of arachnoid cysts are diagnosed in childhood.

TERMINOLOGY

Abbreviations and Synonyms
- Arachnoid cyst (AC), subarachnoid cyst

Definitions
- Pocket of cerebrospinal fluid (CSF) lined by arachnoid that does not directly communicate with ventricular system or subarachnoid space

IMAGING FINDINGS

General Features
- Best diagnostic clue: Extra-axial CSF collection with mass effect
- Location
  - 50-60% middle cranial fossa (MCF)
  - 10% cerebellopontine angle (CPA)
  - 10% suprasellar arachnoid cyst
  - Spinal lesions are uncommon
    - May be a complication of prior trauma, myelography
    - Septations in arachnoid may balloon and mimic AC
- Size: Variable ⇒ likelihood of symptoms increases with cyst size
- Morphology
  - Sharply delineated
  - "Compromised" shape ⇒ partly accommodates to surrounding spaces

CT Findings
- NECT
  - Usually CSF attenuation
    - Intracyst hemorrhage may increase attenuation (rare)
  - Thins or remodels calvaria
- CTA: Displaces vessels

MR Findings
- T1WI
  - Sharply-marginated extra-axial fluid collection isointense with CSF
  - Less than expected mass effect
    - Adjacent brain accommodates cyst
- T2WI
  - Isointense with CSF
  - No edema in adjacent brain
- PD/Intermediate: Isointense with CSF
- FLAIR
  - Suppresses completely with FLAIR
  - Reduced/absent flow artifact compared to subarachnoid CSF
- DWI: No restricted diffusion
- T1 C+: No enhancement
- MRA: Cortical vessels displaced away from calvaria

DDx: Cystic Lesions In Children

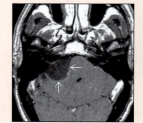
Epidermoid

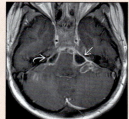
Abscesses

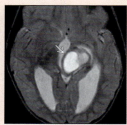
Astrocytoma

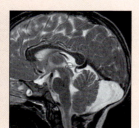
Cisterna Magna

ARACHNOID CYST

Key Facts

Terminology
- Arachnoid cyst (AC), subarachnoid cyst
- Pocket of cerebrospinal fluid (CSF) lined by arachnoid that does not directly communicate with ventricular system or subarachnoid space

Imaging Findings
- Best diagnostic clue: Extra-axial CSF collection with mass effect
- 50-60% middle cranial fossa (MCF)
- Less than expected mass effect
- Adjacent brain accommodates cyst
- Suppresses completely with FLAIR
- Reduced/absent flow artifact compared to subarachnoid CSF
- DWI: No restricted diffusion

Top Differential Diagnoses
- Epidermoid cyst
- Subdural hygroma
- Porencephalic cyst
- Neuroepithelial cyst

Pathology
- 1% of all intracranial masses

Clinical Issues
- Often asymptomatic, found incidentally
- 75% diagnosed in childhood

Diagnostic Checklist
- FLAIR, DWI best sequences for distinguishing etiology of cystic-appearing intracranial masses

---

- MRV: Can demonstrate anomalies of venous drainage
- MR Cine: Can help distinguish AC from enlarged subarachnoid space
- MRS
  - No identifiable resonances
    - Can easily distinguish from other cystic intracranial masses

Ultrasonographic Findings
- Grayscale Ultrasound: Anechoic

Non-Vascular Interventions
- CT cisternography can definitively distinguish arachnoid cyst from enlarged subarachnoid space (mega cisterna magna)

Nuclear Medicine Findings
- SPECT
  - May show hypoperfusion in brain adjacent to cyst

Imaging Recommendations
- Best imaging tool: Non-contrast MR
- Protocol advice: Always use FLAIR, DWI

DIFFERENTIAL DIAGNOSIS

Epidermoid cyst
- Does not follow CSF on all sequences
  - "Brighter" on CT and T1WI
  - Doesn't suppress on FLAIR
  - Shows restricted diffusion (bright) on DWI
- Engulfs vessels and nerves, doesn't displace them

Chronic subdural hematoma
- Signal not identical to CSF
  - Hyperintense to CSF on FLAIR, PD, and T1WI
- May show enhancing membrane

Subdural hygroma
- Leakage of CSF from subarachnoid space into subdural space
  - 2-7 days after trauma
- Crescentic, often bilateral

Porencephalic cyst
- Result of trauma or stroke
- Surrounded by injured, not compressed/distorted, brain

Neuroepithelial cyst
- Benign cysts lined by "epithelium"
- Periventricular, intraventricular, choroid fissure

Epidural abscess
- Enhancing wall
- Elevated lactate on MRS
- Restricted diffusion (bright) on DWI

Pilocytic astrocytoma
- Enhancing mural nodule
- Intra-axial

Mega cisterna magna
- More posterior than retrocerebellar AC

PATHOLOGY

General Features
- General path comments
  - Fluid-containing cyst with translucent membrane
  - Arachnoid layers contain CSF
- Etiology
  - Old concept = "splitting" or diverticulum of developing arachnoid
  - New concept (middle fossa ACs)
    - Frontal, temporal embryonic meninges (endomeninx) fail to merge as sylvian fissure forms
    - Remain separate, forming "duplicated" arachnoid
  - May rarely form as shunt complication
  - Suprasellar AC may reflect upward herniation of an obstructed membrane of Lillequist
  - Possible mechanisms for enlargement
    - Active fluid secretion by cyst wall
    - Slow distention by CSF pulsations
    - CSF accumulates by one-way (ball-valve) flow

ARACHNOID CYST

- Epidemiology
  - 1% of all intracranial masses
    - Likely even more common ⇒ small MCF cysts may be missed
- Associated abnormalities
  - With MCF cysts, adjacent temporal lobe is often hypoplastic
  - Subdural hematoma (increased prevalence, especially MCF)
  - Syndromic ACs
    - Acrocallosal (cysts in 1/3), Aicardi, Pallister-Hall syndromes

Gross Pathologic & Surgical Features
- Bluish-gray arachnoid bulges around CSF-filled cyst

Microscopic Features
- Wall consists of flattened but normal arachnoid cells
- No inflammation or neoplastic changes

Staging, Grading or Classification Criteria
- Galassi classification: ↑ with ↑ size/mass effect and ↓ communication with basal cisterns
  - Type I: Small, spindle shaped, limited to anterior MCF
  - Type II: Superior extent along sylvian fissure; temp lobe displaced
  - Type III: Huge, fills entire MCF; frontal/temp/parietal displacement

CLINICAL ISSUES

Presentation
- Most common signs/symptoms
  - Often asymptomatic, found incidentally
  - Associated symptoms vary with size, location of cyst
    - Headache, dizziness, sensorineural hearing loss, hemifacial spasm/tic
    - Suprasellar ACs may cause obstructive hydrocephalus, "bobble-head doll syndrome", precocious puberty

Demographics
- Age
  - Can be found at any age
  - 75% diagnosed in childhood
- Gender: M:F = 3-5:1 especially middle cranial fossa

Natural History & Prognosis
- May (but usually don't) slowly enlarge

Treatment
- Treatment: Often none
  - Morbidity from treatment may be greater than symptoms attributed to cyst
- Resection/fenestration (may be endoscopic)
- Shunt

DIAGNOSTIC CHECKLIST

Consider
- Think of epidermoid when encountering CPA arachnoid cyst
  - Concept that they are nearly identical is not supported with modern imaging techniques

Image Interpretation Pearls
- FLAIR, DWI best sequences for distinguishing etiology of cystic-appearing intracranial masses

SELECTED REFERENCES

1. Yildiz H et al: evaluation of communication between intracranial arachnoid cysts and cisterns with phase-contrast cine MR imaging. AJNR Am J Neuroradiol. 26(1):145-51, 2005
2. Booth TN et al: Pre- and postnatal MR imaging of hypothalamic hamartomas associated with arachnoid cysts. AJNR Am J Neuroradiol. 25(7):1283-5, 2004
3. Erman T et al: Congenital peripheral facial palsy associated with cerebellopontine angle arachnoid cyst. Pediatr Neurosurg. 40(6):297-300, 2004
4. Huang HP et al: Arachnoid cyst with GnRH-dependent sexual precocity and growth hormone deficiency. Pediatr Neurol. 30(2):143-5, 2004
5. Kulkarni AG et al: Extradural arachnoid cysts: a study of seven cases. Br J Neurosurg. 18(5):484-8, 2004
6. Nakagawa A et al: Usefulness of constructive interference in steady state (CISS) imaging for the diagnosis and treatment of a large extradural spinal arachnoid cyst. Minim Invasive Neurosurg. 47(6):369-72, 2004
7. Orlacchio A et al: A new SPG4 mutation in a variant form of spastic paraplegia with congenital arachnoid cysts. Neurology. 62(10):1875-8, 2004
8. Wang JC et al: Advances in the endoscopic management of suprasellar arachnoid cysts in children. J Neurosurg. 100(5 Suppl Pediatrics):418-26, 2004
9. Alkadhi H et al: Somatomotor functional MRI in a large congenital arachnoid cyst. Neuroradiology. 45(3):153-6, 2003
10. Desai KI et al: Suprasellar arachnoid cyst presenting with bobble-head doll movements: a report of 3 cases. Neurol India. 51(3):407-9, 2003
11. McBride LA et al: Cystoventricular shunting of intracranial arachnoid cysts. Pediatr Neurosurg. 39(6):323-9, 2003
12. Yu Q et al: Differential diagnosis of arachnoid cyst from subarachnoid space enlargement by phase-contrast cine MRI. Chin Med J (Engl). 116(1):116-20, 2003
13. Dutt SN et al: Radiologic differentiation of intracranial epidermoids from arachnoid cysts. Otol Neurotol. (1):84-92, 2002
14. Gosalakkal JA: Intracranial arachnoid cysts in children: a review of pathogenesis, clinical features, and management. Pediatr Neurol. 26(2):93-8, 2002
15. Kirollos RW et al: Endoscopic treatment of suprasellar and third ventricle-related arachnoid cysts. Childs Nerv Syst. 17(12):713-8, 2001
16. Sgouros S et al: Congenital middle fossa arachnoid cysts may cause global brain ischaemia: a study with 99Tc-hexamethylpropyleneamineoxime single photon emission computerised tomography scans. Pediatr Neurosurg. 35(4):188-94, 2001
17. Ibarra R et al: Role of MR imaging in the diagnosis of complicated arachnoid cyst. Pediatr Radiol. 30(5):329-31, 2000
18. Park SH et al: Diffusion-weighted MRI in cystic or necrotic intracranial lesions. Neuroradiology. 42(10):716-21, 2000

ARACHNOID CYST

IMAGE GALLERY

Typical

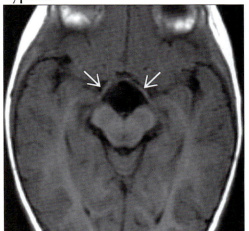
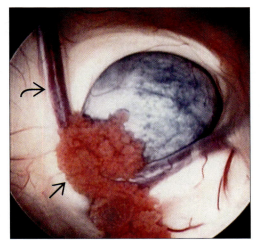

(Left) Axial T1WI MR shows splaying of the optic tracts *(arrows)* by a suprasellar arachnoid cyst. Unlike their effect on adjacent brain, arachnoid cysts displace vessels and nerves significantly. *(Right)* Endoscopic photograph shows characteristic bluish hue of a suprasellar AC projecting into the foramen of Monro, anterior to the choroid *(arrow)*, and thalamostriate vein *(curved arrow)*.

Typical

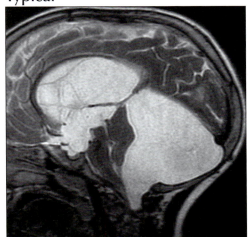
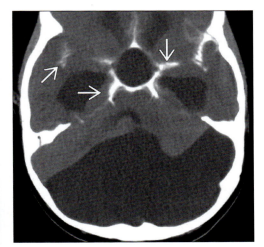

(Left) Sagittal T2WI MR shows mass effect on the vermis from a posterior fossa arachnoid cyst. Mega cisterna magna will typically flatten the posterior margin of the vermis, but not elevate it. *(Right)* Axial CT cisternogram in the same child shows contrast throughout the subarachnoid space *(arrows)*, but not in the cyst.

Variant

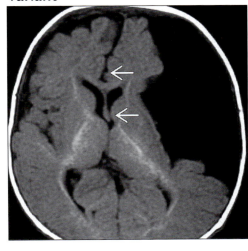
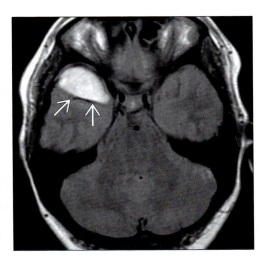

(Left) Axial T1WI MR in a 6 month old shows a large AC projecting superiorly out of the middle cranial fossa. Despite the large size, there is only mild rightward shift of the midline *(arrows)*. *(Right)* Axial PD/Intermediate MR shows bright signal in an otherwise typical MCF cyst *(arrows)*, due to hemorrhage. Less than expected mass effect from a subdural hematoma may indicate bleeding into an AC.

DERMOID AND EPIDERMOID CYSTS

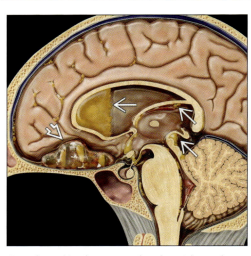

Sagittal graphic shows complex dermoid on planum sphenoidale (open arrow), with fat-fluid levels in cisterns and ventricles (arrows), indicating rupture.

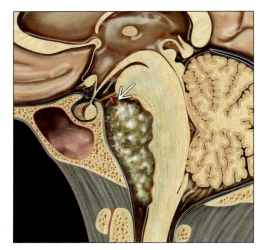

Sagittal graphic shows "mother-of-pearl" sheen of pre-pontine epidermoid cyst. Note encasement of basilar artery (arrow), and irregular interface with brainstem.

TERMINOLOGY

Abbreviations and Synonyms
- Ectodermal inclusion cyst, cholesteatoma, epidermal inclusion cyst, dermolipoma

Definitions
- Dermoids and epidermoids are inclusions of ectodermal tissue within the central nervous system (CNS)
- Epidermoids consist of squamous epithelium
- Dermoids contain squamous epithelium and associated dermal appendages
  ○ Sebaceous glands, dental enamel, hair follicles

IMAGING FINDINGS

General Features
- Best diagnostic clue
  ○ Dermoid ⇒ fat signal/attenuation droplets in cisterns, sulci, ventricles if ruptured
  ○ Epidermoid ⇒ CSF-like mass that envelops vessels and nerves
- Location
  ○ Dermoids are most commonly found in suprasellar and frontonasal regions
    ▪ Less commonly in posterior fossa, midline vermis & 4th ventricle
  ○ Epidermoids are most commonly found in cerebellopontine angle (CPA), around 4th ventricle, parasellar
  ○ Spine ⇒ both can be found in association with neural tube closure defects
    ▪ Acquired lesions from trauma, lumbar puncture (LP)
  ○ Orbit ⇒ "dermolipoma" at zygomatico-frontal suture line
- Morphology
  ○ Dermoids are usually well-circumscribed
  ○ Epidermoids are more amorphous

Radiographic Findings
- Sutural dermoids often incidentally seen on skull radiographs as small lucencies at base of coronal suture or at zygomatico-frontal suture line

CT Findings
- NECT
  ○ Dermoids have striking fat density on NECT ⇒ mimics air
    ▪ With rupture, droplets of fat disseminate in cisterns, may cause fat-fluid level within ventricles
    ▪ Ca++ in 20%
    ▪ Skull/scalp dermoid expands diploe
  ○ Epidermoids usually resemble CSF on NECT

DDx: Lesions That Mimic Dermoids And Epidermoids

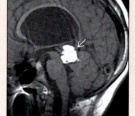
Arachnoid Cyst

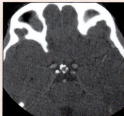
Craniopharyngioma

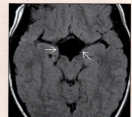
Arachnoid Cyst

DERMOID AND EPIDERMOID CYSTS

Key Facts

Terminology
- Dermoids and epidermoids are inclusions of ectodermal tissue within the central nervous system (CNS)
- Epidermoids consist of squamous epithelium
- Dermoids contain squamous epithelium and associated dermal appendages

Imaging Findings
- Dermoids are typically hyperintense on T1WI
- Epidermoids are only slightly hyperintense to CSF on T1WI
- Distinction of epidermoid from CSF is obvious on FLAIR
- Dermoids/epidermoids have minimal marginal enhancement or none at all

Top Differential Diagnoses
- Craniopharyngioma
- Arachnoid cyst

Pathology
- Dermoids are rare: < 0.5% of primary intracranial tumors
- Epidermoids are 5-10x more common

Diagnostic Checklist
- Use contrast to distinguish suprasellar dermoid from craniopharyngioma
- Fat suppression of dermoid much less "clean" than lipoma
- It is a myth that epidermoids are difficult to distinguish from arachnoid cysts

---

- Ca++ in 10-25%
  - Rare "dense" dermoid/epidermoid is hyperattenuating on CT
- CECT: Generally no enhancement

MR Findings
- T1WI
  - Dermoids are typically hyperintense on T1WI
    - Not as uniformly bright as lipomas
    - Heterogeneous, with striated appearance
    - Go "dark" with fat suppression, but not as cleanly as lipoma
    - Droplets from rupture rise to non-dependent regions (frontal horns, convexities), and appear as fat-fluid levels
  - Epidermoids are only slightly hyperintense to CSF on T1WI
    - Mimic complex arachnoid cyst
    - Small septations or lobules may be visible
    - "White" epidermoids ⇒ hyperintense to brain (rare)
- T2WI
  - Dermoids are typically heterogeneous
    - Striated or "layered" appearance more easily seen
    - Chemical shift artifact in frequency encoding direction
    - Rare "dense" posterior fossa dermoid: Very hypointense
  - Epidermoids are iso- to hyperintense to CSF
    - Rare "dense" epidermoid: Very hypointense
- FLAIR
  - Distinction of epidermoid from CSF is obvious on FLAIR
    - Usually obvious on PD/Intermediate and constructive interference in steady-state (CISS) sequences also
- DWI: Epidermoids have markedly restricted diffusion
- T1 C+
  - Dermoids/epidermoids have minimal marginal enhancement or none at all
  - Exception ⇒ ruptured dermoid will cause chemical ventriculitis and ependymal enhancement
- MRA: Vessels encased by epidermoid may be narrowed
- MRS: Both show very strong and broad resonances from mobile lipids at 0.9 and 1.3 ppm

Non-Vascular Interventions
- Cisternography can be used to distinguish epidermoid from arachnoid cyst
  - Lobular "cauliflower-like" surface of epidermoid becomes apparent
  - FLAIR/CISS/DWI have made cisternography unnecessary

Imaging Recommendations
- Best imaging tool: MR, especially in setting of rupture
- Protocol advice
  - Use fat-suppression, DWI, and FLAIR
  - Use MRA to assess vascular narrowing
  - Look for chemical shift artifact, especially with rupture

DIFFERENTIAL DIAGNOSIS

Craniopharyngioma
- Nearly identical imaging characteristics as suprasellar dermoid
  - Difference is in nature of cells lining walls
- Distinguishing characteristic ⇒ enhancement in over 90%
- Much more common than dermoid

Arachnoid cyst
- Myth ⇒ arachnoid cysts and epidermoids can be identical
- Similar, but epidermoids always have more "character" of signal
- Much more common than epidermoids, except in spine

Lipoma
- Fatty signal/attenuation more homogeneous
- Ca++ less frequent than in dermoids
- Similar etiology ⇒ mesodermal "inclusion"

DERMOID AND EPIDERMOID CYSTS

Teratoma
- Germ cell tumor that contains two or more embryologic layers
- Pituitary and pineal region
- Usually has enhancing components

PATHOLOGY

General Features
- Etiology
  o Inclusion of cutaneous ectoderm during neural tube closure
  o Acquired ⇒ displacement of epithelium into CNS during LP, trauma, surgery
    - Extremely rare
- Epidemiology
  o Dermoids are rare: < 0.5% of primary intracranial tumors
  o Epidermoids are 5-10x more common
- Associated abnormalities
  o 89% of dermal sinuses are associated with inclusion cysts
  o Dermoid/epidermoid is known late complication of spinal dysraphism, with or without surgical repair
  o Goldenhar syndrome (aka oculoauriculovertebral dysplasia) includes cranial lipomas and dermoids

Gross Pathologic & Surgical Features
- Dermoids contain a mixture of greasy lipid, cholesterol debris
  o Often contain hair and may contain enamel
- Epidermoids often have shiny "mother of pearl" appearance to surface
  o Insinuating growth pattern
  o Cyst contents ⇒ soft, waxy flaky material

Microscopic Features
- Dermoid has outer wall of fibrous connective tissue with inner lining of keratinized squamous epithelium, dermal appendages
  o Desquamated keratin, cellular debris in cyst
- Epidermoid has wall of simple stratified cuboidal squamous epithelium
  o Solid crystalline cholesterol, keratin in cyst

CLINICAL ISSUES

Presentation
- Most common signs/symptoms
  o Dermoid: Headache, seizure
    - Rupture ⇒ acute severe headache, collapse
    - Causes chemical meningitis (6.9%)
  o Epidermoid: Headache, cranial nerve neuropathies
    - Chemical meningitis rare
- Other signs/symptoms
  o Hypopituitarism, diabetes insipidus, visual symptoms
  o Spinal lesions associated with symptoms of cord tethering

Demographics
- Age
  o Both lesions more commonly diagnosed in adults
    - Exception ⇒ periorbital/sutural dermoids

Natural History & Prognosis
- Slowly growing, often asymptomatic
- Dermoid rupture can cause significant morbidity/mortality
- Dermoid + dermal sinus may cause infection
- Rare malignant transformation into squamous cell carcinoma (adults)

Treatment
- Complete microsurgical excision
  o Residual capsule may lead to recurrence
  o Subarachnoid dissemination of contents may occur

DIAGNOSTIC CHECKLIST

Image Interpretation Pearls
- Use contrast to distinguish suprasellar dermoid from craniopharyngioma
- Fat suppression of dermoid much less "clean" than lipoma
- It is a myth that epidermoids are difficult to distinguish from arachnoid cysts
  o Use FLAIR, DWI, MRS, CISS

SELECTED REFERENCES

1. Caldarelli M et al: Intracranial midline dermoid and epidermoid cysts in children. J Neurosurg. 100(5 Suppl Pediatrics):473-80, 2004
2. Cummings TJ et al: The pathology of extracranial scalp and skull masses in young children. Clin Neuropathol. 23(1):34-43, 2004
3. Ziv ET et al: Iatrogenic intraspinal epidermoid tumor: two cases and a review of the literature. Spine. 29(1):E15-8, 2004
4. Lacey M et al: Temporal dermoids: three cases and a modified treatment algorithm. Ann Plast Surg. 51(1):103-9, 2003
5. Perry JD et al: Simultaneous ipsilateral temporal fossa and orbital dermoid cysts. Am J Ophthalmol. 135(3):413-5, 2003
6. Brown JY et al: Unusual imaging appearance of an intracranial dermoid cyst. AJNR Am J Neuroradiol. 22(10):1970-2, 2001
7. Calabro F et al: Rupture of spinal dermoid tumors with spread of fatty droplets in the CSF pathways. Neuroradiol. 42: 572-9, 2000
8. Martinez-Lage JF et al: Extradural dermoid tumours of the posterior fossa. Arch Dis Child. 77(5):427-30, 1997
9. Higashi S et al: Occipital dermal sinus associated with dermoid cyst in the fourth ventricle. AJNR Am J Neuroradiol. 16(4 Suppl):945-8, 1995
10. Poptani H et al: Characterization of intracranial mass lesions with in vivo proton MR spectroscopy. AJNR Am J Neuroradiol. 16(8):1593-603, 1995
11. Smirniotopoulos JG et al: Teratomas, dermoids, and epidermoids of the head and neck. RadioGraphics. 15:1437-55, 1995

DERMOID AND EPIDERMOID CYSTS

IMAGE GALLERY

Typical

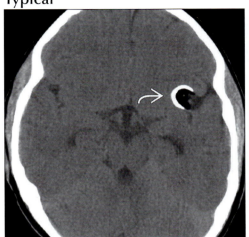
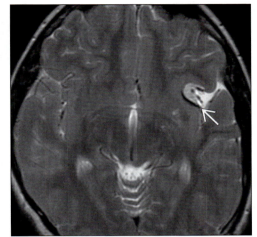

(Left) Axial NECT shows small dermoid cyst of the left sylvian fissure *(arrow)*. Dramatic contrast of smooth calcification and fatty content are a helpful clue to the correct diagnosis. *(Right)* Axial T2WI MR shows chemical shift artifact at posterior margin, along the frequency encoding direction *(arrow)*. Hypointense signal from Ca++ would be expected to continue more anteriorly.

Typical

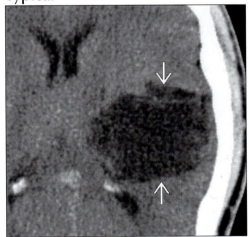
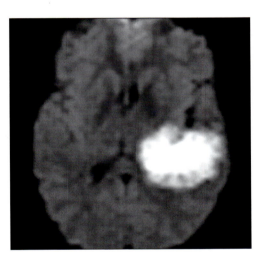

(Left) Axial NECT shows epidermoid in left sylvian fissure *(arrows)*. Note heterogeneous signal compared to CSF in ventricles; lesion margins are also much more irregular than an arachnoid cyst. *(Right)* Axial DWI MR shows restricted diffusion in the same lesion as prominent bright signal. DWI can confidently differentiate between epidermoid and arachnoid cysts.

Typical

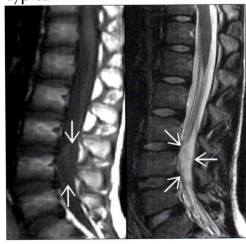
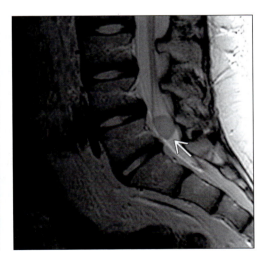

(Left) Sagittal T1WI and T2WI show a dermoid cyst in the lumbar spine *(arrows)*, displacing nerve roots of the cauda equina. Spinal cysts are often less dramatic on imaging than intracranial cysts. *(Right)* Sagittal T2WI MR shows an epidermoid cyst at L5, displacing nerve roots *(arrow)*. To prove causation by prior LP would require negative imaging before or shortly after the original procedure.

PILOCYTIC ASTROCYTOMA

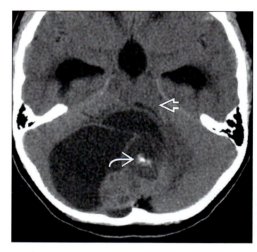

Axial NECT shows cystic and solid right cerebellar mass compressing the 4th ventricle (open arrow). Calcification (curved arrow) is seen in 20% of pilocytic astrocytomas.

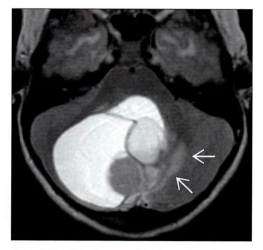

Axial T2WI MR in the same child shows clear distinction between cystic and solid components. Despite the large size, the tumor incites very little vasogenic edema (arrows).

TERMINOLOGY

Abbreviations and Synonyms
- Pilocytic astrocytoma (PA), juvenile pilocytic astrocytoma (JPA)
- "Spongioblastoma polare" ⇒ archaic

Definitions
- Pilocytic astrocytoma = typically well-circumscribed tumor, often cystic, slow growing
- Characterized by Rosenthal fibers and/or eosinophilic granular bodies at microscopy

IMAGING FINDINGS

General Features
- Best diagnostic clue
  ○ Cystic cerebellar mass with enhancing mural nodule
  ○ Enlarged optic nerve/chiasm/tract with variable enhancement
- Location: Cerebellum (60%) > optic nerve/chiasm (25-30%) > adjacent to 3rd ventricle > brainstem
- Size
  ○ Cerebellar lesions are large (> 3 cm)
  ○ Optic nerve lesions typically smaller
- Morphology
  ○ Overall morphology often determined by cystic component
  ○ Optic nerve tumors elongate and widen nerve, causing buckling in orbit: "Dotted i"

CT Findings
- NECT
  ○ Mixed cystic/solid mass
  ○ Often has little surrounding edema
  ○ Solid component hypo- to isodense to gray matter (GM)
  ○ Ca++ 20%, hemorrhage rare
  ○ Often causes obstructive hydrocephalus
    ▪ May be a greater clinical management problem than tumor itself
- CECT
  ○ > 95% enhance (patterns vary)
    ▪ 50% nonenhancing cyst, strongly enhancing mural nodule
    ▪ 40% solid with necrotic center, heterogeneous enhancement
    ▪ 10% solid, homogeneous
    ▪ Cyst may accumulate contrast on delayed images

MR Findings
- T1WI
  ○ Solid portions iso/hypointense to GM
  ○ Cyst contents iso- to slightly hyperintense to cerebrospinal fluid (CSF)

DDx: Optic Nerve Enhancement In Children

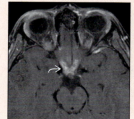
Sarcoidosis

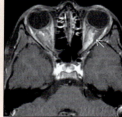
Optic Neuritis (MS)

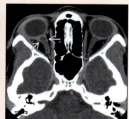
Orbital Pseudotumor

PILOCYTIC ASTROCYTOMA

Key Facts

Terminology
- Pilocytic astrocytoma (PA), juvenile pilocytic astrocytoma (JPA)

Imaging Findings
- Cystic cerebellar mass with enhancing mural nodule
- Enlarged optic nerve/chiasm/tract with variable enhancement
- Paradoxical finding: MRS does not accurately reflect clinical behavior of tumor

Top Differential Diagnoses
- Medulloblastoma (PNET-MB)
- Ependymoma
- Optic neuritis in acute multiple sclerosis (MS), acute disseminated encephalomyelitis, pseudotumor, or sarcoid can mimic optic nerve glioma

Pathology
- 15% of NF1 patients develop PAs, most commonly in optic pathway
- Up to 1/3 of patients with optic pathway PAs have NF1
- Most common primary brain tumor in children

Clinical Issues
- Peak incidence: 5-15 years of age
- Older than children with medulloblastoma

Diagnostic Checklist
- Differentiate cerebellar lesions from medulloblastoma
- Medulloblastoma arises from vermis and fills/expands 4th ventricle
- PA arises from hemisphere, compresses 4th ventricle
- Aggressive appearance of tumor is misleading

- T2WI
  - Solid portions hyperintense to GM
  - Cyst contents iso- to slightly hyperintense to CSF
- FLAIR
  - Solid portions hyperintense to GM
  - Cyst contents do not suppress: Hyperintense to CSF
  - Margins of chiasmatic/hypothalamic tumors in patients with NF1 difficult to resolve
    - May blend into nonspecific signal abnormalities of NF1
- T1 C+
  - Intense but heterogeneous enhancement of solid portion
  - Cyst wall occasionally enhances
  - Rare: Leptomeningeal metastases
- MRS
  - Aggressive-appearing metabolite pattern
    - High choline, low NAA, high lactate
  - Paradoxical finding: MRS does not accurately reflect clinical behavior of tumor

Ultrasonographic Findings
- Grayscale Ultrasound
  - Solid components are hyperechoic relative to brain parenchyma
  - Cysts may contain debris

Angiographic Findings
- Conventional
  - Avascular mass
    - Occasional neovascularity seen in solid portion

Nuclear Medicine Findings
- PET
  - 18F-fluorodeoxyglucose (FDG) studies show increased tumor metabolism
  - Paradoxical finding: PET does not accurately reflect historical behavior of tumor

Imaging Recommendations
- Best imaging tool: Contrast-enhanced MR
- Protocol advice
  - Multiplanar or 3D volume post contrast imaging key to showing point of origin and degree of extension
  - MRS pattern is contradictory to clinical behavior
- Small residual tumor on post-operative studies may not negatively impact prognosis

DIFFERENTIAL DIAGNOSIS

Medulloblastoma (PNET-MB)
- Hyperdense enhancing midline mass fills 4th ventricle
- Younger patient age (2-6 years)

Ependymoma
- "Plastic" tumor, extends out 4th ventricle foramina
- Ca++, cysts, hemorrhage common; heterogeneous enhancement

Pilomyxoid astrocytoma
- Chiasmatic/hypothalamic tumor in infants
- Solid and enhancing
- More likely to disseminate, more aggressive

Atypical teratoid-rhabdoid tumor
- Large mass with cyst or necrosis
- Variable enhancement pattern
- PNET-MB mimic

Ganglioglioma
- Solid/cystic, cortically-based enhancing mass
- Ca++ common

Dysembryoplastic neuroepithelial tumor (DNET)
- Cortical lesion
- May remodel overlying skull

Pleomorphic xanthoastrocytoma (PXA)
- Enhancing nodule abuts pia
- May remodel overlying skull

Hemangioblastoma
- Large cyst with small enhancing mural nodule
- Adult tumor

PILOCYTIC ASTROCYTOMA

- Associated with von Hippel Lindau disease

Demyelination/inflammation
- Optic neuritis in acute multiple sclerosis (MS), acute disseminated encephalomyelitis, pseudotumor, or sarcoid can mimic optic nerve glioma
- Will not cause "dotted i" sign

PATHOLOGY

General Features
- General path comments: Gross appearance and clinical impact varies with location
- Genetics
  - Syndromic: Association with neurofibromatosis (NF1)
    - 15% of NF1 patients develop PAs, most commonly in optic pathway
    - Up to 1/3 of patients with optic pathway PAs have NF1
  - Sporadic: No definite loss of tumor suppressor gene identified
- Etiology: Astrocytic precursor cell
- Epidemiology
  - Most common primary brain tumor in children
    - Close to 25% of total
  - Analysis often divides into subtypes based on location
- Associated abnormalities
  - Major source of morbidity in NF1
  - Frequently causes obstructive hydrocephalus

Gross Pathologic & Surgical Features
- Well-circumscribed, soft, gray mass +/- cyst

Microscopic Features
- Classic "biphasic" pattern of two astrocyte populations
  - Compacted bipolar cells with Rosenthal fibers
    - Rosenthal fibers = electron dense glial fibrillary acidic protein (GFAP) staining cytoplasmic inclusions
  - Loose-textured multipolar cells with microcysts, eosinophilic granular bodies
- MIB-1 (histological marker of cellular proliferation) = 0-3.9% (mean 1.1%)
- May infiltrate into parenchyma
- Rare development of malignant features
  - Some association with prior radiation therapy

Staging, Grading or Classification Criteria
- WHO grade I

CLINICAL ISSUES

Presentation
- Most common signs/symptoms
  - Headache, nausea and vomiting
  - Visual loss (optic pathway lesions)
  - Ataxia, cerebellar signs (cerebellar lesions)
  - Cranial nerve palsies, diplopia
- Other signs/symptoms
  - "Middle-aged" child, 5-15 years old
  - Prolonged duration of symptoms on close inquiry: Months to years

Demographics
- Age
  - > 80% under 20 y
  - Peak incidence: 5-15 years of age
    - Older than children with medulloblastoma
- Gender: M = F

Natural History & Prognosis
- Slowly growing
  - Mass effect tolerated due to accommodation
  - Rarely involute without treatment or after partial resection or biopsy
- Tumor may spread through subarachnoid space in rare cases (but is still WHO grade I)
- > 94% survival at 10 years

Treatment
- Cerebellar or hemispheric: Resection
  - Adjuvant chemotherapy or radiation only if residual progressive unresectable tumor
- Opticochiasmatic/hypothalamic: Often none
  - Stable or slowly progressive tumors watched
  - Debulking or palliative surgery considered after vision loss
  - Radiation or chemotherapy for rapidly progressive disease

DIAGNOSTIC CHECKLIST

Consider
- May rarely present with subarachnoid metastatic disease or as a hemorrhagic mass

Image Interpretation Pearls
- Differentiate cerebellar lesions from medulloblastoma
  - Medulloblastoma arises from vermis and fills/expands 4th ventricle
  - PA arises from hemisphere, compresses 4th ventricle
- Aggressive appearance of tumor is misleading
  - An enhancing intra-axial tumor with cystic change in a "middle-age" child is more likely to be PA than anything else

SELECTED REFERENCES

1. Koeller KK et al: From the archives of the AFIP: pilocytic astrocytoma: radiologic-pathologic correlation. Radiographics. 24(6):1693-708, 2004
2. Arslanoglu A et al: MR imaging characteristics of pilomyxoid astrocytomas. AJNR Am J Neuroradiol. 24(9):1906-8, 2003
3. Bernaerts A et al: Juvenile pilocytic astrocytoma. JBR-BTR. 86(3):142-3, 2003
4. Fernandez C et al: Pilocytic astrocytomas in children: prognostic factors--a retrospective study of 80 cases. Neurosurgery. 53(3):544-53; discussion 554-5, 2003
5. Hwang JH et al: Proton MR spectroscopic characteristics of pediatric pilocytic astrocytomas. AJNR. 19:535-540, 1998
6. Kaschten B et al: Preoperative evaluation of 54 gliomas by PET with fluorine-18-fluorodeoxyglucose and/or carbon-11-methionine. J Nucl Med. 39(5):778-85, 1998

PILOCYTIC ASTROCYTOMA

IMAGE GALLERY

Typical

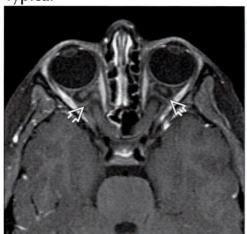
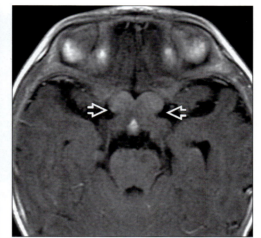

(Left) Axial T1 C+ MR with fat-saturation shows characteristic "dotted i" appearance of intra-orbital optic nerves (arrows), caused by buckling of the elongated nerve proximal to the globe. *(Right)* Axial T1 C+ MR shows marked enlargement and mild enhancement of the optic chiasm (arrows) in a 4 month old. Not all optic pathway gliomas are pilocytic, but the vast majority are.

Typical

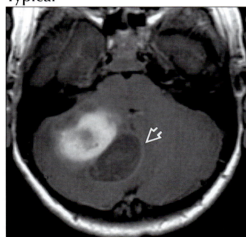
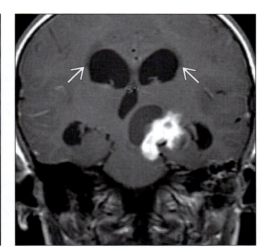

(Left) Axial T1 C+ MR shows characteristic "cyst with mural nodule" appearance of cerebellar pilocytic astrocytoma. Note the fluid in the cyst (arrow) is hyperintense relative to CSF. *(Right)* Coronal T1 C+ MR shows classic-appearing PA centered in the cerebral peduncle. Mass effect on the aqueduct is causing obstructive hydrocephalus with transependymal edema (arrows).

Variant

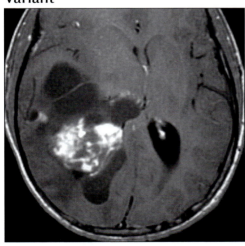
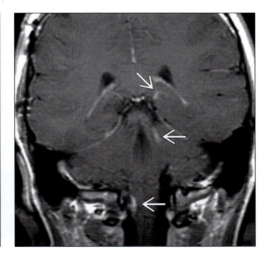

(Left) Axial T1 C+ MR in a teenager shows a large parietal lobe pilocytic astrocytoma. Although the most common type of pediatric brain tumor, it is unusual to see PA in the cerebral hemisphere. *(Right)* Coronal T1 C+ MR shows 3 enhancing metastases (arrows) from a pilocytic astrocytoma of the temporal lobe. < 5% of PAs will have subarachnoid spread of tumor.

MEDULLOBLASTOMA

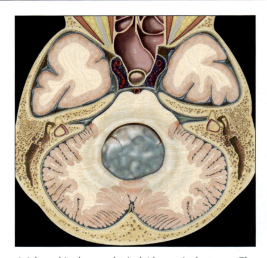

Axial graphic shows spherical 4th ventricular tumor. The homogeneous appearance of PNET-MB at both pathology and imaging reflects the lack of differentiation of the tumor cells.

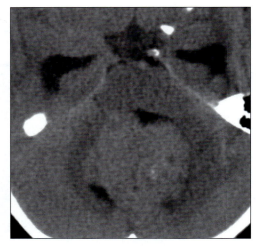

Axial NECT shows a hyperdense 4th ventricular mass that is higher in attenuation than brain parenchyma. The scant cytoplasm of PNET-MB at histology results in a greater density on CT.

TERMINOLOGY

Abbreviations and Synonyms
- Medulloblastoma (MB), posterior fossa PNET, PNET-MB

Definitions
- Malignant, invasive, highly cellular embryonal tumor

IMAGING FINDINGS

General Features
- Best diagnostic clue: Round, dense, 4th ventricle mass
- Location
  - 4th ventricle tumor, arises from roof (superior medullary velum)
    - Distinguished from ependymoma which typically arises from floor of 4th ventricle
  - Lateral origin (cerebellar hemisphere) more common in older children and adults
    - May indicate desmoplastic sub-type
- Size: 1-3 cm
- Morphology: Spherical, pushes brain away on all sides

Radiographic Findings
- Radiography: Hyperdense bone metastases may occur late in disease course (rare)

CT Findings
- NECT
  - Solid mass in 4th ventricle (V)
    - 90% hyperdense
    - Ca++ in up to 20%; hemorrhage rare
    - Small intratumoral cysts/necrosis in 40-50%
  - Hydrocephalus common (95%)
- CECT
  - > 90% enhance
    - Relatively homogeneous
    - Occasionally patchy (may fill in slowly)

MR Findings
- T1WI: Hypointense to gray matter (GM)
- T2WI: Near GM signal intensity
- PD/Intermediate: Hyperintense to GM
- FLAIR
  - Hyperintense to brain
  - Good differentiation of tumor from CSF in 4th V
- DWI: Restricted diffusion
- T1 C+
  - > 90% enhance
  - Often heterogeneous
  - Contrast essential to detect CSF dissemination
    - Linear icing-like enhancement over brain surface: "Zuckerguss"
    - Extensive "grape-like" tumor nodules less common
  - Contrast-enhanced MR of spine (entire neuraxis)

DDx: 4th Ventricular Masses In Children

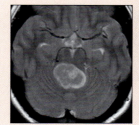

Ependymoma

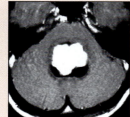

CPP

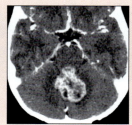

AT/RhT

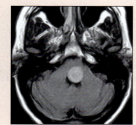

Brainstem Glioma

MEDULLOBLASTOMA

Key Facts

Terminology
- Medulloblastoma (MB), posterior fossa PNET, PNET-MB
- Malignant, invasive, highly cellular embryonal tumor

Imaging Findings
- 4th ventricle tumor, arises from roof (superior medullary velum)
- > 90% enhance
- Contrast essential to detect CSF dissemination
- Up to a third have subarachnoid metastatic disease at presentation

Top Differential Diagnoses
- Cerebellar pilocytic astrocytoma (PA)
- Ependymoma

Pathology
- 15-20% of all pediatric brain tumors
- 30-40% of posterior fossa tumors in children
- WHO grade IV

Clinical Issues
- Ataxia, signs of increased intracranial pressure
- Relatively short (< 1 month) duration of symptoms
- Most diagnosed by 5 years
- Rapid growth with early subarachnoid spread
- Surgical excision, adjuvant chemotherapy

Diagnostic Checklist
- Remember AT/RhT in patients under 3 years
- 4th V tumor arising from roof = PNET-MB
- 4th V tumor arising from floor = ependymoma

- Up to a third have subarachnoid metastatic disease at presentation
- Image pre-op to avoid false (+) post-op: Blood in spinal canal may mimic or mask metastases
- MRS
  - ↓↓ NAA
  - ↑↑ Choline
  - Lactate usually present

Angiographic Findings
- Conventional: Avascular or hypovascular posterior fossa mass

Non-Vascular Interventions
- Myelography
  - May be helpful in identifying "drop" mets
  - Largely replaced by spinal MR with contrast

Nuclear Medicine Findings
- PET
  - Increased uptake on FDG PET
    - Negative correlation with survival

Imaging Recommendations
- Best imaging tool: Contrast-enhanced MR
- Protocol advice
  - Sagittal images pre- and post-contrast to show site of origin (roof vs. floor)
  - Quality of spine MR better if performed as a separate exam

DIFFERENTIAL DIAGNOSIS

Cerebellar pilocytic astrocytoma (PA)
- Older children
- Hemispheric lesion
- Cyst with enhancing nodule

Ependymoma
- Older children
- More heterogeneous, Ca++ and hemorrhage more common
- Extension through 4th V foramina/foramen magnum: "Plastic tumor"

Choroid plexus papilloma (CPP)
- Much less common in 4th V
- Vigorous and homogeneous enhancement
- Less mass effect

Atypical teratoid/rhabdoid tumor (AT/RhT)
- Indistinguishable by imaging
- Younger children

Dorsally exophytic brainstem glioma
- Use MR to show origin from brainstem

PATHOLOGY

General Features
- General path comments
  - Most common posterior fossa tumor in children
  - Four major PNET-MB subtypes recognized
    - Classic
    - Desmoplastic
    - Extensively nodular with advanced neuronal differentiation
    - Large cell
- Genetics
  - "Patched-1" and "smoothened" genes implicated in tumor development
  - Neoplasm and germline mutations (isochromosomes 17q, p53)
  - Sonic hedgehog (SHH) activation in desmoplastic MB
- Etiology
  - Two cell lines suspected as source
    - Cell rests of posterior medullary velum (roof of 4th V)
    - External granular layer of cerebellum
- Epidemiology
  - 15-20% of all pediatric brain tumors
  - 30-40% of posterior fossa tumors in children
  - Rare in adults

MEDULLOBLASTOMA

- Associated abnormalities
  - Association with familial cancer syndromes
    - Gorlin (nevoid basal cell carcinoma) syndrome
    - Li-Fraumeni syndrome
    - Turcot syndrome
    - Gardner syndrome
    - Cowden syndrome
  - Also associated with Taybi and Coffin-Siris syndromes

Gross Pathologic & Surgical Features
- Firm/discrete to soft/less well-defined

Microscopic Features
- Densely packed hyperchromatic cells with scanty cytoplasm
- Frequent mitoses
- Anaplasia 24%
- Neuronal/neuroblastic differentiation manifests as pale islands or Homer-Wright rosettes
  - Homer Wright rosette = central stellate zone of fibrillar processes coming from tumor cells
  - Neuronal/neuroblastic differentiation often causes nodular growth pattern
- Desmoplastic subtype has abundant connective tissue between tumor cells
- Immunohistochemistry: +/- Synaptophysin, vimentin
  - Some have glial differentiation (+ GFAP staining)

Staging, Grading or Classification Criteria
- WHO grade IV

CLINICAL ISSUES

Presentation
- Most common signs/symptoms
  - Ataxia, signs of increased intracranial pressure
  - Macrocephaly in infants with open sutures
- Other signs/symptoms
  - Relatively short (< 1 month) duration of symptoms
  - Symptoms reflect local mass effect and/or increased ICP
    - Nausea and vomiting
    - Ataxia
    - Cranial nerve palsies (less common than in brainstem astrocytomas)

Demographics
- Age
  - 75% < 10 years
  - Most diagnosed by 5 years
- Gender: M > F = 2-4:1

Natural History & Prognosis
- Rapid growth with early subarachnoid spread
- Initial positive response to treatment reflects high mitotic activity
- "Standard risk" clinical profile
  - No metastases or gross residual tumor s/p resection
  - With ERBB-2 tumor protein negative = high 5 year survival rate (100%)
  - With ERBB-2 tumor protein positive = low 5 year survival rate (54%)
- "High risk" clinical profile
  - 5 year survival rate is ≈ 20%
  - Gross residual tumor after surgery
  - Documented metastatic disease
- Adult presentation slightly better outcome
  - May reflect greater resectability of lateral lesions, desmoplastic variant

Treatment
- Surgical excision, adjuvant chemotherapy
- Craniospinal irradiation if > 3 years
- Complications of treatment
  - Endocrinopathy, growth failure
  - Leukoencephalopathy
  - Mineralizing microangiopathy
  - Hearing loss

DIAGNOSTIC CHECKLIST

Consider
- Remember AT/RhT in patients under 3 years
- Pre-operative evaluation of entire neuraxis and post-operative evaluation of surgical bed are keys to prognosis

Image Interpretation Pearls
- 4th V tumor arising from roof = PNET-MB
- 4th V tumor arising from floor = ependymoma

SELECTED REFERENCES

1. Chojnacka M et al: Medulloblastoma in childhood: Impact of radiation technique upon the outcome of treatment. Pediatr Blood Cancer. 42(2):155-60, 2004
2. Gajjar A et al: Clinical, histopathologic, and molecular markers of prognosis: toward a new disease risk stratification system for medulloblastoma. J Clin Oncol. 22(6):984-93, 2004
3. Gururangan S et al: [18F]Fluorodeoxyglucose-Positron Emission Tomography in Patients with Medulloblastoma. Neurosurgery. 55(6):1280-9, 2004
4. Ray A et al: A clinicobiological model predicting survival in medulloblastoma. Clin Cancer Res. 10(22):7613-20, 2004
5. Suresh TN et al: Medulloblastoma with extensive nodularity: a variant occurring in the very young-clinicopathological and immunohistochemical study of four cases. Childs Nerv Syst. 20(1):55-60, 2004
6. Eberhart CG et al: Anaplasia and grading in medulloblastoma. Brain Pathol. 13:376-85, 2003
7. Koeller K et al: Medulloblastoma: a comprehensive review with radiologic-pathologic correlation. RadioGraphics 23:1613-37, 2003
8. Pramanik P et al: A comparative study of classical vs. desmoplastic medulloblastomas. Neurol India. 51(1):27-34, 2003
9. Sarkar C et al: Are childhood and adult medulloblastomas different? A comparative study of clinicopathological features, proliferation index and apoptotic index. J Neurooncol. 59(1):49-61, 2002
10. Huber H et al: Angiogenic profile of childhood primitive neuroectodermal brain tumours/medulloblastomas. Eur J Cancer. 37(16):2064-72, 2001
11. Meyers SP et al: Postoperative evaluation for disseminated medulloblastoma involving the spine. Am J Neuroradiol. 21:1757-65, 2000

MEDULLOBLASTOMA

IMAGE GALLERY

Typical

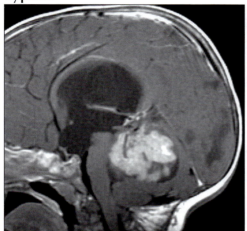
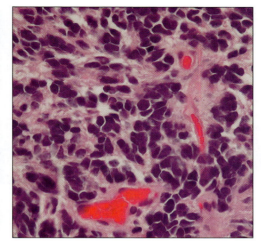

(Left) Sagittal T1 C+ MR shows a diffusely enhancing tumor projecting into the fourth ventricle from the superior medullary velum, a growth pattern typical of PNET-MB. *(Right)* Micropathology, high power shows typical "sheets of round blue cells" seen in PNET-MB. The high nucleus to cytoplasm ratio accounts for high density on CT and blue monotony on H & E stain.

Variant

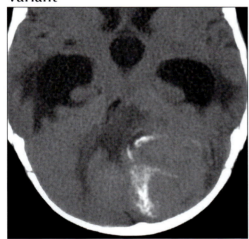
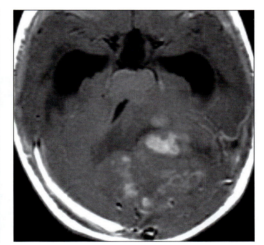

(Left) Axial NECT shows a Ca++ mass in the cerebellar hemisphere, with mass effect on the 4th ventricle. This is a desmoplastic medulloblastoma, a variant that often has atypical imaging features. *(Right)* Axial T1 C+ MR of the same tumor shows a more heterogeneous pattern of enhancement than typically seen in PNET-MB. The desmoplastic sub-type appears to have a better long-term prognosis.

Typical

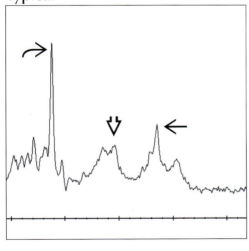
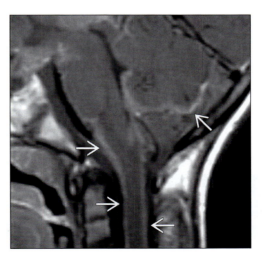

(Left) MRS shows the high-grade spectrum characteristically seen in medulloblastoma, with markedly elevated Choline (curved arrow), reduced NAA (open arrow), and elevated lactate (arrow). *(Right)* Sagittal T1 C+ MR shows characteristic icing-like enhancement (arrows) over the pial surface: "Zuckerguss".

EPENDYMOMA

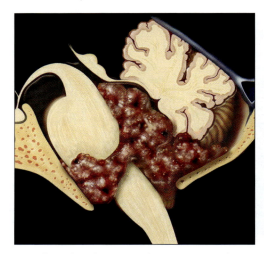

Sagittal graphic shows ependymoma as a red mass growing out of fourth ventricle foramina. Although usually low-grade, difficult surgical resection decreases 5 year survival rates.

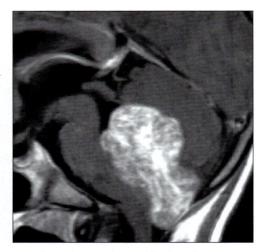

Sagittal T1 C+ MR shows diffusely enhancing mass obstructing 4th V. Interface with the floor of the ventricle is less distinct than with the roof, typical of ependymoma as opposed to PNET-MB.

TERMINOLOGY

Abbreviations and Synonyms
- Ependymoma
- Subtypes: Cellular, myxopapillary, subependymoma

Definitions
- Slow-growing tumor of ependymal cells

IMAGING FINDINGS

General Features
- Best diagnostic clue
  - Heterogeneous signal
  - Soft or "plastic" tumor: Squeezes out through 4th ventricle foramina into cisterns
  - Indistinct interface with floor of 4th ventricle
- Location
  - Intracranial
    - 2/3rd infratentorial, 4th ventricle (V)
    - 1/3rd supratentorial, majority periventricular white matter
  - Spinal
    - Much less common in children
    - Myxopapillary: Filum terminale, conus, cauda equina
    - Cellular: Cervical cord > thoracic cord > conus
- Size
  - Intracranial: 2-4 cm
  - Spinal: 2-4 segments
- Morphology
  - Irregular shape in posterior fossa
    - Accommodates to shape of ventricle or cisterns
  - Spherical in cerebral hemisphere
  - Well-circumscribed in spinal cord and filum

Radiographic Findings
- Radiography: Spinal tumors may cause canal widening or vertebral scalloping
- Myelography
  - May be helpful in showing "drop" mets from intracranial tumors
    - Largely replaced by contrast-enhanced MR
  - Intramedullary tumors demonstrate fusiform cord enlargement
  - Conus lesions have cauda equina nerve roots draped around mass

CT Findings
- NECT
  - Ca++ common (50%); +/- cysts, hemorrhage
  - Hydrocephalus common with 4th V tumors
  - Supratentorial typically large heterogeneous periventricular mass
- CECT
  - Variable heterogeneous enhancement

DDx: Pediatric Posterior Fossa Masses

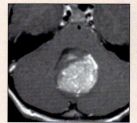
Medulloblastoma

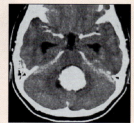
CPP

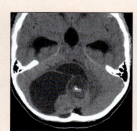
Pilocytic Astrocytoma

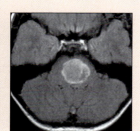
Pontine Glioma

EPENDYMOMA

Key Facts

Terminology
- Slow-growing tumor of ependymal cells

Imaging Findings
- Soft or "plastic" tumor: Squeezes out through 4th ventricle foramina into cisterns
- 2/3rd infratentorial, 4th ventricle (V)
- 1/3rd supratentorial, majority periventricular white matter
- Ca++ common (50%); +/- cysts, hemorrhage
- High quality sagittal imaging can distinguish point of origin as floor vs. roof of 4th ventricle

Top Differential Diagnoses
- Medulloblastoma (PNET-MB)
- Cerebellar pilocytic astrocytoma (PA)

Pathology
- Third most common posterior fossa tumor in children (after PA and PNET-MB)
- 20-30% of intramedullary spinal tumors in children

Clinical Issues
- Usually older than medulloblastoma
- Gross total resection + XRT correlates with improved survival

Diagnostic Checklist
- Surveillance imaging to detect asymptomatic recurrence can increase survival
- Indistinct interface with floor of 4th ventricle = ependymoma
- Indistinct interface with roof of 4th ventricle = PNET-MB

- Myxopapillary tumors enhance vigorously

MR Findings
- T1WI
  - Heterogeneous, usually iso- to hypointense
  - Cystic foci slightly hyperintense to cerebrospinal fluid (CSF)
  - Hyperintense Ca++, blood products
  - Spinal tumor isointense to hypointense with cord
- T2WI
  - Heterogeneous, usually iso- to hyperintense
  - Hyperintense cystic foci
  - Hypointense Ca++, blood products
  - Spinal tumors hyperintense to cord
    - Often have rim of hypointense signal from hemosiderin: "Cap sign"
    - Often have associated syrinx
- FLAIR
  - Can show sharp interface between tumor and CSF
  - Tumor cysts very hyperintense to CSF
- T2* GRE: "Blooming" of hypointense Ca++ foci
- DWI: May see hyperintensity (rare)
- T1 C+
  - Mild to moderate, heterogeneous enhancement
  - Spinal tumors typically have intense enhancement
- MRS
  - NAA ↓, Cho ↑
    - NAA: Cho ratio higher than in PNET-MB
  - Lactate ↑
  - MR spectroscopy alone does not reliably differentiate ependymoma from astrocytoma or PNET-MB

Nuclear Medicine Findings
- PET
  - Increased 18F-fluorodeoxyglucose (FDG) uptake
  - May help differentiate recurrent tumor from radiation necrosis

Imaging Recommendations
- Best imaging tool: MR with contrast
- Protocol advice
  - MR with contrast, CT, MRS before surgery

- Need a combination of imaging & clinical findings to distinguish from PNET-MB
- High quality sagittal imaging can distinguish point of origin as floor vs. roof of 4th ventricle

DIFFERENTIAL DIAGNOSIS

Medulloblastoma (PNET-MB)
- Hyperdense homogeneous mass on NECT
- Arises from roof of 4th ventricle
  - More distinct interface with floor

Cerebellar pilocytic astrocytoma (PA)
- Cyst with mural nodule
- Solid portion enhances vigorously

Brainstem glioma
- Infiltrating mass expanding brainstem
- May project into 4th ventricle

Choroid plexus papilloma (CPP)
- 4th ventricle location more common in adults

Oligodendroglioma
- Heterogeneous supratentorial mass with Ca++ in young adults

Spinal cord astrocytoma
- More common in children than ependymoma
- Less well-defined

Spinal cord hemangioblastoma
- Associated with von Hippel-Lindau syndrome (VHL)

Spinal cord cavernous malformation
- Minimal enhancement

PATHOLOGY

General Features
- General path comments
  - 4 subtypes encountered in brain

EPENDYMOMA

- Cellular: Most common type in 4th ventricle and in spinal cord
- Papillary: Extensive epithelial surface
- Clear-cell: Microscopic features of oligodendroglioma
- Tanycytic: Elongated cells resembling pilocytic astrocytoma
  - Myxopapillary ependymoma nearly exclusive to filum terminale
- Genetics
  - Intracranial tumors associated with aberrations on chromosomes 1q, 6q, 9, 13, 16, 17, 19, 20, 22
  - Spinal lesions associated with chromosome 7, 22 abnormalities
    - Chromosome 22 abnormalities associated with neurofibromatosis 2 (NF2) (multiple spinal ependymomas)
- Etiology
  - Arise from ependymal cells or ependymal rests
    - Periventricular ependymal rests account for supratentorial tumors
- Epidemiology
  - 15% of posterior fossa tumors in children
    - Third most common posterior fossa tumor in children (after PA and PNET-MB)
  - 20-30% of intramedullary spinal tumors in children
- Associated abnormalities
  - Spinal ependymoma known component of NF2
  - Myxopapillary tumors associated with superficial siderosis

Gross Pathologic & Surgical Features
- Well demarcated soft, lobulated, grayish-red mass
- +/- Cysts, necrosis, hemorrhage
- Extrudes through 4th V outlet foramina

Microscopic Features
- Ependymoma
  - Perivascular pseudorosettes
  - Moderately cellular with low mitotic activity and occasional nuclear atypia
  - Immunohistochemistry: S-100, glial fibrillary acidic protein (GFAP), vimentin +
- Anaplastic ependymoma
  - High cellularity, nuclear atypia, hyperchromatism
  - Occasional pseudopalisading or necrosis in most malignant lesions

Staging, Grading or Classification Criteria
- Standard cellular type: WHO grade II
- Anaplastic: WHO grade III
- Subependymoma: WHO grade I
- Myxopapillary: WHO grade I

CLINICAL ISSUES

Presentation
- Most common signs/symptoms
  - Brain: Headache, nausea, vomiting
  - Spine: Back pain, radiculopathy
- Other signs/symptoms
  - Ataxia, hemiparesis, visual disturbances, neck pain, torticollis, dizziness
  - Infants: Irritability, lethargy, developmental delay, vomiting, macrocephaly

Demographics
- Age
  - Usually older than medulloblastoma
    - Peak at 1-5 years, but many cases in adolescents
  - Spinal tumors much more common in adults
- Gender: Slight male predominance

Natural History & Prognosis
- 3-17% CSF dissemination
- Overall 5 year survival for brain lesions: 60-70%
  - Worse with ↑ grade
- 5 year survival for cellular spinal cord tumors: 85%
- Excellent prognosis with complete resection for myxopapillary type

Treatment
- Surgical resection is key element of treatment
  - +/- Chemo, radiation therapy (XRT)
  - Gross total resection + XRT correlates with improved survival
  - 5 year survival after recurrence = 15%
- Surgical resection of 4th V tumors often difficult due to adherence and infiltrating nature

DIAGNOSTIC CHECKLIST

Consider
- Much less common than PNET-MB or PA
- Gross total resection has greater impact on survival than in PNET-MB or PA
- Surveillance imaging to detect asymptomatic recurrence can increase survival

Image Interpretation Pearls
- Indistinct interface with floor of 4th ventricle = ependymoma
- Indistinct interface with roof of 4th ventricle = PNET-MB

SELECTED REFERENCES

1. Jaing TH et al: Multivariate analysis of clinical prognostic factors in children with intracranial ependymomas. J Neurooncol. 68(3):255-61, 2004
2. Korshunov A et al: Gene expression patterns in ependymomas correlate with tumor location, grade, and patient age. Am J Pathol. 163(5):1721-7, 2003
3. Good CD et al: Surveillance neuroimaging in childhood intracranial ependymoma: how effective, how often, and for how long? J Neurosurg. 94(1):27-32, 2001
4. Akyuz C et al: Intracranial ependymomas in childhood--a retrospective review of sixty-two children. Acta Oncol. 39(1):97-100, 2000
5. Merchant TE et al: Pediatric low-grade and ependymal spinal cord tumors. Pediatr Neurosurg. 32(1):30-6, 2000
6. Palma L et al: The importance of surgery in supratentorial ependymomas. Long-term survival in a series of 23 cases. Childs Nerv Syst. 16(3):170-5, 2000
7. Lonjon M et al: Intramedullary spinal cord ependymomas in children: treatment, results and follow-up. Pediatr Neurosurg. 29(4):178-83, 1998

EPENDYMOMA

IMAGE GALLERY

Typical

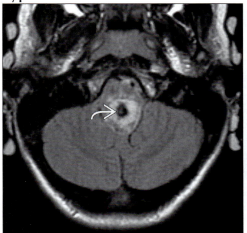
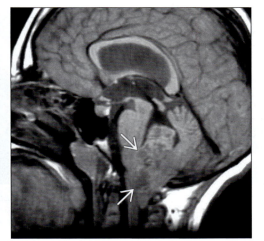

(Left) Axial FLAIR MR shows central hypointensity in this 4th ventricle ependymoma (arrow), caused by calcification within the tumor. 50% of intracranial ependymomas have Ca++. *(Right)* Sagittal T1WI MR shows typical pattern of growth of posterior fossa ependymoma, with tumor projecting up into the 4th ventricle from its origin on the dorsal brainstem (arrows).

Typical

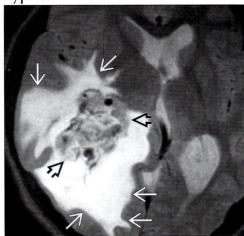
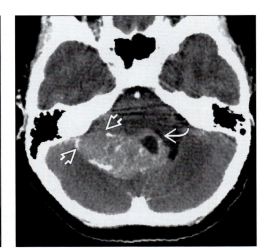

(Left) Axial T2WI MR shows a heterogeneous parietal lobe mass (open arrows) with extensive surrounding edema (arrows) in this 17 year old. Supratentorial ependymomas are usually quite large at diagnosis. *(Right)* Axial CECT shows an irregular shaped enhancing tumor with Ca++ and a cyst (curved arrow) that extends from the 4th ventricle into the right cerebellopontine angle cistern (open arrows).

Variant

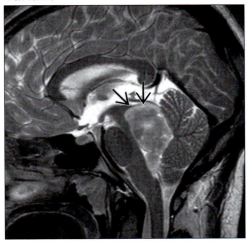
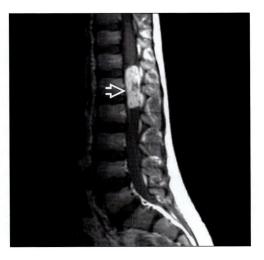

(Left) Sagittal T2WI MR shows an exophytic subependymoma projecting dorsally off the back of the tectum (arrows) into the superior 4th ventricle, an appearance more typical of exophytic glioma. *(Right)* Sagittal T1 C+ MR in an 11 year old shows brightly enhancing and slightly lobulated myxopapillary ependymoma (arrow) of the filum terminale, a subtype almost exclusively seen in adults.

BRAINSTEM GLIOMA

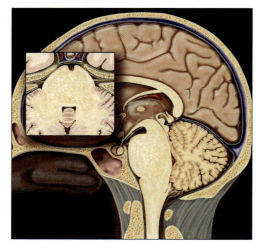

Sagittal graphic with axial insert shows diffuse enlargement of the pons typical of brainstem glioma. Insert shows the infiltrating tumor narrowing the fourth ventricle without obstruction.

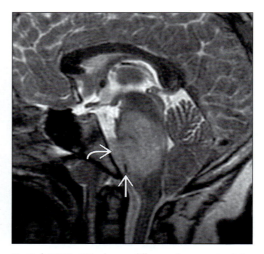

Sagittal T2WI MR shows diffuse enlargement of the pons caused by a glioma. Note exophytic component (curved arrow) that extends anterior to basilar artery (arrow).

TERMINOLOGY

Abbreviations and Synonyms
- Brainstem glioma (BSG), pontine glioma, diffuse pontine glioma (DPG), midbrain glioma

Definitions
- Infiltrating fibrillary astrocytoma of the pons and brainstem
  - Share many clinical features with thalamic gliomas
- Distinct from well-defined pilocytic astrocytomas (PA)
  - PA more likely to be exophytic
  - PA more likely to be centered at cervico-medullary junction
  - PA has considerably better prognosis than brainstem glioma
- Distinct from benign-behaving tectal gliomas
  - Tectal gliomas are rarely progressive lesions
  - Tectal gliomas present with hydrocephalus in 6-10 year olds
  - Shunting is often only treatment required

IMAGING FINDINGS

General Features
- Best diagnostic clue: Expansion of pons with abnormal signal on MR
- Location
  - Ponto-medullary junction to cerebral peduncles
    - Exclusive of tectal plate
- Size: Typically large, encompassing entire pons
- Morphology
  - Infiltrating tumor accommodates to pontine morphology
    - Sometimes exophytic

CT Findings
- NECT
  - Decreased attenuation and enlargement of pons
  - Flattening of anterior border of 4th ventricle
    - Streak artifact from petrous pyramids can hamper detection
- CECT: Mild to absent enhancement

MR Findings
- T1WI
  - Mildly to moderately hypo-intense
  - Central areas of preserved signal may reflect preserved white matter (WM) tracts
- T2WI
  - Bright signal, slightly heterogeneous
  - Edema vs. infiltrating tumor
  - Exophytic component can engulf basilar artery, vertebral arteries
- FLAIR
  - High signal

DDx: Infiltrating Brainstem Lesions In Children

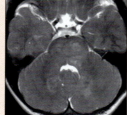
NF1

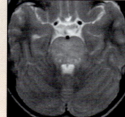
Encephalitis

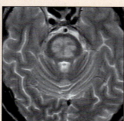
Osmotic DM

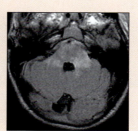
HLH

BRAINSTEM GLIOMA

Key Facts

Terminology
- Infiltrating fibrillary astrocytoma of the pons and brainstem
- Distinct from well-defined pilocytic astrocytomas (PA)
- Distinct from benign-behaving tectal gliomas

Imaging Findings
- Best diagnostic clue: Expansion of pons with abnormal signal on MR
- Exophytic component can engulf basilar artery, vertebral arteries
- Foci of restricted diffusion may reflect necrosis or higher grade
- Enhancement at presentation ⇒ worse prognosis
- Include sagittal T2 and/or FLAIR images

Top Differential Diagnoses
- Brainstem encephalitis, rhombencephalitis
- Acute disseminated encephalomyelitis (ADEM)
- Neurofibromatosis type 1 (NF1)
- Osmotic demyelination (osmotic DM)

Pathology
- ≈ 15% of pediatric brain tumors

Clinical Issues
- Age: Peak incidence ≈ 3-10 years old
- Median survival ≈ 1 yr

Diagnostic Checklist
- Flattening of floor of 4th ventricle on CT ⇒ proceed to MR with contrast

---

    - Sometimes better defined than on T2WI
- DWI
  - Most infiltrating gliomas do not have restricted diffusion
    - Hampers distinction of tumor from surrounding edema
  - Foci of restricted diffusion may reflect necrosis or higher grade
  - Diffusion tractography (DTI) can show displacement of white matter tracts by tumor
    - Caveat ⇒ infiltrating BSG can have some central preservation of white matter tracts
- T1 C+
  - Variable enhancement, usually minimal
  - Enhancement at presentation ⇒ worse prognosis
  - Development of enhancement during treatment ⇒ response to therapy?
    - Remember that decrease in enhancement during therapy may reflect effects of steroids on blood-brain barrier only; not necessarily a decrease in tumor burden
  - Exophytic component often enhances
- MRA: Basilar artery engulfed by tumor but not typically narrowed
- MRS
  - Preservation of NAA may indicate less aggressive course
  - Elevated choline: NAA ratio typically implies more aggressive tumor
  - Presence of lactate implies necrosis

Imaging Recommendations
- Best imaging tool: MRI with contrast
- Protocol advice
  - Include sagittal T2 and/or FLAIR images
  - Consider use of DTI, but be cautious with conclusions

DIFFERENTIAL DIAGNOSIS

Brainstem encephalitis, rhombencephalitis
- Listeria monocytogenes often implicated
  - Viral agents ⇒ West Nile virus, adenovirus, Epstein-Barr
- More acute clinical course
  - Often more ill at presentation
  - More dramatic onset of symptoms
- Febrile

Acute disseminated encephalomyelitis (ADEM)
- Will usually have other sites of demyelination
  - Supratentorial, spinal cord (transverse myelitis)
- Delayed onset after viral prodrome or vaccination

Neurofibromatosis type 1 (NF1)
- Asymptomatic poorly defined foci of bright signal on T2WI
- Increase in early childhood and diminish as adolescence approaches
- Dentate nuclei involvement more common than pons
  - Globus pallidus very frequently affected
- Occasionally expansile ⇒ cannot exclude glioma
  - Glioma in NF1 may progress more slowly

Osmotic demyelination (osmotic DM)
- Pontine myelinolysis
- Associated with rapid correction of hyponatremia
- Preservation of descending pyramidal tracts ⇒ "trident configuration"

Histiocytosis
- Langerhans cell histiocytosis (LCH)
- Hemophagocytic lymphohistiocytosis (HLH)
- May cause signal abnormalities in pons and cerebellum
  - Cerebellar hemisphere involvement more typical
- Often associated with other sites of disease

Presumed hamartoma
- Rare cases of asymptomatic lesions resembling pontine glioma on MR
  - Presumed diagnosis of BSG
  - No progression despite lack of treatment
  - May regress over time

CRANIOPHARYNGIOMA

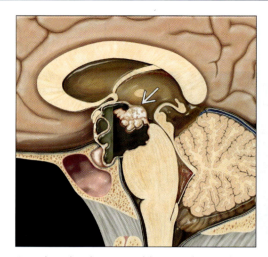

Sagittal graphic shows typical features of a mixed intra- and suprasellar craniopharyngioma, with a nodule of solid tissue (arrow) in the wall of a complex cyst that projects into the sella.

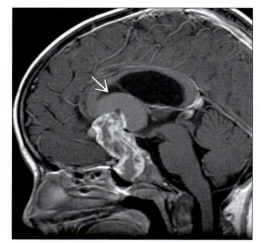

Sagittal T1 C+ MR shows a markedly heterogeneous craniopharyngioma projecting out of the sella turcica into the anterior third ventricle. Arrow points to non-enhancing cystic component.

TERMINOLOGY

Abbreviations and Synonyms
- Craniopharyngioma (CrP), craniopharyngeal duct tumor, Rathke pouch tumor, adamantinoma

Definitions
- Histologically benign epithelial tumor arising from squamous rests along involuted hypophyseal-Rathke duct

IMAGING FINDINGS

General Features
- Best diagnostic clue: Cystic suprasellar mass with calcifications and enhancing mural nodule or cyst wall
- Location
  - Suprasellar ⇒ 75%
  - Mixed suprasellar + intrasellar ⇒ 21%
  - Intrasellar ⇒ 4%
  - Larger tumors can extend into multiple cranial fossae
    - The term "monstrous craniopharyngioma" has been proposed for these
  - Rare ectopic locations
    - Third ventricle, nasopharynx, sphenoid sinus
  - Distinction of retro-chiasmatic versus pre-chiasmatic key for surgical approach
- Size
  - Often large at presentation (> 5 cm)
    - Cyst is typically largest component
- Morphology: Complex cystic mass, often lobulated

Radiographic Findings
- Skull radiographs
  - Sellar enlargement, erosion of clinoids
  - Suprasellar calcifications (Ca++)

CT Findings
- Ninety percent rule
  - 90% are cystic
  - 90% have calcifications
  - 90% enhance (wall and solid portions)
- May present with obstructive hydrocephalus from compression on 3rd ventricle and foramen of Monro

MR Findings
- T1WI
  - Cyst contents hyperintense to cerebrospinal fluid (CSF)
    - Often very bright ⇒ reflects protein, cholesterol, and/or blood products in fluid
  - Solid component heterogeneous
- T2WI
  - Solid component heterogeneous

DDx: Sellar-Parasellar Masses In Children

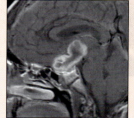

Chiasm Glioma

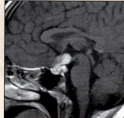

Germinoma

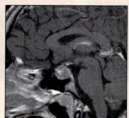

Pituitary Adenoma

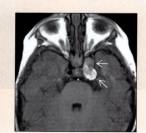

Aneurysm

CRANIOPHARYNGIOMA

Key Facts

Terminology
- Histologically benign epithelial tumor arising from squamous rests along involuted hypophyseal-Rathke duct

Imaging Findings
- Best diagnostic clue: Cystic suprasellar mass with calcifications and enhancing mural nodule or cyst wall
- 90% are cystic
- 90% have calcifications
- 90% enhance (wall and solid portions)
- Most vessels displaced by cysts
- Circle of Willis vessels encased by solid components
- Rarely narrowed
- Important to identify displacement of chiasm

Top Differential Diagnoses
- Rathke cleft cyst (RCC)
- Germinoma, brain
- Arachnoid cyst

Pathology
- Two clinically and pathologically distinct subtypes
- Adamantinous ⇒ classic calcified cyst with mural nodule seen in children
- Squamous-papillary ⇒ mostly solid tumor almost exclusively found in adults
- Most common non-glial pediatric intracranial tumor

Clinical Issues
- Recurrence much more frequent with adamantinous histology than with papillary
- Treatment associated with high rate of morbidity

- Hypointensity from Ca++, blood products, cholesterol
  - ± Hyperintense signal in adjacent brain
    - Tumor invasion, reactive gliosis/edema
- FLAIR: Cyst contents typically hyperintense
- T2* GRE: Ca++ components markedly hypointense
- DWI: Variable depending upon the character of cyst fluid
- T1 C+
  - Solid portions enhance heterogeneously
  - Cyst wall enhances
- MRA
  - Most vessels displaced by cysts
  - Circle of Willis vessels encased by solid components
    - Rarely narrowed
- MRS: Cyst contents show broad lipid spectrum at 0.9-1.5 ppm

Imaging Recommendations
- Best imaging tool: Thin sagittal and coronal T1 C+ MR
- Protocol advice
  - Contrast enhanced MR, with thin post-contrast sagittal and coronal imaging
  - MRA to aid in surgical planning
  - Important to identify displacement of chiasm

DIFFERENTIAL DIAGNOSIS

Rathke cleft cyst (RCC)
- Not calcified, generally non-enhancing
- No solid component
- Cyst more homogeneous

Pituitary adenoma
- Solid tumor that is isointense with brain, enhances strongly
- Cystic adenomas very rare in children

Germinoma, brain
- Solid components larger than cystic
- Associated with diabetes insipidus

Hypothalamic-chiasmatic glioma
- More solid and homogeneous
- Extension into prechiasmatic optic nerves, optic tracts/radiations
- Infiltrate/enlarge chiasm instead of displacing it

Arachnoid cyst
- Thin/imperceptible wall
- Cyst contents follow CSF

Dermoid and epidermoid cysts
- Epidermoids are solid lesions that mimic cysts
- Suprasellar lesions are rare in children
- Minimal enhancement

Aneurysm
- "Onion-skin" layers of aging blood products
- Bright enhancement of residual lumen

PATHOLOGY

General Features
- General path comments
  - Two clinically and pathologically distinct subtypes
    - Adamantinous ⇒ classic calcified cyst with mural nodule seen in children
    - Squamous-papillary ⇒ mostly solid tumor almost exclusively found in adults
    - 15% of tumors have mixed histology ⇒ behave like adamantinous
- Etiology
  - Arise from rests of epithelial cells
  - Two proposed sites of origin
    - In the pars tuberalis at the distal aspect of infundibulum
    - Along tract of involuted craniopharyngeal duct
- Epidemiology
  - Most common non-glial pediatric intracranial tumor
  - 6 to 9% of all pediatric intracranial tumors
  - 0.5 to 2.5 new cases per million per year
  - Comprise over half of all pediatric suprasellar region tumors

CRANIOPHARYNGIOMA

- Second peak of incidence in 5th-7th decade
  - Squamous-papillary subtype
- Embryology
  - Rathke pouch (hypophyseal duct) is an invagination of the primitive stomatodeum
  - Rathke pouch forms the pars tuberalis and adenohypophysis

Gross Pathologic & Surgical Features
- Cyst fluid is usually straw-colored and thick ⇒ "crankcase oil"
- Adamantinous
  - Mixed cystic and solid tumor
  - Cysts >> solid components
- Papillary
  - Solid >> cysts
- Epithelial fronds invade adjacent structures, hampering resection

Microscopic Features
- Adamantinous
  - Cyst walls of simple stratified squamous epithelium, with a collagenous basement membrane
  - Peripheral cellular palisading and stellate reticulum
  - Nodules of "wet" keratin
  - Dystrophic Ca++
- Papillary
  - Formation of papillae
  - Ca++ or necrotic debris rare

Staging, Grading or Classification Criteria
- Both adamantinous and squamous-papillary are WHO Grade I

CLINICAL ISSUES

Presentation
- Most common signs/symptoms
  - Headache, vomiting
  - Hydrocephalus and papilledema
  - Visual disturbance (bitemporal hemianopsia), decline in school performance
- Other signs/symptoms
  - Hormonally-mediated symptoms in at least 1/3 of cases
    - Due to mass effect on pituitary/hypothalamus
    - Growth hormone deficiency, hypothyroidism, diabetes insipidus

Demographics
- Age
  - Peak at 8-12 years
    - Peak for squamous-papillary at 40-60 years
- Gender: M = F

Natural History & Prognosis
- Slow-growing and benign tumor
- High rate of recurrence
  - 20% recurrence rate if < 5 cm
  - 83% recurrence rate if > 5 cm
  - Can recur up to 30 years after resection
  - Occasional ectopic sites of recurrence
- 64-96% overall 10-year survival
- Recurrence much more frequent with adamantinous histology than with papillary

Treatment
- Surgical
  - Gross total resection
    - Limited by tumor size, adherence to vessels and hypothalamus
  - Limited resection
    - Radiation therapy
    - Intracavitary radiation
- Treatment associated with high rate of morbidity
  - Peri-operative hyperthermia
  - Vascular injury and pseudoaneurysm
  - Hypopituitarism
  - Long-term hypothalamic syndrome
    - Morbid obesity from compulsive eating

DIAGNOSTIC CHECKLIST

Consider
- Rathke cleft cyst can be identical to small CrP
  - RCC has no Ca++ and is more homogeneous
  - Use NECT to identify Ca++ in CrP
- Be sure to identify displacement of chiasm for surgical planning

SELECTED REFERENCES

1. Chakrabarti I et al: Long-term neurological, visual, and endocrine outcomes following transnasal resection of craniopharyngioma. J Neurosurg. 102(4):650-7, 2005
2. Karavitaki N et al: Craniopharyngiomas in children and adults: systematic analysis of 121 cases with long-term follow-up. Clin Endocrinol (Oxf). 62(4):397-409, 2005
3. Ullrich NJ et al: Craniopharyngioma therapy: long-term effects on hypothalamic function. Neurologist. 11(1):55-60, 2005
4. Tavangar SM et al: Craniopharyngioma: a clinicopathological study of 141 cases. Endocr Pathol. 15(4):339-44, 2004
5. Sartoretti-Schefer S et al: MR differentiation of adamantinous and squamous-papillary craniopharyngiomas. AJNR Am J Neuroradiol. 18(1):77-87, 1997
6. Sutton LN et al: Proton spectroscopy of suprasellar tumors in pediatric patients. Neurosurgery. 41(2):388-94; discussion 394-5, 1997
7. Eldevik OP et al: Craniopharyngioma: radiologic and histologic findings and recurrence. AJNR Am J Neuroradiol. 17(8):1427-39, 1996

CRANIOPHARYNGIOMA

IMAGE GALLERY

Typical

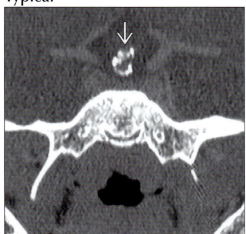
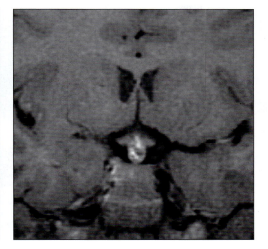

(Left) Coronal CECT shows an incidentally discovered suprasellar craniopharyngioma. This calcified lesion (arrow) was identified on a CT performed for peri-orbital cellulitis. *(Right)* Coronal T1WI MR in the same child shows the entirely suprasellar location of the tumor, impinging on the inferior aspect of the chiasm. Location relative to chiasm is a key factor in determining surgical approach.

Variant

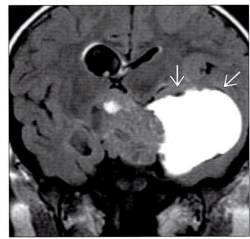
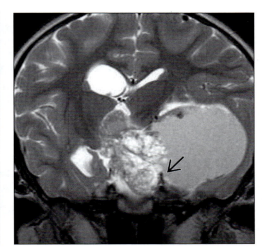

(Left) Coronal FLAIR MR shows a suprasellar CrP with a large cyst projecting into the left middle cranial fossa (arrows). CrP cyst contents are almost always hyperintense on FLAIR images. *(Right)* Coronal T2WI MR in the same child. Note encasement of internal carotid artery (arrow). The term "monstrous" CrP has been proposed for tumors that project into multiple cranial fossae.

Typical

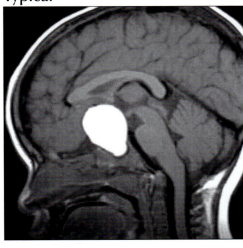
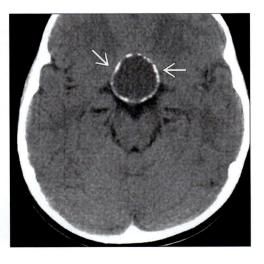

(Left) Sagittal T1WI MR shows hyperintense cyst contents in this simple intra- and suprasellar adamantinous CrP. Cyst contents are frequently, but not invariably, hyperintense on T1WI. *(Right)* Axial NECT in the same child shows typical calcifications in the cyst wall (arrows). The adamantinous subtype is found in children; > 90% have identifiable calcifications on imaging.

GERMINOMA, BRAIN

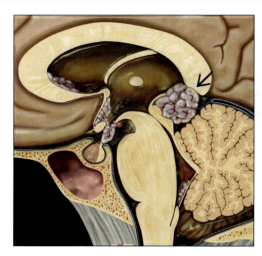

Sagittal graphic shows pineal region germinoma (arrow) with subarachnoid spread of tumor to hypothalamus, anterior 3rd ventricle, frontal horn, and 4th ventricle.

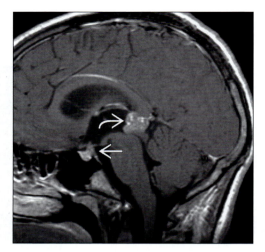

Sagittal T1 C+ MR shows avidly enhancing mass (curved arrow) protruding into 3rd ventricle from the pineal region. Second focus of tumor can be seen in the hypothalamus (arrow).

TERMINOLOGY

Abbreviations and Synonyms
- Dysgerminoma, extra-gonadal seminoma, formerly called atypical teratoma

Definitions
- Tumor of primordial germs cells, essentially identical to seminoma or dysgerminoma in the gonads or mediastinum

IMAGING FINDINGS

General Features
- Best diagnostic clue
  - Suprasellar mass with diabetes insipidus (DI)
  - Pineal region mass that "engulfs" the pineal gland
- Location
  - Central nervous system (CNS) germinomas have a propensity to hug the midline near the 3rd ventricle
    - Suprasellar ~ 50-60%
    - Pineal region ~ 30-40%
  - Large thalamic or basal ganglia tumors uncommon in children
- Size
  - 1-3 cm
  - Relatively small pineal region germinoma may present with ventricular obstruction
  - Tiny or inapparent suprasellar germinoma may cause DI
- Morphology: Often well-delineated, lobular

Radiographic Findings
- Radiography
  - Pineal Ca++ on skull radiographs before age 10?
    - Not a useful sign in CT era
    - Physiologic pineal Ca++ reported in children younger than 6
    - If no associated mass, pineal Ca++ of doubtful significance

CT Findings
- NECT
  - Sharply circumscribed dense mass (hyperdense to gray matter)
    - Drapes around posterior 3rd ventricle or "engulfs" pineal gland
    - Suprasellar mass without calcifications or dominant cysts
- CECT
  - Avid enhancement
  - Enhancing subarachnoid metastases

MR Findings
- T1WI

DDx: Enhancing Suprasellar Masses In Children

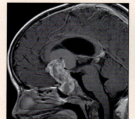
Craniopharyngioma

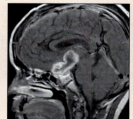
Optic Glioma

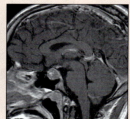
Macroadenoma

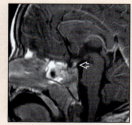
LCH

GERMINOMA, BRAIN

Key Facts

Terminology
- Tumor of primordial germs cells, essentially identical to seminoma or dysgerminoma in the gonads or mediastinum

Imaging Findings
- Central nervous system (CNS) germinomas have a propensity to hug the midline near the 3rd ventricle
- Suprasellar ~ 50-60%
- Pineal region ~ 30-40%
- Avid enhancement
- Often "speckled"

Top Differential Diagnoses
- Craniopharyngioma
- Hypothalamic/chiasmatic astrocytoma
- Other germ cell tumors (nongerminomatous germ cell tumors, NGGCTs)
- Pineoblastoma (pineal PNET)

Clinical Issues
- DI can be present for an extended period prior to MR abnormalities
- Germinomas are most commonly seen in adolescents
- Intracranial NGGCTs are more common in younger children
- Very radiosensitive

Diagnostic Checklist
- Child or adolescent with DI
- Expect absence of posterior pituitary bright spot
- Repeat MR imaging with contrast in 3-6 months in children with DI and no identified lesion

---

  - Isointense or hyperintense to GM
  - Absent posterior pituitary bright spot in children with DI
    - No tumor may be apparent at presentation
- T2WI
  - Iso- to hyperintense to GM
  - Hyperintense cystic or necrotic foci
    - Hypointense foci from blood or Ca++ rare
- FLAIR: Hyperintense to GM
- DWI: Restricted diffusion
- T1 C+
  - Avid enhancement
    - Often "speckled"
  - Enhancing subarachnoid metastases
- MRS: ↑ Choline, ↓ NAA, ± lactate

Imaging Recommendations
- Best imaging tool: Enhanced MR of brain and spine
- Protocol advice
  - MR evaluation of entire neuraxis before surgery
  - Negative MR exam in a child with DI does not exclude germinoma
    - Repeat study in 3-6 months to assess for growing suprasellar tumor

DIFFERENTIAL DIAGNOSIS

Craniopharyngioma
- Cystic, solid, and Ca++ components

Hypothalamic/chiasmatic astrocytoma
- Rarely associated with DI

Langerhans cell histiocytosis (LCH)
- Thickened infundibulum
- Small enhancing lesion

Pituitary macroadenoma
- Unlikely to cause DI

Hypothalamic hamartoma
- Isointense to GM
- No enhancement

Other germ cell tumors (nongerminomatous germ cell tumors, NGGCTs)
- Malignant mixed germ cell, teratoma (mature, immature), yolk sac tumor, choriocarcinoma, embryonal carcinoma
  - Heterogeneous, Ca++, fat, hemorrhage

Pineoblastoma (pineal PNET)
- Mass "explodes" rather than "engulfs" pineal Ca++
  - Less helpful finding in pediatrics
  - Many children develop tumors well before developing physiologic pineal Ca++

Pineal cyst
- Atypical features (> 1 cm, heterogeneous enhancement, ± tectal compression)
- Repeat imaging in 9-12 months to show stability if no other findings

Tectal astrocytoma
- Little or no enhancement
- Blends into tectal plate

PATHOLOGY

General Features
- General path comments
  - Unencapsulated solid mass, soft and friable, tan-white coloration, ± cystic foci
  - Necrosis, calcification and hemorrhage uncommon
- Genetics
  - Cytogenetics ~ ↑ risk of CNS germ cell neoplasms
    - Extra X chromosome (Klinefelter syndrome)
    - Alterations of chromosomes 1 (1q21-1qter region)
    - Over-representation of chromosome 12 (12p duplication)
    - Other chromosomes: 8q, 13q, 18q, 9q, 11q
  - Molecular genetics ~ ↑ risk of CNS germ cell neoplasms
    - TP53 tumor suppressor gene mutations (exons 5-8)

GERMINOMA, BRAIN

- MDM2 gene amplification
- Etiology
  - Germ cell tumors are found in the gonads, mediastinum, parasellar, and pineal regions
    - Regions where primordial germ cells migrate during embryogenesis
  - Primordial germ cells persist, maldifferentiate into germinoma
- Epidemiology
  - Germinomas ⇒ 3-8% of pediatric CNS tumors
    - 9-15% of CNS tumors in Japanese children
  - Germinomas ⇒ 65-70% of all CNS germ cell tumors (GCTs)
  - Germinomas ~ 40% of pineal region neoplasms
- Associated abnormalities
  - Klinefelter syndrome (47XXY)
  - Down syndrome
  - Neurofibromatosis type I (NF1)
  - Laboratory derangements
    - Elevated placental alkaline phosphatase (PLAP)
    - ± Elevation of serum and cerebrospinal fluid (CSF) human chorionic gonadotropin (HCG)

Gross Pathologic & Surgical Features
- Soft and friable, tan-white mass, ± necrosis

Microscopic Features
- Sheets of large polygonal primitive germ cells
  - Large vesicular nuclei & prominent nucleoli
  - Clear, glycogen-rich cytoplasm (PAS-positive)
- Lymphocytic infiltrates along fibrovascular septa

Staging, Grading or Classification Criteria
- Staging multiple site involvement (pineal, suprasellar, basal ganglia, thalamus) is considered metastatic in USA but synchronous in Canada and Europe

CLINICAL ISSUES

Presentation
- Most common signs/symptoms
  - Suprasellar germinoma
    - Diabetes insipidus
    - Visual loss
    - Hypothalamic-pituitary dysfunction (↓ growth, precocious puberty)
  - Pineal region germinoma
    - Parinaud syndrome (upward gaze paralysis and altered convergence)
    - Headache due to tectal compression and hydrocephalus
    - Precocious puberty or DI (associated with infiltration into 3rd ventricle floor)
- Other signs/symptoms
  - DI can be present for an extended period prior to MR abnormalities
  - DI may be present with germinomas of pineal, suprasellar, or basal ganglia origin

Demographics
- Age
  - Germinomas are most commonly seen in adolescents
    - Peak age: 10-12 years
  - Intracranial NGGCTs are more common in younger children
    - Teratoma is the most common congenital brain tumor
- Gender
  - Pineal region germinoma has strong male predominance
  - Suprasellar germinoma may be slightly more common in females
- Ethnicity
  - CNS GCTs much more prevalent in Asia
    - 9-15% of all CNS tumors in Japan
    - Basal ganglia and thalamic germinomas more common in Japan and Korea

Natural History & Prognosis
- Pure germinoma has favorable prognosis
  - Low secretion of HCG (< 50) ⇒ favorable
  - Very radiosensitive
- Malignant but relatively benign prognosis due to radiation and chemotherapy sensitivity
- CSF dissemination and invasion of adjacent brain common

Treatment
- Biopsy to confirm histology, "pure" germinomas have best outcome
- Radiotherapy +/- adjuvant chemotherapy
- 5 year survival > 90%

DIAGNOSTIC CHECKLIST

Consider
- Child or adolescent with DI
  - Expect absence of posterior pituitary bright spot
  - Thickened and enhancing infundibulum ⇒ LCH or germinoma
  - Lobular enhancing mass ⇒ germinoma
  - No enhancing lesion ⇒ could still be germinoma
- Adolescent with pineal mass ⇒ germinoma
- Child with pineal mass
  - Heterogeneous and complex ⇒ NGGCT or PNET
  - Homogeneous ⇒ germinoma or PNET

Image Interpretation Pearls
- Repeat MR imaging with contrast in 3-6 months in children with DI and no identified lesion

SELECTED REFERENCES

1. Wellons JC 3rd et al: Neuroendoscopic findings in patients with intracranial germinomas correlating with diabetes insipidus. J Neurosurg Spine. 100(5):430-6, 2004
2. Halbauer GE et al: Cytogenetic profile of primary pituitary germinoma. J Neurooncol. 50(3): 251-5, 2000
3. Akyuz C et al: Primary intracranial germ cell tumors in children: a report of eight cases and review of the literature. Turk J Pediatr. 41(2):161-72, 1999
4. Sano K: Pathogenesis of intracranial germ cell tumors reconsidered. J Neurosurg. 90:258-64, 1999
5. Jennings MT et al: Intracranial germ-cell tumors: natural history and pathogenesis. J Neurosurg. 63(2):155-67, 1985

GERMINOMA, BRAIN

IMAGE GALLERY

Typical

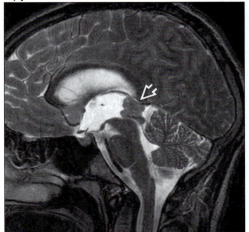
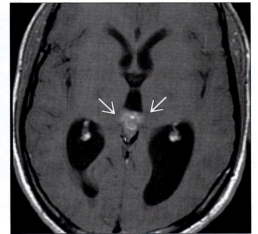

(Left) Sagittal T2WI MR shows germinoma compressing the tectum (arrow), causing expansion of the third and lateral ventricles. Germinoma is the most commonly encountered pineal tumor in children. *(Right)* Axial T1 C+ MR shows moderate and heterogeneous pattern of enhancement of the same tumor (arrows).

Typical

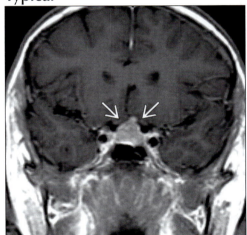
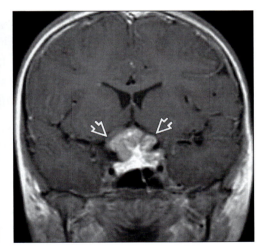

(Left) Coronal T1 C+ MR shows an intrasellar and suprasellar germinoma (arrows), mimicking a macroadenoma. This same boy had a pineal teratoma resected seven years earlier. *(Right)* Coronal T1 C+ MR shows lobular enhancing suprasellar mass (arrows) in a child with diabetes insipidus. The heterogeneous "speckled" pattern of enhancement is commonly seen in germinoma.

Typical

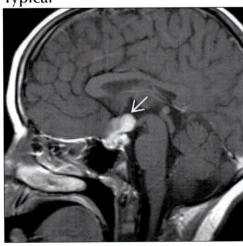
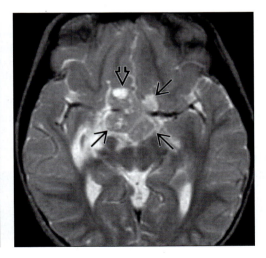

(Left) Sagittal T1 C+ MR shows suprasellar germinoma infiltrating through the hypothalamus into the floor of the third ventricle (arrow), a location allowing biopsy through a ventriculoscope. *(Right)* Axial T2WI MR shows hyperintense germinoma encasing circle of Willis arteries (arrows). Small cysts (open arrow) can be seen in germinoma, but this tumor is usually solid and homogeneous on imaging.

CHOROID PLEXUS PAPILLOMA

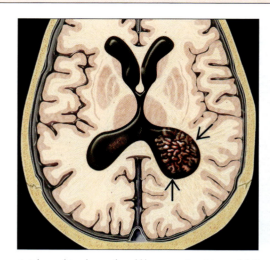 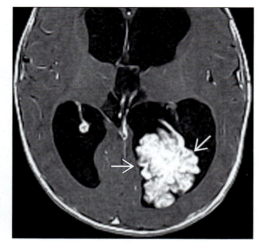

Axial graphic shows frond-like mass in atrium of left lateral ventricle (arrows). In children, choroid plexus tumors are much more common in the lateral ventricles than in the 3rd or 4th ventricles.

Axial T1 C+ MR shows avid enhancement of CPP (arrows). Hydrocephalus can be a result of ventricular obstruction, or from overproduction or decreased resorption of cerebrospinal fluid (CSF).

TERMINOLOGY

Abbreviations and Synonyms
- Choroid plexus papilloma (CPP), choroid plexus tumor (CPT)
- Choroid plexus carcinoma (CPCa)

Definitions
- Intraventricular, papillary neoplasm derived from choroid plexus epithelium

IMAGING FINDINGS

General Features
- Best diagnostic clue: Strongly enhancing, lobulated intraventricular mass
- Location
  - 70% ⇒ atrium of lateral ventricle, left > right
  - 20% ⇒ fourth ventricle
    - Most common site of origin in adults
- Size: Often large at diagnosis
- Morphology: Lobulated fronds, some accommodation to ventricular morphology

CT Findings
- NECT
  - Intraventricular lobular mass
  - 75% iso- or hyper-attenuating
  - 25% have calcification (Ca++)
  - Hydrocephalus
- CECT
  - Intense, homogeneous enhancement
    - Heterogeneous enhancement may suggest CPCa

MR Findings
- T1WI
  - Well-delineated, lobulated mass
  - Iso- to hypointense
- T2WI
  - Iso- to hyperintense
  - ± Internal linear and branching vascular flow voids
  - Large CPP may invade into brain parenchyma
    - Extensive invasion suggests CPCa
  - Hydrocephalus
  - Foci of diminished signal representing Ca++ or hemorrhage
- FLAIR
  - Bright periventricular signal
    - Transependymal interstitial edema due to ventricular obstruction
- T2* GRE: ± Foci of diminished signal if Ca++ and/or blood products are present
- T1 C+
  - Robust homogeneous enhancement
  - Occasional cysts and small foci of necrosis

DDx: Intraventricular Masses In Children

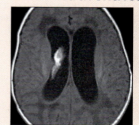 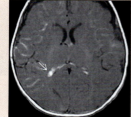 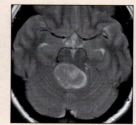 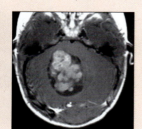

Hematoma | Sturge-Weber | Subependymoma | Medulloblastoma

CHOROID PLEXUS PAPILLOMA

Key Facts

Terminology
- Choroid plexus papilloma (CPP), choroid plexus tumor (CPT)
- Choroid plexus carcinoma (CPCa)
- Intraventricular, papillary neoplasm derived from choroid plexus epithelium

Imaging Findings
- Best diagnostic clue: Strongly enhancing, lobulated intraventricular mass
- 70% ⇒ atrium of lateral ventricle, left > right

Top Differential Diagnoses
- Sturge-Weber
- Medulloblastoma
- Ependymoma

Pathology
- CPP or CPCa may both show invasion into brain parenchyma
- Both may also have subarachnoid spread of tumor
- CPP ⇒ WHO grade I
- CPCa ⇒ WHO grade III-IV

Clinical Issues
- One of the more common brain tumors in children less than 2 years of age
- 86% present by 5 years
- 5 year survival close to 100%

Diagnostic Checklist
- Imaging alone cannot reliably distinguish CPP from CPCa

  - May have subarachnoid spread
    - Scan entire neuraxis
- MRA
  - Flow related signal within mass
  - Enlarged choroidal artery (trigonal mass)
- MRV: Flow related signal
- MRS
  - ↓ NAA, ↑ choline
  - Lactate indicates necrosis ⇒ not necessarily more aggressive

Ultrasonographic Findings
- Grayscale Ultrasound
  - Hyperechoic mass with frond-like projections
  - Echo texture similar to normal choroid plexus

Angiographic Findings
- Conventional
  - Enlarged choroidal artery
  - Prolonged vascular stain
  - Arteriovenous shunting

Nuclear Medicine Findings
- PET: 11C-Methionine ⇒ ↑ tumor-to-normal brain ratios in CPP compared to gliomas

Imaging Recommendations
- Best imaging tool: MRI with contrast
- Protocol advice: Perform contrast-enhanced MR of entire neuraxis before surgery

DIFFERENTIAL DIAGNOSIS

Hematoma
- Intraventricular hemorrhage (IVH) can be a consequence of germinal matrix hemorrhage in the neonate
- Clot adherent to the choroid can be mass-like in appearance

Sturge-Weber
- Enlargement of the choroid glomus ipsilateral to the pial venous malformation

Medulloblastoma
- Most common 4th ventricular neoplasm in a child
- More spherical than CPP

Ependymoma
- Ependymoma and medulloblastoma are more common 4th ventricular masses than CPP
- More heterogeneous than CPP

Xanthogranuloma or xanthoma
- Benign tumor of lipid laden cells in choroid glomus
  - Similar to epidermoid inclusion
- More common in adults
- Unrelated to juvenile xanthogranuloma (histiocytic skin lesion)

Meningioma
- Intraventricular lesions uncommon in children
- Consider NF2

Arteriovenous malformation
- Can present as a ventricular mass or with IVH

Subependymoma
- Adult tumor, rare in children

PATHOLOGY

General Features
- General path comments
  - Well-circumscribed lobulated intraventricular mass
  - CPP or CPCa may both show invasion into brain parenchyma
    - Both may also have subarachnoid spread of tumor
- Genetics
  - Li-Fraumeni and Aicardi syndromes (possible TP53 germline mutation)
  - Association of CPP and duplication of short arm of chromosome 9
- Etiology: DNA sequences from simian virus 40 (SV40), have been found in CPTs
- Epidemiology

CHOROID PLEXUS PAPILLOMA

- 2-4% of all pediatric brain tumors
- CPCa comprise < 20% of choroid plexus tumors
- Associated abnormalities
  - Hydrocephalus
    - Mechanical obstruction
    - CSF overproduction or impaired resorption (due to hemorrhage)

Gross Pathologic & Surgical Features
- Pink or reddish-tan intraventricular mass
- Cauliflower-like surface
- ± Cysts, necrosis, and hemorrhage

Microscopic Features
- CPP
  - Fibrovascular connective tissue fronds, covered by cuboidal or columnar epithelium
  - Mitotic activity, necrosis, and brain invasion typically absent
  - Resembles non-neoplastic choroid plexus
- CPCa
  - Highly cellular
  - Loss of normal architecture
  - High mitotic index and cellular atypia
- Immunohistochemistry
  - Cytokeratin and vimentin are expressed by CPPs
  - S-100 protein in 90% of CPPs
  - Some are positive for GFAP (glial fibrillary acidic protein)

Staging, Grading or Classification Criteria
- CPP ⇒ WHO grade I
- CPCa ⇒ WHO grade III-IV

CLINICAL ISSUES

Presentation
- Most common signs/symptoms
  - Child in first two years of life with signs and symptoms of elevated ICP
    - Focal neurologic signs and symptoms suggests CPCa
- Other signs/symptoms: Macrocrania, bulging fontanelle, vomiting, headache, ataxia, seizure

Demographics
- Age
  - One of the more common brain tumors in children less than 2 years of age
  - 86% present by 5 years
  - CPCa tend to be older at presentation
- Gender
  - CPP: M > F
  - CPCa: M = F

Natural History & Prognosis
- Benign, slowly growing
  - May seed CSF pathways (both CPP & CPCa)
- May become anaplastic over time
  - Reports of benign tumors at first surgery having malignant degeneration at second surgery

Treatment
- Total surgical resection

- 5 year survival close to 100%

DIAGNOSTIC CHECKLIST

Consider
- Although relatively rare, CPP is still most likely enhancing mass in lateral ventricle of a child < 2
- 4th ventricular CPP is much less likely than ependymoma or medulloblastoma

Image Interpretation Pearls
- Imaging alone cannot reliably distinguish CPP from CPCa
  - Final diagnosis is histologic

SELECTED REFERENCES

1. Kumar R et al: Childhood choroid plexus papillomas: operative complications. Childs Nerv Syst. 21(2):138-43, 2005
2. Fujimura M et al: Hydrocephalus due to cerebrospinal fluid overproduction by bilateral choroid plexus papillomas. Childs Nerv Syst. 20(7):485-8, 2004
3. Noguchi A et al: Choroid plexus papilloma of the third ventricle in the fetus. Case illustration. J Neurosurg. 100(2 Suppl Pediatrics):224, 2004
4. Phi JH et al: Temporal lobe epilepsy caused by choroid plexus papilloma in the temporal horn. Clin Neuropathol. 23(3):95-8, 2004
5. Strojan P et al: Choroid plexus tumors: a review of 28-year experience. Neoplasma. 51(4):306-12, 2004
6. D'Ambrosio AL et al: Villous hypertrophy versus choroid plexus papilloma: a case report demonstrating a diagnostic role for the proliferation index. Pediatr Neurosurg. 39(2):91-6, 2003
7. Heese O et al: Diffuse arachnoidal enhancement of a well differentiated choroid plexus papilloma. Acta Neurochir (Wien). 144(7):723-8, 2002
8. Koeller KK et al: From the archives of the AFIP. Cerebral intraventricular neoplasms: radiologic-pathologic correlation. Radiographics. 22(6):1473-505, 2002
9. Murphy M et al: Presentation of a choroid plexus papilloma mimicking an extradural haematoma after a head injury. Childs Nerv Syst. 18(8):457-9, 2002
10. Pianetti Filho G et al: Choroid plexus papilloma and Aicardi syndrome: case report. Arq Neuropsiquiatr. 60(4):1008-10, 2002
11. Sunada I et al: 18F-FDG and 11C-methionine PET in choroid plexus papilloma--report of three cases. Radiat Med. 20(2):97-100, 2002
12. Horska A et al: Proton magnetic resonance spectroscopy of choroid plexus tumors in children. J Magn Reson Imaging. 14(1):78-82, 2001
13. Levy ML et al: Choroid plexus tumors in children: significance of stromal invasion. Neurosurgery. 48(2):303-9, 2001
14. Shin JH et al: Choroid plexus papilloma in the posterior cranial fossa: MR, CT, and angiographic findings. J Clin Imaging. 25: 154-62, 2001
15. Aguzzi A et al: Choroid plexus tumors. In Kleihues P, Cavenee WK (eds): Tumors of the Nervous System, IARC Press, 84-6, 2000
16. Sarkar C et al: Choroid plexus papilloma: a clinicopathological study of 23 cases. Surg Neurol. 52: 37-39, 1999

CHOROID PLEXUS PAPILLOMA

IMAGE GALLERY

Variant

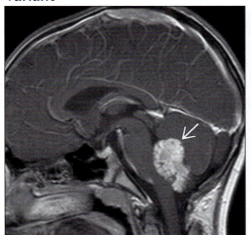
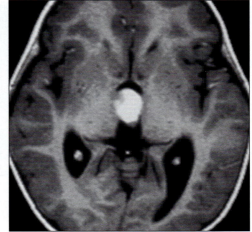

(Left) Sagittal T1 C+ MR shows brightly enhancing 4th ventricle CPP *(arrow)*. This location is more common in adults; in children, medulloblastoma or ependymoma are much more common in the 4th ventricle. *(Right)* Axial T1 C+ MR shows an enhancing CPP in the anterior 3rd ventricle. This is the least common location for choroid plexus tumors.

Typical

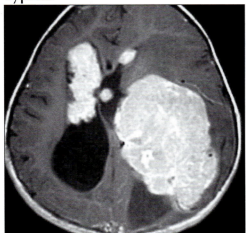
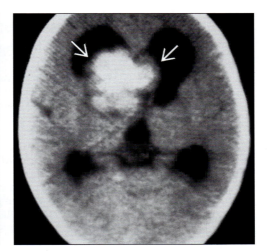

(Left) Axial T1 C+ MR shows multiple enhancing masses in a child with CPCa. Multicentricity and brain invasion are suggestive of the more aggressive histology, but can also be seen in CPP. *(Right)* Axial CECT shows a very unusual frontal horn location of a CPP *(arrows)*. This tumor grew anteriorly out of the foramen of Monro, deviating the septum pellucidum to the left.

Variant

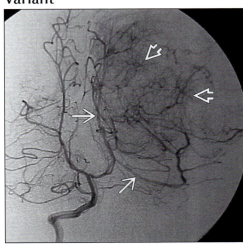
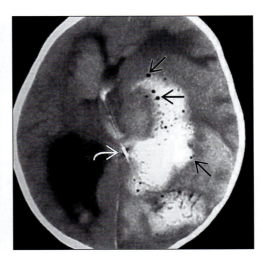

(Left) Anteroposterior catheter angiography shows displacement of posterior cerebral artery branches *(arrows)* and extensive neovascularity *(open arrows)* supplying the left ventricular tumor. *(Right)* Axial NECT after pre-operative embolization shows contrast staining in tumor, with air-density polyvinyl alcohol particles *(arrows)* and streak from platinum coils *(curved arrow)*.

SPINAL CORD ASTROCYTOMA

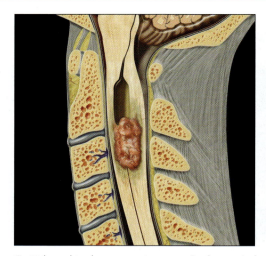

Sagittal graphic shows an astrocytoma in the cervical cord with a cephalad syrinx. Intramedullary cord tumors can cause syrinx in the same manner that brain tumors cause hydrocephalus.

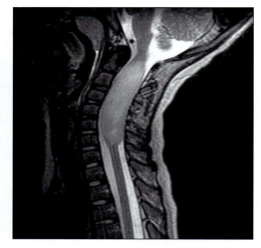

Sagittal T2WI MR shows a hyperintense intramedullary mass expanding the cervical cord in a 5 year old with arm weakness. Homogeneous signal is typical of cord astrocytoma in children.

TERMINOLOGY

Abbreviations and Synonyms
- Spinal glioma, intramedullary glioma

Definitions
- Primary intramedullary neoplasm of spinal cord originating from astrocytes

IMAGING FINDINGS

General Features
- Best diagnostic clue: Enhancing infiltrating cord mass in child
- Location: Cervical > thoracic > lumbar
- Size: Usually 1-3 cm, less than 4 segments
- Morphology: Oblong, fusiform expansion of cord

CT Findings
- NECT
  - Enlargement of cord difficult to appreciate on axial images
    - Obliteration of cerebrospinal fluid (CSF) around cord
  - Sagittal or coronal reformats key
  - Occasional expansion and remodeling of bony canal
    - Medial erosion of pedicles
- CECT: Mild enhancement, may be difficult to appreciate

MR Findings
- T1WI
  - Cord expansion
    - Usually < 4 segments
    - Occasionally multisegmental, even holocord (more common with pilocytic astrocytoma)
  - 40% have tumor cysts or syringohydromyelia
    - Cyst fluid slightly hyperintense to CSF
  - Solid portion hypo/isointense
- T2WI
  - Hyperintense to normal cord
  - Not as hyperintense as cyst/syrinx contents
- T2* GRE: Rarely hemorrhagic
- T1 C+
  - Great majority enhance moderately
  - May aid in differentiating edema from solid tumor
  - Fat-saturation not essential
    - May ease windowing of images by decreasing bright signal from subcutaneous fat

Ultrasonographic Findings
- Grayscale Ultrasound
  - Can be used intraoperatively to delineate extent of tumor
  - Hyperechoic to normal cord

DDx: Intramedullary Spinal Cord Lesions In Children

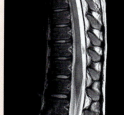
Transverse Myelitis

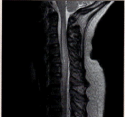
Contusion

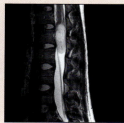
Ependymoma

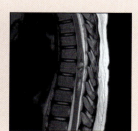
Cavernous Angioma

SPINAL CORD ASTROCYTOMA

Key Facts

Terminology
- Spinal glioma, intramedullary glioma
- Primary intramedullary neoplasm of spinal cord originating from astrocytes

Imaging Findings
- Location: Cervical > thoracic > lumbar
- Morphology: Oblong, fusiform expansion of cord
- 40% have tumor cysts or syringohydromyelia
- Great majority enhance moderately

Top Differential Diagnoses
- Ependymoma
- Less common in children
- Ganglioglioma
- Multiple sclerosis
- Cord contusion

Pathology
- Most common spinal cord tumor in children
- Two histologic sub-types ⇒ pilocytic and fibrillary
- 80-90% low grade

Clinical Issues
- Pain
- Myelopathy
- Survival varies with tumor histology/grade and degree of tumor resection
- Gross total resection is goal in pilocytic and low grade tumors

Diagnostic Checklist
- Remember inflammatory lesions in differential
- Image entire spinal cord

Non-Vascular Interventions
- Myelography: Expanded cord (nonspecific)

Nuclear Medicine Findings
- PET: Increased uptake of [18F]-fluorodeoxyglucose (FDG) or 11C-methionine

Imaging Recommendations
- Best imaging tool: Contrast-enhanced MR
- Protocol advice: Image entire spinal cord

DIFFERENTIAL DIAGNOSIS

Ependymoma
- Less common in children
- Sharply delineated tumor
- Hemorrhage common
  - May present with superficial siderosis

Ganglioglioma
- Similar imaging features
- Comprise up to 30% of cord tumors in children < 3 years

Schwannoma
- Rarely presents as intramedullary mass
- More likely intradural-extramedullary

Paraganglioma
- Cauda equina lesion

Syringohydromyelia
- No enhancement
- No solid component

Multiple sclerosis
- Multiple lesions
- Dorsal aspect of cord

Transverse myelitis
- Acute disseminated encephalomyelitis (ADEM) of cord
- Absent or mild enhancement
- Preceding vaccine or viral prodrome

Cavernous angioma
- Hemorrhagic lesion
- Heterogeneous

Cord infarct
- Rare lesion in children
- Symptoms more acute and severe than astrocytoma

Cord contusion
- History leads to correct diagnosis
- Look for associated disk or ligament injury

PATHOLOGY

General Features
- General path comments
  - Bony canal may be remodeled
    - Implies long-term growth
- Genetics
  - Astrocytoma development associated with abnormalities of chromosome 17p
    - TP53 gene
- Etiology: No specific cause known
- Epidemiology
  - Most common spinal cord tumor in children
    - 30-35% of intraspinal neoplasms in children
    - 60% of primary spinal cord tumors in children
- Associated abnormalities
  - Some increased risk in patients with neurofibromatosis (NF1, NF2)
  - Ependymoma and extramedullary tumors more common in NF2

Gross Pathologic & Surgical Features
- Expanded cord

Microscopic Features
- Two histologic sub-types ⇒ pilocytic and fibrillary
- Pilocytic astrocytoma
  - Rosenthal fibers, glomeruloid/hyalinized vessels
  - Low prevalence of nuclear atypia/mitoses
- Fibrillary astrocytoma

SPINAL CORD ASTROCYTOMA

  - Increased cellularity, variable atypia/mitoses
  - Parenchymal infiltration

Staging, Grading or Classification Criteria
- 80-90% low grade
  - Pilocytic astrocytoma = WHO I
  - Fibrillary astrocytoma = WHO II
- 10-15% high grade
  - Anaplastic astrocytomas = WHO III

CLINICAL ISSUES

Presentation
- Most common signs/symptoms
  - Pain
  - Myelopathy
- Other signs/symptoms
  - Scoliosis
  - Muscle wasting
  - Bony remodeling
  - Lesions at cervical-medullary junction can cause hydrocephalus

Demographics
- Age
  - Typically pre-adolescent, 5-10 years old
  - Small number in infants
- Gender
  - M > F overall 1.3:1
  - No gender difference in children

Natural History & Prognosis
- Most are slow-growing
- Malignant tumors may cause rapid neurologic deterioration
- Survival varies with tumor histology/grade and degree of tumor resection
  - 80% 5 year survival for low grade
  - 30% 5 year survival for high grade
  - 13 month average survival with high grade lesions in children
- Post-operative neurologic function determined largely by degree of preoperative deficit

Treatment
- Obtain tissue diagnosis
- Gross total resection is goal in pilocytic and low grade tumors
  - Definitive treatment for pilocytic tumors
  - Intraoperative evoked potentials helpful
  - Intraoperative ultrasound can show extent of tumor versus syrinx
- Adjuvant therapy
  - No evidence that radiation therapy, chemotherapy improve long-term outcome

DIAGNOSTIC CHECKLIST

Consider
- Remember inflammatory lesions in differential

Image Interpretation Pearls
- Sagittal images are more helpful than axial
- Image entire spinal cord
- Subtotal surgical resection may be unimpressive on imaging
  - Residual lesion "fills in" resection cavity

SELECTED REFERENCES

1. Peraud A et al: Recurrent spinal cord astrocytoma with intraventricular seeding. Childs Nerv Syst. 20(2):114-8, 2004
2. Colby C et al: Rapid deterioration of a newborn with congenital spinal cord astrocytoma. Med Pediatr Oncol. 36(4):500-2, 2001
3. Ng HK et al: Spinal cord pilocytic astrocytoma with cranial meningeal metastases. J Clin Neurosci. 8(4):374-7, 2001
4. Chacko AG et al: Favorable outcome after radical excision of a 'Holocord' astrocytoma. Clin Neurol Neurosurg. 102(4):240-242, 2000
5. Constantini S et al: Radical excision of intramedullary spinal cord tumors: surgical morbidity and long-term follow-up evaluation in 164 children and young adults. J Neurosurg. (Spine 2) 93: 183-93, 2000
6. Houten JK et al: Pediatric intramedullary spinal cord tumors: special considerations. J Neurooncol. 47(3):225-30, 2000
7. Houten JK et al: Spinal cord astrocytomas: presentation, management and outcome. J Neurooncol. 47: 219-4, 2000
8. Merchant TE et al: Pediatric low-grade and ependymal spinal cord tumors. Pediatr Neurosurg. 32(1):30-6, 2000
9. Ng A et al: Congenital spinal astrocytoma: how favourable is the long-term outcome? Br J Neurosurg. 14(4):366-70, 2000
10. Nishio S et al: Spinal cord gliomas: management and outcome with reference to adjuvant therapy. J Clin Neurosci. 7(1):20-3, 2000
11. Wilmshurst JM et al: Positron emission tomography in imaging spinal cord tumors. J Child Neurol. 15(7):465-72, 2000
12. Abdel-Wahab M et al: Prognostic factors and survival in patients with spinal cord gliomas after radiation therapy. Am J Clin Oncol. 22(4):344-51, 1999
13. Kulkarni AV et al: MR characteristics of malignant spinal cord astrocytomas in children. Can J Neurol Sci. 26(4):290-3, 1999
14. Merchant TE et al: High-grade pediatric spinal cord tumors. Pediatr Neurosurg. 30(1):1-5, 1999
15. Bouffet E et al: Prognostic factors in pediatric spinal cord astrocytoma. Cancer. 83(11):2391-9, 1998
16. Lowis SP et al: Chemotherapy for spinal cord astrocytoma: can natural history be modified? Childs Nerv Syst. 14(7):317-21, 1998
17. Yagi T et al: Intramedullary spinal cord tumour associated with neurofibromatosis type 1. Acta Neurochir (Wien). 139(11):1055-60, 1997

SPINAL CORD ASTROCYTOMA

IMAGE GALLERY

Typical

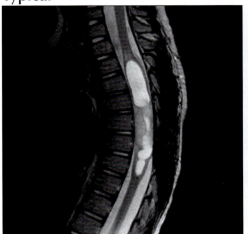 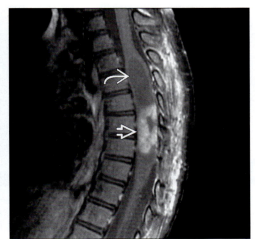

(Left) Sagittal T2WI MR shows a mixed solid and cystic astrocytoma in the thoracic cord of a 5 year old girl. Cord astrocytomas can cause a syrinx or form intrinsic tumor cysts. *(Right)* Sagittal T1 C+ MR in the same child shows irregular enhancement of the mass (open arrow), but not the cyst walls (curved arrow). The cyst was a syrinx, not lined by tumor cells.

Typical

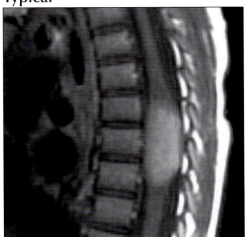 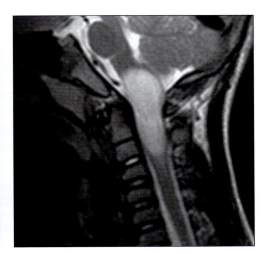

(Left) Sagittal T1 C+ MR in a 2 year old with abdominal pain shows a homogeneously enhancing mass expanding the mid-thoracic spinal cord. Most cord astrocytomas demonstrate enhancement on MR. *(Right)* Sagittal T2WI MR shows hyperintense signal of a cervicomedullary junction astrocytoma in a 7 year old boy with neck pain. Despite the crucial location, these tumors are often mildly symptomatic.

Variant

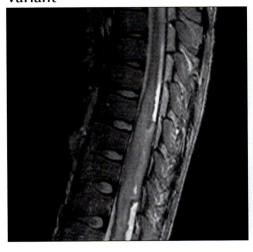 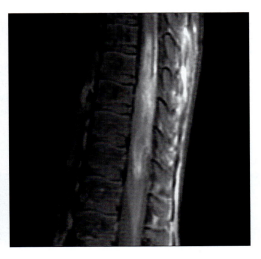

(Left) Sagittal T2WI MR shows a heterogeneous and poorly defined intramedullary tumor with a dorsal exophytic component. This demonstrates an anaplastic astrocytoma. *(Right)* Sagittal T1 C+ MR in the same patient shows the more infiltrative pattern of enhancement that distinguishes this tumor from the more commonly encountered low-grade cord astrocytoma.

GERMINAL MATRIX HEMORRHAGE

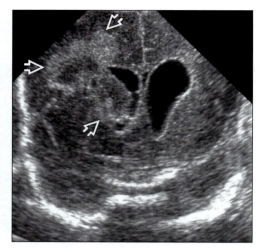

Graphic shows blood in highly vascular germinal matrix, between caudate nucleus and thalamus, extending into occipital horns.

Coronal ultrasound shows mixed echogenicity blood in the right periventricular region (arrows), compressing the frontal horn, in this premature infant with a grade IV bleed.

TERMINOLOGY

Abbreviations and Synonyms
- Germinal matrix hemorrhage (GMH), germinal matrix bleed, preterm caudothalamic hemorrhage, intracranial bleed, germinal matrix-intraventricular hemorrhage (GMH-IVH)

Definitions
- Hemorrhage which occurs in a very specific, richly vascular, but stress sensitive area of the brain in premature infants

IMAGING FINDINGS

General Features
- Best diagnostic clue: Echogenic area in the caudothalamic groove which may extend into the lateral ventricle(s) or periventricular brain parenchyma
- Location
  - Between the caudate nucleus and thalamus
  - Look for extension into ventricular system
- Size: Variable
- Morphology: Echogenic when acute, changing to iso- and hypo- echoic with time

CT Findings
- CT scan preferred over ultrasound when trauma is suspected
- Excellent at detecting intracranial hemorrhage: Parenchymal, subdural, subarachnoid, intraventricular
- CT has higher sensitivity and is more reproducible than ultrasound, but not always feasible

MR Findings
- Usually reserved for infants with complex congenital anomalies who are stable enough to travel to the MR suite
- Germinal matrix has low signal intensity on T2 weighted images, which corresponds to its highly cellular histologic appearance
- Periventricular and subcortical layers of white matter have high signal intensity on T2 weighted images
- Acute hemorrhage has low signal intensity on T2 weighted images
- MR is more sensitive, specific, and reproducible than ultrasound, but is not always practical in critically ill premies

Ultrasonographic Findings
- Grayscale Ultrasound
  - Carefully assess the caudothalamic groove for evidence of blood on both sagittal and coronal images

DDx: Other Neonatal Abnormalities

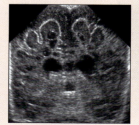
Cystic PVL

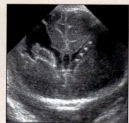
Porencephaly & Shunt

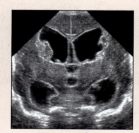
Ventriculitis

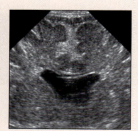
Subarachnoid Heme

GERMINAL MATRIX HEMORRHAGE

Key Facts

Terminology
- Hemorrhage which occurs in a very specific, richly vascular, but stress sensitive area of the brain in premature infants

Imaging Findings
- Best diagnostic clue: Echogenic area in the caudothalamic groove which may extend into the lateral ventricle(s) or periventricular brain parenchyma

Top Differential Diagnoses
- Porencephaly or cystic periventricular leukomalacia
- Choroid plexus cysts or hematoma
- Ventriculitis
- Ischemia or infarction
- Intraventricular hemorrhage

Pathology
- Most GMHs occur in the first week of life
- Related to perinatal stresses: Labile blood pressure, hypoxia, hypercarbia, etc.
- Most common in infants < 32 weeks gestation and < 1500 grams
- Grade I: Confined to the caudothalamic groove
- Grade II: Extends into the ventricle but does not expand it
- Grade III: Fills and distends the adjacent ventricle
- Grade IV: Parenchymal hemorrhage/edema/ischemia beyond the germinal matrix

---

- Acute blood is echogenic, later clot retracts and becomes iso- to hypo- echoic
- Fluid-debris levels may be visible in the ventricles
- Secondary hydrocephalus (communicating) is common
- If hemorrhage extends into the ventricles, chemical ventriculitis ensues in 2-3 days
  - Ependymal lining becomes thick and echogenic
- Examine the rest of the brain for
  - Congenital anomalies
  - Extra-axial fluid collections
  - Ventricular size & symmetry
- Color Doppler
  - Useful to differentiate avascular hematoma from vascular choroid plexus
  - Useful demonstrating bridging veins in the extra-axial spaces, thereby differentiating subdural from subarachnoid location of fluid collections
  - Attempts to use Doppler to predict premies at risk for GMH have not been successful

Imaging Recommendations
- Best imaging tool
  - Ultrasound is ideal
    - High sensitivity and specificity for germinal matrix abnormalities
    - Portability
    - Available sonographic window of anterior fontanelle
    - And lack of ionizing radiation
- Protocol advice: Small footprint, high frequency transducer, using multiple focal zones

DIFFERENTIAL DIAGNOSIS

Porencephaly or cystic periventricular leukomalacia
- Hypo or anechoic spaces reflecting brain parenchymal loss
- Often follows a hypoxic, ischemic event or high grade germinal matrix bleed
- Most common in watershed zone between deep and superficial vessels
- Can occur in utero or perinatally
- Often bilateral but asymmetric

Choroid plexus cysts or hematoma
- Cysts and hematoma may both occur in the choroid plexus, sparing the germinal matrix area

Ventriculitis
- Thickening and increased echoes in the ependyma lining the ventricles
- Often associated with intraventricular hemorrhage or GMH
- But also seen in infectious, toxic, and metabolic disorders without bleeding
- Re-image to determine if communicating hydrocephalus develops after ventriculitis
  - Serial head circumference is not reliable
  - Bulging fontanelle is a late sign of hydrocephalus

Ischemia or infarction
- Ischemic areas show increased echogenicity
- Lack mass effect of hematoma
- Tend to occur in different areas of the brain, periventricular white matter

Periventricular calcifications
- Not typically seen in the caudothalamic groove
- Related to TORCH infections most commonly

Intraventricular hemorrhage
- Hematoma may be confined to the ventricle without involvement of germinal matrix
- Consider this diagnosis in patients who are older than 34 weeks gestation

PATHOLOGY

General Features
- General path comments

GERMINAL MATRIX HEMORRHAGE

- The germinal matrix is only transiently present as a region of thin-walled vessels, migrating neuronal components and vessel precursors
- It has matured or "involuted" by 34 weeks gestation, such that hemorrhage becomes very unlikely after this age
- Most GMHs occur in the first week of life
- Genetics: Not inherited
- Etiology
  - Related to perinatal stresses: Labile blood pressure, hypoxia, hypercarbia, etc.
  - Probably potentiated by poor or underdeveloped cerebral perfusion autoregulation
- Epidemiology
  - Most common in infants < 32 weeks gestation and < 1500 grams
  - Higher risk of GMH in premies who have congenital heart disease, surgical procedures, severe respiratory distress
  - Rate of severe grade III or IV GMH decreased from 70% in 1986 to 23% in 1995 & mortality rate decreased by 30% in the same period

Gross Pathologic & Surgical Features
- Areas of hemorrhagic necrosis, liquefaction, and gliosis

Microscopic Features
- Bleeding occurs from venous leak or rupture
- Arteriole sources and arteriovenous shunts have not been found

Staging, Grading or Classification Criteria
- Germinal Matrix Grading system created by Burstein et al in 1979
- Grade I: Confined to the caudothalamic groove
- Grade II: Extends into the ventricle but does not expand it
- Grade III: Fills and distends the adjacent ventricle
- Grade IV: Parenchymal hemorrhage/edema/ischemia beyond the germinal matrix
  - Unclear if Grade IV hemorrhage results from subependymal bleeding into the adjacent brain or venous infarction

CLINICAL ISSUES

Presentation
- Most common signs/symptoms: Variable: Hypotonia, seizures, hyperreflexia, falling hematocrit, irritability, failure to thrive, paresis, acidosis, feeding difficulties
- Other signs/symptoms: GMH may occur in utero and follow the same pathway of evolution & complications

Demographics
- Age
  - Premature infants in the first week of life
  - Half of all GMHs occur on the first day of life
- Gender: M = F
- Ethnicity: No predisposition

Natural History & Prognosis
- GMHs may progress or re-bleed and increase in severity of grade
- Secondary hydrocephalus occurring several days after a grade II bleed should not be mislabeled as grade III hemorrhage
- In general, the clot retracts, lyses, and becomes hypoechoic leaving behind a cyst or area of porencephaly
- Prognosis
  - Grade I & II bleeds generally have a good prognosis
  - Grade III & IV bleeds have variable long-term deficits
    - Including spastic diplegia, seizures, developmental delay
    - Many patients require ventriculoperitoneal shunting or endoscopic third ventriculostomy for communicating hydrocephalus

Treatment
- Supportive in the acute phase
- CSF shunting may be needed in higher grade bleeds

SELECTED REFERENCES
1. Ballabh P et al: Anatomic analysis of blood vessels in germinal matrix, cerebral cortex, and white matter in developing infants. Pediatr Res. 56(1):117-24, 2004
2. Vasileiadis GT et al: Uncomplicated intraventricular hemorrhage is followed by reduced cortical volume at near-term age. Pediatrics. 114(3):e367-72, 2004
3. Roland EH et al: Germinal matrix-intraventricular hemorrhage in the premature newborn: management and outcome. Neurol Clin. 21(4):833-51, vi-vii, 2003
4. Smyth MD et al: Endoscopic third ventriculostomy for hydrocephalus secondary to central nervous system infection or intraventricular hemorrhage in children. Pediatr Neurosurg. 39(5):258-63, 2003
5. Vollmer B et al: Predictors of long-term outcome in very preterm infants: gestational age versus neonatal cranial ultrasound. Pediatrics. 112(5):1108-14, 2003
6. Fukui K et al: Fetal germinal matrix and intraventricular haemorrhage diagnosed by MRI. Neuroradiology. 43(1):68-72, 2001
7. Blankenberg FG et al: Sonography, CT, and MR imaging: a prospective comparison of neonates with suspected intracranial ischemia and hemorrhage. AJNR Am J Neuroradiol. 21(1):213-8, 2000
8. Tsuji M et al: Cerebral intravascular oxygenation correlates with mean arterial pressure in critically ill premature infants. Pediatrics. 106(4):625-32, 2000
9. Felderhoff-Mueser U et al: Relationship between MR imaging and histopathologic findings of the brain in extremely sick preterm infants. AJNR Am J Neuroradiol. 20(7):1349-57, 1999
10. Volpe JJ: Brain injury in the premature infant: overview of clinical aspects, neuropathology, and pathogenesis. Semin Pediatr Neurol. 5(3):135-51, 1998
11. Levy ML et al: Outcome for preterm infants with germinal matrix hemorrhage and progressive hydrocephalus. Neurosurgery. 41(5):1111-7; discussion 1117-8, 1997
12. Ghazi-Birry HS et al: Human germinal matrix: venous origin of hemorrhage and vascular characteristics. AJNR Am J Neuroradiol. 18(2):219-29, 1997
13. Burstein J et al: Intraventricular hemorrhage and hydrocephalus in premature newborns: a prospective study with CT. AJR Am J Roentgenol. 132(4):631-5, 1979

GERMINAL MATRIX HEMORRHAGE

IMAGE GALLERY

Typical

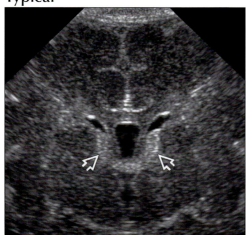
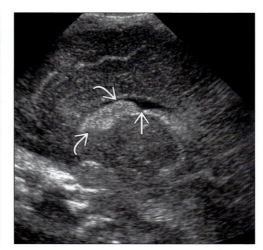

(Left) Coronal ultrasound shows echogenic blood in the germinal matrix bilaterally *(arrows)* in a premature infant with grade I bleeds. Note the normal midline cavum septi pellucidi. *(Right)* Sagittal ultrasound in the same patient shows ovoid echogenic blood *(curved arrows)* confined to the germinal matrix region, not extending into the ventricle. Note the notch between GMH and choroid *(arrow)*.

Typical

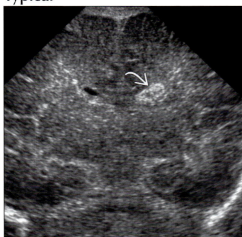
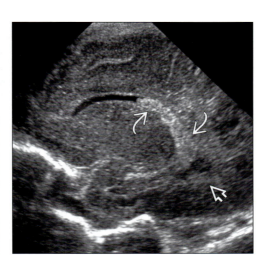

(Left) Coronal ultrasound shows echogenic blood *(arrow)* in the germinal matrix extending into the left lateral ventricle, but not expanding the ventricle, in this case of a grade II GMH. *(Right)* Sagittal ultrasound shows a similar grade II bleed in different patient. Note the echogenic blood blending with the choroid plexus posteriorly *(curved arrows)* and some blood in the occipital horn *(open arrow)*.

Typical

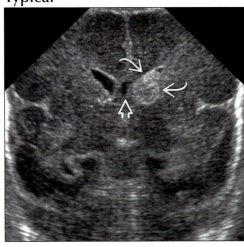
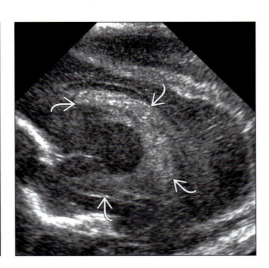

(Left) Coronal ultrasound shows a grade III germinal matrix hemorrhage *(curved arrows)* distending the left frontal horn and effacing the cavum septi pellucidi *(open arrow)*. *(Right)* Sagittal ultrasound in the same patient shows echogenic blood filling and distending the lateral ventricle *(arrows)*. No anechoic CSF is visible.

HYPOXIC ISCHEMIC ENCEPHALOPATHY

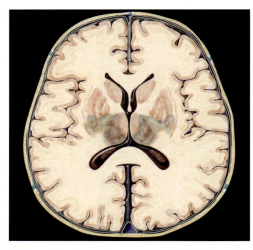

Axial graphic shows deep pattern of HIE injury, with edema in ventrolateral thalamus and posterior putamen. This pattern is associated with profound hypotension or circulatory arrest.

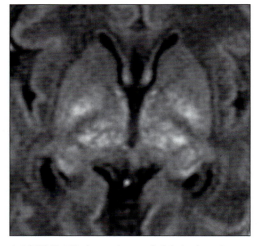

Axial T1WI MR shows abnormal globular hyperintense signal in a similar distribution in a neonate with profound HIE. The irregularity of signal distinguishes it from normal myelination.

TERMINOLOGY

Abbreviations and Synonyms
- Hypoxic ischemic encephalopathy (HIE), perinatal or birth asphyxia, asphyxia neonatorium

Definitions
- An acquired condition in neonates generally attributed to cerebral hypoperfusion
  - Physiology leading to injury incompletely understood
- Several patterns of brain injury can be seen; differences attributed to several clinical variables
  - Degree of infant development/maturity
  - Severity of insult
  - Duration of insult
  - Superimposed infection, metabolic derangement
- Clear correlation with clinical factors difficult due to inability to detect/monitor all relevant physiologic parameters in perinatal period
- Considered distinct from focal infarction due to arterial or venous occlusion/compromise, intracranial hemorrhage (ICH), inborn errors of metabolism

IMAGING FINDINGS

General Features
- Best diagnostic clue
  - Three general patterns of injury can be identified
    - Deep ⇒ abnormalities in ventrolateral thalamus (VLT), basal ganglia (BG)
    - Periventricular ⇒ abnormalities in periventricular white matter (WM) of hemispheres, parietal/occipital > frontal
    - Peripheral ⇒ abnormalities in peripheral cortex and/or subcortical white matter
  - Not exclusive of each other
- Pattern of injury is presumed to be affected by age at time of insult, not at time of delivery
  - Very difficult to know exact timing of injury
- Deep pattern of injury is characteristically seen with profound degrees of insult
  - Seen in both pre-term and full-term infants!
    - May be accompanied by more diffuse peripheral cortical insult
- Periventricular injury is seen almost exclusively in pre-term infants
  - Prior to 34-35 weeks gestation
  - If seen in full-term, presumed to reflect in utero insult
- Subcortical or "watershed" injury is seen almost exclusively in full-term infants

DDx: Evolution Of Periventricular Injury

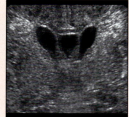
Early PVL On US

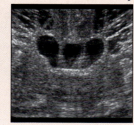
Cystic PVL On US

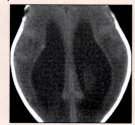
Early PVL On CT

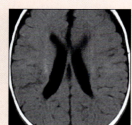
Late PVL On MR

HYPOXIC ISCHEMIC ENCEPHALOPATHY

Key Facts

Terminology
- An acquired condition in neonates generally attributed to cerebral hypoperfusion
- Several patterns of brain injury can be seen; differences attributed to several clinical variables
- Clear correlation with clinical factors difficult due to inability to detect/monitor all relevant physiologic parameters in perinatal period

Imaging Findings
- Deep pattern of injury is characteristically seen with profound degrees of insult
- Seen in both pre-term and full-term infants!
- Periventricular injury is seen almost exclusively in pre-term infants
- Subcortical or "watershed" injury is seen almost exclusively in full-term infants
- Deep injury can appear normal on DWI
- If lactate peak approaches NAA or creatine peak in size, it is abnormal
- Periventricular ⇒ characteristic increased echogenicity in periventricular WM
- US ideal in initial evaluation, but limited
- Use T1WI and PD/Intermediate for identification of deep and periventricular injury

Pathology
- Reasons for differing patterns of injury not completely understood
- Likely factors include metabolic demand, vascular regulation, neurotransmitter distribution, oligodendrocyte distribution
- Placental pathologic analysis often very helpful in understanding clinical picture

---

  - Watershed ⇒ brain regions at periphery of arterial bed, lowest perfusion pressure with compromise of flow

CT Findings
- NECT
  - Deep ⇒ loss of distinction of BG/internal capsules early
    - Later: Volume loss, ↑ density ⇒ calcification (Ca++), hemorrhage
  - Periventricular: ± Decreased density foci in periventricular WM early
    - Periventricular cysts in subacute stage
    - Characteristic angular enlargement of trigones and occipital horns of lateral ventricles late ⇒ periventricular leukomalacia (PVL)
  - Peripheral ⇒ diffuse loss of GM/WM distinction, or focal loss in watershed zones
    - Diffuse volume loss and cystic encephalomalacia develop in severe insults
    - Watershed or limited insults result in ulegyria ⇒ mushroom-shaped gyri due to loss of subcortical WM

MR Findings
- T1WI
  - Deep ⇒ abnormal hyperintense signal in VLT and BG early
    - May be difficult to distinguish from normal bright signal in these regions
    - Normal ⇒ smooth, poorly-defined, similar to peripheral cortical ribbon in intensity
    - Pathology ⇒ globular, irregular, brighter than cortical ribbon
  - Periventricular ⇒ globular foci of bright signal (gliosis, hemorrhage?)
  - Peripheral ⇒ ↑ signal in focal regions of cortical ribbon
  - Cerebellar insults often accompany deep or periventricular insults
- T2WI
  - Deep ⇒ poor definition of BG; abnormally hyperintense
    - Hypo-intense if Ca++ or hemorrhage
  - Periventricular ⇒ bright signal corresponding to abnormalities on T1WI reflects gliosis
    - Dark signal corresponding to abnormalities on T1WI reflects hemorrhage
  - Peripheral ⇒ discontinuity of cortical ribbon in region of injury
    - May have hypointense signal reflecting laminar necrosis, petechial hemorrhage
- PD/Intermediate: Deep ⇒ signal abnormality more apparent than on T2WI
- T2* GRE: Often reveals subtle germinal matrix hemorrhage
- DWI
  - Deep injury can appear normal on DWI
    - Explanations: Injury not truly ischemic, injury evolves over time (becomes like cellular ischemia only after 24-48 hours), injury occurred more than 7 days prior to imaging, "wet" WM has limited ability to have effect on water diffusion
  - Helpful if positive; use caution if negative
    - Limited window of opportunity to document injury, underestimates damage if performed at wrong time
  - Normalizes around 7 days, even in damaged areas
- MRS
  - Lactate doublet at 1.33 ppm is marker for anaerobic metabolism
    - Normal neonate cerebrospinal fluid (CSF) has measurable lactate on MRS
    - If voxel contains part of ventricle, spurious lactate detection
    - "Wet" immature white matter will also show small lactate peak
    - Be sure to distinguish from propanediol, a phenobarbital solvent with a peak at 1.5 ppm
  - If lactate peak approaches NAA or creatine peak in size, it is abnormal
  - ↑ Glutamate/glutamine peaks in BG correlate with ↑ severity of injury
    - Difficult to resolve at 1.5T

HYPOXIC ISCHEMIC ENCEPHALOPATHY

Ultrasonographic Findings
- Grayscale Ultrasound
  - Periventricular ⇒ characteristic increased echogenicity in periventricular WM
    - Develops into cystic change over time ⇒ PVL
    - Associated with germinal matrix hemorrhage (Gr III)

Imaging Recommendations
- Best imaging tool
  - US ideal in initial evaluation, but limited
  - MR with MRS and DWI at 24-72 hours
    - FLAIR, MRA not helpful
  - Detrimental effects of radiation outweigh diagnostic utility of CT
- Protocol advice
  - MR environment is noxious to unstable neonate, especially pre-term
    - Temperature instability, noise intolerance, diminished monitoring capabilities
    - Use of MR-compatible incubator has potential to decrease detrimental effects of diagnostic imaging in perinatal period
  - Use T1WI and PD/Intermediate for identification of deep and periventricular injury
    - Correlate/verify with DWI and MRS
    - Recognize false negatives

DIFFERENTIAL DIAGNOSIS

Kernicterus
- Mimics profound injury on acute T1WI

Metabolic disorders
- Mitochondrial encephalopathy, methylmalonic acidemia

Normal
- Myelin in thalamus and corticospinal tracts can mimic deep injury on T1WI

PATHOLOGY

General Features
- General path comments
  - Reasons for differing patterns of injury not completely understood
  - Likely factors include metabolic demand, vascular regulation, neurotransmitter distribution, oligodendrocyte distribution
  - Metabolic demand ⇒ concept that regions of highest energy use are most susceptible
    - Correspond to regions of deep brain injury
  - Vascular regulation ⇒ poorly developed autoregulation in pre-term and neonate
    - Cannot adapt to wide swings in cerebral perfusion pressure ⇒ "pressure passive flow"
    - More pronounced in pre-term, exacerbated by hypercarbia and hypoxemia
    - Explains watershed-type injury
  - Neurotransmitter distribution ⇒ glutamate release in response to asphyxia sets off cascade of harmful free radicals
    - Distribution of glutamate receptors in neonate parallels pattern of deep injury
    - May explain diffusion-negative injury
  - Oligodendrocyte distribution ⇒ these cells are particularly sensitive to hypoxic ischemic injury
    - Concentrated in periventricular region in pre-term
  - Placental pathologic analysis often very helpful in understanding clinical picture
- Epidemiology
  - 11% of US births are < 2500 g
  - 0.2% of term births have HIE
- Associated abnormalities: Maternal: Infection (chorioamnionitis), pre-eclampsia, diabetes, cocaine

Staging, Grading or Classification Criteria
- "Profound partial", "profound acute" categorization
  - Presumes a clear picture of inciting insult

CLINICAL ISSUES

Presentation
- Most common signs/symptoms
  - Sarnat I: Hyperalert, irritable, normal EEG
  - Sarnat II: Lethargy, hypotonia, seizure
  - Sarnat III: Flaccid, absent reflexes, seizure

Natural History & Prognosis
- PVL ⇒ > 50% have cerebral palsy
- Severe HIE: 50% mortality, 80% severe morbidity

Treatment
- Correct hypoxia, metabolic disturbances
- Hypothermia can blunt insult if applied early in course

DIAGNOSTIC CHECKLIST

Consider
- Impact of MR imaging findings on clinical management still limited

Image Interpretation Pearls
- Keep reference normal for T1WI and MRS for comparison

SELECTED REFERENCES
1. Thoresen M et al: Therapeutic hypothermia for hypoxic-ischaemic encephalopathy in the newborn infant. Curr Opin Neurol. 18(2):111-6, 2005
2. Barkovich AJ et al: Proton spectroscopy and diffusion imaging on the first day of life after perinatal asphyxia: Preliminary report. AJNR. 22(9):1786-94, 2001
3. Groenendaal F et al: Glutamate in cerebral tissue of asphyxiated neonates during the first week of life demonstrated in vivo using proton MRS. Biol Neonate. 79(3-4):254-257, 2001

HYPOXIC ISCHEMIC ENCEPHALOPATHY

IMAGE GALLERY

Typical

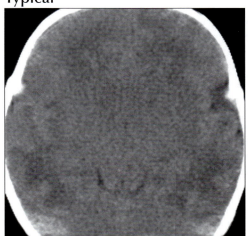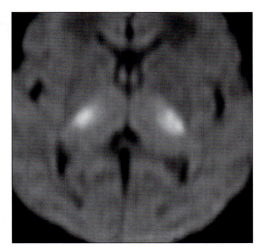

(Left) Axial NECT shows loss of distinction of basal ganglia in a term neonate with HIE. Note preservation of peripheral gray-white differentiation. *(Right)* Axial DWI MR shows restricted diffusion in ventrolateral thalamus in pre-term infant with HIE. DWI can be falsely negative, in part due to difficulty in timing of MR relative to insult.

Typical

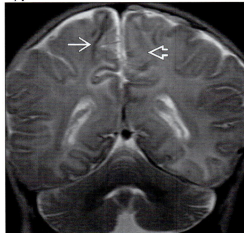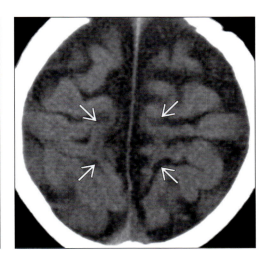

(Left) Coronal T2WI MR shows hypointense signal and loss of volume in parasagittal gyrus (arrow), and focal loss of cortical ribbon (open arrow) in a term neonate with moderate injury. *(Right)* Axial NECT in the same child several year later shows loss of volume in affected parasagittal gyri, with ulegyria (arrows).

Typical

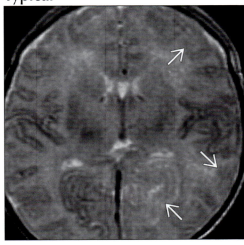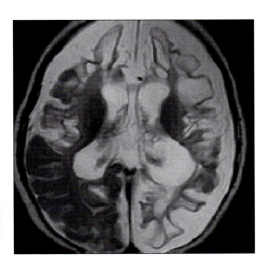

(Left) Axial T2WI MR shows several areas with loss of cortical ribbon continuity (arrows), poor definition of basal ganglia, and subtle increased signal in WM. *(Right)* Axial T2WI MR several months later in the same infant shows extensive cystic encephalomalacia throughout the brain.

CHILDHOOD STROKE

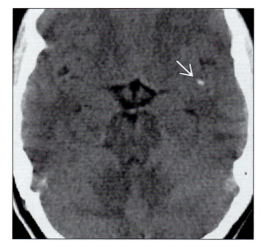

Axial NECT in a 14 yo male with acute right hemiparesis shows HMCAS (arrow), indicating hyperdense thrombus in proximal middle cerebral artery branch.

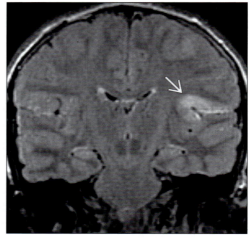

Coronal FLAIR MR in same patient shows edema in insular cortex supplied by affected MCA branch (arrow). He had complete recovery without direct treatment, and no etiology was found.

TERMINOLOGY

Abbreviations and Synonyms
- Cerebrovascular accident (CVA), cerebral infarct, cerebral ischemia

Definitions
- Acute alteration of neurologic function due to loss of vascular integrity
- This discussion addresses insults occurring outside of the perinatal period

IMAGING FINDINGS

General Features
- Best diagnostic clue: Edema, restricted diffusion in affected territory
- Location: Proximal and distal middle cerebral artery (MCA) territory most commonly affected
- Morphology
  ○ Stroke caused by arterial occlusion often conforms to arterial territory
  ○ Venous territories typically less well recognized

CT Findings
- NECT
  ○ Decreased attenuation of affected gray matter (GM)
    ▪ Often wedge-shaped and corresponding to arterial territory
    ▪ Diffuse ischemic injury can result in "reversal sign", with GM diffusely decreased in attenuation relative to white matter (WM), poor distinction of basal ganglia
  ○ Insular ribbon sign ⇒ loss of distinction of insular cortex
  ○ Hyperdense MCA sign (HMCAS) ⇒ increased density of thrombosed MCA
  ○ Hemorrhagic conversion of stroke
    ▪ Cortical hemorrhage often petechial
    ▪ WM or deep nuclear hemorrhage often mass-like ⇒ hematoma within infarcted tissue
  ○ Hyperdense dural sinus ⇒ "delta" sign
- CECT
  ○ Enhancement of infarcted territory typically occurs after 5-7 days
  ○ Enhancement of sagittal sinus wall around non-enhancing clot ⇒ "empty delta" sign
- CTA: Invaluable for demonstrating focal vascular abnormalities in acute setting

MR Findings
- T1WI
  ○ Gyral swelling and hypointensity in affected territory
  ○ Loss of normal vascular flow void

DDx: Vasculopathy In Children

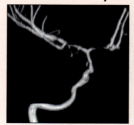
Vasculitis

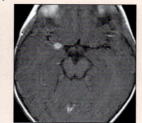
Varicella

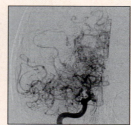
Moyamoya

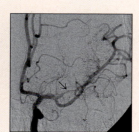
Radiation

CHILDHOOD STROKE

Key Facts

Terminology
- Acute alteration of neurologic function due to loss of vascular integrity

Imaging Findings
- Location: Proximal and distal middle cerebral artery (MCA) territory most commonly affected
- Hyperdense MCA sign (HMCAS) ⇒ increased density of thrombosed MCA
- Enhancement of infarcted territory typically occurs after 5-7 days
- Use of fat-saturation allows confident identification of crescent of mural hematoma in dissected vessel
- "Climbing ivy" ⇒ bright vessels in sulci distal to arterial occlusion
- Restriction of diffusion seen within 45 minutes of arterial occlusion
- MRS: ↑ Lactate hallmark of ischemia/infarct
- Catheter angiography rarely necessary in acute evaluation of childhood stroke

Pathology
- Anterior circulation > posterior, left > right
- Etiology: No underlying cause is discovered in > 33% of cases
- Associated abnormalities: Cardiac disease (25-50%), sickle cell (200-400x increased risk), trauma

Clinical Issues
- Under-recognized as significant source of morbidity in pediatric population
- Capacity for recovery much greater than in adults
- Greater capacity for compensatory mechanisms, collateral recruitment

---

- Entry slice artifact can cause false positive!
- Irregular signal can be seen in normal veins due to slow flow ⇒ thrombosed veins are typically enlarged
- T1WI FS
  - Use of fat-saturation allows confident identification of crescent of mural hematoma in dissected vessel
    - Use in combination with MRA (2D or 3D)
- T2WI: Edema evident in affected territory after 4-6 hours of arterial occlusion
- FLAIR
  - More sensitive than T2WI for ischemia-induced cytotoxic edema
  - Also shows loss of normal arterial flow voids
    - "Climbing ivy" ⇒ bright vessels in sulci distal to arterial occlusion
    - Same effect is seen with T1 C+, classically seen in moyamoya
  - Excellent for detection of venous thrombosis
    - Iso/hyperintense thrombus compared to hypointense flowing blood in sinus
- DWI
  - Most sensitive imaging sequence for ischemic injury
  - Restriction of diffusion seen within 45 minutes of arterial occlusion
  - Apparent diffusion coefficient (ADC) mapping essential to avoid false positive from "T2 shine through"
- T1 C+
  - Can provide earliest sign of proximal arterial occlusion ⇒ enhancement of arteries in territory distal to occlusion
    - Collateral flow to distal vascular bed is slower
    - Normal flow void caused by rapid arterial flow is out-weighed by T1 shortening effect of contrast
  - Beware! Contrast effect increased on 3T and gradient echo acquisitions ⇒ normal arteries/veins may show enhancement
- MRA: Sensitive in detection of arterial occlusion and stenosis in large and medium sized cerebral vessels
- MRV: Can demonstrate focal occlusion, response to treatment
- MRS: ↑ Lactate hallmark of ischemia/infarct
- MR perfusion
  - Can provide valuable information regarding region at risk in setting of acute stroke
    - Ischemic penumbra ⇒ region with diminished perfusion not yet infarcted (perfusion-diffusion mismatch)
    - May define brain salvageable with acute stroke therapy
  - Arterial spin-labeling techniques hold promise for standardized perfusion imaging without contrast administration

Ultrasonographic Findings
- Grayscale Ultrasound: Affected territory hyperechoic in acute/subacute stage
- Color Doppler
  - Direct Doppler evaluation ideal for surveillance of vascular occlusion in neonate with open sutures
  - Transcranial Doppler evaluation of circle of Willis through temporal squamosa
    - Increased velocities can predict stenoses detectable by MRA
    - Used as screening tool in children with sickle cell anemia

Angiographic Findings
- Catheter angiography rarely necessary in acute evaluation of childhood stroke
  - Only justified if contemplating endovascular therapy
- Best modality for detailed evaluation of primary arteriopathies

Nuclear Medicine Findings
- PET and SPECT techniques can be used to investigate normal development, effects of therapy, and subclinical pathology
  - Can identify salvageable regions at risk (ischemic penumbra)
  - Can demonstrate effects of synangiosis surgery in moyamoya

CHILDHOOD STROKE

Imaging Recommendations
- Best imaging tool: MR with diffusion, MRA, and MRV
- Protocol advice: Contrast can help in assessing timing of injury and in performing perfusion imaging

DIFFERENTIAL DIAGNOSIS

Primary arteriopathies
- Moyamoya vascularity, idiopathic, syndromic, or acquired
- Radiation vasculopathy
- Infectious vasculitis ⇒ bacterial, viral (varicella, chicken-pox vasculitis)
- Primary arteritis of the CNS ⇒ rare, often involves vessels too small to image by angiography

Embolic disease
- Proximal sources ⇒ cardiac (congenital heart disease)
- Paradoxical emboli ⇒ venous source passing through patent foramen ovale

Hypoperfusion
- Cardiopulmonary collapse

Metabolic encephalopathies
- Mitochondrial encephalopathies, organic acidurias

Vascular lesions
- Aneurysms, vascular malformations

Trauma
- Cervical dissections ⇒ vertebral > carotid
- Penetrating trauma causing direct vascular injury

Venous occlusion
- High association with sepsis or adjacent infection (mastoiditis)

Coagulopathies
- Factor deficiencies, lupus anticoagulant, protein C, protein S

PATHOLOGY

General Features
- General path comments
  - Pathologic findings similar to adults
  - Anterior circulation > posterior, left > right
- Etiology: No underlying cause is discovered in > 33% of cases
- Epidemiology
  - Incidence 2-3/100,000 per year in US
    - Mortality 0.6/100,000
  - "Stroke belt" ⇒ higher incidence in southeastern states
- Associated abnormalities: Cardiac disease (25-50%), sickle cell (200-400x increased risk), trauma

CLINICAL ISSUES

Presentation
- Most common signs/symptoms
  - Under-recognized as significant source of morbidity in pediatric population
  - Children with stroke typically present in delayed fashion (> 24 hours)
    - Poor recognition/understanding of symptoms by child, caregiver, physician
  - Seizure ⇒ deficit often attributed to post-ictal state (Jacksonian paralysis)
  - Speech difficulties, gait abnormality
  - Focal deficit often masked by lethargy, coma, irritability
  - Preceding transient events occur in 25%

Demographics
- Age: Incidence/mortality greatest < 1 year
- Gender: Boys > girls

Natural History & Prognosis
- Canadian registry ⇒ 61% abnormal, 27% normal
- Recurrence 20-40%
- Capacity for recovery much greater than in adults
  - Fewer concomitant risk factors
  - Greater capacity for compensatory mechanisms, collateral recruitment

Treatment
- No randomized trials of therapies
  - Clinical window of opportunity/benefit much narrower than in adults
    - Acute aggressive therapy may not improve on outcome in large population based on experience in adults
    - Exception ⇒ perinatal
- Aspirin is mainstay of chronic therapy for fixed vascular lesions and vasculopathies
- Transfusion therapy for at-risk children with sickle cell disease

DIAGNOSTIC CHECKLIST

Image Interpretation Pearls
- Use same imaging signs as in adults
- Have low threshold for use of CTA

SELECTED REFERENCES

1. Abboud MR et al: Magnetic resonance angiography in children with sickle cell disease and abnormal transcranial Doppler ultrasonography findings enrolled in the STOP study. Blood. 103(7):2822-6, 2004
2. Fullerton HJ et al: Pediatric Stroke Belt: geographic variation in stroke mortality in US children. Stroke. 35(7):1570-3, 2004
3. Scott RM et al: Long-term outcome in children with moyamoya syndrome after cranial revascularization by pial synangiosis. J Neurosurg. 100(2 Suppl Pediatrics):142-9, 2004
4. Golomb MR et al: Cranial ultrasonography has a low sensitivity for detecting arterial ischemic stroke in term neonates. J Child Neurol. 18(2):98-103, 2003
5. Carvalho KS et al: Arterial strokes in children. Neurol Clin. 20(4):1079-100, vii, 2002
6. Lynch JK et al: Report of the National Institute of Neurological Disorders and Stroke workshop on perinatal and childhood stroke. Pediatrics. 109(1):116-23, 2002

CHILDHOOD STROKE

IMAGE GALLERY

Typical

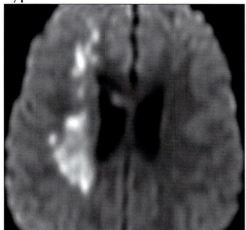
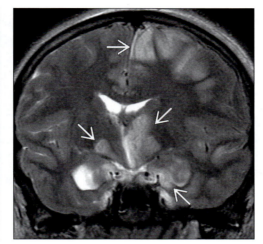

(Left) Axial DWI MR shows characteristic "watershed" distribution of infarction in right cerebral hemisphere from carotid terminus stenosis stemming from bacterial meningitis and vasculitis. *(Right)* Coronal T2WI MR shows multiple areas of infarction (arrows) resulting from left hemisphere herniation. Secondary infarction from herniation often causes more morbidity than initial insult.

Typical

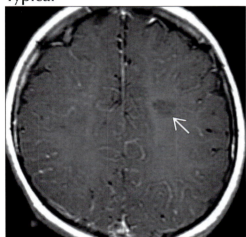
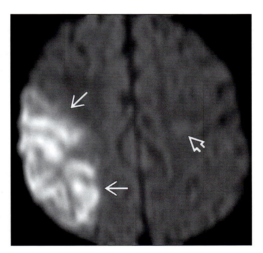

(Left) Axial T1 C+ MR shows typical "climbing ivy" pattern of arterial enhancement in distal territories caused by proximal occlusion in moyamoya disease. Note WM infarct on left (arrow). *(Right)* DWI MR in the same child shows acute infarct on the right (arrows), with T2 shine-through in old left-sided stroke (open arrow). DWI is essential in MR of children with multiple infarcts.

Typical

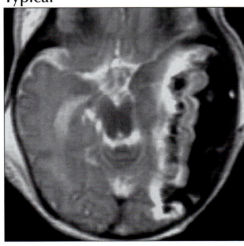
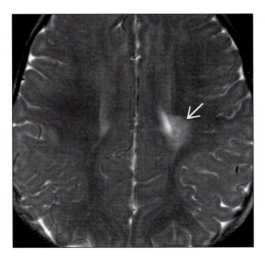

(Left) Axial T2WI MR shows typical appearance of hemorrhagic infarct resulting from thrombosis of the vein of Labbe on the left. Despite dramatic appearance, there is typically very good recovery. *(Right)* Axial T2WI MR shows small periventricular infarct (arrow) in a 6 month old. MRA revealed left carotid aneurysm. Proximal arterial pathology should always be investigated at presentation.

VEIN OF GALEN ANEURYSMAL MALFORMATION

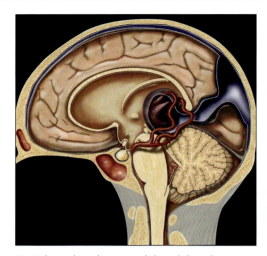

Sagittal graphic shows medial and lateral posterior choroidal arteries connected directly to an enlarged midline vein, which drains through an anomalous venous channel to the sagittal sinus.

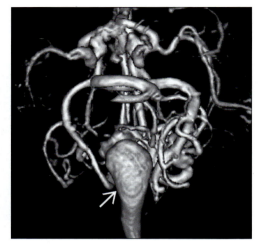

Inferior projection from 3D MRA reconstruction shows multiple choroidal vessels surrounding varix (arrow). MRA is very valuable in showing location of feeding vessels prior to treatment.

TERMINOLOGY

Abbreviations and Synonyms
- Vein of Galen malformation (VGAM, VGM), vein of Galen "aneurysm", Galenic varix

Definitions
- Arteriovenous fistula (AVF) between deep choroidal arteries and the median prosencephalic vein (MPV) of Markowski
  - There is no aneurysm of the true vein of Galen, which fails to form because of fistula

IMAGING FINDINGS

General Features
- Best diagnostic clue: Large midline varix in neonate/infant
- Location: Quadrigeminal plate cistern
- Size: Varix can be several centimeters in diameter
- Morphology: Spherical or tubular varix

Radiographic Findings
- Radiography: Cardiomegaly and edema from heart failure (CHF) evident on chest X-ray

CT Findings
- NECT
  - Venous pouch mildly hyperdense to brain
  - Hydrocephalus
  - Subcortical white matter (WM) Ca++ from chronic venous ischemia
  - Streak artifact from coils or glue make CT a poor choice for post-treatment imaging
- CECT: Strong enhancement of feeding arteries and varix
- CTA: Excellent pre-angiographic delineation

MR Findings
- T1WI
  - Pulsation artifact from varix
  - Varix contents hypointense and heterogeneous (turbulent flow)
  - Herniation of cerebellar tonsils
  - Compression of tectum
  - Prominent sulci
    - Elevated venous pressures cause decreased resorption of cerebrospinal fluid (CSF)
- T2WI
  - Varix homogeneously hypointense
  - Prominent flow voids from feeding arteries around varix
  - Sharp delineation of malformation
- DWI
  - Restricted diffusion in areas of acute ischemia or infarction

DDx: Pediatric Vascular Lesions

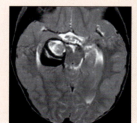

Giant Aneurysm

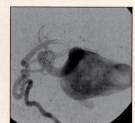

Dural AVF

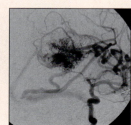

Pial AVM

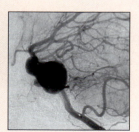

Basilar Aneurysm

VEIN OF GALEN ANEURYSMAL MALFORMATION

Key Facts

Terminology
- Arteriovenous fistula (AVF) between deep choroidal arteries and the median prosencephalic vein (MPV) of Markowski
- There is no aneurysm of the true vein of Galen, which fails to form because of fistula

Imaging Findings
- Pulsation artifact from varix
- Elevated venous pressures cause decreased resorption of cerebrospinal fluid (CSF)
- Key for pre-treatment assessment of feeders to malformation
- Unaffected by coils or acrylic embolic material
- Frequent venous abnormalities
- Diagnostic arteriography performed in concert with embolization

Top Differential Diagnoses
- Arteriovenous malformation (AVM) with drainage into true vein of Galen
- Childhood dural arteriovenous fistula (dAVF)

Pathology
- Up to 30% of all pediatric vascular malformations
- "Choroidal" or "mural" classification based on angioarchitecture of VGM

Clinical Issues
- Delay in treatment until 4-6 months associated with better outcome
- Transcatheter embolization (TCE) at 4-6 months
- May require staged embolizations
- Shunt placement associated with exacerbation of venous ischemia

---

   - Valuable in immediate post-treatment studies
- MRA
   - Key for pre-treatment assessment of feeders to malformation
   - Unaffected by coils or acrylic embolic material
- MRV
   - Essential in initial and follow-up evaluation
   - Presence and degree of venous stenosis can have major influence on prognosis
- Fetal MR
   - Can identify malformation in 2nd and 3rd trimester
   - Can identify presence or absence of brain or other end-organ injury
      - Significant antenatal end-organ injury is a contradiction to aggressive treatment

Ultrasonographic Findings
- Prenatal studies identify malformation in 3rd trimester
- Cardiac dilatation, hydrops fetalis = poor prognosis

Echocardiographic Findings
- Dilatation of right heart, superior vena cava, ascending aorta and great vessels
- Poor prognostic indicators
   - Descending aorta diastolic flow reversal
   - Suprasystemic pulmonary artery hypertension
   - Persistent ductus arteriosus with significant right to left shunt

Angiographic Findings
- Conventional
   - "Choroidal" or "mural" classification based on angioarchitecture
      - Classification has limited value in predicting prognosis or response to treatment
   - Frequent venous abnormalities
      - Embryonic falcine sinus drains MPV in 50%
      - Frequent stenoses at sigmoid-jugular junction

Imaging Recommendations
- Best imaging tool
   - MR with MRA and MRV
   - Diagnostic arteriography performed in concert with embolization
- Protocol advice
   - Maximize MRA evaluation
      - 3D reconstruction can provide valuable insight

DIFFERENTIAL DIAGNOSIS

Vein of Galen aneurysmal dilation (VGAD)
- Arteriovenous malformation (AVM) with drainage into true vein of Galen
- Looks like choroidal type of VGAM
   - Much less common than VGAM

Childhood dural arteriovenous fistula (dAVF)
- High-flow fistulas with venous varices
   - Typically in transverse sinuses
- Massive torcular enlargement may thrombose spontaneously after delivery
   - Especially when supplied exclusively by external carotid artery branches

Giant aneurysm
- Not associated with venous abnormalities
- "Onion skin" layers in wall

Complex developmental venous anomaly (DVA)
- Dilatation of veins draining normal brain parenchyma
- Associated with blue rubber-bleb nevus syndrome

Pial AVM
- Distinguished by true nidus at transition
- Rarely present before 3 years of age

PATHOLOGY

General Features
- General path comments
   - Embryology

NORMAL MYELINATION

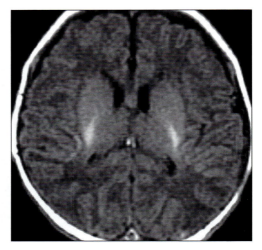

Axial NECT shows accentuated gray-white differentiation in a normal newborn. High water content of the white matter accounts for the clear distinction of the cortical ribbon in neonates.

Axial T1WI MR shows hyperintense signal in posterior limb of internal capsules in a neonate. Dorsal aspect of the corticospinal tracts are one of the few myelinated structures in the newborn.

TERMINOLOGY

Abbreviations and Synonyms
- Myelin maturation, white matter development

Definitions
- Organized and predetermined pattern of development and distribution of myelin sheaths on axons
- Begins in 5th fetal month and continues throughout life

IMAGING FINDINGS

General Features
- Best diagnostic clue: Myelin development correlates with functional milestones
- Location: Myelin maturation proceeds caudal to rostral, central to peripheral, dorsal to ventral
- Size: White matter (WM) tracts increase in size with myelin formation, especially corpus callosum
- Morphology: Diffusion tractography may provide insight on morphology of developing tracts

CT Findings
- NECT
  - Unmyelinated white matter is hypodense relative to gray matter and to myelinated white matter
  - Gray-white differentiation is accentuated in neonate due to high water content of white matter
  - Density increase with myelination is relatively subtle, making CT insensitive in detecting delays in myelination

MR Findings
- T1WI
  - T1WI is key sequence in assessing normal myelination in children < 1 year
  - Inversion recovery (IR) technique can accentuate T1 shortening of myelin
  - Detection of myelination progresses in a predictable fashion
  - Neonate has hyperintense signal in
    - Dorsal brainstem
    - Dentate nucleus
    - Optic tracts
    - Anterior commissure
    - Posterior limb internal capsule
    - Rolandic and perirolandic gyri
    - Pyramidal tracts
  - 2 months
    - Splenium of corpus callosum
    - Anterior limb internal capsule
    - Early optic radiations
  - 4 months
    - Genu of corpus callosum

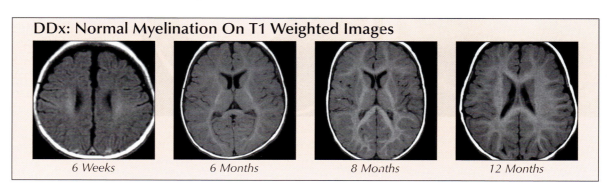

DDx: Normal Myelination On T1 Weighted Images

6 Weeks | 6 Months | 8 Months | 12 Months

NORMAL MYELINATION

Key Facts

Terminology
- Organized and predetermined pattern of development and distribution of myelin sheaths on axons
- Begins in 5th fetal month and continues throughout life

Imaging Findings
- Best diagnostic clue: Myelin development correlates with functional milestones
- Location: Myelin maturation proceeds caudal to rostral, central to peripheral, dorsal to ventral
- Gray-white differentiation is accentuated in neonate due to high water content of white matter
- Inversion recovery (IR) technique can accentuate T1 shortening of myelin
- Use both T1WI and T2WI to assess myelination

- T1WI under 12 months
- T2WI from 12-24 months
- Conventional double spin-echo sequences preferred for T2WI
- PD/Intermediate echo images especially valuable < 24 months

Clinical Issues
- Age: All children should achieve adult appearance of WM by 36-40 months

Diagnostic Checklist
- Know gestational age before assigning myelination stage

- Optic radiations become more apparent
- Peripheral rami in pyramidal tracts (perirolandic gyri)
  - 6 months
    - Genu and splenium are equally hyperintense
    - Peripheral rami in parietal and occipital lobes become hyperintense
  - 8 months
    - All but most peripheral rami of frontal gyri are hyperintense
  - 10-12 months
    - Adult appearance of myelin achieved on T1WI
- T2WI
  - T2WI is key sequence in assessing normal myelination in children 1-2 years
  - As myelin sheaths tighten peri-axonal water is displaced
    - Hypointense signal on T2WI
  - This process is delayed relative to changes seen on T1WI, but follows same pattern
  - Neonate has hypointense signal in
    - Dorsal brainstem
    - Part of posterior limb of internal capsule
    - Perirolandic gyri
  - 4 months
    - More hypointense signal in rolandic and perirolandic gyri
    - Splenium of corpus callosum
    - More anterior extension in internal capsule
  - 8 months
    - Genu and splenium of corpus callosum
    - Anterior limb of internal capsule
    - Decreasing signal in centrum semiovale and optic radiations
    - Decreasing signal in basal ganglia and thalamus
  - 12 months
    - External capsule hypointense signal becomes apparent
    - Expansion of centrum semiovale hypointensity
    - Clearly defined peripheral rami around central sulcus and in occipital poles
  - 16 months
    - Better definition of deep nuclei in brainstem and basal ganglia
    - Peripheral rami in parietal lobes become hypointense
  - 18 months
    - All but most peripheral frontal white matter rami are now hypointense
    - Some residual hyperintense signal around trigones of lateral ventricles; "terminal zones"
  - 36 months
    - Adult appearance of myelin achieved on T2WI
- PD/Intermediate
  - Very helpful in distinguishing gliosis from lack of myelination
    - Gliosis appears more hyperintense on PD/Intermediate than normal unmyelinated white matter
    - Brighter than "terminal zones"
- FLAIR
  - FLAIR generates relatively "flat" images in immature brains
  - Signal changes associated with myelination (hyperintense to hypointense) similar to T2WI
  - Tend to occur 2-3 months after changes visible on T2WI
    - Smaller amounts of interaxonal water may exert greater influence on FLAIR sequences
- DWI
  - ADC values predate T1 and T2 weighted signal changes
  - Presence of myelin has significant effect on ability of water to diffuse
    - Fractional anisotropy increases with brain maturation
    - Diffusion perpendicular to myelin sheaths is restricted with decline in extra-axonal water
    - Diffusivity along the axon increases
  - Diffusion tractography (DTI) has capability to identify fiber tracts as they become myelinated
    - Correlate with functional milestones
    - May allow more specific identification of developing functional tracts

NORMAL MYELINATION

- MRS
  - Changes in relative metabolite concentrations in first two years of life may reflect myelination
  - Myoinositol and choline are high in neonate
    - Choline declines with myelination
  - NAA increases with myelination in the first year of life

Ultrasonographic Findings
- Grayscale Ultrasound: White matter becomes more echogenic as myelination progresses

Other Modality Findings
- Magnetization transfer increases with brain myelination

Imaging Recommendations
- Best imaging tool
  - Use both T1WI and T2WI to assess myelination
    - T1WI under 12 months
    - T2WI from 12-24 months
- Protocol advice
  - IR may increase sensitivity to T1 shortening
  - FSE sequences may minimize abnormal hyperintensity
  - Conventional double spin-echo sequences preferred for T2WI
    - PD/Intermediate echo images especially valuable < 24 months

PATHOLOGY

General Features
- General path comments
  - Oligodendrocytes form, maintain axon myelin sheath
  - One oligodendrocyte may invest up to 50 axons
- Genetics
  - Two major structural proteins of myelin are myelin basic protein (MBP) and proteolipid protein (PLP)
    - MBP gene is encoded on chromosome 18q
    - PLP gene is encoded on chromosome Xq21-q22
- Etiology
  - Embryology
    - Oligodendrocyte precursors proliferate in germinal matrix
    - Neuron induces myelinization by electrical impulse

Gross Pathologic & Surgical Features
- Pre-myelinated brain "soft" due to high water content

Microscopic Features
- Myelin sheath formed of multiple layers wrapped around axon
  - Form a protein-lipid-protein-lipid-protein stack

Staging, Grading or Classification Criteria
- Myelination is assessed as "appropriate" for age or delayed
- Delay in myelination should prompt investigation for possible causes

CLINICAL ISSUES

Presentation
- Most common signs/symptoms
  - MR demonstration of normal myelination closely parallels developmental functional milestones
  - Assessment of myelination is an essential aspect of MR in children
    - Analogous to documentation of developmental milestones by pediatrician

Demographics
- Age: All children should achieve adult appearance of WM by 36-40 months
- Gender: No significant male/female difference

Natural History & Prognosis
- Myelination progresses throughout life

Treatment
- Acquired disorders causing myelin delay can sometimes be treated

DIAGNOSTIC CHECKLIST

Consider
- Know gestational age before assigning myelination stage

Image Interpretation Pearls
- Use IR for T1WI < 10 months
- Use conventional double spin-echo sequences for T2WI

SELECTED REFERENCES

1. Jellison BJ et al: Diffusion tensor imaging of cerebral white matter: A pictorial review of physics, fiber tract anatomy, and tumor imaging patterns. AJNR. 25:356-69, 2004
2. McGraw P et al: Evaluation of normal age-related changes in anisotropy during infancy and childhood as shown by diffusion tensor imaging. AJR Am J Roentgenol. 179(6):1515-22, 2002
3. Mukherjee P et al: Diffusion-tensor MR imaging of gray and white matter development during normal human brain maturation. AJNR Am J Neuroradiol. 23(9):1445-56, 2002
4. Barkovich AJ: Concepts of myelin and myelination in neuroradiology. AJNR. 21:1099-1109, 2000
5. Murakami JW et al: Normal myelination of the pediatric brain imaged with fluid-attenuated inversion-recovery (FLAIR) MR imaging. AJNR Am J Neuroradiol. 20(8):1406-11, 1999
6. Nakagawa H et al: Normal myelination of anatomic nerve fiber bundles: MR analysis. AJNR. 19: 1129-36, 1998
7. Van der Knaap MS, Valk J: Chapter 1 Myelin and white matter. In: Magnetic resonance of myelin, myelination, and myelin disorders, 2nd ed. Springer, Berlin, 1-17, 1995

NORMAL MYELINATION

IMAGE GALLERY

Typical

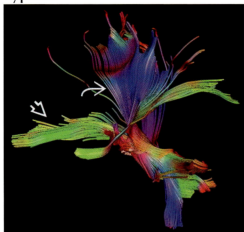
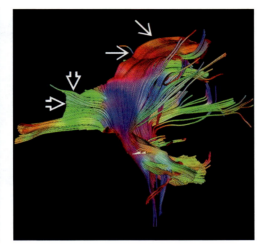

(Left) Sagittal oblique diffusion tractography in a 3 month old shows anterior-posterior oriented fibers in green (open arrow) and vertical fibers in blue (curved arrow). *(Right)* Sagittal oblique tractography at 8 months with same color scheme shows interval development of additional frontal lobe anterior-posterior (open arrows) and red transverse tracts (arrows).

Typical

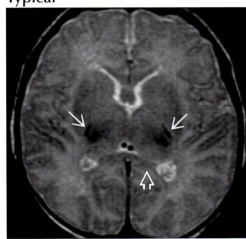
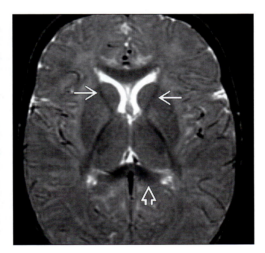

(Left) Axial T2WI MR in a normal neonate shows hypointense signal in dorsal limbs of internal capsules only (arrows). Note how thin splenium appears (open arrow). *(Right)* Axial T2WI MR at 8 months shows hypointense signal in myelinated anterior limb of internal capsule (arrows) and thickening of splenium (open arrow). No evidence of myelin in frontal gyri.

Typical

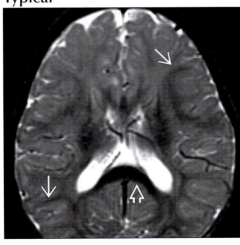
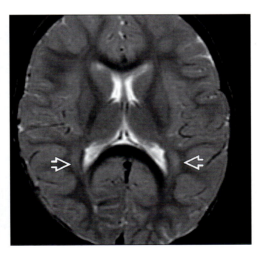

(Left) Axial T2WI MR at 12 months shows peripheral extension of hypointense signal in parietal greater than frontal lobes (arrows). Splenium now appears mature (open arrow). *(Right)* Axial T2WI MR at 18 months shows near-adult degree of myelin maturation. Bright signal in peri-trigonal WM (arrows) reflects incomplete compaction and prominent centripetal cerebrospinal fluid flow.

HYDROCEPHALUS

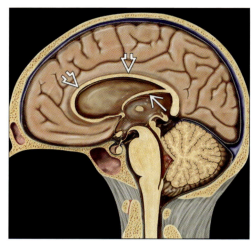

Sagittal graphic shows enlargement of 3rd and lateral ventricles with normal-sized 4th ventricle. Note exaggerated convexity of fornix (arrow) and the thinned corpus callosum (open arrows).

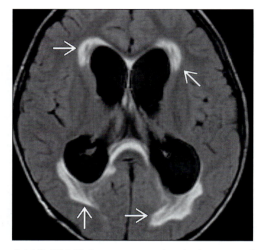

Axial FLAIR MR shows transependymal edema around the margins of the frontal and occipital horns (arrows) in this child with an obstructing fourth ventricle tumor.

TERMINOLOGY

Abbreviations and Synonyms
- Obstructive hydrocephalus, intraventricular obstructive hydrocephalus (IVOH)
- Communicating hydrocephalus, external hydrocephalus, extraventricular obstructive hydrocephalus (EVOH)

Definitions
- Excess volume of intracranial cerebrospinal fluid (CSF)
  o Due to obstruction of CSF flow within ventricular system IVOH
  o Due to decreased resorption into dural sinuses EVOH
  o Due to overproduction ⇒ controversial
- Ventriculomegaly does not equal hydrocephalus!

IMAGING FINDINGS

General Features
- Best diagnostic clue
  o IVOH ⇒ enlarged ventricles with decreased extra-axial spaces
  o EVOH ⇒ enlarged ventricles with enlarged extra-axial spaces
  o In children with open sutures, hydrocephalus always causes macrocrania
  o In children with closed sutures, hydrocephalus always causes increased intracranial pressure (ICP)
  o Open sutures may limit compression of extra-axial spaces
    ▪ Macrocrania compensates for increasing volume without increasing pressure
- Location
  o IVOH ⇒ obstructing lesions at key points in ventricular system
    ▪ Foramen of Monro: Subependymal giant cell astrocytoma, colloid cyst
    ▪ Posterior 3rd ventricle: Pineal germinoma
    ▪ Cerebral aqueduct: Tectal glioma, aqueductal stenosis
    ▪ Fourth ventricle: Medulloblastoma, cerebellar pilocytic astrocytoma
    ▪ "Trapped" temporal horn by mass effect on trigone
  o EVOH ⇒ obstruction at level of arachnoid granulations
    ▪ Prior intracranial hemorrhage (ICH) or meningitis
    ▪ Elevated pressure in venous sinuses
- Size: Ventriculomegaly does not equal hydrocephalus!
- Morphology
  o As ventricles enlarge, they lose angular margins
    ▪ Frontal horns and third ventricle become rounder

DDx: Complications Of Ventriculoperitoneal Shunts

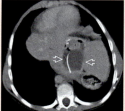
Pseudocyst

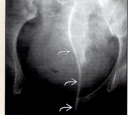
Erosion Into Rectum

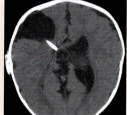
Intracranial Leak

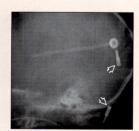
Disconnection

HYDROCEPHALUS

Key Facts

Terminology
- Excess volume of intracranial cerebrospinal fluid (CSF)
- Due to obstruction of CSF flow within ventricular system IVOH
- Due to decreased resorption into dural sinuses EVOH
- Ventriculomegaly does not equal hydrocephalus!

Imaging Findings
- Trigones enlarge first when lateral ventricles obstructed
- Shunt series is mainstay of evaluating integrity of ventricular drainage systems
- Isotope cisternography can show intraventricular reflux and delayed isotope resorption in EVOH
- NECT is most repeatable, efficient, and consistent means of evaluating ventricle size

Top Differential Diagnoses
- Benign macrocrania
- A self-limited form of EVOH common in children 6-24 months of age
- Shunt malfunction

Pathology
- Epidemiology: Most common neurosurgical procedure in children = CSF shunting for hydrocephalus
- Associated abnormalities: Common sequela of congenital brain malformations

Diagnostic Checklist
- Always correlate ventriculomegaly with head circumference measurements

---

- ○ LaPlace law applies ⇒ as pressure increases, regions with larger radius are under more tension and preferentially dilate
  - Trigones enlarge first when lateral ventricles obstructed

Radiographic Findings
- Shunt series is mainstay of evaluating integrity of ventricular drainage systems
  - ○ Anteroposterior (AP) and lateral skull, AP chest, and AP abdomen radiographs

CT Findings
- NECT
  - ○ Enlarged and rounded ventricles
  - ○ Periventricular halo of low attenuation ⇒ transependymal edema
  - ○ Basal cisterns and sulci compressed in IVOH
  - ○ Basal cisterns and sulci enlarged in EVOH
- CECT: May help show subarachnoid vessels in enlarged extra-axial spaces in EVOH

MR Findings
- T1WI
  - ○ Enlarged and rounded ventricles
  - ○ Corpus callosum thinned, stretched upward
  - ○ Optic recess of 3rd ventricle herniated into expanded sella
  - ○ Bright signal in frontal horns or posterior third ventricle may reflect pulsatile CSF flow
- T2WI
  - ○ Morphologic findings like T1WI
  - ○ Transependymal edema
    - Hyperintense "stain" spreading from acute ventricular margins
    - Accentuated at corners, minimized at lateral walls
    - May reduce or resolve in chronic obstruction (compensated)
- FLAIR: Best modality for showing transependymal edema
- MRV
  - ○ Dural sinus thrombosis can cause EVOH
    - More likely to cause pseudotumor cerebri
- MR Cine
  - ○ Ideal for demonstrating patency of 3rd ventriculostomy defects
    - Third ventriculostomy ⇒ hole created in floor of third ventricle via ventriculoscope
    - Allows passage of CSF from 3rd ventricle into subarachnoid space

Ultrasonographic Findings
- Transcranial US ideal for identifying ventriculomegaly in infants with macrocrania and patent anterior fontanelle
- Clearly distinguishes enlarged extra-axial spaces as subarachnoid or subdural

Nuclear Medicine Findings
- Isotope cisternography can show intraventricular reflux and delayed isotope resorption in EVOH

Other Modality Findings
- Contrast-enhanced ventriculography (CT or MR) can identify webs and other subtle obstructing lesions

Imaging Recommendations
- Best imaging tool
  - ○ NECT is most repeatable, efficient, and consistent means of evaluating ventricle size
  - ○ Fast and motion-reducing MR sequences may replace CT
    - No radiation
    - Less well tolerated by non-sedated children
  - ○ Cine MR invaluable for assessing CSF flow through regions of interest
  - ○ Nuclear medicine cisternography required for diagnosis of communicating hydrocephalus (EVOH)
- Protocol advice
  - ○ All CT studies must be acquired at consistent levels and angles
  - ○ Cardiac-gated phase-contrast cine MR

HYDROCEPHALUS

DIFFERENTIAL DIAGNOSIS

Benign macrocrania
- A self-limited form of EVOH common in children 6-24 months of age
- Large-headed child with large-headed parents
- Head circumference measurements abnormal, but parallel normal growth curve
- No associated symptoms

Ventriculomegaly from parenchymal volume loss
- Diffuse enlargement of sulci, cisterns
- Normal to small head circumference
- Thickened cranium with closed sutures (chronic)

Choroid plexus papilloma (CPP)
- Usually located in the trigones of the lateral ventricles
- Said to "over-produce" CSF
- More frequently obstruction from tumor or associated hemorrhage

Hemimegalencephaly
- Causes increase in volume of parenchyma and ventricle on same side
- Gray matter is dysplastic and thickened

Shunt malfunction
- Kinked or disrupted catheter tubing
  - In head, soft tissue of neck, thorax, abdomen
  - Intracranial cracks can cause pseudocysts in brain
- Faulty or misapplied valve
  - Pressure too high, facing wrong direction
- Pseudocyst around distal tubing
  - US ideal modality to show pseudocysts
- Erosion of distal tube into viscus
  - May precipitate meningitis
- Occluded proximal catheter
  - More common in former premature infants

PATHOLOGY

General Features
- General path comments: Large ventricles without loss/dysgenesis of brain tissue
- Genetics: Cell adhesion molecule L1 (L1CAM) located on X chromosome (Xq28)
- Etiology
  - CSF comes from two sources
    - Produced by choroid
    - Seeps into ventricles from interstitium
  - Migrates from ventricles into subarachnoid spaces
  - Transported into dural sinuses via arachnoid granulations
    - Energy-dependent active transport
  - Obstruction or failure at any point causes hydrocephalus
  - Inflammatory processes can render arachnoid granulations impaired
    - ICH, meningitis
- Epidemiology: Most common neurosurgical procedure in children = CSF shunting for hydrocephalus
- Associated abnormalities: Common sequela of congenital brain malformations

Gross Pathologic & Surgical Features
- Ependyma and adjacent white matter secondarily injured

Microscopic Features
- Ependymal lining damaged or lost

CLINICAL ISSUES

Presentation
- Most common signs/symptoms: Macrocrania, headache, papilledema
- Other signs/symptoms: Nausea, irritability, seizures

Demographics
- Age
  - All ages
  - Tectal gliomas typically present in school-age or older children
    - CSF diversion may be only treatment necessary
- Gender
  - Both genders affected
  - Some congenital causes or tumors are gender biased (x-linked aqueductal stenosis, germinoma)

Natural History & Prognosis
- Typically fatal if untreated and sutures closed
- Untreated hydrocephalus may become compensated
- Massive macrocrania can result if begins when sutures are open

Treatment
- CSF diversion (shunt), third ventriculostomy, septation fenestration

DIAGNOSTIC CHECKLIST

Consider
- Consider MR for routine assessment to reduce life-long radiation dose to patients with shunts
- Tectal glioma can be very subtle on CT
  - Use MR to evaluate unexplained lateral and third ventriculomegaly

Image Interpretation Pearls
- Always correlate ventriculomegaly with head circumference measurements
- Size of ventricles generally correlates poorly with intracranial pressure
- Pulsatile CSF may create confusing signal intensity, even mimic intraventricular mass
- Ventricular asymmetry is normal

SELECTED REFERENCES
1. Grunert P et al: The role of third ventriculostomy in the management of obstructive hydrocephalus. Minim Invasive Neurosurg. 46(1):16-21, 2003
2. Joseph VB et al: MR ventriculography for the study of CSF flow. AJNR Am J Neuroradiol. 24(3):373-81, 2003

HYDROCEPHALUS

IMAGE GALLERY

Typical

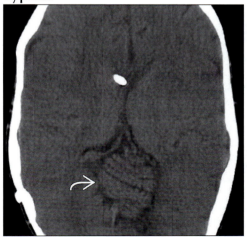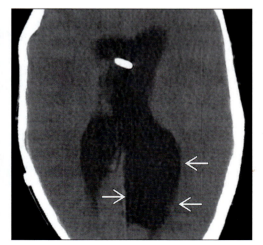

(Left) Axial NECT in a child with shunted hydrocephalus as a consequence of Chiari I malformation shows slit-like morphology of lateral ventricles at baseline. Note towering cerebellum *(arrow)*. *(Right)* Axial NECT in the same patient shows marked enlargement of the lateral ventricles with stable catheter position. Note preferential enlargement of trigone *(arrows)*.

Typical

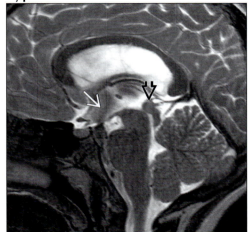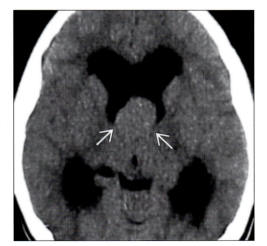

(Left) Sagittal T2WI MR shows a "jet" of CSF flow *(arrow)* through 3rd ventriculostomy defect connecting 3rd ventricle and pre-pontine cistern. Open arrow points to tectal glioma causing IVOH. *(Right)* Axial NECT shows hyperdense colloid cyst *(arrows)* at foramen of Monro causing bilateral ventricular enlargement.

Variant

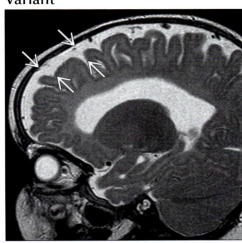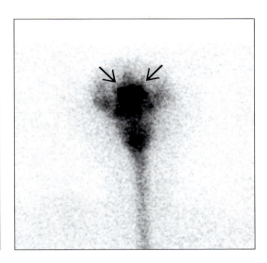

(Left) Sagittal T2WI MR shows enlarged extra-axial spaces *(arrows)* and lateral ventricle in an asymptomatic child with enlarged head circumference. Benign macrocrania. *(Right)* Anteroposterior view from cisternogram 4 hours after injection of isotope in a teenager with EVOH from trauma shows reflux into lateral ventricles *(arrows)*. Prominent and persistent reflux is typical of EVOH.

NASAL DERMAL SINUS

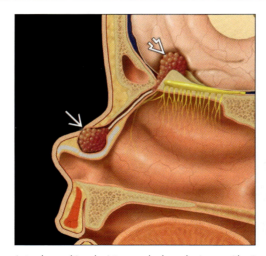

Lateral graphic depicts nasal dermal sinus with 2 dermoids. Extracranial dermoid is present just below nasal pit (arrow). Intracranial dermoid (open arrow) splits bifid crista galli.

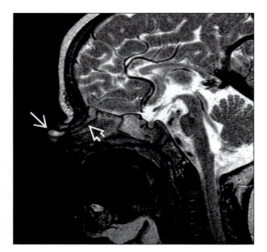

Sagittal T2WI MR shows small hyperintense subcutaneous nasal mass (arrow) with a small tract (open arrow) leading to the region of the foramen cecum in a child with nasal dermoid.

TERMINOLOGY

Abbreviations and Synonyms
- Abbreviation: Nasal dermal sinus (NDS)
- Synonyms: Nasal dermoid sinus; nasal dermoid sinus cyst; anterior neuropore anomaly

Definitions
- NDS: Defective embryogenesis of anterior neuropore resulting in any mixture of dermoid, epidermoid ± sinus tract in frontonasal region

IMAGING FINDINGS

General Features
- Best diagnostic clue
  - Bone CT: Bifid crista galli with large foramen cecum
  - Sagittal T1 MR: Focal low signal (epidermoid or dermoid) or high signal (dermoid) mass found between tip of nose & apex of crista galli
- Location: Epidermoid or dermoid seen from nose tip to apex of crista galli
- Size: 5 mm to 2 cm dermoid or epidermoid
- Morphology: Ovoid mass ± tubular sinus tract

CT Findings
- NECT
  - Bone CT indirect signs of intracranial extension
    - Large foramen cecum with bifid or deformed crista galli
    - Cribriform plate deformity also suggests intracranial extension
  - NECT findings of epidermoid-dermoid
    - Focal mass (epidermoid or dermoid) within or deep to nasal bridge or along sinus tract to crista galli
    - Fluid density mass = epidermoid (or dermoid)
    - Fat density mass = dermoid

MR Findings
- T1WI
  - Sagittal may show epidermoid or dermoid as focal mass from tip of nose to apex of crista galli
    - Fluid intensity mass = epidermoid (or dermoid)
    - Fat intensity mass = dermoid
    - Intracranial mass is seen in region of foramen cecum in a minority of patients
- T2WI
  - Focal high signal if epidermoid/dermoid present
  - If sinus tract associated, tract seen passing from tip of nose through enlarged foramen cecum on sagittal MR
- DWI
  - Focal area of diffusion restriction (high signal) if epidermoid present

DDx: Anterior Neuropore Area Lesions

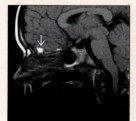
Fatty Marrow CG

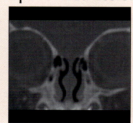
Normal FC 8 Mo

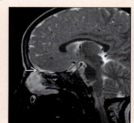
Meningocele

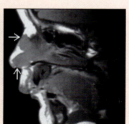
Nasal Glioma

NASAL DERMAL SINUS

Key Facts

Terminology
- Synonyms: Nasal dermoid sinus; nasal dermoid sinus cyst; anterior neuropore anomaly
- NDS: Defective embryogenesis of anterior neuropore resulting in any mixture of dermoid, epidermoid ± sinus tract in frontonasal region

Imaging Findings
- Bone CT: Bifid crista galli with large foramen cecum
- Thin-section MR imaging focused to frontonasal area best delineates underlying pathology

Top Differential Diagnoses
- Fatty marrow in crista galli (CG)
- Non-ossified foramen cecum (FC)
- Nasofrontal or nasoethmoidal cephalocele
- Nasal glioma

Pathology
- Failure of involution of neuropore in 4th gestational week may leave neuroectoderm along tract of dural stalk
- Dermoid or epidermoid alone or in concert with nasal dermal tract
- 80% have no intracranial extension

Clinical Issues
- Clinical Profile: Child (mean age = 32 months) with nasal pit ± nasoglabellar mass

Diagnostic Checklist
- Nasoglabellar mass or pit on nose sends clinician in search of NDS with intracranial extension
- Beware! Foramen cecum closes postnatally in first 5 years of life

---

  - Susceptibility artifacts at skull base may obscure signal from epidermoid

Imaging Recommendations
- Imaging "sweet spot" is small & anterior
  - Focus imaging from tip of nose to back of crista galli
  - Inferior end of axial imaging is hard palate
- Thin-section MR imaging focused to frontonasal area best delineates underlying pathology
  - Sagittal plane important
  - Axial & coronal 3 mm thick T1 & T2 sequences needed
  - Contrast does not help make or delineate this diagnosis
  - DWI imaging important additional sequence
- If intracranial extension, add NECT
  - Thin-section (1-2 mm) bone & soft tissue axial & coronal CT nasofrontal region region

DIFFERENTIAL DIAGNOSIS

Fatty marrow in crista galli (CG)
- No nasoglabellar mass or pit on nose
- CT & MR otherwise normal

Non-ossified foramen cecum (FC)
- Closes postnatally in first 5 years of life
- Crista galli not deformed or bifid
- If nasal dermoid present, may mistakenly suggest intracranial extension

Nasofrontal or nasoethmoidal cephalocele
- Bone dehiscence is larger, involving a broader area of midline cribriform plate or frontal bone
- Direct extension of meninges, subarachnoid space ± brain can be seen projecting into cephalocele on sagittal MR

Nasal glioma
- Solid mass of glial tissue separated from brain by subarachnoid space & meninges
- Most commonly found projecting extranasally into paramedian bridge of nose

- Less commonly in anterior nasal septum

PATHOLOGY

General Features
- General path comments
  - Embryology-anatomy: Normal development of anterior neuropore
    - Dural stalk passes from area of future foramen cecum to area of osteocartilaginous nasal junction, then regresses completely
    - Failure of involution creates anterior neuropore anomalies
  - Anterior neuropore anomaly = general term for anomalous anterior neuropore regression; 3 main types
    - Type 1: Nasal dermal sinus
    - Type 2: Anterior cephalocele
    - Type 3: Nasal glioma
- Genetics: Familial clustering
- Etiology
  - Failure of involution of neuropore in 4th gestational week may leave neuroectoderm along tract of dural stalk
  - Dermoid or epidermoid alone or in concert with nasal dermal tract
- Epidemiology
  - 80% have no intracranial extension
  - Intracranial extension of nasal dermal sinus seen in 20%
- Associated abnormalities: Craniofacial anomalies (15%)

Gross Pathologic & Surgical Features
- If sinus tract is present, tube of tissue can be followed through bones

Microscopic Features
- Nasal sinus tract is a midline epithelial-lined tract
- Epidermoid cyst contains desquamated epithelium
- Dermoid cyst contains epithelium, keratin debris, skin adnexa

CHOANAL ATRESIA

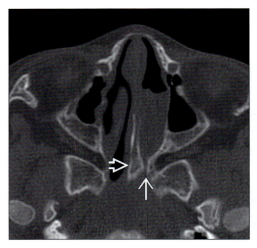

Axial NECT shows an enlarged vomer (open arrow) and thick posterior lateral wall of the nasal cavity nearly occluding the left choana (arrow).

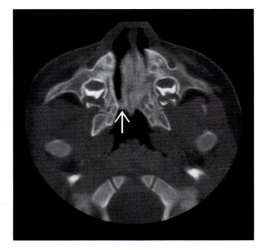

Axial shows bilateral choanal atresia with a large atretic bony plate occluding the left choana and majority of the nasal passage and a small bony bridge occluding the right choana (arrow).

TERMINOLOGY

Definitions
- Atresia of the posterior nasal cavity (choana)

IMAGING FINDINGS

General Features
- Best diagnostic clue: Narrowing of the posterior nasal cavity with medial bowing and thickening of the lateral wall of the nasal cavity and enlargement of the posterior portion of the vomer
- Location
  - Posterior nasal cavity (choana)
  - 50-60% unilateral, 40-50% bilateral (BL)
- Size
  - Choanal atresia
    - Choanal airspace < 0.34 cm in newborn
    - Vomer > 0.34 cm in children less than 8 years
  - Normal mean width of posterior choanal air space
    - Newborns 0.67 cm (+/- 2 SD = 0.34 - 1.01 cm)
    - 6 years is 0.86 cm (+/- 2 SD = 0.53 - 1.19 cm)
    - 16 years 1.13 cm (+/- 2 SD = 0.79 - 1.46 cm)
  - Normal vomer width
    - Children less than 8 years of age usually less than 0.23 cm, should not exceed 0.34 cm
    - Children over 8 years of age 0.28 cm, should not exceed 0.55 cm
- Morphology
  - Purely bony atresia in 29%
  - Mixed bony-membranous malformation in 71%
  - Purely membranous rare, true existence disputed by some authors
  - Older literature bony 90%, membranous 10%

CT Findings
- NECT
  - Thin-section axial bone CT
    - Narrowing of posterior choanae < 0.34 cm in newborn
    - Medial bowing and thickening of the posterior medial maxilla which may be fused with lateral margin of vomer
    - Thickening of vomer
    - Membranes may be thin or thick
    - Retained fluid in nasal cavity

Imaging Recommendations
- Best imaging tool: High-resolution unenhanced bone CT
- Protocol advice
  - Suction secretions and apply topical nasal vasoconstriction agents prior to scan
  - Supine 1-1.5 mm contiguous axial images through nasopharynx

DDx: Nasal Obstruction In Infants

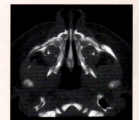

CNPAS

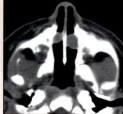

BL NLD Mucoceles

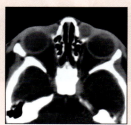

BL NLD Mucoceles

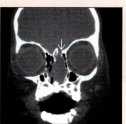

Nasal Cephalocele

CHOANAL ATRESIA

Key Facts

Terminology
- Atresia of the posterior nasal cavity (choana)

Imaging Findings
- Best diagnostic clue: Narrowing of the posterior nasal cavity with medial bowing and thickening of the lateral wall of the nasal cavity and enlargement of the posterior portion of the vomer
- 50-60% unilateral, 40-50% bilateral (BL)
- Choanal airspace < 0.34 cm in newborn
- Vomer > 0.34 cm in children less than 8 years
- Purely bony atresia in 29%
- Mixed bony-membranous malformation in 71%

Top Differential Diagnoses
- Congenital nasal pyriform aperture stenosis (CNPAS)
- Nasolacrimal duct (NLD) mucocele
- Nasoethmoid cephalocele
- Nasal dermoid

Pathology
- Most common congenital abnormality of nasal cavity
- 75% with bilateral atresia have other congenital anomalies

Clinical Issues
- Bilateral choanal atresia: Severe respiratory distress with cyanosis in newborn
- Unilateral choanal atresia: Chronic purulent rhinorrhea, mild airway symptoms in older child

---

- o Imaging plane parallel or 5-10 degrees cephalad to hard palate
- o High-resolution, edge-enhancement bone filters
- o Multiplanar reformations as needed
- o 3D volume rendering techniques at times helpful in clinical decision making

DIFFERENTIAL DIAGNOSIS

Congenital nasal pyriform aperture stenosis (CNPAS)
- Clinical: Obstructed nasal inlet (pyriform aperture)
- Axial bone CT appearance
  - o Thickened anteromedial maxilla
  - o Narrowing of anterior & inferior nasal passage
  - o Small triangular shaped hard palate
- Isolated or in association with other anomalies
  - o Solitary central maxillary incisor
  - o Holoprosencephaly
  - o Hypopituitarism
  - o Chromosomal deletion short arm of chromosome 18

Nasolacrimal duct (NLD) mucocele
- Round, cystic masses in inferior meatus
- Enlargement of nasolacrimal canal which houses nasolacrimal duct
- Cystic enlargement of lacrimal sac
- Unilateral or bilateral

Nasoethmoid cephalocele
- Associated findings
  - o Extension of mass through bony defect in cribriform plate

Nasal dermoid
- Associated findings
  - o Bifid crista galli
  - o Large foramen cecum

PATHOLOGY

General Features
- General path comments
  - o 50-60% unilateral
  - o Mixed bony-membranous (71%), bony atresias (29%)
- Genetics
  - o May be seen in isolation
  - o Familial form exists
- Etiology
  - o Proposed theories
    - Persistence of buccopharyngeal membrane or failure of bucconasal membrane to perforate
    - Mesodermal defect caused by faulty neural crest cell migration-best explains association with other craniofacial malformation
- Epidemiology
  - o Most common congenital abnormality of nasal cavity
  - o 1:5,000 to 10,000 live births
- Associated abnormalities
  - o 75% with bilateral atresia have other congenital anomalies
  - o CHARGE syndrome
    - Coloboma
    - Heart/cardiovascular anomalies
    - Atresia of choana
    - Retarded growth and development
    - Genital hypoplasia
    - Ear anomalies
  - o Other associated syndromes
    - Apert syndrome
    - Crouzon syndrome
    - de Lange syndrome
    - Fetal alcohol syndrome
    - Di George syndrome
    - Treacher-Collins syndrome
  - o Associated with chromosome 18, 12, 22, XO abnormalities

CHOANAL ATRESIA

Gross Pathologic & Surgical Features
- Membranous soft tissue or bony plate occludes choanal opening

CLINICAL ISSUES

Presentation
- Most common signs/symptoms
  - Bilateral choanal atresia: Severe respiratory distress with cyanosis in newborn
    - Aggravated by feeding
    - Relieved by crying
    - Infants are obligate nasal breathers up to 6 months of age
  - Unilateral choanal atresia: Chronic purulent rhinorrhea, mild airway symptoms in older child
    - Less than one year of age: Less severe airway and feeding issues than bilateral involvement
- Other signs/symptoms
  - Inability to pass nasoenteric tube through nasal cavity or absence of nasal mirror misting
  - Nasal stuffiness
  - Grunting, snorting, low-pitched stridor
- Clinical Profile
  - Bilateral: Infant with severe respiratory distress
  - Unilateral: Child with unilateral purulent rhinorrhea

Demographics
- Age
  - Bilateral atresia presents at birth
  - Unilateral choanal atresia may present in older child

Natural History & Prognosis
- Bilateral choanal atresia
  - Diagnosed and treated in newborn period
- Unilateral choanal atresia/stenosis
  - May present later in childhood
  - Once diagnosed, prognosis is excellent after surgical therapy
- Some patients prone to re-stenosis

Treatment
- Establish oral airway immediately to ensure proper breathing
- Membranous atresias may be perforated upon passage of nasoenteric tube
- Surgical correction of bilateral atresia performed as soon as possible after diagnosis
- Transnasal endoscopic approaches frequently used for simple membranous & bony atresias
  - May be combined with laser or stenting
- Bilateral bony atresias require transpalatal resection of vomer with choanal reconstruction
- Post-operative scar & incomplete resection of atresia plate best evaluated with bone CT

DIAGNOSTIC CHECKLIST

Consider
- Respiratory distress & nasal obstruction in newborn establish patent airway

- Thin-section axial bone CT is imaging modality of choice

Image Interpretation Pearls
- Determine unilateral or bilateral
- Describe as mixed bony-membranous, purely bony or rarely purely membranous
- Comment on thickness of bony atresia plate
- Look for any associated anomalies in head & neck

SELECTED REFERENCES

1. Koch BL: Case 73: Nasolacrimal duct mucocele. Radiology. 232(2):370-2, 2004
2. Samadi DS et al: Choanal atresia: a twenty-year review of medical comorbidities and surgical outcomes. Laryngoscope. 113(2):254-8, 2003
3. Triglia JM et al: Choanal atresia: therapeutic management and results in a series of 58 children. Rev Laryngol Otol Rhinol. 124(3):139-43, 2003
4. Holzmann D et al: Unilateral choanal atresia: surgical technique and long-term results. J Laryngol Otol. 116(8):601-4, 2002
5. Sanlaville D et al: A CGH study of 27 patients with CHARGE association. Clin Genet. 61(2):135-8, 2002
6. Van Den Abbeele T et al: Transnasal endoscopic treatment of choanal atresia without prolonged stenting. Arch Otolaryngol Head Neck Surg. 128(8):936-40, 2002
7. Vanzieleghem BD et al: Imaging studies in the diagnostic workup of neonatal nasal obstruction. J Comput Assist Tomogr. 25(4):540-9, 2001
8. Behar PM et al: Paranasal sinus development and choanal atresia. Arch Otolaryngol Head Neck Surg. 126(2):155-7, 2000
9. Keller JL et al: Choanal atresia, CHARGE association, and congenital nasal stenosis. Otolaryngol Clin North Am. 33(6):1343-51, viii, 2000
10. Lowe LH et al: Midface anomalies in children. Radiographics. 20(4):907-22; quiz 1106-7, 1112, 2000
11. Park AH et al: Endoscopic versus traditional approaches to choanal atresia. Otolaryngol Clin North Am. 33(1):77-90, 2000
12. Garabedian EN et al: Nasal fossa malformations and paramedian facial cleft: new perspectives. J Craniofac Genet Dev Biol. 19(1):12-9, 1999
13. Black CM et al: Potential pitfalls in the work-up and diagnosis of choanal atresia. AJNR Am J Neuroradiol. 19(2):326-9, 1998
14. Sadek SA: Congenital bilateral choanal atresia. Int J Pediatr Otorhinolaryngol. 42(3):247-56, 1998
15. Brown OE et al: Choanal atresia: a new anatomic classification and clinical management applications. Laryngoscope. 106(1 Pt 1):97-101, 1996
16. Rand PK et al: Congenital nasolacrimal mucoceles: CT evaluation. Radiology. 173(3):691-4, 1989
17. Ey EH et al: Bony inlet stenosis as a cause of nasal airway obstruction. Radiology. 168(2):477-9, 1988
18. Slovis TL et al: Choanal atresia: precise CT evaluation. Radiology. 155(2):345-8, 1985
19. Hengerer AS et al: Choanal atresia: a new embryologic theory and its influence on surgical management. Laryngoscope. 92(8 Pt 1):913-21, 1982
20. Pagon RA et al: Coloboma, congenital heart disease, and choanal atresia with multiple anomalies: CHARGE association. J Pediatr. 99(2):223-7, 1981

CHOANAL ATRESIA

IMAGE GALLERY

Typical

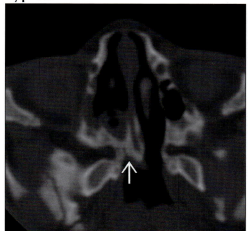
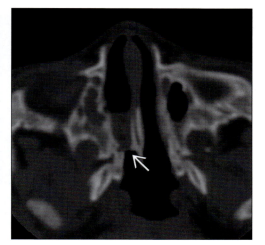

(Left) Axial NECT shows thick posterior wall of the right nasal cavity and vomer with a small bony bridge occluding the superior aspect of the right choana *(arrow)*. The left choana is patent. *(Right)* Axial NECT shows mixed bony-membranous occlusion of the right choana *(arrow)* 3 mm more inferior than the image on the left in the same patient.

Typical

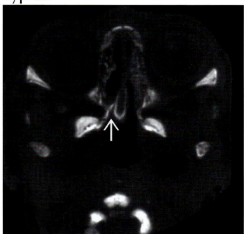
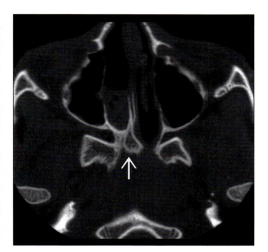

(Left) Axial NECT shows right choanal obstruction by a small bony bridge *(arrow)* and enlarged vomer. *(Right)* Axial NECT shows occlusion of the right choana *(arrow)* with bony atresia and an air-fluid level in the right nasal passage.

Variant

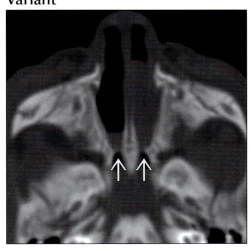
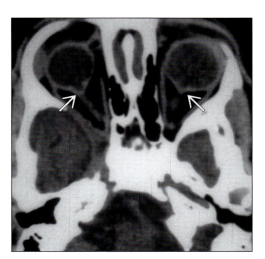

(Left) Axial NECT shows bilateral membranous atresia *(arrows)*, complete opacification of the left nasal cavity and air-fluid level in the right nasal cavity. *(Right)* Axial NECT shows conical protrusions at the posterior aspect of both globes *(arrows)* consistent with coloboma in a child with bilateral choanal atresia and CHARGE syndrome.

OTIC CAPSULE DYSPLASIAS

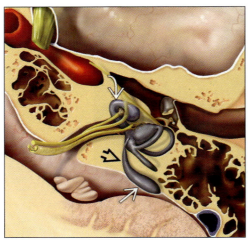

Axial graphic shows large endolymphatic sac and duct, intracranial (arrow) and intraosseous (open arrow) components. Notice the associated mild cochlear dysplasia (curved arrow).

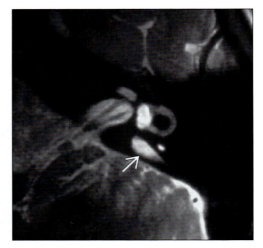

Axial T2WI MR shows magnified view of the left inner ear with large endolymphatic sac (arrow) in a patient with large endolymphatic sac anomaly.

TERMINOLOGY

Abbreviations and Synonyms
- Large vestibular aqueduct syndrome (LVAS)
- Large endolymphatic sac anomaly (LESA)
- Semicircular canal (SSC) dysplasia (SSCD)
- Sensorineural hearing loss (SNHL), conductive hearing loss (CHL)
- Vestibular aqueduct (VA), endolymphatic sac (ES), incomplete partition (IP)
- Cystic cochleovestibular (CCV) anomaly

Definitions
- Otic capsule dysplasia: Inner ear anomalies
  - Cochlea, vestibule, SSCs and VA
  - Most common: LVA and SSCD

IMAGING FINDINGS

General Features
- Best diagnostic clue
  - LESA/LVAS: MRI - large ES, CT - VA > than 1.5 mm midpoint
  - SSCD: Dilated lateral SCC and vestibule form single cavity - most common
- Location
  - LESA/LVAS: Posterior wall of temporal bone
    - ES: Intracranial and intraosseous components
    - Endolymphatic duct - short connection - vestibule (or crus commune) to intraosseous ES
  - SSCD: Membranous labyrinth
    - Nonsyndromic: Lateral SCC most often involved
- Size
  - LESA/LVAS
    - Visible ES on axial T2 MR: Top normal or enlarged
    - VA > 1.5 mm at midpoint abnormal on bone CT
  - SSCD: Short and dilated, hypoplastic or aplastic

CT Findings
- Bone CT
  - LESA/LVAS: Most common congenital anomaly on imaging studies in patients with SNHL
    - VA > 1.5 mm midway
    - Cochlear dysplasia with apical turn dysmorphism and modiolar deficiency
  - SSCD
    - Vestibule and dilated lateral SCC form single cavity: Most common
    - Posterior and superior SCC may be normal, dilated or hypoplastic, +/- ossicular anomalies and/or oval window atresia

DDx: Inner Ear Anomalies

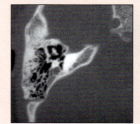
Inner Ear Aplasia

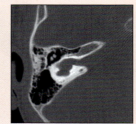
Cochlear Aplasia

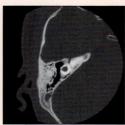
Otocyst

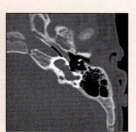
CCV Anomaly

OTIC CAPSULE DYSPLASIAS

Key Facts

Terminology
- Otic capsule dysplasia: Inner ear anomalies
- Cochlea, vestibule, SSCs and VA
- Most common: LVA and SSCD

Imaging Findings
- LESA/LVAS: MRI - large ES, CT - VA > than 1.5 mm midpoint
- SSCD: Dilated lateral SCC and vestibule form single cavity - most common
- Second most common form with CHARGE syndrome: Bilateral absence of all SCCs, small dysmorphic vestibule, oval window atresia (+/- overlying tympanic segment facial nerve), cochlear anomalies (isolated cochlea with lack of cochlear aperture most common)

Top Differential Diagnoses
- Labyrinthine aplasia
- Cochlea aplasia
- Common cavity deformity
- CCV anomaly = IP type I

Pathology
- Jackler classification congenital inner ear malformation: 1987

Diagnostic Checklist
- When see LESA/LVAS, check for associated cochlear dysplasia
- CHARGE syndrome expect findings of severe SCCD

- Second most common form with CHARGE syndrome: Bilateral absence of all SCCs, small dysmorphic vestibule, oval window atresia (+/- overlying tympanic segment facial nerve), cochlear anomalies (isolated cochlea with lack of cochlear aperture most common)

MR Findings
- LESA/LVAS
  - T2WI
    - High signal enlarged ES obvious
    - Associated cochlear dysplasia: Bulbous apical turn, modiolar deficiency or absence, scalar chamber asymmetry with anterior scala vestibuli larger than posterior
- SSCD
  - T2WI
    - Sporadic SCCD: Dilated vestibule and short, wide lateral SCC +/- mild dysplasia posterior and lateral SCC
    - Syndromic SCCD: All SCCs absent, small dysmorphic vestibule, isolated cochlea with dysplastic aperture (black bony bar across cochlear base and absent cochlear nerve)

Imaging Recommendations
- LESA/LVAS
  - Thin section axial CT (1 mm or 0.625 mm)
  - High resolution thin-section T2 MR: To detect modiolar deficiency and scalar chamber asymmetry
- SSCD
  - Thin-section CT best to identify SCCs
    - Axial and coronal to confirm oval window atresia
  - High resolution thin section T2 MR: To detect presence or absence of cochlear nerve

DIFFERENTIAL DIAGNOSIS

Labyrinthine aplasia
- Inner ear aplasia, old term Michel anomaly
- Complete absence of cochlea, vestibule and SCCs

Cochlea aplasia
- Absent cochlea with dysmorphic vestibule and SSCs

Common cavity deformity
- Cochlea/vestibule/SCC = single featureless cavity
  - SCC occasionally normal or dysplastic
- Persistent otocyst = very small featureless cavity

CCV anomaly = IP type I
- "Figure of 8" cystic cochlea and vestibule
- SCC normal, dilated and dysmorphic or absent

PATHOLOGY

General Features
- Genetics
  - LESA/LVAS
    - 15% have Pendrin gene mutation (SLC26A4) = Pendred syndrome
    - 85% no Pendrin gene mutation
  - SSCD may be part of genetic syndrome
    - CHARGE syndrome: Coloboma, heart anomaly, atresia of choana, retardation, genital hypoplasia, ear anomalies
    - Alagille (arteriohepatic dysplasia), Waardenburg, Crouzon (craniofacial dysostosis), Apert (acrocephalosyndactylism type I), Goldenhar syndromes
- Etiology
  - LESA/LVAS: Arrested inner ear development 7th week
    - SNHL hypothesis: Secondary to "fragile" cochlea susceptible to injury from mild trauma as a result of microscopic infrastructural deficiencies
  - SSCD: Arrest or insult at 6-8 weeks
    - Lateral SCC forms last, most commonly affected
- Associated abnormalities
  - LESA/LVAS
    - Cochlear dysplasia (75%): Often mild incomplete partitioning, more severe in Pendred syndrome
    - Vestibular and/or SCC anomalies (50%)

OTIC CAPSULE DYSPLASIAS

- ○ SSCD
  - +/- Labyrinthine aplasia, cochlear hypoplasia, common cavity deformity, mild cochlear dysplasia, oval window atresia, dehiscent and/or inferiorly displaced tympanic portion facial nerve canal or ossicular chain anomalies

Staging, Grading or Classification Criteria
- Sennaroglu classification of cochleovestibular malformations: 2002 (from severe to mild)
  - ○ Inner ear aplasia (Michel deformity): 3rd week arrest
  - ○ Cochlear aplasia: Late 3rd week arrest
  - ○ Common cavity: 4th week arrest
  - ○ CCV anomaly (IP type 1): 5th week arrest
  - ○ Cochlear hypoplasia: 6th week arrest
  - ○ LESA/LVA (IP type 2): 7th week arrest
- Jackler classification congenital inner ear malformation: 1987
  - ○ With an absent or malformed cochlea
    - Complete labyrinthine aplasia = Michel deformity
    - Cochlear aplasia: Normal or malformed vestibule and SCCs
    - Common cavity: Cochlea and vestibule form common cavity without internal architecture, normal or malformed SCCs
    - Incomplete partition: Small cochlea with incomplete or no interscalar septum, normal or malformed vestibule and SCCs
  - ○ With a normal cochlea
    - Vestibule-lateral SSCD
    - Enlarged VA with normal SCCS, normal or enlarged vestibule

CLINICAL ISSUES

Presentation
- Most common signs/symptoms
  - ○ LESA/LVAS
    - SNHL: Usually normal at birth, then deterioration
    - Fluctuating or "cascading" SNHL, often with post-traumatic decrease
    - Severe bilateral SNHL +/- goiter and/or hypothyroidism in Pendred syndrome
  - ○ SSCD
    - SNHL: Sporadic mild to profound, syndromic usually profound
    - CHL when oval window atresia and ossicular chain anomalies present

Natural History & Prognosis
- LESA/LVAS
  - ○ When bilateral, ultimately leads to severe SNHL
  - ○ Prognosis better when unilateral or late development of SNHL

Treatment
- LESA/LVAS
  - ○ No contact sports, limit "headers" in soccer, helmet for skiing, bicycling, skating, etc.
  - ○ Cochlear implant when bilateral and severe SNHL, best prognosis in postlingual deafness group
- SSCD: Bilateral syndromic may benefit from cochlear implant, unilateral sporadic no treatment

DIAGNOSTIC CHECKLIST

Image Interpretation Pearls
- When see LESA/LVAS, check for associated cochlear dysplasia
- CHARGE syndrome expect findings of severe SCCD

SELECTED REFERENCES

1. Naganawa S et al: Enlarged endolymphatic duct and sac syndrome: relationship between MR findings and genotype of mutation in Pendred syndrome gene. Magn Reson Imaging. 22(1):25-30, 2004
2. Madden C et al: Enlarged vestibular aqueductsyndrome in the pediatric population. Otol Neurotol. 24(4):625-32, 2003
3. Ceruti S et al: Temporal bone anomalies in the branchio-oto-renal syndrome: detailed computed tomographic and magnetic resonance imaging findings. Otol Neurotol. 23(2):200-7, 2002
4. Miyamoto RT et al: Cochlear implantation with large vestibular aqueduct syndrome. Laryngoscope. 112(7 Pt 1):1178-82, 2002
5. Naganawa S et al: Serial MR imaging studies in enlarged endolymphatic duct and sac syndrome. Eur Radiol. 12 Suppl 3:S114-7, 2002
6. Sennaroglu L et al: A new classification for cochleovestibular malformations. Laryngoscope. 112(12):2230-41, 2002
7. Benton C et al: Imaging of congenital anomalies of the temporal bone. Neuroimaging Clin N Am. 10(1):35-53, vii-viii, 2000
8. Pyle GM: Embryological development and large vestibular aqueduct syndrome. Laryngoscope. 110(11):1837-42, 2000
9. Davidson HC et al: MR evaluation of vestibulocochlear anomalies associated with large endolymphatic duct and sac. AJNR Am J Neuroradiol. 20(8):1435-41, 1999
10. Naganawa S et al: MR imaging of the cochlear modiolus: area measurement in healthy subjects and in patients with a large endolymphatic duct and sac. Radiology. 213(3):819-23, 1999
11. Phelps PD et al: Radiological malformations of the ear in Pendred syndrome. Clin Radiol. 53(4):268-73, 1998
12. Tong KA et al: Large vestibular aqueduct syndrome: a genetic disease? AJR Am J Roentgenol. 168(4):1097-101, 1997
13. Harnsberger HR et al: Advanced techniques in magnetic resonance imaging in the evaluation of the large endolymphatic duct and sac syndrome. Laryngoscope. 105(10):1037-42, 1995
14. Jackler RK et al: Congenital malformations of the inner ear: a classification based on embryogenesis. Laryngoscope. 97(40):2-14, 1987

OTIC CAPSULE DYSPLASIAS

IMAGE GALLERY

Typical

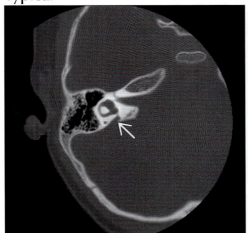
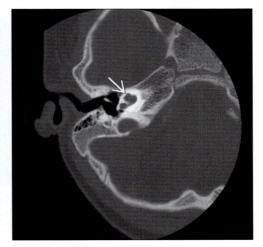

(Left) Axial bone CT shows enlarged bony vestibular aqueduct *(arrow)* in a patient with severe bilateral SNHL and left VA similar in size (not shown). *(Right)* Axial bone CT shows associated cochlear dysplasia with incomplete partitioning *(arrow)* in the same child with Pendred syndrome (2 copies Pendrin gene mutation).

Typical

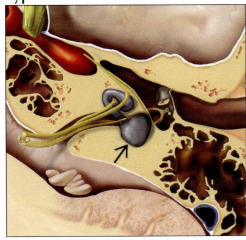
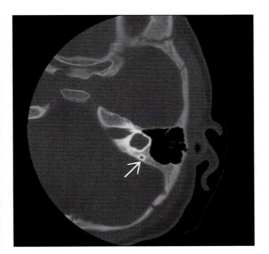

(Left) Axial graphic shows severe semicircular canal dysplasia with complete absence of all semicircular canals, cochlear dysplasia and dysmorphic, small vestibule *(arrow)*. *(Right)* Axial bone CT shows dilated vestibule fused to the lateral semicircular canal, lack of normal bone island in center of vestibule and hypoplastic posterior semicircular canal *(arrow)*.

Typical

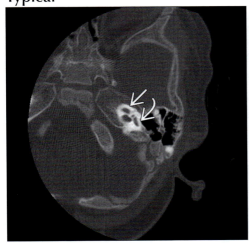
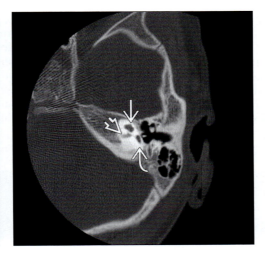

(Left) Axial bone CT shows hypoplastic, dysmorphic cochlea *(arrow)*, hypoplastic vestibule *(curved arrow)* with absent SCCs in a child with CHARGE syndrome. *(Right)* Axial bone CT shows small, dysplastic cochlea *(arrow)*, tiny vestibule *(curved arrow)*, hypoplastic IAC *(open arrow)* and absent semicircular canals in another child with CHARGE syndrome.

AURAL ATRESIA

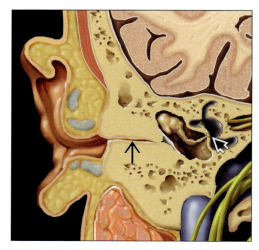

Coronal graphic of EAC shows deformed auricle & bony EAC atresia (arrow). Ossicular fusion & rotation with oval window atresia (open arrow) are also present.

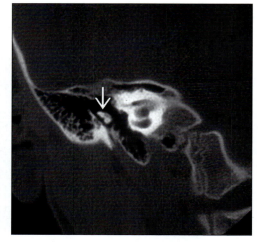

Coronal NECT shows atresia of the EAC with moderate size of middle ear cavity and mastoid air cells. Note dysmorphic appearance of the fused malleus and incus (arrow).

TERMINOLOGY

Abbreviations and Synonyms
- External auditory canal (EAC) atresia
- Congenital aural dysplasia (CAD)

Definitions
- Dysplasia of the outer ear (auricle and EAC)
  - Stenosis or atresia of EAC

IMAGING FINDINGS

General Features
- Best diagnostic clue: Soft tissue or bony atretic plate occluding the EAC where tympanic membrane (TM) should be
- Location
  - EAC, middle ear & mastoid complex
  - Inner ear spared in most cases
- Size: Stenosis usually extends from external opening of canal to tympanic membrane
- Morphology
  - Dysplastic auricle (microtia)
  - Mildest form has narrowed EAC
  - More severe has no identifiable EAC
  - Hypoplasia or underpneumatization of middle ear cavity & mastoid complex
  - Dysmorphic ossicular chain, especially malleus & incus
    - Hypoplastic, absent, abnormal joint or fusion to attic wall

CT Findings
- NECT
  - External ear & EAC
    - Small, dysmorphic pinna
    - Bony, soft tissue, or mixed stenosis/atresia of membranous and bony portions of EAC
    - Variable thickness of atretic plate
  - Middle ear findings depend on severity of atresia
    - Small middle ear cavity (especially hypotympanum)
    - Fusion, abnormal rotation, hypoplasia or absence of malleus & incus
    - Abnormal malleoincudal or incudostapedial articulation
    - Oval window atresia may be associated
    - Normal morphology & location of stapes important for surgical reconstruction of ossicular function
    - Congenital or acquired cholesteatoma in EAC or behind atresia plate (< 10%)
  - Facial nerve canal findings
    - Aberrant course of tympanic & mastoid portions of facial nerve common

DDx: EAC Occlusion

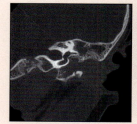
Rhabdomyosarcoma

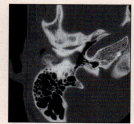
Exostosis

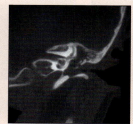
Cholesteatoma

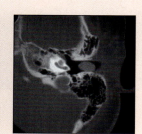
FB Kidney Bean

AURAL ATRESIA

Key Facts

Terminology
- External auditory canal (EAC) atresia
- Congenital aural dysplasia (CAD)
- Dysplasia of the outer ear (auricle and EAC)

Imaging Findings
- Small, dysmorphic pinna
- Bony, soft tissue, or mixed stenosis/atresia of membranous and bony portions of EAC
- Small middle ear cavity (especially hypotympanum)
- Fusion, abnormal rotation, hypoplasia or absence of malleus & incus
- Congenital or acquired cholesteatoma in EAC or behind atresia plate (< 10%)
- Aberrant course of tympanic & mastoid portions of facial nerve common

Top Differential Diagnoses
- Rhabdomyosarcoma
- EAC osteoma or exostosis
- EAC cholesteatoma
- Foreign body (FB)

Pathology
- Failure of canalization leads to EAC atresia
- Inner ear forms earlier during gestation, so anomalies of labyrinth & IAC rarely associated with EAC atresia

Diagnostic Checklist
- Severity of auricular dysplasia parallels degree of deformity of middle ear & ossicles

---

- Tympanic segment may be dehiscent and or caudally displaced, overlying oval or round windows
- Mastoid segment usually anteriorly and laterally displaced
- May exit skull base into glenoid fossa, between glenoid fossa and styloid process or lateral to styloid process
○ Inner ear findings
- Inner ear & IAC normal in most cases
- 12% abnormal: Hypoplastic cochlea, hypoplastic or large lateral semicircular canal, large vestibule or large vestibular aqueduct

MR Findings
- Unnecessary for initial imaging
- Of use if large associated cholesteatoma

Imaging Recommendations
- High-resolution axial & coronal plane bone CT is best imaging approach

DIFFERENTIAL DIAGNOSIS

Rhabdomyosarcoma
- Enhancing soft tissue mass, usually with associated osseous erosion

EAC osteoma or exostosis
- Usually unilateral
- Benign bony growth obliterating EAC

EAC cholesteatoma
- Unilateral with normal auricle
- Soft tissue mass protrudes into EAC
- Underlying bony EAC scalloping
- May have bone fragments in soft tissue mass

Foreign body (FB)
- May see surgical packing in adults
- Small toys, beans & beads in children

PATHOLOGY

General Features
- General path comments
  ○ Non-syndromal EAC atresia usually unilateral
  ○ Bilateral atresia common when EAC malformation is syndromal
  ○ Atresia is membranous, bony or mixed
  ○ Embryology-anatomy
    - 1st & 2nd branchial arches & 1st pharyngeal pouch develop at same time during embryogenesis
    - Associated middle ear & mastoid anomalies are commonly seen with auricular dysplasia & EAC atresia
    - Branchial groove & 1st pharyngeal pouch give rise to EAC
    - Initially, core of epithelial cells solid in future EAC location, 3rd trimester core canalizes to form EAC
    - Failure of canalization leads to EAC atresia
    - 1st branchial arch forms malleus head, incus body & short process & tensor tympani tendon
    - 2nd branchial arch forms manubrium of malleus, long process of incus, stapes (except footplate) & stapedial muscle and tendon
    - Inner ear forms earlier during gestation, so anomalies of labyrinth & IAC rarely associated with EAC atresia
- Genetics
  ○ 14% have positive prior family history
  ○ May be associated with inherited syndromes
    - Crouzon, Goldenhar or Pierre Robin syndromes
- Etiology: Presumed to be in utero insult, epithelial cells of 1st branchial groove fail to split & canalize
- Epidemiology
  ○ 1 in 10,000 births
    - 1 in 900 births in the era of thalidomide embryopathy
  ○ Bony >> membranous atresia
- Associated abnormalities
  ○ Inner ear anomaly occurs in up to 12%
  ○ May be isolated malformation, or part of craniofacial syndrome

AURAL ATRESIA

Gross Pathologic & Surgical Features
- Pinna is malformed & abnormally positioned
- Atresia plate can be membranous or bony and of variable thickness

Microscopic Features
- Cholesteatoma may occur in rudimentary middle ear cavity

Staging, Grading or Classification Criteria
- Mild anomaly may have normal pinna, minimal deformity of malleus & incus, hypoplastic middle ear cavity
- Moderate malformation has rudimentary auricle, more severe ossicular anomalies & aberrant facial nerve course
- Severe anomaly may have no pinna, rudimentary middle ear cleft, absent ossicles & inner ear malformations

CLINICAL ISSUES

Presentation
- Most common signs/symptoms
  - Conductive hearing loss
  - Physical exam
    - Dysplastic auricle, EAC absent or stenotic

Demographics
- Age: Congenital lesion
- Gender: Occurs more commonly in males

Natural History & Prognosis
- Status at birth remains unchanged through life, unless there is associated middle ear cholesteatoma
- In unilateral atresia, other ear has normal hearing
- Bilateral atresia may present as bilateral conductive hearing loss
  - Surgical success depends on degree of associated middle and inner ear anomalies
- Auricle reconstruction may require 4-5 staged surgeries

Treatment
- Unilateral atresia usually treated with auricle reconstruction and bone anchored hearing aid if other ear is normal
- Course of facial nerve, status of oval and round window, ossicles, inner ear structures, and IAC should be established by CT prior to surgery
- Bilateral atresia is treated at 5-8 years of age, when mastoid development is complete
  - Reconstruction of auricle precedes surgical treatment of middle ear & ossicular deformities
  - Surgical reconstruction on side with mildest EAC atresia if bilateral
  - Both auricles are repaired for cosmetic reasons

DIAGNOSTIC CHECKLIST

Consider
- EAC atresia = clinical diagnosis
  - CT provides pre-operative roadmap
- Severity of auricular dysplasia parallels degree of deformity of middle ear & ossicles
- Temporal bone CT later in life to exclude associated cholesteatoma

Image Interpretation Pearls
- Pre-operative T-bone CT checklist essential for surgical planning
  - Type (bony or membranous) & thickness of atresia plate
  - Size of mastoid complex & middle ear cavity helps determine surgical approach
  - Status of ossicular chain, including presence, morphology, & fusion to lateral middle ear cavity wall
  - Carefully assess malleoincudal and incudostapedial articulations
  - Status of oval window & stapes inspected for oval window atresia
  - Trace course of facial nerve, as aberrant and/or dehiscent nerve may be at risk during surgery
  - Hypoplastic or aplastic IAC with deficient cochlear nerve, and hypoplastic cochlea may be a surgical contraindication

SELECTED REFERENCES

1. Blevins NH et al: External auditory canal duplication anomalies associated with congenital aural atresia. J Laryngol Otol. 117(1):32-8, 2003
2. Klingebiel R et al: Multislice computed tomographic imaging in temporal bone dysplasia. Otol Neurotol. 23(5):715-22, 2002
3. Benton C et al: Imaging of congenital anomalies of the temporal bone. Neuroimaging Clin N Am. 10(1):35-53, vii-viii, 2000
4. Calzolari F et al: Clinical and radiological evaluation in children with microtia. Br J Audiol. 33(5):303-12, 1999
5. Declau F et al: Diagnosis and management strategies in congenital atresia of the external auditory canal. Study Group on Otological Malformations and Hearing Impairment. Br J Audiol. 33(5):313-27, 1999
6. Karhuketo TS et al: Visualization of the middle ear with high resolution computed tomography and superfine fiberoptic videomicroendoscopy. Eur Arch Otorhinolaryngol. 255(6):277-80, 1998
7. Selesnick S et al: Surgical treatment of acquired external auditory canal atresia. Am J Otol. 19(2):123-30, 1998
8. Mayer TE et al: High-resolution CT of the temporal bone in dysplasia of the auricle and external auditory canal. AJNR Am J Neuroradiol. 18(1):53-65, 1997
9. Nishizaki K et al: A computer-assisted operation for congenital aural malformations. Int J Pediatr Otorhinolaryngol. 36(1):31-7, 1996
10. Yeakley JW et al: CT evaluation of congenital aural atresia: what the radiologist and surgeon need to know. J Comput Assist Tomogr. 20(5):724-31, 1996
11. Chandrasekhar SS et al: Surgery of congenital aural atresia. Am J Otol. 16(6):713-7, 1995
12. Andrews JC et al: Three-dimensional CT scan reconstruction for the assessment of congenital aural atresia. Am J Otol. 13(3):236-40, 1992
13. Jahrsdoerfer RA et al: Grading system for the selection of patients with congenital aural atresia. Am J Otol. 13(1):6-12, 1992

AURAL ATRESIA

IMAGE GALLERY

Typical

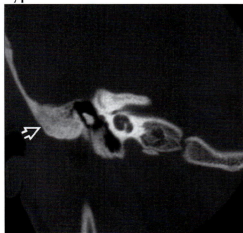
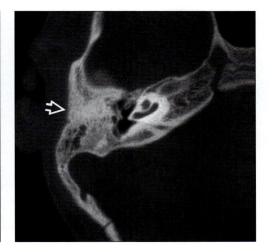

(Left) Coronal NECT shows bony atresia (arrow) of the right EAC, underpneumatization of the mastoid air cells and a small middle ear cavity with dysmorphic middle ear ossicles. *(Right)* Axial NECT shows bony atresia (arrow) of the EAC, underpneumatization of the mastoid air cells and a small middle ear cavity in the same child as shown on the left.

Variant

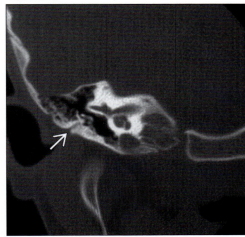
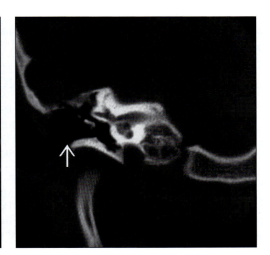

(Left) Coronal NECT shows near complete atresia of the EAC with only a diminutive remnant filled with soft tissue (arrow). The middle ear cavity and inner ear structures are normal. *(Right)* Coronal NECT shows widely patent newly constructed EAC (arrow) in this patient status post repair of aural atresia (same patient as image on the left).

Typical

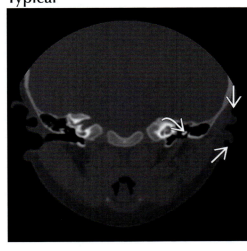
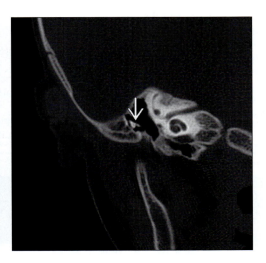

(Left) Coronal NECT shows deformed left pinna (arrows), atresia of the left EAC, malformed ossicles (curved arrow), and small mastoid complex. Contralateral normal included for comparison. *(Right)* Coronal NECT shows small, dysmorphic ossicles (arrow) fused to the lateral attic wall.

FIRST BRANCHIAL APPARATUS ANOMALIES

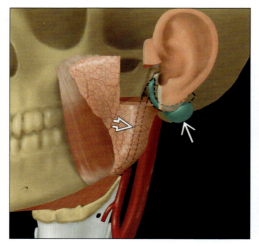 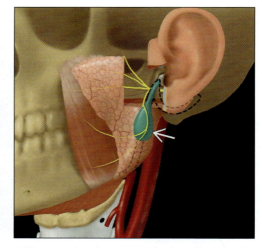

Oblique graphic shows work type I first BAC (arrow) along tract from bony-cartilaginous junction of EAC situated just posteroinferior to auricle. Open arrow demonstrates type II.

Oblique graphic shows example of work type II first BAC (arrow) along course of tract from bony-cartilaginous EAC to angle of mandible. Note intimate relationship to facial nerve.

TERMINOLOGY

Abbreviations and Synonyms
- Abbreviation: First branchial apparatus cyst (BAC) or branchial apparatus anomaly (BAA)
- External auditory canal (EAC)
- Synonyms: Cervicoaural cyst, 1st branchial cleft cyst (BCC)

Definitions
- 1st branchial apparatus anomalies most commonly cysts or sinuses
- 1st BAC: Benign, congenital cyst that occurs in or adjacent to parotid gland, EAC or pinna
  - Remnant of 1st branchial apparatus: Two most commonly used classifications
    - Work type I: Duplication of membranous EAC; ectodermal (cleft) origin
    - Work type II: Duplication of membranous EAC and cartilaginous pinna; skin (ectodermal cleft) and cartilage (mesodermal arch) origin; may also have contribution from the second arch
    - Arnot type I: Derived from buried rests of 1st branchial cleft results in intraparotid cyst or sinus
    - Arnot type II: Secondary to incomplete closure of the 1st branchial cleft results in cyst or sinus in anterior triangle of neck +/- communication with EAC
- 1st branchial apparatus sinus tract opens in region of parotid gland, EAC, parapharyngeal space or anterior triangle of the neck

IMAGING FINDINGS

General Features
- Best diagnostic clue: Cystic mass around pinna and EAC (type I) or extending from EAC to angle of mandible (type II)
- Location
  - Type I: Periauricular cyst or sinus tract
    - Anterior, inferior or posterior to pinna and concha
  - Type II: Periparotid
    - More intimately associated with parotid gland, medial or lateral to the facial nerve
    - Superficial, parotid & parapharyngeal spaces
- Size: Variable, but usually less than 3 cm
- Morphology: Well-circumscribed, unilocular ovoid cyst

CT Findings
- NECT
  - Low density cyst
  - If previously infected, can be isodense
- CECT
  - Well-circumscribed, non-enhancing or rim-enhancing, low-density mass

DDx: Cystic Parotid And Periparotid Masses

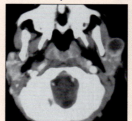 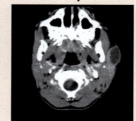 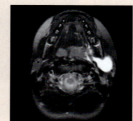 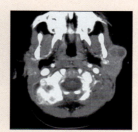

Epithelial Cyst   Parotid Abscess   LM   MAI

FIRST BRANCHIAL APPARATUS ANOMALIES

Key Facts

Terminology
- Abbreviation: First branchial apparatus cyst (BAC) or branchial apparatus anomaly (BAA)
- Synonyms: Cervicoaural cyst, 1st branchial cleft cyst (BCC)

Imaging Findings
- Best diagnostic clue: Cystic mass around pinna and EAC (type I) or extending from EAC to angle of mandible (type II)
- Well-circumscribed, non-enhancing or rim-enhancing, low-density mass
- If infected, may have thick enhancing rim

Top Differential Diagnoses
- Benign lymphoepithelial cysts
- Suppurative adenopathy/abscess
- Lymphatic malformation (LM)
- Nontuberculous mycobacterial adenitis

Pathology
- Remnant of 1st branchial apparatus
- Accounts for 8% of all branchial apparatus remnants

Clinical Issues
- Soft, painless, compressible periauricular or periparotid suprahyoid neck mass

Diagnostic Checklist
- Think of 1st BAC in patient with chronic unexplained otorrhea or recurrent parotid gland abscess
- Look for cyst in or adjacent to parotid gland, EAC or pinna, or rarely parapharyngeal

---

  - If infected, may have thick enhancing rim
    - Surrounding induration suggests infection
  - 1st BAC, type I
    - Cyst can be found anterior, inferior or posterior to EAC
    - Lesion may "beak" toward bony-cartilaginous junction of EAC
    - Often runs parallel to EAC
  - 1st BAC, type II
    - Cyst can be found in superficial, parotid or parapharyngeal space
    - May be found as far inferior as posterior submandibular space
    - Deep projection may "beak" to bony-cartilaginous junction of EAC

MR Findings
- T1WI: Low signal intensity unilocular cyst
- T2WI
  - High signal intensity cyst
  - May see sinus tract to skin, EAC or rarely parapharyngeal space
- T1 C+
  - No wall enhancement on T1 C+ MR images is typical
  - Previous or concurrent infection may result in thick enhancing rim

Ultrasonographic Findings
- Anechoic mass in periauricular or periparotid area

Imaging Recommendations
- CECT usually adequate for evaluation of cyst
- Direct coronal or reformatted images (multidetector CT) helpful for evaluating relationship to EAC
- MRI better to evaluate small lesions and associated sinus tract (particularly T2WI)

DIFFERENTIAL DIAGNOSIS

Benign lymphoepithelial cysts
- Single or multiple
- When multiple and bilateral, suspect HIV
  - Rare in children
  - Usually associated with cervical adenopathy and Waldeyer ring hypertrophy

Suppurative adenopathy/abscess
- Clinical: Presents with marked tenderness and fever
- Imaging: Thick-walled, ovoid, cystic mass within parotid

Lymphatic malformation (LM)
- Multilocular, frequently trans-spatial, rarely unilocular within or superficial to parotid gland

Nontuberculous mycobacterial adenitis
- Mycobacterium avium intracellulare (MAI)
- Rim enhancing with low attenuation nonenhancing center
- May lack surrounding inflammatory change
- May lack signs and symptoms of acute infection

Primary parotid neoplasms
- Uncommon in children
- Solid much more common than cystic

PATHOLOGY

General Features
- General path comments
  - Embryology-anatomy
    - Remnant of 1st branchial apparatus
    - Cleft (ectoderm) of 1st apparatus gives rise to external auditory canal
    - Arch (mesoderm) gives rise to mandible, muscles of mastication, CN5, incus body, head of malleus
    - Pouch (endoderm) gives rise to eustachian tube, middle ear cavity, & mastoid air cells
    - Branchial remnant occurs if there is incomplete obliteration of 1st branchial apparatus
    - Isolated branchial cleft cyst has no internal (pharyngeal) or external (cutaneous) communication

FIRST BRANCHIAL APPARATUS ANOMALIES

- Branchial cleft fistula has both internal & external connections, from EAC lumen to skin
- Branchial cleft sinus opens either externally or (rarely) internally, closed portion ends as blind pouch
- 2/3 of 1st branchial cleft remnants are isolated cysts
- Epidemiology
  - Accounts for 8% of all branchial apparatus remnants
  - Type II >> type I 1st BAC
- Associated abnormalities: May be seen in association with other first branchial apparatus anomalies

Gross Pathologic & Surgical Features
- Cystic neck mass, easily dissected at surgery unless there has been repeated infection
- Contents of cyst usually thick mucus
- Type II has variable relationship to parotid gland & facial nerve
  - Cystic remnant may split facial nerve trunk
  - Facial nerve may be medial or lateral to 1st BAC
  - Close proximity to CN7 makes surgery more difficult
- Most common location for 1st BAC to terminate is in EAC between cartilaginous & bony portions

Microscopic Features
- Thin outer layer - fibrous pseudocapsule
- Inner layer - flat squamoid epithelium
- +/- Germinal centers & lymphocytes in cyst wall

CLINICAL ISSUES

Presentation
- Most common signs/symptoms
  - Soft, painless, compressible periauricular or periparotid suprahyoid neck mass
  - Other signs/symptoms
    - Recurrent preauricular or periparotid swelling
    - Tender neck mass, fever if infected
    - EAC or skin sinus tract rare
    - Chronic purulent ear drainage if ear sinus tract

Demographics
- Age
  - Age of presentation: Majority present < 10 years old
  - If associated with a sinus, presents earlier
  - When cyst only, may present later, even as adult
- Gender: No gender predilection

Natural History & Prognosis
- May enlarge with upper respiratory tract infection
  - Lymph follicles in wall react, wall secretes
- Often incised & drained as an "abscess," only to recur
- Prognosis is excellent if completely resected
- May recur if residual cyst wall remains

Treatment
- Complete surgical resection
- Proximity to facial nerve puts nerve at risk during surgery
  - Type I: Proximal facial nerve
  - Type II: More distal facial nerve branches

DIAGNOSTIC CHECKLIST

Consider
- Think of 1st BAC in patient with chronic unexplained otorrhea or recurrent parotid gland abscess
- Look for cyst in or adjacent to parotid gland, EAC or pinna, or rarely parapharyngeal

SELECTED REFERENCES

1. Koch BL: Cystic malformations of the neck in children. Pediatr Radiol. 35(5):463-77, 2005
2. Daniel SJ et al: Surgical management of nonmalignant parotid masses in the pediatric population: the Montreal Children's Hospital's experience. J Otolaryngol. 32(1):51-4, 2003
3. Gritzmann N et al: Sonography of soft tissue masses of the neck. J Clin Ultrasound. 30(6):356-73, 2002
4. Nusbaum AO et al: Recurrence of a deep neck infection: a clinical indication of an underlying congenital lesion. Arch Otolaryngol Head Neck Surg. 125(12):1379-82, 1999
5. Robson CD et al: Nontuberculous mycobacterial infection of the head and neck in immunocompetent children: CT and MR findings. AJNR Am J Neuroradiol. 20(10):1829-35, 1999
6. Sichel JY et al: Clinical update on type II first branchial cleft cysts. Laryngoscope. 108(10):1524-7, 1998
7. Triglia JM et al: First branchial cleft anomalies: a study of 39 cases and a review of the literature. Arch Otolaryngol Head Neck Surg. 124(3):291-5, 1998
8. Nofsinger YC et al: Periauricular cysts and sinuses. Laryngoscope. 107(7):883-7, 1997
9. Van der Goten A et al: First branchial complex anomalies: report of 3 cases. Eur Radiol. 7(1):102-5, 1997
10. Arndal H et al: First branchial cleft anomaly. Clin Otolaryngol. 21(3):203-7, 1996
11. Choi SS et al: Branchial anomalies: a review of 52 cases. Laryngoscope. 105(9 Pt 1):909-13, 1995
12. Mukherji SK et al: Evaluation of first branchial anomalies by CT and MR. J Comput Assist Tomogr. 17(4):576-81, 1993
13. Benson MT et al: Congenital anomalies of the branchial apparatus: embryology and pathologic anatomy. RadioGraphics. 12:943-60, 1992
14. Doi O et al: Branchial remnants: a review of 58 cases. J Pediatr Surg. 23(9):789-92, 1988
15. Finn DG et al: First branchial cleft cysts: clinical update. Laryngoscope. 97(2):136-40, 1987
16. Graham MD et al: First branchial cleft cyst presenting as a mass within the external auditory canal. Am J Otol. 6(6):500-2, 1985
17. Sherman NH et al: Ultrasound evaluation of neck masses in children. J Ultrasound Med. 4(3):127-34, 1985
18. Harnsberger HR et al: Branchial cleft anomalies and their mimics: computed tomographic evaluation. Radiology. 152(3):739-48, 1984
19. Olsen KD et al: First branchial cleft anomalies. Laryngoscope. 90(3):423-36, 1980

FIRST BRANCHIAL APPARATUS ANOMALIES

IMAGE GALLERY

Typical

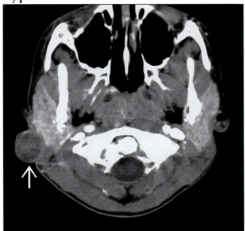
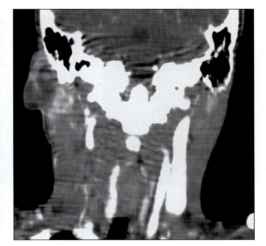

(Left) Axial CECT demonstrates low attenuation first BAC (arrow) superficial to the right parotid gland with minimal peripheral contrast-enhancement. *(Right)* Coronal CECT demonstrates mild enhancement of the superior margin and a septation at the mid portion, changes related to superimposed infection in the same patient with first BAC.

Typical

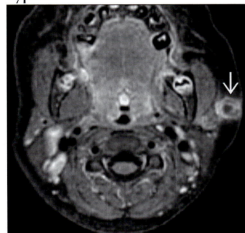
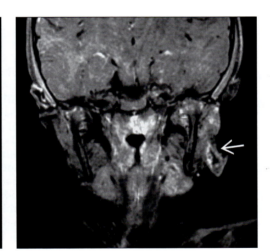

(Left) Axial T1 C+ MR demonstrates a first branchial apparatus cyst (arrow) superficial to the left parotid gland with irregular rim enhancement secondary to superimposed infection. *(Right)* Coronal T1 C+ MR demonstrates the anomaly in the same patient with a pointed proximal margin extending towards the EAC (arrow).

Variant

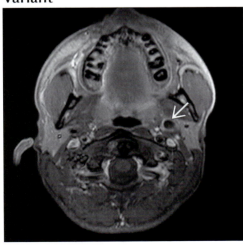
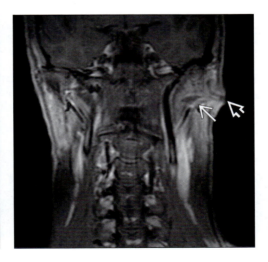

(Left) Axial T1 C+ MR shows a small parapharyngeal first branchial apparatus cyst (arrow) in teenager with recurrent periauricular draining sinus tract. *(Right)* Coronal T1 C+ MR shows a fluid-filled sinus tract (arrow) leading to the cutaneous opening (open arrow) in the same patient.

SECOND BRANCHIAL APPARATUS ANOMALIES

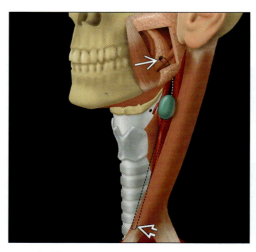

Sagittal oblique graphic shows 2nd BAC anterior to sternomastoid muscle and anterolateral to carotid space. Fistula tract may extend from faucial tonsil (arrow) to low neck (open arrow).

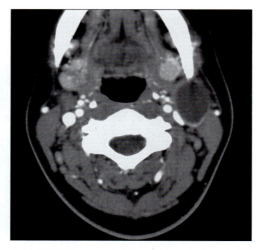

Axial CECT shows well-defined thin-walled cystic left neck mass posterolateral to submandibular gland, lateral to carotid sheath and anteromedial to SCM, typical location of 2nd BAC.

TERMINOLOGY

Abbreviations and Synonyms
- Second branchial apparatus anomaly (BAA)
- Second branchial cleft cyst (BCC) or branchial apparatus cyst (BAC)
- Second branchial cleft remnant or anomaly

Definitions
- 2nd BAC: Most common branchial apparatus anomaly
  - Cystic remnant of cervical sinus of His: Derivative of 2nd, 3rd and 4th branchial clefts; and second branchial arch
- Sinus: Usually communicate externally along anterior margin of sternocleidomastoid muscle (SCM)
- Fistula: Communicate externally and internally
  - Secondary to persistence of both branchial cleft and pharyngeal pouch remnant
- Combination of cyst and sinus or fistula

IMAGING FINDINGS

General Features
- Best diagnostic clue: Cystic neck mass posterolateral to submandibular gland, lateral to carotid space, anterior (or anteromedial) to SCM
- Location
  - Bailey classification of second branchial apparatus cysts
    - Type I: Deep to the platysma muscle and anterior to the SCM
    - Type II: Anterior to SCM, posterior to submandibular gland, lateral to carotid sheath
    - Type III: Protrudes between the internal and external carotid arteries, may extend to the lateral wall of pharynx or superiorly to skull base
    - Type IV: Adjacent to pharyngeal wall, probably remnant of second pharyngeal pouch
  - 2nd branchial apparatus fistula extends from anterior to the SCM, through carotid artery bifurcation & terminates in tonsillar fossa
- Size: Variable, may range from several cm to > 5 cm
- Morphology
  - Ovoid or rounded well-circumscribed cyst
  - Focal rim of cyst extending to carotid bifurcation
    - "Notch sign" pathognomonic for 2nd BCC

CT Findings
- NECT: Low density unilocular cyst with no discernible wall
- CECT
  - Low density cyst with nonenhancing wall
  - If infected, wall is thicker & enhances with surrounding soft tissue cellulitis

DDx: Cystic Neck Masses

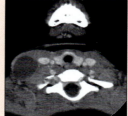
LM

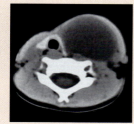
Thymic Cyst

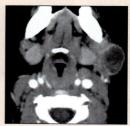
Abscess

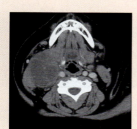
Necrotic Node-PTC

SECOND BRANCHIAL APPARATUS ANOMALIES

Key Facts

Terminology
- Second branchial apparatus anomaly (BAA)
- 2nd BAC: Most common branchial apparatus anomaly
- Cystic remnant of cervical sinus of His: Derivative of 2nd, 3rd and 4th branchial clefts; and second branchial arch

Imaging Findings
- Best diagnostic clue: Cystic neck mass posterolateral to submandibular gland, lateral to carotid space, anterior (or anteromedial) to SCM
- If infected, wall is thicker & enhances with surrounding soft tissue cellulitis

Top Differential Diagnoses
- Lymphatic malformation (LM)
- Cervical thymic cyst
- Suppurative lymphadenopathy/abscess
- Cystic malignant adenopathy

Pathology
- Epidemiology: 2nd branchial apparatus anomalies account for up to 95% of all branchial apparatus anomalies

Diagnostic Checklist
- Beware an adult with first presentation of "2nd BCC": Mass may be metastatic node from head & neck SCCa primary tumor or papillary thyroid carcinoma

MR Findings
- T1WI
  - Cyst is usually isointense to CSF
  - Infection may increase signal intensity secondary to increased protein content
- T2WI: Hyperintense cyst, no discernible wall
- FLAIR: Cyst is iso- or slightly hyperintense to CSF
- T1 C+
  - No intrinsic contrast-enhancement
  - Peripheral wall enhancement if infected

Ultrasonographic Findings
- Anechoic or hypoechoic thin-walled cyst with through transmission
- When hypoechoic, may give "pseudo-solid" US appearance
  - Real time will demonstrate mobile internal echoes to differentiate from solid lesion
- Thickened cyst wall if infected

Imaging Recommendations
- CT, US or MRI clearly demonstrate location of Bailey type I, II and III cysts
- May be difficult to visualize Bailey type IV cysts with US
- CT or MRI best demonstrate associated findings of infection and rare type IV cysts

DIFFERENTIAL DIAGNOSIS

Lymphatic malformation (LM)
- Unilocular or multilocular
- Frequently trans-spatial
- Fluid-fluid levels if intralesional hemorrhage
- Isolated to same location as 2nd branchial apparatus anomalies is uncommon

Cervical thymic cyst
- Remnant of thymopharyngeal duct, derivative of 3rd pharyngeal pouch
- Left side more common than right
- Up to 50% extend into superior mediastinum

Suppurative lymphadenopathy/abscess
- Present with signs and symptoms of infection
- Irregular thick enhancing wall with nonenhancing central cavity
- Surrounding soft tissue induration
- Associated ipsilateral nonsuppurative adenopathy

Cystic malignant adenopathy
- Necrotic mass with thick, enhancing wall
- Rare in children, occasional in teenagers, most in adults
- Squamous cell carcinoma (SCCa) metastasis
- Papillary thyroid carcinoma (PTC) metastasis
- Others: Neuroblastoma, hepatoblastoma, testicular neoplasms

PATHOLOGY

General Features
- General path comments
  - Embryology
    - 2nd branchial arch overgrows 2nd, 3rd & 4th branchial clefts, forming the ectodermally lined cervical sinus of His
    - Remnant of second, third and fourth branchial clefts open into cervical sinus of His via cervical vesicles
    - Normal development cervical sinus of His and vesicles involute
    - Remnants of second branchial apparatus may form cyst, sinus or fistula
- Etiology
  - Remnants of cervical sinus of His or second branchial apparatus
    - 2nd BAC, sinus or fistulae
- Epidemiology: 2nd branchial apparatus anomalies account for up to 95% of all branchial apparatus anomalies
- Associated abnormalities
  - Usually isolated lesion
  - May be part of branchio-otorenal (BOR) syndrome

SECOND BRANCHIAL APPARATUS ANOMALIES

- Autosomal dominant inheritance
- Bilateral branchial fistulas or cysts
- Profound mixed hearing loss: Cochlear and semicircular canal malformations, stapes fixation
- Renal anomalies: Dysplasia, aplasia, polycystic kidney
- Patulous eustachian tubes

Gross Pathologic & Surgical Features
- Well-defined cyst in the locations described by Bailey
- Filled with cheesy material or serous, mucoid or purulent fluid
- If associated with fistula, cutaneous opening typically at anterior border of SCM near mid or lower portion

Microscopic Features
- Squamous epithelial-lined cyst
- Lymphoid infiltrate in wall, often in form of germinal centers
  - Lymphoid tissue suggests epithelial rests may be entrapped within cervical lymph nodes during embryogenesis

CLINICAL ISSUES

Presentation
- Most common signs/symptoms
  - Painless, compressible lateral neck mass in child or young adult
  - May enlarge during upper respiratory tract infection, probably due to response of lymphoid tissue
  - Fever, tenderness and erythema if infected

Demographics
- Age: Majority less than 5 years of age, second peak 2nd or 3rd decade

Natural History & Prognosis
- If untreated, may become repeatedly infected & inflamed
- Recurrent inflammation makes surgical resection more difficult
- Excellent prognosis if lesion is completely resected

Treatment
- Complete surgical resection is treatment of choice
- Surgeon must dissect around cyst bed to exclude the possibility of an associated fistula or sinus
  - If a tract goes superomedially, it passes through carotid bifurcation into crypts of faucial palatine tonsil
  - If a tract goes inferiorly, it passes along anterior carotid space, reaching skin in supraclavicular area
    - If fistula present, usually identified at birth
    - Mucoid secretions are emitted from skin opening

DIAGNOSTIC CHECKLIST

Consider
- Infection if cyst wall enhances or surrounding cellulitis
- Does cyst appear adherent to internal jugular vein or carotid sheath?

Image Interpretation Pearls
- Beware an adult with first presentation of "2nd BCC": Mass may be metastatic node from head & neck SCCa primary tumor or papillary thyroid carcinoma

SELECTED REFERENCES

1. Koch BL: Cystic malformations of the neck in children. Pediatr Radiol. 35(5):463-77, 2005
2. Kemperman MH et al: Evidence of progression and fluctuation of hearing impairment in branchio-oto-renal syndrome. Int J Audiol. 43(9):523-32, 2004
3. Ceruti S et al: Temporal bone anomalies in the branchio-oto-renal syndrome: detailed computed tomographic and magnetic resonance imaging findings. Otol Neurotol. 23(2):200-7, 2002
4. Choo MJ et al: A case of second branchial cleft cyst with oropharyngeal presentation. J Korean Med Sci. 17(4):564-5, 2002
5. Kemperman MH et al: Inner ear anomalies are frequent but nonobligatory features of the branchio-oto-renal syndrome. Arch Otolaryngol Head Neck Surg. 128(9):1033-8, 2002
6. Shin JH et al: Parapharyngeal second branchial cyst manifesting as cranial nerve palsies: MR findings. AJNR Am J Neuroradiol. 22(3):510-2, 2001
7. Stinckens C et al: The presence of a widened vestibular aqueduct and progressive sensorineural hearing loss in the branchio-oto-renal syndrome. A family study. Int J Pediatr Otorhinolaryngol. 59(3):163-72, 2001
8. Lev S et al: Imaging of cystic lesions. Radiol Clin North Am. 38(5):1013-27, 2000
9. Nusbaum AO et al: Recurrence of a deep neck infection: a clinical indication of an underlying congenital lesion. Arch Otolaryngol Head Neck Surg. 125(12):1379-82, 1999
10. Ahuja A et al: Solitary cystic nodal metastasis from occult papillary carcinoma of the thyroid mimicking a branchial cyst: a potential pitfall. Clin Radiol. 53(1):61-3, 1998
11. McDermott ID et al: Metastatic papillary thyroid carcinoma presenting as a typical branchial cyst. J Laryngol Otol. 110(5):490-2, 1996
12. Choi SS et al: Branchial anomalies: a review of 52 cases. Laryngoscope. 105(9 Pt 1):909-13, 1995
13. Gatot A et al: Branchial cleft cyst manifesting as hypoglossal nerve palsy. Head Neck. 13(3):249-50, 1991
14. Benson MT et al: Congenital anomalies of the branchial apparatus: embryology and pathologic anatomy. Radiographics. 12(5):943-60, 1992
15. Doi O et al: Branchial remnants: a review of 58 cases. J Pediatr Surg. 23(9):789-92, 1988
16. Salazar JE et al: Second branchial cleft cyst: unusual location and a new CT diagnostic sign. AJR Am J Roentgenol. 145(5):965-6, 1985
17. Harnsberger HR et al: Branchial cleft anomalies and their mimics: computed tomographic evaluation. Radiology. 152(3):739-48, 1984
18. Gold BM: Second branchial cleft cyst and fistula. AJR Am J Roentgenol. 134(5):1067-9, 1980
19. Poswillo D: The pathogenesis of the first and second branchial arch syndrome. Oral Surg Oral Med Oral Pathol. 35(3):302-28, 1973
20. Bailey:Branchial cysts and other essays on surgical subjects in the faciocervical region The clinical aspect of branchial cysts.London, Lewis.1-18, 1929

SECOND BRANCHIAL APPARATUS ANOMALIES

IMAGE GALLERY

Typical

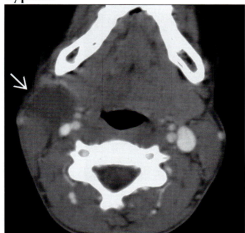
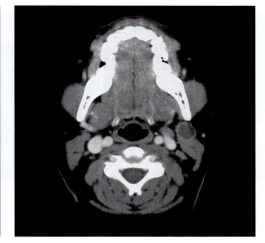

(Left) Axial CECT shows cystic right neck mass in the most common location of 2nd BACs with mild induration of the adjacent subcutaneous fat (arrow) consistent with associated cellulitis. (Right) Axial CECT shows small 2nd branchial apparatus cyst. Notice smooth thick wall secondary to prior infection. Cyst was clinically much larger prior to treatment with antibiotics.

Typical

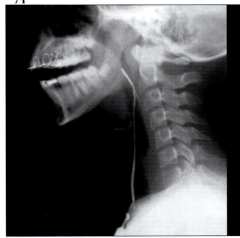
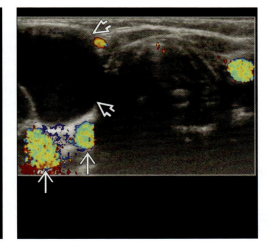

(Left) Lateral fistulagram shows classic demonstration of the location of the entire second branchial apparatus tract. (Right) Axial ultrasound shows 2nd branchial cleft cyst as well-defined anechoic cyst (open arrows) with increased through transmission and deviation of carotid sheath vessels (arrows). Trachea is to left of lesion.

Variant

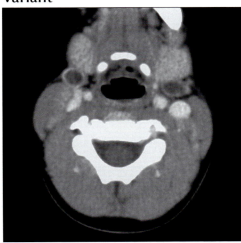
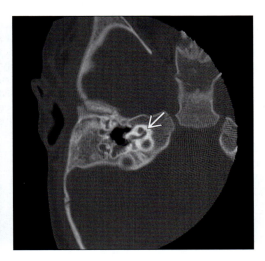

(Left) Axial CECT shows small bilateral cystic masses in the classic location of Bailey type II second branchial apparatus cysts in a child with branchio-otorenal syndrome. (Right) Axial NECT shows hypoplastic, incompletely partitioned right cochlea (arrow) in the same patient with branchio-otorenal syndrome.

THIRD BRANCHIAL APPARATUS ANOMALIES

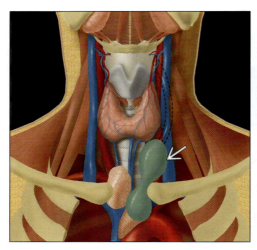 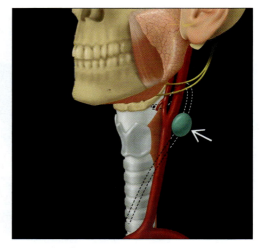

Coronal graphic shows typical cervical thymic cyst (arrow) along the course of the thymopharyngeal duct (dashes).

Lateral graphic illustrates course of 3rd branchial anomaly (dashes) along which 3rd branchial cleft cysts arise, most commonly in the upper posterior triangle (arrow).

TERMINOLOGY

Abbreviations and Synonyms
- Cervical thymic cyst (CTC)
  - Thymopharyngeal duct cyst
- 3rd branchial cleft cyst (BCC) or branchial apparatus cyst (BAC)

Definitions
- Cervical thymic cyst: Cystic remnant of thymopharyngeal duct, derivative of 3rd pharyngeal pouch
- 3rd BCC: Cystic remnant of 3rd branchial cleft or cervical sinus of His

IMAGING FINDINGS

General Features
- Best diagnostic clue
  - Cervical thymic cyst: Cystic lateral neck mass closely associated with carotid sheath
  - 3rd branchial cleft cyst: Unilocular cyst in upper posterior cervical space or lower anterior neck
- Location
  - Cervical thymic cyst
    - Anywhere along the tract of the thymopharyngeal duct from the pyriform sinus to the anterior mediastinum
    - Left more common than right
    - Up to 50% continuous with mediastinal thymus: Direct extension of cyst or via fibrous cord
    - Intimate association with carotid sheath, frequently splay the carotid artery and jugular vein
  - 3rd branchial cleft cyst
    - Upper neck posterior cervical space, lower neck anterior border sternocleidomastoid muscle
    - Rarely can be in submandibular space, just lateral to cephalad hypopharynx

CT Findings
- CECT
  - Rounded or ovoid sharply marginated lesions with central fluid attenuation
  - Cyst wall thin, no calcifications
  - If infected, cyst wall thickens, enhances and adjacent soft tissues show evidence of cellulitis
  - CTC
    - Closely associated with carotid sheath
    - With or without continuation of cyst to the mediastinal thymus
    - Solid components rare = aberrant thymic tissue, lymphoid aggregates or parathyroid tissue

DDx: Cystic Neck Masses In Children

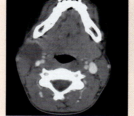 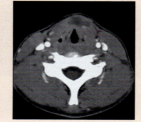 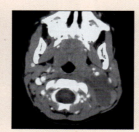 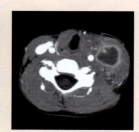

Second BAC   *TGD Cyst*   *LM*   *Abscess*

THIRD BRANCHIAL APPARATUS ANOMALIES

Key Facts

Terminology
- Cervical thymic cyst: Cystic remnant of thymopharyngeal duct, derivative of 3rd pharyngeal pouch
- 3rd BCC: Cystic remnant of 3rd branchial cleft or cervical sinus of His

Imaging Findings
- Cervical thymic cyst: Cystic lateral neck mass closely associated with carotid sheath
- 3rd branchial cleft cyst: Unilocular cyst in upper posterior cervical space or lower anterior neck

Top Differential Diagnoses
- 2nd branchial apparatus cyst
- Thyroglossal duct (TGD) cyst
- Lymphatic malformation
- Abscess

Pathology
- Lymphoid tissue in walls of cyst with reactive lymphoid follicles

Diagnostic Checklist
- If the cyst is intimately associated with the anterior carotid sheath, think CTC
- If the cyst extends from the anterior neck to the upper mediastinum, consider CTC
- If the cyst is in the posterior triangle of the upper neck, think 3rd BCC

- 3rd BCC
  - Sternocleidomastoid muscle displaced laterally when cyst in high posterior neck
  - Sternocleidomastoid muscle displaced posterolaterally when cyst in low anterior neck
  - May contain air if cyst communicates with pyriform sinus via patent tract (3rd pharyngeal pouch derivative)

MR Findings
- T1WI
  - Homogeneous T1 hypointense fluid contents
  - Cyst wall thin or imperceptible
- T2WI: Homogeneous T2 hyperintense fluid contents
- T1 C+
  - Thin, uniform minimally enhancing cyst wall
  - If infected
    - Cyst wall thickened & enhancing
    - Fluid contents hyperintense relative to CSF
    - Strandy enhancement in surrounding soft tissues

Ultrasonographic Findings
- Thin walled hypoechoic mass

Imaging Recommendations
- Best imaging tool: CECT or MRI
- Protocol advice: Include upper mediastinum to demonstrate mediastinal extension in CTC

DIFFERENTIAL DIAGNOSIS

2nd branchial apparatus cyst
- Most common branchial apparatus anomaly
- Usually lateral to carotid space, posterior to submandibular gland & anteromedial to sternomastoid muscle

Thyroglossal duct (TGD) cyst
- Midline cyst in child or young adult
- Anywhere along TGD from base of tongue (foramen cecum) to lower anterior neck in region of thyroid bed
- Embedded in strap muscles when infrahyoid

Lymphatic malformation
- Majority diagnosed under 2 years of age
- Unilocular or multilocular; focal or infiltrative
- Fluid-fluid levels if intralesional hemorrhage

Abscess
- Present with signs and symptoms of infection
- Irregular thick enhancing wall, low attenuation center
- Surrounding soft tissue induration
- If associated with thyroid gland, think 4th brachial pouch anomaly

PATHOLOGY

General Features
- Etiology
  - CTC
    - Failure of obliteration of thymopharyngeal duct - remnant of 3rd pharyngeal pouch
  - 3rd BCC
    - Failure of obliteration of third branchial cleft or portion of cervical sinus of His
- Epidemiology
  - CTC
    - Rare
  - 3rd BCC
    - Rare lesion
    - 3rd branchial cleft anomalies account for only 3% of all branchial anomalies
- Associated abnormalities
  - 3rd branchial cleft sinus
    - Single opening: Endopharyngeal in high lateral hypopharynx or cutaneous in supraclavicular area anterior to carotid artery
  - 3rd branchial cleft fistula
    - 2 openings: Endopharyngeal in high lateral hypopharynx & cutaneous in supraclavicular area anterior to carotid artery

Gross Pathologic & Surgical Features
- Smooth thin-walled cysts

THIRD BRANCHIAL APPARATUS ANOMALIES

- CTC may have cystic extension or fibrous cord to mediastinal thymus

Microscopic Features
- CTC
  - Hassall corpuscles in cyst wall diagnostic but not always present if prior infection or hemorrhage
  - Cholesterol crystals and granulomas in cyst wall common, possibly related to prior hemorrhage
- 3rd BCC
  - Lined by squamous epithelium (occasionally by columnar epithelium)
  - Lymphoid tissue in walls of cyst with reactive lymphoid follicles

CLINICAL ISSUES

Presentation
- Most common signs/symptoms
  - CTC
    - Enlarging, compressible mid to lower cervical mass
    - Other signs/symptoms: If large, may cause dysphagia or respiratory distress
  - 3rd BAC
    - Fluctuant mass in posterolateral neck
    - May enlarge rapidly following an upper respiratory tract infection
    - Other signs/symptoms: Recurrent lateral neck or retropharyngeal abscesses, draining sinus along anterior margin of sternocleidomastoid muscle

Demographics
- Age
  - CTC
    - Most diagnosed between 2 and 15 years of age
  - 3rd BAC
    - Frequently present in adulthood
    - Presentation of cysts in neonates & infants unusual
    - When sinus or fistula present, early presentation more common

Natural History & Prognosis
- CTC and 3rd BCC: Good prognosis if completely resected

Treatment
- CTC and 3rd BCC
  - Surgical resection

DIAGNOSTIC CHECKLIST

Consider
- If the cyst is intimately associated with the anterior carotid sheath, think CTC
- If the cyst extends from the anterior neck to the upper mediastinum, consider CTC
- If the cyst is in the posterior triangle of the upper neck, think 3rd BCC

SELECTED REFERENCES

1. Koch BL: Cystic malformations of the neck in children. Pediatr Radiol. 35(5):463-77, 2005
2. Khariwala SS et al: Cervical presentations of thymic anomalies in children. Int J Pediatr Otorhinolaryngol. 68(7):909-14, 2004
3. Pereira KD et al: Management of anomalies of the third and fourth branchial pouches. Int J Pediatr Otorhinolaryngol. 68(1):43-50, 2004
4. Hsieh YY et al: Pathological analysis of congenital cervical cysts in children: 20 years of experience at Chang Gung Memorial Hospital. Chang Gung Med J. 26(2):107-13, 2003
5. Tsai CC et al: Branchial-cleft sinus presenting with a retropharyngeal abscess for a newborn: a case report. Am J Perinatol. 20(5):227-31, 2003
6. De Caluwe D et al: Cervical thymic cysts. Pediatr Surg Int. 18(5-6):477-9, 2002
7. Liberman M et al: Ten years of experience with third and fourth branchial remnants. J Pediatr Surg. 37(5):685-90, 2002
8. Huang RY et al: Third branchial cleft anomaly presenting as a retropharyngeal abscess. Int J Pediatr Otorhinolaryngol. 54(2-3):167-72, 2000
9. Mandell DL: Head and neck anomalies related to the branchial apparatus. Otolaryngol Clin North Am. 33(6):1309-32, 2000
10. Mukherji SK et al: Imaging of congenital anomalies of the branchial apparatus. Neuroimaging Clin N Am. 10(1):75-93, viii, 2000
11. Nicolias R et al: Congenital cysts and fistulas of the neck. Int J Pediatr Otorhinolaryngol. 55(2):117-24, 2000
12. Koeller KK et al: Congenital cystic masses of the neck: radiologic-pathologic correlation. Radiographics. 19(1):121-46; quiz 152-3, 1999
13. Millman B et al: Cervical thymic anomalies. Int J Pediatr Otorhinolaryngol. 47(1):29-39, 1999
14. Mouri N et al: Reappraisal of lateral cervical cysts in neonates: pyriform sinus cysts as an anatomy-based nomenclature. J Pediatr Surg. 33(7):1141-4, 1998
15. Edmonds JL et al: Third branchial anomalies. Avoiding recurrences. Arch Otolaryngol Head Neck Surg. 123(4):438-41, 1997
16. Kelley DJ et al: Cervicomediastinal thymic cysts. Int J Pediatr Otorhinolaryngol. 39(2):139-46, 1997
17. Nguyen Q et al: Cervical thymic cyst: case reports and review of the literature. Laryngoscope. 106(3 Pt 1):247-52, 1996
18. Benson MT et al: Congenital anomalies of the branchial apparatus: embryology and pathologic anatomy. Radiographics. 12(5):943-60, 1992
19. Cressman WR et al: Pathologic quiz case 1. Cervical thymic cyst. Arch Otolaryngol Head Neck Surg. 118(7):772-4, 1992
20. Zarbo RJ et al: Thymopharyngeal duct cyst: a form of cervical thymus. Ann Otol Rhinol Laryngol. 92(3 Pt 1):284-9, 1983
21. Guba AM Jr et al: Cervical presentation of thymic cysts. Am J Surg. 136(4):430-6, 1978

THIRD BRANCHIAL APPARATUS ANOMALIES

IMAGE GALLERY

Typical

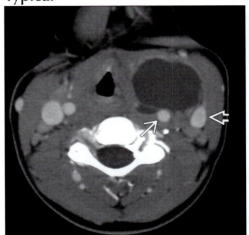
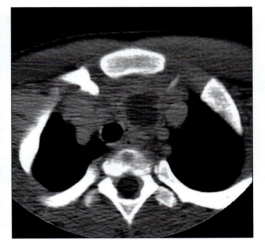

(Left) Axial CECT shows nonenhancing unilocular cyst splaying the left carotid artery (arrow) and jugular vein (open arrow) and mild deviation of the airway to the right. **(Right)** Axial CECT shows extension of the cyst into the upper mediastinum in the same patient with cystic remnant of the thymopharyngeal duct, i.e. CTC.

Typical

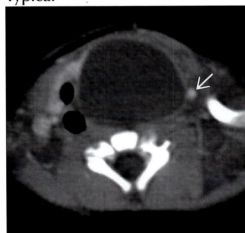
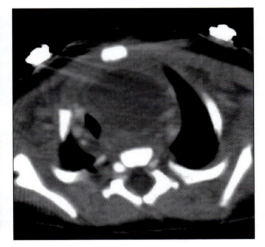

(Left) Axial CECT shows a large unilocular nonenhancing left anterior neck cyst medial to the left carotid artery (arrow), with significant rightward deviation of the airway and thyroid gland. **(Right)** Axial CECT in the same patient shows inferior extension of the cyst into the upper anterior mediastinum consistent with thymic cyst, a remnant of the thymopharyngeal duct.

Typical

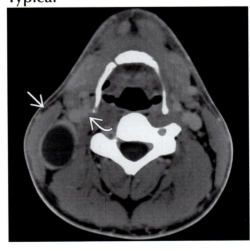
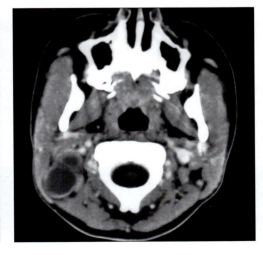

(Left) Axial CECT demonstrates a mildly thick-walled, infected third branchial cleft cyst deep to the sternocleidomastoid muscle (arrow) and posterolateral to the carotid sheath (curved arrow). **(Right)** Axial CECT demonstrates a third branchial cleft cyst in the posterior triangle of the upper neck. Mild enhancement and internal septation are consistent with superimposed infection.

FOURTH BRANCHIAL APPARATUS ANOMALIES

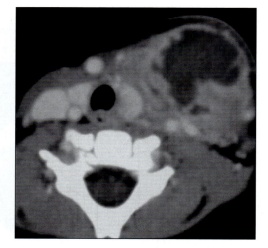

Oblique graphic illustrates 4th branchial tract (arrow) along which 4th branchial cysts arise. A typical cyst site (open arrow) and associated thyroiditis are shown.

Axial CECT shows large abscess anterior to the left thyroid lobe in a child with recurrent neck abscess and intermittent drainage of oral contents through fistulous opening in the skin.

TERMINOLOGY

Abbreviations and Synonyms
- 4th branchial apparatus anomaly (BAA)
- 4th branchial apparatus cyst (BAC)
- 4th branchial cleft cyst (BCC): Misnomer because remnant of pharyngeal pouch, not branchial cleft

Definitions
- 4th BAC epithelial-lined cystic remnant of the fourth branchial pouch, course from apex of pyriform sinus to upper aspect of the left thyroid lobe
- Branchial sinus tract: One opening-to-skin surface, external auditory canal, pharynx or hypopharynx
- Branchial fistula: Congenital anomaly that connects the skin to the lumen of the foregut; two openings
  ○ Arises as an epithelial-lined tract left behind when there is persistence of both a branchial cleft and its corresponding pharyngeal pouch

IMAGING FINDINGS

General Features
- Best diagnostic clue
  ○ Sinus tract extending from the apex of the pyriform sinus to the lower anterior neck after barium swallow
  ○ Cyst or abscess in or adjacent to anterior left thyroid lobe
- Location
  ○ May occur anywhere from LEFT pyriform sinus apex to thyroid lobe
    ▪ Commonly against or within superior aspect of the LEFT lobe of thyroid gland or attached to thyroid cartilage
    ▪ Upper end may communicate with or be adherent to pyriform sinus
- Size: Variable
- Morphology: Thin walled if not infected, thick enhancing wall if infected

Fluoroscopic Findings
- Barium swallow
  ○ Barium filled sinus tract extending from the apex of the pyriform sinus to the anterior lower neck
  ○ If performed during acute infection, may not fill portions of sinus tract

CT Findings
- CECT
  ○ Thin-walled cyst without significant enhancement
  ○ Thick enhancing wall with surrounding cellulitis if infected
- NECT after barium swallow
  ○ Barium filled tract extending from the apex of the pyriform sinus to the lower anterior neck

DDx: Peri-Thyroidal Cystic Masses

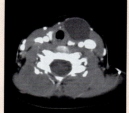
Thyroglossal Duct Cyst

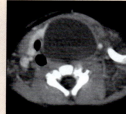
Thymic Cyst

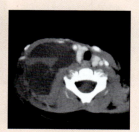
LM

FOURTH BRANCHIAL APPARATUS ANOMALIES

Key Facts

Terminology
- 4th BAC epithelial-lined cystic remnant of the fourth branchial pouch, course from apex of pyriform sinus to upper aspect of the left thyroid lobe

Imaging Findings
- Sinus tract extending from the apex of the pyriform sinus to the lower anterior neck after barium swallow
- Cyst or abscess in or adjacent to anterior left thyroid lobe
- Morphology: Thin walled if not infected, thick enhancing wall if infected
- CECT best demonstrates cyst or abscess
- Fluoroscopically guided barium swallow followed by noncontrast CT best demonstrates sinus tract

Top Differential Diagnoses
- Thyroglossal duct (TGD) cyst
- Cervical thymic cyst
- Lymphatic malformation
- Thyroid colloid cyst

Clinical Issues
- Recurrent neck abscesses
- Recurrent suppurative thyroiditis

Diagnostic Checklist
- Left thyroid lobe abscess in pediatric patient should strongly suggest diagnosis of 4th BAA

MR Findings
- Thin-walled fluid signal intensity cyst if not infected
- Thick wall with increased signal intensity of fluid and surrounding cellulitis if infected

Ultrasonographic Findings
- Thin walled echolucent cyst if not infected
- Internal echoes seen when infection or hemorrhage
- Thick walled abscess with hyperemic wall anterior to thyroid if infected

Nuclear Medicine Findings
- Cold nodule on thyroid scan

Imaging Recommendations
- Best imaging tool
  - CECT best demonstrates cyst or abscess
  - Fluoroscopically guided barium swallow followed by noncontrast CT best demonstrates sinus tract
  - Direct injection of fistula best demonstrates course of fistula
- Protocol advice: Thin section postcontrast helical CT with multiplanar reconstructions very helpful

DIFFERENTIAL DIAGNOSIS

Thyroglossal duct (TGD) cyst
- Anywhere along TGD from base of tongue (foramen cecum) to lower anterior neck in region of thyroid bed
- Infrahyoid TGD cyst
  - Off-midline, anterior to thyroid lobe itself
  - Closely related to thyroid cartilage or strap muscles

Cervical thymic cyst
- Congenital cyst: Remnant of thymopharyngeal duct, derivative of 3rd pharyngeal pouch
- Left side more common than right
- When confined to visceral space, may closely mimic 4th BAA
- Up to 50% of cervical thymic cysts extend into superior mediastinum

Lymphatic malformation
- Unilocular or multilocular
- Focal or infiltrative
- Fluid-fluid levels if intralesional hemorrhage

Thyroid colloid cyst
- Uncommon in young children, most occur in older children and adults
- True thyroid cysts are rare
- Most "thyroid cysts" are degenerating adenomas
- May appear bright on T1 MR due to hemorrhage, colloid or high protein content

PATHOLOGY

General Features
- Etiology
  - Controversial
    - Failure of obliteration of 4th branchial pouch (? or 3rd pouch)
    - Failure of obliteration of distal cervical sinus of His
- Epidemiology
  - Rarest of all forms of branchial apparatus anomalies (1-2% of all branchial anomalies)
  - Most cases arise on LEFT
- Associated abnormalities
  - 4th branchial sinus
    - When sinus connection with apex of pyriform sinus is maintained, infection is likely
    - Thyroiditis ± thyroid abscess possible in such circumstances
  - 4th branchial fistula
    - Term fistula denotes 2 openings, one in low anterior neck, 2nd into pyriform sinus apex

Gross Pathologic & Surgical Features
- Anterolateral neck cyst or abscess; mostly found within anterior thyroid lobe
- Direct probing of the pyriform apex frequently demonstrates the fistula or sinus tract

FOURTH BRANCHIAL APPARATUS ANOMALIES

Microscopic Features
- Typically lined by non-keratinizing squamous epithelium, but occasionally by columnar epithelium
- Lymphoid tissue in cyst walls with reactive lymphoid follicles
- Thyroid follicles may be found in walls of cyst

CLINICAL ISSUES

Presentation
- Most common signs/symptoms
  - Recurrent neck abscesses
  - Recurrent suppurative thyroiditis
  - Fluctuant mass in lower third of neck anteromedial to sternocleidomastoid muscle; tender if infected
  - Throat pain, dysphagia, stridor

Demographics
- Age
  - Most branchial sinuses & fistulae (all types) present in childhood
  - Most 4th branchial apparatus anomalies are diagnosed in infants and young children
- Gender: More common in females

Natural History & Prognosis
- If sinus connection to pyriform sinus unrecognized & untreated, recurrent suppurative thyroiditis
- Recurrence likely if tract not resected & contains secretory epithelium

Treatment
- Complete resection of cyst & any associated sinus or fistula
- Surgery after antibiotic therapy if infected
- Thyroid lobectomy is required for lesions in thyroid lobe to prevent recurrence
- Pyriform sinus opening must be obliterated

DIAGNOSTIC CHECKLIST

Consider
- In any child with phlegmon or abscess in or anterior to left thyroid lobe or recurrent suppurative thyroiditis

Image Interpretation Pearls
- Left thyroid lobe abscess in pediatric patient should strongly suggest diagnosis of 4th BAA

SELECTED REFERENCES

1. Koch BL: Cystic malformations of the neck in children. Pediatr Radiol. 35(5):463-77, 2005
2. Pereira KD et al: Management of anomalies of the third and fourth branchial pouches. Int J Pediatr Otorhinolaryngol. 68(1): 43-50, 2004
3. Chaudhary N et al: Fistula of the fourth branchial pouch. Am J Otolaryngol. 24(4): 250-2, 2003
4. Wang HK et al: Imaging studies of pyriform sinus fistula. Pediatr Radiol. 33(5):328-33, 2003
5. Liberman M et al: Ten years of experience with third and fourth branchial remnants. J Pediatr Surg. 37(5): 685-90, 2002
6. Link TD et al: Fourth branchial pouch sinus: a diagnostic challenge. Plast Reconstr Surg. 108(3): 695-701, 2001
7. Minhas SS et al: Fourth branchial arch fistula and suppurative thyroiditis: a life-threatening infection. J Laryngol Otol. 115(12): 1029-31, 2001
8. Cases JA et al: Recurrent acute suppurative thyroiditis in an adult due to a fourth branchial pouch fistula. J Clin Endocrinol Metab. 85(3): 953-6, 2000
9. Mandell DL: Head and neck anomalies related to the branchial apparatus. Otolaryngol Clin North Am. 33(6): 1309-32, 2000
10. Nicollas R et al: Congenital cysts and fistulas of the neck. Int J Pediatr Otorhinolaryngol. 55(2): 117-24, 2000
11. Park SW et al: Neck infection associated with pyriform sinus fistula: imaging findings. AJNR Am J Neuroradiol. 21(5):817-22, 2000
12. Stone ME et al: A new role for computed tomography in the diagnosis and treatment of pyriform sinus fistula. Am J Otolaryngol. 21(5):323-5, 2000
13. Yang C et al: Fourth branchial arch sinus: clinical presentation, diagnostic workup, and surgical treatment. Laryngoscope. 109(3): 442-6, 1999
14. Nicollas R et al: Fourth branchial pouch anomalies: a study of six cases and review of the literature. Int J Pediatr Otorhinolaryngol. 44(1): 5-10, 1998
15. Cote DN et al: Fourth branchial cleft cysts. Otolaryngol Head Neck Surg. 114(1): 95-7, 1996
16. Choi SS et al: Branchial anomalies: a review of 52 cases. Laryngoscope. 105(9 Pt 1): 909-13, 1995
17. Benson MT et al: Congenital anomalies of the branchial apparatus: embryology and pathologic anatomy. Radiographics. 12(5):943-60, 1992
18. Rosenfeld RM et al: Fourth branchial pouch sinus: diagnosis and treatment. Otolaryngol Head Neck Surg. 105(1): 44-50, 1991
19. Godin MS et al: Fourth branchial pouch sinus: principles of diagnosis and management. Laryngoscope. 100(2 Pt 1): 174-8, 1990
20. Lucaya J et al: Congenital pyriform sinus fistula: a cause of acute left-sided suppurative thyroiditis and neck abscess in children. Pediatr Radiol. 21(1):27-9, 1990
21. Taylor WE Jr et al: Acute suppurative thyroiditis in children. Laryngoscope. 92(11):1269-73, 1982

FOURTH BRANCHIAL APPARATUS ANOMALIES

IMAGE GALLERY

Typical

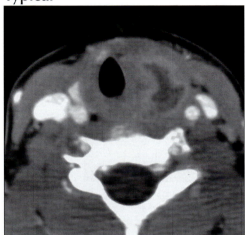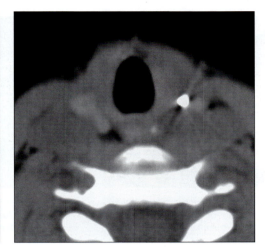

(Left) Axial CECT shows left lobe thyroid abscess with surrounding cellulitis, myositis and rightward deviation of the trachea in a child with an infected 4th branchial apparatus anomaly. *(Right)* Axial fistulagram shows contrast within the 4th branchial pouch remnant, post barium swallow NECT obtained in the same patient one month after treatment with antibiotics.

Typical

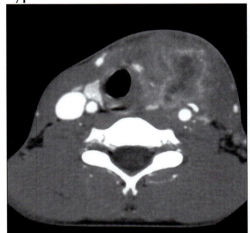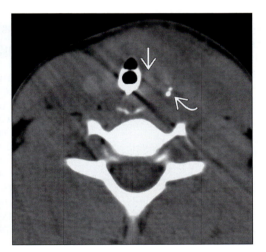

(Left) Axial CECT shows ill-defined left anterior neck abscess, surrounding cellulitis, myositis and involvement of the left thyroid lobe in patient with 4th branchial pouch sinus tract and recurrent thyroid abscess. *(Right)* Axial fistulagram shows contrast (curved arrow) adjacent to the left thyroid lobe (arrow) at the site of 4th pharyngeal pouch remnant, source of anterior neck infection.

Typical

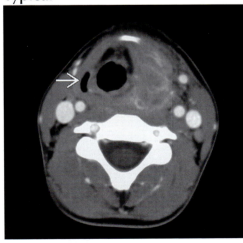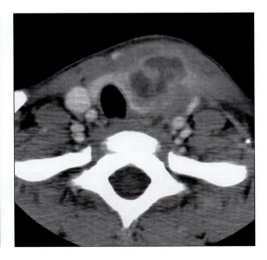

(Left) Axial CECT shows heterogeneous enhancement of phlegmonous tissue compressing the right pyriform sinus apex. Compare to normal left pyriform sinus (arrow). *(Right)* Axial CECT shows abscess involving the left lobe of the thyroid gland in the same patient with infection secondary to sinus tract extending from the left pyriform sinus apex.

CONGENITAL CHOLESTEATOMA

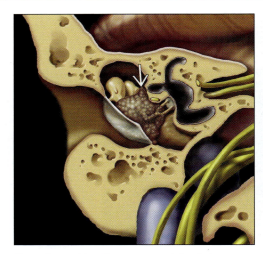

Coronal graphic shows congenital cholesteatoma involving the middle ear. Notice the lesion has extended medial to ossicles (arrow) as it engulfs the entire ossicle chain. TM is intact.

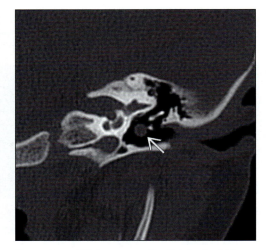

Coronal bone CT shows a small well-defined middle ear congenital cholesteatoma (arrow) abutting the malleus, without ossicular erosion.

TERMINOLOGY

Abbreviations and Synonyms
- Abbreviation: Congenital cholesteatoma (CCh), middle ear (ME), tympanic membrane (TM), external auditory canal (EAC)
- Synonyms: Primary cholesteatoma, epidermoid, "skin in the wrong place"

Definitions
- Aberrant rest of epithelial cells

IMAGING FINDINGS

General Features
- Best diagnostic clue: Smooth, well-circumscribed middle ear mass ± ossicular erosions
- Location
  - Majority middle ear (CCh-ME)
    - Anterosuperior tympanic cavity near eustachian tube or stapes: Most common
    - Posterior epitympanum at tympanic isthmus (area between middle ear cavity & attic)
  - Other locations: EAC, middle ear-mastoid, petrous apex, CP angle, geniculate ganglion
- Size
  - Usually small, identified on otoscopic exam
  - Rarely fills entire middle ear cavity
- Morphology: Lobular, discrete ME mass

CT Findings
- Bone CT
  - Appearance depends on size of lesion and location
  - Small CCh-ME: Detected early, appears as well-circumscribed ME lesion
  - Large CCh-ME: Larger mass may erode ossicles, middle ear wall, lateral semicircular canal or tegmen tympani
    - Bone erosion less common than in acquired cholesteatoma
    - Occurs late in disease
    - Ossicular erosion unusual with anterior mesotympanum involvement
    - Long process of incus & stapes superstructure most commonly destroyed ossicles
    - Labyrinthine extension may occur but only late in disease process
    - If aditus ad antrum occluded, mastoid air cells opacify with retained secretions
  - Common locations of CCh-ME
    - Anterosuperior middle ear, adjacent to eustachian tube & anterior tympanic ring, medial to ossicular structures

DDx: Middle Ear Masses

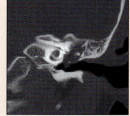

Acq Cholesteatoma

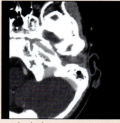

Rhabdomyosarcoma

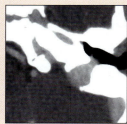

Dehiscent Jugular Bulb

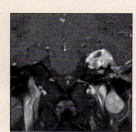

Facial Schwannoma

CONGENITAL CHOLESTEATOMA

Key Facts

Terminology
- Synonyms: Primary cholesteatoma, epidermoid, "skin in the wrong place"

Imaging Findings
- Best diagnostic clue: Smooth, well-circumscribed middle ear mass ± ossicular erosions
- Other locations: EAC, middle ear-mastoid, petrous apex, CP angle, geniculate ganglion

Top Differential Diagnoses
- Acquired cholesteatoma
- Rhabdomyosarcoma, middle ear
- Dehiscent jugular bulb
- Facial nerve schwannoma, middle ear

Pathology
- Congenital abnormal ectodermal rest
- Epidemiology: 2-5% of cholesteatomas are congenital
- Early or "closed" CCh: Small, encapsulated focal anterior tympanic cavity mass
- Late or "open" CCh: Large ME mass, extends throughout cavity & mastoid complex

Clinical Issues
- Most common signs/symptoms: Avascular ME mass behind intact TM without prior history of inflammation or trauma
- Unilateral conductive hearing loss (CHL)

- Inferior but adjacent to tensor tympani muscle, mimics pars tensa acquired middle ear cholesteatoma that also often ends up medial to ossicles
  - Near stapes
  - Posterior epitympanum, at tympanic isthmus

MR Findings
- T1WI: Iso- to hypointense ME mass
- T2WI
  - Intermediate intensity ME mass
  - With larger lesions, aditus ad antrum obstruction seen as high signal retained secretions in mastoid air cells
- T1 C+
  - Peripherally-enhancing ME mass
    - CCh-ME is nonenhancing material surrounded by thin subtle rim-enhancement
  - If lesion is long-standing, associated scar may be seen as thickened area of enhancement adjacent to CCh-ME

Imaging Recommendations
- Temporal bone CT is examination of choice
- T1 C+ MR is complimentary exam in certain circumstances, recommended if
  - Recurrent or large CCh-ME
  - Diagnosis uncertain

DIFFERENTIAL DIAGNOSIS

Acquired cholesteatoma
- Clinical: Otoscopy reveals retraction pocket, pars flaccida or pars tensa TM perforation
- CT findings
  - Pars flaccida cholesteatoma, acquired
    - Scutum erosion with lesion in Prussak space of lateral epitympanum
    - Ossicular chain & lateral semicircular canal more likely eroded
    - Chronic inflammatory changes present
  - Pars tensa cholesteatoma, acquired
    - Lesion enlarges medial to ossicles
    - Ossicular erosion common

Rhabdomyosarcoma, middle ear
- Parameningeal type
- Imaging findings
  - Aggressive, destructive mass in middle ear and mastoid
  - Potential extension
    - Lateral extension into EAC
    - Medial extension into internal auditory canal
    - Cephalad extension into middle cranial fossa
    - Posterior extension into posterior cranial fossa
    - Inferior extension into nasopharyngeal, temporal mandibular joint, masticator or parotid space

Dehiscent jugular bulb
- Clinical: Usually asymptomatic, incidental finding in imaging studies
  - May present with blue mass behind intact tympanic membrane on otoscopic exam
- CT findings
  - Superior and lateral extension of jugular bulb into middle ear cavity via dehiscent jugular plate of sigmoid sinus

Facial nerve schwannoma, middle ear
- Clinical: Otoscopy shows avascular mass behind intact TM
  - Rare in children
- Imaging findings
  - Tubular mass emanating from tympanic facial nerve canal, enhancing on T1 C+ MR
  - Enlarged bony facial nerve canal and geniculate fossa
  - Extends from geniculate ganglion along tympanic segment of facial nerve

PATHOLOGY

General Features
- Etiology

CONGENITAL CHOLESTEATOMA

- ○ Congenital abnormal ectodermal rest
  - ▪ In middle ear: Abnormal migration of external canal ectoderm beyond tympanic ring, becomes a mass-like middle ear accumulation of stratified epithelial squamous cells
- Epidemiology: 2-5% of cholesteatomas are congenital
- Associated abnormalities
  - ○ EAC atresia can present with associated CCh
  - ○ Rarely associated with 1st branchial cleft remnant

Gross Pathologic & Surgical Features
- Circumscribed, pearly-white mass with capsular sheen
- When detected early, no associated inflammatory changes

Microscopic Features
- Identical to epidermoid inclusion cyst
- Stratified squamous epithelium, with progressive exfoliation of keratinous material
- Contents rich in cholesterol crystals

Staging, Grading or Classification Criteria
- Early or "closed" CCh: Small, encapsulated focal anterior tympanic cavity mass
- Late or "open" CCh: Large ME mass, extends throughout cavity & mastoid complex

CLINICAL ISSUES

Presentation
- Most common signs/symptoms: Avascular ME mass behind intact TM without prior history of inflammation or trauma
- Other symptoms
  - ○ Unilateral conductive hearing loss (CHL)
  - ○ Large lesions can obstruct eustachian tube with resultant ME effusion & infection
  - ○ May be discovered surgically after chronic ME effusion unresponsive to tympanostomy tubes
  - ○ EAC mass if arises in EAC (rare)

Demographics
- Age
  - ○ Average age of presentation or detection
    - ▪ Anterior or anterosuperior: 4 years
    - ▪ Posterosuperior & mesotympanum: 12 years
    - ▪ Attic & mastoid antrum involvement: 20 years
- Gender: M:F = 3:1

Natural History & Prognosis
- CCh-ME: Smaller, anterior lesions have better outcome, with complete surgical resection
- If untreated, keratin debris accumulates over time, with resultant larger lesion
  - ○ Enlarging, cyst-like CCh may rupture, extending throughout ME
  - ○ If eustachian tube obstructed, ME effusions & otitis occur
  - ○ Larger lesions with infection may be difficult to differentiate from acquired cholesteatoma
- Large lesions or posterior epitympanic CCh have recurrence rates as high as 20%
  - ○ Staged surgical resection often used for large lesions

- Temporal bone CT to assess for recurrence

Treatment
- Complete surgical extirpation = treatment of choice
- Ossicle chain reconstruction may be necessary

DIAGNOSTIC CHECKLIST

Consider
- CCh-ME mass is seen behind intact TM
- No history of prior TM perforation
- ME is opacified with wall erosion in patient with external auditory canal atresia

SELECTED REFERENCES

1. El-Bitar MA et al: Congenital middle ear cholesteatoma: need for early recognition--role of computed tomography scan. Int J Pediatr Otorhinolaryngol. 67(3):231-5, 2003
2. Darrouzet V et al: Congenital middle ear cholesteatomas in children: our experience in 34 cases. Otolaryngol Head Neck Surg. 126(1):34-40, 2002
3. El-Bitar MA et al: Bilateral occurrence of congenital middle ear cholesteatoma. Otolaryngol Head Neck Surg. 127(5):480-2, 2002
4. Koltai PJ et al: The natural history of congenital cholesteatoma. Arch Otolaryngol Head Neck Surg. 128(7):804-9, 2002
5. Nelson M et al: Congenital cholesteatoma: classification, management, and outcome. Arch Otolaryngol Head Neck Surg. 128(7):810-4, 2002
6. Potsic WP et al: A staging system for congenital cholesteatoma. Arch Otolaryngol Head Neck Surg. 128(9):1009-12, 2002
7. Potsic WP et al: Congenital cholesteatoma: 20 years' experience at The Children's Hospital of Philadelphia. Otolaryngol Head Neck Surg. 126:409-14, 2002
8. Shohet JA et al: The management of pediatric cholesteatoma. Otolaryngol Clin North Am. 35(4):841-51, 2002
9. Yammine FG et al: Anterior and posterior middle ear congenital cholesteatomas in children. J Otolaryngol. 30(1):29-33, 2001
10. Yeo SW et al: The clinical evaluations of pathophysiology for congenital middle ear cholesteatoma. Am J Otolaryngol. 22(3):184-9, 2001
11. Liu JH et al: Congenital cholesteatoma of the middle ear. Clin Pediatr (Phila). 39(9):549-51, 2000
12. Melero GA et al: Facial paralysis: An unusual presentation of congenital cholesteatoma. Otolaryngol Head Neck Surg. 122(4):615-6, 2000
13. Tos M: A new pathogenesis of mesotympanic (congenital) cholesteatoma. Laryngoscope. 110(11):1890-7, 2000
14. De la Cruz A et al: Detection and management of childhood cholesteatoma. Pediatr Ann. 28(6):370-3, 1999
15. Friedberg J: Congenital cholesteatoma. Laryngoscope. 104:1-24, 1994

CONGENITAL CHOLESTEATOMA

IMAGE GALLERY

Typical

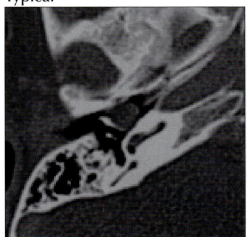
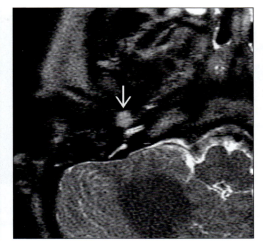

(Left) Axial bone CT shows well-defined middle ear congenital cholesteatoma abutting the malleus and cochlear promontory without osseous erosion. *(Right)* Axial T2WI MR in the same patient shows the middle ear congenital cholesteatoma as an intermediate signal intensity well-defined middle ear mass *(arrow)*.

Typical

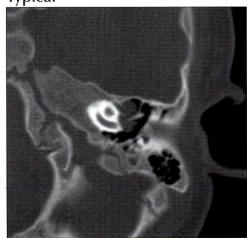
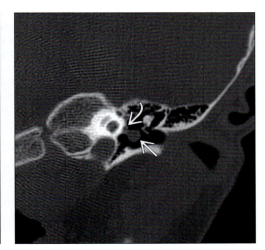

(Left) Axial bone CT shows a medium sized congenital cholesteatoma in the middle ear without osseous destruction. The mastoid air cells are clear without evidence of chronic inflammatory disease. *(Right)* Coronal bone CT in the same patient shows well-defined middle ear cholesteatoma *(arrow)* abutting the lateral aspect of the horizontal facial nerve canal *(curved arrow)*, without osseous erosion.

Variant

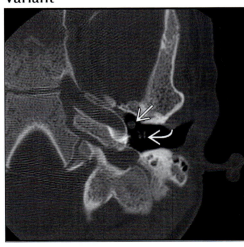
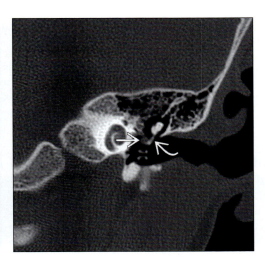

(Left) Axial bone CT shows small well-defined middle ear cholesteatoma *(arrow)* at the eustachian tube orifice, noticed in the operating room during placement of myringotomy tube *(curved arrow)*. *(Right)* Coronal bone CT in the same patient shows a second well-defined middle ear congenital cholesteatoma *(arrow)* abutting the medial aspect of the long process of the malleus *(curved arrow)*.

ACQUIRED CHOLESTEATOMA

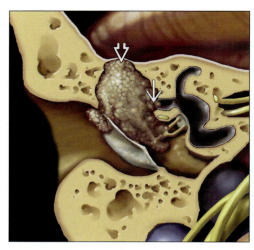

Coronal graphic shows large pars flaccida acquired cholesteatoma. Complications include erosion of ossicles, lateral semicircular canal (arrow) and thinning of tegmen tympani (open arrow).

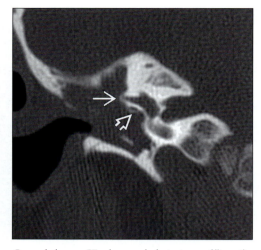

Coronal bone CT shows cholesteatoma filling the middle ear cavity with erosion of the ossicles. The lateral semicircular canal (arrow), facial nerve canal (open arrow) and tegmen tympani are intact.

TERMINOLOGY

Abbreviations and Synonyms
- Secondary or acquired cholesteatoma (ACh)
  - "Attic" or "Prussak space" cholesteatoma = pars flaccida cholesteatoma (PFC)
  - Pars tensa cholesteatoma (PTC)
    - "Sinus" cholesteatoma = PTC involving sinus tympani
- Tympanic membrane (TM)

Definitions
- Stratified squamous epithelium-lined sac filled with exfoliated keratin debris

IMAGING FINDINGS

General Features
- Best diagnostic clue
  - PFC: Nonenhancing soft tissue mass in Prussak space with scutum erosion
    - +/- Tegmen tympani, lateral semicircular canal, facial nerve canal or sigmoid sinus plate dehiscence
  - PTC: Nonenhancing mass in posterior tympanum medial to ossicles
- Location
  - Pars flaccida ACh: 82% of all cholesteatomas
    - Secondary to TM perforation or retraction pocket involving the anterior superior pars flaccida portion of the TM (also called Shrapnell membrane)
  - Pars tensa ACh: 18% of all cholesteatomas
    - Secondary to TM perforation or retraction pocket in the inferior pars tensa portion of TM
  - Mural = automastoidectomy, atypical cholesteatoma shell
    - Residual cholesteatoma rind left behind after middle ear-mastoid acquired cholesteatoma extrudes central matrix through TM or EAC bony wall
  - Other: Petrous apex, cerebellopontine angle
- Size: Few mm to several cm

CT Findings
- CECT
  - No enhancement of cholesteatoma
  - Surrounding granulation tissue may enhance
- Bone CT
  - Pars flaccida ACh
    - Soft tissue mass in Prussak space, LATERAL to malleus head, scutum erosion characteristic
    - Ossicles displaced medially

DDx: Temporal Bone Masses With Bony Destruction

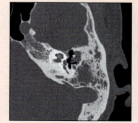
Cong Cholesteatoma

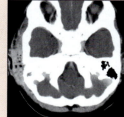
Mastoiditis

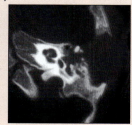
LCH

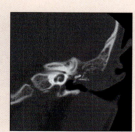
Rhabdomyosarcoma

ACQUIRED CHOLESTEATOMA

Key Facts

Terminology
- Secondary or acquired cholesteatoma (ACh)
- "Attic" or "Prussak space" cholesteatoma = pars flaccida cholesteatoma (PFC)
- Pars tensa cholesteatoma (PTC)

Imaging Findings
- PFC: Nonenhancing soft tissue mass in Prussak space with scutum erosion
- PTC: Nonenhancing mass in posterior tympanum medial to ossicles

Top Differential Diagnoses
- Congenital cholesteatoma
- Chronic otitis media with ossicular erosion
- Acute coalescent otomastoiditis (ACOM) with abscess
- Langerhan cell histiocytosis (LCH)
- Rhabdomyosarcoma

Pathology
- TM retraction or TM perforation results in accumulation of stratified squamous epithelial cells in middle ear cavity
- Squamous epithelial cells produce mass-like ball of keratin
- Continually enlarges, may cause erosion of adjacent bone

Diagnostic Checklist
- When middle ear and mastoid opacified, difficult to differentiate effusion from cholesteatoma
- Presence of ossicular erosion supports diagnosis of cholesteatoma but may also occur in non-cholesteatomatous chronic otitis media

---

- Ossicular erosion in 70%: Most commonly incus long process, less commonly incus body & malleus head
- May extend posterolateral to aditus ad antrum and mastoid antrum or inferiorly to posterior middle ear recesses
- May also erode lateral semicircular canal, facial nerve canal, tegmen tympani and/or sigmoid sinus plate
  - Pars tensa ACh
    - Erosive mass in posterior tympanum MEDIAL to ossicles
    - May involve sinus tympani, facial recess, aditus ad antrum and/or mastoid
    - Ossicular erosion common (90%), especially medial aspect of incus long process, stapes suprastructure and malleus manubrium
    - +/- Posterior tegmen tympani dehiscence
  - Mural ACh
    - "Hollowed out" middle ear-mastoid with residual cholesteatoma rind along walls of cavity
  - Radiologists search pattern and report should include
    - Location of mass
    - Relationship to ossicles
    - Integrity of ossicles, scutum, lateral semicircular canal, tegmen tympani, facial nerve canal and sigmoid sinus plate
    - Extension into mastoid antrum
    - Assessment of mastoid air cells: Aerated or opaque, coalescent or non-coalescent, may be small and underpneumatized with sclerotic septations secondary to chronic infection

MR Findings
- T1WI: Middle ear mass hypointense
- T2WI: Mildly hyperintense, usually less than trapped secretions
- T1 C+
  - PFC or PTC does not enhance
  - Associated granulation tissue or scar may enhance
  - If tegmen tympani dehiscent, coronal may show dural enhancement, adjacent to bony defect

Imaging Recommendations
- Best imaging tool
  - Noncontrast bone CT: Axial and coronal
    - Prussak space mass, scutum and tegmen tympani best evaluated on coronal images
    - Ossicular erosion, lateral semicircular canal and facial nerve canal erosion: Need to view axial and coronal images
    - Sigmoid plate erosion best evaluated on axial images
  - Coronal T1 C+ MR useful adjunct when cephalocele, intracranial extension or intracranial infection suspected

DIFFERENTIAL DIAGNOSIS

Congenital cholesteatoma
- 2% of all cholesteatomas
- Well-defined middle ear mass behind intact TM
- Osseous erosion similar to ACh if large
- Usually lacks history of recurrent infection or TM perforation

Chronic otitis media with ossicular erosion
- Non-cholesteatomatous ossicular erosion: Distal incus most common
- TM often retracted
- Often without surrounding inflammatory debris
- Mastoid may be sclerotic secondary to chronic otitis media during mastoid formation
- May be indistinguishable from ACh on CT

Acute coalescent otomastoiditis (ACOM) with abscess
- Clinical presentation: Fever, periauricular erythema, pain, fluctuance
- Rim-enhancing fluid collection adjacent to opacified mastoid air cells = abscess
  - May be intracranial or extracranial
- Variable trabecular & cortical erosions, erosion may be difficult to detect

ACQUIRED CHOLESTEATOMA

- Regional complications of acute coalescent mastoiditis
  - Subperiosteal abscess
  - Meningitis, brain abscess, epidural abscess
  - Sigmoid sinus thrombosis secondary to thrombophlebitis
  - Bezold abscess around sternocleidomastoid muscle
  - Labyrinthitis
  - Petrous apicitis
  - Communicating hydrocephalus secondary to obstruction of arachnoid granulations

Langerhan cell histiocytosis (LCH)
- Enhancing soft tissue mass with bone destruction
- Locations in head and neck: orbit, maxilla, mandible, temporal bone, cervical spine, skull

Rhabdomyosarcoma
- Parameningeal = middle ear, paranasal sinus, nasopharynx
- Soft tissue mass with variable contrast-enhancement
- Aggressive osseous destruction common

PATHOLOGY

General Features
- Etiology
  - TM retraction or TM perforation results in accumulation of stratified squamous epithelial cells in middle ear cavity
  - Squamous epithelial cells produce mass-like ball of keratin
  - Continually enlarges, may cause erosion of adjacent bone
  - Associated chronic inflammation may cause further bone erosion
- Associated abnormalities: Increased risk in patients with cleft palate

Gross Pathologic & Surgical Features
- Pearly white mass

Microscopic Features
- Collection of stratified squamous epithelium filled with exfoliated keratin debris, rich in cholesterol crystals
- Chronic inflammatory changes usually present

CLINICAL ISSUES

Presentation
- Most common signs/symptoms
  - Conductive hearing loss (CHL)
  - Recurrent or chronic middle ear infections with TM perforation or retraction pocket
  - Foul-smelling aural discharge
  - Middle ear mass with TM perforation on otologic examination
- Other signs/symptoms: Painless otorrhea, vertigo, otalgia, facial nerve paralysis

Demographics
- Age
  - Occurs in children and adults
  - Unusual in children less than 4 years of age

Natural History & Prognosis
- Natural history
  - Small cholesteatoma forms within retraction pocket, progressive increase in size results in destruction of surrounding structures (ossicles, semicircular canals, tegmen tympani, facial nerve canal, transverse sinus invasion)
  - If untreated: CN 7 involvement, venous sinus thrombosis and intracranial extension are late complications
- Prognosis
  - Excellent if complete removal of small lesions
  - Residual CHL, sensorineural hearing loss and peripheral facial nerve paralysis possible
  - Sinus tympani extension associated with high post-surgical recurrence rate

Treatment
- Surgical excision, mastoidectomy and ossicular chain reconstruction if needed

DIAGNOSTIC CHECKLIST

Image Interpretation Pearls
- When middle ear and mastoid opacified, difficult to differentiate effusion from cholesteatoma
- Presence of ossicular erosion supports diagnosis of cholesteatoma but may also occur in non-cholesteatomatous chronic otitis media

SELECTED REFERENCES

1. Shohet JA et al: The management of pediatric cholesteatoma. Otolaryngol Clin North Am. 35(4):841-51, 2002
2. Watts S et al: A systematic approach to interpretation of computed tomography scans prior to surgery of middle ear cholesteatoma. J Laryngol Otol. 114(4):248-53, 2000
3. Fageeh NA et al: Surgical treatment of cholesteatoma in children. J Otolaryngol. 28(6):309-12, 1999
4. Mafee MF et al: Epidermoid cyst (cholesteatoma) and cholesterol granuloma of the temporal bone and epidermoid cysts affecting the brain. Neuroimaging Clin N Am. 4(3):561-78, 1994
5. Mafee MF: MRI and CT in the evaluation of acquired and congenital cholesteatomas of the temporal bone. J Otolaryngol. 22(4):239-48, 1993
6. Vartiainen E et al: Long-term results of surgical treatment in different cholesteatoma types. Am J Otol. 14(5):507-11, 1993
7. Schuring AG et al: Staging for cholesteatoma in the child, adolescent, and adult. Ann Otol Rhinol Laryngol. 99(4 Pt 1):256-60, 1990
8. Mafee MF et al: Cholesteatoma of the middle ear and mastoid. A comparison of CT scan and operative findings. Otolaryngol Clin North Am. 21(2):265-93, 1988
9. Nardis PF et al: Unusual cholesteatoma shell: CT findings. J Comput Assist Tomogr. 12(6):1084-5, 1988
10. Swartz JD: Cholesteatomas of the middle ear. Diagnosis, etiology, and complications. Radiol Clin North Am. 22(1):15-35, 1984
11. Michaels L: Biology of cholesteatoma. Otolaryngol Clin North Am. 22(5):869-81, 1989

ACQUIRED CHOLESTEATOMA

IMAGE GALLERY

Typical

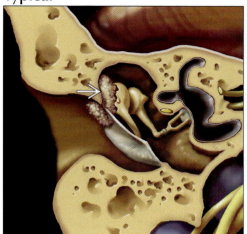
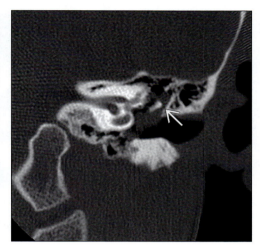

(Left) Coronal graphic shows small cholesteatoma originating at pars flaccida portion of the tympanic membrane, filling Prussak space (arrow), with slight medial displacement of the ossicles. *(Right)* Coronal bone CT shows cholesteatoma lateral to the ossicles, filling Prussak space (arrow), the mesotympanum and to a lesser extent the hypotympanum without bone erosion.

Typical

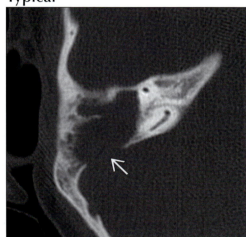
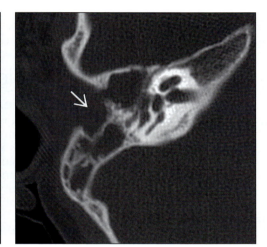

(Left) Axial bone CT shows complete opacification of right tympanic cavity and mastoid complex. There is destruction of mastoid septations and focal dehiscence of the sigmoid sinus plate (arrow). *(Right)* Axial bone CT in the same patient shows mastoid and middle ear opacification, ossicular erosions and erosion of the anterior suprameatal mastoid cortex (arrow).

Typical

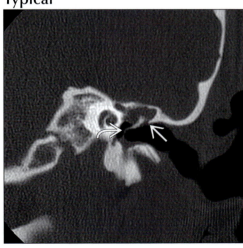
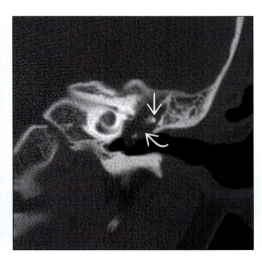

(Left) Coronal bone CT shows retraction of the TM (curved arrow) and cholesteatoma filling the epitympanic cavity and Prussak's space, without erosion of the scutum (arrow). *(Right)* Coronal bone CT shows cholesteatoma filling the mesotympanum, epitympanum and attic. There is partial erosion of the malleus head (arrow) and manubrium (curved arrow).

ORBITAL CELLULITIS

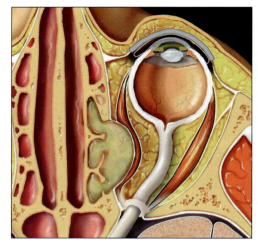

Axial graphic shows the spread of infection from the ethmoid sinuses through the lamina papyracea into the medial orbit. Subperiosteal abscess results, putting the optic nerve at risk.

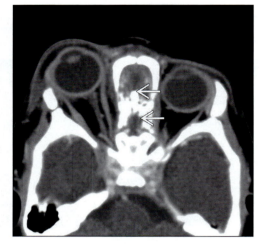

Axial CECT shows right preseptal and postseptal (arrows) soft tissue inflammation. The medial rectus muscle is elevated, the lateral rectus muscle is enlarged and there is proptosis.

TERMINOLOGY

Abbreviations and Synonyms
- Extraocular muscle (EOM)
- Subperiosteal abscess (SPA)

Definitions
- Orbital septum
  - Periosteal reflection from the bony orbit to the tarsal plates of the eyelids
- Chandler classification: Orbital complications of sinusitis
  - Preseptal cellulitis
    - Inflammation anterior to the orbital septum
    - Eyelid edema
    - Without tenderness, visual loss or limited EOM motility (ophthalmoplegia)
  - Orbital cellulitis without abscess
    - Diffuse postseptal edema of orbital fat
  - Orbital cellulitis with subperiosteal abscess
    - +/- Proptosis
    - +/- Decreased vision
    - +/- Limited EOM motility
  - Orbital cellulitis with abscess in orbital fat
    - Usually severe proptosis
    - Decreased vision
    - Limited EOM motility
  - Cavernous sinus thrombosis secondary to orbital phlebitis
    - Unilateral or bilateral

IMAGING FINDINGS

General Features
- Best diagnostic clue
  - Thickening and edema of orbital soft tissues = cellulitis and/or phlegmon
  - Low attenuation rim enhancing subperiosteal collection
    - Majority are drainable abscess (SPA)
    - 20% phlegmon without drainable abscess
- Location
  - Preseptal: Disease anterior to the orbital septum
  - Postseptal: Disease posterior to the orbital septum
    - Intraconal: Within the cone formed by the EOMs
    - Extraconal: Postseptal disease between the bony orbit and the EOMs
    - Subperiosteal: Between the bony orbit and the orbital periosteum
  - Associated myositis
    - Swollen EOMs, may have abnormal contrast-enhancement
  - Beware of associated extraorbital complications of sinusitis

DDx: Extra-Orbital Complications Of Sinusitis

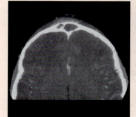
PPT

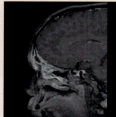
PPT/Meninigitis

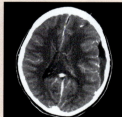
Empyema

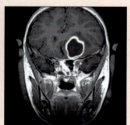
Cerebral Abscess

ORBITAL CELLULITIS

Key Facts

Terminology
- Chandler classification: Orbital complications of sinusitis
- Preseptal cellulitis
- Orbital cellulitis without abscess
- Orbital cellulitis with subperiosteal abscess
- Orbital cellulitis with abscess in orbital fat
- Cavernous sinus thrombosis secondary to orbital phlebitis

Imaging Findings
- Thickening and edema of orbital soft tissues = cellulitis and/or phlegmon
- Low attenuation rim enhancing subperiosteal collection
- Preseptal: Disease anterior to the orbital septum
- Postseptal: Disease posterior to the orbital septum
- Associated myositis
- CECT: Axial and direct coronal or coronal reformatted images (multidetector CT)
- MRI: Best for evaluation of intracranial complications of sinusitis

Diagnostic Checklist
- May be difficult to distinguish subperiosteal abscess from phlegmon
- Cavernous sinus thrombosis may be subtle: Compare size, shape and enhancement to contralateral side if unilateral
- Beware of extraorbital complications sinusitis
- MRI indicated if suspect intracranial complication

- Frontal osteomyelitis, meningitis, empyema, cerebritis, parenchymal abscess

Imaging Recommendations
- Best imaging tool
  - CECT: Axial and direct coronal or coronal reformatted images (multidetector CT)
  - MRI: Best for evaluation of intracranial complications of sinusitis

DIFFERENTIAL DIAGNOSIS

Frontal osteomyelitis - Pott puffy tumor (PPT)
- Forehead cellulitis, phlegmon and/or subgaleal abscess
- Frontal bone lytic lesion may be difficult to detect acutely

Meningitis
- Abnormal meningeal contrast enhancement

Empyema
- Epidural (lenticular) or subdural (crescent) extra-axial collection of pus
- Restricted diffusion DWI (increased signal intensity)
- Usually with peripheral dural contrast-enhancement
- Nonenhancing collections may be sterile, i.e. effusions rather than pus

Cerebritis
- Amorphous intra-axial edema without rim-enhancement

Abscess
- Round or ovoid collection of pus within the brain
- Ring enhancing wall with uniform thickness
- Hyperintense DWI, hypointense ADC

PATHOLOGY

General Features
- Etiology
  - Sinusitis: Most common cause of orbital cellulitis
    - Other causes: Trauma, foreign body, skin infection, rarely retinoblastoma may present as orbital cellulitis
  - Beware of underlying cause of sinusitis
    - Nasolacrimal duct mucocele
    - Antrochoanal polyp
    - Sinonasal foreign body
    - Odontogenic sinusitis
  - Orbital cellulitis: Most common complication of sinusitis
    - Up to 3% of patients with sinusitis
    - May precede signs and symptoms of sinusitis
    - Usually secondary to ethmoiditis
  - Spread of sinus infection to the orbit
    - Direct extension via thin, acquired dehiscence, and/or normal foramina in the lamina papyracea
    - Valveless venous system (diploic veins of Breschet) connects orbital circulation with ethmoid, frontal and maxillary sinus circulation
    - Lymphatic seeding unlikely - no lymph vessels in the orbit
- Associated abnormalities
  - Potential intracranial spread of infection via diploic veins
    - Meningitis
    - Subdural or epidural effusion or empyema
    - Cerebritis
    - Brain abscess

Microscopic Features
- Microbiology
  - Under 10 years; usually single aerobe
    - Majority Streptococcus pneumoniae, Hemophilus influenza, Moraxella catarrhalis, Streptococcus pyogenes
  - 10-15; years mixed, mostly aerobes
  - Over 15 years; mixed, aerobes and anaerobes

ORBITAL CELLULITIS

CLINICAL ISSUES

Presentation
- Most common signs/symptoms
  - Depends on degree of inflammation
    - Eyelid swelling, erythema, tenderness
    - Proptosis
    - Ophthalmoplegia results in diplopia
    - Decreased visual acuity
    - Relative afferent pupillary defect (Marcus Gunn pupil) if pressure on optic nerve, dural sheath or vascular supply
- Other signs/symptoms
  - Cranial nerve palsies (CN III, IV, V, VI) with cavernous sinus thrombosis
  - Seizures, mental status change if associated with intracranial complications

Demographics
- Age: 50% of children are less than 4 years of age

Natural History & Prognosis
- Good with appropriate treatment
- Rare cause of blindness if untreated

Treatment
- Imaging indications
  - Significant impairment in visual acuity or ophthalmoplegia: Contrast-enhanced orbit CT
  - No improvement or worsening of symptoms on appropriate antibiotics
  - Suspect subperiosteal or orbital abscess in a patient with severe eyelid edema that prohibits evaluation of vision and EOM motility
- Medical management = intravenous antibiotics
  - Broad spectrum polymicrobial coverage: 2nd or 3rd generation cephalosporins, B-lactamase resistant penicillin combinations, carbapenems
  - Add clindamycin for anaerobic coverage particularly if 10-15 years of age
- Surgical management indications
  - Subperiosteal abscess (not absolute indication)
    - Younger children may only require antibiotics
    - More aggressive surgical drainage in older children
    - Emergent if visual disturbance from optic nerve or retinal compromise
  - Orbital abscess
  - Frontal sinus drainage in osteomyelitis
  - Rarely intracranial drainage of empyemas: Majority resolve with antibiotic therapy

DIAGNOSTIC CHECKLIST

Image Interpretation Pearls
- May be difficult to distinguish subperiosteal abscess from phlegmon
- Cavernous sinus thrombosis may be subtle: Compare size, shape and enhancement to contralateral side if unilateral
- Beware of underlying cause of sinusitis
- Beware of extraorbital complications sinusitis
- MRI indicated if suspect intracranial complication

SELECTED REFERENCES

1. Pelton RW et al: Cosmetic considerations in surgery for orbital subperiosteal abscess in children: experience with a combined transcaruncular and transnasal endoscopic approach. Arch Otolaryngol Head Neck Surg. 129(6):652-5, 2003
2. Givner LB: Periorbital versus orbital cellulitis. Pediatr Infect Dis J. 21(12):1157-8, 2002
3. Sobol SE et al: Orbital complications of sinusitis in children. J Otolaryngol. 31(3):131-6, 2002
4. Younis RT et al: Orbital infection as a complication of sinusitis: are diagnostic and treatment trends changing? Ear Nose Throat J. 81(11):771-5, 2002
5. Management of orbital subperiosteal abscess in children: Arch Otolaryngol Head Neck Surg. 127(3):281-6, 2001
6. Starkey CR et al: Medical management of orbital cellulitis. Pediatr Infect Dis J. 20(10):1002-5, 2001
7. Ambati BK et al: Periorbital and orbital cellulitis before and after the advent of Haemophilus influenzae type B vaccination. Ophthalmology. 107(8):1450-3, 2000
8. Garcia GH et al: Criteria for nonsurgical management of subperiosteal abscess of the orbit: analysis of outcomes 1988-1998. Ophthalmology. 107(8):1454-6; discussion 1457-8, 2000
9. Mehra P et al: Odontogenic sinusitis causing orbital cellulitis. J Am Dent Assoc. 130(7):1086-92, 1999
10. Donahue SP et al: Preseptal and orbital cellulitis in childhood. A changing microbiologic spectrum. Ophthalmology. 105(10):1902-5; discussion 1905-6, 1998
11. Nelson LB et al: Managing orbital cellulitis. J Pediatr Ophthalmol Strabismus. 35(2):68, 1998
12. Pereira KD et al: Management of medial subperiosteal abscess of the orbit in children--a 5 year experience. Int J Pediatr Otorhinolaryngol. 38(3):247-54, 1997
13. Babu RP et al: Pott's puffy tumor: the forgotten entity. Case report. J Neurosurg. 84(1):110-2, 1996
14. Harris GJ: Subperiosteal abscess of the orbit: computed tomography and the clinical course. Ophthal Plast Reconstr Surg. 12(1):1-8, 1996
15. Harris GJ: Subperiosteal abscess of the orbit. Age as a factor in the bacteriology and response to treatment. Ophthalmology. 101(3):585-95, 1994
16. Arjmand EM et al: Pediatric sinusitis and subperiosteal orbital abscess formation: diagnosis and treatment. Otolaryngol Head Neck Surg. 109(5):886-94, 1993
17. Andrews TM et al: The role of computed tomography in the diagnosis of subperiosteal abscess of the orbit. Clin Pediatr (Phila). 31(1):37-43, 1992
18. Handler LC et al: The acute orbit: differentiation of orbital cellulitis from subperiosteal abscess by computerized tomography. Neuroradiology. 33(1):15-8, 1991
19. Patt BS et al: Blindness resulting from orbital complications of sinusitis. Otolaryngol Head Neck Surg. 104(6):789-95, 1991
20. Shields JA et al: Retinoblastoma manifesting as orbital cellulitis. Am J Ophthalmol. 112(4):442-9, 1991
21. Chandler JR et al: The pathogenesis of orbital complications in acute sinusitis. Laryngoscope. 80(9):1414-28, 1970

ORBITAL CELLULITIS

IMAGE GALLERY

Typical

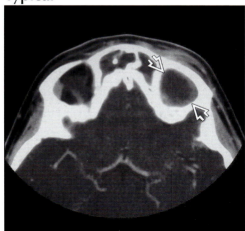
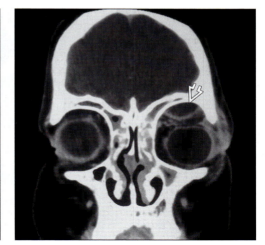

(Left) Axial CECT shows frontal sinus opacification, left forehead cellulitis and low attenuation collection in superior aspect of left orbit (arrows) which simulates appearance of the globe. *(Right)* Coronal CECT shows clearly that low attenuation collection (arrow) in superior left orbit is a rim-enhancing subperiosteal abscess causing inferior displacement of left globe.

Typical

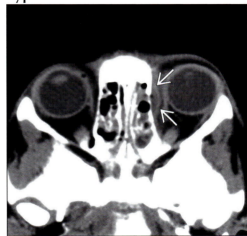
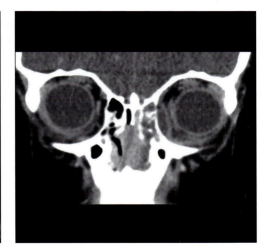

(Left) Axial CECT shows a small rim-enhancing subperiosteal collection (arrows) with a small bubble of gas in the medial extra-conal space of the left orbit. Associated ethmoid sinusitis. *(Right)* Coronal CECT better demonstrates the rim-enhancing subperiosteal collection in the medial extra-conal space of the left orbit. The left medial rectus muscle is elevated and there is strandy edema in the medial and inferior extra-conal space.

Typical

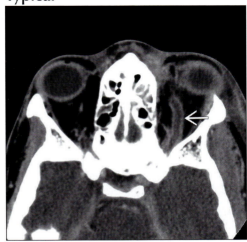
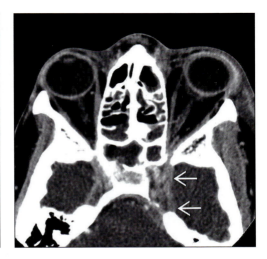

(Left) Axial CECT shows diffuse enlargement and lack of central enhancement in the left superior ophthalmic vein (arrow), associated ethmoid sinus disease, preseptal and postseptal orbital cellulitis. *(Right)* Axial CECT shows enlargement and heterogeneous contrast-enhancement in the partially thrombosed left cavernous sinus (arrows).

RETINOBLASTOMA

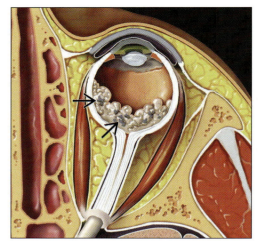

Axial graphic depicts retinoblastoma, with lobulated tumor extending through the limiting membrane into the vitreous. Punctate calcifications (arrows) are characteristic.

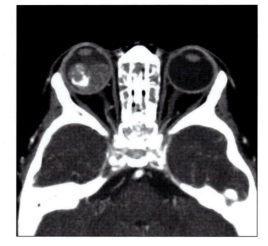

Axial CECT shows a large bilobed, partially calcified right intraocular mass typical of retinoblastoma. The noncalcified portion demonstrates mild fairly homogeneous contrast enhancement.

TERMINOLOGY

Abbreviations and Synonyms
- Retinoblastoma (RB)

Definitions
- Malignant retinal neoplasm, arises from neuroectodermal cells
- Trilateral RB: Bilateral ocular tumors plus midline intracranial neuroblastic tumor, pineal >> suprasellar
- Quadrilateral (tetralateral) RB: Bilateral disease plus pineal and suprasellar tumor
- Retinocytoma: Rare benign variant, similar genetics

IMAGING FINDINGS

General Features
- Best diagnostic clue: Calcified intraocular mass
- Location
  o Unilateral in 70-75%
  o Bilateral in 25-40%
  o Trilateral or quadrilateral disease rare
    ▪ 5-15% of familial lesions
  o Optic nerve or intraorbital extension uncommon
    ▪ 10-15% of patients, poor prognostic factor
  o Leptomeningeal metastasis rare
    ▪ 15-20% of patients with recurrent disease
  o Hematogenous metastasis rare
- Growth patterns
  o Endophytic form: Inward growth into vitreous
    ▪ Associated with vitreous seeding
  o Exophytic form: Outward growth into subretinal space
    ▪ Associated with retinal detachment
  o Diffuse infiltrating form: Plaque-like growth along retina
    ▪ Rare (1-2%); often no Ca++; older children
    ▪ Simulates inflammatory or other conditions

CT Findings
- NECT: Calcified intraocular mass 90-95%
- CECT: Variable enhancement of noncalcified portion

MR Findings
- T1WI: Variable, mildly hyperintense relative to vitreous
- T2WI
  o Hypointense relative to vitreous
  o Helps distinguish from other congenital lesions
  o Useful for demonstrating retinal detachment
- T1 C+
  o Moderate to marked heterogeneous enhancement
  o Best evaluates optic nerve and transscleral extension
  o Anterior segment enhancement more aggressive tumor behavior

DDx: Leukocoria

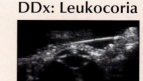
PHPV

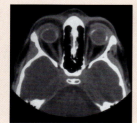
ROP

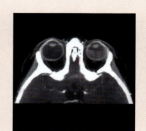
Coat Disease

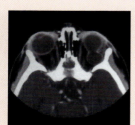
Coloboma

RETINOBLASTOMA

Key Facts

Terminology
- Malignant retinal neoplasm, arises from neuroectodermal cells

Imaging Findings
- Best diagnostic clue: Calcified intraocular mass
- Unilateral in 70-75%
- Hypointense relative to vitreous
- Moderate to marked heterogeneous enhancement
- CT for demonstrating calcification
- MR for assessing extraocular and intracranial disease

Top Differential Diagnoses
- Persistent hyperplastic primary vitreous (PHPV)
- Retinopathy of prematurity (ROP)
- Coat disease
- Coloboma of choroid or optic disc

Pathology
- RB1 gene codes for pRB tumor suppressor protein
- Sporadic nonfamilial form: 60%
- Familial hereditary form: 40%
- Most common malignant intraocular tumor of childhood; 3% of cancers in children under 15

Clinical Issues
- Most common signs/symptoms: Leukocoria (white pupillary reflex): 60%
- 90-95% diagnosed by age 5 years
- 90% cure for noninvasive intraocular RB

Diagnostic Checklist
- Check for intracranial trilateral or quadrilateral disease in pineal and suprasellar regions

---

Ultrasonographic Findings
- A-scan: Highly reflective spikes at calcifications
- B-scan: Echogenic, irregular mass with focal shadows
- Limited visualization of extra-ocular extension

Imaging Recommendations
- Best imaging tool
  - CT for demonstrating calcification
  - MR for assessing extraocular and intracranial disease
- Protocol advice: Include whole brain for trilateral disease and CSF seeding; FSE T2 and FS T1W MRI orbit

DIFFERENTIAL DIAGNOSIS

Persistent hyperplastic primary vitreous (PHPV)
- Failure of primary vitreous to undergo normal regression
- Proliferation of embryonic connective tissue
- Small globe, hyperdense; no Ca++
- Hyperintense T2WI retrolental fibrovascular stalk

Retinopathy of prematurity (ROP)
- Retrolental fibroplasia
- Secondary to prolonged exposure to supplemental oxygen
- Vitreous hemorrhage and retinal detachments
- Small globe, hyperdense, bilateral; Ca++ if advanced

Coat disease
- Primary retinal telangiectasia and exudative retinopathy
- Results in intraretinal/subretinal exudates/detachment
- Normal or small globe, hyperdense; no Ca++
- Hyperintense on T1WI and T2WI
- Usually boys older than 4 years of age

Coloboma of choroid or optic disc
- Congenital anomaly; focal posterior outpouching
- Normal size or small globe may have associated cyst

Ocular toxocariasis
- Sclerosing endophthalmitis due to Toxocara canis
- Uveoscleral enhancement; no Ca++ acutely

Other causes of leukocoria
- Retinal dysplasia, congenital cataract, retinal hamartoma, choroidal osteoma, choroidal hemangioma, nonspecific retinal detachment

PATHOLOGY

General Features
- Genetics
  - RB1 gene on Chromosome 13 at q14 locus
    - RB1 gene codes for pRB tumor suppressor protein
    - Regulates cell growth, division, and apoptosis
    - Two hit theory: Lack of both RB1 alleles in embryonic retinoblast leads to absence of pRB, resulting in malignancy
    - Other cell line malignancies also related to RB1
  - Somatic mosaicism in 10-20% of RB patients
- Etiology
  - Sporadic nonfamilial form: 60%
    - Spontaneous somatic mutation or deletion of both copies of RB1 in a retinoblast
    - Majority (85%) of unilateral disease
  - Familial hereditary form: 40%
    - Germline mutation or deletion of one copy of RB1, spontaneous mutation of other copy
    - Autosomal dominant
    - Positive family history in 5-10%
    - New germline mutations in 30-35%
    - Essentially all bilateral and multilateral disease
    - Minority (15%) of unilateral disease
- Epidemiology
  - Most common malignant intraocular tumor of childhood; 3% of cancers in children under 15
  - 1% of cancer deaths; 5% of childhood blindness
  - Incidence of 1:15,000-30,000 live births
    - Has increased in past 60 years
- Associated abnormalities

RETINOBLASTOMA

- Risk of other nonocular malignancies in patients with familial form
  - 20-30% in non-irradiated patients; 50-60% in irradiated patients
  - Within 30 years, average 10-13 years
  - Osteosarcoma, soft tissue sarcomas, melanoma
- 13q deletion syndrome: RB plus multiple organ system anomalies

Gross Pathologic & Surgical Features
- Yellowish-white to pink irregular retinal mass

Microscopic Features
- Small round cells, scant cytoplasm and large nuclei
- Flexner-Wintersteiner rosettes and fleurettes

Staging, Grading or Classification Criteria
- Reese-Ellsworth classification
  - Groups I through V; based on size, location, and multifocality
  - More useful in radiation therapy management
- Murphree classification (newer)
  - Groups A through E; based on size, retinal location, subretinal or vitreous seeding, and several specific prognostic features
  - More useful in chemotherapy management

CLINICAL ISSUES

Presentation
- Most common signs/symptoms: Leukocoria (white pupillary reflex): 60%
- Other signs/symptoms
  - Strabismus, severe vision loss, inflammatory signs (10%)
  - Less common: Anisocoria, heterochromia, glaucoma, cataract, nystagmus, proptosis

Demographics
- Age
  - RB is congenital but usually not apparent at birth
  - Average age 13 months at diagnosis in US
    - Earlier if family history with routine screening
  - 90-95% diagnosed by age 5 years

Natural History & Prognosis
- 90% cure for noninvasive intraocular RB
- Degree of nerve involvement correlates with survival
  - Superficial or no invasion: 90%; invasion to lamina cribrosa: 70%; invasion beyond lamina cribrosa: 60%; involvement at surgical margin: 20%
- Poor prognosis for extraocular disease
  - > 90% mortality
- Dismal prognosis for trilateral disease or CSF spread
  - < 24 month survival

Treatment
- Chemotherapy (chemoreduction)
  - Recent advance; limits need for external radiation
  - Currently favored first line therapy for lower grade intraocular tumors
  - Used in conjunction with other local modalities to achieve cure
- External beam radiation therapy (EBRT)
  - Indicated for bulky tumors with seeding
  - Unfavorable complications, e.g., arrested bone growth and radiation-induced tumors
- Plaque radiotherapy
  - Locally directed, I-215 or other isotope
  - Selected solitary or small tumors
- Enucleation
  - Indicated when no chance of preserving useful vision due to tumor spread or retinal detachments
- Cryotherapy
  - Primary local treatment of small anterior tumors
- Photocoagulation
  - Primary local treatment of small posterior tumors

DIAGNOSTIC CHECKLIST

Consider
- Early diagnosis is crucial for good outcome
- Regular screening for children with family history
- Close surveillance until age 7 for development of metachronous multilateral tumors
- RB can mimic inflammatory disease, particularly diffuse form

Image Interpretation Pearls
- Biopsy carries significant risk of seeding; therefore imaging diagnosis is crucial
- Check for intracranial trilateral or quadrilateral disease in pineal and suprasellar regions

SELECTED REFERENCES

1. Galluzzi P et al: Retinoblastoma: Abnormal gadolinium enhancement of anterior segment of eyes at MR imaging with clinical and histopathologic correlation. Radiology. 228(3):683-90, 2003
2. Schueler AO et al: High resolution magnetic resonance imaging of retinoblastoma. Br J Ophthalmol. 87(3):330-5, 2003
3. Tateishi U et al: CT and MRI features of recurrent tumors and second primary neoplasms in pediatric patients with retinoblastoma. AJR Am J Roentgenol. 181(3):879-84, 2003
4. De Potter P: Current treatment of retinoblastoma. Curr Opin Ophthalmol. 13(5):331-6, 2002
5. Brisse HJ et al: Sonographic, CT, and MR imaging findings in diffuse infiltrative retinoblastoma: report of two cases with histologic comparison. AJNR Am J Neuroradiol. 22(3):499-504, 2001
6. Shields CL et al: Recent developments in the management of retinoblastoma. J Pediatr Ophthalmol Strabismus. 36(1):8-18; quiz 35-6, 1999
7. Kaufman LM et al: Retinoblastoma and simulating lesions. Role of CT, MR imaging and use of Gd-DTPA contrast enhancement. Radiol Clin North Am. 36(6):1101-17, 1998
8. Skulski M et al: Trilateral retinoblastoma with suprasellar involvement. Neuroradiology. 39(1):41-3, 1997
9. Wong FL et al: Cancer incidence after retinoblastoma. Radiation dose and sarcoma risk. JAMA. 278(15):1262-7, 1997
10. Provenzale JM et al: Radiologic-pathologic correlation. Bilateral retinoblastoma with coexistent pineaoblastoma (trilateral retinoblastoma). AJNR Am J Neuroradiol. 16(1):157-65, 1995

RETINOBLASTOMA

IMAGE GALLERY

Variant

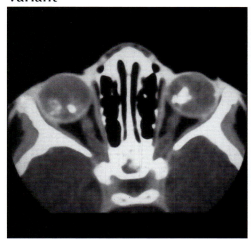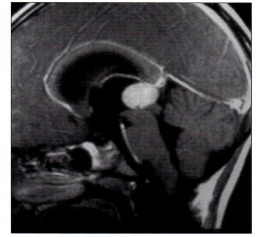

(Left) Axial CECT shows bilateral partially calcified intraocular retinoblastomas. *(Right)* Sagittal T1 C+ MR shows an enhancing pineal region mass consistent with trilateral RB in a child with bilateral retinoblastoma diagnosed 2 years prior. (Courtesy B. Ey, MD).

Typical

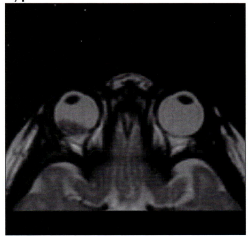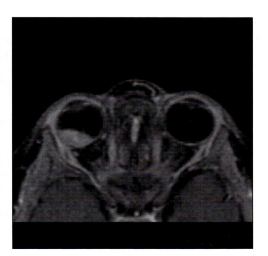

(Left) Axial T2WI MR shows a right intraocular mass, hypointense relative to the vitreous secondary to dense calcifications. *(Right)* Axial T1 C+ MR shows moderate diffuse postcontrast enhancement in the same patient with retinoblastoma.

Typical

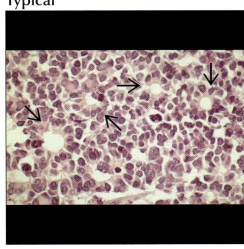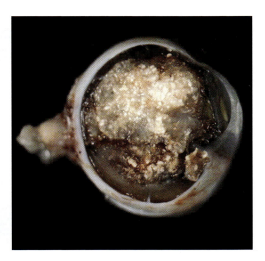

(Left) Micropathology, high power shows several Flexner-Wintersteiner rosettes (arrows) in a sea of bluish-red cells with scant cytoplasm. (Courtesy B. Ey, MD). *(Right)* Gross pathology shows the macroscopic appearance of the eye after exenteration. Retinoblastoma fills the vitreous. (Courtesy B. Ey, MD).

JUVENILE NASOPHARYNGEAL ANGIOFIBROMA

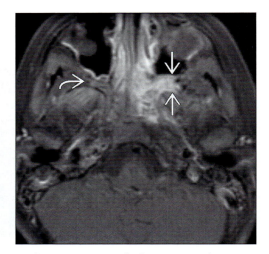

Graphic of skull base shows JNA origin in SPF, extending laterally into infratemporal fossa (arrow), superiorly into sphenoid (open arrow), and anteriorly into nasal cavity (curved arrow).

Axial T1 C+ MR with fat-saturation shows JNA expanding the pterygopalatine fossa (arrows) and extending into nasopharynx. Note normal appearance of contralateral PPF (curved arrow).

TERMINOLOGY

Abbreviations and Synonyms
- Juvenile nasal angiofibroma (JNA), juvenile angiofibroma (JAF), angiofibromatous hamartoma

Definitions
- Benign but aggressive hypervascular mass arising from sphenopalatine foramen (SPF) on lateral nasopharyngeal wall

IMAGING FINDINGS

General Features
- Best diagnostic clue: Enhancing mass arising from SPF in an adolescent male
- Location
  o Characteristic origin at SPF
  o Extends laterally into pterygopalatine fossa (PPF, pterygomaxillary fossa) in 90% of cases
  o Extends posteromedially into nasopharynx
  o Extends anteriorly into nasal cavity
  o Extends superiorly into sphenoid sinus, orbit, skull base and middle cranial fossa
- Size: Usually > 1 cm at diagnosis, can be very large
- Morphology: Usually appears well-defined at imaging

Radiographic Findings
- Anterior displacement (bowing) of posterior wall of maxillary sinus evident on lateral radiographs
  o Posterior wall may merely appear indistinct
- Soft tissue mass in nasal cavity or nasopharynx
- Erosion of medial pterygoid plate

CT Findings
- NECT
  o Soft tissue mass at SPF
  o Erosion/destruction of pterygoid plate
  o Displacement/destruction of posterior wall of maxillary sinus
  o Obliteration of normal fat attenuation in PPF
    ▪ Enlargement of PPF
- CECT: Avid and diffuse enhancement of mass
- CTA
  o Can show enlargement of ipsilateral external carotid artery (ECA) feeders to tumor
  o Can identify internal carotid artery (ICA) supply
  o Helpful in pre-angiographic planning

MR Findings
- T1WI
  o Generally isointense to muscle/brain
  o Contains foci of hypointensity ⇒ flow voids
- T2WI

DDx: Nasopharyngeal Masses In Children

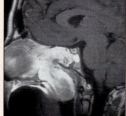
Vascular Polyp

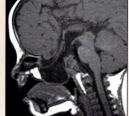
Encephalocele

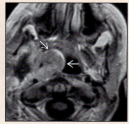
Rhabdomyosarcoma

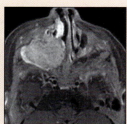
Germ Cell Tumor

JUVENILE NASOPHARYNGEAL ANGIOFIBROMA

Key Facts

Terminology
- Benign but aggressive hypervascular mass arising from sphenopalatine foramen (SPF) on lateral nasopharyngeal wall

Imaging Findings
- Extends laterally into pterygopalatine fossa (PPF, pterygomaxillary fossa) in 90% of cases
- Obliteration of normal fat attenuation in PPF
- Enlarged ECA branches supply tumor that has dense capillary blush and delayed wash out
- Distal branches of internal maxillary artery invariably involved
- MR with contrast and fat-saturation essential for identifying intracranial invasion
- Multiplanar reformatting and volume rendering can help in surgical planning

Top Differential Diagnoses
- Hypervascular polyp
- Rhabdomyosarcoma

Pathology
- Pathologic characteristics indicate it may be a vascular malformation rather than a tumor
- Associated abnormalities: Gardner syndrome (familial adenomatous polyposis) ⇒ 25x increased incidence

Clinical Issues
- Local recurrence after surgery in up to 25%
- Surgical resection with pre-operative embolization
- Particles or liquid embolics to reduce blood loss
- Surgery in 24-72 hours

  - Heterogeneous with flow voids more prominent than on T1WI
  - Ideal sequence to distinguish sinus secretions and mucosal thickening from tumor
- T1 C+ FS
  - Use of fat-saturation key in post contrast imaging of head and neck
  - Best sequence for defining extent of tumor
  - Multiplanar imaging essential to identify intracranial extension
- MRA
  - Can identify ECA and ICA supply to tumor
  - Helpful in pre-angiographic planning

Angiographic Findings
- Enlarged ECA branches supply tumor that has dense capillary blush and delayed wash out
  - Distal branches of internal maxillary artery invariably involved
  - Ascending pharyngeal artery, facial artery
- Tumor vessels are tortuous and sometimes irregular
- Important to identify any supply from contralateral ECA
- Essential to identify any supply from ICA
  - Ethmoidal branches of ophthalmic artery, vidian artery
  - Almost invariably present with tumors invading the skull base

Imaging Recommendations
- Best imaging tool
  - MR with contrast and fat-saturation essential for identifying intracranial invasion
    - Extension through skull base foramina (foramen ovale, foramen rotundum) and dural enhancement best shown on coronal T1 C+ FS
  - CT not always essential, but often first exam obtained
    - Defines bone erosion and remodeling best
    - Multiplanar reformatting and volume rendering can help in surgical planning
- Protocol advice
  - All JNA should be evaluated with MR
    - 3 planes post-contrast with fat-saturation
  - MRA to outline arterial supply for angiographic and surgical planning
  - Catheter angiography with bilateral ECA injection and at least ipsilateral ICA injection
  - Endovascular therapy (embolization) as pre-operative adjunct
    - Decrease intraoperative blood loss
    - May allow endoscopic removal of smaller tumors
    - Particles (polyvinyl alcohol), liquid embolic agents

DIFFERENTIAL DIAGNOSIS

Hypervascular polyp
- Angiomatous polyp ⇒ nasopharyngeal polyp that becomes hypervascular due to repeated injury
- Does not involve SPF, PPF
- Not as vascular as JNA, easier to resect

Rhabdomyosarcoma
- Most common primary malignant head and neck tumor in children
- Does not typically involve SPF, PPF

Germ cell tumors
- Nasopharyngeal teratoma ⇒ epignathus
- More primitive germ cell tumors can arise from same location

Nasopharyngeal carcinoma
- Associated with Epstein-Barr virus infection
- Higher incidence in south-east Asia
- Early peak incidence in second decade

Encephalocele
- Congenital herniation of intracranial contents into posterior nasopharynx
- Not hypervascular

Fibrous dysplasia
- Can mimic more aggressive lesions on MR
- Ground-glass appearance on CT diagnostic

VASCULAR MALFORMATIONS, HEAD AND NECK

Axial T2WI MR Multiloculated trans-spatial LM in the anterior neck. Multiple loculations contain fluid levels (arrows) and hyperintense T1 signal consistent with blood product.

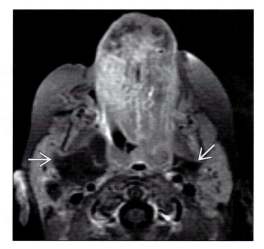

Axial T1 C+ MR shows bilateral cystic parapharyngeal masses (arrows), diffuse enlargement and heterogeneous contrast-enhancement of the tongue in a mixed venous and lymphatic malformation.

TERMINOLOGY

Abbreviations and Synonyms
- Synonyms
  - Lymphatic malformation (preferred term); cystic hygroma, lymphangioma
  - Venous malformation (preferred term); cavernous malformation, cavernous hemangioma (latter term should be avoided)
- Abbreviations
  - Lymphatic malformation (LM)
  - Venous malformation (VM)
  - Arteriovenous malformation (AVM)

Definitions
- Vascular malformations: Congenital malformation; not a neoplasm; grow commensurate with the child
  - Lymphatic malformation
  - Venous malformation
  - Arteriovenous malformation
  - Capillary malformation
  - Mixed malformations: Most common venous and lymphatic = lymphaticovenous or venolymphatic

IMAGING FINDINGS

General Features
- Best diagnostic clue
  - Lymphatic malformation: Trans-spatial multicystic mass with fluid-fluid levels
    - Unilocular or multilocular nonenhancing cystic mass with imperceptible wall
    - Microcystic or macrocystic
    - Trans-spatial = cross multiple contiguous spaces
    - Fluid-fluid levels typical if intralesional hemorrhage
    - Septations may enhance
    - If infected, wall and surrounding tissues may enhance
  - Venous malformation: Lobulated soft tissue "mass" of venous channels with phleboliths
    - May appear cystic on precontrast images
    - Variable contrast enhancement: Homogeneous, heterogeneous, mild or intense, may be delayed
    - Osseous remodeling adjacent bone
    - Fat hypertrophy in adjacent soft tissues
    - May have enlarged draining veins
  - Arteriovenous malformation: Tangle of high flow vessels without significant soft tissue mass
    - High flow large feeding arteries, nidus and large draining veins
    - Focal or diffuse

DDx: Non-Inflammatory Head And Neck Masses

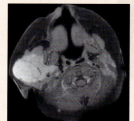 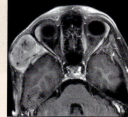 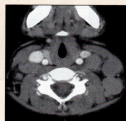 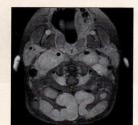

Hemangioma   *Rhabdomyosarcoma*   *Hodgkin Lymphoma*   *NF1*

VASCULAR MALFORMATIONS, HEAD AND NECK

Key Facts

Terminology
- Lymphatic malformation
- Venous malformation
- Arteriovenous malformation
- Capillary malformation
- Mixed malformations: Most common venous and lymphatic = lymphaticovenous or venolymphatic

Imaging Findings
- Lymphatic malformation: Trans-spatial multicystic mass with fluid-fluid levels
- Venous malformation: Lobulated soft tissue "mass" of venous channels with phleboliths
- Arteriovenous malformation: Tangle of high flow vessels without significant soft tissue mass
- Mixed venolymphatic malformation: Mixed cystic and enhancing venous trans-spatial mass
- Capillary malformation: In Sturge-Weber syndrome leptomeningeal enhancement, ipsilateral choroid plexus enlargement, +/- cerebral atrophy

Diagnostic Checklist
- Trans-spatial nonenhancing cystic mass in the head and neck, primary consideration lymphatic malformation
- Enhancing "mass" in the neck associated with calcifications, primary consideration venous malformation
- Mixed cystic and enhancing trans-spatial lesion in the head and neck, primary consideration mixed venous/lymphatic vascular malformation
- High flow vascular mass without significant soft tissue component consider arteriovenous malformation

---

- +/- Bone destruction or overgrowth
- Intense contrast-enhancement
- Pulsed Doppler: High systolic flow, arteriovenous shunting and arterial wave forms in venous structures
  - Mixed venolymphatic malformation: Mixed cystic and enhancing venous trans-spatial mass
  - Capillary malformation: In Sturge-Weber syndrome leptomeningeal enhancement, ipsilateral choroid plexus enlargement, +/- cerebral atrophy
- Location
  - Lymphatic malformation
    - Submandibular space, parotid space, masticator space, posterior cervical space, orbit
    - Frequently trans-spatial
  - Venous vascular malformation
    - Masticator space, sublingual space, buccal space, tongue, orbit
- Morphology
  - Lymphatic malformation and venous vascular malformation
    - Solitary or multiple
    - Well-circumscribed or infiltrative

Imaging Recommendations
- Best imaging tool
  - Lymphatic malformation
    - MRI T2 best demonstrates extent of lesion and presence of fluid-fluid levels
    - Post-contrast T1WI with fat-saturation best demonstrates enhancing septations and enhancing venous component in mixed venolymphatic malformations
  - Venous vascular malformation
    - CT best demonstrates phleboliths
    - MRI best demonstrates extent of lesion and best characterizes mixed venolymphatic malformations
  - Arteriovenous malformation
    - MRI with gradient recalled echo sequence to demonstrate high flow vessels
    - Doppler ultrasound
    - Conventional arteriography and transarterial embolization for therapy

DIFFERENTIAL DIAGNOSIS

Infantile hemangioma
- Diffuse contrast-enhancement with intralesional high flow vessels
- Benign neoplasm with cellular proliferation
- Present shortly after birth, proliferative phase and spontaneous involutional phase

Sarcoma
- Enhancing soft tissue mass, usually less enhancement than infantile hemangioma
- +/- Osseous destruction
- Usually lacks high flow vessels (exception = alveolar soft part sarcoma)

Lymphoma
- Hodgkin or non-Hodgkin lymphoma (NHL): Imaging can not differentiate
- Unilateral or bilateral nodal masses
- NHL more frequently extranodal (30%)

Neurofibroma
- Variable contrast-enhancement
  - Suspect neurofibromatosis type 1 (NF1) if multiple or plexiform
- "Target sign" highly suggestive

PATHOLOGY

General Features
- Genetics
  - LMs associated with Noonan syndrome, Turner syndrome and fetal alcohol syndrome
  - VMs associated with Blue rubber bleb nevus syndrome, Turner syndrome, trisomy 13, 18 and 21
- Etiology
  - Lymphatic malformation

VASCULAR MALFORMATIONS, HEAD AND NECK

- Failure of primordial lymphatic sacs to drain into the adjacent veins, abnormal sequestration of lymphatic tissue or abnormal budding of lymphatics
- Venous vascular malformation
  - Anomalous congenital venous vascular rests
- Arteriovenous malformation
  - Congenital abnormal direct connection between arterial and venous vessels, without intervening capillary bed
- Associated abnormalities
  - Klippel-Trenaunay syndrome
    - Capillary-lymphaticovenous malformation of extremity
    - Bony overgrowth of extremity

Microscopic Features
- Lymphatic malformation
  - Composed of primitive embryonic lymph sacs of varying sizes separated by connective tissue stroma - increasing size of endothelial lined channels
    - Lymphangioma simplex
    - Cavernous lymphangioma
    - Cystic hygroma
- Venous malformation
  - Composed of venous channels of varying sizes and wall thickness, absent internal elastic lamina
  - Luminal thrombi = phleboliths

CLINICAL ISSUES

Presentation
- Most common signs/symptoms
  - Lymphatic malformation
    - Nontender, compressible soft tissue mass
    - May rapidly increase in size in association with viral respiratory infection or intralesional hemorrhage
  - Venous malformation
    - Pain, soft tissue mass
  - Arteriovenous malformation
    - Pulsatile mass, less commonly thrill, bruit, hyperthermia, skeletal overgrowth, pain, bleeding secondary to ulceration, congestive heart failure, embolism
  - Capillary malformation
    - Port-wine stain - most common; usually isolated; occasionally associated with Sturge-Weber syndrome; distinguish from more common fading macular stains of infancy (stork bite, angel's kiss, salmon patch)
    - Telangiectasias- essential telangiectasia, Rendu-Osler-Weber syndrome, ataxia telangiectasia (Louis-Bar syndrome)
    - Cutis marmorata telangiectasia congenita

Demographics
- Age
  - Most LM and VM identified at birth
  - 90% of LM diagnosed before age 2 years

Treatment
- Lymphatic malformation
  - Surgical resection and/or percutaneous sclerotherapy
- Venous malformation
  - Aimed at reduction of symptoms rather than total elimination of lesion
    - Aspirin to prevent thrombosis, elastic compression garments, percutaneous sclerotherapy, surgical resection
- Arteriovenous malformation
  - Transarterial embolization

DIAGNOSTIC CHECKLIST

Image Interpretation Pearls
- Trans-spatial nonenhancing cystic mass in the head and neck, primary consideration lymphatic malformation
- Enhancing "mass" in the neck associated with calcifications, primary consideration venous malformation
- Mixed cystic and enhancing trans-spatial lesion in the head and neck, primary consideration mixed venous/lymphatic vascular malformation
- High flow vascular mass without significant soft tissue component consider arteriovenous malformation

SELECTED REFERENCES

1. Koch BL: Cystic malformations of the neck in children. Pediatr Radiol. 35(5):463-77, 2005
2. Marler JJ et al: Current management of hemangiomas and vascular malformations. Clin Plast Surg. 32(1):99-116, ix, 2005
3. Lee BB et al: Advanced management of venous malformation with ethanol sclerotherapy: mid-term results. J Vasc Surg. 37(3):533-8, 2003
4. Donnelly LF et al: Vascular malformations and hemangiomas: a practical approach in a multidisciplinary clinic. AJR Am J Roentgenol. 174(3):597-608, 2000
5. Donnelly LF et al: Combined sonographic and fluoroscopic guidance: a modified technique for percutaneous sclerosis of low-flow vascular malformations. AJR Am J Roentgenol. 173(3):655-7, 1999
6. Burrows PE et al: Diagnostic imaging in the evaluation of vascular birthmarks. Dermatol Clin. 16(3):455-88, 1998
7. Fishman SJ et al: Vascular anomalies. A primer for pediatricians. Pediatr Clin North Am. 45(6):1455-77, 1998
8. Kohout MP et al: Arteriovenous malformations of the head and neck: natural history and management. Plast Reconstr Surg. 102(3):643-54, 1998
9. Barnes PD et al: Hemangiomas and vascular malformations of the head and neck: MR characterization. AJNR Am J Neuroradiol. 15(1):193-5, 1994
10. Fishman SJ et al: Hemangiomas and vascular malformations of infancy and childhood. Pediatr Clin North Am. 40(6):1177-200, 1993
11. Zadvinskis DP et al: Congenital malformations of the cervicothoracic lymphatic system: embryology and pathogenesis. Radiographics. 12(6):1175-89, 1992
12. Meyer JS et al: Biological classification of soft-tissue vascular anomalies: MR correlation. AJR Am J Roentgenol. 157(3):559-64, 1991
13. Mulliken JB et al: Hemangiomas and vascular malformations in infants and children: a classification based on endothelial characteristics. Plast Reconstr Surg. 69(3):412-22, 1982

VASCULAR MALFORMATIONS, HEAD AND NECK

IMAGE GALLERY

Typical

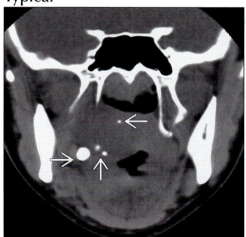
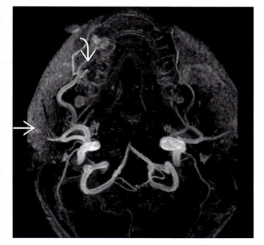

(Left) Coronal NECT demonstrates multiple phleboliths (arrows) in a right palatine tonsil mass. *(Right)* Axial MRA demonstrates enlarged arterial feeder (arrow) and intra-osseous component (curved arrow) of right face and mandible AVM.

Typical

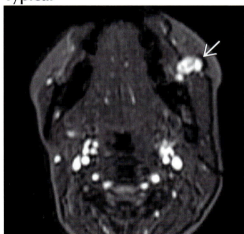
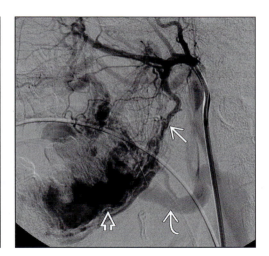

(Left) Axial T2* GRE MR shows high flow vessels within a left cheek and mandible AVM (arrow). *(Right)* Sagittal oblique angiography shows large arterial feeder (arrow), intra-osseous venous lakes (open arrow) and large draining vein (curved arrow) in the same child as on left with AVM.

Typical

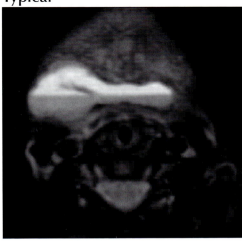
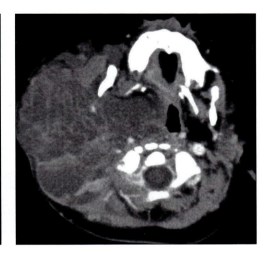

(Left) Axial T2WI MR shows fluid levels (secondary to intralesional hemorrhage) within a lobulated anterior neck lymphatic malformation. *(Right)* Axial CECT shows multiloculated, infiltrative, primarily nonenhancing trans-spatial lymphatic malformation involving the right neck, parotid, parapharyngeal, masticator and carotid spaces.

RHABDOMYOSARCOMA, PEDS HEAD AND NECK

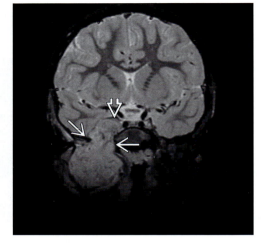

Axial CECT shows a large right masticator space RMS with destruction of the right mandibular ramus (arrow) and the right lateral pterygoid plate (open arrow).

Coronal STIR MR shows right masticator space RMS in the same patient, with perineural spread along CN V3 through enlarged foramen ovale (arrows) and cavernous sinus invasion (open arrow).

TERMINOLOGY

Abbreviations and Synonyms
- Rhabdomyosarcoma (RMS)

Definitions
- Malignant neoplasm of striated muscle, most common childhood soft tissue sarcoma

IMAGING FINDINGS

General Features
- Best diagnostic clue: Soft tissue mass with variable contrast enhancement and bone destruction
- Location
  - Up to 40% occur in H & N
    - Orbit
    - Parameningeal: Middle ear, paranasal sinus, nasopharynx
    - All other head and neck sites including cervical neck, nasal cavity
  - Up to 55% of parameningeal rhabdomyosarcomas have intracranial extension
- Size: Variable, may present earlier in orbit secondary to small space and early proptosis

CT Findings
- Soft tissue mass with variable contrast-enhancement
- Osseous erosion common but does not occur in all cases

MR Findings
- Relative to muscle; isointense T1WI, hyperintense T2WI
- Variable contrast-enhancement, +/- intracranial extension in parameningeal

Imaging Recommendations
- Best imaging tool
  - CT best to evaluate osseous erosion
  - MRI best to evaluate intracranial and perineural spread
- Protocol advice
  - Coronal postcontrast fat-saturation T1 imaging for intracranial disease assessment
  - Axial and coronal thin section bone algorithm for osseous erosion
  - Include neck to rule out cervical metastatic adenopathy

DDx: Non-Inflammatory H & N Masses With Osseous Erosion

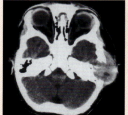
LCH

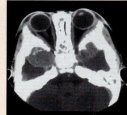
Metastatic NBL

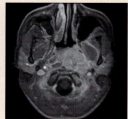
NP Carcinoma

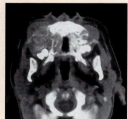
AML

RHABDOMYOSARCOMA, PEDS HEAD AND NECK

Key Facts

Terminology
- Rhabdomyosarcoma (RMS)
- Malignant neoplasm of striated muscle, most common childhood soft tissue sarcoma

Imaging Findings
- Best diagnostic clue: Soft tissue mass with variable contrast enhancement and bone destruction
- Up to 40% occur in H & N
- Orbit
- Parameningeal: Middle ear, paranasal sinus, nasopharynx
- All other head and neck sites including cervical neck, nasal cavity
- Soft tissue mass with variable contrast-enhancement
- Osseous erosion common but does not occur in all cases
- Relative to muscle; isointense T1WI, hyperintense T2WI
- CT best to evaluate osseous erosion
- MRI best to evaluate intracranial and perineural spread

Top Differential Diagnoses
- Langerhan cell histiocytosis (LCH)
- Metastatic neuroblastoma (NBL)
- Nasopharyngeal (NP) carcinoma
- Leukemia
- Lymphoma
- Juvenile nasopharyngeal angiofibroma

DIFFERENTIAL DIAGNOSIS

Langerhan cell histiocytosis (LCH)
- Enhancing soft tissue mass with smooth osseous erosion
- In head and neck: Orbit, maxilla, mandible, temporal bone, cervical spine, calvaria

Metastatic neuroblastoma (NBL)
- The most common malignant tumor in children less than one year of age
- Cervical primary lesions rare, most cervical disease is metastatic
- Metastatic disease to skull base frequently bilateral with enhancing masses, intracranial and/or extracranial extension, aggressive osseous erosion with spiculated periosteal reaction

Nasopharyngeal (NP) carcinoma
- NP mass with variable contrast-enhancement
- Central skull base erosion, widening of the petroclival fissure, extension to pterygopalatine fossa, masticator space, parapharyngeal space, unilateral or bilateral cervical adenopathy, lateral retropharyngeal adenopathy
- In children, most are 10-19 years of age
- In the United States, more common in African Americans than in Caucasians

Leukemia
- Granulocytic sarcoma = chloroma
- Soft tissue mass +/- aggressive bone destruction
- Rare complication acute myeloid leukemia (AML) or chronic myeloid leukemia (CML)
- Most in adults, most in patients with AML
- In CML, ominous sign, usually heralds blast crisis
- In AML, does not affect overall prognosis
- Locations in H & N: Skull, face, orbit, paranasal sinuses, nasal cavity, nasopharynx, tonsil, mouth, lacrimal gland, salivary glands

Lymphoma
- Accounts for approximately 50% of all head and neck malignancies in children
  - 50% Hodgkin disease (HD), 50% non-Hodgkin lymphoma (NHL)
  - Imaging characteristics similar, can not differentiate between HD and NHL
- Sinonasal, orbital or nasopharyngeal may cause osseous erosion
- Unilateral or bilateral cervical adenopathy, usually without osseous erosion

Juvenile nasopharyngeal angiofibroma
- Presents with epistaxis or nasal obstruction in adolescent males
- Intensely enhancing mass with bone destruction and intralesional high flow vessels
  - Originates at sphenopalatine foramen on lateral nasopharyngeal wall, potential spread
    - Pterygopalatine and pterygomaxillary fissures into infratemporal fossa
    - Orbit via inferior orbital fissure
    - Intracranial
    - Sphenoid or ethmoid sinus

PATHOLOGY

General Features
- Genetics
  - Increased incidence in children with p53 tumor suppressor gene mutation
  - Most embryonal RMS have loss of heterozygosity (LOH) at 11p15 locus
  - PAX3-FKHR and variant PAX7-FKHR gene fusions in some with alveolar RMS
    - PAX3-FKHR gene fusion better prognosis
- Etiology: Originates from primitive mesenchymal cells committed to skeletal muscle differentiation (rhabdomyoblasts)
- Associated abnormalities

RHABDOMYOSARCOMA, PEDS HEAD AND NECK

- Rarely associated with neurofibromatosis type I, Li-Fraumeni syndrome and Beckwith-Wiedemann syndrome
- Rarely associated with hereditary retinoblastoma
- May occur as radiation induced second primary neoplasm

Microscopic Features
- Rhabdomyoblasts in varying stages of differentiation
- Immunohistochemistry: Positive for desmin, vimentin and antibody to muscle-specific actin
- Histologic subtypes
  - Embryonal RMS: Most common
    - Primitive cellular structure
    - Round or elongated cells with hyperchromic, irregular nuclei and frequent mitoses
    - Account for more that 50% of all RMS, 70-90% of which occur in H & N or genitourinary tract
    - Botryoid RMS gross appearance similar to cluster of grapes, 75% arise in vagina, prostate or bladder, 25% in H & N or bile ducts, most patients 2-5 years of age
  - Alveolar RMS: Second most common
    - Most common in extremities and trunk
    - Usually occurs in patients 15-25 years of age
  - Pleomorphic RMS: Least common
    - Usually in adults 40-60 years of age, rarely less than 15 years of age
    - Most arise in extremities, rarely in H & N

Staging, Grading or Classification Criteria
- Intergroup Rhabdomyosarcoma Study Group (IRSG)
  - Group I: Localized tumor completely resected
  - Group II: Gross total resection with microscopic residual disease
  - Group III: Incomplete resection with gross residual disease
  - Group IV: Distant metastases
- WHO Classification: 6 histologic subtypes
- TNM: Tumor site, size (5 cm), local invasion, lymph nodes, distant metastases

CLINICAL ISSUES

Presentation
- Most common signs/symptoms
  - Variable, depends on location
    - Orbit: Orbital mass, proptosis, decreased vision
    - Sinonasal: Nasal obstruction, epistaxis, may present late with soft tissue facial mass
    - Temporal bone: Postauricular mass, otitis media, external auditory canal mass
    - Neck: Neck mass, pain, rarely airway compromise

Demographics
- Age: 70% under 12 years, 43% under 5 years of age
- Ethnicity: More common in Caucasians

Natural History & Prognosis
- Variable, depends on location and cell type
  - Orbit : Best prognosis (80-90% disease-free survival)
  - Parameningeal: Worst prognosis (40-50% disease free survival)
  - Alveolar worse prognosis than embryonal and pleomorphic

Treatment
- Surgical debulking, chemotherapy, and/or radiation therapy

DIAGNOSTIC CHECKLIST

Consider
- Not always associated with bone destruction
  - Beware of enhancing soft tissue mass without bone destruction, may simulate infantile hemangioma
    - Infantile hemangioma usually more intensely and homogeneously enhancing, with intralesional high flow vessels
    - Flow voids usually absent in sarcomas with the exception of alveolar soft part sarcomas

SELECTED REFERENCES

1. Stambuk HE et al: Nasopharyngeal carcinoma: recognizing the radiographic features in children. AJNR Am J Neuroradiol. 26(6):1575-9, 2005
2. Breneman JC et al: Prognostic factors and clinical outcomes in children and adolescents with metastatic rhabdomyosarcoma--a report from the Intergroup Rhabdomyosarcoma Study IV. J Clin Oncol. 21(1):78-84, 2003
3. Tateishi U et al: CT and MRI features of recurrent tumors and second primary neoplasms in pediatric patients with retinoblastoma. AJR Am J Roentgenol. 181(3):879-84, 2003
4. Sorensen PH et al: PAX3-FKHR and PAX7-FKHR gene fusions are prognostic indicators in alveolar rhabdomyosarcoma: a report from the children's oncology group. J Clin Oncol. 20(11):2672-9, 2002
5. McCarville MB et al: Rhabdomyosarcoma in pediatric patients: the good, the bad, and the unusual. AJR Am J Roentgenol. 176(6):1563-9, 2001
6. Koch BL: Langerhans histiocytosis of temporal bone: role of magnetic resonance imaging. Top Magn Reson Imaging. 11(1):66-74, 2000
7. Kraus DH et al: Pediatric rhabdomyosarcoma of the head and neck. Am J Surg. 174(5):556-60, 1997
8. Pappo AS et al: Biology and therapy of pediatric rhabdomyosarcoma. J Clin Oncol. 13(8):2123-39, 1995
9. Quraishi MS et al: Langerhans' cell histiocytosis: head and neck manifestations in children. Head Neck. 17(3):226-31, 1995
10. Castillo M et al: Rhabdomyosarcoma of the middle ear: imaging features in two children. AJNR Am J Neuroradiol. 14(3):730-3, 1993
11. Yousem DM et al: Rhabdomyosarcomas in the head and neck: MR imaging evaluation. Radiology. 177(3):683-6, 1990
12. Wiatrak BJ et al: Rhabdomyosarcoma of the ear and temporal bone. Laryngoscope. 99(11):1188-92, 1989
13. Latack JT et al: Imaging of rhabdomyosarcomas of the head and neck. AJNR Am J Neuroradiol. 8(2):353-9, 1987
14. Schwartz RH et al: Rhabdomyosarcoma of the middle ear: a wolf in sheep's clothing. Pediatrics. 65(6):1131-3, 1980
15. Abramson DH et al: Second tumors in nonirradiated bilateral retinoblastoma. Am J Ophthalmol. 87(5):624-7, 1979

RHABDOMYOSARCOMA, PEDS HEAD AND NECK

IMAGE GALLERY

Typical

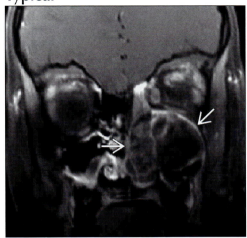
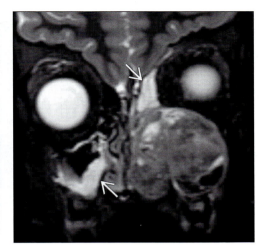

(Left) Coronal T1 C+ MR shows heterogeneous left nasal and maxillary sinus RMS (arrows), difficult to separate from adjacent inflammatory disease. *(Right)* Coronal T2WI MR shows heterogeneous relatively hypointense RMS in the same patient. Hyperintense T2 inflammatory paranasal sinus disease (arrows) clearly separated from the neoplasm.

Typical

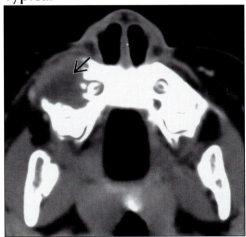
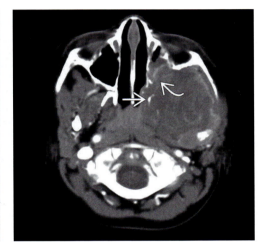

(Left) Axial CECT shows left maxillary RMS with bone destruction and central area of decreased attenuation (arrow) consistent with central necrosis. *(Right)* Axial CECT shows a large heterogeneously enhancing left masticator space RMS. Note destruction of the left pterygoid plate (arrow) and posterior maxillary sinus wall (curved arrow).

Variant

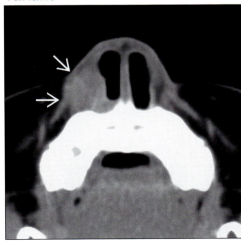
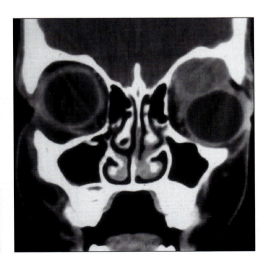

(Left) Axial CECT shows homogeneous mildly enhancing RMS of the right nasal ala (arrows) without significant osseous erosion. *(Right)* Coronal CECT shows a relatively low attenuation, nonenhancing left extraconal superior orbital RMS, without osseous destruction, deviating the left globe inferiorly.

INFANTILE HEMANGIOMA, HEAD AND NECK

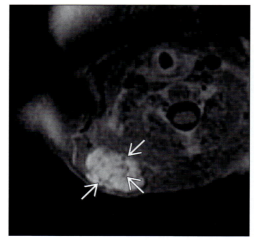 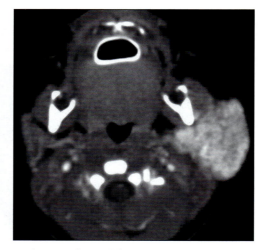

Axial T1WI MR shows lobulated diffusely enhancing mass in the right posterior neck with intralesional flow voids (arrows).

Axial CECT shows diffuse enlargement and intense contrast-enhancement of the superficial and deep portions of the left parotid gland.

TERMINOLOGY

Abbreviations and Synonyms
- Hemangioma of infancy (HI), capillary hemangioma, infantile hemangioma

Definitions
- Benign neoplasm of proliferating endothelial cells
- Not congenital vascular malformation

IMAGING FINDINGS

General Features
- Best diagnostic clue
  - Well-defined mass with diffuse post-contrast enhancement
  - High flow vessels in and adjacent to mass during proliferative phase (PP)
  - Decrease size with fatty replacement during involutional phase (IP)
- Location
  - 60% occur in head and neck (any space including parotid glands, orbit, nasal cavity, subglottic airway)
  - Parotid gland and orbital involvement may by bilateral
  - Other locations: Extremities, trunk
- Size
  - Variable; small to very large
  - Depends on clinical phase: PP or IP
- Morphology
  - Majority single in the subcutaneous tissues
  - Occasionally multiple, trans-spatial or deep
  - Associated abnormalities in PHACES syndrome
    - Posterior fossa brain malformations (Dandy Walker malformation)
    - Hemangiomas of the head and neck
    - Arterial abnormalities (stenosis, occlusion, aneurysm)
    - Cardiovascular defects (aortic coarctation, cardiac anomalies)
    - Eye abnormalities
    - Supra-umbilical and Sternal clefts
- CT Findings
  - NECT
    - Intermediate attenuation without calcification
    - Rarely remodeling of adjacent osseous structures, no osseous erosion
    - Fatty infiltration during involutional phase
  - CECT
    - Diffuse and prominent contrast enhancement
    - Prominent vessels in and adjacent to mass during proliferative phase
- MR Findings
  - T1WI: Isointense to muscle proliferative phase; fatty replacement involutional phase

DDx: Enhancing Masses In The Head And Neck

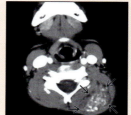 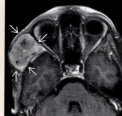 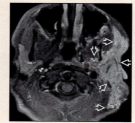 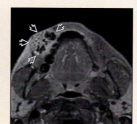

VM   Rhabdomyosarcoma   Plexiform NF   AVM

INFANTILE HEMANGIOMA, HEAD AND NECK

Key Facts

Terminology
- Hemangioma of infancy (HI), capillary hemangioma, infantile hemangioma
- Benign neoplasm of proliferating endothelial cells
- Not congenital vascular malformation

Imaging Findings
- Well-defined mass with diffuse post-contrast enhancement
- High flow vessels in and adjacent to mass during proliferative phase (PP)
- Decrease size with fatty replacement during involutional phase (IP)

Top Differential Diagnoses
- Venous malformation (VM)
- Sarcoma
- Plexiform neurofibroma (NF)
- Arteriovenous malformation (AVM)

Pathology
- Incidence is 1-2% of neonates and up to 12% by age 1 year

Clinical Issues
- Majority don't require treatment; expectant waiting

Diagnostic Checklist
- Visible shortly after birth
- Phleboliths suggest venous malformation
- Older child or osseous destruction consider sarcoma
- Trans-spatial mass with cafe au lait skin lesions suggest plexiform neurofibroma
- Large vessels with little or ill-defined parenchymal mass suggest AVM

- T2WI: Mildly hyperintense relative to muscle
- T1WI C+
  - Intense contrast-enhancement
  - Best appreciated on fat-saturation T1WI
  - Serpiginous flow voids in and adjacent to mass
- MR GRE: High flow vessels in and adjacent to mass
- MRA: Stenosis, occlusion, aneurysm in PHACES syndrome
- Sonographic Findings
  - Soft tissue mass with prominent vessels
  - Arterial and venous waveforms
  - Mean venous peak velocities NOT elevated as might be identified in true arteriovenous malformation (AVM)
- Angiographic Findings
  - Not a primary imaging tool for diagnosis
  - Hypervascular mass with prolonged capillary blush, without arteriovenous shunting

Imaging Recommendations
- Best imaging tool
  - MRI or CT with contrast to identify diffuse contrast-enhancement
  - Gradient-recalled echo sequences to identify intralesional and perilesional high flow vessels
  - MRA to identify associated vascular abnormalities
  - Imaging indications (most not imaged, diagnosed by history and physical examination)
    - Suspect deep extension to identify total extent of lesion (particularly orbit and airway)
    - Pretreatment if considering medical or surgical/laser treatment
    - Assess response to treatment
    - Atypical history, older patient or suspect neoplasm
- Protocol advice
  - MRI
    - Pre-contrast T1, FSE, STIR and SPGR images
    - Post-contrast T1 images with fat-suppression
    - MRA to identify associated vascular anomalies: Stenosis, occlusions, moya moya, aneurysms
  - CT
    - Post-contrast, pre-contrast if considering venous malformation in DDx to identify phleboliths
    - CTA to identify associated vascular anomalies in suspected PHACES syndrome

DIFFERENTIAL DIAGNOSIS

Venous malformation (VM)
- Congenital vascular malformation composed of large venous lakes
- Hyperintense T2, hypointense T1, diffuse postcontrast enhancement, phleboliths
- Present often at birth and grow proportionally to child

Sarcoma
- Older child
  - Suspect if age, appearance, growth history, or imaging does not fit for hemangioma
  - Marked enhancement with prominent vessels suspect alveolar soft part sarcoma (ASPS)
  - Mild to moderate enhancement frequently with osseous erosion suspect rhabdomyosarcoma

Plexiform neurofibroma (NF)
- Infiltrative, ill-defined margins frequently with trans-spatial involvement
- Associated with additional stigmata of neurofibromatosis type 1

Arteriovenous malformation (AVM)
- Congenital vascular malformation
- High flow feeding arteries, arteriovenous shunting and large draining veins

PATHOLOGY

General Features
- Genetics
  - Majority sporadic
  - Rare association with chromosome 5q31-q33

INFANTILE HEMANGIOMA, HEAD AND NECK

- Etiology: Proposed theory = clonal expansion of angioblasts with high expression of basic fibroblast growth factors and other angiogenesis markers
- Epidemiology
  - Most common head and neck tumor in infants
  - Incidence is 1-2% of neonates and up to 12% by age 1 year
  - More common in preterm infants, as high as 29% in infants weighing less than 1 kg

Microscopic Features
- Prominent endothelial cells, pericytes, mast cells with mitotic figures and multi-laminated endothelial basement membrane

CLINICAL ISSUES

Presentation
- Most common signs/symptoms
  - During the proliferative phase (usually lasts up to 12 months), there is increase in size of soft tissue mass, typically with warm, reddish or "strawberry-like" cutaneous discoloration
  - Occasionally deep, present with overlying bluish coloration of the skin secondary to prominent draining veins
  - Spontaneous involution over the next 9-12 years
- Other signs/symptoms
  - Ulceration if associated breakdown of overlying subcutaneous fat
  - Airway obstruction with airway involvement
  - Proptosis if large orbital lesion
  - Associated abnormalities in PHACES syndrome

Demographics
- Age: Typically inapparent at birth, usually presents with rapid growth within first few months of life
- Gender: More common in females than males, male to female 1:2.5
- Ethnicity
  - Most frequent in Caucasians

Natural History & Prognosis
- Proliferative phase during first year of life
- Involutional phase may last up to 12 years

Treatment
- Majority don't require treatment; expectant waiting
- Treatment indications
  - Compromise vital structures such as optic nerve or airway obstruction
  - Significant skin ulceration
- Medical therapy
  - Steroids (systemic or intralesional injection), alpha interferon
- Procedural therapy
  - Laser, rarely surgical excision and embolization

DIAGNOSTIC CHECKLIST

Consider
- Visible shortly after birth
- Phleboliths suggest venous malformation
- Older child or osseous destruction consider sarcoma
- Trans-spatial mass with cafe au lait skin lesions suggest plexiform neurofibroma
- Large vessels with little or ill-defined parenchymal mass suggest AVM

SELECTED REFERENCES

1. Bhattacharya JJ et al: PHACES syndrome: a review of eight previously unreported cases with late arterial occlusions. Neuroradiology. 46(3):227-33, 2004
2. Aiken AH et al: Alveolar soft-part sarcoma of the tongue. AJNR Am J Neuroradiol. 24(6):1156-8, 2003
3. Hein KD et al: Venous malformations of skeletal muscle. Plast Reconstr Surg. 110(7):1625-35, 2002
4. Pang LM et al: Alveolar soft-part sarcoma: a rare soft-tissue malignancy with distinctive clinical and radiological features. Pediatr Radiol. 31(3):196-9, 2001
5. Fordham LA et al: Imaging of congenital vascular and lymphatic anomalies of the head and neck. Neuroimaging Clin N Am. 10(1):117-36, viii, 2000
6. Koch BL: Imaging extracranial masses of the pediatric head and neck. Neuroimaging Clin N Am. 10(1):193-214, ix, 2000
7. Mulliken JB et al: Vascular anomalies. Curr Probl Surg. 37(8):517-84, 2000
8. Dubois J et al: Imaging and therapeutic approach of hemangiomas and vascular malformations in the pediatric age group. Pediatr Radiol. 29(12):879-93, 1999
9. Jones BV et al: Magnetic resonance imaging of the pediatric head and neck. Top Magn Reson Imaging. 10(6):348-61, 1999
10. Robertson RL et al: Head and neck vascular anomalies of childhood. Neuroimaging Clin N Am. 9(1):115-32, 1999
11. Burrows PE et al: Diagnostic imaging in the evaluation of vascular birthmarks. Dermatol Clin. 16(3):455-88, 1998
12. Fishman SJ et al: Vascular anomalies. A primer for pediatricians. Pediatr Clin North Am. 45(6):1455-77, 1998
13. Laor T et al: Congenital anomalies and vascular birthmarks of the lower extremities. Magn Reson Imaging Clin N Am. 6(3):497-519, 1998
14. Yang WT et al: Sonographic features of head and neck hemangiomas and vascular malformations: review of 23 patients. J Ultrasound Med. 16(1):39-44, 1997
15. Barnes PD et al: Hemangiomas and vascular malformations of the head and neck: MR characterization. AJNR Am J Neuroradiol. 15(1):193-5, 1994
16. Mulliken JB: Cutaneous vascular anomalies. Semin Vasc Surg. 6(4):204-18, 1993
17. Meyer JS et al: Biological classification of soft-tissue vascular anomalies: MR correlation. AJR Am J Roentgenol. 157(3):559-64, 1991
18. Burrows PE et al: Childhood hemangiomas and vascular malformations: angiographic differentiation. AJR Am J Roentgenol. 141(3):483-8, 1983
19. Finn MC et al: Congenital vascular lesions: clinical application of a new classification. J Pediatr Surg. 18(6):894-900, 1983
20. Mulliken JB et al: Hemangiomas and vascular malformations in infants and children: a classification based on endothelial characteristics. Plast Reconstr Surg. 69(3):412-22, 1982

INFANTILE HEMANGIOMA, HEAD AND NECK

IMAGE GALLERY

Typical

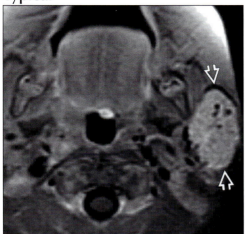 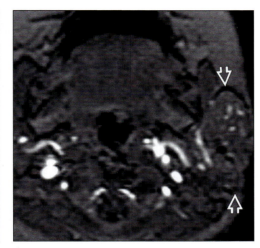

(Left) Axial T1 C+ MR shows prominent vessels within and deep to a diffusely and intensely enhancing large left parotid gland (arrows). *(Right)* Axial T2* GRE MR shows high flow vessels within and deep to the large left parotid gland (arrows).

Typical

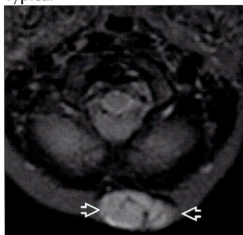 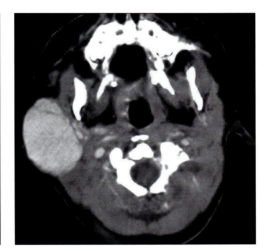

(Left) Axial T2WI MR shows well defined mildly hyperintense mass (arrows) in the midline suboccipital subcutaneous fat with serpiginous flow voids consistent with high flow vessels. *(Right)* Axial CECT shows well-defined large right parotid mass with diffuse post-contrast enhancement.

Variant

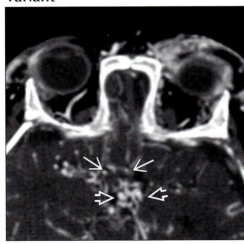 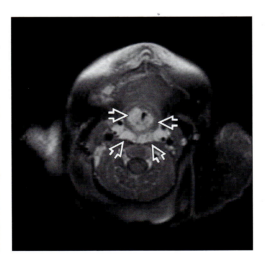

(Left) Axial CECT shows enhancing left orbital mass, diminutive carotid terminus bilaterally (arrows) and multiple serpiginous suprasellar collateral vessels (open arrows) in a child with moya moya and PHACES syndrome. *(Right)* Axial T1 C+ MR shows enhancing masses (arrows) surrounding the subglottic airway and in the retropharyngeal space in the same child with PHACES syndrome.

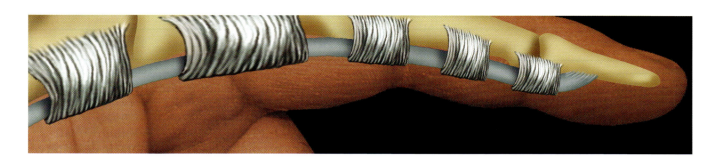

INDEX

A

Abdominal distension, 2:44
Abscess
    Brodie. *See also* Osteomyelitis
        Langerhans cell histiocytosis vs., **6:86i**
        stress fracture vs., **6:18i**, 6:19
    cerebral, 7:58–60, **7:61i**
        differential diagnosis, **7:58i**, 7:59
        orbital cellulitis vs., **7:190i**, 7:191
    epidural, **7:86i**, 7:87
    fungal, **4:134i**, 4:135
    hepatic
        Caroli disease vs., 4:101
        choledochal cyst vs., 4:97
        liver trauma vs., **4:122i**, 4:123
    lung
        parapneumonic effusion and empyema vs., **2:70i**, 2:72
        pneumonia with cavitary necrosis vs., 2:75
    mesenteric lymphatic malformation vs., **4:112i**, 4:113
    parotid, **7:166i**, 7:167
    pelvic
        hydrometrocolpos vs., 5:67
        rhabdomyosarcoma vs., 5:83
        sacrococcygeal teratoma vs., 5:87
    renal
        angiomyolipoma vs., **5:62i**, 5:63
        calyceal diverticulum vs., **5:48i**, 5:49
    retropharyngeal. *See* Retropharyngeal abscess
    second branchial apparatus anomalies vs., **7:170i**, 7:171
    splenic, **4:126i**, 4:127
    third branchial apparatus anomalies vs., **7:174i**, 7:175
    tubo-ovarian, 5:91
Achalasia
    chronic esophageal foreign body vs., **2:134i**, 2:135
    cricopharyngeal, **4:162i**, 4:163
    esophageal strictures vs., **4:162i**, 4:163
    gastroesophageal reflux vs., **4:48i**, 4:49
Achondroplasia, 6:114–116, **6:117i**
    Chiari type I vs., 7:12
    differential diagnosis, **6:114i**, 6:115–116
    homozygous, **6:114i**, 6:116
    osteopetrosis vs., **6:126i**
Aciduria, glutaric, **7:78i**, 7:80
Acute chest syndrome, 2:114–116, **2:117i**
    differential diagnosis, **2:114i**, 2:115
Adamantinoma. *See* Craniopharyngioma
Adenoids, enlarged
    encephalocele vs., **7:18i**, 7:19–20
    glossoptosis vs., 1:24
Adenoma. *See also* Cystic adenomatoid malformation
    cystadenoma. *See* Nephroma, multilocular cystic
    pituitary
        colloid cyst vs, 7:83
        craniopharyngioma vs., **7:110i**, 7:111
        macroadenoma, vs. germinoma, **7:114i**, 7:115
Adenoma sebaceum, **7:50i**, 7:51
Adenopathy, cystic malignant, 7:171
Adrenal cysts
    adrenal hemorrhage vs., 5:75
    normal adrenal gland vs., **5:70i**, 72
Adrenal gland, neonatal
    hemorrhage, 5:74–76, **5:77i**
        differential diagnosis, **5:74i**, 5:75
        neuroblastoma vs., **5:78i**, 5:79
        normal adrenal gland vs., **5:70i**, 5:72
        shock vs., **5:74i**, 5:75
        traumatic vs. neonatal, **5:74i**, 5:75
    hyperplasia, congenital
        adrenal hemorrhage vs., **5:74i**, 5:75
        normal adrenal gland vs., 5:71
    normal, 5:70–72, **5:72i**
        differential diagnosis, **5:70i**, 5:71–72
Adrenal insufficiency, 5:71–72
Adrenocortical carcinoma, **5:78i**, 5:79
Adrenoleukodystrophy, X-linked, **7:66i**, 7:67–68
Aicardi-Goutieres syndrome, 7:55
Airway compression, with thoracic deformity, 1:54–55
    differential diagnosis, **1:54i**, 1:55
    midline descending aorta vs., **1:46i**, 1:47
Airway imaging, 1:6–67
    airway compression with thoracic deformity, 1:54–55
    asthma, 1:64–66, **1:67i**

INDEX

    differential diagnosis, **4:92i**, 4:93
Biliary cyst, **4:100i**, 4:102
Biliary drain, percutaneous, **4:104i**, 4:106
Biliary hypoplasia, **4:92i**, 4:93
Birth trauma, 2:99
Bladder
    cyst. *See* Ureterocele
    diverticula, 5:122–124, **5:125i**
        differential diagnosis, **5:122i**, 5:123
            ureterocele vs., 5:19
    duplex, **5:14i**
    exstrophy vs. gastroschisis, 4:67
    hematoma vs. rhabdomyosarcoma, 5:83
    neurogenic. *See* Neurogenic bladder
Blalock-Taussig shunt, 3:90, **3:90i**
Bland-Garland-White syndrome. *See* Coronary artery, left, anomalous origin of
Blastoma, pleuropulmonary. *See* Pleuropulmonary blastoma
Bochdalek hernia. *See* Diaphragmatic hernia, congenital
Body stalk anomaly, 4:67
Bolande tumor. *See* Nephroma, mesoblastic
Bone cysts
    aneurysmal
        discitis vs., 2:108
        fibroxanthoma vs., **6:90i**, 6:91
        osteosarcoma vs., **6:78i**, 6:79
        tarsal coalition vs., 6:148
    unicameral, fibroxanthoma vs., **6:90i**, 6:91
Bones
    bent, **6:14i**, 6:15–16
    dysplasia
        incomplete fractures vs., **6:14i**, 6:15–16
        osteosclerotic, 6:128
    tumors vs. stress fracture, 6:19
Bourneville syndrome. *See* Tuberous sclerosis
Bowel injury, 4:118–120, **4:121i**
    differential diagnosis, **4:118i**, 4:120
    hypoperfusion complex vs., **4:114i**, 4:115
Brain
    abscess, 7:58–60, **7:61i**
        differential diagnosis, **7:58i**, 7:59
        orbital cellulitis vs., **7:190i**, 7:191
    injuries
        accidental, child abuse vs., 7:80
        child abuse and, 7:78–80, **7:81i**
            differential diagnosis, **7:78i**, 7:80
Brainstem glioma, 7:106–108, **7:109i**
    differential diagnosis, **7:106i**, 7:107–108
    ependymoma vs., **7:102i**, 7:103
    medulloblastoma vs., **7:98i**, 7:99
Branchial apparatus anomalies
    first, 7:166–168, **7:169i**
        differential diagnosis, **7:166i**, 7:167

    second, 7:170–172, **7:173i**
        cysts vs. third branchial apparatus anomalies, **7:174i**, 7:175
        differential diagnosis, **7:170i**, 7:171
    third, 7:174–176, **7:177i**
        differential diagnosis, **7:174i**, 7:175
        second branchial apparatus anomalies vs., **7:170i**, 7:171
        fourth branchial apparatus anomalies vs., **7:178i**, 7:179
    fourth, 7:178–180, **7:181i**
        differential diagnosis, **7:178i**, 7:179
Branchial cleft anomalies, 6:164
Brodie abscess. *See also* Osteomyelitis
    Langerhans cell histiocytosis vs., **6:86i**
    stress fracture vs., **6:18i**, 6:19
Bronchial atresia, 2:26–28, **2:29i**
    congenital lobar emphysema vs., 2:19
    differential diagnosis, **2:26i**, 2:27–28
Bronchial obstruction, chronic, 2:12
Bronchiolitis
    asthma vs., **1:64i**, 1:65
    tracheomalacia vs., **1:56i**, 1:57
Bronchiolitis obliterans, 1:62
Bronchogenic cyst, 2:14–16, **2:17i**
    bronchial atresia vs., **2:26i**, 2:27
    differential diagnosis, **2:14i**, 2:15–16
    discitis vs., 2:108
    innominate artery compression syndrome vs., 1:43
    pleuropulmonary blastoma vs., 2:91
    pneumonia with cavitary necrosis vs., **2:74i**, 2:76
    pulmonary sequestration vs., **2:10i**, 2:12
    pulmonary sling vs., **1:34i**, 1:35
    round pneumonia vs., **2:66i**, 2:67
    thoracic neuroblastoma vs., **2:102i**, 2:103
Bronchopulmonary aspergillosis, allergic
    bronchial atresia vs., 2:27
    cystic fibrosis vs., **2:110i**, 2:111
Bronchopulmonary dysplasia, 2:50–52, **2:53i**
    differential diagnosis, **2:50i**, 2:51
    pulmonary interstitial emphysema vs., **2:46i**, 2:47
Bruck syndrome, 6:123
Bucket-handle tear, **6:150i**, 6:151
Burkitt lymphoma
    hydrometrocolpos vs., **5:66i**, 5:67
    rhabdomyosarcoma vs., **5:82i**, 5:83
    sacrococcygeal teratoma vs., **5:86i**, 5:87
Bursitis, infrapatellar
    Osgood-Schlatter lesion vs., 6:35

INDEX

C

Caffey-Kempe syndrome. *See* Child abuse
Calcaneal fractures, 6:148
Calcaneus, vertical, 6:139
Calcifications, periventricular, 7:127
Callosal dysgenesis, 7:26–28, **7:29i**
    differential diagnosis, **7:26i**, 7:27
    holoprosencephaly vs., **7:22i**, 7:23
Callosotomy, prior, 7:27
Callus formation, hyperplastic, 6:124
Calyceal diverticulum, 5:48–49
    differential diagnosis, **5:48i**, 5:49
    multilocular cystic nephroma vs., **5:56i**, 5:57
Canavan disease, **7:66i**, 7:68
Candida infections
    esophagitis vs. chronic foreign body, **2:134i**, 2:135
    lymphoproliferative disorder vs., 4:135
Capillary hemangioma. *See* Hemangioma, infantile
Carbohydrate deficient glycoprotein syndrome type 1a, 7:7
Carcinoid tumor
    bronchial atresia vs., 2:27
    pulmonary inflammatory pseudotumor vs., 2:96
Carcinoma, 7:171
    adrenocortical, neuroblastoma vs., **5:78i**, 5:79
    choroid plexus. *See* Choroid plexus papilloma
    epithelial, ovarian teratoma vs., 5:91
    hepatocellular
        hemangioendothelioma vs., 4:88
        hepatoblastoma vs., 4:83
    nasopharyngeal
        encephalocele vs., **7:18i**, 7:20
        juvenile nasopharyngeal angiofibroma vs., 7:199
        rhabdomyosarcoma vs., **7:206i**, 7:207
    papillary thyroid, necrotic node, **7:170i**, 7:171
    renal cell. *See* Renal cell carcinoma
    squamous cell, 7:171
Cardiac arrhythmias
    hypoplastic left heart syndrome vs., 3:51
    transient tachypnea of newborn vs., **2:42i**, 2:43
Cardiac imaging, 3:6–111. *See also* Heart disease
    aortic coarctation, 3:78–80, **3:81i**
    aortic stenosis, 3:82–84, **3:85i**
    cardiomyopathy, 3:62–64, **3:65i**
    double outlet right ventricle, 3:66–68, **3:69i**
    Ebstein anomaly, 3:30–32, **3:33i**
    great arteries
        D-transposition of, 3:34–36, **3:37i**
        L-transposition of, 3:70–72, **3:73i**
    heterotaxia syndromes, 3:74–76, **3:78i**
    hypoplastic left heart syndrome, 3:50–52, **3:53i**
    Kawasaki disease, 3:104–106, **3:107i**
    left coronary artery anomalous origin, 3:54–56, **3:57i**
    myocarditis, 3:58–60, **3:61i**
    operative CHD procedures, 3:90–92, **3:93i**
    patent ductus arteriosus, 3:18–20, **3:21i**
    pulmonary artery stenosis, 3:86–88, **3:89i**
    pulmonary atresia, 3:26–28, **3:29i**
    rhabdomyoma, 3:102–103
    rheumatic heart disease, 3:108–110, **3:111i**
    right ventricular dysplasia, 3:94–96, **3:97i**
    scimitar syndrome, 3:98–100, **3:101i**
    septal defects
        atrial, 3:10–12, **3:13i**
        atrioventricular, 3:14–16, **3:17i**
        ventricular, 3:6–8, **3:9i**
    tetralogy of Fallot, 3:22–24, **3:25i**
    total anomalous pulmonary venous return, 3:46–48, **3:49i**
    tricuspid atresia, 3:38–40, **3:41i**
    truncus arteriosus, 3:42–44, **3:45i**
Cardiac tumors, malignant, 3:103
Cardiogenic shock, 3:59
Cardiomyopathy, 3:62–64, **3:65i**
    differential diagnosis, **3:62i**, 3:63
    dilated
        rheumatic heart disease vs., **3:108i**, 3:109
        right ventricular dysplasia vs., **3:94i**, 3:95
    hypertrophic, **3:94i**, 3:95
    hypoplastic left heart syndrome vs., 3:51
    idiopathic, 3:63
    left coronary artery anomalous origin vs., **3:54i**, 3:55
    myocarditis vs., 3:59
Cardiopulmonary resuscitation, trauma from, **2:98i**, 2:100
Caroli disease, 4:100–102, **4:103i**
    choledochal cyst vs., **4:96i**, 4:97
    differential diagnosis, **4:100i**, 4:101–102
Cataract, congenital, 7:195
Catheterization complications, **2:54i**, 2:55
Caudal regression syndrome, 7:40
Cavernous angioma, **7:122i**, 7:123
Cavernous malformation, 7:103
Cavitary necrosis with pneumonia. *See* Pneumonia, with cavitary necrosis
Cecoureterocele. *See* Ureterocele
Celiac disease, 4:168
Cellulitis
    orbital, 7:190–192, **7:193i**
        differential diagnosis, **7:190i**, 7:191
    scrotal
        epididymoorchitis vs., **5:98i**, 5:99
        torsion of testicular appendage vs., **5:106i**, 5:107
Central incisor syndrome, 7:23

INDEX

Cephalocele. *See* Encephalocele
Cerebellar hypoplasia, 7:7
Cerebral infarction or ischemia. *See* Stroke
Cerebral palsy, 6:99
Cerebritis, 7:191
Cerebrocostomandibular syndrome, **2:98i**, 2:100
Cerebrovascular accident. *See* Stroke
Cervical arch anomalies, 6:164
Cervicoaural cyst. *See* Branchial apparatus anomalies, first
Chest imaging, 2:6–137
    acute chest syndrome, 2:114–116, **2:117i**
    arteriovenous malformation, pulmonary, 2:118–120, **2:121i**
    bronchial atresia, 2:26–28, **2:29i**
    bronchogenic cyst, 2:14–16, **2:17i**
    bronchopulmonary dysplasia, 2:50–52, **2:53i**
    child abuse, rib fractures, 2:98–100, **2:101i**
    chylothorax, 2:58–60, **2:61i**
    cystic adenomatoid malformation, 2:6–8, **2:9i**
    cystic fibrosis, lung, 2:110–112, **2:113i**
    diaphragmatic hernia, congenital, 2:22–24, **2:25i**
    discitis, 2:106–108, **2:109i**
    emphysema
        lobar, congenital, 2:18–20, **2:21i**
        pulmonary interstitial, 2:46–48, **2:49i**
    esophageal foreign body, chronic, 2:134–136, **2:137i**
    germ cell tumors, mediastinum, 2:86–88, **2:89i**
    inflammatory pseudotumor, pulmonary, 2:94–96, **2:97i**
    lung contusion and laceration, 2:122–124, **2:125i**
    lymphoma, thoracic, 2:82–84, **2:85i**
    meconium aspiration syndrome, 2:38–40, **2:41i**
    neuroblastoma, thoracic, 2:102–104, **2:105i**
    normal thymus, 2:78–80, **2:81i**
    papillomatosis, 2:126–128, **2:129i**
    parapneumonic effusion and empyema, 2:70–72, **2:73i**
    pectus excavatum, 2:130–132, **2:133i**
    pleuropulmonary blastoma, 2:90–92, **2:93i**
    pneumonia
        neonatal, 2:34–36, **2:37i**
        round, 2:66–68, **2:69i**
        with cavitary necrosis, 2:74–76, **2:77i**
    pulmonary sequestration, 2:10–12, **2:13i**
    sickle cell disease, 2:114–116, **2:117i**
    surfactant deficient disease, 2:30–32, **2:33i**
    transient tachypnea of the newborn, 2:42–44, **2:45i**
    umbilical catheter complications, 2:54–56, **2:57i**
    viral lung infection, 2:62–64, **2:65i**
Chiari malformations
    type I, 7:10–12, **7:13i**
        differential diagnosis, **7:10i**, 7:11–12
    type II
        Chiari I vs., **7:10i**, 7:11–12
        differential diagnosis, **7:14i**, 7:15
        with myelomeningocele, 7:14–16, **7:17i**
    type III, vs. type II, **7:14i**, 7:15
    type IV
        Chiari II vs., **7:14i**, 7:15
        Dandy Walker malformation vs., 7:7
Child abuse
    brain injuries, 7:78–80, **7:81i**
        differential diagnosis, **7:78i**, 7:80
    fractures vs., in toddlers, 6:28
    Henoch-Schönlein purpura vs., **4:170i**, 4:171
    metaphyseal fractures, 6:10–12, **6:13i**
        differential diagnosis, **6:10i**, 6:11–12
    osteogenesis imperfecta vs., 6:124
    rib fractures, 2:98–100, **2:101i**
        differential diagnosis, **2:98i**, 2:99–100
Choanal atresia, 7:154–156, **7:157i**
    differential diagnosis, **7:154i**, 7:155
Cholangitis
    ascending, 4:101
    chronic, **4:96i**, 4:97
    primary sclerosing, **4:100i**, 4:101
    recurrent pyogenic, **4:100i**, 4:101–102
Choledochal cyst, 4:96–98, **4:99i**
    Caroli disease vs., **4:100i**, 4:101–102
    differential diagnosis, **4:96i**, 4:97
Choledochocele, 4:53
Cholelithiasis, **4:92i**
Cholelithiasis, obstructing, **4:96i**, 4:97
Cholesteatoma. *See also* Epidermoid cyst
    acquired, 7:186–188, **7:189i**
        congenital vs., **7:182i**, 7:183
        differential diagnosis, **7:186i**, 7:187–188
    aural atresia vs., **7:162i**, 7:163
    congenital, 7:182–184, **7:185i**
        acquired vs., **7:186i**, 7:187
        differential diagnosis, **7:182i**, 7:183
Chondroblastoma
    Langerhans cell histiocytosis vs., 6:87
    tarsal coalition vs., 6:148
Chondroma, 2:95
Chondromatosis, synovial, **6:130i**, 6:132
Choriomeningitis, congenital lymphocytic, 7:55
Choroid plexus cyst
    colloid cyst vs, 7:83
    germinal matrix hemorrhage vs., 7:127
Choroid plexus papilloma, 7:118–120, **7:121i**
    colloid cyst vs, **7:82i**, 7:83
    differential diagnosis, **7:118i**, 7:119
    ependymoma vs., **7:102i**, 7:103
    hydrocephalus vs., 7:148
    medulloblastoma vs., **7:98i**, 7:99
    tuberous sclerosis vs., 7:51

INDEX

Chylothorax, 2:58–60, **2:61i**
   differential diagnosis, **2:58i**, 2:59
   parapneumonic effusion and empyema vs., 2:72
Cisterna magna
   arachnoid cyst vs., **7:86i**, 7:87
   Dandy Walker malformation vs., 7:7
Cloacal exstrophy
   anorectal malformation vs., 4:41–42
   gastroschisis vs., 4:67
Club foot (talipes equinovarus), 6:138–140, **6:141i**
   differential diagnosis, **6:138i**, 6:139
Coagulopathy
   bowel injury vs., 4:120
   stroke vs., 7:136
Coarctation
   abdominal, **3:78i**, 3:79
   aortic, 3:78–80, **3:81i**
      aortic stenosis vs., **3:82i**, 3:83
      differential diagnosis, **3:78i**, 3:79
   preductal
      D-transposition of great arteries vs., 3:34
      hypoplastic left heart syndrome vs., **3:50i**, 3:51
      patent ductus arteriosus with, **3:14i**
Coat disease, **7:194i**, 7:195
Cochlea aplasia, **7:158i**, 7:159
Cochleovestibular anomaly, cystic, **7:158i**, 7:159
Cole-Carpenter syndrome, 6:123
Colitis. *See also* Enterocolitis
   allergic
      Hirschsprung disease vs., **4:22i**, 4:23
      necrotizing enterocolitis vs., **4:36i**, 4:37
   granulomatous. *See* Crohn disease
   Henoch-Schönlein purpura vs., **4:170i**, 4:171
   infectious
      Crohn disease vs., **4:150i**, 4:152
      neutropenic colitis vs., **4:142i**, 4:143
      pseudomembranous colitis vs., **4:138i**, 4:139
      ulcerative colitis vs., **4:154i**, 4:156
   inflammatory, 4:147
   lymphoproliferative disorder vs., **4:134i**, 4:135
   neutropenic. *See* Neutropenic colitis
   pseudomembranous. *See* Pseudomembranous colitis
   ulcerative. *See* Ulcerative colitis
Collateral ligaments, **6:30i**, 6:31
Colloid cyst, 7:82–84, **7:85i**
   differential diagnosis, **7:82i**, 7:83
   thyroid, 7:179
Coloboma, **7:194i**, 7:195
Colon
   atresia, **4:26i**, 4:27
   immature. *See also* Meconium plug syndrome
      Hirschsprung disease vs., **4:22i**, 4:23
      jejunoileal atresia vs., **4:18i**, 4:19
      necrotizing enterocolitis vs., **4:36i**, 4:37
   sigmoid, normal position vs. ileocolic intussusception, **4:74i**, 4:75
Column of Bertin, 5:15
Compartment syndromes, 6:135
Conduit thrombosis, **3:26i**
Cor triatriatum, 3:47
Corner fracture, metaphyseal, **6:154i**, 6:156
Coronary artery
   fistula, **3:54i**, 3:55
   left, anomalous origin of, 3:54–56, **3:57i**
      cardiomyopathy vs.., 3:63
      differential diagnosis, **3:54i**, 3:55
      myocarditis vs., 3:59
   single, **3:54i**, 3:55
Corpus callosum
   attenuation of, 7:27
   injuries, **7:26i**, 7:27
   normal neonatal, **7:26i**, 7:27
Cortical defects
   fibrous. *See* Fibroxanthoma
   subperiosteal. *See* Femur, distal metaphyseal irregularity
Cortical dysplasia, 7:52
Corticosteroids, **6:170i**, 6:172
Cowper syringocele, **5:28i**
Coxa valga, **6:98i**, 6:99
Coxa varum, **6:102i**, 6:103
Craniodiaphyseal dysplasia, 6:127
Craniometaphyseal dysplasia, autosomal dominant, 6:127
Craniopharyngioma, 7:110–112, **7:113i**
   colloid cyst vs, **7:82i**, 7:83
   dermoid cyst vs., **7:90i**, 7:91
   differential diagnosis, **7:110i**, 7:111
   germinoma vs., **7:114i**, 7:115
Crista galli, fatty marrow in, **7:150i**, 7:151
Crohn disease, 4:150–152, **4:153i**
   appendicitis vs., 4:71
   cystic fibrosis vs., **4:174i**, 4:175
   differential diagnosis, **4:150i**, 4:151–152
   duodenal hematoma vs., 4:131
   hypoperfusion complex vs., 4:115
   juvenile rheumatoid arthritis vs., 6:131
   Meckel diverticulum vs., 4:79
   mesenteric adenitis vs., **4:108i**, 4:109
   neutropenic colitis vs., **4:142i**, 4:143
   pseudomembranous colitis vs., **4:138i**, 4:139
   spondylolysis vs., 6:179
   ulcerative colitis vs., **4:154i**, 4:155
Croup, 1:10–12, **1:13i**
   differential diagnosis, **1:10i**, 1:11
   epiglottitis vs., **1:6i**, 1:7
   esophageal foreign body vs., 2:135
   exudative tracheitis vs., **1:14i**, 1:15
   membranous. *See* Exudative tracheitis
   retropharyngeal abscess vs., **1:18i**, 1:19

INDEX

        differential diagnosis, **7:158i**, 7:159
        retinal, 7:195
        right ventricular, 3:94–96, **3:97i**
            arrhythmogenic, 3:31
            differential diagnosis, **3:94i**, 3:95
        septo-optic, 7:23
        spondylodysplasia, **6:126i**
        spondyloepiphyseal, **6:118i**, 6:119
        spondylometaphyseal
            child abuse-related metaphyseal fractures vs., **6:10i**, 6:12
            mucopolysaccharidoses vs., **6:118i**, 6:119
        Taylor, 7:52
        thanatophoric, **6:114i**, 6:116
Dysraphism, occult spinal, 7:38–40, **7:41i**
        differential diagnosis, **7:38i**, 7:39–40
Dyssynergia, detrusor-sphincter, **5:118i**, 5:119

E

Ebstein anomaly, 3:30–32, **3:33i**
        differential diagnosis, **3:30i**, 3:31
        pulmonary atresia vs., **3:26i**, 3:27
        right ventricular dysplasia vs., **3:94i**
        tricuspid atresia vs., **3:38i**, 3:39
Ectodermal inclusion cyst. *See* Epidermoid cyst
Edema, postoperative, **4:52i**, 4:53
Ehlers-Danlos syndrome
        aortic stenosis vs., 3:83
        neurogenic bladder vs., 5:119
Ellis van Creveld syndrome, 6:11, **6:114i**
Embolism
        childhood stroke vs., 7:136
        septic emboli vs. papillomatosis, **2:126i**, 2:127
Emphysema. *See* Lobar emphysema; Pulmonary interstitial emphysema
Empyema. *See* Parapneumonic effusion and empyema
Encephalitis
        brainstem, **7:106i**, 7:107
        chronic focal, **7:30i**, 7:31
        mitochondrial encephalopathies vs., **7:70i**, 7:71–72
Encephalocele, 7:18–20, **7:21i**
        differential diagnosis, **7:18i**, 7:19–20
        juvenile nasopharyngeal angiofibroma vs., **7:198i**, 7:199
        nasal, **7:154i**, 7:155
        nasal dermal sinus vs., **7:150i**, 7:151
        nasoethmoid
            choanal atresia vs., 7:155
            nasal dermal sinus vs., 7:151
        nasofrontal, 7:151
Encephalomyelitis, acute disseminated, 7:62–64, **7:65i**
        brain abscess vs., 7:59
        brainstem glioma vs., 7:107
        differential diagnosis, **7:62i**, 7:63
        pilocytic astrocytoma vs., 7:96
Encephalopathy
        hypoxic ischemic, 7:130–132, **7:133i**
            differential diagnosis, **7:130i**, 7:132
            mitochondrial encephalopathies vs., 7:71
        metabolic, stroke vs., 7:136
        mitochondrial, 7:70–72, **7:73i**
            child abuse vs., **7:78i**, 7:80
            differential diagnosis, **7:70i**, 7:71–72
Endocardial cushion defect. *See* Septal defects, atrioventricular
Endocardial fibroelastosis, 3:51
Endocarditis
        papillomatosis vs., 2:127
        rheumatic heart disease vs., **3:108i**, 3:109
Endometrioma, 5:91
Endometriosis, 5:95
Enteric tube malpositions, **2:54i**, 2:55
Enteritis
        infectious, **4:108i**, 4:109
        radiation-induced, 4:147
        regional. *See* Crohn disease
Enterocolitis
        infectious, 4:115
        necrotizing, 4:36–38, **4:39i**
            differential diagnosis, **4:36i**, 4:37
        of term infants, 4:37
Eosinophilic fasciitis, **6:134i**, 6:135
Ependymoma, 7:102–104, **7:105i**
        choroid plexus papilloma vs., 7:119
        differential diagnosis, **7:102i**, 7:103
        medulloblastoma vs., **7:98i**, 7:99
        pilocytic astrocytoma vs., 7:95
        spinal cord astrocytoma vs., **7:122i**, 7:123
Epicondyle avulsion, medial, 6:30–32, **6:33i**
        differential diagnosis, **6:30i**, 6:31–32
Epidermoid cyst, 7:90–92, **7:93i**. *See also* Teratoma, ovarian
        arachnoid cyst vs., **7:86i**, 7:87
        craniopharyngioma vs., 7:111
        differential diagnosis, **7:90i**, 7:91–92
Epidermolysis bullosa, **2:134i**, 2:135
Epididymitis, 5:99
Epididymoorchitis, 5:98–100, **5:101i**
        differential diagnosis, **5:98i**, 5:99
        testicular torsion vs., **5:102i**, 5:103
        torsion of testicular appendage vs., **5:106i**, 5:107
Epiglottis
        exudative tracheitis vs., **1:14i**, 1:15
        omega, **1:6i**, 1:7
        retropharyngeal abscess vs., **1:18i**, 1:19
Epiglottitis, 1:6–9, **1:9i**
        croup vs., **1:10i**, 1:11
        differential diagnosis, **1:6i**, 1:7

INDEX

Epiloia. *See* Tuberous sclerosis
Epiphyseal dysplasia, multiple
    mucopolysaccharidoses vs., 6:119
    osteogenesis imperfecta vs., **6:122i**, 6:123
    osteopetrosis vs., **6:126i**
Epiphysiolysis, femoral capital, traumatic, 6:103
Epithelial carcinoma, 5:91
Epithelial cyst, **7:166i**, 7:167
Esophageal disorders
    atresia with tracheoesophageal fistula, 4:44–46, **4:47i**
        differential diagnosis, **4:44i**, 4:45
    duplication cyst, 1:35
    perforation, **4:44i**, 4:45
    strictures, 4:162–164, **4:165i**
        chronic esophageal foreign body vs., **2:134i**, 2:135
        differential diagnosis, **4:162i**, 4:163
Esophagitis
    chronic foreign body vs., **2:134i**, 2:135
    esophageal strictures and, 4:163
    gastroesophageal reflux and, 4:49
Ewing sarcoma, 6:74–76, **6:78i**
    differential diagnosis, **6:74i**, 6:75–76
    extraosseous, **6:70i**, 6:71
    Langerhans cell histiocytosis vs., **6:86i**, 6:87
    leukemia vs., **6:82i**, 6:83
    osteomyelitis vs., **6:42i**, 6:43
    osteosarcoma vs., **6:78i**, 6:79
    pleuropulmonary blastoma vs., **2:90i**, 2:91
    pulmonary inflammatory pseudotumor vs., 2:95
    sickle cell disease vs., **2:114i**
Exostosis, **7:162i**, 7:163
Extrapulmonary sequestration, of mesoblastic nephroma, 5:59
Exudative tracheitis, 1:14–16, **1:17i**
    croup vs., **1:10i**, 1:11
    differential diagnosis, 1:14–15, **1:14i**
    epiglottitis vs., **1:6i**, 1:7
    retropharyngeal abscess vs., **1:18i**, 1:19
    subglottic hemangioma vs., **1:38i**, 1:39

F

Fahr disease, **7:54i**, 7:55
Fallopian tube disorders, 5:67
Fasciitis
    eosinophilic, **6:134i**, 6:135
    necrotizing, 6:135
Fat, normal epicardial, 3:95
Fat necrosis, post-traumatic, **6:38i**, 6:39–40
Feeding tubes, **2:54i**, 2:55
Femur
    bowing of, **6:102i**
    distal metaphyseal irregularity, 6:154–156, **6:157i**
        differential diagnosis, **6:154i**, 6:155–156
        fibroxanthoma vs., 6:91
    short, 6:103
Fibroelastosis, endocardial, 3:51
Fibroma
    cardiac, **3:102i**, 3:103
    chondromyxoid, **6:90i**, 6:91
    nonossifying. *See* Fibroxanthoma
    renal. *See* Nephroma, mesoblastic
Fibromatosis
    aggressive, 6:66–68, **6:69i**
        differential diagnosis, **6:66i**, 6:68
    chronic foreign body vs., **6:38i**, 6:39
    infantile desmoid, 6:164
Fibromatosis colli, 6:162–164, **6:165i**
    differential diagnosis, **6:162i**, 6:163–164
Fibrosarcoma
    aggressive fibromatosis vs., **6:66i**, 6:68
    distal femoral metaphyseal irregularity vs., 6:155–156
    infantile hemangioma vs., **6:50i**, 6:51
    rhabdomyosarcoma vs., 6:71
Fibrous dysplasia
    fibroxanthoma vs., 6:91
    incomplete fractures vs., **6:14i**, 6:15
    juvenile nasopharyngeal angiofibroma vs., 7:199
    osteogenesis imperfecta vs., **6:122i**, 6:123
Fibrous histiocytoma
    benign. *See* Fibroxanthoma
    malignant
        aggressive fibromatosis vs., 6:68
        rhabdomyosarcoma vs., 6:71
Fibroxanthoma, 6:90–92, **6:93i**
    differential diagnosis, **6:90i**, 6:91
    distal femoral metaphyseal irregularity vs., **6:154i**, 6:156
Fluoroscopic mimics, **5:6i**, 5:7
Fontan procedure, 3:90
Foramen cecum, non-ossified, **7:150i**, 7:151
Foreign bodies
    bronchial, 1:60–62, **1:63i**
        airway compression with thoracic deformity vs., 1:55
        croup vs., 1:11
        differential diagnosis, **1:60i**, 1:61–62
        epiglottitis vs., 1:7
        exudative tracheitis vs., 1:14
        midline descending aorta vs., 1:47
        retropharyngeal abscess vs., 1:19
        viral infection vs., **2:62i**, 2:63
    chronic, 6:38–40, **6:41i**
        differential diagnosis, **6:38i**, 6:39–40
    in ear, **7:162i**, 7:163
    esophageal
        asthma vs., **1:64i**, 1:65
        chronic, 2:134–136, **2:137i**

INDEX

      differential diagnosis, **2:134i**, 2:135
      esophageal strictures vs., **4:162i**, 4:163
    pulmonary inflammatory pseudotumor vs., 2:96
Fractures
    calcaneal, 6:148
    condyle, lateral, **6:22i**, 6:23
    of distal humerus, 6:23
    incomplete, 6:14–16, **6:17i**
      differential diagnosis, **6:14i**, 6:15–16
    Jefferson, **7:74i**, 7:75
    metaphyseal, 6:10–12, **6:13i**
      corner, **6:154i**, 6:156
      differential diagnosis, **6:10i**, 6:11–12
    odontoid, 7:76
    olecranon, **6:22i**, 6:23
    open, **6:22i**, 6:23
    physeal, 6:6–8, **6:9i**
      differential diagnosis, **6:6i**, 6:7
    of rib, 2:98–100, **2:101i**
      differential diagnosis, **2:98i**, 2:99–100
    stress, 6:18–20, **6:21i**
      differential diagnosis, **6:18i**, 6:19–20
      osteochondritis dissecans vs., **6:166i**
      osteogenesis imperfecta vs., 6:124
      osteoid osteoma vs., 6:95
      osteosarcoma vs., **6:78i**, 6:79
      physeal fractures vs., **6:6i**, 6:7
    subtalar, **6:146i**, 6:148
    supracondylar, 6:22–24, **6:25i**
      differential diagnosis, **6:22i**, 6:23
    talar, **6:146i**, 6:148
    Tillaux, **6:6i**, 6:7
    in toddlers, 6:26–28, **6:29i**
      differential diagnosis, **6:26i**, 6:28
    triplane, **6:6i**, 6:7
    vertebral
      diastematomyelia vs., **7:42i**, 7:43
      spondylolysis vs., **6:178i**, 6:179
Fukuyama muscular dystrophy, 7:31
Fungal diseases, 2:127
Funnel chest (pectus excavatum), 2:130–132, **2:133i**
differential diagnosis, **2:130i**, 2:132

G

Galenic varix. *See* Vein of Galen aneurysmal malformation
Gallbladder, small, **4:92i**
Ganglioglioma
    pilocytic astrocytoma vs., 7:95
    spinal cord astrocytoma vs., 7:123
Ganglioneuroma
    mesoblastic nephroma vs., **5:58i**, 5:59
    normal adrenal gland vs., **5:70i**, 5:72
    scoliosis vs., **6:174i**, 6:176
Gartland fracture. *See* Fractures, supracondylar

Gastroenteritis, 4:75
Gastroesophageal reflux, 4:48–50, **4:51i**
    differential diagnosis, **4:48i**, 4:49
    esophageal strictures vs., 4:163
    midgut volvulus vs., **4:6i**, 4:7–8
    pyloric stenosis vs., **4:52i**, 4:53
Gastrointestinal imaging, 4:6–177
    anorectal malformation, 4:40–42, **4:43i**
    appendicitis, 4:70–72, **4:73i**
    bezoar, 4:60–61
    biliary atresia, 4:92–94, **4:95i**
    bowel injury, 4:118–120, **4:121i**
    Caroli disease, 4:100–102, **4:103i**
    choledochal cyst, 4:96–98, **4:99i**
    colitis
      necrotizing enterocolitis, 4:36–38, **4:39i**
      neutropenic, 4:142–144, **4:145i**
      pseudomembranous, 4:138–140, **4:141i**
      ulcerative, 4:154–156, **4:157i**
    Crohn disease, 4:150–152, **4:153i**
    cystic fibrosis, 4:174–176, **4:177i**
    duodenal atresia or stenosis, 4:10–12, **4:13i**
    duodenal hematoma, 4:130–132, **4:133i**
    duodenal web, 4:14–16, **4:17i**
    duplication cysts, 4:158–160, **4:161i**
    esophageal atresia, 4:44–46, **4:47i**
    esophageal strictures, 4:162–164, **4:165i**
    gastroesophageal reflux, 4:48–50, **4:51i**
    gastroschisis, 4:66–68, **4:69i**
    graft-versus-host disease, 4:146–148, **4:149i**
    hemangioendothelioma, 4:86–88, **4:89i**
    Henoch-Schönlein purpura, 4:170–172, **4:173i**
    hepatoblastoma, 4:82–84, **4:85i**
    Hirschsprung disease, 4:22–24, **4:25i**
    hypertrophic pyloric stenosis, 4:52–54, **4:55i**
    hypoperfusion complex, 4:114–116, **4:117i**
    intussusception
      ileocolic, 4:74–76, **4:77i**
      small bowel, 4:166–168, **4:169i**
    jejunoileal atresia, 4:18–20, **4:21i**
    liver transplant complications, 4:104–106, **4:107i**
    liver trauma, 4:122–124, **4:125i**
    lymphoproliferative disorder, 4:134–136, **4:137i**
    Meckel diverticulum, 4:78–80, **4:81i**
    meconium ileus, 4:30–32, **4:33i**
    meconium peritonitis, 4:34–35
    meconium plug syndrome, 4:26–28, **4:29i**
    mesenchymal hamartoma, 4:90–91
    mesenteric adenitis, 4:108–110, **4:111i**
    mesenteric lymphatic malformations, 4:112–113
    omphalocele, 4:62–64, **4:65i**
    spleen trauma, 4:126–128, **4:129i**
    tracheoesophageal fistula, 4:44–46, **4:47i**
    volvulus
      gastric, 4:56–58, **4:59i**

INDEX

midgut, 4:6–8, **4:9i**
Gastroschisis, 4:66–68, **4:69i**
   differential diagnosis, **4:66i**, 4:67
   omphalocele vs., **4:62i**, 4:63
Gaucher disease, **6:106i**
Genitourinary imaging, 5:6–123
   adrenal gland, neonatal
      hemorrhage of, 5:74–76, **5:77i**
      normal, 5:70–72, **5:72i**
   angiomyolipoma, 5:62–64, **5:65i**
   bladder diverticula, 5:122–124, **5:125i**
   calyceal diverticulum, 5:48–49
   epididymoorchitis, 5:98–100, **5:101i**
   hydrometrocolpos, 5:66–68, **5:69i**
   megaureter, primary, 5:26–27
   multicystic dysplastic kidney, 5:36–38, **5:39i**
   nephroblastomatosis, 5:54–55
   nephroma
      mesoblastic, 5:58–60, **5:61i**
      multilocular cystic, 5:56–57
   neuroblastoma, 5:78–80, **5:81i**
   neurogenic bladder, 5:118–120, **5:121i**
   ovarian torsion, 5:94–96, **5:97i**
   polycystic renal disease
      dominant, 5:44–46, **5:47i**
      recessive, 5:40–42, **5:43i**
   pyelonephritis, 5:110–112, **5:113i**
   renal ectopia and fusion, 5:22–24, **5:25i**
   renal injury, 5:114–116, **5:117i**
   rhabdomyosarcoma, genitourinary, 5:82–84, **5:85i**
   teratoma
      ovarian, 5:90–92, **5:93i**
      sacrococcygeal, 5:86–88, **5:89i**
   testicular torsion, 5:102–104, **5:105i**
   torsion of testicular appendage, 5:106–108,
      urachal abnormalities, 5:32–34, **5:35i**
   ureterocele, 5:18–20, **5:21i**
   ureteropelvic duplications, 5:14–16, **5:17i**
   ureteropelvic junction obstruction, 5:10–12, **5:13i**
   urethral valves, posterior, 5:28–30, **5:31i**
   vesicoureteral reflux, 5:6–8, **5:9i**
   Wilm tumor, 5:50–52, **5:53i**
GERDS. *See* Gastroesophageal reflux
Germ cell tumors
   germinoma of brain vs., 7:115
   juvenile nasopharyngeal angiofibroma vs., **7:198i**, 7:199
   of mediastinum, 2:86–88, **2:89i**
      differential diagnosis, **2:86i**, 2:87
   ovarian teratoma vs., 5:91
   thoracic lymphoma vs., **2:82i**, 2:84
Germinal matrix hemorrhage, 7:126–128, **7:129i**
   differential diagnosis, **7:126i**, 7:127
Germinoma, 7:114–116, **7:117i**
   craniopharyngioma vs., **7:110i**, 7:111
   differential diagnosis, **7:114i**, 7:115
Giant aneurysm, **7:138i**, 7:139
Glenn shunt, 3:90, **3:90i**
Gliocele. *See* Encephalocele
Glioma
   brainstem. *See* Brainstem glioma
   fornix, **7:82i**, 7:83
   hypothalamic-chiasmatic, **7:110i**, 7:111
   intramedullary. *See* Spinal cord, astrocytoma
   nasal
      dermal sinus vs., **7:150i**, 7:151
      encephalocele vs., 7:20
   optic, **7:114i**
   spinal. *See* Spinal cord, astrocytoma
Gliomatosis cerebri, **7:30i**, 7:31
Glomerulonephritis, 5:45
Glossoptosis, 1:26–28, **1:29i**
   differential diagnosis, **1:26i**, 1:27
Glucose-6-phosphate dehydrogenase deficiency, 6:172
Glutaric aciduria, **7:78i**, 7:80
Glycoprotein syndrome type 1a, carbohydrate deficient, 7:7
Gonadoblastoma, 5:91
Graft-versus-host disease, 4:146–148, **4:149i**
   bowel injury vs., **4:118i**, 4:120
   differential diagnosis, **4:146i**, 4:147
   hypoperfusion complex vs., **4:114i**, 4:115
   lymphoproliferative disorder vs., **4:134i**, 4:135
   neutropenic colitis vs., 4:144
Granuloma
   pulmonary arteriovenous malformation vs., **2:118i**, 2:119
   tracheal, vs. subglottic hemangioma, **1:38i**, 1:39
Granulomatous disease
   chronic, **2:110i**, 2:111
   pulmonary inflammatory pseudotumor vs., 2:95
Great arteries
   D-transposition of, 3:34–36, **3:37i**
      differential diagnosis, **3:34i**, 3:35
      double outlet right ventricle vs., **3:66i**, 3:68
      patent ductus arteriosus with, **3:18i**
   L-transposition of, 3:70–72, **3:73i**
      differential diagnosis, **3:70i**, 3:71
   transposition of
      Ebstein anomaly vs., **3:30i**, 3:31
      pulmonary atresia vs., 3:27
      total anomalous pulmonary venous return vs., **3:46i**
      tricuspid atresia vs., **3:38i**, 3:39
      truncus arteriosus vs., **3:42i**, 3:43
Grisel syndrome, 7:76
Gymnast wrist, **6:158i**, 6:160

INDEX

H

Hamartoma
    biliary, 4:102
    hypothalamic, 7:115
    leiomyomatous. *See* Nephroma, mesoblastic
    mesenchymal. *See* Mesenchymal hamartoma
    presumed, vs. brainstem glioma, 7:107–108
    pulmonary inflammatory pseudotumor vs., 2:95
    retinal, 7:195
Heart disease. *See also* Cardiac *terms;* Myocarditis
    cardiac tumors, malignant vs. rhabdomyoma, 3:103
    congenital
        chylothorax vs., 2:59
        innominate artery compression syndrome vs., 1:43
        meconium aspiration syndrome vs., **2:38i**, 2:39
        neonatal pneumonia vs., **2:30i**, 2:31
        surfactant deficient disease vs., **2:30i**, 2:31
        transient tachypnea of newborn vs., **2:42i**, 2:43
        with left to right shunt, **3:86i**, 3:87
    congestive heart failure, 3:50–65
        aortic coarctation vs., 3:79
        cardiomyopathy. *See* Cardiomyopathy
        hypoplastic left heart syndrome. *See* Hypoplastic left heart syndrome
        L-transposition of great arteries vs., 3:71
        left coronary artery anomalous origin. *See* Coronary artery, left, anomalous origin of myocarditis. *See* Myocarditis
    cyanotic, vs. necrotizing enterocolitis, 4:37
    endocarditis
        papillomatosis vs., 2:127
        rheumatic heart disease vs., **3:108i**, 3:109
    rheumatic. *See* Rheumatic heart disease
Hemangioblastoma
    pilocytic astrocytoma vs., 7:95–96
    spinal cord, 7:103
Hemangioendothelioma, 4:86–88, **4:89i**
    differential diagnosis, **4:86i**, 4:87–88
    hepatoblastoma vs., **4:82i**, 4:83
    mesenchymal hamartoma vs., **4:90i**, 4:91
Hemangioma
    arteriovenous malformation vs., **6:62i**, 6:63
    of chest wall, **2:130i**, 2:132
    choroidal, 7:195
    chronic foreign body vs., 6:39
    croup vs., **1:10i**
    exudative tracheitis vs., **1:14i**
    gastrointestinal duplication cyst vs., 4:160
    infantile, 6:50–52, **6:53i**
        differential diagnosis, **6:50i**, 6:51, **7:210i**, 7:211
    encephalocele vs., 7:19
    of head and neck, 7:210–212, **7:213i**
    vascular malformations vs., **7:202i**, 7:203
    lymphatic malformations vs., **6:58i**, 6:59
    Meckel diverticulum vs., 4:79
    pulmonary inflammatory pseudotumor vs., 2:96
    rhabdomyoma vs., **3:102i**, 3:103
    rhabdomyosarcoma vs., 6:71
    subglottic, 1:38–40, **1:41i**
        differential diagnosis, **1:38i**, 1:39
        papillomatosis vs., 2:127
    of umbilical cord, 5:33
    venous malformations vs., **6:54i**, 6:55
Hematoma
    adrenal cortical. *See* Adrenal gland, neonatal, hemorrhage
    brain abscess vs., **7:58i**, 7:59
    Chiari type I vs., 7:11
    choroid plexus, 7:127
    choroid plexus papilloma vs., **7:118i**, 7:119
    rhabdomyosarcoma vs., 6:71
    subdural, 7:87
    ureterocele vs., 5:19
Hematometrocolpos
    rhabdomyosarcoma vs., 5:83
    sacrococcygeal teratoma vs., 5:87
Hemimegalencephaly, 7:30–32, **7:33i**
    differential diagnosis, **7:30i**, 7:31
    hydrocephalus vs., 7:148
Hemolytic uremic syndrome, **4:170i**, 4:171
Hemophagocytic lymphohistiocytosis
    acute disseminated encephalomyelitis vs., **7:62i**, 7:63
    brainstem glioma vs., **7:106i**, 7:107
Hemophilia
    bowel injury vs., 4:120
    juvenile rheumatoid arthritis vs., **6:130i**, 6:132
Hemorrhage
    adrenal. *See* Adrenal gland, neonatal, hemorrhage
    germinal matrix, 7:126–128, **7:129i**
        differential diagnosis, **7:126i**, 7:127
    intraventricular, **7:126i**, 7:127
Hemothorax, 2:59
Henoch-Schönlein purpura, 4:170–172, **4:173i**
    bowel injury vs., **4:118i**, 4:120
    differential diagnosis, **4:170i**, 4:171
    hypoperfusion complex vs., **4:114i**, 4:115
    small bowel intussusception vs., **4:166i**, 4:167
Hepatic abscess
    Caroli disease vs., 4:101
    choledochal cyst vs., 4:97
    liver trauma vs., **4:122i**, 4:123
Hepatic vein stenosis, **4:104i**, 4:106
Hepatitis, neonatal, **4:92i**, 4:93
Hepatoblastoma, 4:82–84, **4:85i**

INDEX

differential diagnosis, **4:82i**, 4:83
 hemangioendothelioma vs., **4:86i**, 4:87
 liver trauma vs., **4:122i**, 4:123
 mesenchymal hamartoma vs., **4:90i**, 4:91
 second branchial apparatus anomalies vs., 7:171
Hepatocellular carcinoma
 hemangioendothelioma vs., 4:88
 hepatoblastoma vs., 4:83
Hernia
 diaphragmatic. *See* Diaphragmatic hernia, congenital
 hiatal, **4:56i**, 4:57
 mesenteric, 4:35
 physiologic gut, 4:67
 scrotal, 5:99
 testicular torsion vs., 5:103
 tonsillar, acquired, 7:11
 torsion of testicular appendage vs., 5:107
 umbilical, **4:62i**, 4:63
Heterotaxia syndromes, 3:74–76, **3:78i**
 differential diagnosis, **3:74i**, 3:75
Heterotopia
 hemimegalencephaly vs., 7:31
 trans-mantle, 7:35
 X-linked subependymal, 7:52
Hip
 dislocation, congenital. *See* Developmental dysplasia of hip
 irritable, 6:111
 joint inflammation, **6:110i**, 6:111
 septic
  developmental dysplasia of hip vs., **6:98i**
  Legg-Calve-Perthes disease vs., 6:107
Hirschsprung disease, 4:22–24, **4:25i**
 anorectal malformation vs., **4:40i**, 4:41
 differential diagnosis, **4:22i**, 4:23
 jejunoileal atresia vs., **4:18i**, 4:19
 meconium ileus vs., **4:30i**, 4:31
 meconium plug syndrome vs., **4:26i**, 4:27
 necrotizing enterocolitis vs., **4:36i**, 4:37
Histiocytoma, fibrous. *See* Fibrous histiocytoma
Histiocytosis syndromes. *See also* Langerhans cell histiocytosis
 acute disseminated encephalomyelitis vs., **7:62i**, 7:63
 brainstem glioma vs., 7:107
Hodgkin lymphoma, **7:202i**, 7:203
Holoprosencephaly, 7:22–24, **7:25i**
 differential diagnosis, **7:22i**, 7:23
 schizencephaly vs., **7:34i**, 7:35
Holt-Oram syndrome, 6:143
Horseshoe kidney. *See* Renal ectopia and fusion
Humerus fractures, distal, 6:23
Huntington disease, juvenile, **7:70i**, 7:71
Hyaline membrane disease. *See* Surfactant deficient disease

Hydatid cyst, 4:97
Hydranencephaly
 holoprosencephaly vs., **7:22i**, 7:23
 schizencephaly vs., **7:34i**, 7:35
Hydrocephalus, 7:146–148, **7:149i**
 child abuse vs., 7:80
 congenital, 7:15
 differential diagnosis, **7:146i**, 7:148
 holoprosencephaly vs., **7:22i**, 7:23
Hydrometrocolpos, 5:66–68, **5:69i**
 differential diagnosis, **5:66i**, 5:67
 gastrointestinal duplication cyst vs., 4:159
Hydronephrosis
 multicystic dysplastic kidney vs., **5:36i**, 5:37
 ureteropelvic junction obstruction vs., 5:11
Hydroureter, secondary, 5:27
Hygroma
 cystic, 4:160
 subdural, 7:87
Hyperostosis, infantile cortical (Caffey disease), 6:47
Hyperparathyroidism
 incomplete fractures vs., 6:16
 osteogenesis imperfecta vs., 6:123
Hyperphosphatasia, 6:123
Hyperphosphatemia, 6:16
Hypertension. *See also* Pulmonary hypertension
 systemic, vs. aortic stenosis, **3:82i**, 3:83
Hypochondroplasia, **6:114i**, 6:115
Hypogenetic lung syndrome. *See* Scimitar syndrome
Hypoperfusion complex, 4:114–116, **4:117i**
 bowel injury vs., **4:118i**, 4:120
 differential diagnosis, **4:114i**, 4:115
 graft-versus-host disease vs., **4:146i**, 4:147
 stroke vs., 7:136
Hypopharynx collapse
 enlarged pharyngeal tonsils vs., **1:22i**, 1:24
 glossoptosis vs., **1:26i**, 1:27
Hypophosphatasia
 incomplete fractures vs., 6:16
 syphilis vs., 6:47
Hypoplasia
 biliary, **4:92i**, 4:93
 cerebellar, 7:7
 pulmonary. *See* Pulmonary hypoplasia
 pulmonary artery
  congenital lobar emphysema vs., **2:18i**, 2:19
  tetralogy of Fallot vs., **3:22i**, 3:23
Hypoplastic left heart syndrome, 3:50–52, **3:53i**
 aortic coarctation vs., **3:78i**, 3:79
 differential diagnosis, **3:50i**, 3:51
 patent ductus arteriosus with, **3:18i**
 total anomalous pulmonary venous return vs., **3:46i**, 3:47
Hypotension, intracranial, spontaneous, 7:11

INDEX

I

Ileal atresia (stenosis). *See* Jejunoileal atresia
Ileitis, terminal. *See* Crohn disease
Ileocecal syndrome. *See* Neutropenic colitis
Ileocolitis. *See* Crohn disease
Immotile cilia syndrome, **2:110i**, 2:111
Immunodeficiency disorders, 2:111
Imperforate anus. *See* Anorectal malformation
Infarction
    cerebral. *See* Stroke
    liver, **4:122i**, 4:123
    omental, 4:71
    renal, 5:111
    right ventricular, 3:95
    spinal cord, 7:123
    splenic, **4:126i**, 4:127
Inflammation, intra-abdominal, 4:167
Inflammatory bowel disease. *See* Crohn disease
Innominate artery compression syndrome, 1:42–44, **1:45i**
    differential diagnosis, **1:42i**, 1:43
    double aortic arch vs., 1:31
Intestines, duplication of, 4:79
Intubation errors and malpositions, **2:54i**, 2:55
Intussusception
    ileocolic, 4:74–76, **4:77i**
        differential diagnosis, **4:74i**, 4:75
        small bowel intussusception vs., **4:166i**, 4:167
    mesenteric adenitis vs., **4:108i**, 4:109
    renal ectopia vs., **5:22i**, 5:24
    small bowel, 4:166–168, **4:169i**
        differential diagnosis, **4:166i**, 4:167–168
        hypoperfusion complex vs., **4:114i**, 4:115
Ischemia
    cerebral. *See* Stroke
    myocardial, **3:62i**, 3:63
    neutropenic colitis vs., 4:143
    subcortical, infarction and, 7:52
    venous, **7:54i**, 7:55

J

Jarcho-Levin syndrome, 6:143
Jatene procedure, 3:90–91
Jejunoileal atresia, 4:18–20, **4:21i**
    anorectal malformation vs., **4:40i**, 4:41
    differential diagnosis, **4:18i**, 4:19
    meconium ileus vs., **4:30i**, 4:31
    meconium peritonitis vs., **4:34i**, 4:35
    meconium plug syndrome vs., **4:26i**, 4:27
Joubert anomaly, **7:6i**, 7:7
Jugular bulb, dehiscent, **7:182i**, 7:183

K

Kawasaki disease, 3:104–106, **3:107i**
    cardiomyopathy vs., **3:62i**, 3:63
    differential diagnosis, **3:104i**, 3:105
    left coronary artery anomalous origin vs., **3:54i**, 3:55
    myocarditis vs., **3:58i**, 3:59
    rheumatic heart disease vs., **3:108i**, 3:109
Kempe-Silverman syndrome. *See* Child abuse
Kernicterus
    hypoxic ischemic encephalopathy vs., 7:132
    mitochondrial encephalopathies vs., 7:71
Kidney. *See also* Nephro- *terms*; Renal *terms*
    duplicated. *See* Ureteropelvic duplications
    infarction, 5:111
    multicystic dysplastic. *See* Multicystic dysplastic kidney
    pelvic
        hydrometrocolpos vs., **5:66i**, 5:67
        ovarian teratoma vs., **5:90i**, 5:91
Kidney calculi, 5:7
Kippel-Feil anomaly, 7:76
Krabbe disease, **7:66i**, 7:67
Kyphoscoliosis, **5:22i**, 5:24

L

Labyrinthine aplasia, **7:158i**, 7:159
Lactobezoar, 4:61
Langerhans cell histiocytosis, 6:86–88, **6:89i**
    acquired cholesteatoma vs., **7:186i**, 7:188
    acute disseminated encephalomyelitis vs., 7:63
    brainstem glioma vs., 7:107
    differential diagnosis, **6:86i**, 6:87
    discitis vs., **2:106i**, 2:108
    Ewing sarcoma vs., **6:74i**, 6:76
    germinoma vs., **7:114i**, 7:115
    leukemia vs., **6:82i**, 6:83
    normal thymus vs., **2:78i**, 2:80
    osteoid osteoma vs., **6:94i**, 6:95
    osteomyelitis vs., **6:42i**, 6:43
    papillomatosis vs., 2:127
    rhabdomyosarcoma vs., **7:206i**, 7:207
    sickle cell anemia vs., **6:170i**, 6:172
    spondylolysis vs., 6:179
Laryngotracheal cleft, **4:44i**, 4:45
Laryngotracheobronchitis
    acute. *See* Croup
    asthma vs., 1:65
    membranous. *See* Exudative tracheitis
LeCompte procedure, 3:91
Legg-Calve-Perthes disease, 6:106–108, **6:109i**
    differential diagnosis, **6:106i**, 6:107
    mucopolysaccharidoses vs., **6:118i**, 6:119
    osteochondritis dissecans vs., **6:166i**, 6:167

INDEX

slipped capital femoral epiphysis vs., **6:110i**, 6:111
Lemierre syndrome, 2:127
Leukemia, 6:82–84, **6:85i**
    acute myelogenic, vs. rhabdomyosarcoma, **7:206i**, 7:207
    child abuse-related metaphyseal fractures vs., **6:10i**, 6:12
    differential diagnosis, **6:82i**, 6:83
    discitis vs., 2:108
    distal femoral metaphyseal irregularity vs., **6:154i**, 6:156
    fractures vs., in toddlers, **6:26i**, 6:28
    juvenile rheumatoid arthritis vs., 6:132
    Langerhans cell histiocytosis vs., 6:87
    nephroblastomatosis vs., 5:54
    osteomyelitis vs., **6:42i**, 6:43
    rickets vs., **6:158i**, 6:160
    sickle cell anemia vs., **6:170i**, 6:172
    spondylolysis vs., 6:179
    syphilis vs., **6:46i**, 6:47
Leukocoria, 7:195
Leukodystrophies, 7:66–68, **7:69i**
    differential diagnosis, **7:66i**, 7:67–68
    globoid, **7:66i**, 7:67
    metachromatic, **7:66i**, 7:67
Leukomalacia, periventricular
    callosal dysgenesis vs., **7:26i**, 7:27
    germinal matrix hemorrhage vs., **7:126i**, 7:127
    hypoxic ischemic encephalopathy vs., **7:130i**, 7:132
Ligaments, instability of, 7:76
Lingual tonsils, enlarged, **1:26i**, 1:27
Lipoma
    dermoid cyst vs., 7:91
    spinal. *See* Dysraphism, occult spinal
Liposarcoma
    angiomyolipoma vs., 5:63
    myxoid, 6:71
Liver. *See also* Hepat- *terms*
    infarction, **4:122i**, 4:123
    transplant complications, 4:104–106, **4:107i**
        treatment of, **4:104i**, 4:106
    trauma, 4:122–124, **4:125i**
        differential diagnosis, **4:122i**, 4:123
Lobar emphysema
    congenital, 2:18–20, **2:21i**
        bronchial atresia vs., **2:26i**, 2:27
        bronchopulmonary dysplasia vs., 2:51
        congenital diaphragmatic hernia vs., **2:22i**, 2:23
        differential diagnosis, **2:18i**, 2:19–20
        pulmonary interstitial emphysema vs., **2:46i**, 2:47
        transient tachypnea of newborn vs., 2:43
    pulmonary sling vs., **1:34i**, 1:35

Loose bodies
    discoid meniscus vs., **6:150i**, 6:151
    medial epicondyle avulsion vs., 6:32
Lumbo-peritoneal shunt, **7:10i**, 7:11
Lung. *See also* Pulmonary *terms*
    abscess
        parapneumonic effusion and empyema vs., **2:70i**, 2:72
        pneumonia with cavitary necrosis vs., 2:75
    agenesis. *See* Pulmonary agenesis
    contusions and lacerations, 2:122–124, **2:125i**
        differential diagnosis, **2:122i**, 2:123
    disease of prematurity. *See* Surfactant deficient disease
    hypoplasia. *See* Pulmonary hypoplasia
Lupus erythematosus, systemic
    bowel injury vs., **4:118i**, 4:120
    Kawasaki disease vs., 3:105
Lymphadenopathy
    bronchogenic cyst vs., **2:14i**, 2:16
    cervical, **6:162i**, 6:163
    pulmonary sling vs., **1:34i**, 1:35
    suppurative, **7:170i**, 7:171
Lymphangiectasia
    bronchopulmonary dysplasia vs., 2:51
    transient tachypnea of newborn vs., **2:42i**, 2:43
Lymphangioleiomyomatosis, **7:50i**, 7:51
Lymphatic malformations, 6:58–60, **6:61i**
    arteriovenous malformation vs., **6:62i**, 6:63
    branchial apparatus anomalies vs.
        first, **7:166i**, 7:167
        second, **7:170i**, 7:171
        third, **7:174i**, 7:175
        fourth, **7:178i**, 7:179
    chronic foreign body vs., 6:39
    differential diagnosis, **6:58i**, 6:59
    gastrointestinal duplication cyst vs., 4:159
    infantile hemangioma vs., **6:50i**, 6:51
    mesenteric, 4:112–113
        differential diagnosis, 4:112–113, **4:112i**
    musculoskeletal, 6:58–60, **6:61i**
    pectus excavatum vs., **2:130i**, 2:132
    retropharyngeal abscess vs., 1:19
    venous malformations vs., **6:54i**, 6:55
Lymphatic mass, **1:42i**, 1:43
Lymphoepithelial cysts, benign, 7:167
Lymphohistiocytosis, hemophagocytic
    acute disseminated encephalomyelitis vs., **7:62i**, 7:63
    brainstem glioma vs., **7:106i**, 7:107
Lymphoma. *See also* Non-Hodgkin lymphoma
    anterior mediastinum, 1:43
    Crohn disease vs., **4:150i**, 4:152
    double aortic arch vs., **1:30i**, 1:31
    encephalocele vs., 7:20
    germ cell tumor vs., **2:86i**, 2:87

INDEX

Hodgkin, vascular malformations vs., **7:202i**, 7:203
Langerhans cell histiocytosis vs., **6:86i**, 6:87
leukemia vs., **6:82i**, 6:83
nephroblastomatosis vs., 5:54
normal thymus vs., **2:78i**, 2:80
osteomyelitis vs., 6:43
parapneumonic effusion and empyema vs., **2:70i**, 2:71
pelvic, 5:83
pulmonary inflammatory pseudotumor vs., **2:94i**, 2:95
pyelonephritis vs., **5:110i**, 5:111
renal
    angiomyolipoma vs., 5:63
    dominant polycystic renal disease vs., **5:44i**, 5:45
rhabdomyosarcoma vs., 5:83, 7:207
small bowel intussusception vs., 4:168
spondylolysis vs., 6:179
thoracic, 2:82–84, **2:85i**
    differential diagnosis, **2:82i**, 2:83–84
thoracic neuroblastoma vs., **2:102i**, 2:103
Lymphoproliferative disorder, 4:134–136, **4:137i**
differential diagnosis, **4:134i**, 4:135
graft-versus-host disease vs., **4:146i**, 4:147

M

Macroadenoma, pituitary, **7:114i**, 7:115
Macrocrania, benign
    child abuse vs., 7:80
    hydrocephalus vs., 7:148
Malabsorption syndromes, 4:168
Malpositioned tubes and catheters, **2:54i**, 2:55
Marble bone disease. *See* Osteopetrosis
Marfan disease, **3:82i**, 3:83
Mastoiditis, acute coalescent, **7:186i**, 7:187–188
Meckel diverticulum, 4:78–80, **4:81i**
    appendicitis vs., **4:70i**, 4:71
    differential diagnosis, **4:78i**, 4:79
    ileocolic intussusception vs., **4:74i**, 4:75
    meconium peritonitis vs., 4:35
    small bowel intussusception vs., **4:166i**, 4:167
Meckel-Gruber syndrome, 5:41
Meconium aspiration syndrome, 2:38–40, **2:41i**
    bronchopulmonary dysplasia vs., **2:50i**, 2:51
    differential diagnosis, **2:38i**, 2:39
    neonatal pneumonia vs., **2:30i**, 2:31
    surfactant deficient disease vs., **2:30i**, 2:31
    transient tachypnea of newborn vs., 2:43
Meconium ileus, 4:30–32, **4:33i**
    anorectal malformation vs., **4:40i**, 4:41
    differential diagnosis, **4:30i**, 4:31
    jejunoileal atresia vs., **4:18i**, 4:19
    meconium peritonitis vs., **4:34i**, 4:35
    meconium plug syndrome vs., **4:26i**, 4:27
Meconium peritonitis, 4:34–35
    differential diagnosis, **4:34i**, 4:35
Meconium plug syndrome, 4:26–28, **4:29i**
    anorectal malformation vs., **4:40i**, 4:41
    differential diagnosis, **4:26i**, 4:27
    Hirschsprung disease vs., **4:22i**, 4:23
    jejunoileal atresia vs., **4:18i**, 4:19
    meconium ileus vs., **4:30i**, 4:31
Meconium pseudocyst
    gastrointestinal duplication cyst vs., **4:158i**, 4:159
    Meckel diverticulum vs., **4:78i**, 4:79
Mediastinal mass
    airway compression with thoracic deformity vs., 1:55
    midline descending aorta vs., 1:51
Medulloblastoma, 7:98–100, **7:101i**
    choroid plexus papilloma vs., **7:118i**, 7:119
    differential diagnosis, **7:98i**, 7:99
    ependymoma vs., **7:102i**, 7:103
    pilocytic astrocytoma vs., 7:95
Megacalycosis, **5:10i**, 5:11
Megalencephaly, unilateral. *See* Hemimegalencephaly
Megalourethra, 5:29
Megaureter
    nonrefluxing, **5:26i**, 5:27
    primary, **5:26i**, 5:27
    refluxing, **5:26i**, 5:27
    ureteropelvic junction obstruction vs., **5:10i**, 5:12
Membranous croup. *See* Exudative tracheitis
Meningioma, 7:119
Meningitis
    child abuse vs., 7:80
    orbital cellulitis vs., **7:190i**, 7:191
Meningocele. *See* Encephalocele
Meniscus
    bucket-handle tear, **6:150i**, 6:151
    discoid, 6:150–152, **6:153i**
        differential diagnosis, **6:150i**, 6:151
    flipped, **6:150i**, 6:151
Menkes syndrome
    abuse-related metaphyseal fractures vs., 6:12
    abuse-related rib fractures vs., 2:99
    neurogenic bladder vs., 5:119
Mesenchymal hamartoma, 4:90–91. *See also* Nephroma, mesoblastic
    differential diagnosis, **4:90i**, 4:91
    hemangioendothelioma vs., **4:86i**, 4:88
    hepatoblastoma vs., **4:82i**, 4:83
Mesenteric adenitis, 4:108–110, **4:111i**
    appendicitis vs., **4:70i**, 4:71
    Crohn disease vs., **4:150i**, 4:151–152
    differential diagnosis, **4:108i**, 4:109–110

INDEX

Mesenteric cyst, **4:158i**, 4:159
Metastasis (metastatic disease)
    liver trauma vs., 4:123
    neuroblastoma
        Ewing sarcoma vs., **6:74i**, 6:76
        hemangioendothelioma vs., **4:86i**, 4:87
        hepatoblastoma vs., **4:82i**, 4:83
        Langerhans cell histiocytosis vs., 6:87
        leukemia vs., 6:83
        mesenchymal hamartoma vs., **4:90i**, 4:91
        rhabdomyosarcoma vs., **7:206i**, 7:207
    normal adrenal gland vs., **5:70i**, 5:71–72
    osteosarcoma
        pulmonary arteriovenous malformation vs., **2:118i**, 2:119
        pulmonary inflammatory pseudotumor vs., **2:94i**
    papillomatosis vs., **2:126i**, 2:127
    rhabdomyosarcoma vs., **5:82i**
    second branchial apparatus anomalies vs., 7:171
    spondylolysis vs., 6:179
    squamous cell carcinoma, 7:171
Metatarsus adductus, **6:138i**, 6:139
Metatropic dysplasia, 6:115
Methylmalonic acidemia, 7:132
Meyer dysplasia, **6:106i**, 6:107
Microcolon, **4:22i**, 4:23
Mid-aortic syndrome
    hypoplastic left heart syndrome vs., **3:50i**
Midline descending aorta, 1:50–52, **1:53i**
    airway compression with thoracic deformity vs., **1:54i**, 1:55
    carina compression syndrome vs. pulmonary sling, 1:35
    differential diagnosis, **1:50i**, 1:51
Milk allergy colitis, **4:22i**, 4:23
Mononucleosis, 3:105
Morgagni hernia. *See* Diaphragmatic hernia, congenital
Morquio disease, **6:114i**, 6:116
Moyamoya disease
    Kawasaki disease vs., **3:104i**, 3:105
    stroke vs., **7:134i**, 7:136
Mucocele, **7:154i**, 7:155
Mucocutaneous lymph node syndrome. *See* Kawasaki disease
Mucoepidermoid tumor, 2:96
Mucopolysaccharidoses, 6:118–120, **6:121i**
    differential diagnosis, **6:118i**, 6:119
Mucoviscidosis. *See* Cystic fibrosis
Multicystic dysplastic kidney, 5:36–38, **5:39i**
    differential diagnosis, **5:36i**, 5:37–38
    mesoblastic nephroma vs., 5:59
    multilocular cystic nephroma vs., 5:57
    recessive polycystic renal disease vs. differential diagnosis, **5:40i**, 5:41–42
    segmental, 5:15
    ureteropelvic junction obstruction vs., **5:10i**, 5:11
Multiple sclerosis
    acute disseminated encephalomyelitis vs., **7:62i**, 7:63
    brain abscess vs., **7:58i**, 7:59
    optic neuritis vs. pilocytic astrocytoma, **7:94i**, 7:96
    spinal cord astrocytoma vs., 7:123
Muscle-eye-brain disease, 7:31
Muscle injuries
    dermatomyositis vs., **6:134i**, 6:135
    discitis vs., 2:107
Muscular dystrophy
    Duchenne
        cardiomyopathy vs., **3:62i**, 3:63
        myocarditis vs., **3:58i**
    Fukuyama, vs. hemimegalencephaly, 7:31
    transient tachypnea of the newborn vs., 2:44
Musculoskeletal imaging, 6:6–181
    achondroplasia, 6:114–116, **6:117i**
    arteriovenous malformations, 6:62–64, **6:65i**
    child abuse, metaphyseal fracture in, 6:10–12, **6:13i**
    club foot (talipes equinovarus), 6:138–140, **6:141i**
    dermatomyositis, 6:134–136, **6:137i**
    developmental dysplasia of hip, 6:98–100, **6:101i**
    discoid meniscus, 6:150–152, **6:153i**
    distal femoral metaphyseal irregularity, 6:154–156, **6:157i**
    Ewing sarcoma, 6:74–76, **6:78i**
    fibromatosis, aggressive, 6:66–68, **6:69i**
    fibromatosis colli, 6:162–164, **6:165i**
    fibroxanthoma, 6:90–92, **6:93i**
    foreign body, chronic, 6:38–40, **6:41i**
    fractures
        incomplete, 6:14–16, **6:17i**
        metaphyseal, 6:10–12, **6:13i**
        physeal, 6:6–8, **6:9i**
        stress, 6:18–20, **6:21i**
        supracondylar, 6:22–24, **6:25i**
        in toddlers, 6:26–28, **6:29i**
    infantile hemangioma, 6:50–52, **6:53i**
    Langerhans cell histiocytosis, 6:86–88, **6:89i**
    Legg-Calve-Perthes disease, 6:106–108, **6:109i**
    leukemia, 6:82–84, **6:85i**
    lymphatic malformations, 6:58–60, **6:61i**
    medial epicondyle avulsion, 6:30–32, **6:33i**
    mucopolysaccharidoses, 6:118–120, **6:121i**
    Osgood-Schlatter lesion, 6:34–36, **6:37i**
    osteochondritis dissecans, 6:166–168, **6:169i**
    osteogenesis imperfecta, 6:122–124, **6:125i**
    osteoid osteoma, 6:94–96, **6:97i**

INDEX

osteomyelitis, 6:42–44, **6:45i**
osteopetrosis, 6:126–128, **6:129i**
osteosarcoma, 6:78–80, **6:81i**
proximal focal femoral deficiency, 6:102–104, **6:105i**
rhabdomyosarcoma, 6:70–72, **6:73i**
rheumatoid arthritis, juvenile, 6:130–132, **6:133i**
rickets, 6:158–160, **6:161i**
scoliosis, 6:174–176, **6:177i**
sickle cell anemia, of bone, 6:170–172, **6:173i**
slipped capital femoral epiphysis, 6:110–112, **6:113i**
spondylolysis, 6:178–180, **6:181i**
syphilis, 6:46–48, **6:49i**
tarsal coalition, 6:146–148, **6:149i**
VACTERL association, 6:142–144, **6:145i**
venous malformations, 6:54–56, **6:57i**
Mustard/Senning procedure, 3:90
Mycobacterial adenitis, nontuberculous, **7:166i**, 7:167
Mycobacterium avium intracellulare, **7:166i**, 7:167
Myelination, normal, 7:142–144, **7:145i**
hypoxic ischemic encephalopathy vs., 7:132
T1 weighted images of, **7:142i**
Myelinolysis, pontine, 7:107
Myelitis, transverse, **7:122i**, 7:123
Myelocystocele
occult spinal dysraphism vs., **7:38i**, 7:39
sacrococcygeal teratoma vs., **5:86i**, 5:87
Myelodysplasia, 5:119
Myelomeningocele
abuse-related metaphyseal fractures vs., 6:11
Chiari type II with, 7:14–16, **7:17i**
neurogenic bladder vs., **5:118i**, 5:119
occult spinal dysraphism vs., **7:38i**, 7:39
sacrococcygeal teratoma vs., 5:87
Myocardial ischemia, **3:62i**, 3:63
Myocarditis, 3:58–60, **3:61i**
cardiomyopathy vs., 3:63
differential diagnosis, **3:58i**, 3:59
rheumatic heart disease vs., 3:109
viral
Kawasaki disease vs., **3:104i**, 3:105
right ventricular dysplasia vs., **3:94i**, 3:95
Myocardium, normal epicardial fat in, 3:95
Myositis, infectious, **6:134i**, 6:135
Myositis ossificans
dermatomyositis vs., 6:135
osteogenesis imperfecta vs., 6:124
osteosarcoma vs., 6:80
Myxoma, 3:103

N

Nasal pyriform aperture stenosis, congenital, **7:154i**, 7:155
Nasopharyngeal angiofibroma. *See* Angiofibroma, juvenile nasopharyngeal
Nasopharyngeal carcinoma
encephalocele vs., **7:18i**, 7:20
juvenile nasopharyngeal angiofibroma vs., 7:199
rhabdomyosarcoma vs., **7:206i**, 7:207
Near drowning, **7:70i**, 7:71
Necrosis, avascular. *See* Legg-Calve-Perthes disease
Necrotizing fasciitis, 6:135
Neoplasms. *See* Tumor(s)
Nephritis, radiation-induced, 5:45
Nephroblastomatosis, 5:54–55
differential diagnosis, **5:54i**
dominant polycystic renal disease vs., **5:44i**, 5:45
pyelonephritis vs., **5:110i**, 5:111
Wilm tumor vs., **5:50i**, 5:51
Nephroma
mesoblastic, 5:58–60, **5:61i**
differential diagnosis, **5:58i**, 5:59
multicystic dysplastic kidney vs., 5:37–38
Wilm tumor vs., **5:50i**, 5:51
multilocular cystic, 5:56–57
differential diagnosis, **5:56i**, 5:57
mesenteric lymphatic malformation vs., **4:112i**, 4:113
ovarian teratoma vs., 5:91
Wilm tumor vs., **5:50i**, 5:51
Nerve sheath tumor, malignant peripheral, **6:70i**, 6:71
Neuroblastoma, 5:78–80, **5:81i**
abuse-related rib fractures vs., **2:98i**, 2:100
adrenal hemorrhage vs., **5:74i**, 5:75
bronchogenic cyst vs., **2:14i**, 2:15–16
child abuse vs., **7:78i**
congenital, vs. fibromatosis colli, **6:162i**, 6:163
differential diagnosis, **5:78i**, 5:79
discitis vs., **2:106i**, 2:108
fractures vs., in toddlers, **6:26i**, 6:28
mesoblastic nephroma vs., **5:58i**, 5:59
metastasis. *See* Metastasis (metastatic disease), neuroblastoma
normal adrenal gland vs., **5:70i**, 5:72
osteomyelitis vs., **6:42i**, 6:43
pelvic
hydrometrocolpos vs., 5:67
rhabdomyosarcoma vs., 5:83
pleuropulmonary blastoma vs., 2:91
rhabdomyosarcoma vs., 6:71
round pneumonia vs., **2:66i**, 2:67
sacrococcygeal teratoma vs., 5:87
second branchial apparatus anomalies vs., 7:171

INDEX

syphilis vs., 6:47
thoracic, 2:102–104, **2:105i**
    differential diagnosis, **2:102i**, 2:103
Wilm tumor vs., 5:51
Neurocysticercosis
    colloid cyst vs, 7:83
    TORCH infections vs., **7:54i**, 7:55
Neurocytoma, central
    colloid cyst vs, 7:83
    tuberous sclerosis vs., 7:51
Neuroectodermal tumor, primitive (PNET)
    pleuropulmonary blastoma vs., 2:91
    rhabdomyosarcoma vs., 6:71
Neuroepithelial cyst, 7:87
Neuroepithelial tumor, dysembryoplastic (DNET)
    brain abscess vs., **7:58i**, 7:59
    pilocytic astrocytoma vs., 7:95
    tuberous sclerosis vs., 7:51
Neurofibroma
    innominate artery compression syndrome vs., 1:43
    orbital, 7:20
    plexiform, **7:210i**, 7:211
    rhabdomyosarcoma vs., **6:70i**, 6:71
    vascular malformations vs., 7:203
Neurofibromatosis
    incomplete fractures vs., **6:14i**, 6:16
    osteogenesis imperfecta vs., **6:122i**, 6:123
    type 1, 7:46–48, **7:49i**
        brainstem glioma vs., **7:106i**, 7:107
        differential diagnosis, **7:46i**, 7:47–48
        encephalocele vs., 7:20
        mitochondrial encephalopathies vs., **7:70i**, 7:71
        vascular malformations of head and neck vs., **7:202i**, 7:203
    type 2, **7:46i**, 7:47
Neurogenic bladder, 5:118–120, **5:121i**
    differential diagnosis, **5:118i**, 5:119
    vesicoureteral reflux vs., **5:6i**, 5:7
Neuroimaging, 7:6–213
    arachnoid cyst, 7:86–88, **7:89i**
    astrocytoma
        pilocytic, 7:94–96, **7:97i**
        spinal cord, 7:122–124, **7:125i**
    atlanto-axial injuries, 7:74–76, **7:77i**
    aural atresia, 7:162–164, **7:165i**
    brain abscess, 7:58–60, **7:61i**
    brainstem glioma, 7:106–108, **7:109i**
    branchial apparatus anomalies
        first, 7:166–168, **7:169i**
        second, 7:170–172, **7:173i**
        third, 7:174–176, **7:177i**
        fourth, 7:178–180, **7:181i**
    callosal dysgenesis, 7:26–28, **7:29i**
    Chiari malformations
        type I, 7:10–12, **7:13i**
        type II, with myelomeningocele, 7:14–16, **7:17i**
    child abuse, brain and, 7:78–80, **7:81i**
    childhood stroke, 7:134–136, **7:137i**
    choanal atresia, 7:154–156, **7:157i**
    cholesteatoma
        acquired, 7:186–188, **7:189i**
        congenital, 7:182–184, **7:185i**
    choroid plexus papilloma, 7:118–120, **7:121i**
    colloid cyst, 7:82–84, **7:85i**
    craniopharyngioma, 7:110–112, **7:113i**
    Dandy Walker malformation, 7:6–8, **7:9i**
    dermoid and epidermoid cysts, 7:90–92, **7:93i**
    diastematomyelia, 7:42–44, **7:45i**
    encephalocele, 7:18–20, **7:21i**
    encephalomyelitis, acute disseminated, 7:62–64, **7:65i**
    encephalopathy
        hypoxic ischemic, 7:130–132, **7:133i**
        mitochondrial, 7:70–72, **7:73i**
    ependymoma, 7:102–104, **7:105i**
    germinal matrix hemorrhage, 7:126–128, **7:129i**
    germinoma, 7:114–116, **7:117i**
    hemangioma, infantile, of head and neck, 7:210–212, **7:213i**
    hemimegalencephaly, 7:30–32, **7:33i**
    holoprosencephaly, 7:22–24, **7:25i**
    hydrocephalus, 7:146–148, **7:149i**
    leukodystrophies, 7:66–68, **7:69i**
    medulloblastoma, 7:98–100, **7:101i**
    myelination, normal, 7:142–144, **7:145i**
    nasal dermal sinus, 7:150–152, **7:153i**
    nasopharyngeal angiofibroma, juvenile, 7:198–200, **7:201i**
    neurofibromatosis type 1, 7:46–48, **7:49i**
    occult spinal dysraphism, 7:38–40, **7:41i**
    orbital cellulitis, 7:190–192, **7:193i**
    otic capsule dysplasias, 7:158–160, **7:161i**
    retinoblastoma, 7:194–196, **7:197i**
    rhabdomyosarcoma, head and neck, 7:206–208, **7:209i**
    schizencephaly, 7:34–36, **7:37i**
    TORCH infections, 7:54–56, **7:57i**
    tuberous sclerosis, 7:50–52, **7:53i**
    vascular malformations, head and neck, 7:202–204, **7:205i**
    vein of Galen aneurysmal malformation, 7:138–140, **7:141i**
Neuromuscular disorders, 6:99
Neuronal migration, disorders of, **7:30i**, 7:31
Neutropenic colitis, 4:142–144, **4:145i**
    differential diagnosis, **4:142i**, 4:143–144
    graft-versus-host disease vs., **4:146i**, 4:147
        pseudomembranous colitis vs., **4:138i**, 4:139

INDEX

ulcerative colitis vs., **4:154i**, 4:155–156
Non-Hodgkin lymphoma
    pseudomembranous colitis vs., 4:139
    small bowel intussusception vs., 4:168
    vascular malformations of head and neck vs., 7:203
Nonaccidental trauma. See Child abuse
Nonvascular masses, 1:31
Norwood procedure, 3:91

O

Obstructive sleep apnea
    causes of, **1:22i**
    enlarged pharyngeal tonsils and, 1:22–24, **1:25i**
Olecranon
    fracture, **6:22i**, 6:23
    stress injury vs. medial epicondyle avulsion, **6:30i**, 6:31
Oligodendroglioma, 7:103
Olivopontocerebellar degeneration, 7:7
Omega epiglottis, **1:6i**, 1:7
Omental infarction, 4:71
Omovertebral bone, **6:162i**, 6:164
Omphalitis, **5:32i**, 5:33
Omphalocele, 4:62–64, **4:65i**
    differential diagnosis, **4:62i**, 4:63
    gastroschisis vs., **4:66i**, 4:67
Oncocytoma, 5:64
Operative procedures, cardiac, 3:90–92, **3:90i**, **3:93i**
Optic neuritis, **7:94i**, 7:96
Orbital cellulitis, 7:190–192, **7:193i**
    differential diagnosis, **7:190i**, 7:191
Orchitis. See Epididymoorchitis
Os odontoideum, 7:76
Osgood-Schlatter lesion, 6:34–36, **6:37i**
    differential diagnosis, **6:34i**, 6:35
Ossification, normal, **6:166i**, 6:167
Osteoblastoma
    discitis vs., 2:108
    Langerhans cell histiocytosis vs., 6:87
    osteoid osteoma vs., **6:94i**, 6:95
    spondylolysis vs., 6:179
Osteochondral injuries, **6:166i**, 6:167
Osteochondritis coxae juvenilis. See Legg-Calve-Perthes disease
Osteochondritis dissecans, 6:166–168, **6:169i**
    capitellar
        medial epicondyle avulsion vs., **6:30i**, 6:31
        supracondylar fracture vs., 6:23
    differential diagnosis, **6:166i**, 6:167
    discoid meniscus vs., **6:150i**, 6:151
    tarsal coalition vs., **6:146i**, 6:147–148
Osteochondroma, 6:124
Osteochondrosis, tibial. See Osgood-Schlatter lesion
Osteogenesis imperfecta, 6:122–124, **6:125i**
    abuse-related metaphyseal fractures vs., **6:10i**, 6:11
    abuse-related rib fractures vs., **2:98i**, 2:99
    differential diagnosis, **6:122i**, 6:123–124
    incomplete fractures vs., **6:14i**, 6:15
Osteoid osteoma, 6:94–96, **6:97i**
    differential diagnosis, **6:94i**, 6:95
    discitis vs., **2:106i**, 2:108
    fractures vs., in toddlers, **6:26i**, 6:28
    Langerhans cell histiocytosis vs., **6:86i**, 6:87
    Legg-Calve-Perthes disease vs., 6:107
    scoliosis vs., **6:174i**, 6:176
    slipped capital femoral epiphysis vs., **6:110i**, 6:111
    spondylolysis vs., **6:178i**, 6:179
    stress fracture vs., **6:18i**, 6:19
Osteolysis, 6:172
Osteoma. See also Osteoid osteoma
    aural atresia vs., 7:163
    choroidal, 7:195
    osteoid osteoma vs., 6:95
Osteomyelitis, 6:42–44, **6:45i**. See also Brodie abscess
    differential diagnosis, **6:42i**, 6:43
    distal femoral metaphyseal irregularity vs., 6:155
    Ewing sarcoma vs., **6:74i**, 6:75
    fractures vs., in toddlers, **6:26i**, 6:28
    frontal, **7:190i**, 7:191
    Langerhans cell histiocytosis vs., 6:87
    leukemia vs., **6:82i**, 6:83
    osteogenesis imperfecta vs., 6:124
    osteoid osteoma vs., **6:94i**, 6:95
    osteosarcoma vs., **6:78i**, 6:80
    scoliosis vs., **6:174i**, 6:176
    spondylolysis vs., **6:178i**, 6:179
    syphilis vs., **6:46i**, 6:47
    tarsal coalition vs., **6:146i**, 6:147
Osteonecrosis, juvenile, 6:107
Osteopathia striata, 6:128
Osteopenia
    abuse-related rib fractures vs., 2:99
    sickle cell anemia vs., 6:172
Osteopetrosis, 6:126–128, **6:129i**
    bisphosphonate-induced, 6:127
    differential diagnosis, **6:126i**, 6:127–128
    with renal tubular acidosis, 6:127
Osteoporosis, idiopathic juvenile, 6:123
Osteoporosis-pseudoglioma syndrome, 6:123
Osteosarcoma, 6:78–80, **6:81i**
    chronic foreign body vs., **6:38i**, 6:39
    differential diagnosis, **6:78i**, 6:79–80
    distal femoral metaphyseal irregularity vs., **6:154i**, 6:155
    encephalocele vs., 7:20
    Ewing sarcoma vs., **6:74i**, 6:76
    metastasis

INDEX

pulmonary arteriovenous malformation vs., **2:118i**, 2:119
pulmonary inflammatory pseudotumor vs., **2:94i**
osteogenesis imperfecta vs., 6:124
scoliosis vs., **6:174i**, 6:176
stress fracture vs., **6:18i**, 6:19
Osteosclerotic bone dysplasia, lethal, 6:128
Ostium primum defect. *See* Septal defects, atrioventricular
Otic capsule dysplasias, 7:158–160, **7:161i**
    differential diagnosis, **7:158i**, 7:159
Otocyst, **7:158i**, 7:159
Ovarian disorders
    cysts
        gastrointestinal duplication cyst vs., 4:159
        teratoma vs., **5:90i**, 5:91, **5:94i**, 5:95
        torsion vs., **5:94i**, 5:95
    hydrometrocolpos vs., 5:67
    ileocolic intussusception vs., **4:74i**, 4:75
    teratoma. *See* Teratoma, ovarian
    torsion. *See* Torsion, ovarian
    tumors
        rhabdomyosarcoma vs., 5:83
        sacrococcygeal teratoma vs., 5:87
        torsion vs., 5:95
Overshunting, **7:78i**, 7:80

P

Pachygyria, **7:30i**, 7:31
Palatine tonsils, enlarged, 1:27
Pancake kidney. *See* Renal ectopia and fusion
Pancreas
    annular
        duodenal atresia or stenosis vs., 4:11
        duodenal hematoma vs., 4:132
        duodenal web vs., 4:15
        midgut volvulus vs., 4:8
        pyloric stenosis vs., 4:53
    tumors
        duodenal hematoma vs., 4:132
Pancreatitis
    duodenal hematoma vs., 4:132
    small bowel intussusception vs., **4:166i**, 4:167
Papilloma, chorioid plexus. *See* Choroid plexus papilloma
Papillomatosis, 2:126–128, **2:129i**
    differential diagnosis, **2:126i**, 2:127
    tracheal, 1:39
Paraganglioma, 7:123
Parapneumonic effusion and empyema, 2:70–72, **2:73i**
    differential diagnosis, **2:70i**, 2:71–72
    orbital cellulitis vs., **7:190i**, 7:191
    pleuropulmonary blastoma vs., **2:90i**, 2:91
    subdural, **7:78i**, 7:80
Paravertebral soft tissues, widening of
    discitis vs., 2:108
    neuroblastoma vs., 2:103
Parotid abscess, **7:166i**, 7:167
Paroxysmal supraventricular tachycardia, 3:51
Parvovirus infections, 4:35
Patellar tendonitis, 6:35
Patent ductus arteriosus, 3:18–20, **3:21i**
    atrioventricular septal defect vs., **3:14i**, 3:16
    differential diagnosis, **3:18i**, 3:19
    ventricular septal defect vs., **3:6i**, 3:7
Pectus carinatum (pigeon chest), **2:130i**, 2:132
Pectus excavatum (funnel chest), 2:130–132, **2:133i**
    differential diagnosis, **2:130i**, 2:132
Pelizaeus-Merzbacher disease, 7:68
Pelvic abscess
    hydrometrocolpos vs., 5:67
    rhabdomyosarcoma vs., 5:83
    sacrococcygeal teratoma vs., 5:87
Pelvic inflammatory disease
    mesenteric adenitis vs., 4:109–110
    ovarian torsion vs., 5:95
    rhabdomyosarcoma vs., 5:83
    spondylolysis vs., 6:179
Pericardial effusion, 3:31
Perisylvian syndrome, congenital bilateral, 7:31
Peritoneal cyst, 5:91
Peritonitis, meconium, 4:34–35
    differential diagnosis, **4:34i**, 4:35
Persistent fetal circulation syndrome
    patent ductus arteriosus vs., 3:19
    total anomalous pulmonary venous return vs., 3:47
Persistent hyperplastic primary vitreous, **7:194i**, 7:195
PHACES, **7:46i**, 7:47
Pharyngeal tonsils, enlarged, 1:22–24, **1:25i**
    differential diagnosis, **1:22i**, 1:24
PHAVER syndrome, 6:143
Pheochromocytoma, 5:79
Phytobezoar, 4:61
    pyloric stenosis vs., 4:53
Pigeon chest (pectus carinatum), **2:130i**, 2:132
Pilocytic astrocytoma, 7:94–96, **7:97i**
    arachnoid cyst vs., **7:86i**, 7:87
    brain abscess vs., **7:58i**, 7:59
    differential diagnosis, **7:94i**, 7:95–96
    ependymoma vs., **7:102i**, 7:103
    medulloblastoma vs., 7:99
Pineal cyst, 7:115
Pineoblastoma, 7:115
Pitcher's elbow. *See* Epicondyle avulsion, medial
Pituitary adenoma
    colloid cyst vs, 7:83
    craniopharyngioma vs., **7:110i**, 7:111

INDEX

    macroadenoma vs. germinoma, **7:114i**, 7:115
Pleomorphic xanthoastrocytoma, 7:95
Pleural effusion, **2:70i**, 2:71
Pleuropulmonary blastoma, 2:90–92, **2:93i**
    bronchogenic cyst vs., 2:16
    differential diagnosis, **2:90i**, 2:91
    pulmonary inflammatory pseudotumor vs., **2:94i**, 2:95
    pulmonary sequestration vs., 2:12
Pneumatoceles, 2:127
Pneumonia
    bacterial, **2:62i**, 2:63
    esophageal atresia with tracheoesophageal fistula vs., 4:45
    group B streptococcal, **2:30i**, 2:31
    interstitial, 2:59
    neonatal, 2:34–36, **2:37i**
        bronchopulmonary dysplasia vs., **2:50i**, 2:51
        chylothorax vs., **2:58i**, 2:59
        differential diagnosis, **2:34i**, 2:35
        meconium aspiration syndrome vs., **2:38i**, 2:39
        transient tachypnea of newborn vs., 2:43
    pre-existing, **2:122i**, 2:123
    round. *See* Round pneumonia
    thoracic neuroblastoma vs., **2:102i**, 2:103
    with cavitary necrosis, 2:74–76, **2:77i**
        congenital diaphragmatic hernia vs., **2:22i**, 2:23
        cystic adenomatoid malformation vs., **2:6i**, 2:7–8
        differential diagnosis, **2:74i**, 2:75–76
        parapneumonic effusion and empyema vs., **2:70i**, 2:72
        pulmonary sequestration vs., **2:10i**, 2:12
Pneumoperitoneum
    surfactant deficient disease vs., **2:30i**, 2:31
    transient tachypnea of the newborn vs., 2:44
Pneumothorax
    acute chest syndrome vs., **2:114i**, 2:115
    congenital lobar emphysema vs., **2:18i**, 2:20
Polyarteritis nodosa, 3:105
Polychondritis
    innominate artery compression syndrome vs., **1:42i**, 1:43
    tracheomalacia vs., **1:56i**, 1:57
Polycystic liver disease, 4:101
Polycystic renal disease
    dominant, 5:44–46, **5:47i**
        differential diagnosis, **5:44i**, 5:45
        recessive vs., **5:40i**, 5:41
    recessive, 5:40–42, **5:43i**
        differential diagnosis, **5:40i**, 5:41–42
        dominant vs., **5:44i**, 5:45
        mesoblastic nephroma vs., 5:59
Polymicrogyria, focal, 7:31

Polymyositis, 6:135
Polyps, antral, 4:53
Pontine glioma. *See* Brainstem glioma
Porencephalic cyst, 7:87
Porencephaly
    agenetic. *See* Schizencephaly
    encephaloclastic, 7:35
    germinal matrix hemorrhage vs., **7:126i**, 7:127
Portal vein
    preduodenal
        duodenal atresia or stenosis vs., 4:11
        duodenal web vs., 4:15
    stenosis, **4:104i**, 4:106
Posterior reversible encephalopathy syndrome, **7:62i**, 7:63
Postoperative complications
    cavities vs. schizencephaly, **7:34i**, 7:35
    gastric volvulus vs., **4:56i**, 4:57
    small bowel obstruction vs. cystic fibrosis, **4:174i**, 4:175
Posttransplantation lymphoproliferative disorder. *See* Lymphoproliferative disorder
Pott puffy tumor, **7:190i**, 7:191
Preductal coarctation
    D-transposition of great arteries vs., 3:34
    hypoplastic left heart syndrome vs., **3:50i**, 3:51
    patent ductus arteriosus with, **3:14i**
Pregnancy
    cocaine abuse and infant enterocolitis, 4:37
    ectopic, **5:94i**, 5:95
    ovarian teratoma vs., **5:90i**, 5:91
Primitive neuroectodermal tumor
    pleuropulmonary blastoma vs., 2:91
    rhabdomyosarcoma vs., 6:71
Pringle disease. *See* Tuberous sclerosis
Proximal focal femoral deficiency, 6:102–104, **6:105i**
    developmental dysplasia of hip vs., **6:98i**, 6:99
    differential diagnosis, **6:102i**, 6:103
Prune belly syndrome, **5:28i**
Pseudo-achondroplasia, 6:115
Pseudo-TORCH syndromes, 7:55
Pseudocoarctation, **3:78i**, 3:79
Pseudocyst
    hydrocephalus vs., **7:146i**, 7:148
    meconium, **4:78i**, 4:79
    mesenteric lymphatic malformation vs., 4:112–113, **4:112i**
    pancreatic, 4:97
Pseudomembranous colitis, 4:138–140, **4:141i**
    differential diagnosis, **4:138i**, 4:139
    graft-versus-host disease vs., **4:146i**, 4:147
    hypoperfusion complex vs., 4:115
    lymphoproliferative disorder vs., **4:134i**, 4:135
    mesenteric adenitis vs., 4:109
    neutropenic colitis vs., **4:142i**, 4:143

INDEX

ulcerative colitis vs., **4:154i**, 4:155
Pseudosubluxation, 7:75
Pseudothalidomide syndrome, 6:143
Pseudotruncus. See Pulmonary atresia
Pseudotumor
    orbital, **7:94i**, 7:96
    pulmonary inflammatory, 2:94–96, **2:97i**
        arteriovenous malformation vs., 2:119
        differential diagnosis, **2:94i**, 2:95–96
        lymphoma vs., **2:82i**, 2:83
        pleuropulmonary blastoma vs., 2:91
Pseudotumor cerebri, 7:11
Pulmonary agenesis
    bronchial atresia vs., 2:27
    parapneumonic effusion and empyema vs., **2:70i**
    transient tachypnea of newborn vs., 2:43
Pulmonary artery
    agenesis, 2:27
    hypoplasia
        congenital lobar emphysema vs., **2:18i**, 2:19
        tetralogy of Fallot vs., **3:22i**, 3:23
    normal chest, **3:10i**, 3:12
        stenosis vs., **3:86i**, 3:87
    operative procedures for, 3:90, **3:90i**
    stenosis, 3:86–88, **3:89i**
        differential diagnosis, **3:86i**, 3:87
Pulmonary atresia, 3:26–28, **3:29i**
    differential diagnosis, **3:26i**, 3:27
    Ebstein anomaly vs., **3:30i**, 3:31
    patent ductus arteriosus with, **3:18i**
    tetralogy of Fallot vs., **3:22i**, 3:23
    total anomalous pulmonary venous return vs., **3:46i**
Pulmonary edema with effusions, 2:59
Pulmonary hypertension
    atrial septal defect vs., **3:10i**, 3:12
    pulmonary artery stenosis vs., **3:86i**, 3:87
    total anomalous pulmonary venous return vs., 3:47
Pulmonary hypoplasia
    bronchial atresia vs., **2:26i**, 2:27–28
    congenital lobar emphysema vs., **2:18i**, 2:19
    Scimitar syndrome vs., 3:99
Pulmonary interstitial emphysema, 2:46–48, **2:49i**
    bronchopulmonary dysplasia vs., **2:50i**, 2:51
    congenital lobar emphysema vs., **2:18i**, 2:19
    differential diagnosis, **2:46i**, 2:47
Pulmonary nodule, solitary, 2:27
Pulmonary sequestration, 2:10–12, **2:13i**
    bronchial atresia vs., 2:28
    bronchogenic cyst vs., 2:16
    cystic adenomatoid malformation vs., **2:6i**, 2:7
    differential diagnosis, **2:10i**, 2:12
    discitis vs., 2:108
    pleuropulmonary blastoma vs., 2:91
    pneumonia with cavitary necrosis vs., **2:74i**, 2:75
    pulmonary inflammatory pseudotumor vs., 2:95
    renal ectopia vs., **5:22i**, 5:24
    round pneumonia vs., **2:66i**, 2:67
    Scimitar syndrome vs., **3:98i**, 3:99
    subdiaphragmatic, 5:75
    thoracic neuroblastoma vs., **2:102i**, 2:103
    viral infection vs., **2:62i**, 2:63
Pulmonary sling, 1:34–36, **1:37i**
    airway compression with thoracic deformity vs., **1:54i**, 1:55
    bronchial foreign body vs., 1:62
    differential diagnosis, **1:34i**, 1:35
    double aortic arch vs., **1:30i**, 1:31
    midline descending aorta vs., **1:46i**, 1:47
Pulmonary varix, **2:118i**, 2:119
Pulmonary vein agenesis, 2:28
Pulmonary venolobar syndrome, congenital. See Scimitar syndrome
Pulmonary venous return, anomalous
    partial, **3:98i**, 3:99
    total, 3:46–48, **3:49i**
        chylothorax vs., **2:58i**, 2:59
        differential diagnosis, **3:46i**, 3:47
        Scimitar syndrome vs., **3:98i**, 3:99
        transient tachypnea of newborn vs., **2:42i**, 2:43
        tricuspid atresia vs., **3:38i**, 3:39
Pycnodysostosis, 6:128
Pyelonephritis, 5:110–112, **5:113i**
    differential diagnosis, **5:110i**, 5:111
    nephroblastomatosis vs., **5:54i**
    renal injury vs., **5:114i**, 5:116
    spondylolysis vs., 6:179
Pyle disease, 6:128
Pyloric stenosis
    gastroesophageal reflux vs., **4:48i**, 4:49
    hypertrophic, 4:52–54, **4:55i**
        differential diagnosis, **4:52i**, 4:53
Pylorospasm, 4:53
Pyruvate kinase deficiency, 6:171

R

Radiation injury, vs. stroke, **7:134i**, 7:136
Radiation therapy, vs. dermatomyositis, 6:135
Radius, absent, **6:142i**, 6:143
Ranulum, 4:160
Rasmussen syndrome, 7:31
Rastelli procedure, **3:90i**, 3:91
Rathke cleft cyst, 7:111
Rathke pouch tumor. See Craniopharyngioma
RDS (respiratory distress syndrome). See Surfactant deficient disease
Re-tethering, 7:40

INDEX

Rectal malformation, 4:40–42, **4:43i**
   differential diagnosis, **4:40i**, 4:41–42
Refsum disease, 7:68
Reiter's syndrome, 6:131
Renal cell carcinoma
   angiomyolipoma vs., **5:62i**, 5:63
   calyceal diverticulum vs., **5:48i**, 5:49
   cystic, **5:56i**, 5:57
   renal injury vs., **5:114i**, 5:116
   Wilm tumor vs., **5:50i**, 5:51
Renal disease
   abscess
      angiomyolipoma vs., **5:62i**, 5:63
      calyceal diverticulum vs., **5:48i**, 5:49
   cysts. *See also* Polycystic renal disease
      calyceal diverticulum vs., **5:48i**, 5:49
      multilocular cystic nephroma vs., **5:56i**, 5:57
      multiple simple, 5:45
   dysplasia, cystic, **5:40i**, 5:41
   end-stage, **5:36i**, 5:37
   failure, chronic, 6:127
   infarction, 5:111
   scarring vs. pyelonephritis, 5:111
   tumors. *See also* Renal cell carcinoma
      fibroma. *See* Nephroma, mesoblastic
      medullary carcinoma, 5:51
      ossifying, of infancy, 5:59
Renal ectopia and fusion, 5:22–24, **5:25i**
   differential diagnosis, **5:22i**, 5:24
Renal injury, 5:114–116, **5:117i**
   differential diagnosis, **5:114i**, 5:116
   pyelonephritis vs., **5:110i**, 5:111
Renal vein thrombosis, 5:45
Repetitive stress injury, 6:32
Respiratory distress syndrome. *See* Surfactant deficient disease
Retinal detachment, 7:195
Retinal dysplasia, 7:195
Retinoblastoma, 7:194–196, **7:197i**
   differential diagnosis, **7:194i**, 7:195
Retinopathy of prematurity, **7:194i**, 7:195
Retroperitoneal varices, **2:118i**, 2:119
Retropharyngeal abscess, 1:18–20, **1:21i**
   chronic esophageal foreign body vs., 2:135
   differential diagnosis, **1:18i**, 1:19
      epiglottitis vs., **1:6i**, 1:7
      esophageal strictures vs., 4:163
Retropharyngeal soft tissues, pseudothickening of, **1:18i**, 1:19
Rhabdoid tumor, 5:51
Rhabdomyolysis, **6:134i**, 6:135
Rhabdomyoma, 3:102–103
   differential diagnosis, **3:102i**, 3:103
   tuberous sclerosis vs., **7:50i**, 7:51
Rhabdomyosarcoma
   genitourinary, 5:82–84, **5:85i**
      differential diagnosis, **5:82i**, 5:83
      hydrometrocolpos vs., **5:66i**, 5:67
      neurogenic bladder vs., 5:119
      sacrococcygeal teratoma vs., **5:86i**, 5:87
      ureterocele vs., **5:18i**, 5:19
   of head and neck, 7:206–208, **7:209i**
      acquired cholesteatoma vs., **7:186i**, 7:188
      aural atresia vs., **7:162i**, 7:163
      differential diagnosis, **7:206i**, 7:207
      encephalocele vs., 7:20
      infantile hemangioma vs., **7:210i**, 7:211
      juvenile nasopharyngeal angiofibroma vs., **7:198i**, 7:199
      of middle ear, **7:182i**, 7:183
      vascular malformations vs., **7:202i**, 7:203
   musculoskeletal, 6:70–72, **6:73i**
      aggressive fibromatosis vs., **6:66i**, 6:68
      differential diagnosis, **6:70i**, 6:71
      fibromatosis colli vs., 6:163
      infantile hemangioma vs., **6:50i**, 6:51
      Langerhans cell histiocytosis vs., 6:87
   pleuropulmonary blastoma vs., 2:91
Rheumatic heart disease, 3:108–110, **3:111i**
   aortic stenosis vs., 3:83
   cardiomyopathy vs., **3:62i**, 3:63
   differential diagnosis, **3:108i**, 3:109
   Kawasaki disease vs., **3:104i**, 3:105
   myocarditis vs., **3:58i**
Rheumatoid arthritis, juvenile, 6:130–132, **6:133i**
   differential diagnosis, **6:130i**, 6:131–132
   fractures vs., in toddlers, 6:28
   Henoch-Schönlein purpura vs., 4:171
   Legg-Calve-Perthes disease vs., 6:107
   tarsal coalition vs., **6:146i**, 6:148
Rhombencephalitis, **7:106i**, 7:107
Rhombencephalosynapsis, 7:7
Rib fractures, 2:98–100, **2:101i**
   differential diagnosis, **2:98i**, 2:99–100
Rickets, 6:158–160, **6:161i**
   abuse-related metaphyseal fractures vs., 6:11
   differential diagnosis, **6:158i**, 6:160
   incomplete fractures vs., 6:16
   osteogenesis imperfecta vs., 6:123
   syphilis vs., **6:46i**, 6:47
Rockerbottom foot, **6:138i**, 6:139
Ross-Konno procedure, 3:91
Rotary fixation, atlantoaxial, 7:75
Round pneumonia, 2:66–68, **2:69i**
   bronchogenic cyst vs., **2:14i**, 2:15
   differential diagnosis, **2:66i**, 2:67
   pulmonary sequestration vs., **2:10i**, 2:12

S

Sacrococcygeal teratoma, 5:86–88, **5:89i**
   differential diagnosis, **5:86i**, 5:87

INDEX

hydrometrocolpos vs., 5:67
rhabdomyosarcoma vs., 5:83
Sacroiliitis, 6:179
Sacrum, agenesis of, **6:142i**, 6:143
Salmonella infections
    Crohn disease vs., **4:150i**, 4:152
    mesenteric adenitis vs., **4:108i**, 4:109
    neutropenic colitis vs., **4:142i**, 4:143
    pseudomembranous colitis vs., **4:138i**, 4:139
    ulcerative colitis vs., **4:154i**, 4:156
Salter fractures. *See* Fractures, physeal
Sarcoidosis, **7:94i**, 7:96
Sarcoma
    clear cell
        multilocular cystic nephroma vs., 5:57
        Wilm tumor vs., 5:51
    infantile hemangioma of head and neck vs., **7:210i**, 7:211
    osteogenic. *See* Osteosarcoma
    pulmonary inflammatory pseudotumor vs., **2:94i**, 2:95
    soft tissue
        arteriovenous malformation vs., **6:62i**, 6:63–64
        chronic foreign body vs., **6:38i**, 6:39
        infantile hemangioma vs., **6:50i**, 6:51
        lymphatic malformations vs., **6:58i**, 6:59
        venous malformations vs., **6:54i**, 6:56
    synovial cell
        aggressive fibromatosis vs., **6:66i**, 6:68
        rhabdomyosarcoma vs., **6:70i**, 6:71
    undifferentiated, **2:90i**, 2:91
    vascular malformations of head and neck vs., **7:202i**, 7:203
Scheuermann disease
    discitis vs., 2:107
    spondylolysis vs., **6:178i**, 6:179
Schizencephaly, 7:34–36, **7:37i**
    differential diagnosis, **7:34i**, 7:35
    hemimegalencephaly vs., 7:31
    holoprosencephaly vs., **7:22i**, 7:23
Schwannoma
    of facial nerve, **7:182i**, 7:183
    spinal cord astrocytoma vs., 7:123
Scimitar syndrome, 3:98–100, **3:101i**
    atrial septal defect vs., **3:10i**, 3:12
    bronchial atresia vs., 2:28
    differential diagnosis, **3:98i**, 3:99
Sclerosis. *See also* Multiple sclerosis; Tuberous sclerosis
    Balo concentric, **7:62i**, 7:63
Sclerosteosis, 6:128
Scoliosis, 6:174–176, **6:177i**
    differential diagnosis, **6:174i**, 6:176
    gastroschisis vs., 4:67
    spondylolysis vs., 6:179

Scrotal cellulitis
    epididymoorchitis vs., **5:98i**, 5:99
    torsion of testicular appendage vs., **5:106i**, 5:107
Scrotum, acute. *See* Epididymoorchitis
Scurvy (vitamin C deficiency), 6:47
Seminoma. *See* Germ cell tumors; Germinoma
Sepsis, **2:30i**, 2:31
Septal defects
    atrial, 3:10–12, **3:13i**
        differential diagnosis, **3:10i**, 3:12
        Ebstein anomaly vs., 3:31
    atrioventricular, 3:14–16, **3:17i**
        differential diagnosis, **3:14i**, 3:15–16
        patent ductus arteriosus vs., 3:19
        ventricular septal defect vs., **3:6i**, 3:7
    ventricular, 3:6–8, **3:9i**
        atrial septal defect vs., **3:10i**, 3:12
        atrioventricular septal defect vs., **3:14i**, 3:15
        differential diagnosis, **3:6i**, 3:7–8
        double outlet right ventricle vs., **3:66i**, 3:67–68
        L-transposition of great arteries vs., **3:70i**, 3:71
        right ventricular dysplasia vs., 3:95
Septic emboli, **2:126i**, 2:127
Septic hip
    developmental dysplasia of hip vs., **6:98i**
    Legg-Calve-Perthes disease vs., 6:107
Septic shock syndrome, 3:105
Septo-optic dysplasia, 7:23
Shaken baby syndrome. *See* Child abuse
Shinsplints (medial tibial stress syndrome), 6:19–20
Shock abdomen. *See* Hypoperfusion complex
Shock bowel. *See* Hypoperfusion complex
Sickle cell disease
    acute chest syndrome, 2:114–116, **2:117i**
        differential diagnosis, **2:114i**, 2:115
    of bone, 6:170–172, **6:173i**
        differential diagnosis, **6:170i**, 6:171–172
        spondylolysis vs., 6:179
    myocarditis vs., **3:58i**
Sickle cell trait, 6:172
Sigmoid colon
    mass effect vs. ureterocele, 5:19
    normal position, **4:74i**, 4:75
Sinding-Larsen-Johansson disease, **6:34i**, 6:35
Single ventricle, with unobstructed pulmonary flow, **3:34i**, 3:35
Sinus venosus atrial septal defect, **3:14i**, 3:16
Sinusitis, 7:80
Situs ambiguous, **3:74i**, 3:75
Situs inversus, 3:75
Sjögren syndrome, 2:127
Skull and scalp tumors, 7:20
Sleep apnea, obstructive
    causes of, **1:22i**

INDEX

enlarged pharyngeal tonsils and, 1:22–24, **1:25i**
Slipped capital femoral epiphysis, 6:110–112, **6:113i**
    differential diagnosis, **6:110i**, 6:111
    Legg-Calve-Perthes disease vs., **6:106i**, 6:107
    traumatic, 6:111
Small bowel obstruction, postoperative, **4:174i**, 4:175
Small left colon syndrome. See Meconium plug syndrome
Soft palate, 1:24
Sonographic mimics, **5:6i**, 5:7
Spherocytosis, hereditary, 6:171
Spina bifida occulta. See Dysraphism, occult spinal
Spinal cord
    astrocytoma, 7:122–124, **7:125i**
        differential diagnosis, **7:122i**, 7:123
        ependymoma vs., 7:103
    duplicated, 7:43
    infarction, 7:123
    injuries, **7:122i**, 7:123
Spinal fusion anomalies, **6:162i**, 6:164
Spinocerebellar ataxia, 7:7
Spleen trauma, 4:126–128, **4:129i**
    differential diagnosis, **4:126i**, 4:127
Splenic abscess, **4:126i**, 4:127
Splenic cleft, **4:126i**, 4:127
Splenic infarction, **4:126i**, 4:127
Split cord malformation. See Diastematomyelia
Spondylitis
    ankylosing, 6:131
    infectious. See Discitis
Spondyloarthropathies, juvenile, 6:131
Spondylodysplasia, **6:126i**
Spondyloepiphyseal dysplasia, **6:118i**, 6:119
Spondylolysis, 6:178–180, **6:181i**
    differential diagnosis, **6:178i**, 6:179
    discitis vs., **2:106i**, 2:107–108
Spondylometaphyseal dysplasia
    abuse-related metaphyseal fractures vs., **6:10i**, 6:12
    mucopolysaccharidoses vs., **6:118i**, 6:119
Sprains and strains, **6:30i**, 6:31
Squamous cell carcinoma, metastasis, 7:171
Still disease. See Rheumatoid arthritis, juvenile
Stomach, midline, **3:74i**
Stridor, **1:6i**, **1:10i**, **1:14i**, **1:18i**
Stroke
    childhood, 7:134–136, **7:137i**
        differential diagnosis, **7:134i**, 7:136
        germinal matrix hemorrhage vs., 7:127
    prenatal, **7:34i**, 7:35
Stromal tumors, 5:91
Sturge-Weber syndrome
    choroid plexus papilloma vs., **7:118i**, 7:119
    neurofibromatosis type 1 vs., **7:46i**, 7:47
Subarachnoid cyst. See Arachnoid cyst

Subependymoma
    choroid plexus papilloma vs., **7:118i**, 7:119
    tuberous sclerosis vs., 7:51
Subglottic stenosis
    croup vs., **1:10i**, 1:11
    exudative tracheitis vs., **1:14i**, 1:15
    hemangioma vs., 1:39
Subtalar fractures, **6:146i**, 6:148
Surfactant deficient disease, 2:30–32, **2:33i**
    differential diagnosis, **2:30i**, 2:–31
    neonatal pneumonia vs., **2:30i**, 2:31
    pulmonary interstitial emphysema vs., 2:47
Swyer-James syndrome, 1:62
Synovial chondromatosis, **6:130i**, 6:132
Synovitis
    pigmented villonodular, 6:132
    slipped capital femoral epiphysis vs., **6:110i**, 6:111
    toxic
        fractures vs., in toddlers, 6:28
        Legg-Calve-Perthes disease vs., 6:107
    transient, 6:132
Syphilis, 6:46–48, **6:49i**
    differential diagnosis, **6:46i**, 6:47
    Langerhans cell histiocytosis vs., 6:87
    leukemia vs., **6:82i**, 6:83
    rickets vs., **6:158i**, 6:160
Syringohydromyelia, 7:123
Syringomyelia, **7:42i**, 7:43
Syrinx
    diastematomyelia vs., **7:42i**, 7:43
    spondylolysis vs., 6:179
Systemic artery to pulmonary vein shunt, **2:118i**, 2:119
Systemic lupus erythematosus
    bowel injury vs., **4:118i**, 4:120
    Kawasaki disease vs., 3:105

T

Tachycardia, paroxysmal supraventricular, 3:51
Tachypnea, transient. See Transient tachypnea of newborn
Takayasu arteritis
    aortic coarctation vs., 3:79
    Kawasaki disease vs., **3:104i**, 3:105
Talar fractures, **6:146i**, 6:148
Talipes equinovarus (club foot), 6:138–140, **6:141i**
    differential diagnosis, **6:138i**, 6:139
Talus, vertical, **6:138i**, 6:139
Tarsal coalition, 6:146–148, **6:149i**
    differential diagnosis, **6:146i**, 6:147–148
Taylor dysplasia, 7:52
Tendonitis, patellar, 6:35
Tennis elbow, medial. See Epicondyle avulsion, medial

INDEX

Teratoid-rhabdoid tumor, atypical
    medulloblastoma vs., **7:98i**, 7:99
    pilocytic astrocytoma vs., 7:95
Teratoma. *See also* Germ cell tumors
    atypical. *See* Germinoma
    cervical, 6:164
    lymphoma vs., **2:82i**, 2:84
    malignant, 5:91
    nasopharyngeal, **7:18i**, 7:20
    ovarian, 5:90–92, **5:93i**, 7:90–92, **7:93i**. *See also* Epidermoid cyst
        craniopharyngioma vs., 7:111
        differential diagnosis, **5:90i**, 5:91, **7:90i**, 7:91–92
        gastrointestinal duplication cyst vs., **4:158i**, 4:159
        rhabdomyoma vs., 3:103
    sacrococcygeal. *See* Sacrococcygeal teratoma
Testicular disorders
    rupture, 5:99
    torsion. *See* Torsion, testicular
    trauma
        testicular torsion vs., **5:102i**, 5:103
        torsion of testicular appendage vs., 5:107
    tumors
        second branchial apparatus anomalies vs., 7:171
        testicular torsion vs., **5:102i**, 5:103
        torsion of testicular appendage vs., 5:107
Tethered cord syndrome. *See* Dysraphism, occult spinal
Tetralogy of Fallot, 3:22–24, **3:25i**
    differential diagnosis, **3:22i**, 3:23
    double outlet right ventricle vs., **3:66i**, 3:68
    Ebstein anomaly vs., **3:30i**, 3:31
    L-transposition of great arteries vs., **3:70i**, 3:71
    pulmonary atresia vs., **3:26i**, 3:27
    tricuspid atresia vs., **3:38i**, 3:39
Thalassemia, 6:171
Thanatophoric dysplasia, **6:114i**, 6:116
Thoracic deformity, airway compression with, 1:54–55
    differential diagnosis, **1:54i**, 1:55
    midline descending aorta vs., **1:46i**, 1:47
Thrombocytopenia absent-radius syndrome, 6:143
Thrombocytopenia purpura, idiopathic
    bowel injury vs., 4:120
    Henoch-Schönlein purpura vs., **4:170i**, 4:171
Thymic cyst
    cervical. *See* Branchial apparatus anomalies, third
    germ cell tumor vs., **2:86i**, 2:87
    innominate artery compression syndrome vs., 1:43
Thymic sail sign. *See* Thymus, normal
Thymolipoma, 2:87

Thymoma
    germ cell tumor vs., 2:87
    thoracic lymphoma vs., 2:84
Thymus
    aberrant, **1:42i**, 1:43
    mediastinal, cervical extension of, 6:164
    normal, 2:78–80, **2:81i**
        differential diagnosis, **2:78i**, 2:80
        germ cell tumor vs., **2:86i**, 2:87
        lymphoma vs., **2:82i**, 2:83
Thyroglossal duct cyst
    fibromatosis colli vs., **6:162i**, 6:163–164
    third branchial apparatus anomalies vs., **7:174i**, 7:175
    fourth branchial apparatus anomalies vs., **7:178i**, 7:179
Thyroid
    colloid cyst, 7:179
    lingual, 4:160
    papillary carcinoma, necrotic node, **7:170i**, 7:171
Tibia
    fractures, distal, **6:6i**, 6:7
    tubercle avulsion of, **6:34i**
Tibiofibular joint, inferior, congenital diastasis of, 6:139
Toddlers, fractures in, 6:26–28, **6:29i**
    differential diagnosis, **6:26i**, 6:28
Tonsil(s)
    herniation, acquired, 7:11
    lingual, **1:26i**, 1:27
    palatine, 1:27
    pharyngeal, 1:22–24, **1:25i**
TORCH infections, 7:54–56, **7:57i**
    differential diagnosis, **7:54i**, 7:55
    tuberous sclerosis vs., 7:51
Torsion
    ovarian, 5:94–96, **5:97i**
        appendicitis vs., **4:70i**, 4:71
        differential diagnosis, **5:94i**, 5:95
        gastrointestinal duplication cyst vs., 4:159
        Meckel diverticulum vs., **4:78i**, 4:79
        teratoma vs., **5:90i**, 5:91
    testicular, 5:102–104, **5:105i**
        differential diagnosis, **5:102i**, 5:103
        epididymoorchitis vs., **5:98i**, 5:99
        Henoch-Schönlein purpura vs., 4:171
        torsion of testicular appendage vs., **5:106i**, 5:107
    of testicular appendage, 5:106–108, **5:109i**
        differential diagnosis, **5:106i**, 5:107
        epididymoorchitis vs., **5:98i**
    tubo-ovarian, **5:82i**
Torticollis. *See* Fibromatosis colli
Toxocariasis, ocular, 7:195
Tracheal compression, extrinsic, 1:62

INDEX

Tracheal stenosis
    chronic esophageal foreign body vs., **2:134i**, 2:135
    differential diagnosis, **1:30i**
    tracheomalacia vs., **1:56i**, 1:57
Tracheitis, exudative. *See* Exudative tracheitis
Tracheoesophageal fistula. *See* Esophageal disorders, atresia with tracheoesophageal fistula
Tracheomalacia, 1:56–58, **1:59i**
    differential diagnosis, **1:56i**, 1:57
    double aortic arch vs., **1:30i**, 1:31
Transient tachypnea of newborn, 2:42–44, **2:45i**
    chylothorax vs., **2:58i**, 2:59
    differential diagnosis, **2:42i**, 2:43–44
    extrathoracic causes of, 2:43
    meconium aspiration syndrome vs., **2:38i**, 2:39
    neonatal pneumonia vs., **2:30i**, 2:31
    systemic causes of, 2:44
Trauma, nonaccidental. *See* Child abuse
Trichobezoar, 4:61
    pyloric stenosis vs., **4:52i**, 4:53
Tricuspid atresia, 3:38–40, **3:41i**
    D-transposition of great arteries vs., **3:34i**, 3:35
    differential diagnosis, **3:38i**, 3:39
    Ebstein anomaly vs., **3:30i**, 3:31
    L-transposition of great arteries vs., **3:70i**, 3:71
    pulmonary atresia vs., **3:26i**, 3:27
    tetralogy of Fallot vs., **3:22i**, 3:23
Trisomy 13, **6:142i**, 6:143
Trisomy 18, **6:142i**, 6:143
Truncus arteriosus, 3:42–44, **3:45i**
    D-transposition of great arteries vs., **3:34i**, 3:35
    differential diagnosis, **3:42i**, 3:43
    double outlet right ventricle vs., 3:68
    total anomalous pulmonary venous return vs., **3:46i**
    transient tachypnea of newborn vs., **2:42i**, 2:43
    type 4. *See* Pulmonary atresia
Tuberous sclerosis, 7:50–52, **7:53i**
    colloid cyst vs, **7:82i**, 7:83
    differential diagnosis, **7:50i**, 7:51–52
    dominant polycystic renal disease vs., **5:44i**, 5:45
    hemimegalencephaly vs., 7:31
    multicystic dysplastic kidney vs., **5:36i**, 5:37
    neurofibromatosis type 1 vs., **7:46i**, 7:47
    papillomatosis vs., **2:126i**, 2:127
    recessive polycystic renal disease vs., **5:40i**, 5:42
    TORCH infections vs., **7:54i**, 7:55
Tubo-ovarian abscess, 5:91
Tubo-ovarian torsion, **5:82i**
Tumor(s). *See also* Metastasis (metastatic disease); *specific tumor type*
    Askin, **2:130i**, 2:132
    Bolande. *See* Nephroma, mesoblastic
    bone, vs. stress fracture, 6:19
    carcinoid
        bronchial atresia vs., 2:27
        pulmonary inflammatory pseudotumor vs., 2:96
    cardiac, malignant, 3:103
    germ cell. *See* Germ cell tumors
    nasopharyngeal, **7:18i**, 7:20
    nerve sheath, malignant peripheral, **6:70i**, 6:71
    posterior fossa, 7:11
    renal
        calyceal diverticulum vs., **5:48i**, 5:49
        ossifying, of infancy, 5:59
    rhabdoid, of kidney, 5:51
    of skull and scalp, 7:20
    of small bowel, 4:131–132
    soft tissue, **6:38i**, 6:39
    stromal, 5:91
    teratoid-rhabdoid, atypical
        medulloblastoma vs., **7:98i**, 7:99
        pilocytic astrocytoma vs., 7:95
    testicular
        testicular torsion vs., **5:102i**, 5:103
        torsion of testicular appendage vs., 5:107
    Wilm. *See* Wilm tumor
Typhlitis. *See* Neutropenic colitis

U

Uhl anomaly
    Ebstein anomaly vs., 3:31
    right ventricular dysplasia vs., 3:95
Ulcer, duodenal, 4:131
Ulcerative colitis, 4:154–156, **4:157i**
    Crohn disease vs., **4:150i**, 4:151
    differential diagnosis, **4:154i**, 4:155–156
    mesenteric adenitis vs., 4:109
    pseudomembranous colitis vs., **4:138i**, 4:139
Ulnar neuritis, 6:31
Umbilical catheter complications, 2:54–56, **2:57i**
    differential diagnosis, **2:54i**, 2:55
Umbilical cord
    hemangioma of, 5:33
    stump granulation tissue, **5:32i**, 5:33
Umbilical hernia, **5:32i**, 5:33
Urachal abnormalities, 5:32–34, **5:35i**
    differential diagnosis, **5:32i**, 5:33
Urachal cyst, **4:158i**, 4:159
Urachal diverticulum, **5:122i**, 5:123
Ureter, cobra head. *See* Ureterocele
Ureteral calculus, distal, 5:95
Ureteral stump, **5:122i**, 5:123
Ureterocele, 5:18–20, **5:21i**
    bladder diverticula vs., **5:122i**, 5:123
    differential diagnosis, **5:18i**, 5:19
    posterior urethral valves vs., **5:28i**, 5:29
    rhabdomyosarcoma vs., 5:83

INDEX

Ureteropelvic duplications, 5:14–16, **5:17i**
    differential diagnosis, **5:14i**, 5:15–16
Ureteropelvic junction obstruction, 5:10–12, **5:13i**
    differential diagnosis, **5:10i**, 5:11–12
    multicystic dysplastic kidney vs., **5:36i**, 5:37
    ureterocele vs., **5:18i**, 5:19
Urethra
    caruncle of, 5:19
    duplex, **5:14i**
    prolapse of, 5:19
    strictures of, 5:30
Urethral valves
    anterior, 5:29
    posterior, 5:28–30, **5:31i**
        differential diagnosis, **5:28i**, 5:29–30
        neurogenic bladder vs., **5:118i**, 5:119
        primary megaureter vs., **5:26i**, 5:27
        ureterocele vs., **5:18i**, 5:19
Urogenital imaging. See Genitourinary imaging
Urticle, prostatic, **5:28i**, 5:30
Uterine fibroid, pedunculated, 5:91
Uterus, septate
    hydrometrocolpos vs., **5:66i**, 5:67
    rhabdomyosarcoma vs., **5:82i**, 5:83

V

VACTERL association, 6:142–144, **6:145i**
    differential diagnosis, **6:142i**, 6:143
Vacuum phenomenon, 6:151
Vagina, duplex, **5:14i**
Valgus injury, 6:23
Van Buchem disease, type 2, 6:128
Van Buchem hyperostosis corticalis generalisata, 6:128
Varicella infections, **7:134i**, 7:136
Vascular injuries, 7:136
Vascular malformations. See also Arteriovenous malformations; Lymphatic malformations; Venous malformations
    asthma vs., **1:64i**, 1:65
    bronchogenic cyst vs., 2:16
    chronic foreign body vs., 6:39
    esophageal strictures vs., **4:162i**, 4:163
    germ cell tumor vs., **2:86i**, 2:87
    of head and neck, 7:202–204, **7:205i**
        differential diagnosis, **7:202i**, 7:203
    high-flow. See Arteriovenous malformations
    innominate artery compression syndrome vs., **1:42i**, 1:43
    pectus excavatum vs., **2:130i**, 2:132
    pulmonary arteriovenous malformation vs., **2:118i**, 2:119
    stroke vs., 7:136
    tracheomalacia vs., **1:56i**
Vascular polyp, nasopharyngeal, **7:198i**, 7:199

Vasculitis
    autoimmune-mediated, 7:63
    bowel injury vs., **4:118i**, 4:120
    stroke vs., **7:134i**, 7:136
Vein of Galen aneurysmal malformation, 7:138–140, **7:141i**
    aneurysmal dilation vs., 7:139
    differential diagnosis, **7:138i**, 7:139
Venous anomaly, complex developmental, 7:139
Venous malformations, 6:54–56, **6:57i**
    aggressive fibromatosis vs., **6:66i**, 6:68
    arteriovenous malformation vs., **6:62i**, 6:63
    chronic foreign body vs., 6:39
    differential diagnosis, **6:54i**, 6:55–56
    infantile hemangioma vs., **6:50i**, 6:51, **7:210i**, 7:211
    lymphatic malformations vs., **6:58i**, 6:59
    musculoskeletal, 6:54–56, **6:57i**
    rhabdomyosarcoma vs., **6:70i**, 6:71
Venous occlusion, 7:136
Venous return, anomalous pulmonary. See Pulmonary venous return, anomalous
Ventricular disorders
    double outlet. See Double outlet right ventricle
    right ventricular dysplasia, 3:94–96, **3:97i**
        arrhythmogenic, 3:31
        differential diagnosis, **3:94i**, 3:95
    right ventricular infarction
        right ventricular dysplasia vs., 3:95
    septal. See Septal defects, ventricular
    single ventricle, with unobstructed pulmonary flow, **3:34i**, 3:35
Ventriculitis, **7:126i**, 7:127
Ventriculomegaly, 7:148
Ventriculoperitoneal shunts, **7:146i**, 7:148
Vertebral anomalies, **7:42i**, 7:43
Vesicoureteral reflux, 5:6–8, **5:9i**
    differential diagnosis, **5:6i**, 5:7
    ureteropelvic junction obstruction vs., **5:10i**, 5:11
Viral infections, of lung, 2:62–64, **2:65i**
    bronchial foreign body vs., **1:60i**, 1:61
    differential diagnosis, **2:62i**, 2:63
Vitreous, persistent hyperplastic primary, **7:194i**, 7:195
Volvulus
    gastric, 4:56–58, **4:59i**
        differential diagnosis, **4:56i**, 4:57
    midgut, 4:6–8, **4:9i**
        differential diagnosis, **4:6i**, 4:7–8
        duodenal atresia or stenosis vs., **4:10i**, 4:11
        duodenal hematoma vs., **4:130i**, 4:131
        duodenal web vs., **4:14i**, 4:15
        meconium peritonitis vs., **4:34i**, 4:35
        meconium plug syndrome vs., **4:26i**, 4:27
        pyloric stenosis vs., 4:53

INDEX

Von Hippel Lindau disease, 7:47
von Recklinghausen disease. *See* Neurofibromatosis, type 1

W

Walker-Warburg syndrome, **7:6i**, 7:7
Wegener granulomatosis, **2:126i**, 2:127
Weismann-Netter syndrome, 6:47
Werdnig Hoffman disease, 2:44
Wet lung disease. *See* Transient tachypnea of newborn
Williams syndrome
    hypoplastic left heart syndrome vs., **3:50i**
    neurogenic bladder vs., **5:118i**, 5:119
Wilm tumor, 5:50–52, **5:53i**
    angiomyolipoma vs., **5:62i**, 5:63
    differential diagnosis, **5:50i**, 5:51
    mesoblastic nephroma vs., **5:58i**, 5:59
    multicystic dysplastic kidney vs., **5:36i**, 5:37
    multilocular cystic nephroma vs., 5:57
    nephroblastomatosis vs., **5:54i**
    neuroblastoma vs., **5:78i**, 5:79
    pyelonephritis vs., 5:111
    renal injury vs., **5:114i**, 5:116
Wilson disease, 7:72
Wolman disease
    adrenal hemorrhage vs., 5:75
    normal adrenal gland vs., 5:72
Wry neck. *See* Fibromatosis colli

X

Xanthoastrocytoma, pleomorphic, 7:95
Xanthogranuloma, 7:119
Xanthoma, 7:119
Xanthomatosis, primary familial
    adrenal hemorrhage vs., 5:75
    normal adrenal gland vs., 5:72